MAYO INTERNAL MEDICINE
BOARD REVIEW
1996 - 97

MAYO
INTERNAL MEDICINE
BOARD REVIEW
1996 - 97

Udaya B. S. Prakash, M.D.

Editor-in-Chief

Mayo Foundation for Medical Education and Research

Rochester, Minnesota

THIS VOLUME IS

DEDICATED TO

Residents and Fellows, past and present, of

Mayo Clinic and Mayo Foundation and

Mayo Graduate School of Medicine

FOREWORD

We welcome the opportunity to once again serve as a resource for physicians preparing to take the American Board of Internal Medicine Certification and Recertification Board Examinations. Because of the overwhelming response to the first edition of our book, we have published this new edition, *Mayo Internal Medicine Board Review 1996-97*.

As an educational institution, Mayo holds a commitment to share knowledge and thus contribute to a broader understanding of health and disease. It is our intent that this book enhance the medical profession's quest for continuous improvement in the standard of care that people today expect and deserve.

Thirty Mayo physicians contributed to this comprehensive study guide, which also can serve as a reference to help you keep abreast of the latest information in internal medicine and other specialties.

We hope we have made the experience of preparing for the board examination easier for you, and we wish you success on the examination. Also, we hope that our service as an information resource will continue to be valuable to your quest for excellence in medical practice.

Robert R. Waller, M.D.
President and Chief Executive Officer
Mayo Foundation

EDITORIAL AND PRODUCTION STAFF

Editor-in-Chief   Udaya B. S. Prakash, M.D.

Managing Editor   Mary L. Rysavy

Editorial Production   LeAnn M. Stee

    O. E. Millhouse, Ph.D.

Art Director   Karen E. Barrie

Editorial Assistants   Mary K. Horsman

    Margery J. Lovejoy

Proofreader   Dorothy L. Tienter

Design Assistants   Cheryl K. Ashelin

    Constance M. Batt

Computer Scientific Illustrators   Marcia W. Blackburn

    Diane M. Knight

    Chantal N. Lichaa

Marketing Manager   Marne J. M. Gade

Digital Printing Coordinator   Thomas F. Flood

Printing Coordinator   Stephen Q. Sponsel

Customer Service Manager   Christie L. Herman

Administrative Secretaries   Joanne M. Souhrada

    Monica J. Farrell

Administrative Advisers   David E. Larson, M.D.

    Vicki L. Moore

    Ronald R. Ward

CONTRIBUTORS

Charles F. Abboud, M.D.
Consultant, Division of Endocrinology/ Metabolism and Internal Medicine,* Associate Professor of Medicine†

Thomas F. Bugliosi, M.D.
Consultant, Division of Emergency Medical Services and Internal Medicine,* Assistant Professor of Medicine†

Darryl S. Chutka, M.D.
Consultant, Section of Geriatric Medicine,* Assistant Professor of Medicine†

William F. Dunn, M.D.
Consultant, Division of Pulmonary and Critical Care Medicine and Internal Medicine,* Assistant Professor of Medicine†

William W. Ginsburg, M.D.
Consultant, Division of Rheumatology,‡ Associate Professor of Medicine†

Thomas M. Habermann, M.D.
Consultant, Division of Hematology and Internal Medicine,* Assistant Professor of Medicine†

Philip T. Hagen, M.D.
Consultant, Division of Preventive Medicine and Internal Medicine,* Assistant Professor of Preventive Medicine†

Stephen C. Hammill, M.D.
Consultant, Division of Cardiovascular Diseases and Internal Medicine,* Professor of Medicine†

Lynn C. Hartmann, M.D.
Consultant, Division of Medical Oncology,* Associate Professor of Oncology†

Barry L. Karon, M.D.
Consultant, Division of Cardiovascular Diseases and Internal Medicine,* Instructor in Medicine†

James T. Li, M.D.
Consultant, Division of Allergic Diseases and Internal Medicine,* Associate Professor of Medicine†

Scott C. Litin, M.D.
Consultant, Division of Area General Internal Medicine,* Assistant Professor of Medicine†

William F. Marshall, M.D.
Consultant, Division of Infectious Diseases and Internal Medicine,* Assistant Professor of Medicine†

Marian T. McEvoy, M.D.
Consultant, Department of Dermatology,* Assistant Professor of Dermatology†

Virginia V. Michels, M.D.
Chair, Department of Medical Genetics,* Professor of Medical Genetics†

Deborah C. Newman, M.D.
Consultant, Section of General and Community Psychiatry,* Assistant Professor of Psychiatry†

*Mayo Clinic and Mayo Foundation, Rochester, Minnesota.
†Mayo Medical School, Rochester, Minnesota.
‡Mayo Clinic Jacksonville, Jacksonville, Florida.

Rick A. Nishimura, M.D.
Consultant, Division of Cardiovascular Diseases and Internal Medicine,* Professor of Medicine†

Douglas R. Osmon, M.D.
Consultant, Division of Infectious Diseases and Internal Medicine,* Assistant Professor of Medicine†

Steve G. Peters, M.D.
Consultant, Division of Pulmonary and Critical Care Medicine and Internal Medicine,* Associate Professor of Medicine†

John J. Poterucha, M.D.
Consultant, Division of Gastroenterology and Internal Medicine,* Assistant Professor of Medicine†

Udaya B. S. Prakash, M.D.
Consultant, Division of Pulmonary and Critical Care Medicine and Internal Medicine,* Professor of Medicine†

Thom Rooke, M.D.
Consultant, Division of Cardiovascular Diseases and Internal Medicine,* Associate Professor of Medicine†

Frank A. Rubino, M.D.
Consultant, Department of Neurology,‡ Associate Professor of Neurology†

Thomas R. Schwab, M.D.
Consultant, Division of Nephrology and Internal Medicine,* Associate Professor of Medicine†

Gary L. Schwartz, M.D.
Consultant, Division of Hypertension and Internal Medicine,* Assistant Professor of Medicine†

Marshall S. Stanton, M.D.
Consultant, Division of Cardiovascular Diseases and Internal Medicine,* Assistant Professor of Medicine†

Zelalem Temesgen, M.D.
Fellow in Infectious Diseases,§ Instructor in Medicine†

Robert M. Valente, M.D.
Consultant, Division of Rheumatology and Internal Medicine,* Assistant Professor of Medicine†

Thomas R. Viggiano, M.D.
Consultant, Division of Gastroenterology and Internal Medicine,* Associate Professor of Medicine†

Carole A. Warnes, M.D.
Consultant, Division of Cardiovascular Diseases and Internal Medicine,* Associate Professor of Medicine†

*Mayo Clinic and Mayo Foundation, Rochester, Minnesota.
†Mayo Medical School, Rochester, Minnesota.
‡Mayo Clinic Jacksonville, Jacksonville, Florida.
§Mayo Graduate School of Medicine.

TABLE OF CONTENTS

PREFACE

The tremendous reception accorded to *Mayo Internal Medicine Board Review 1994-95* prompted the publication of this revised edition, *Mayo Internal Medicine Board Review 1996-97*. The results of the informal survey of candidates who used the 1994-95 edition of this volume demonstrated that the contents and format of the book were extremely helpful to them in preparing for and passing the board examination. The authors are grateful to readers who provided many valuable ideas for improvement. It is gratifying to recognize that *Mayo Internal Medicine Board Review 1994-95* was used as a course syllabus by several board review courses in the United States. My coauthors and I hope that this volume also will provide assistance to physicians preparing for not only the certifying and recertifying board examinations in 1996 and 1997 but also other certifying medical examinations.

Several points from the first edition need reiteration. This volume is not a comprehensive textbook of internal medicine. It should be used as a guide or notebook containing selected topics deemed important for physicians preparing for either the certifying or the recertifying examinations offered by the American Board of Internal Medicine (ABIM) or other examining institutions. All chapters are prepared under the assumption that readers will have studied at length one of the standard textbooks of internal medicine before studying this review. The first chapter includes further instructions regarding the other study materials and methods of preparation for the board examinations.

The chapters are divided by subspecialties in internal medicine. Readers of the previous edition found that the bulleted "pearls" were extremely helpful during their preparation for the examination. As a result, more pearls were added to many chapters in this edition. The repetition of important points in the form of pearls is intentional and is aimed at stressing the clinical and "board-eligible" aspects of the subjects. The questions at the end of each chapter contain both the multiple-choice *single-best-answer* format and the multiple *true/false* format. This volume contains more than 400 questions (answers are also provided). Candidates for the 1996 examination should note that all questions in the 1995 ABIM examination were of the *single-best-answer* format. The multiple true/false questions should be helpful to those taking non-ABIM examinations. The inclusion of an index in this volume should make it easier for readers to find the various topics. (The material in the questions and answers is not included in the index.)

I personally thank several authors of the previous edition who were not involved in this edition for allowing us to use some of their material in this volume. My gratitude goes to all authors for their prompt completion of the manuscripts. My coauthors and I gratefully acknowledge the hard labor of the editorial and production staff in bringing forth this volume.

My coauthors and I hope that this volume will be as well received as its predecessor. We look forward to suggestions and comments from the readers.

Udaya B. S. Prakash, M.D.
Editor-in-Chief

CHAPTER 1

THE BOARD EXAMINATION

Udaya B. S. Prakash, M.D.

A substantial number of physicians take the American Board of Internal Medicine (ABIM) certifying examination in internal medicine (IM) annually. Indeed, the total number of candidates who applied for the ABIM certification examination in IM for August 22-23, 1995, was 14,997, of whom 7,591 were first-time takers and 7,406 were repeaters. The discussion in this chapter is primarily aimed at candidates preparing for the ABIM's certifying or recertifying examinations in IM. However, candidates preparing for non-ABIM examinations may also benefit from the discussion, which covers various aspects of preparation for an examination, strategies to answer the questions effectively, and avoidance of pitfalls.

AIM OF THE EXAMINATION

The ABIM has stated that the certifying examination tests the breadth and depth of a candidate's knowledge in IM to ensure that the candidate has attained the necessary proficiency required for the practice of IM. According to the ABIM, the examination has two goals: the first is to ensure competence in the diagnosis and treatment of common disorders that have important consequences for patients, and the second is to ensure excellence in the broad domain of IM.

EXAMINATION FORMAT

The examination for ABIM certification in IM requires 2 days to complete and is divided into four sections; morning sessions are 4 hours and afternoon sessions are 3.5 hours. The dates of the next five examinations are as follows: August 20-21, 1996, August 19-20, 1997, August 25-26, 1998, August 24-25, 1999, and August 22-23, 2000. More details regarding the examination, training requirements, eligibility requirements, application forms, and other related information can be obtained from the American Board of Internal Medicine, 3624 Market Street, Philadelphia, PA 19104-2675

(telephone numbers: 215-243-1500 or 800-441-ABIM; fax number: 215-382-5515).

- Examination dates: August 20-21, 1996, and August 19-20, 1997.

Several hundred questions are used. Candidates should know that several questions known as field questions or pretest questions are included for experimental purposes only. These cannot be identified during the examination, and the answers to these are not scored. Because there is no penalty for guessing the answers, candidates should *answer every question.* Marking multiple answers for a single question is incorrect. Most questions (75%) are based on the presentations of patients. Among these, 75% are in the setting of outpatient or emergency room encounters, and the remaining 25% are in the inpatient setting, including critical care unit and nursing home. The ability to answer these questions requires integration of information provided from several sources (such as history, physical examination, laboratory test results, and consultations), prioritization of alternatives, or use of clinical judgment in reaching a correct conclusion. The overall ability to manage the patient in the most cost-effective fashion is stressed. Questions that require simple recall of medical facts are in the minority. The question format and examples are shown below.

- Candidates should answer every question; there is no penalty for guessing.
- Most questions (75%) are based on presentations of patients.
- Questions that require simple recall of medical facts are in the minority.

A list of normal laboratory values and illustrative materials (electrocardiograms, blood smears, Gram stains, urine sediments, chest radiographs, and photomicrographs) necessary to answer questions are provided in a separate atlas. Candidates should interpret the abnormal values on the basis of the normal values provided in the atlas and not on the basis of the normal values to which they are accustomed in their practice or training. Candidates for the 1995 certifying examination received a 57-page information booklet several weeks before the examination. The booklet provided a detailed description of the examination, including the types of questions used. Although much of the information in this chapter is borrowed from the 1995 booklet, the candidates for ABIM examinations in 1996 and 1997 should read the booklet that will be sent several weeks before each examination because the ABIM may change the format of the examination.

- A list of normal laboratory values and illustrative materials necessary to answer questions is provided.
- Read the information booklet sent several weeks before the examination by the ABIM.

SCORING

The passing scores reflect standards set by the ABIM. The core and non-core questions are scored separately. To pass, candidates have to pass both sections. Those who fail in either will have to pass both sections in any subsequent examination. Passing scores are set before the examination and therefore are not dependent on the performance of any group of candidates taking the examination.

- Passing scores are set before the examination.

THE CONTENT

The questions in the examination cover a broad area of IM, as listed below. They are divided into "primary" and "cross-content" groups and into "core" and "non-core" questions (see next paragraph). In the past few years, the subspecialties included in the primary content areas have included cardiovascular diseases, gastroenterology, pulmonary diseases, infectious diseases, rheumatology/orthopedics, endocrinology/metabolism, oncology, hematology, nephrology/urology, neurology, psychiatry, allergy and immunology, dermatology, obstetrics/gynecology, ophthalmology, otolaryngology, and miscellaneous. The specialties in the cross-content group have included adolescent medicine, critical care medicine, clinical epidemiology, ethics, geriatrics, nutrition, occupational medicine, preventive medicine, and substance abuse. Approximately 75% of the questions test knowledge in the following major specialties in IM: cardiology, endocrinology, gastroenterology, hematology, infectious disease, nephrology, oncology, pulmonary diseases, and rheumatology. The remaining 25% of questions cover allergy/immunology, dermatology, gynecology, neurology, ophthalmology, and psychiatry.

Independent of primary content, about 40% of the questions encompass the cross-content topics.

- About 75% of the questions test knowledge in the major specialties.
- About 25% of the questions cover allergy/immunology, dermatology, gynecology, neurology, ophthalmology, and psychiatry.
- About 40% of all questions encompass the cross-content topics: adolescent medicine, critical care medicine, clinical epidemiology, ethics, geriatrics, nutrition, occupational medicine, preventive medicine, and substance abuse.

CORE AND NON-CORE QUESTIONS

The various contents of the examination as outlined notwithstanding, the questions are broadly divided into core (35%) and non-core (65%) questions. The core questions assess whether the candidate possesses a minimal level of clinical competence. In other words, the core questions are aimed at evaluating knowledge and judgment about patients' problems that are frequent in practice and for which physician intervention makes a significant difference. Obviously, the non-core questions are more difficult to answer because they are structured to reflect excellence in clinical competence rather than just minimal competence. For example, a core question on hypertension might address treatment of uncomplicated essential hypertension; a non-core question might address the workup of secondary hypertension or the management of hypertensive cardiomyopathy. It is important for candidates to recognize that core and non-core questions are scored separately and that all candidates must achieve a passing score in both core and non-core questions to become ABIM-certified. Those who pass only one or the other will have to take both portions in the subsequent examination. Candidates cannot compensate for poor performance in core questions with a good performance in non-core questions. More than 80% of all candidates pass the core portion, but only 65% of first-time takers pass the non-core portion of the examination. Core and non-core questions are not labeled as such in the question book. It is a waste of time for the candidate to attempt to separate the core questions from the non-core questions during the examination because the questions judged to be non-core by the candidate may be considered a core question by the examiners.

- Questions: core (35%) and non-core (65%).
- Core questions assess a minimal level of clinical competence.
- Non-core questions are more difficult to answer; they are structured to reflect excellence in clinical competence.
- All candidates must pass both core and non-core questions.

Table 1-1 shows the distribution of the contents for the 1995 ABIM certification examination in IM.

Table 1-1.--Contents of the 1995 Certification Examination of the American Board of Internal Medicine

	Core and non-core components, %	
	Non-core	Core
Primary content areas		
Cardiovascular diseases	14	14
Gastroenterology	10	10
Pulmonary diseases	10	10
Infectious diseases	9	9
Rheumatology/orthopedics	8	8
Endocrinology/metabolism	7	8
Oncology	7	7
Hematology	6	5
Nephrology/urology	6	5
Neurology	4	4
Psychiatry	4	5
Allergy and immunology	3	2
Dermatology	3	3
Obstetrics/gynecology	2	2
Ophthalmology	2	2
Otolaryngology	2	2
Miscellaneous	3	3
Total	100	100
Cross-content areas		
Critical care medicine	10	12
Geriatrics	10	12
Preventive medicine	6	8
Clinical epidemiology	3	2
Ethics	3	2
Nutrition	3	3
Adolescent medicine	2	2
Occupational medicine	2	0
Substance abuse	2	3

From ABIM News Update: 1995 Internal Medicine Certification Examination. American Board of Internal Medicine, Philadelphia, Summer 1995. By permission.

QUESTION FORMAT

All questions will be of the *single-best-answer* type. This format reflects a change beginning with the 1995 examination. The question may be in the form of a case history, a brief statement, an roentgenogram, a graph, or a picture (such as a blood smear or Gram stain). Each question has five possible answers, and the candidates should identify the single best answer. It is essential to realize that more than one answer may appear correct or partially correct for a question. In this situation, the one answer that is better than the others should be selected. As noted above, most questions are based on encounters with patients. Some questions are progressive; that is, more than one question is based on the same patient. The examples in this chapter, the questions at the end of each chapter in this book, and the examples included in the ABIM's information booklet should help candidates become familiar with the ques-

tion format. Furthermore, the national in-training examination taken by about 90% of all second-year residents in IM provides ample opportunity to become familiar with the question format. The questions at the end of each chapter in this book contain both the single-best-answer format and the multiple true/false format. The latter is included to aid candidates preparing for examinations other than that given by the ABIM.

- *All* questions are of the *single-best-answer* type (this format was used in 1995).
- Become familiar with the question format by using various study guides.

Examples
Select *one best answer* for each of the following questions (answers are provided on page 5).

1. A 56-year-old woman is referred to you for an evaluation of dyspnea and chest pain of 6 weeks in duration. The chest pain is nonpleuritic, nonexertional, and located along the lower right lateral chest cage. She has no fever, cough, or chills. During the past few weeks, she has been experiencing constant low back pain. The patient underwent right mastectomy 4 years ago because of carcinoma of the breast with metastatic involvement of the right axillary lymph nodes. She received radiotherapy followed by chemotherapy for 24 months. Examination now reveals diminished breath sounds in the right lower lung field. The remainder of the examination is unremarkable. A chest radiograph suggests a moderate right pleural effusion. Which of the following is most likely to be helpful in confirming the suspected diagnosis?
   a. Bone scan with [99]technetium diphosphonate
   b. Bone marrow aspirate and biopsy
   c. Scalene fat pad biopsy
   d. Thoracentesis
   e. Mammography

2. A 20-year-old male military recruit returns home from several weeks of summer training in boot camp. He appears in your office the following day with a 12-day history of fever (≤38°C), coryza, pharyngitis, and cough. Physical examination discloses a bullous lesion over the right tympanic membrane and scattered crackles in both lung fields. Blood cell count reveals mild thrombocytopenia. A chest radiograph demonstrates patchy alveolar-interstitial infiltrates in both lungs. Which of the following is the best treatment for this patient?
   a. Erythromycin
   b. Penicillin
   c. Trimethoprim
   d. Clindamycin
   e. Ceftazidime

3. A 49-year-old male executive comes to your office with a 6-month history of cough, shortness of breath, and chest tightness soon after significant exertion. He notices these symptoms soon after he finishes a game of racquetball. He is a nonsmoker and has no risk factors for coronary artery disease. Results of physical examination in your office are normal. His weight is normal for his height. The chest radiograph is normal. Treadmill test for ischemic heart disease is negative. Which of the following diagnostic tests is indicated?
   a. Computed tomography of the chest
   b. Arterial blood gas studies at rest and after exercise
   c. Spirometry before and after exercise
   d. Ventilation-perfusion lung scan
   e. Cardiopulmonary exercise testing

4. Which of the following is not a clinical feature of infection caused by *Pneumocystis carinii* in adult patients with acquired immunodeficiency syndrome (AIDS) when compared with immunosuppressed patients without AIDS?
   a. Longer duration of symptoms
   b. Higher arterial oxygen tension
   c. Greater incidence of side effects from trimethoprim-sulfamethoxazole
   d. Recurrence or persistence of *P. carinii* infection
   e. The number of organisms seen microscopically is usually scanty

5. A hospitalized patient with AIDS dies of disseminated infection caused by *Mycobacterium avium* complex. Cough develops in the 28-year-old resident physician who cared for this patient. A chest radiograph reveals a nodular infiltrate in the right upper lobe. Tuberculin skin test (PPD) is positive (12 mm). Which of the following is the most appropriate next step?
   a. Begin antituberculous therapy with at least four drugs because *M. avium* is resistant to two-drug therapy
   b. Obtain sputum and gastric washings for stain and culture of tubercle bacilli
   c. Order human immunodeficiency virus (HIV) serologic testing now and in 6 months
   d. Begin prophylactic isoniazid therapy 300 mg/day for 12 months
   e. Treat with isoniazid 300 mg/day and rifampin 600 mg/day for 9 months

6. A 37-year-old woman presents with a history of recurrent palpebral swelling, laryngospasm, and urticaria-like skin lesions. A similar history is present among three family members. Which one of the following is not true of this disease?
   a. It can be mediated by IgE and IgG
   b. The precise cause is not identifiable in most patients
   c. It may be precipitated by drugs, contrast dye, or

   surgical procedures
   d. It is associated with a high mortality
   e. C1-esterase inhibitor is always absent

7. Which of the following pulmonary diagnoses cannot be established by bronchoalveolar lavage?
   a. Pulmonary alveolar proteinosis
   b. *Pneumocystis carinii* infection
   c. Pulmonary tuberculosis
   d. Idiopathic pulmonary fibrosis
   e. Lymphangitic pulmonary metastasis

8. A 68-year-old woman, nonsmoker, presents with an 8-week history of low-grade fever, malaise, myalgias, sore throat, hoarseness, and cough. She also complains of headaches, cramps in the jaws, and intermittent visual blurring. The leukocyte count is normal, and the erythrocyte sedimentation rate is 86 mm/hr. A chest radiograph is normal. Which of the following treatments is likely to resolve these symptoms?
   a. Cranial radiation and chemotherapy
   b. Itraconazole
   c. Corticosteroid
   d. Amantadine
   e. Antiplatelet therapy (aspirin)

9. A 34-year-old woman comes to your office with a 4-week history of hemoptysis, intermittent wheeze, and generalized weakness. Examination reveals that her blood pressure is 186/112 mm Hg. She appears cushingoid and has noted these changes taking place during the past 12 weeks. Auscultation discloses localized wheezing in the left mid-lung area. The chest radiograph indicates partial atelectasis of left upper lobe. She is referred to you for further evaluations. Which of the following is least likely to provide useful information in the diagnosis and treatment?
   a. Serum adrenocorticotropic hormone (ACTH) level
   b. 24-Hour urine test for 5-hydroxyindoleacetic acid (5-HIAA) level
   c. Bronchoscopy
   d. Computed tomography of chest
   e. Serum potassium level

10. A lung biopsy in a middle-aged man with a diffuse lung process is interpreted as showing lymphocytic interstitial pneumonitis. This abnormality may be encountered in all of the following except
   a. Diffuse alveolar cell carcinoma
   b. Chronic lymphocytic leukemia
   c. Sjögren's syndrome
   d. Patients with acquired immunodeficiency syndrome (AIDS)
   e. Lymphomatoid granulomatosis

11. A 42-year-old man who is an office worker presents to the emergency room with acute dyspnea. He has smoked 1 1/2 packs per day for 25 years and had been relatively asymptomatic except for a smoker's cough and mild dyspnea on exertion. Physical examination findings were not remarkable except for slightly diminished intensity of breath sounds over the right lung and some prolonged expiratory slowing, consistent with obstructive lung disease. The chest radiograph is shown below.

(Chest radiograph courtesy of Edward C. Rosenow III, M.D.)

Which of the following entities is most likely responsible for this patient's symptoms?
a. Pulmonary alveolar proteinosis
b. Silicosis
c. Pulmonary eosinophilic granuloma (histiocytosis X)
d. Idiopathic pulmonary fibrosis
e. Sarcoidosis

12. In a 34-year-old man with acute myelomonocytic leukemia, fever and progressive respiratory distress develop, and the chest radiograph shows diffuse alveolar infiltrates. The patient completed intensive chemotherapy 6 weeks earlier. The total leukocyte count has remained <900/mm^3 for more than 3 weeks. He is currently (for at least 10 days) receiving a cephalosporin (ceftazidime). Which of the following is the most appropriate therapy for this patient?
a. Clindamycin

b. Blood transfusion to increase the number of circulating leukocytes
c. Antituberculous (triple-drug) therapy
d. Amphotericin intravenously
e. Pentamidine aerosol

The answers to the questions are as follows: 1, d (metastatic pleural effusion); 2, a (*Mycoplasma* infection); 3, c (exercise-induced asthma); 4, e; 5, b; 6, e (hereditary angioneurotic edema); 7, d; 8, c (giant cell arteritis); 9, b (bronchial carcinoid); 10, a; 11, c (pulmonary eosinophilic granuloma with spontaneous pneumothorax); 12, d (disseminated aspergillosis in a leukopenic patient).

Questions 1 through 3 are examples of core questions because they are aimed at evaluating knowledge and judgment about problems that are encountered frequently in practice and for which physician intervention makes a significant difference. These core questions judge the candidate's minimal level of clinical competence. Questions 1 through 3 include descriptions of typical clinical features of metastatic breast carcinoma, *Mycoplasma* pneumonia, and exercise-induced asthma, respectively. Therefore, the decision making is relatively easy and straightforward. Questions 4 through 12 are non-core questions. They are more difficult to answer because they are structured to reflect excellence in clinical competence rather than just minimal competence. In other words, they require more extensive knowledge (that is, knowledge beyond that required for minimal competence) in IM and its subspecialties. Although most of the questions above are based on encounters with patients, some (questions 4, 7, and 10) require recall of well-known medical facts. A minority of questions in the ABIM examination are in this category.

PREPARATION FOR THE TEST

Training during medical school forms the foundation on which advanced clinical knowledge is accumulated during residency training. However, the serious preparation for the examination actually starts at the beginning of the residency training in IM. Most candidates, however, require a minimum of 6 to 8 months of intense preparation for the examination. Cramming just before the examination is counterproductive. Some of the methods for preparation for the board examination are described below. Additionally, each candidate may develop her or his own system.

● Preparation for the ABIM examination starts at the beginning of the residency training in IM.

It is essential that each candidate study a standard textbook of medicine from beginning to end. Any of the standard textbooks on IM should provide a good basic knowledge in all areas of IM. Ideally, the candidate should read one good textbook and not jump from one to another, except for reading certain chapters that are outstanding in a particular textbook (see below). This book and similar board review syllabi are excellent tools for brushing up on important board-relevant information several weeks to months before the examination. They, however, cannot take the place of comprehensive textbooks of medicine. This book is designed as only a study guide rather than a comprehensive textbook of medicine. Therefore, it should not be used as the sole source of medical information for the examination.

- Candidates should thoroughly study a standard textbook of medicine.
- This book is designed as only a study guide.

The Medical Knowledge Self-Assessment Program (MKSAP) prepared by the American College of Physicians is valuable for obtaining practice in answering multiple-choice questions and multiple true/false questions. The text contents, however, are uneven in the coverage of topics. By design, the MKSAP is prepared for the continuing medical education of practicing (presumably ABIM-certified) internists rather than for those preparing for initial certification by the ABIM. For recertification purposes, MKSAP is a reasonable aid.

Formation of study groups, three to five candidates per group, permits study of different textbooks and review articles in journals. It is important that the group meet regularly and that each candidate be assigned reading materials. Selected review papers and state-of-the-art articles on common and important topics in IM should be included in the study materials. Indiscriminate reading of articles from many journals should be avoided. In any case, most candidates who begin preparation 6 to 8 months before the examination will not find time for extensive study of journal materials. The newer information in the recent (within 6 to 9 months of the examination) medical journals is unlikely to be included in the examination. Notes and other materials the candidates have gathered during their residence training are also good sources of information. These clinical "pearls" gathered from mentors will be of help in remembering certain important points.

- Study groups may help cover large amounts of information.
- Avoid indiscriminate reading of articles from many journals.
- Information in the recent (within 6 to 9 months of the examination) medical journals is unlikely to be included in the examination.

Certain diseases are more important because they are topical (for example, AIDS, tuberculosis, lipid disorders, and recent increase in morbidity and mortality due to asthma). Try to remember some of the uncommon manifestations of the most common diseases (such as polycythemia in common obstructive pulmonary disease) and common manifestations of uncommon diseases (such as pneumothorax in eosinophilic granuloma). Certain diseases, many peculiar and uncommon, are eminently "board-eligible," meaning that they may appear in the board examinations more frequently than in clinical practice. They are usually in the non-core category. Most of these are covered in this book. Certain formulas and points should be memorized (such as the alveolar gas equation). Most significantly, the clinical training obtained and the regular study habits formed during residency training are the most important aspects of preparing for the boards.

- Study as much as possible about board-eligible topics.
- Learn about the uncommon manifestations of common diseases and the common manifestations of uncommon diseases.

DAY OF THE EXAMINATION

Plenty of time is allowed to read and answer all the questions; therefore, there is no need to rush or become anxious. Start by answering the first question and continue sequentially (do not skip too many--see below). Do not be alarmed by lengthy questions; look for the salient points in the question. When faced with a lengthy or confusing question, do not become distracted by that question. Mark it so you can find it later, then go to the next question and come back to the unanswered ones at the end. Extremely lengthy stem statements or case presentations are apparently intended to test the candidate's ability to separate the essential from the unnecessary or unimportant information. Carry a simple ruler (make sure it is allowed) to the examination. It can be used, for instance, to estimate the P50 point on the oxyhemoglobin dissociation curve or for drawing nomograms from memory.

- Look for the salient points in each question.
- Do not skip questions.

Some candidates may fail the examination despite the possession of an immense amount of knowledge and the clinical competence necessary to pass the examination. Their failure to pass the examination may be caused by the lack of ability to understand or interpret the questions properly. The ability to understand the nuances of the question format is sometimes referred to as "boardsmanship." Intelligent interpretation of the questions is very important for candidates who are not well versed in the format of multiple-choice questions. It is very critical to read the final sentence (that appears just before the multiple answers) several times to understand how an answer should be selected. For example, the question may ask you to select the *correct* or *incorrect* answer. It is very likely that the questions will no longer have wording such as "all of the following are true except." Nevertheless, it is advisable to recheck the question format before selecting the correct answer.

Another hint for selecting the correct answers is to avoid answers that contain absolute or very restrictive words such as "always," "never," or "must." For example, if an answer states that "pneumonia vaccine must (or always, or never) be given to all patients with chronic obstructive pulmonary disease," then it is obviously a wrong answer. Another means to ensure that you know the correct answer is to cover the answers with a piece of paper before tackling the question; read the question and then try to write the answer on a piece of paper before looking at the list of potential answers. If the answer you had formulated is not among the list of answers provided, then it may indicate a problem in the interpretation of the question. When a patient's case is presented, write down the diagnosis before looking at the list of answers. It will be reassuring to realize (particularly if your diagnosis is supported by the answers) that you are on the "right track."

- Develop "boardsmanship."
- Do not select answers with absolute or very restrictive words such as "always," "never," or "must."
- Try to formulate your own answer before looking at the answers provided.

Candidates are well advised to use the basic fund of knowledge accumulated from clinical experience and reading to solve the questions. Approaching the questions as "real-life" encounters with patients is far better than trying to second-guess the examiners or trying to analyze whether the question is "tricky." As indicated above, the questions are never "tricky," and there is no reason for the ABIM to trick the candidates into choosing wrong answers.

- Approach questions as "real-life" encounters with patient.
- There are no "trick" questions.

It is better not to discuss the questions or answers (after the examination) with other candidates. Such discussions usually cause more consternation, although some candidates may derive a false sense of having performed well in the examination. In any case, the candidates are bound by their oath to the ABIM not to discuss or disseminate the questions.

CONNECTIONS

Associations, causes, complications, and other relationships between a phenomenon or disease and clinical features are important to remember and recognize. I call these "connections." For example, Table 1-2 lists some of the "connections" in infectious and occupational entities in pulmonary medicine. Each subspecialty has many similar connections, and candidates

for the ABIM and other examinations may want to prepare lists like this for different areas.

RECERTIFICATION

The diplomate certificates issued to successful candidates who have passed the ABIM examination in IM in 1990 and thereafter are valid for 10 years. The ABIM has announced plans for the newly devised recertification examination in IM. The first final examination under the new guidelines will be administered annually beginning November 20, 1996 (see details below). In its Recertification Program Application Information Booklet 1995-96, the ABIM has stated that the recertification program is dedicated to promoting clinical excellence within the specialty of IM. The goals of the recertification program are to 1) improve the quality of patient care, 2) set high standards of clinical competence, and 3) foster the continuing scholarship required for professional excellence over a lifetime of practice.

- Certificates issued to successful candidates who have passed the ABIM examination in IM in 1990 and thereafter are valid for 10 years.
- The first recertification examination under the new guidelines will be administered on November 20, 1996.

Registration for the recertification examination opened on July 1, 1995. The recertification program consists of three steps:

1. Completion of the Self-Evaluation Process (SEP), the at-home, open-book examination. The SEP modules became available on October 1, 1995, and they must be returned to ABIM by August 1, 1996 (those who do not want to take the final examination in 1996 can take the SEP modular examination on a self-determined schedule over 5 years).
2. Submission of application for the final examination by September 1, 1996. This includes verification of clinical competence and possession of a valid certificate in either Basic Life Saving (BLS) or Advanced Cardiac Life Support (ACLS).
3. A proctored, written final examination on November 20, 1996, and annually thereafter. The format of the final examination is somewhat similar to that of the certifying examination discussed above (three modules, and each module consists of 60 multiple-choice questions).

- All recertification candidates must have valid certificate in either BLS or ACLS.
- October 1, 1995: SEP modules became available.
- August 1, 1996: deadline for returning completed SEP

modules to ABIM.
- September 1, 1996: deadline for submission of application for the final examination.
- November 20, 1996: final examination (a written, proctored examination).

Details of the recertification program can be obtained by writing to the ABIM offices at the American Board of Internal Medicine, 3624 Market Street, Philadelphia, PA 19104-2675 (telephone numbers: 215-243-1500 or 800-441-ABIM; fax number: 215-382-5515).

Table 1-2.--Example of "Connections" Between Etiologic Factors and Diseases

Etiologic factor	Agent, disease
Cattle, swine, horses, wool, hide	Anthrax
Abattoir worker, veterinarian	Brucellosis
Travel to Southeast Asia, South America	Melioidosis
Squirrels, chipmunks, rabbits, rats	Plague
Rabbits, squirrels, infected flies, or ticks	Tularemia
Birds	Psittacosis, histoplasmosis
Rats, dogs, cats, cattle, swine	Leptospirosis
Goats, cattle, swine	Q-fever
Soil, water-cooling tower	Legionellosis
Military camps	Mycoplasmosis
Chicken coop, starling roosts, caves	Histoplasmosis
Soil	Blastomycosis
Travel in Southwestern United States	Coccidioidomycosis
Ohio and Mississippi river valleys	Histoplasmosis
Decaying wood	Histoplasmosis
Gardeners, florists, straw, plants	Sporotrichosis
Progressive, massive fibrosis	Silicosis, coal, hematite, kaolin, graphite, asbestosis
Autoimmune mechanism	Silicosis, asbestosis, berylliosis
Monday morning sickness	Byssinosis, bagassosis, metal fume fever
Metals and fumes producing asthma	Baker's asthma, meat wrapper's asthma, printer's asthma, nickel, platinum, toluene diisocyanate (TDI), cigarette cutter's asthma
Increased incidence of tuberculosis	Silicosis, hematite lung
Increased incidence of carcinoma	Asbestos, hematite, arsenic, nickel, uranium, chromate
Welder prone to develop	Siderosis, pulmonary edema, bronchitis, emphysema
Centrilobar emphysema	Coal, hematite
Generalized emphysema	Cadmium, bauxite
Silo filler's lung produced by	Nitrogen dioxide
Farmer's lung produced by	*Thermoactinomyces, Micropolyspora*
Asbestos exposure	Mesothelioma, bronchogenic carcinoma, gastrointestinal cancer
Eggshell calcification	Silicosis, sarcoid
Sarcoid-like disease	Berylliosis
Diaphragmatic calcification	Asbestosis (also ankylosing spondylitis)
Nonfibrogenic pneumoconioses	Tin, emery, antimony, titanium, barium
Minimal pathology in lungs	Siderosis, baritosis, stannosis
Bullous emphysema	Bauxite lung

CHAPTER 2
ALLERGY

James T. Li, M.D.

ASTHMA

History

Allergic asthma can be mild and self-limiting or potentially debilitating, but intrinsic asthma tends to be progressive, to result in hospitalization for status asthmaticus, and to require continuous steroid therapy for suppression. Some patients have both intrinsic and allergic asthma. You can be reasonably certain someone has allergic asthma if the symptoms are sporadic and consistently related to exposure to animal dander (e.g., visiting the house of someone who has cats) or are seasonal (e.g., correspond to hay fever season). You can be reasonably certain someone does not have it if allergy skin test results are negative.

- In allergic asthma, symptoms are sporadic and consistently related to exposure or are seasonal.

If a patient has either form of asthma, nonspecific bronchial hyperresponsiveness tends to blur the distinctions between allergic and intrinsic aspects, with allergic patients likely responding also to many nonimmunologic triggers, e.g., airborne particulates (however inert), temperature change, air pollutants, and strong odors (including "fragrances"). Cold dry air is very provocative, especially under conditions of hyperpnea, e.g., physical exercise.

- Allergic patients are likely to respond to many nonimmunologic triggers.
- Cold dry air is very provocative.

Assessment of Severity

Asthma is mild if the symptoms are sporadic, continuous treatment is not needed, and the flow-volume curve during formal pulmonary function testing is normal between episodes of symptoms. Even in patients fitting this description, inflammation (albeit patchy) in airways is significant, and glucocorticoid inhaled on a regular basis diminishes bronchial hyperresponsiveness.

- Glucocorticoid inhaled on a regular basis diminishes bronchial hyperresponsiveness.

Asthma is moderate when 1) the symptoms occur with some regularity or daily, 2) there is some nocturnal occurrence of symptoms, or 3) medication is required on a regularly scheduled basis for asthma control. For many of these patients, the flow-volume curve is rarely normal, and complete pulmonary function testing may show evidence of hyperinflation, as indicated by increased residual volume or an increase above expected levels for the diffusing capacity of the lung for CO_2.

Asthma is severe when symptoms are present almost continuously and when the upper end of the dose range of the usual medications is needed to control the asthma. Most patients require either large doses of inhaled glucocorticoids or oral prednisone daily for adequate control. Most of them have been hospitalized more than once and for more than overnight observation. Occasionally, patients move from one form of asthma to another. Someone may have severe asthma for a couple of years which finally is adequately controlled. Their status then changes to moderate asthma. Note that one of the first signs that asthma is not well-controlled is the emergence of the nocturnal symptoms.

- Nocturnal symptoms suggest that asthma is worsening.

Pathophysiology

Asthmatics tend to have abnormalities in β-adrenergic responsiveness throughout the body and not just in the lung. Peripheral blood leukocytes and adrenergic neural pathways behave as though signal transduction is impaired in adrenergic receptors. How this relates to histologic changes in asthma is unclear.

9

- Abnormalities in β-adrenergic responsiveness.

Common to all forms of asthma is bronchial hyperresponsiveness. Bronchial hyperresponsiveness is measured by assessing pulmonary function before and after exposure to methacholine, histamine, cold air, or exercise. Prolonged glucocorticoid therapy reduces bronchial hyperresponsiveness. Prolonged therapy with certain other anti-inflammatory drugs, e.g., sodium cromolyn, also reduces bronchial hyperresponsiveness, as shown in study of long-term (1-year) therapy with nedocromil, a cromolyn congener. Note that although cromolyn and nedocromil both were originally touted as "anti-allergic" (they inhibited mast cell activation), they affect most cells involved in inflammation; also, the effects on these cells occur at lower doses than those that inhibit mast cell activation.

- Bronchial hyperresponsiveness generally is present in all forms of asthma.
- Prolonged glucocorticoid therapy reduces bronchial responsiveness.
- Cromolyn and nedocromil affect most cells involved in inflammation.

Asthmatics with allergic asthma probably have mast cell and basophil mediators that have significant roles in the development of the endobronchial inflammation and smooth muscle changes that occur after acute exposure to allergen. Polymorphonuclear leukocytes are prominent during the immediate reaction.

- In the immediate-phase reaction, mast cells and basophils are important.

In the so-called late-phase reaction to allergen exposure, the bronchi have histologic features of chronic inflammation, and eosinophils become prominent in the reaction.

- In the late-phase reaction, eosinophils become prominent.

Patients with negative allergy skin test results and chronic asthma seem to have an inflammatory infiltrate in the bronchi and a histologic picture dominated by eosinophils when asthma is active. Patients with sudden asphyxic asthma may have a neutrophilic rather than an eosinophilic infiltration of the airway.

Various hypotheses explain the development of nonallergic asthma. One proposal is that the initial inflammation represents an autoimmune reaction arising from a viral or other microbial infection in the lung and, for reasons unknown, inflammation becomes chronic and characterized by a lymphocyte cytokine profile in which interleukin-5 (IL-5) is prominent. The intense eosinophilic inflammation is thought to come from IL-5 influence of T cells in the chronic inflamma-

tory infiltrate. Consistent with this hypothesis is recent evidence implicating chlamydial infection as an inciting factor in several postinfectious adult-onset asthmatics. Airway macrophages and platelets have low-affinity IgE receptors on their membranes and are activated by cross-linking of these receptors by allergen, suggesting that some phases of lung inflammation in allergy may involve the macrophage as a primary responder cell.

- IL-5 stimulates eosinophils.
- Airway macrophages and platelets have low-affinity IgE receptors.

The two types of helper T cells are TH1 and TH2. In general, TH1 cells produce interferon-γ (IFN-γ) and IL-2, and TH2 cells produce IL-4 and IL-5. IL-4 stimulates IgE synthesis. Hence, many clinical scientists believe that atopic asthma is caused by a preferential activation of TH2 lymphocytes.

- IL-4 stimulates IgE synthesis.
- TH2 lymphocytes produce IL-4 and IL-5.

Important characteristics of cytokines are summarized in Table 2-1.

Spirometry

Peak flow rate (PFR) changes little during loss of a large fraction of expiratory flow rate in mid-regions of the flow-volume curve. PFR occurs when little more than anatomical dead space volume has been expired and is only an approximate measure of airway obstruction.

Asthma chiefly affects medium- and small-sized airways; expired air from these airways generates the mid-expiratory flow rates. The flow-volume curve of asthmatics is often concave.

- Medium- and small-sized airways are affected in asthma.
- The flow-volume curve in asthmatics is often concave.

As asthma progresses, the flow-volume curve declines and for the same reason that PFR eventually declines: hyperinflation induces acute restrictive change in pulmonary function. Because of air-trapping, there is no room to expire a normal volume of air.

- As asthma progresses, flow-volume curve declines.
- Hyperinflation is secondary to air-trapping.

Pathology

The pathologic features of asthma have been studied chiefly in fatal cases; some bronchoscopic data are available about mild and moderate asthmatics. The amount of variation between mild and fatal asthma is unknown, but it probably is not large.

Table 2-1.--Characteristics of Cytokines

Cytokine	Major actions	Primary sources
IL-1	Lymphocyte activation	Macrophages
	Fibroblast activation	Endothelial cells
	Fever	Lymphocytes
IL-2	T- and B-cell activation	T cells (TH1)
IL-3	Mast cell proliferation	T cells
	Neutrophil, macrophage maturation	Mast cells
IL-4	IgE synthesis	T cells (TH2)
IL-5	Eosinophil proliferation and differentiation	T cells (TH2)
IL-6	IgG synthesis	Fibroblasts
	Lymphocyte activation	T cells
IL-8	Neutrophil chemotaxis	Fibroblasts
		Endothelial cells
		Monocytes
IL-10	Inhibits IFN-γ, IL-1 production	T cells
		Macrophages
IFN-α	Antiviral activity	Leukocytes
IFN-γ	Activates macrophages	T cells (TH1)
	Stimulates MHC expression	
	Inhibits TH2 activity	
TNF-γ	Antitumor cell activity	Lymphocytes
		Macrophages
TNF-β	Antitumor cell activity	T cells
GM-CSF	Stimulates mast cells, granulocytes, macrophages	Lymphocytes
		Mast cells
		Macrophages

GM-CSF, granulocyte-macrophage colony-stimulating factor; IFN, interferon; IL, interleukin; MHC, major histocompatibility complex; TH, helper T cell; TNF, tumor necrosis factor.

The histologic hallmarks of asthma are listed in Table 2-2.

● Histologic hallmarks of asthma: mucus gland hypertrophy, mucus hypersecretion, epithelial desquamation, widening of basement membrane, infiltration by eosinophils.

Airway Inflammation

Glucocorticoids applied topically to asthmatic bronchi can decrease the inflammation and control the disease. Glucocorticoids given systemically prevent eosinophil release from the bone marrow, making them unavailable for the inflammatory response. This mechanism is not operative with topical therapy because topical therapy has little or no systemic effect.

● Inhaled glucocorticoids decrease airway inflammation.
● Inhaled glucocorticoids have little systemic effect.

The maintenance of round-cell lymphocyte/monocyte inflammatory infiltrate in the bronchial submucosa likely depends on lymphokine secretory patterns. Glucocorticoids may interfere at several levels in the lymphokine cascade.

Bronchioalveolar lavage and biopsy studies show that glucocorticoids inhibit IL-4, IL-5, and granulocyte-macrophage colony-stimulating factor (GM-CSF) in asthma.

● Glucocorticoids reduce airway inflammation by modulating cytokines.

Table 2-2.--Histologic Hallmarks of Asthma

Mucus gland hypertrophy
Mucus hypersecretion
Alteration of tinctorial and viscoelastic properties of mucus
Widening of basement membrane zone of bronchial epithelial membrane
Increased number of intraepithelial leukocytes and mast cells
Round cell infiltration of bronchial submucosa
Intense eosinophilic infiltration of submucosa
Widespread damage to bronchial epithelium
    Large areas of complete desquamation of epithelium into airway lumen
    Mucus plugs filled with eosinophils and their products

Finally, monocytes or platelets may be important in the asthmatic process. Glucocorticoids modify self-activation pathways for monocytes and activation properties of platelets (probably by modulating arachidonate metabolism).

- Glucocorticoids can inhibit the inflammatory properties of monocytes and platelets.

Furthermore, glucocorticoids have vasoconstrictive properties, which reduce vascular congestive changes in the mucosa, and they tend to reduce mucus gland secretion (principally, proteoglycan components).

- Glucocorticoids have vasoconstrictive properties.
- Glucocorticoids reduce mucus gland secretion.

Corticosteroid Therapy

Because of long-term benefits in reduced bronchial hyper-responsiveness with little or no side effects, the trend is to prescribe inhaled glucocorticoids earlier in mild asthma, sometimes as the only therapeutic agent, even without antecedent bronchodilators. Long-term use of β-agonist bronchodilators may adversely affect asthma; this also argues for earlier use of inhaled glucocorticoids. Asthma mortality has been linked to heavy use of β-agonist inhalers. This association may simply reflect that patients with more severe asthma (who are more likely to die of an asthma attack) use more β-agonist inhalers. However, prolonged and heavy use of inhaled β-agonists may have a direct deleterious effect on asthma, but this has not been proven. Certainly, asthmatics with regularly recurring symptoms probably should have inhaled steroid (or cromolyn or nedocromil) as part of the treatment. When the steroid requirement is unknown, it is reasonable to start with two puffs of beclomethasone (Beclovent or Vanceril, 84 μg per puff) or triamcinolone acetonide (Azmacort, 100 μg per puff) four times daily, or flunisolide (Aerobid, 250 μg per puff) twice daily. In very mild cases, starting with an inhaled β-agonist alone may be reasonable.

- Prescribe inhaled glucocorticoids earlier in mild asthma.
- Long-term use of β-agonist bronchodilators may worsen asthma.

The most common adverse effects of inhaled corticosteroids are dysphonia and thrush. These unwanted effects occur in about 10% of patients and can be reduced by using a spacer device and rinsing the mouth after administration. Usually, oral thrush can be treated successfully with antifungal troches. Dysphonia, when persistent, should be treated by reducing or discontinuing the use of inhaled corticosteroids.

Detailed study of the systemic effects of inhaled corticosteroids show that these agents are much safer than oral corticosteroids. Nevertheless, there is biochemical evidence that inhaled corticosteriods can affect the hypothalamic-pituitary-adrenal axis and bone metabolism. Inhaled corticosteroids can also decrease growth velocity in children and adolescents.

In patients with significant symptoms, it probably is best to induce as complete a remission in airway inflammation as possible with a 10-day course of oral prednisone concomitant with initiating inhaled steroid. If the patient has not taken corticosteroids in the last 3 months or more, a reasonable prednisone course is 10 mg four times daily for the first 7 days, tapering by 10 mg daily for the next 3 days. If the patient has taken corticosteroids recently, particularly systemic corticosteroids, then the starting dose of inhaled corticosteroids should be increased to four puffs four times daily, and the oral prednisone dose schedule needs to be increased. The most common cause of poor results in asthma therapy is poor inhaler technique by patients taking inhaled steroid. Poor technique can make a powerful and effective therapy worthless. Therefore, all patients using a metered-dose inhaler should be taught the proper technique of using these devices. Most patients using inhaled corticosteroids should be using a spacer device with the inhaler.

- The most common cause of poor results is poor inhaler technique.
- Patients should use a spacer device with inhaled corticosteroids.

Goals of Asthma Management

The goals of asthma management are listed in Table 2-3.

Medications for Asthma

Medications for asthma are listed in Table 2-4. Currently, the only anticholinergic drug available in the U.S.A. for treating asthma is ipratropium bromide (Atrovent), although it is approved for only chronic obstructive pulmonary disease. Many β-adrenergic compounds are available, but albuterol (Proventil,

Table 2-3.--Goals of Asthma Management

Patient understands the disease

Hospitalizations for asthma are rare because patient understands step-care and has plan for responding to flares of the disease

Physician fosters independence of patient and accurate/appropriate self-care

Asthma has low impact on patient's life-style

Patient micromanages and physician provides guidance on broad issues and in setting goals

Treatment program makes adequate use of glucocorticoids and appropriately de-emphasizes β₂-agonist drugs

Pulmonary function test results are normal, nearly normal, or at patient's best documented level

---

Table 2-4.--Medications for Asthma

Bronchodilator compounds
    Anticholinergic drugs (ipratropium bromide)
    β_2-agonist drugs
    Methylxanthines (theophylline + congeners)
"Anti-allergic" compounds
    Cromolyn
    Nedocromil
Glucocorticoids
    Systemic
        Prednisone
        Methylprednisolone
        Hydrocortisone
        Triamcinolone
        Dexamethasone
    Topical
        Triamcinolone acetonide
        Beclomethasone
        Flunisolide

Ventolin), pirbuterol (Maxair), and metaproterenol (Alupent) are probably prescribed most. All these agents are available in oral rather than inhaled form, and more side effects occur when they are given orally. Nebulized β-agonists are infrequently used chronically in adult asthma, although they may be lifesaving in acute attacks. For home use, the metered-dose inhaler is the preferred delivery system. Theophylline is effective for asthma but has a narrow therapeutic index. Note drug interactions (cimetidine, erythromycin, and quinolone antibiotics can increase the serum level of theophylline).

- Theophylline has a narrow therapeutic index.
- β-agonists are best delivered by the inhaler route.

Management of Chronic Asthma

A step-care approach is shown in the accompanying algorithm (Fig. 2-1). Baseline spirometry is recommended for all patients with asthma, and home peak flow monitoring is recommended for patients with moderate and severe asthma.

- Spirometry is recommended for all asthma patients.
- Home peak flow monitoring is recommended for those with moderate and severe asthma.

Environmental triggers should be discussed with all patients with asthma, and allergy testing should be offered to patients with suspected allergic asthma or to those whose asthma is not well controlled. Although allergy immunotherapy is effective, it is recommended only for patients with allergic asthma who have undergone a careful evaluation by an asthma specialist.

Management of Acute Asthma

Inhaled β-agonists, measurements of lung function, and systemic corticosteroids (for most patients) are the cornerstones of managing acute asthma (Fig. 2-2). Generally, nebulized albuterol, administered repeatedly if necessary, is the first line of treatment. Delivery of β-agonist by metered-dose inhaler can be substituted in less severe asthma attacks. Inhaled β-agonist delivered by continuous nebulization may be appropriate for more severe patients.

- Inhaled β-agonist can be delivered by intermittent nebulization, continuous nebulization, or metered-dose inhaler.

It is important to measure lung function (usually PEFR but also FEV whenever possible) at presentation and after administration of bronchodilator. These measurements provide invaluable information that allows the physician to assess the severity of the asthma attack and the response (if any) to treatment.

Patients who do not respond promptly and fully to inhaled β-agonists should receive a course of systemic corticosteroids. The most severe and poorly responsive patients should be treated in the hospital or intensive care unit.

- Measure pulmonary function at presentation and after giving bronchodilators.
- Most patients with acute asthma need a course of systemic corticosteroids.

Asthma-Provoking Drugs

It is important to recognize the potentially severe adverse response asthmatics may show to β-blocking drugs; propranolol leads the list of agents causing severe adverse responses. Severe asthma can be provoked in some asthmatics who have been asymptomatic for long periods, so vigilance is necessary in all clinical circumstances. These remarks apply to asthmatics with glaucoma treated with ophthalmic preparations of timolol and betaxolol (betaxolol is much less likely to cause problems but is not completely innocent).

- β-blocking drugs, including eyedrops, can cause severe adverse responses.
- Note that so-called β_1 selective agents such as atenolol may also provoke asthma.

A significant fraction of asthmatics *cough* when given angiotensin converting enzyme (ACE) inhibitor drugs, and the asthma of some worsens. Because pulmonary function testing does not show decrement in many of these asthmatics and many nonasthmatics may also cough after taking ACE inhibitors, the coughing may not be additional bronchospasm, as it often seems to be when asthmatics cough.

- ACE inhibitors can cause coughing.

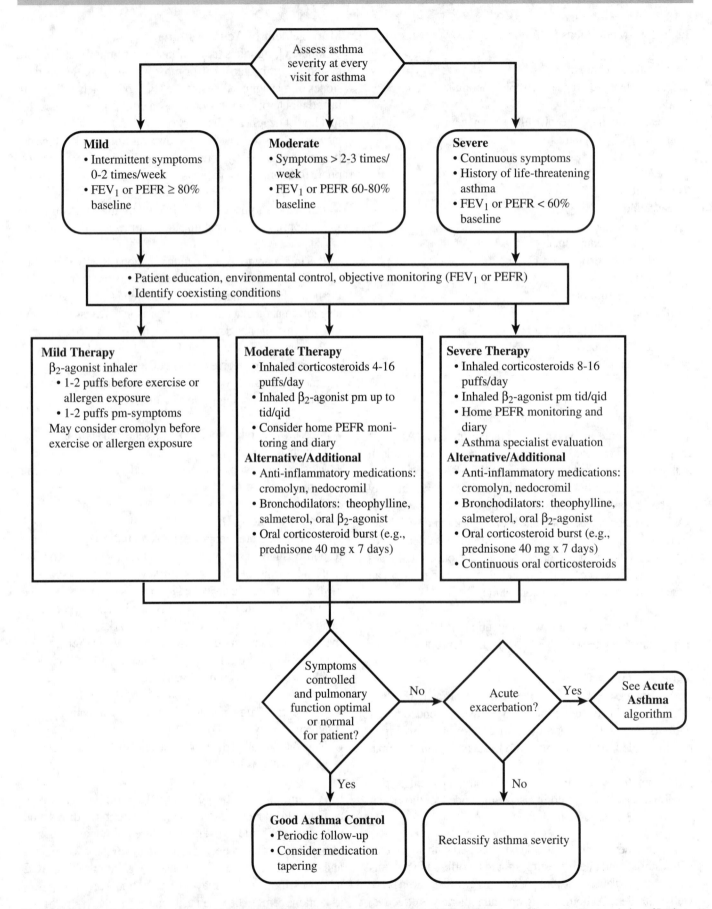

Fig. 2-1. Management of chronic asthma in adults. FEV_1, 1-second forced expiratory volume; PEFR, peak expiratory flow rate. (By permission of Institute of Clinical Systems Integration.)

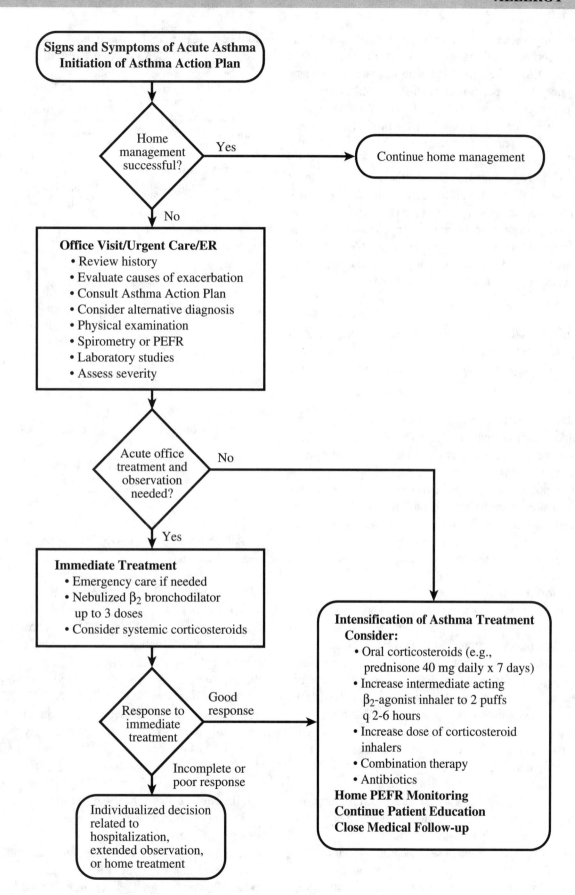

Fig. 2-2. Management of acute asthma in adults. ER, emergency room; PEFR, peak expiratory flow rate. (By permission of Institute of Clinical Systems Integration.)

Aspirin ingestion can cause acute, severe, and fatal asthma in a small subset of asthmatics. The cause of the reaction is unknown. Most of the affected patients have nasal polyposis and hyperplastic pansinus mucosal disease and are steroid-dependent for control of asthma. However, not all asthmatics with this reaction to aspirin fit the profile; thus, physicians should be aware of this possibility. Many nonsteroidal anti-inflammatory drugs can trigger the reaction to aspirin; the likelihood of a drug causing the reaction correlates with its potency of inhibiting cyclooxygenase enzyme in vitro. Structural aspects of the drug seem unrelated to its tendency to provoke the reaction. Thus, enolic acid agents and carboxylic acids are capable of provoking reactions. Table 2-5 lists specific drugs. Only nonacetylated salicylates such as choline salicylate (a weak cyclooxygenase inhibitor) seem not to provoke the reaction.

- Aspirin and other nonsteroidal anti-inflammatory agents can cause acute, severe asthma.
- Asthma, nasal polyposis, and aspirin sensitivity form the aspirin triad.

Traditionally, asthmatics have been warned not to use antihistamines, because anticholinergic activity of some antihistamines was thought to cause drying of lower respiratory tract secretions, further worsening the asthma. However, antihistamines do not worsen asthma. On occasion, we specifically prescribe antihistamine for allergic asthmatics, because the drug may have some beneficial effect on asthmatic inflammation.

- Antihistamines are not contraindicated in asthma.

Occupational Asthma

Every patient interviewed about a history of allergy or asthma must also provide an adequate occupational history. A large fraction of occupational asthma probably escapes diagnosis because physicians obtain an inadequate (or no) history. An enormous range of possible industrial circumstances may lead to exposure and resultant disease. Table 2-6 lists the most widely recognized types of occupational asthma.

- Inquiry into a possible occupational cause of asthma is important in all asthmatics.

As new industrial processes and products evolve, occupational asthma may become more common. An example of a potentially huge problem is latex-induced asthma among medical workers, with the widespread use in the last 3-4 years of latex gloves for medical workers. Another new problem is asthma in airline pilots exposed to cockpit communications equipment that uses TDI-based inks. Incidence of occupational asthma is estimated to be 6%-15% of all adult-onset asthmatics.

Table 2-5.--Common Nonsteroidal Anti-Inflammatory Drugs That Can Provoke Bronchospasm in Aspirin-Sensitive Asthmatics

	Generic (tradename)
Enolic acid	Piroxicam (Feldene)
Carboxylic acid	
Acetic group	Indomethacin (Indocin)
	Sulindac (Clinoril)
	Tolmetin (Tolectin)
Propionic acid group	Ibuprofen (Advil, Rufen)
	Naproxen (Naprosyn, Anaprox)
	Fenoprofen (Nalfon)
Fenamate group	Meclofenamate (Meclomen)
	Mefenamic acid (Ponstel)

- Allergy to latex is a newly discovered cause of occupational asthma.

Gastroesophageal Reflux and Asthma

The role of gastroesophageal reflux in asthma is not known. Two mechanistic hypotheses are 1) reflux bronchospasm from acid in the distal esophagus and 2) recurrent aspiration of gastric contents. A well-documented reflex in dogs links acid in the distal esophagus to vagally mediated bronchospasm, but no such reflex had been identified in humans. Thus, the hypothesis that gastric contents reach the tracheobronchial tree by ascending to the hypopharynx is apparently the mechanism by which gastroesophageal reflux causes human asthma (if it does).

Methacholine Bronchial Challenge

Do not perform a methacholine challenge in patients with severe expiratory obstruction.

Stringent cutoff values for the percentage fall in 1-second forced expiratory volume (FEV_1) after methacholine were established by and are useful mainly in epidemiologic studies. Usually, a 20% decrease in FEV_1 is considered a positive result.

Table 2-6.--Industrial Agents That Can Cause Asthma

Metals
   Salts of platinum, nickel, chrome
Wood dusts
   Mahogany
   Oak
   Redwood
   Western red cedar (plicatic acid)
Vegetable dusts
   Castor bean
   Cotton dust
   Cottonseed
   Flour
   Grain (mite, weevil antigens)
   Green coffee
   Gums
Industrial chemicals and plastics
   Ethylenediamine
   Phthalic and trimellitic anhydrides
   Polyvinyl chloride
   Toluene diisocyanate
Pharmaceutical agents
   Phenylglycine acid chloride
   Penicillins
   Spiramycin
Food industry agents
   Egg protein
   Polyvinylchloride
Biologic enzymes
   Bacillus subtilis (laundry detergent workers)
   Pancreatic enzymes
Animal emanations
   Canine or feline saliva
   Horse dander (racing workers)
   Rodent urine (laboratory animal workers)

A patient with a history suggestive of episodic asthma but who on the day of the examination has normal pulmonary function test results is a reasonable candidate for study. Much has been made of "cough"-variant asthma, but its pathophysiology is uncertain, as is its relationship to typical asthma. The methacholine bronchial challenge is useful in evaluating patients for cough in whom baseline pulmonary function appears normal. Positive results do not always mean asthma but represent more information to be weighed in the clinical evaluation (Table 2-7). Some consider isocapneic hyperventilation with subfreezing dry air (by either exercise or breathing CO_2/air mixture) or exercise as alternatives to methacholine challenge.

Table 2-7.--Medical Conditions Associated With Positive Findings on Methacholine Challenge

Current asthma
Past history of asthma
Chronic obstructive pulmonary disease
Smoking
Recent respiratory infection
Chronic cough
Allergic rhinitis

- Patients with suspected asthma and normal results on pulmonary function tests can benefit from methacholine testing.

Cigarette-Smoking and Asthma

A combination of asthma and cigarette smoking leads to accelerated chronic obstructive pulmonary disease. Because of accelerated decline in irreversible obstruction, all asthmatics who smoke should be told to stop smoking.

Environmental tobacco smoke is an important asthma trigger. In particular, asthmatic children exposed to second-hand smoke have more respiratory infections and asthma attacks.

Differential Diagnosis

The differential diagnosis of wheezing is given in Table 2-8.

Table 2-8.--Differential Diagnosis of Wheezing

Pulmonary embolism
Cardiac failure
Foreign body
Central airway tumors
Aspiration
Carcinoid syndrome
Chondromalacia/polychondritis
Loeffler's syndrome
Bronchiectasis
Tropical eosinophilia
Hyperventilation syndrome
Laryngeal edema
Vascular ring affecting trachea
Factitious (including psychophysiologic vocal cord
   adduction)
α_1-antitrypsin deficiency
Immotile cilia syndrome
Bronchopulmonary dysplasia
Bronchiolitis (including bronchiolitis obliterans), croup
Cystic fibrosis

Allergic Bronchopulmonary Aspergillosis

Allergic bronchopulmonary aspergillosis is an obstructive lung disease caused by an allergic reaction to *Aspergillus* in the lower airway. The typical clinical presentation is severe steroid-dependent asthma. Most of the patients with this condition have coexisting asthma or cystic fibrosis.

- Allergic bronchopulmonary aspergillosis develops in patients with asthma or chronic obstructive pulmonary disease.

The diagnostic features of allergic bronchopulmonary aspergillosis are summarized in Table 2-9. Fungi other than *Aspergillus fumigatus* can cause an allergic bronchopulmonary mycosis similar to allergic bronchopulmonary aspergillosis.

The chest radiograph can show transient or permanent infiltrates and central bronchiectasis, usually affecting the upper lobes (Fig. 2-3). Advanced cases show extensive pulmonary fibrosis.

Allergic bronchopulmonary aspergillosis is treated with systemic corticosteroids. Total serum IgE may be helpful in following the disease course. Antifungal therapy has not been effective.

Fig. 2-3. Chest radiograph in allergic bronchopulmonary aspergillosis shows cylindrical infiltrates involving the upper lobes.

ALLERGY TESTING

Standard allergy testing relies on identifying the allergen-specific IgE antibody. Two classic means of doing this are the immediate wheal-and-flare skin test (a small amount of antigen is introduced into the skin and evaluated at 15 minutes for the presence of an immediate wheal-and-flare reaction) and in vitro testing. The skin test identifies the presence of allergen-specific IgE antibody but *does not indicate whether the person with a positive cutaneous reaction has a mucosal immune response to the same antigen under natural conditions*.

Allergy practices without a clear scientific basis include cytotoxic testing, provocation-neutralization testing or treatment, "yeast allergy," and sublingual immunotherapy.

In Vitro Allergy Testing

In vitro allergy testing involves chemically coupling allergen protein molecules to a solid-phase substance (e.g., micro-

crystalline cellulose) or to activated biologic membranes (e.g., nitrocellulose). The test is conducted by incubating a serum (from patient) that may contain IgE antibody specific for the allergen that has been immobilized to the membrane for a standard period of time. The solid phase is then washed free of nonbinding materials from the serum and incubated in a second solution containing a signal reagent (e.g., radiolabeled anti-IgE antibody). The various wells are counted and the radioactivity is correlated directly with the preparation of a standard curve in which known amounts of allergen-specific IgE antibody were incubated with a set of standard preparations of a solid phase. In vitro allergy testing uses the principles of radioimmunoassay.

It is important to understand that this test only identifies the presence of allergen-specific IgE antibody in the same way that the allergen skin test does. Generally, in vitro allergy testing is not as sensitive as any form of skin testing and has some limitations because of the potential for chemical modification of the protein while coupling it to the solid phase by means of covalent reaction. The advantage of in vitro allergy testing is its use in research as a specific quantifier of allergen-specific IgE antibody. Also, in vitro allergy testing is easier to follow over time than skin tests are. It generally is much more expensive than allergen skin tests and has no advantage in routine clinical work. It has the substantial liability of requiring about 3 days to be reported from our laboratory, but allergen skin

Table 2-9.--Diagnostic Features of Allergic Bronchopulmonary Aspergillosis

Clinical asthma
Bronchiectasis (usually proximal)
Increased total serum IgE
IgE antibody to *Aspergillus* (by skin test or in vitro assay)
Precipitins or IgG antibody to *Aspergillus*
Radiographic infiltrates (often upper lobes)
Peripheral blood eosinophilia

testing results are available within 15 minutes after application to the patient. In vitro allergy testing may be useful clinically for patients 1) who have been taking antihistamines and in whom no positive histamine responsiveness can be induced in the skin and 2) who have primary cutaneous diseases that make allergen skin testing impractical or inaccurate (e.g., severe atopic eczema with most of the skin involved in a flare).

● Skin testing is more sensitive and less expensive than in vitro allergy testing.

Patch Tests and Prick (Cutaneous) Tests

Many people seem confused about the concept of patch testing of skin as opposed to immediate wheal-and-flare skin testing. Patch testing is used to investigate contact dermatitis, a type IV hypersensitivity reaction. Patch tests require about 96 hours for complete evaluation (similar to tuberculin skin reactivity that requires 72 hours). Patch testing is useful only for investigating type IV hypersensitivity reactions leading to contact dermatitis. Most substances that cause contact dermatitis are small organic molecules that can penetrate various barriers inherent in the skin surface. The mechanisms of hypersensitivity postulated to explain these reactions usually involve haptenation of endogenous dermal proteins.

Inhalant allergens generally are sizable intact proteins in which each molecule can be multivalent with respect to IgE binding. Such molecules penetrate skin poorly and are seldom involved in cutaneous type IV hypersensitivity reactions. The exception appears to be house dust mite allergen in damaged skin of patients with severe atopic dermatitis. These patients mount a positive patch test to house dust mite allergen and an immediate wheal-and-flare cutaneous response with prick testing of allergen solutions.

● Patch testing is used to investigate contact dermatitis.
● Prick (immediate) skin testing is used to investigate respiratory allergy to pollens and molds.

Practical Skin Testing

Prick, scratch, and intradermal testing involve introducing allergen to the skin layers below the external keratin layer. Each of these techniques is increasingly sensitive (but less specific) as allergen is introduced more closely to responding cells and at higher doses. We perform allergen skin tests by the prick technique because it adequately identifies patients with significant clinical sensitivities without unduly identifying a large number of those with minimal levels of IgE antibody and no clinical sensitivity. We use scratch or intradermal testing in selective cases, including the protocol for evaluating stinging insect venoms.

● Intradermal skin tests are more sensitive but less specific than prick skin tests.

Double-Blind Placebo-Controlled Food Challenge

Historically, double-blind placebo-controlled food challenges are the standard for evaluating food allergy. We rarely use this challenge for patients with routine complaints of food allergy. Most patients with food allergy are aware of foods that are significant allergens and avoid them, without needing further therapy. The usual end points in food challenge testing are nausea, vomiting, diarrhea, abdominal cramps, and urticaria. Normally, we do not use this test for patients who have had anaphylaxis.

● The double-blind challenge is the standard test for food allergy.

Three other primary types of clinical challenge testing used in allergy are conjunctival challenge in the eye, allergen challenge in the nose, and bronchial challenge by inhalation of allergen aerosols. Common principles of good challenge testing include 1) blinding the tests, 2) using both positive and negative controls (the usual positive control is histamine and the negative control is bland diluent without allergen), and 3) choosing a time course for challenge that allows adequate return of challenged tissue to baseline before a subsequent challenge. For bronchial challenges, basal conditions may not be regained for 3-6 weeks after a positive challenge. Thus, in most instances, investigating sensitivities by direct tissue challenge is a lengthy process.

CHRONIC RHINITIS

History

Vasomotor rhinitis is defined as nasal symptoms occurring in response to nonspecific (in the sense of immunologic specificity) stimuli. One cause is pre-existing inflammation in the nasal mucosa; thus, allergic rhinitis can cause vasomotor rhinitis. However, vasomotor rhinitis does not cause allergic rhinitis. All patients with allergic rhinitis likely have nasal congestion and other nasal symptoms provoked by change in air temperature, inert particulates, irritants, and strong odors (even pleasant ones, e.g., fragrances). For patients with allergic rhinitis who have symptoms caused by such immunologically nonspecific stimuli, we say their allergic rhinitis is complicated by vasomotor rhinitis. Patients who have nasal symptoms but no allergy have (pure) vasomotor rhinitis.

● Vasomotor rhinitis is nasal symptoms in response to nonspecific stimuli.
● Vasomotor rhinitis does not cause allergic rhinitis.

Historical factors favoring allergic rhinitis include a history of nasal symptoms that have a recurrent seasonal pattern (e.g., every August and September) or seem to be provoked by being near animals. Factors favoring vasomotor rhinitis include the weather, soap aisles in supermarkets, strong odors, humidity and temperature changes (independent of "weather," i.e., air conditioning is a potent trigger), and lack of response to previous therapeutic trials of topical glucocorticoid medications flunisolide (Nasalide), beclomethasone (Vancenase, Beconase), triamcinolone (Nasacort), budesonide (Rhinocort) or fluticasone (Flonase).

- Allergic rhinitis has a recurrent seasonal pattern and is provoked by being near animals.
- Triggers of vasomotor rhinitis include the weather, humidity and temperature changes, supermarket soap aisles, and strong odors.

Factors favoring both allergic rhinitis and vasomotor rhinitis (thus, without differential diagnostic value) include perennial symptoms, intolerance of cigarette smoke, and history of "dust" sensitivity. Although "dust" is a widely recognized allergen, allergists and other professionals use the term to mean allergens of a specific arthropod, the house dust mite. These allergens cause allergic rhinitis when in airborne concentrations far below levels necessary for casual observers to detect a particulate load in the air. Therefore, patients are unlikely to offer historical observations that correlate with house dust mite allergen exposure. When patients offer a history of "dust" sensitivity, they mean that when symptoms are provoked the particulate load in the atmosphere is enough to scatter light, appearing grossly "dusty." Because all particulates (inert or otherwise) can trigger vasomotor rhinitis, the observation that "dusty" places cause symptoms is nonspecific. Factors that suggest fixed nasal obstruction (which should prompt physicians to consider other diagnoses) include unilateral nasal obstruction, unilateral facial pain, unilateral nasal purulence, nasal voice but no nasal symptoms, disturbances of olfaction without any nasal symptoms, unilateral nasal bleeding, and reflux of swallowed materials through the nose (Table 2-10).

- Perennial symptoms, intolerance of cigarette smoke, and history of dust sensitivity are common to allergic and vasomotor rhinitis.
- Dust mite sensitivity is a common cause of perennial allergic rhinitis.

Allergy Skin Tests

Allergy skin tests ask an artificial question: "Does the patient have allergen-specific IgE antibody-sensitizing cutaneous mast cells?" Even if the answer is "yes," no allergic disease may arise from the biologic phenomenon represented by the positive skin test. Many persons in the general population (15%) have positive allergy skin tests to one or more allergens and may not have symptoms of an allergy. Because of the statistical frequency of both positive allergy skin tests and chronic

Table 2-10.--Differential Diagnosis of Chronic Rhinitis

Allergic rhinitis
Vasomotor rhinitis
Rhinitis medicamentosus
Sinusitis
Nasal polyposis
Nasal septal deviation
Foreign body
Tumor

nonallergic rhinitis (also called vasomotor rhinitis) in the population, some patients with only vasomotor rhinitis as a clinical problem will also have positive allergy skin tests. How can this be sorted out?

- In the general population, 15% have positive allergy skin tests.

The interpretation of allergy skin test results must be tailored to the unique features of each patient.

1. For patients with perennial symptoms and negative results on allergy skin tests, the diagnosis is vasomotor rhinitis.

2. For patients with seasonal symptoms and appropriately positive allergy skin tests, the diagnosis is seasonal allergic rhinitis.

3. For patients with perennial symptoms and allergy skin tests positive to tree and ragweed pollens, two major possibilities are: a) skin tests are coincidental and unrelated to the perennial symptoms; thus, the diagnosis is vasomotor rhinitis; b) skin tests indicate clinical sensitivity to tree and ragweed pollens.

4. For patients with perennial symptoms, allergy skin tests positive for house dust mite suggest house dust mite allergic rhinitis. Another way to decide whether house dust mite allergen is clinically important is to conduct a clinical trial of dust mite allergen avoidance, e.g., have patient encase bedding appropriately (because the bed probably provides the greatest amount of house dust mite allergen exposure--but wet carpet on concrete is worse).

5. For patients with seasonal (spring and fall) nasal symptoms and negative allergy skin test results, the diagnosis is vasomotor rhinitis.

Sinusitis

Sinusitis is closely associated with edematous obstruction of the sinus osita. Poor drainage of the sinus cavities predispose to infection, particularly by microorganisms that thrive in low oxygen environments (e.g., anaerobes). In adults, *Streptococcus pneumoniae, Haemophilus influenzae,* anaerobes, and viruses are common pathogens. *Branhamella catarrhalis* is an important pathogen in children.

Important clinical features of acute sinusitis are nasal discharge, tooth pain, cough, and poor response to decongestants. Findings on paranasal sinus transillumination may be abnormal.

- Purulent nasal discharge, tooth pain, and abnormal transillumination are important clinical features of sinusitis.

Clinicians should be aware of the complications of sinusitis, which can be life-threatening (Table 2-11). Mucormycosis can cause recurrent or persistent sinusitis refractory to antibiotics. Allergic fungal sinusitis is characterized by persistent sinusitis, eosinophilia, increased total IgE, antifungal (usually *Aspergillus*) IgE and IgE antibodies, and fungal colonization of the sinuses. Wegener's granulomatosis, ciliary dysmotility, and hypogammaglobulinemia are medical conditions that can cause refractory sinusitis (Table 2-12).

Untreated sinusitis can cause osteomyelitis, orbital and periorbital cellulitis, meningitis, and brain abscess. Cavernous sinus thrombosis, an especially serious complication, can lead to retrobulbar pain, extraocular muscle paralysis, and blindness.

Persistent, refractory, and complicated sinusitis should be evaluated by a specialist. Sinus computed tomography (CT) is the preferred imaging study for these patients (Fig. 2-4).

Amoxicillin, 500 mg three times daily, or trimethoprim-sulfamethoxazole (one double-strength capsule twice daily) for 10-14 days is the treatment of choice for uncomplicated maxillary sinusitis.

Some physicians think the sensitivity of plain film radiographs of the sinuses is poor compared with that of CT scan-

Fig. 2-4. Sinus computed tomogram showing opacification of the ostiomeatal complex on the left, subtotal opacification of the right maxillary sinus and an air-fluid level in the left maxillary antrum.

ning (using coronal sectioning technique). Good-quality CT scans with coronal technique do reveal greater detail about sinus mucosal surfaces, but it is debated whether the additional time and cost of CT scans can be justified. However, CT scanning probably is reasonable for patients being considered for a sinus operation and for those failing standard treatment for sinusitis. Be aware that patients with extensive dental restorations that contain metal may generate too much artifact for CT to be useful. For these patients, magnetic resonance imaging (MRI) techniques are better.

- Sinus imaging is indicated for suspected recurrent sinusitis.
- Sinus CT is preferred to sinus radiography for complicated sinusitis.

Corticosteroid Therapy for Rhinitis

The need for systemic corticosteroid treatment for rhinitis is limited. Occasionally, patients with severe symptoms of hay fever may benefit greatly from 5 days of 10-mg prednisone (10 mg four times daily by mouth for 5 days). This may induce sufficient improvement so that topical steroids can penetrate the nose and satisfactory levels of antihistamine can be established in the blood. Taper of such a course is usually not necessary. Some physicians inject intramuscularly a parenteral steroid preparation (such as triamcinolone, 40 mg) that is long-acting; this can be helpful in patients unresponsive to other standard treatment. The proper dose is important if good results are to be obtained, but often too low a dose is given for the treatment

Table 2-11. Complications of Sinusitis

Osteomyelitis
Meningitis
Subdural abscess
Extradural abscess
Orbital infection
Cellulitis
Cavernous sinus thrombosis

Table 2-12. Causes of Persistent or Recurrent Sinusitis

Nasal polyposis
Mucormycosis
Allergic fungal sinusitis
Ciliary dyskinesia
Wegener's granulomatosis
Hypogammaglobulinemia
Tumor

to succeed. Patients with nasal polyposis may warrant 2 weeks of oral prednisone at 10 mg four times daily, because a significant fraction of them have near-miraculous "melting away" of nasal polyps on such a course. Subsequently, their condition may be controllable with topical corticosteroids alone. Some physicians believe that all patients with nasal polyposis contemplating surgical treatment of the polyps should undergo a trial of oral prednisone at this dosage schedule preoperatively, because some of them will have such satisfactory results that surgical treatment is unnecessary. The percentage of polyposis patients who will benefit has not been reliably estimated, and the practice remains controversial among ENT surgeons.

- The need for systemic corticosteroids in rhinitis is limited.
- For very severe hay fever symptoms, 40 mg of oral prednisone daily for 5 days.
- Nasal polyposis may warrant oral prednisone followed by topical corticosteroids.

Physicians proposing courses of systemic corticosteroid at these dose schedules need to counsel patients carefully. The likelihood of any significant side effect is low for these short durations of therapy, but the side effects that are seen can be catastrophic. The following must be specifically mentioned to patients and this disclosure **must** be documented in each patient's record: acute steroid psychosis, aseptic necrosis of the femoral head(s), acute glaucoma, mania, depression, weight gain (both fluid retention and real fat expansion due to appetite stimulation as well as specific pharmacologic effects on certain fat tissues), acceleration of any pre-existing tendency to ocular cataract, and renal stone formation. It is also a good idea to make a summary comment to the patient emphasizing the importance of contacting the physician immediately if anything unusual or unexpected (in the way of medical symptoms) should occur during the course of corticosteroid therapy, just in case a catastrophic complication should occur and not be recognized by the patient.

- Know the important adverse effects of systemic corticosteroid therapy.

In contrast with systemic corticosteroid therapy, topical corticosteroid agents for the nose are easy to use. The only agents considered herein are beclomethasone (available as Beconase and Vancenase), flunisolide (Nasalide), triamcinolone (Nasacort), budesonide (Rhinocort), and fluticasone (Flonase). The only corticosteroid marketed specifically for use in the nose is dexamethasone (Decadron Turbinaire), which has significant systemic effects when used as directed and no therapeutic advantage over beclomethasone and flunisolide.

- Intranasal corticosteroids have few if any systemic effects.

When should topical corticosteroids be prescribed for rhinitis? They are successful in treating hay fever and are safe to use. If therapy is initiated about a week before the start of the relevant pollen season, many patients can be free of allergic rhinitis symptoms for the entire pollen season. In challenge laboratories, these agents are the most potent protection for inhibiting mucosal responses to allergen, even when given only 1 hour before allergen exposure.

- Topical corticosteroids are successful for hay fever.
- Initiate therapy about 1 week before the start of the relevant pollen season.

When intranasal corticosteroids are used in combination with an oral antihistamine, nearly 90% of hay fever patients are satisfied with the relief. However, many patients seek medical advice only after pollen season has started. They must be counseled that nasal spray works slowly and its full benefits will not be realized for 3 weeks. Recall that most people's experience with nasal sprays is that a marked change occurs within 5 to 10 minutes after spraying; thus, if patients are not adequately counseled, they may abandon the spray after 2 or 3 doses, because it did nothing to help their symptoms. (These patients may become angry with the physician because of the expense of the spray.)

- When intranasal corticosteroids are used with antihistamine, 90% of hay fever patients are satisfied.

Most people are aware that treatment with nasal sprays is a bad idea because of the "addictive" potential (a vicious cycle of rhinitis medicamentosa caused by topical vasoconstrictors is common knowledge). Reassure patients that topical corticosteroid does not induce any dependence.

- Unlike decongestant nasal sprays, topical intranasal corticosteroid does not induce tachyphylaxis and rebound congestion.

A significant number of patients with vasomotor rhinitis also have a good response to topical aerosol corticosteroid therapy, especially if the patient has the nasal eosinophilia and/or nasal polyposis form of vasomotor rhinitis. Without eosinophils on nasal smears and nasal polyps, the response is unpredictable. Only nasal smears and nasal polyps permit distinguishing eosinophilic and non-eosinophilic types of vasomotor rhinitis, so a therapeutic trial is the simplest therapeutic approach for nonallergic rhinitis. Some physicians think the answer to "Who should have topical corticosteroid sprays prescribed for rhinitis" is "everyone." Although others think this answer fosters an uncritical attitude and shotgun therapy, it is not inappropriate if the implications of response and non-response to therapeutic trials are considered.

● Many patients with vasomotor rhinitis have a good response to topical aerosol corticosteroid therapy.

If a hay fever patient does not receive adequate relief with topical steroid plus antihistamine therapy, it may indicate the need for systemic corticosteroid and for initiating immunotherapy in the winter so the patient is prepared for the next pollen season.

● If pharmacologic management fails, allergy immunotherapy should be considered for patients with allergic rhinitis.

The only important side effect of intranasal corticosteroids is nasal septal perforation. Dry powder spray cannisters deliver a powerful jet of particulates, and a few patients have misdirected the jet to the nasal septum. Septal perforation occurred because of mechanical irritation. Aqueous preparations avoid this minor complication.

● Nasal topical corticosteroid sprays rarely can cause nasal septal perforation.

For all the foregoing reasons, it appears that rhinitis patients with perennial symptoms can use topical steroids year-round without concern about side effects. There is no evidence that topical corticosteroids adversely affect the natural history of viral upper respiratory tract infections, so such infections are not a reason to discontinue corticosteroid therapy.

● Topical intranasal corticosteroids do not adversely affect the natural history of viral upper respiratory tract infections.

The important point is that internists, when acting as consultants to primary care physicians in cases of recurrent rhinitis, can make a more sophisticated evaluation of the patients and make a substantial contribution to understanding the nature of the clinical condition. In such cases, any course of antibiotic therapy should have a clear evidential rationale.

Antihistamines and Decongestants

Antihistamines antagonize the interaction of histamine with its receptors. If histamine is the cause of the nasal vascular congestion, antihistamines may diminish nasal congestion. However, in cases of rhinitis other than allergic rhinitis, the role of histamine is unclear, and effective antagonism may appear to have little impact on symptoms. Histamine may be more effective than other mediators for nasal itch and sneez-

ing. These are symptoms most often responsive to antihistamine therapy. Almost all the nasal effects of histamine are mediated by H_1 receptors (H_2 receptors are mainly but not exclusively in the gut). More traditional antihistamines also have anticholinergic effects in many patients (mediated mostly via the central nervous system rather than directly in the periphery); the "drying" effects of antihistamines occur primarily by this mechanism rather than by antagonism of histamine receptors locally in the respiratory tract. This is important in considering several newer antihistamines that are designed not to cross the blood-brain barrier. These agents have little or no anticholinergic effect and thus no "drying" effect. Previously, the "drying" effect of some antihistamines was thought useful in managing a "wet" nose. Currently, patients are informed through advertising about nondrowsiness properties of newer antihistamines and usually request them. Terfenadine and astemizole can cause serious cardiac arrhythmias (prolonged QT and torsades de pointes) in patients taking erythromycin or ketoconazole or who have significant liver disease. These adverse effects are rare, but patients should be informed. The nonsedating antihistamine loratidine has not been associated with these adverse effects.

● Histamine is an important mediator in allergic rhinitis.
● The nasal effects of histamine are mediated by H_1 receptors.
● Terfenadine and astemizole can cause serious cardiac arrhythmias in patients taking erythromycin or ketoconazole or who have significant liver disease.

Two decongestants, pseudoephedrine and phenylpropanolamine, are the most common agents in nonprescription drugs for treating cold symptoms/rhinitis and usually are the active agents in widely used proprietary prescription agents. A large number of prescription and nonprescription combination agents combine antihistamine and decongestant. You cannot be familiar with all of them but should be aware that combination drugs dominate the nonprescription market. Decongestant preparations are often the only therapeutic option for patients with vasomotor rhinitis unresponsive to topical glucocorticoids, and they are often helpful for those patients in whom headache is a dominant feature of the symptom complex.

● Pseudoephedrine and phenylpropanolamine are the most common decongestant agents in nonprescription preparations.

Note that middle-aged and older men may have urinary retention caused by antihistamines (principally the older drugs that have anticholinergic effects) and decongestants; these patients should be alerted to this. Although there has been concern for years that decongestants may exacerbate hypertension because they are α-adrenergic agonists, no clinically significant hypertensive response has been seen in stable medicated patients with hypertension. Nevertheless, keep this possibility (or idiosyncrasy) in mind.

- Antihistamines and decongestants may cause urinary retention in men middle-aged and older.

For antihistamines with anticholinergic activity, elderly patients should be warned about exposure to warm summer days, because the elderly seem more sensitive to anticholinergically mediated failure of sweating, thus increasing the danger of heat stroke. Extremely athletic persons of all ages also should be aware of this potential complication.

- The elderly seem more sensitive to anticholinergically mediated failure of sweating.

Immunotherapy for Allergic Rhinitis

Until topical nasal glucocorticoid sprays were introduced, allergen immunotherapy was considered "first-line" therapy for allergic rhinitis when the relevant allergen was seasonal pollen of grass, trees, or weeds. Immunotherapy became "second-line" therapy after topical steroids were introduced because: 1) immunotherapy has no greater efficacy than glucocorticoids (either in number of responders per 100 cases or in degree of symptom relief in individual cases), 2) glucocorticoids are less expensive (in both time and dollars), and 3) immunotherapy has a small but irreducible risk of a serious reaction (anaphylaxis) that may cause death, but topical glucocorticoids have no serious potential complications. However, immunotherapy for allergic rhinitis can be appropriate first-line therapy in selected patients.

- Immunotherapy is about as effective as intranasal glucocorticoids.
- Anaphylaxis is a risk of immunotherapy.
- Immunotherapy for allergic rhinitis is first-line therapy in selected patients.

Immunotherapy is usually reserved for patients who get no satisfactory relief with topical steroids or who cannot tolerate nasal sprays. Occasionally, patients who had a salutary response to immunotherapy but for some reason interrupted it, want to resume it. A trial of topical steroid is often recommended for such patients to make more informed decisions, but immunotherapy may be appropriate for those explicitly requesting it, because compliance with nasal steroids is often poor. Immunotherapy is not given for food allergy and not usually for animal dander allergy. The practice is less uniform with respect to mold allergens, with endorsement divided in the subspecialty.

- Immunotherapy is reserved for patients who get no relief with intranasal glucocorticoids or who cannot tolerate nasal spray.

Environmental Modification

House Dust Mite

House dust mites are so small they cannot maintain their own internal water unless ambient conditions are high humidity. They eat all kinds of organic matter but seem to favor mold and epidermal scale shed by humans. They occur in all human habitations, although the population size varies with local conditions. The only geographic areas free of house dust mites are those at great elevations with extreme dryness.

- House dust mites require high humidity.
- They are found in all human habitations.

Areas in the home harboring the most significant mite populations are bedding and fabric-upholstered furniture (heavily used) and any area where carpeting is on concrete (when concrete is in contact with grade). Although carpeting is often cited as a significant mite-related problem, carpet on wooden floors in the superstructure of a house usually harbors a small population. Dispersion of allergen from this source is not great compared with that from bedding and furniture. To prevent egress of allergen when the mattress and pillows are compressed by occupancy of the bed, encase the bedding (and sometimes, when practical, furniture cushions) in plastic encasements. To some degree, this also prevents infusion of water vapor into the bedding matrix. These two factors combine to significantly reduce the amount of airborne allergen. Measures for controlling dust mites are listed in Table 2-13.

- Dust mite is an important respiratory allergen.
- The most significant mite population is in bedding and fabric-upholstered furniture.
- Plastic encasements prevent egress of allergen.

Recently, fluid sprays capable of either killing mites or denaturing the protein allergens from them have been mar-

Table 2-13.--Dust Mite Control

Encase bedding and pillows in airtight encasements
Remove carpeting in bedroom
Remove upholstered furniture from bedroom
Remove all carpeting laid on concrete
Discontinue use of humidifier
Wash bedding in hot water
Run dehumidifier

keted. Despite immunochemical evidence that the allergen is denatured by denaturant and mites are killed by acaricides, neither one is substantially helpful when applied in the home.

Pollens

Air conditioning, which enables the warm-season home to remain tightly closed, is the principal defense against pollinosis. Most masks purchased at local pharmacies are **not** capable of excluding pollen particles and, thus, are not worth the expense. Some masks can protect the wearer from allergen exposure, such as industrial-quality respirators designed specifically to pass rigorous testing by OSHA and NIOSH that qualify them capable of excluding a wide spectrum of particulates, including radioactive dusts. These masks allow allergic patients to mow the lawn and do yard work otherwise intolerable because of exposure to pollen allergen.

- Only industrial-quality masks are capable of excluding pollen particles.

Animal Danders

No measure can compare with getting the animal completely out of the house. No air filtration scheme feasible for average homeowners to install can eliminate allergen from an actively elaborating animal. If complete removal is not tenable, some partial measure must be considered.

If the house is heated or cooled by a forced-air system with ductwork, confining the pet to a single room in the house is only partially effective in reducing overall exposure, because air from every room is collected through the air-return ductwork and redistributed through a central plenum. If air-return ducts are sealed in the room where the animal is kept and air can escape from the room only by infiltration, exposure may be reduced. The room selected for this measure should be as far as possible from the bedroom of the allergic patient. Naturally, the allergic patient should avoid close contact with the animal and should consider using a mask if animal handling or entry into the room where the animal is kept is necessary. Most animal danders have little or nothing to do with animal hair, so its shedding status is irrelevant. Bathing cats about once every other week may reduce the allergen load in the environment, but overbathing (daily) may cause dry skin and enhance allergen dispersal.

- Complete avoidance is the only entirely effective way to manage allergy to household pets.

URTICARIA AND ANGIOEDEMA

The distinction between acute and chronic urticaria is arbitrary and based on the duration of the urticaria. If it has been present for 6 weeks or more, it is called chronic urticaria.

Secondary Urticaria

The only reason any disease associations were recognized for urticaria is that the disease came first. Urticaria is rarely the presenting sign of more serious internal disease. Most patients simply have urticaria as a skin disease. Urticaria is part of the clinical syndrome of lupus erythematosus and other connective tissue diseases, particularly of more difficult to categorize "overlap" syndromes. Internal malignancy, mainly of the gastrointestinal tract, and lymphoproliferative diseases are associated with urticaria, as occult internal infection may be, particularly of the gallbladder and dentition. Immune-complex disease has been associated with urticaria, usually with urticarial vasculitis, and only hepatitis B virus has been identified as an antigen in the cases of immune-complex disease.

- Urticaria is associated with lupus erythematosus and other connective tissue diseases, internal malignancy, internal infection, and immune-complex disease.

The common cause of urticaria and angioedema other than the idiopathic variety probably is drug reaction. This is uncommon on a chronic basis without the offending drug being recognized and its use stopped.

- Chronic urticaria and angioedema are often idiopathic.
- The common secondary cause of urticaria and angioedema is drug reaction.

Relationship Between Urticaria and Angioedema

There probably is no fundamental difference between urticaria and angioedema. The critical factor is in what type of tissue the capillary leak and mediator release occur. Urticaria occurs when the capillary events are in the tightly welded tissue wall of the skin--the epidermis. Angioedema occurs when capillary events affect vessels in loose, areolar connective tissue of the deeper layers--the dermis. Virtually all patients with the common idiopathic type of urticaria also have angioedema from time to time. When urticaria is caused by allergic reactions, angioedema nearly always occurs, too. The only exception is with hereditary angioneurotic edema type of disease (HANE), which is not related to mast cell mediator release but is a complement disorder. Patients with this form of angioedema rarely have urticaria. Why the molecular events seem confined to the vessels in deeper tissues is unknown.

- Virtually all patients with urticaria also have angioedema from time to time.

C1 Esterase Inhibitor Deficiency

A number of significant clinical differences usually suggest the diagnosis of hereditary angioedema. If HANE is strongly suspected, the diagnosis can be proved by the appropriate measurement of complement factors (C1 esterase inhibitor, quantitative and functional, and C4 [also, C2, if seen during episode of swelling]).

- C1 esterase inhibitor levels and C4 are decreased in hereditary angioedema.

The duration of individual swellings is quite different. Typical idiopathic urticaria and angioedema swellings last 2-6 hours in usual cases and commonly up to 18 hours; HANE-related swellings last 3-5 days. Many HANE patients have had at least one hospitalization for what appeared to be intestinal obstruction. If they avoided laparotomy on these occasions, the obstruction resolved in 3-5 days. Cramps and diarrhea are the usual intestinal symptoms in patients with idiopathic urticaria and angioedema; 3-5 days of obstruction is rare. In common idiopathic urticaria, the lesions itch intensely because histamine is one of the causes of wheal formation.

- Typical urticarial lesions last 2-18 hours and are pruritic.

Lesions in the HANE type do not itch. The response to epinephrine is a useful differential point: HANE lesions do not respond to epinephrine, but common angioedema usually melts away in ≤15 minutes. Laryngeal edema almost never occurs in the common idiopathic type of disease (although it occurs in allergic episodes with measurable frequency, most often in insect-sting anaphylaxis cases); however, it is relatively common in HANE (earlier papers quoted a 30% mortality rate in HANE, with all deaths due to laryngeal edema). Finally, HANE episodes are traceable to local tissue trauma in a high percentage of occurrences, with dental work often regarded as the classic precipitating factor.

- In HANE, swelling lasts 3-5 days.
- Most HANE patients have been hospitalized for "intestinal obstruction."
- HANE lesions do not respond to epinephrine.
- In HANE, laryngeal edema is relatively common.
- Dental work is the classic precipitating factor for HANE.

The common idiopathic form of urticaria and angioedema is usually unrelated to antecedent trauma except in special cases of delayed-pressure urticaria, in which hives and angioedema follow minor trauma (e.g., to the hands while playing golf) of soft tissues. The duration of the lesions distinguishes this special form of physical urticaria from HANE.

Thus, only a small fraction of all cases with episodic swelling are not easily categorized as HANE-like or not, and assays for serum complement factors may be reserved for the few doubtful cases or to prove the diagnosis in cases with a suggestive history.

The five types of HANE-like disorders are:

1. Classic HANE is a genetic dysregulation of gene function for C1 inhibitor that is inherited in an autosomal-dominant pattern. Therapy with androgens (testosterone, stanozolol, danazol) reverses the dysregulation and allows expression of the otherwise normal gene, resulting in half-normal plasma levels of C1, which is sufficient to eliminate the clinical manifestations of the disease.

- Classic HANE is a genetic dysregulation (autosomal dominant).
- Testosterone, stanozolol, and danazol reverse the dysregulation.

2. In some cases of HANE, the gene for the C1 inhibitor mutates, rendering the molecule functionally ineffective. However, plasma levels of the C1 inhibitor molecule may be normal in these cases. This is the basis for requesting immunochemical and functional measures of serum C1 inhibitor (with immunochemical measures only, the diagnosis is missed in cases of normal levels of an inactive molecule). Both classic HANE (low levels of C1 esterase inhibitor) and classic HANE with mutated gene for C1 inhibitor (nonfunctional C1 esterase inhibitor) are inherited forms of the disease (although both may be seen wherein the proband is also the sport that starts the mutational line, so the family history is not invariably positive even in these forms).

- Hereditary angioedema with normal levels of C1 esterase inhibitor but nonfunctional (by esterase assay) indicates a gene mutation.

3. C1 esterase inhibitor deficiency is seen as an acquired disorder with carcinoma or lymphoproliferative disease. It can be suspected only if the associated neoplasm is recognized--it is not worthwhile to search for occult neoplasm if angioedema is diagnosed. The molecular tip for the presence of the disease is that the plasma levels for C1 and for C1 esterase inhibitor are low. The hypothesis for the pathogenesis of this form of angioedema is that the tumor has or releases determinants that fix complement, and with constant *consumption*, a point is reached wherein the biosynthesis of C1 inhibitor cannot keep up with the consumption rate, and the relative deficiency of C1 inhibitor allows episodes of swelling.

- C1 esterase inhibitor deficiency can be an acquired disorder in carcinoma or lymphoproliferative disease.
- C1 levels are low in acquired C1 esterase inhibitor deficiency.

4. and 5. Basically, these two types are autoimmune disorders in which antibody to the catalytic site on C1 inhibitor or to the binding site for C1 inhibitor on C1q interferes with the function of C1 inhibitor, hastening its destruction.

Physical Urticaria

Heat, light, cold, vibration, and trauma/pressure have been reported to cause hives in susceptible persons. Getting the history is the only way to suspect the diagnosis, which is established by applying each of the stimuli to the patient's skin in the laboratory (with the history guiding the selection of stimuli; we do not routinely do any of these tests in all patients with urticaria). Heat can be applied by placing coins (soaked in hot water for a few minutes) on the patient's forearm. Cold can be applied with coins kept in a freezer or with ice cubes. For vibration, use a laboratory vortex mixer or any common vibrator. A pair of sandbags connected by a strap can be draped over the patient to create enough pressure to cause symptoms in the most susceptible persons. Note that unlike most cases of common idiopathic urticaria (in which the lesions affect essentially all skin surfaces), many cases of physical urticarias seem to involve only certain areas of skin. Thus, challenges will be positive only in the areas usually involved and negative in other areas. Directing challenges to the appropriate area depends on the history.

- For physical urticaria, the history is the only way to suspect the diagnosis, which is established by applying stimuli to the patient's skin.

Food Allergy in Chronic Urticaria

Food allergy almost never causes chronic urticaria. Although urticaria can be an acute manifestation of true food allergy, gastrointestinal consequences of food allergy or anaphylactic phenomena usually predominate and urticaria is considered a minor feature. Most patients with chronic urticaria do not have gastrointestinal symptoms or the symptoms are vague dyspepsias that a huge fraction of the general population has occasionally and are probably unrelated to the urticaria.

Conversely, food allergy may cause acute urticaria, angioedema, or anaphylaxis.

- Food allergy almost never causes *chronic* urticaria.
- Food allergy may cause *acute* urticaria, angioedema, or anaphylaxis.

Histopathology of Chronic Urticaria

Chronic urticaria is characterized by mononuclear cell perivascular cuffing around dermal capillaries, particularly involving the capillary loops that interdigitate with the rete pegs of the epidermis. This mononuclear cell cuff is mostly helper T cells, with some monocytes, macrophages, B cells, and mast cells. This is the usual histologic location for most skin mast cells. It appears there is about a tenfold increase in the number of mast cells in the cuff compared with the normal value. However, the number of mast cells is still small compared with that of other round cells in the cuff. This histologic picture is consistent throughout the skin, regardless of recent active urtication. Most pathologists consider "vasculitis" to indicate actual necrosis of the structural elements of blood vessels; thus, the typical picture of chronic urticaria does not meet the criteria for vasculitis. Immunofluorescence studies on chronic urticaria biopsy samples for fibrin, complement, and immunoglobulin deposition in blood vessels are negative.

Urticarial vasculitis occurs, usually with the histologic features of leukocytoclastic vasculitis. A few cases have intermediate features, i.e., leukocytoclastic features (in terms of the cells seen in the tissue) occur with little or no visible vessel damage.

- Characteristic of chronic urticaria: a mononuclear cell perivascular cuff around capillaries.

Management of Urticaria

The history is of utmost importance if the 2%-4% of cases of chronic urticaria actually due to allergic causes are to be discovered. A complete physical examination is needed, with particular attention to the skin (including some test for dermatographism), to evaluate for the vasculitic nature of the lesions, and to the liver, lymph nodes, and mucous membranes. Laboratory testing need not be exhaustive: a complete blood cell count with differential to discover eosinophilia; liver enzymes; erythrocyte sedimentation rate; serum protein electrophoresis to assess acute phase reactants; hepatitis-B serologies; antinuclear antibody; urinalysis; stool exam for parasites; and chest radiography. Only if the patient seems to have a strong allergic diathesis and some element in the history suggests an allergic cause is allergy skin testing indicated medically. However, patients with urticaria often have fixed ideas about an allergy causing their problem, and skin testing often helps to dissuade them of this idea.

- The history is of utmost importance in diagnosing allergic urticaria.
- Laboratory testing may include eosinophil count, liver enzymes level, erythrocyte sedimentation rate, serum protein electrophoresis, hepatitis-B serologies, and stool exam for parasites.

Management of urticaria and angioedema is usually with H_1 antagonists; the addition of H_2 antagonists may be helpful. Tricyclic antidepressants, e.g., doxepin, have potent antihistamine effects and are useful.

- Urticaria and angioedema: management is with H_1 antagonists.

FOOD ALLERGY

Clinical History

The clinical syndrome of food allergy should prompt patients to provide a history containing some or all the following: For very sensitive persons, some tingling, itching, and a metallic taste in the mouth occur while the food is still in the mouth. Within 15 minutes after swallowing the food, some epigastric distress should occur; it may be nonspecific. There may be nausea and, occasionally with marked sensitivity, vomiting. Abdominal cramping is felt chiefly in the periumbilical area (small bowel phase), and lower abdominal cramping and watery diarrhea should occur. Urticaria may occur in any distribution or there may be only itching of the palms and soles. With increasing clinical sensitivity to the offending allergen, anaphylactic symptoms may emerge, including tachycardia, hypotension, generalized flushing, and alterations of consciousness.

In extremely sensitive persons, generalized flushing, hypotension, and tachycardia may occur before the other symptoms. Nonspecific dyspepsia (which does not emerge as a stereotypic syndrome), chronic rhinitis, and chronic asthma are not part of the natural history of food allergy, nor are chronic fatigue, tingling sensation in the limbs, and aching in muscles and joints. Most patients with food allergy know the offending allergenic foodstuffs, so diagnosis entails confirmation by skin testing or other methods for measuring allergen-specific IgE antibody.

- Allergic reactions to food usually include urticaria.

Common Causes of Food Allergy

Table 2-14 lists items considered the most common allergens.

Food-Related Anaphylaxis

Food-induced anaphylaxis is the same process involved in acute hypersensitivity to food allergens except the severity of the reaction is greater in anaphylaxis. Relatively few foodstuffs are involved in food-induced anaphylaxis; the main ones are peanuts, shellfish, and true nuts.

- Anaphylaxis to food can be life-threatening.

Allergy Skin Testing in Food Allergy

In actual practice, if a patient has positive results on one or more skin tests to foodstuffs (reasonable candidates based on clinical history), an open challenge with the foodstuff may be conducted under physician observation. If that challenge is positive, the most compelling evidence is obtained with a double-blind placebo-controlled food challenge. With comparison of double-blind placebo-controlled food challenge with open

Table 2-14.--Common Causes of Food Allergy

Eggs	Shellfish
Milk	Soybean
Nuts	Wheat
Peanuts	

food challenge, the frequency of positive reactions decreases by half. It is reasonable to conduct allergy skin tests on patients with vague symptoms who think they have a food allergy, because the negative test results can be used to assure them that food allergy is not the root of the problem. Patients with food anaphylaxis should strictly avoid offending foods and carry an epinephrine kit.

- Positive results on skin tests and double-blind food challenges can confirm the diagnosis of food allergy.
- If results of food skin tests are negative, food allergy is unlikely.
- Patients with anaphylaxis to food should strictly avoid the offending food and carry an epinephrine kit.

STINGING INSECT ALLERGY

In patients clinically sensitive to stinging Hymenoptera, reactions to a sting are either the large local or the anaphylactic variety. In the large local sting reaction, swelling at the sting site may be dramatic but there are no symptoms distant from that site. Stings of the head, neck, and dorsum of the hands are particularly prone to large local reactions.

Clinical phenomena of stinging insect anaphylaxis are similar to all other forms of anaphylaxis. With stinging insects, antigen is injected parenterally. Thus, the onset of anaphylaxis may be very rapid, often within 1-2 minutes. Pruritus of the palms and soles is the most common initial manifestation and frequently is followed almost immediately by generalized flushing and hypotension. The reason for attaching importance to whether a stinging insect reaction is a large local or a generalized one is that allergy skin testing and, if positive, allergen immunotherapy are recommended only for generalized reactions. A large local reaction is not a harbinger of future anaphylaxis.

- Two varieties of reaction to sting: large local and anaphylactic.

Bee and Vespid Allergy

Yellow jackets, wasps, and hornets are vespids and their venoms cross-react to a substantial degree. The venom of honeybees (order Apidaea) does **not** cross-react with that of vespids. Unless the patient actually captures the insect delivering the sting, uncertainty will likely attend many cases of insect-sting-ing anaphylaxis. Thus, we usually conduct skin testing to hon-eybee and each of the vespids. To interpret skin tests accu-rately, it is helpful to know which insect caused the sting pro-ducing the generalized reaction. Often, the circumstances of the sting can help determine the type of insect responsible. Multiple stings received while mowing the grass or doing other landscape jobs that may disturb yellow-jacket burrows in the ground are likely causes of yellow-jacket stings. A single sting received while near picnic tables or refuse containers at pic-nic areas is likely from a yellow jacket or possibly a hornet. Stings received while working around the house exterior (paint-ing, cleaning eaves and gutters, attic work) are most likely from wasps.

- Yellow jackets, wasps, and hornets are vespids and their venoms cross-react.
- Venom of bees does not cross-react with that of vespids.
- It is helpful to know which insect caused the sting.

Allergy Testing

Patients who have had generalized reaction warrant aller-gen skin testing. Patients who have had a large local reaction to one of the Hymenoptera stings do **not** warrant allergen skin testing because they are not at increased risk for future anaphylaxis.

- Generalized reaction warrants allergen skin testing.
- Large local reaction does not warrant allergen skin testing.

Skin testing should be delayed for at least 1 month after a sting-induced general reaction, because tests conducted clos-er to the time of the sting have a substantial risk of being false-ly negative. Positive results on skin testing that correlate with the clinical history are sufficient evidence for considering Hymenoptera venom immunotherapy. If the patients are select-ed appropriately for skin testing, results of the tests should not be ambiguous. However, random testing of the general pop-ulation turns up positive results in patients without a history of anaphylaxis.

- Skin testing should be delayed for at least 1 month after sting-induced general reaction.
- Patients with clinical anaphylaxis and positive results on venom skin tests may benefit from venom immunotherapy.

Venom Immunotherapy

The decision to undertake venom immunotherapy can be reached only after a discussion between the patient and physi-cian. General indications for venom immunotherapy are list-ed in Table 2-15. Patients must understand that once initiated the immunotherapy injection schedule has to be maintained and that there is a small risk of the immunotherapy inducing

anaphylaxis. It is important that patients understand that despite receiving allergy immunotherapy, **they must carry epineph-rine when outdoors** because of 2%-10% possibility that immunotherapy will not provide suitable protection.

- There is a small risk that immunotherapy will induce anaphylaxis.
- There is a 2%-10% chance that immunotherapy will not provide protection.

Avoidance

Table 2-16 lists the warnings that every patient with sting-ing-insect hypersensitivity should receive.

The circumstances of each patient may provide additional entries to the list in Table 2-16. Also, patients need to know how to use self-injectable epinephrine in its several forms. Many patients wear an anaphylaxis identification bracelet.

- All patients with stinging-insect sensitivity should carry an epinephrine kit.

DRUG ALLERGY

Anaphylaxis

Anaphylaxis is a generalized allergic reaction whose clin-ical hallmarks are flushing, hypotension, and tachycardia. Urticaria and angioedema may occur in many cases, and in patients with moderate-to-severe asthma or rhinitis as a pre-existing condition, the asthma and rhinitis can be made worse. This definition of anaphylaxis is based on its clinical phe-nomena. A cellular and molecular definition of anaphylaxis is "a generalized allergic reaction in which large quantities of both preformed and newly synthesized mediators are released from activated basophils and mast cells." The dominant medi-ators of acute anaphylaxis are histamine and prostaglandin D_2. The serum levels of tryptase may be increased for a few hours after clinical anaphylaxis. Physiologically, the hypotension of anaphylaxis is caused by peripheral vasodilatation and not by an impaired cardiac contractility. In anaphylaxis patients

Table 2-15.--Indications for Venom Immunotherapy

History of anaphylaxis to a sting
Positive results on skin tests to venom implicated historically in the anaphylactic reaction
Patient's level of anxiety disrupts usual habits and activities in warm months
Occupational--higher than usual risk of sting
House painters
Outdoor construction workers
Forestry workers

Table 2-16.--Do's and Don'ts for Patients With
Hypersensitivity to Insect Stings

Avoid looking or smelling like a flower
  Avoid flowered prints for clothes
    Avoid cosmetics and fragrances, especially ones derived
      from flowering plants
Never drink from a soft-drink can out-of-doors during the
  warm months--a yellow jacket can land **on** or **in** the can
  while you are not watching and go inside the can and sting
  the inside of your mouth (one of the most dangerous places
  for a sensitive patient to be stung) when you take a drink
Avoid doing outdoor maintenance and yard work
Never reach into a mailbox without first looking in it
Never go barefoot
Always look at the underside of picnic table benches and park
  benches before sitting down
Never attempt physically to eject a stinging insect from the
  interior of an automobile but pull over, get out, and let
  someone else remove the insect

---

placed flat or in the Trendelenburg position and in whom blood pressure may be extremely low, cardiac output is elevated and circulatory system is characterized by hyperdynamic low-volume, high-flow state. Also, heparinemia may result from heparin release from mast cell granules (heparin provides a polyanionic complex partner for polycationic histamine storage in mast cell granules); this further helps prevent vascular stasis and thrombosis due to low-flow states. For these reasons, anaphylaxis is usually fatal in patients with preexisting fixed vascular obstructive disease in whom a decrease in proximal perfusion pressure leads to a critical reduction in flow (stroke) or in patients in whom laryngeal edema develops and completely occludes the airway.

- The clinical hallmarks of anaphylaxis are flushing, hypotension, and tachycardia.
- Urticaria and angioedema may be present.
- Histamine and prostaglandin D_2 are the dominant mediators of acute anaphylaxis.
- Peripheral vasodilatation causes hypotension of anaphylaxis.

Latex allergy is an important cause of intraoperative anaphylaxis. Patients with intraoperative anaphylaxis should be evaluated for possible latex allergy, usually by skin test or in vitro assay. When persons with known latex allergy undergo invasive procedures, a latex-free environment is necessary. Patients with dermatitis, rhinitis, or asthma caused by latex allergy are at increased risk for anaphylaxis to latex.

- Latex allergy is an important cause of intraoperative anaphylaxis.

Classes of Drug Allergy

Drug Allergy Not Involving IgE or Immediate-Type Reactions

Stevens-Johnson Syndrome

Stevens-Johnson syndrome is a bullous skin and mucosal reaction; very large blisters appear over much of the skin surface, in the mouth, and along the gastrointestinal tract. Because of the propensity of the blisters to break down and become infected, the reaction often is life-threatening. Treatment consists of stopping the drug causing the reaction, giving systemic steroids, and providing intense supportive care. The patients are often treated in burn units. Penicillin, sulfonamides, barbiturates, diphenylhydantoin, warfarin, and phenothiazines are well-known causes (it seems that any drug may be an etiologic agent in a particular patient). A drug-induced Stevens-Johnson reaction is an absolute contraindication to giving a causative drug to the patient, i.e., there are **no** circumstances in which the indications for giving the drug outweigh the hazard.

- Stevens-Johnson syndrome is life-threatening and is an absolute contraindication for rechallenge with the drug.

Toxic Epidermal Necrolysis Syndrome

Clinically, toxic epidermal necrolysis syndrome is almost indistinguishable from Stevens-Johnson syndrome. Histologically, the cleavage plane for the blisters is deeper than in Stevens-Johnson syndrome. The cleavage plane is *at* the basement membrane of the epidermis, so even the basal cell layer is lost. This makes toxic epidermal necrolysis syndrome slightly more devastating than Stevens-Johnson syndrome, because healing occurs with much scarring. Often, healing cannot be accomplished without skin grafting, so the mortality rate is even higher than in Stevens-Johnson syndrome. Patients with toxic epidermal necrolysis are always cared for in a burn unit because of full-thickness burns over 80%-90% of the skin. The mortality rate is very high, as in burn patients with damage of this extent.

- Toxic epidermal necrolysis syndrome is a life-threatening exfoliative dermatitis.

Macular "Drug Red" Syndrome

Macular "drug red" syndrome is a generalized skin rash that is fairly characteristic because it is intensely bright red. It is nonpruritic, flat (macular), and (except for its frightening appearance) usually causes the patient no significant discomfort. It cannot be predicted, and because it potentially is related to the serious syndromes above, most physicians regard this type of rash as a strong contraindication to giving the drug anytime in the future.

- Macular "drug red" rash is intensely bright red, nonpruritic, and flat (macular).

Ampicillin-Mononucleosis Rash

Ampicillin-mononucleosis rash is a unique drug rash occurring when ampicillin is given to an acutely ill febrile patient who has mononucleosis (a viral illness). The rash is papular, nonpruritic, rose-colored, usually on the abdomen, and has a granular feel when the fingers brush lightly over the surface of the involved skin. It is not known why the rash is specific for ampicillin and mononucleosis. The rash does not portend penicillin anaphylaxis or any of the above syndromes.

- Ampicillin-mononucleosis rash is papular, nonpruritic, rose-colored, and on the abdomen.

Fixed Drug Eruptions

Fixed drug eruptions are red to red-brown macules that appear on a certain area of the patient's skin; any part of the body can be affected. The macules do not itch or have other signs of inflammation, although fever is associated with their appearance in a few patients. The unique aspect of this allergic phenomenon is that if a patient is given the drug of cause in the future, exactly the same skin areas have the rash. Resolution of the macules often includes postinflammatory hyperpigmentation. Except for cosmetic problems due to skin discolorations, the phenomenon does not seem serious. Antibiotics and sulfonamides are the most frequently recognized causes. How a systemically distributed drug causes something so sharply restricted anatomically is a mystery. Bilateral symmetry has been seen in patients with noncontiguous areas of disease.

- In fixed drug eruptions, the same area of skin is affected.

Erythema Nodosum

Erythema nodosum is a characteristic rash of red nodules about the size of a quarter, usually nonpruritic and appearing only over the anterior aspects of the lower legs. Histopathologically, the nodules are plaques of infiltrating mononuclear cells. Erythema nodosum is associated with several connective tissue diseases, viral infections, and drug allergy. This drug allergy is a relative contraindication to readministration of the drug.

- Erythema nodosum rash is usually nonpruritic, appearing only over the anterior aspect of the lower legs.

- It is associated with several connective tissue diseases, viral infections, and drug allergy.

Contact Dermatitis

Contact dermatitis can occur with various drugs. Commonly, it is a form of drug allergy that is an occupational disease in medical or healthcare workers. In some patients receiving topical drugs on the skin, allergy develops to the drug or various elements in its pharmaceutical formulation, e.g., excipients, fillers, stabilizers, antibacterials, and emulsifiers. Contact dermatitis is a manifestation of type IV hypersensitivity and clinically appears as an area of reddening on the skin which progresses to a granular weeping eczematous eruption of the skin, with some dermal thickening and a plaque-like quality of the surrounding skin. Histopathologically, the affected area is infiltrated by mononuclear cells. Giant cells and granulomata are usually absent, except in specialized cases, e.g., reactions to emulsions of particulates of metals. When patients receiving treatment for some kind of dermatitis develop contact hypersensitivity to steroid or other drug used in treatment, a particularly difficult diagnostic problem arises, unless the physician is alert to this possibility. When contact hypersensitivity to a drug occurs, it does not increase the probability of acute type I hypersensitivity developing and is not a harbinger of the above serious exfoliative syndromes. However, patients can develop exquisite cutaneous sensitivity of this type so that almost no avoidance technique in the workplace completely eliminates dermatitis. Thus, it can be occupationally disabling.

- Contact dermatitis is a form of drug allergy.
- It is a manifestation of type IV hypersensitivity.

Penicillin Allergy

Penicillin can cause anaphylaxis in sensitive persons. It is an IgE-mediated process that can be evaluated by skin testing to penicillin major and minor determinants. Patients with positive results on skin testing and a clinical history of penicillin allergy can be desensitized to penicillin (usually orally), but the procedure may be hazardous.

- Penicillin can cause anaphylaxis.
- It is an IgE-mediated process diagnosed by penicillin skin testing.
- Patients can be desensitized, but the procedure may be hazardous.

Radiographic Contrast Media Reactions

Radiographic contrast media can cause reactions that have the clinical appearance of anaphylaxis. Estimates of the frequency of these reactions are 2%-6% of procedures involving intravenous contrast media. Incidence of intra-arterial contrast-induced reactions is lower. The anaphylactoid reactions

do not involve IgE antibody (thus, the reason for the term "anaphylact**oid**" reactions). Radiocontrast media appears to induce mediator release on basis of some other property intrinsic to the contrast agent. The tonicity or ionic strength of the media seems particularly related to anaphylactoid reactions. With availability of low ionic strength media, the incidence of reactions has been low.

- The frequency of contrast media reactions is 2%-6% of procedures.
- The reaction does not involve IgE antibody.
- Nonionic or low osmolar contrast media cause fewer anaphylactoid reactions than standard contrast media.

Radiocontrast media reactions can be prevented with the use of low ionic strength media in patients with a history of asthma or atopy. Patients with reactions who subsequently need radiographic contrast media procedures can be pretreated with a protocol of 50 mg oral prednisone every 6 hours for three doses, with the last dose 1 hour before the procedure. At the time of the last dose, also give 50 mg diphenhydramine and 25 mg ephedrine orally.

- Patients with a history of systemic reactions to radiocontrast media a) should be pretreated with prednisone, diphenhydramine, and ephedrine and b) should be offered nonionic contrast agents.

QUESTIONS

Multiple Choice (choose the one best answer)

1. About how long after the onset of exhalation is the peak expiratory flow rate achieved?
   a. 150 milliseconds
   b. 350 milliseconds
   c. 550 milliseconds
   d. 750 milliseconds
   e. 950 milliseconds

2. Which of the following is an important adverse effect of inhaled corticosteroids?
   a. Osteoporosis of the vertebral bodies
   b. Osteoporosis of the femoral head
   c. Diabetes mellitus
   d. Hypokalemia
   e. Dysphonia

3. Which of the following is not approved for use in asthma by the Food and Drug Administration?
   a. Salmeterol
   b. Pirbuterol
   c. Nedocromil
   d. Ipatropium
   e. Flunisolide

4. Which of the following is most likely to inhibit immediate-type skin testing?
   a. Cimetidine
   b. Theophylline
   c. Prednisone
   d. Methylprednisolone
   e. Doxepin

5. Which of the following statements about hereditary angioedema is true?
   a. Inherited in an autosomal recessive pattern
   b. C1q decreased
   c. C4 decreased
   d. C1 esterase inhibitor level decreased in all cases
   e. Associated with lymphoproliferative disease

6. Patients with previous reactions to radiographic contrast media who undergo procedures involving intravenous injection of a radiocontrast agent should be pretreated with
   a. Prednisone, 50 mg, and diphenhydramine, 50 mg, 1 hour before the procedure

b. Prednisone, 50 mg, and diphenhydramine, 50 mg, 6 hours before the procedure

c. Prednisone, 50 mg, diphenhydramine, 50 mg, and cimetidine, 300 mg, 1 hour before the procedure

d. Prednisone, 50 mg 13 hours, 7 hours, and 1 hour before the procedure and diphenhydramine, 50 mg 1 hour before procedure

e. Prednisone, 50 mg 13 hours, 7 hours, and 1 hour before the procedure

7. The National Asthma Education Expert Panel recommends spirometry for:
   a. All patients with asthma, at initial evaluation
   b. Patients with moderate and severe asthma, at initial evaluation
   c. Patients with severe asthma, at initial evaluation
   d. Patients with moderate and severe asthma, every 3 months
   e. Patients with severe asthma, every 3 months

True/False (indicate whether each answer is true or false)

8. Prolonged and regular inhalation reduces nonspecific bronchial hyperresponsiveness:
   a. Albuterol
   b. Pirbuterol
   c. Fenoterol
   d. Nedocromil sodium
   e. Cromolyn sodium
   f. Beclomethasone dipropionate

9. May cause urinary retention:
   a. Phenylpropanolamine
   b. Pseudoephedrine
   c. Brompheniramine
   d. Chlorpheniramine
   e. Fluticasone
   f. Flunisolide

10. Controlled clinical trials have shown that allergen immuno-therapy is effective:
    a. *Alternaria* (mold)
    b. Birch pollen
    c. Bee venom
    d. *Candida* (yeast)
    e. Tobacco smoke
    f. Chocolate

ANSWERS

1. Answer a.

The peak flow rate is achieved when the first few hundred millileters of air is expired. This occurs within about 150 milliseconds. Thus, the peak flow rate reflects large airway obstruction.

2. Answer e.

The most common adverse effects of inhaled corticosteroids are local (i.e., oral thrush and dysphonia). Although systemic biochemical changes from inhaled corticosteroids have been reported, clinically significant hypercortisolism is exceedingly rare.

3. Answer d.

Ipatropium bromide is approved for use in only chronic obstructive pulmonary disease. Nevertheless, ipatropium bromide may be a useful bronchodilator in asthma.

4. Answer e.

H_1 antagonists are potent inhibitors of the immediate-type skin test. Corticosteroids and H_2 antagonists are much less active in this regard. Tricyclic antidepressants, anticholinergic drugs, and phenothiazines have H_1-blocking activity.

5. Answer c.

Hereditary angioedema is an autosomal-dominant genetic disorder. Typically, the serum level of C4 is decreased. The acquired form of C1 esterase inhibitor deficiency is often associated with lymphoproliferative disease, and the serum level of C1q is decreased. Of the patients with hereditary angioedema, 15% have normal levels of inhibitor.

6. Answer d.

H$_2$ antagonists have not been shown to decrease the reaction rate to radiocontrast media. Ephedrine, 25 mg 1 hour before the procedure, may decrease the reaction rate when added to the pretreatment regimen described in answer d.

7. Answer a.

All patients with asthma or suspected asthma should have spirometry at initial evaluation. Spirometry can help make the diagnosis of asthma and estimate its severity. Continued management should be based on symptoms, peak expiratory flow rates, spirometry, or some combination of these.

8. a, false; b, false; c, false; d, true; e, true; f, true.

The inhaled β-agonists do not reduce nonspecific bronchial hyperresponsiveness. In fact, there is evidence that these agents may *increase* bronchial reactivity to histamine or methacholine. In contrast, inhaled corticosteroids, cromolyn, and nedocromil can reduce bronchial hyperresponsiveness.

9. a, true; b, true; c, true; d, true; e, false; f, false.

Antihistamines and decongestants can cause urinary retention in patients at risk for bladder outlet obstruction.

10. a, true; b, true; c, true; d, false; e, false; f, false.

The diagnosis of "*Candida* allergy" should raise suspicion of unproven and unconventional allergy testing. Immunotherapy to *Candida*, tobacco smoke, and chocolate are never appropriate. However, immunotherapy for respiratory allergy (*Alternaria*, birch pollen) or anaphylaxis (bee venom) is clinically effective.

CHAPTER 3
CARDIOLOGY

Carole A. Warnes, M.D.
Stephen C. Hammill, M.D.
Marshall S. Stanton, M.D.
Rick A. Nishimura, M.D.
Barry L. Karon, M.D.

PART I
Carole A. Warnes, M.D.

PHYSICAL EXAMINATION

Jugular Venous Pressure

This pressure is normally 6-8 cm H_2O. The jugular veins will not be visible when the patient is sitting up. When the pressure is elevated, consider not only biventricular failure but also constrictive pericarditis, pericardial tamponade, cor pulmonale (especially pulmonary embolus), and superior vena cava syndrome. The normal waves are *a*, which reflects atrial contraction; *c*, closure of tricuspid valve; and *v*, ventricular filling.

- Normal jugular venous pressure: 6-8 cm H_2O.
- Normal waves: *a*, atrial contraction; *c*, closure of tricuspid valve; *v*, ventricular filling.

Abnormalities of the waves indicate various conditions, as follows:
1) Large "a" wave: tricuspid stenosis, right ventricular hypertrophy, pulmonary hypertension
2) Cannon "a" wave: atria contracting against a closed atrioventricular valve (atrioventricular dissociation)
3) Large cv wave: tricuspid regurgitation
4) Rapid x + y descent: constrictive pericarditis
5) Kussmaul's sign: pericardial tamponade or constriction

- Abnormalities of waves:
    large "a" wave: tricuspid stenosis, right ventricular hypertrophy, pulmonary hypertension.
    cannon "a" wave: atria contracting against closed atrioventricular valve (atrioventricular dissociation).

rapid x + y descent: constrictive pericarditis.

Arterial Pulse

Palpation of the radial pulse is useful only for rate. Check brachial or carotid pulse for contour. "Tardus" describes the rate of rise of upstroke, and "parvus" describes the volume. In hypertension, look for radiofemoral delay (check radial and femoral pulses simultaneously) to determine whether coarctation is present.

Abnormalities of the arterial pulse and their indicated conditions are as follows:
1) parvus and tardus: aortic stenosis
2) parvus only: low output, cardiomyopathy
3) bounding: aortic regurgitation or atrioventricular fistulae
4) bifid: hypertrophic obstructive cardiomyopathy (from midsystolic obstruction)
5) bisferiens: aortic stenosis and regurgitation

- Abnormalities of arterial pulse:
    parvus and tardus: aortic stenosis.
    parvus only: low output, cardiomyopathy.
    bisferiens: aortic stenosis and regurgitation.

Apical Impulse

This is normally a discrete area of localized contraction. It is usually maximal at the fifth intercostal space, midclavicular line.

Abnormalities of the apical impulse and their indicated conditions are as follows:
1) apex displaced, impulse poor and diffuse: cardiomyopathy

2) sustained: left ventricular hypertrophy, aortic steno-sis, often with large "a" wave
3) trifid: hypertrophic cardiomyopathy
4) hyperdynamic and diffuse with rapid filling wave: mitral regurgitation
5) tapping quality, localized: mitral stenosis

- Abnormalities of apical impulse:
  apex displaced, impulse poor and diffuse: cardio-myopathy.
  trifid: hypertrophic cardiomyopathy.
  tapping quality, localized: mitral stenosis.

Thrills

These indicate turbulent flow (e.g., aortic stenosis, ventricular septal defect).

Heart Sounds

First

This consists of mitral valve closure followed shortly by tricuspid valve closure. A *loud* first heart sound occurs with a short P-R interval and mitral stenosis because the mitral valve is wide open when the left ventricle begins to contract and then slaps shut. The intensity of the first sound is *decreased* if mitral valve is heavily calcified (severe mitral stenosis) and also if P-R interval is long (occurs classically with acute rheumatic fever).

- Loud first heart sound: short P-R interval and mitral stenosis.
- Decreased intensity of first heart sound: mitral valve heavily calcified, long P-R interval.

Second

This consists of aortic closure followed by pulmonary closure. Intensity of both is increased by hypertension (loud P_2 with pulmonary hypertension, and P_2 is audible at apex). Intensity is decreased with heavily calcified valves (severe aortic stenosis). Normally, second sound widens on inspiration.

- Intensity of second heart sound increased by hypertension.
- Intensity decreased with heavily calcified valves.

Abnormalities of splitting of the second heart sound and their indicated conditions are as follows:
1) fixed split: atrial septal defect
2) paradoxic split (caused by delay in aortic closure so it closes after pulmonary valve): left bundle branch block, left ventricular hypertrophy

- Abnormalities of splitting of second heart sound:
  fixed split: atrial septal defect.
  paradoxic split: left bundle branch block, left ventricular hypertrophy.

Third

This is probably caused by tensing of the chordae as the blood distends the left ventricle during diastole. It is heard normally in young people and in older adults and is associated with volume load on the left ventricle such as aortic regurgitation, mitral regurgitation, and cardiomyopathy.

- Third heart sound is heard in young people and older adults in association with volume load on left ventricle (e.g., aortic regurgitation, mitral regurgitation, cardiomyopathy).

Fourth

This occurs with the atrial kick as blood is forced into the left ventricle by atrial contraction. It occurs when the left ventricle is stiff and noncompliant, such as in aortic stenosis, systemic hypertension, hypertrophic cardiomyopathy, and ischemia.

- Fourth heart sound occurs in aortic stenosis, systemic hypertension, hypertrophic cardiomyopathy, and ischemia.

Opening Snap

This is virtually always caused by mitral stenosis, and the interval from the second heart sound to the opening snap helps determine the severity. With severe mitral stenosis, the left atrial pressure is very high and thus the valve opens earlier, and the interval is <60 m/second.

- Opening snap is virtually always caused by mitral stenosis.

Murmurs

These are discussed with the individual valvular lesions described later in this chapter, but some broad guidelines follow here.

A systolic ejection murmur occurs when blood is ejected from a ventricle into a vascular structure. It begins after the first heart sound and ends before the second sound. It may have a diamond-shaped quality with crescendo and decrescendo components, but in general the more severe the obstruction, the longer the murmur and there is less decrescendo quality. It may be preceded by an ejection click.

- Systolic ejection murmur: the more severe the obstruction, the longer the murmur.

A holosystolic murmur occurs when blood goes from a high-pressure to a low-pressure system (mitral regurgitation, ventricular septal defect). It engulfs the first and second heart sounds.

- Holosystolic murmur occurs with mitral regurgitation and ventricular septal defect and engulfs first and second heart sounds.

MANEUVERS THAT ALTER CARDIAC MURMURS

- *Inspiration* increases venous return and so increases right-sided murmurs of tricuspid regurgitation, pulmonary stenosis, pulmonary regurgitation.
- *Valsalva* increases intrathoracic pressure, inhibiting venous return to the right side of the heart.
- Most cardiac murmurs and sounds diminish in intensity during Valsalva maneuver because of decreased ventricular filling and decreased cardiac output (except hypertrophic obstructive cardiomyopathy and mitral valve prolapse).
- *Handgrip* increases cardiac output and systemic arterial pressure.
- A change in *posture* from supine to upright causes decrease in venous return; therefore, stroke volume decreases, and this decrease causes a reflex increase in heart rate and peripheral resistance.
- *Squatting* and the *Valsalva maneuver* have opposite hemodynamic effects. Squatting increases peripheral resistance and increases venous return.

The effects of maneuvers are shown in Table 3-1.

VALVULAR HEART DISEASE

Aortic Stenosis

Supravalvular

The two major types of supravalvular aortic stenosis are diaphragmatic and localized hourglass-shaped narrowing immediately above the aortic sinuses, often associated with hypoplasia of the ascending aorta.

Supravalvular aortic stenosis is associated with Williams' syndrome, which is characterized by so-called elfin facies, mental retardation, and hypercalcemia. Systemic hypertension is a common association. An important feature is large, dilated, thick-walled coronary arteries because the coronary ostia are proximal to the obstruction. This lesion also causes premature atherosclerosis.

Physical Examination

Findings include a prominent left ventricle, a thrill in the suprasternal notch and over the carotid artery (thrill is often more marked in right carotid artery and the pulse upstroke is often brisker on right side than left side), systolic murmur without click, and a loud A_2.

- Features of supravalvular aortic stenosis: thrill in suprasternal notch and over carotid artery, systolic murmur without click, loud A_2.

Subvalvular

The types of subvalvular stenosis are discrete ("membranous") and fibromuscular (fixed or dynamic). These two types can coexist.

Physical Examination

Findings include a prominent left ventricle, reduced pulse pressure, no click, and arterial thrill when the stenosis is severe. Subvalvular aortic stenosis is commonly associated with aortic regurgitation because there is a jet lesion on the aortic valve cusps.

- Features of subvalvular aortic stenosis: prominent left ventricle, reduced pulse pressure, no click, arterial thrill when the stenosis is severe.
- Commonly associated with aortic regurgitation.

Table 3-1.--Effects of Physical Maneuvers and Other Factors on Valvular Diseases

Maneuver	Result	Mitral regurgitation	Aortic stenosis	HOCM
Amyl nitrite	↓ afterload	↓	↑	↑
Valsalva	↓ preload	↓	↓	↑
Handgrip	↑ afterload	↑	↓	↓
Post-PVC	↑ contractility ↓ afterload	=	↑	↑*

*Although the murmur ↑, the peripheral pulse ↓ because of the increase in outflow obstruction.
HOCM, hypertrophic obstructive cardiomyopathy; PVC, premature ventricular complex.

Diagnosis

The diagnosis can usually be made with two-dimensional and Doppler echocardiography, often without the need for cardiac catheterization. Two-dimensional echocardiography can determine the severity of the stenosis and the site and presence or absence of additional valvular abnormality. In addition, it determines the presence or absence of left ventricular hypertrophy. If cardiac catheterization is performed, when the catheter is pulled back from the left ventricle toward the aorta there is a low subvalvular left ventricular pressure tracing before the aortic valve is crossed.

- Diagnosis of subvalvular aortic stenosis is made with two-dimensional and Doppler echocardiography.
- Echocardiography determines presence or absence of left ventricular hypertrophy.

Valvular

Types

The *congenital bicuspid* type occurs in 1% of the population. It may be associated with obstruction in infancy through early adulthood. It is the most common cause of aortic stenosis in adults <55 years old. Even in young adults the valve is frequently still pliable and auscultation is thus different from that of degenerative aortic valve disease. An ejection click often precedes the systolic murmur. The earlier the click (i.e., the closer to the first sound), the more severe the stenosis. A_2 becomes later with increasing stenosis, and when severe there may be paradoxic splitting of the second sound. The lesion may be associated with coarctation. The diagnosis can usually be made successfully with two-dimensional and Doppler echocardiography without the need for cardiac catheterization in young people.

- Congenital bicuspid valvular aortic stenosis occurs in 1% of population.
- It is most common cause of aortic stenosis in adults <55 years old.
- Ejection click often precedes the systolic murmur.
- The earlier the click (closer to first heart sound), the more severe the stenosis.
- A_2 becomes later with increasing stenosis; when severe, there may be paradoxic splitting of second sound.

Degenerative aortic valve disease is the most common cause of aortic stenosis in adults >55 years old. The valve is three-cuspid and calcified. When calcification is extensive, A_2 becomes inaudible.

- Degenerative aortic valve disease is most common cause of aortic stenosis in adults >55 years old.

- When calcification is extensive, A_2 becomes inaudible.

The *rheumatic* type is less common. It is associated with thickening and fusion of the aortic cusps at the commissures. It always occurs with a rheumatic mitral valve, although important mitral stenosis or regurgitation may not always be evident. It usually occurs in early adulthood (age 40-60 years).

- Rheumatic type is less common cause of valvular aortic stenosis.
- Usually occurs at 40-60 years of age.

Symptoms

The classic triad of symptoms includes exertional dyspnea, syncope, and angina; however, most patients are symptom-free. The presence of angina does not necessarily indicate coexisting coronary disease.

- Symptoms of valvular type of aortic stenosis: exertional dyspnea, syncope, angina.
- Angina does not necessarily indicate coexisting coronary disease.

Physical Examination

The pulse is parvus and tardus. The left ventricular impulse is localized and sustained. There may be a palpable fourth sound. Arterial thrills may be palpable in the carotid, suprasternal notch, second intercostal space, or left and right sternal borders. A fourth heart sound may be present. A_2 is diminished or absent. The ejection systolic murmur becomes longer with increasing severity, radiating to the carotid arteries and the apex.

- Pulse is parvus and tardus.
- Ejection systolic murmur becomes longer with increasing severity.

Diagnosis

Electrocardiography may show left ventricular hypertrophy (although it is not a sensitive index, and echocardiography is better), but the results often are normal in young patients. Left bundle branch block is common, and in later stages of the condition conduction abnormalities may develop (e.g., complete heart block) if the calcium impinges on the conducting system. On chest radiography, the heart size is usually normal, even when the stenosis is severe. The aortic root may show post-stenotic dilatation. In degenerative aortic valve disease, calcium in the valve leaflets may be seen, especially on a penetrated lateral view.

- Electrocardiography is often normal in young patients.
- Left bundle branch block is common on electrocardiogram.

- Aortic root may show post-stenotic dilatation on chest radiograph.

Differential diagnoses include 1) hypertrophic cardiomyopathy (note different carotid upstroke and changing murmur with maneuvers) and 2) mitral regurgitation (murmur may radiate anteriorly and upward, particularly if there is rupture of a posterior mitral valve leaflet).

Aortic stenosis can be diagnosed with bedside physical examination. The most important physical finding is the parvus and tardus pulse. However, the degree of aortic stenosis can be difficult to determine, particularly in older patients. Doppler echocardiography is particularly useful for assessing gradient and correlates well with cardiac catheterization. Severe aortic stenosis is present when the mean Doppler gradient is >50 mm Hg and the valve area is <0.75 cm^2. Patients being considered for operation should also have coronary angiography if they are older than 50 years.

- Aortic stenosis can be diagnosed with bedside physical examination.
- Most important physical finding: parvus and tardus pulse.
- Doppler echocardiography is useful for diagnosis.
- Severe aortic stenosis: gradient is >50 mm Hg, valve area is <0.75 cm^2.

Aortic Regurgitation

Etiology

Valvular

Causes of valvular aortic regurgitation include 1) congenital bicuspid valve, 2) rheumatic fever, 3) endocarditis, 4) degenerative aortic valve disease, 5) seronegative arthritis, 6) ankylosing spondylitis, and 7) rheumatoid arthritis.

Aortic Root Dilatation

Various conditions have been associated with aortic root dilatation. Marfan syndrome can be associated with progressive dilatation of the aortic root and sinuses (so-called cystic medial necrosis). Prophylactic β-adrenergic blocker therapy is effective in slowing the rate of aortic dilatation and reducing the development of aortic complications in some patients with Marfan syndrome. When the aortic root reaches ≥5.5 cm in diameter, it should be replaced. Syphilis is an uncommon cause of aortic regurgitation and usually causes aortic root dilatation above the sinuses (syphilis spares the sinuses). Remember that syphilis is associated with calcium in the aortic root on chest radiography. Age is also a related factor. With advancing age, the aorta dilates, and hypertension also tends to accelerate this process. Acute aortic regurgitation may be associated with an aortic dissection.

- Marfan syndrome can be associated with aortic root dilatation.
- Syphilis is uncommon cause of aortic regurgitation.

Symptoms

The symptoms of aortic regurgitation include fatigue, dyspnea, palpitations, and exertional angina.

Physical Examination

A bounding, collapsing Corrigan's pulse resulting from wide pulse pressure is found. Other findings are de Musset's head nodding, Durozier's sign over the femoral artery, and Quincke's sign (pulsatile capillary nail bed). The left ventricular impulse is diffuse and hyperdynamic, and the apex beat is often displaced. A diastolic decrescendo murmur is heard at either the left or the right sternal border, and the second heart sound may be paradoxically split because of increased left ventricular volume. The loudness of the murmur does not correlate with the severity of aortic regurgitation, particularly in acute aortic regurgitation (e.g., with dissection). There may be little or no murmur when there is an abrupt rise in left ventricular end-diastolic pressure. A systolic flow murmur is common. It does not necessarily indicate coexistent aortic stenosis, and so the pulse upstroke should be checked.

- Findings indicative of aortic regurgitation: bounding, collapsing Corrigan's pulse, diastolic decrescendo murmur, second heart sound may be paradoxically split.

Diagnosis

On electrocardiography, features of left ventricular hypertrophy may be found. Ruptured sinus of Valsalva should be considered in the differential diagnosis. The diagnosis can be made at bedside clinical examination, but it can be missed if a patient with acute aortic regurgitation presents with little or no murmur. Doppler echocardiography is useful and also helps evaluate left ventricular size and function. If dissection is suspected, transthoracic echocardiography may be insufficient, and computed tomography, transesophageal echocardiography, or even aortography may be needed.

- Electrocardiography may show left ventricular hypertrophy.
- Differential diagnosis: ruptured sinus of Valsalva.
- Doppler echocardiography is useful.

Timing of Surgery

The timing of surgical management is still controversial. Despite a large volume load on the left ventricle and compensatory left ventricular enlargement, patients with aortic regurgitation may remain asymptomatic for several years. The development of symptoms, however, usually reflects left ventricular dysfunction, and survival is limited unless surgical intervention is prompt. Once left ventricular dysfunction is established, patients are less likely to have a return of normal function after aortic valve replacement. There is still controversy, however, regarding the timing of operation for patients who are asymptomatic or who have very mild symptoms. Certainly when the ejection fraction decreases below normal, operation is needed. Other factors that have been used include echocardiographic data: a systolic dimension >55 mm or a diastolic dimension >80 mm. Asymptomatic patients with large left ventricles need to be followed carefully; therefore, if there is evidence of resting left ventricular dysfunction or of rapidly progressive left ventricular dilatation, they should have operation. Prophylactic angiotensin converting enzyme inhibitors help prevent ventricular dilation in patients with severe aortic regurgitation. This benefit may help to delay operation.

- Timing of operation for aortic regurgitation is controversial.
- Patients can be asymptomatic for several years.
- If symptoms develop, survival is limited unless surgical intervention is prompt.
- If ejection fraction decreases below normal, operation is needed.

When the cause of aortic regurgitation is acute infective endocarditis, antibiotic therapy should always be instituted first. Surgery is indicated for uncontrolled infection, development of left ventricular dysfunction, or pulmonary congestion. Conduction abnormalities suggest an aortic root abscess.

- If cause of aortic regurgitation is acute infective endocarditis, antibiotic therapy should be given first.
- Indications for operation: uncontrolled infection, left ventricular dysfunction, pulmonary congestion.
- Conduction abnormalities suggest aortic root abscess.

Mitral Stenosis

Mitral stenosis is almost always due to rheumatic heart disease causing leaflet thickening with fusion of the commissures and later calcification. Symptoms do not usually develop for several years after mitral stenosis is apparent on physical examination. These symptoms are usually dyspnea and later orthopnea with paroxysmal nocturnal dyspnea. Atrial fibrillation usually causes significant deterioration of symptoms. Other symptoms include hemoptysis, and later pulmonary hypertension may cause signs of right-sided failure with ascites and peripheral edema. Systemic emboli may also result from atrial fibrillation.

- Mitral stenosis is almost always due to rheumatic heart disease.

- Symptoms do not develop for several years after mitral stenosis is found on physical examination.
- Symptoms: dyspnea, orthopnea with paroxysmal nocturnal dyspnea.
- Atrial fibrillation causes significant deterioration of symptoms.

Physical Examination

The first heart sound is loud. The shorter the interval from the second heart sound (A_2) to the opening snap, the more severe the mitral stenosis. An opening snap occurs only with a pliable valve, and it disappears when the valve calcifies. The stenosis is mild if this interval is >90 ms, moderate if it is 80 ms, and severe if it is <60 ms. The diastolic murmur is a low-pitched apical rumble, and the longer it is, the more severe the stenosis. The murmur has presystolic accentuation. Right ventricular lift and increased P_2 are associated with pulmonary hypertension.

- Physical exam in mitral stenosis:
    loud first heart sound.
    the shorter the interval from A_2 to the opening snap, the more severe the stenosis.
    diastolic murmur is low-pitched apical rumble.
    the longer the murmur, the more severe the stenosis.

Diagnosis

Electrocardiography shows P mitrale and later right ventricular hypertrophy. Chest radiography (Fig. 3-1) shows straightening of the left heart border with a large left atrial shadow and dilated upper lobe pulmonary veins. With pulmonary hypertension, the central pulmonary arteries become prominent. In severe stenosis, Kerley B lines may be present.

- Electrocardiography shows P mitrale and later right ventricular hypertrophy.
- Chest radiography shows straightening of the left heart border, a large left atrial shadow, and dilated upper lobe pulmonary veins.
- In severe stenosis, Kerley B lines may be present.

Two-dimensional and Doppler echocardiography is the tool of choice to diagnose mitral stenosis and determine its severity. Information is gained about valve gradient and valve area (Table 3-2), and pulmonary artery pressures can be noninvasively assessed. Cardiac catheterization is usually unnecessary unless the coronary arteries need to be studied or the echocardiographic findings do not concur with the clinical situation. Severe stenosis usually correlates with a mean gradient >12 mm Hg.

- Two-dimensional and Doppler echocardiography is used

Fig. 3-1. Chest radiograph from a patient with severe mitral stenosis, show-ing a typical straight left heart border, prominent pulmonary artery, large left atrium, right ventricular contour, and pulmonary venous hypertension.

to diagnose mitral stenosis and determine severity.
- For diagnosis of mitral stenosis, cardiac catheterization is usually unnecessary.
- Severe stenosis correlates with a mean gradient >12 mm Hg.

Indications for Surgery

Because there is no concern about left ventricular dys-function (left ventricle is small and underfilled) in mitral steno-sis, operation is not needed until there are symptoms of exer-tional dyspnea or pulmonary edema. Atrial fibrillation does not necessarily indicate the need for operation because it can often be controlled medically. With a pliable valve that is noncalcified and has no regurgitation, a commissurotomy can be performed without valve replacement, and this may preclude the need for valve replacement for at least 10 years. Another considera-tion is a percutaneous balloon valvuloplasty if the valve is pli-able and there is no regurgitation. This is probably the proce-dure of choice, and results compare favorably with those of surgical commissurotomy.

Table 3-2.--Severity of Mitral Stenosis, by Valve Area

Severity	Valve area, cm^2
Mild	1.5-2
Moderate	1-1.5
Severe	<1

- Operation for mitral stenosis is indicated with exertional dyspnea or pulmonary edema.
- Atrial fibrillation is not necessarily indicative of operation (can be controlled medically).
- Percutaneous balloon valvuloplasty is probably procedure of choice.

Mitral Regurgitation

Etiology

Causes of mitral regurgitation include the following: 1) rheumatic; 2) mitral valve prolapse (with or without ruptured chordae); 3) infective endocarditis; 4) papillary muscle dys-function--as a result of ischemia, fibrosis, or rupture (note that the posteromedial papillary muscle with its single blood supply from the right coronary artery becomes infarcted more frequently than the anterior papillary muscle); 5) dilat-ed left ventricle; 6) hypertrophic cardiomyopathy; 7) cleft mitral valve associated with primum atrial septal defect; 8) trauma; and 9) systemic lupus erythematosus. Mitral annu-lar calcification, when severe, can also cause mitral regurgi-tation. This may be accelerated by systemic hypertension, diabetes, and hypercalcemic states (e.g., resulting from chron-ic renal failure).

- In mitral regurgitation, the posteromedial papillary muscle becomes infarcted more often than the anterior papillary muscle.
- Mitral annular calcification may be accelerated by systemic hypertension, diabetes, hypercalcemic states.

Symptoms

Fatigue, dyspnea (due to increased left atrial pressure), and pulmonary edema can be present. Symptoms worsen with atrial fibrillation.

Physical Examination

The findings include a diffuse and hyperdynamic left ven-tricular impulse, which may be visible, and a palpable rapid filling wave. The first heart sound is usually obliterated, and there is a holosystolic murmur. The second heart sound is widely split (early A$_2$), and there is a third heart sound. A low-pitched early diastolic rumble is significant for severe regur-gitation, but does not mean there is coexistent mitral stenosis. In acute mitral regurgitation, the murmur may be short because of increased left atrial pressure. The left atrium may be palpable with systole, and the left ventricle with diastole; there may be both third and fourth heart sounds. If the cause is ruptured chordae, an anterior leaflet murmur radiates to the axilla and back, and a posterior leaflet murmur radiates to the base and carotids. Consider acute mitral regurgitation with a normal-sized heart and pulmonary edema.

- Physical examination in mitral regurgitation:
  first heart sound is usually obliterated.
  holosystolic murmur is present.
  second heart sound is widely split (early A_2).
  low-pitched early diastolic rumble is significant for severe regurgitation, but does not mean coexistent mitral stenosis.

Diagnosis

Chest radiography may first show a dilated left atrium and then, as mitral regurgitation increases, dilatation of the left ventricle.

Pathophysiology

Mitral regurgitation "offloads" the left ventricle, so filling volume must increase to maintain adequate forward output. This results in a hyperdynamic ventricle, and thus many patients with significant mitral regurgitation remain asymptomatic for many years. A low or low-normal ejection fraction therefore suggests significant ventricular dysfunction. Left atrial compliance may determine the hemodynamic picture. The left atrium may enlarge slightly and the pressure will increase significantly within it; conversely, it may markedly enlarge and permit a near-normal pressure.

- Many patients with mitral regurgitation remain asymptomatic for many years.
- Low or low-normal ejection fraction suggests significant ventricular dysfunction.

Timing of Surgery

Asymptomatic patients with an ejection fraction >50% can continue to undergo regular observation. Operation should be considered for symptomatic patients (note that ventricular function significantly influences the postoperative outcome), and because "afterload is removed" when the mitral valve is replaced, left ventricular function may actually deteriorate. Mildly symptomatic patients may be considered for operation, particularly if serial examinations reveal progressive cardiac enlargement. Earlier operation may be indicated in those who are obviously suitable for mitral valve repair rather than replacement.

- Symptomatic patients with mitral regurgitation should be considered for operation.
- Mildly symptomatic patients, particularly with progressive cardiac enlargement, may be considered for operation.

Tricuspid Stenosis

The cause of tricuspid stenosis is almost always rheumatic, and it is never an isolated lesion. Carcinoid syndrome may cause tricuspid stenosis, and in rare cases atrial tumors may be the cause.

- Cause of tricuspid stenosis is almost always rheumatic; rarely, carcinoid syndrome and atrial tumors may be the cause.

Tricuspid Regurgitation

This is usually caused by dilatation of the right ventricle. When there is right ventricular hypertension, tricuspid regurgitation is also common. It often results from mitral valve disease, but it may be related to 1) biventricular infarction, 2) primary pulmonary hypertension, 3) congenital heart disease (e.g., Ebstein's anomaly), or 4) carcinoid syndrome--more commonly associated with tricuspid regurgitation than tricuspid stenosis.

- Tricuspid regurgitation is usually caused by dilatation of the right ventricle.
- If often results from mitral valve disease.

Tricuspid Valve Prolapse

This may occur as an isolated entity or in association with other connective tissue abnormalities. The tricuspid valve may prolapse or become flail as a result of trauma or endocarditis (commonly fungal or staphylococcal in drug addicts).

Physical Examination

Findings on physical examination include jugular venous distention with a prominent v wave, a prominent right ventricular impulse, a pansystolic murmur at the left sternal edge increasing with inspiration, possibly a right-sided third heart sound, and peripheral edema, ascites, and hepatomegaly.

Surgical Therapy

Tricuspid annuloplasty may be helpful if regurgitation is a result of right ventricular dilatation; however, if there is significant pulmonary hypertension, tricuspid valve replacement is usually required. This can be done with either a biologic or a mechanical valve. Biologic prostheses in the tricuspid position do not degenerate as quickly as prostheses in the left side of the heart. In patients with endocarditis, the tricuspid valve can be removed completely, and patients may tolerate this well for several years.

CONGENITAL HEART DISEASE

Atrial Septal Defect

Secundum

Patients with secundum atrial septal defect often survive to adulthood and may be asymptomatic. The condition is often detected on routine examination with the finding of a murmur. If the defect has gone undetected, atrial fibrillation frequently develops in patients in their 50s with onset of symptoms, usually dyspnea with subsequent tricuspid regurgitation and right-sided heart failure. The condition may present with a neurologic event.

- Patients with secundum atrial septal defect often survive to adulthood and may be asymptomatic.
- Condition is found on routine examination with finding of murmur.
- Atrial fibrillation often develops in patients in their 50s with onset of symptoms.
- Condition may present with a neurologic event.

Physical Examination

Findings include a normal or slightly prominent jugular venous pressure, a right ventricular heave, an ejection systolic murmur in the pulmonary artery (never more than grade 3/6), a fixed splitting of the second sound, and a tricuspid diastolic flow rumble if the shunt is large.

- Findings of secundum atrial septal defect:
  ejection systolic murmur in pulmonary artery (never more than grade 3/6).
  fixed splitting of second sound.
  tricuspid diastolic flow rumble if shunt is large.

Diagnosis

Electrocardiography usually shows right bundle branch block. Chest radiography shows pulmonary plethora, a prominent pulmonary artery, and right ventricular enlargement (Fig. 3-2). Young patients (<40 years) with secundum atrial septal defect and sinus rhythm do not have left atrial enlargement. If the chest radiograph shows left atrial enlargement, consider another lesion, particularly primum atrial septal defect with mitral regurgitation.

- If chest radiograph shows left atrial enlargement, consider primum atrial septal defect with mitral regurgitation.

Two-dimensional and color Doppler echocardiography can usually demonstrate the defect and right ventricular enlargement with volume overload. If visualization is poor, transesophageal echocardiography can be performed. Cardiac catheterization is usually unnecessary, unless coexisting coronary disease is suspected.

Sinus Venosus

An uncommon condition, this occurs in the superior portion of the atrial septum. It is often associated with anomalous pulmonary veins, usually the right upper. If echocardiography shows right ventricular volume overload and no secundum defect, consider sinus venosus atrial septal defect or anomalous pulmonary veins.

Fig. 3-2. Chest radiograph from a patient with a large left-to-right shunt due to a secundum atrial septal defect. Notice cardiac enlargement with right ventricular contour, very prominent pulmonary artery, and pulmonary plethora.

Primum (Partial Atrioventricular Canal)

This is a defect in the lower portion of the septum. The mitral valve is usually cleft and produces various degrees of regurgitation.

Diagnosis

On electrocardiography, findings are different from those of secundum type with left-axis deviation and right bundle branch block. More than 75% of patients have first-degree atrioventricular block. The chest radiographic findings are the same as those for secundum atrial septal defect, although there may be left atrial enlargement because of mitral regurgitation. Atrioventricular defects are the most common cardiac anomaly associated with Down's syndrome.

- Electrocardiography shows left-axis deviation with right bundle branch block and, commonly, first-degree atrioventricular block.
- Atrioventricular defects are most common cardiac anomaly of Down's syndrome.

Ventricular Septal Defect

Ventricular septal defect occurs in different parts of the ventricular septum, most commonly either in the membranous septum or in the muscular septum. Small defects produce a loud noise, and patients are often asymptomatic. The size of the hole determines the degree of left-to-right shunting. Small defects may have a long holosystolic murmur, often with a thrill at the left sternal edge, usually around the fourth interspace. Large defects may produce a mitral diastolic flow rumble at the apex, especially when the shunt is more than 2.5:1.

- Ventricular septal defects are most common in membranous septum or muscular septum.
- Small defects produce loud noise.
- Size of hole determines the degree of left-to-right shunting.

Patent Ductus Arteriosus

This condition is associated with maternal rubella. It produces essentially an "arteriovenous fistula." A small ductus is compatible with a normal lifespan. The ductus may calcify in adult life. A continuous "machinery" murmur envelops the second heart sound around the second interspace beneath the left clavicle. A large patent ductus arteriosus may produce ventricular failure. Surgical ligation is curative. Patients then do not need endocarditis prophylaxis.

All of the above-described shunt lesions, when large, may produce elevated pulmonary pressures and subsequently pulmonary vascular disease.

- Patent ductus arteriosus is associated with maternal rubella.
- Small ductus is compatible with normal lifespan.
- Continuous "machinery" murmur is present.
- Surgical ligation is curative, and endocarditis prophylaxis then is not needed.
- All described shunt lesions, when large, may produce elevated pulmonary pressures and subsequently pulmonary vascular disease.

Eisenmenger's Syndrome

This syndrome develops in the first few years of life when a large shunt (usually a ventricular septal defect or patent ductus arteriosus) produces pulmonary hypertension and irreversible pulmonary vascular disease. This condition causes the shunt to reverse so that blood flows from the right to the left, and subsequent cyanosis occurs. Patients are then inoperable. Death commonly occurs in the third or fourth decade of life as a result of exercise-induced syncope, arrhythmia, hemoptysis, and stroke. The cyanosis produces significant erythrocytosis, often with hemoglobin values in the teens or 20s. There is no need to phlebotomize patients with a hemoglobin value <20 g/dL or a hematocrit value <65%. Also, repeated phlebotomies frequently lead to iron deficiency, and iron-deficient erythrocytes are more rigid than ordinary ones, and the risk of stroke is thereby increased. Phlebotomy may be necessary in symptomatic patients with a hemoglobin value >20 g/dL. Always remember to replace fluid concomitantly in patients with Eisenmenger's syndrome because hypotension and syncope may be fatal.

- Eisenmenger's syndrome develops in first few years of life.
- Syndrome produces pulmonary hypertension and irreversible pulmonary vascular disease.
- Death is common in the third or fourth decade of life.
- Associated conditions: exercise-induced syncope, arrhythmia, hemoptysis, stroke.
- Cyanosis produces significant erythrocytosis.

Pulmonary Stenosis

This may occur as an isolated lesion or in association with a ventricular septal defect. Valvular pulmonary stenosis often causes few or no symptoms. The valve is frequently pliable, and it may be bicuspid. Thickened dysplastic valves, often stenotic, occur in association with Noonan's syndrome.

- Thickened dysplastic valves, often stenotic, occur with Noonan's syndrome.

Physical Examination

Findings include a prominent "a" wave in the jugular venous pulse; right ventricular heave; ejection click--the earlier the click, the more severe the stenosis (the click indicates that the valve is pliable and noncalcified); ejection systolic murmur--the longer the murmur and the later peaking, the more severe the stenosis; and soft and late P_2 (with severe stenosis P_2 becomes inaudible).

- Findings of pulmonary stenosis:
    prominent "a" wave in the jugular venous pulse.
    ejection click (the earlier the click, the more severe the stenosis).
    soft and late P_2.

Diagnosis

Electrocardiography shows right ventricular hypertrophy. On chest radiography, pulmonary oligemia is found only with *very severe* pulmonary stenosis. There is poststenotic pulmonary dilatation, especially of the left pulmonary artery (Fig. 3-3).

The diagnosis can be reliably made with two-dimensional echocardiography, and Doppler reliably predicts the gradient and estimates right ventricular pressure. In asymptomatic patients, no treatment is indicated unless the right ventricular pressure approaches two-thirds that of the systemic pressure. Later in life, the valve may become calcified when the ejection click disappears. The treatment of choice for a pliable valve is percutaneous balloon valvuloplasty. This has essentially replaced surgical valvotomy.

- Diagnosis of pulmonary stenosis is made with two-dimensional and Doppler echocardiography.
- Treatment for pliable valve is percutaneous balloon valvuloplasty.

Fig. 3-3. Typical chest radiograph of valvular pulmonary stenosis, showing normal cardiac size and marked prominence of main and left pulmonary arteries, representing poststenotic dilatation. This does not occur with infundibular pulmonary stenosis. Lung fields appear mildly oligemic.

Coarctation of the Aorta

This is usually either a discrete or a long segment of narrowing adjacent to the left subclavian artery. It is more common in males and frequently is associated with a bicuspid aortic valve. Most cases of coarctation are diagnosed in childhood; only about 20% are diagnosed in adulthood. This is the most common cardiac anomaly associated with Turner's syndrome. Other associations include aneurysms of the circle of Willis and aortic dissection or rupture. There is an increased incidence of aortic dissection or rupture in Turner's syndrome even in the absence of coarctation. As a result of the coarctation, systemic collaterals develop from the subclavian and axillary arteries through the internal mammary, scapular, and intercostal arteries.

- Coarctation of aorta is more common in males.
- Condition is frequently associated with a bicuspid aortic valve.
- Only 20% of cases are diagnosed in adulthood.
- It is the most common cardiac anomaly associated with Turner's syndrome.
- Incidence of aortic dissection or rupture is increased in Turner's syndrome even in the absence of coarctation.

There are five major complications of coarctation of the aorta: 1) cardiac failure, 2) aortic valve disease, 3) rupture or dissection, 4) endarteritis, and 5) rupture of an aneurysm of the circle of Willis--this is exacerbated by the presence of hypertension, which occurs in the upper limbs. Systemic hypertension may be the presenting feature in adults. Some patients complain of pain in the legs on exercise.

Physical Examination

Findings include an easily palpable brachial pulse; the femoral pulse is weak and delayed. There are differences in systolic pressure between the upper and lower extremities. Exercise may exaggerate the systemic hypertension. An ejection click is present when there is an associated bicuspid valve. A_2 may be loud as a result of hypertension. A fourth heart sound may be present with associated left ventricular hypertrophy and hypertension. Murmurs may originate from 1) the coarctation, which can produce a systolic murmur over the left sternal edge and over the spine in the mid-thoracic region, and it sometimes extends into diastole in the form of a continuous murmur; 2) arterial collaterals, which are spread widely over the thorax; and 3) the bicuspid aortic valve, which may generate a systolic murmur.

- Findings of coarctation of aorta: easily palpable brachial pulse, weak and delayed femoral pulse, differences in systolic pressure between upper and lower extremities.
- Coarctation can produce a systolic murmur over the left sternal edge and over the spine in mid-thorax.
- Arterial collaterals are spread widely over thorax.

Diagnosis

Electrocardiography may be normal. With more severe coarctation or hypertension, left ventricular hypertrophy with or without repolarization changes is found. Chest radiography may show rib notching from the dilated and pulsatile intercostal arteries and a "3" configuration of the aortic knob, which represents the coarctation site with proximal and distal dilatations.

- Chest radiographic findings in coarctation of aorta are rib notching and a "3" configuration of the aortic knob.

The condition may be demonstrated by echocardiography and Doppler, although imaging may be difficult in this area, and additional visualization may be necessary with digital subtraction angiography, magnetic resonance imaging, or computed tomography. Angiography can also be performed.

Treatment

Balloon angioplasty has been performed in some patients, although it is associated with aneurysm formation and re-coarctation. Surgical treatment has been an accepted approach since 1945. However, there is a significant rate of hypertension after coarctation repair. As many as 75% of patients are hypertensive at 30-year follow-up. Surgically treated patients still often die prematurely of coronary disease, heart failure, stroke, or ruptured aorta. Age at operation is important. The 20-year survival rate is 91% in patients who have operation when they are <14 years old and 79% in patients who have operation when they are >14 years old.

- Surgical repair of coarctation of aorta is associated with significant rate of hypertension; 75% of patients are hypertensive at 30-year follow-up.
- Surgically treated patients often die prematurely of coronary disease, heart failure, stroke, or ruptured aorta.

Ebstein's Anomaly

This unusual congenital lesion is thought to be associated with maternal lithium ingestion during pregnancy. It has a variable spectrum. It involves an inferior displacement of the tricuspid valve ring into the right ventricular cavity. The degree of displacement is variable, as is the degree of abnormality of the tricuspid valve. The inferior displacement results in "atrialization" of the right ventricle, the small contractile chamber beneath.

- Ebstein's anomaly is thought to be associated with maternal lithium ingestion during pregnancy.
- Anomaly involves inferior displacement of the tricuspid valve ring into the right ventricular cavity.

Physical Examination

The extremities are usually cool, often with peripheral cyanosis (a reflection of low cardiac output). There may be an "a" wave in the jugular venous pressure (although this is variable because the large right atrium may accommodate a large tricuspid regurgitant volume). A subtle right ventricular lift is noted. The first heart sound has a loud T_1 component. A holosystolic murmur increases on inspiration at the left sternal edge from tricuspid regurgitation. One or more systolic clicks are noted (may be multiple). Common associated conditions are secundum atrial septal defect and preexcitation syndrome. Patients with secundum atrial septal defects are often very cyanotic because of the right-to-left shunting. They may present with neurologic events.

- Findings of Ebstein's anomaly include cool extremities, often with peripheral cyanosis, and a holosystolic murmur that increases on inspiration.
- One or more systolic clicks are noted (may be multiple).
- Associated conditions: secundum atrial septal defect, and preexcitation syndrome.

- Patients with secundum atrial septal defects are often very cyanotic.
- They may present with neurologic events.

Diagnosis

Chest radiography shows a narrow pedicle with enlarged globular silhouette and right atrial enlargement. The lung fields are normal or oligemic. On electrocardiography, a tall P wave (Himalayan P waves) and right bundle branch block are found.

Two-dimensional and Doppler echocardiography delineates the anatomy precisely, and cardiac catheterization is unnecessary. Electrophysiology study may be necessary to delineate the bypass tract, if present.

PREGNANCY AND CARDIAC DISEASE

Physiologic Changes of Pregnancy

Plasma volume starts to increase in the first trimester, peaking around the second trimester to almost 50% above normal. An increase in red cell mass also begins early and peaks in the second trimester, but not to the same degree as the plasma volume; thus, there is a relative anemia. The cardiac output increases, and peripheral resistance decreases. Increased venous pressure in the lower extremities leads to pedal edema in 80% of healthy pregnant women.

- Physiologic changes of pregnancy include increased plasma volume, red cell mass, and cardiac output.
- Peripheral resistance decreases.

Because of these changes, the physical examination may suggest cardiac abnormalities to the unwary. Normal results of physical examination in a healthy pregnant woman include elevation of the jugular venous pressure, bounding carotid pulses, and an ejection systolic murmur in the pulmonary area (never more than grade 3/6). The second heart sound is loud, and there is a third heart sound or diastolic filling sound. A fourth heart sound occasionally may be heard.

- Ejection systolic murmur in the pulmonary area (never more than grade 3/6) is a normal finding in pregnancy.

Although a third heart sound or diastolic filling sound is common, a long rumble should raise the possibility of mitral stenosis. Because of the decrease in peripheral resistance and increased output changes, stenotic lesions are less well tolerated than regurgitant ones; for example, a patient with aortic stenosis has exaggeration of the aortic valve gradient, whereas a patient with mitral regurgitation experiences "afterload reduction" with peripheral vasodilatation and so tolerates pregnancy better.

Functional class of the patient is a consideration in terms of whether pregnancy is possible. Patients who are in functional class III or IV have a maternal mortality rate approaching 7%.

- Third heart sound or diastolic filling sound is common in pregnancy, but a long rumble should raise the possibility of mitral stenosis.
- In patients in functional class III or IV, maternal mortality rate approaches 7%.

Pregnancy is *absolutely contraindicated* in patients with the following conditions: 1) Marfan syndrome with a dilated aortic root--increased risk of dissection and rupture because hormonal changes soften the connective tissue (unpredictable risk of dissection and rupture in Marfan syndrome and pregnancy even when aortic root has normal size), 2) Eisenmenger's syndrome (maternal mortality rate is 50%), 3) primary pulmonary hypertension, 4) symptomatic severe aortic stenosis, 5) symptomatic severe mitral stenosis, and 6) symptomatic dilated cardiomyopathy.

Although not absolute contraindications, the following conditions are also of concern in pregnancy: 1) atrial septal defect (deep venous thrombosis may lead to paradoxical embolus) and 2) coarctation (increased risk of dissection and rupture).

Patients at risk during pregnancy should minimize activity (decreases cardiac output), reduce sodium in the diet, and minimize anemia with iron and vitamin supplements.

If symptoms deteriorate and congestive heart failure supervenes, bed rest may need to be instituted. Arrhythmias such as atrial fibrillation need to be treated promptly in these situations. If necessary, cardioversion can be performed with apparently low risk to the fetus. Fetal cardiac monitoring should be performed at the same time. Occasionally patients need operative intervention. Operation during the first trimester is associated with a significantly increased rate of fetal loss. Percutaneous aortic, mitral, and pulmonary balloon valvuloplasty have been performed during pregnancy and may obviate bypass. Careful lead shielding of the fetus is needed during these procedures.

Drugs

Many cardiac drugs cross the placenta into the fetus but yet can be used safely when necessary and are not absolutely contraindicated in pregnancy. These include digoxin, quinidine, procainamide, β-adrenergic blockers, and verapamil. The β-adrenergic blockers can be associated with growth retardation of the fetus, neonatal bradycardia, and hypoglycemia. They may need to be used, however, in large doses in patients with hypertrophic cardiomyopathy, and fetal growth must be monitored.

Drugs that should be avoided are captopril, which causes fetal renal dysgenesis; phenytoin, which causes hydantoin syn-

drome and teratogenicity; and warfarin, which causes teratogenicity and abortion. One noncardiac drug to avoid is tetracycline, which stains fetal teeth.

- Drugs to avoid in pregnancy: captopril, phenytoin, warfarin, and tetracycline.

Delivery

Delivery is a time of rapid hemodynamic swings. With each uterine contraction, about 500 mL of blood is released into the circulation. Cardiac output goes up with advancing labor. High-risk patients need careful monitoring with Swan-Ganz catheterization to maintain preload at an optimal level, maternal and fetal electrocardiography monitoring, careful analgesia and anesthesia to avoid hypotension, delivery in the left lateral position so the fetus is not lying on the inferior vena cava (this position maintains venous return), and a short second stage (delivery may need to be facilitated if labor progresses slowly).

Vaginal delivery is safer for most women because the average blood loss is 500-800 mL; with cesarean section it is 800 mL. Usually, cesarean section is performed only for obstetric indications. The new guidelines of the American Heart Association state there is no need for antibiotic prophylaxis in an uncomplicated vaginal delivery.

- With each uterine contraction, 500 mL of blood is released into circulation.
- No need for antibiotic prophylaxis in uncomplicated vaginal delivery.

Prosthetic Valves and Pregnancy

Most women of childbearing age who need a valve replacement will receive a biologic valve, and if they are in sinus rhythm they will usually not be receiving anticoagulants. Women with mechanical valves will be taking warfarin, and this poses a problem with teratogenicity and increased risk of abortion. In general, diagnose pregnancy as soon as possible and switch the therapy to subcutaneous heparin, monitoring the activated partial thromboplastin time, and continue this approach throughout pregnancy. This agent is also associated with increased fetal loss, however, and an increased risk of maternal valve thrombosis.

- In pregnant patients with mechanical valves, switch therapy from warfarin to subcutaneous heparin.
- Heparin is associated with increased fetal loss.

PERICARDIAL DISEASE

The pericardium has an inner layer, the visceral pericardium, and an outer layer, the parietal pericardium. Space between the two layers contains approximately 15-25 mL of clear fluid. The pericardium has three main functions: prevent cardiac distention, limit cardiac displacement because of its attachment to neighboring structures, and protect the heart from nearby inflammation.

Acute or Subacute Inflammatory Pericarditis

Presenting Symptoms

The chest pain of pericarditis is often aggravated by movement of the trunk, by inspiration, and by coughing. The pain is often relieved by sitting up. *Low-grade fever* and malaise are other findings.

Diagnosis

Pericardial friction rub may be variable. Chest radiography is usually normal. It may show globular enlargement if pericardial effusion is significant (at least 250 mL). Occasionally, pulmonary infiltrate or small pleural effusion is noted. Left pleural effusion predominates, and the cause is unknown. Electrocardiography shows acute concave ST elevation in all ventricular leads. The PR segment is also depressed in the early stages. Echocardiography allows easy diagnosis of pericardial effusion.

- Chest pain is the presenting symptom of pericarditis.
- Electrocardiography shows concave ST elevation and depressed PR segment.

Causes

The causes of pericarditis include viral pericarditis, idiopathic pericarditis, autoimmune and collagen diseases (systemic lupus erythematosus, rheumatoid arthritis, scleroderma), and postmyocardial infarction. The postcardiotomy syndrome follows open heart procedures. It presents with pyrexia, increased sedimentation rate, and pleural or pericardial chest pain. It occurs weeks to months after operation. Its incidence decreases with age, and it usually responds to anti-inflammatory agents. Pericarditis is also associated with radiation and neoplasm, namely, Hodgkin's disease, leukemia, and lymphoma. Breast, thyroid, and lung tumors can metastasize to the pericardium and cause pericarditis or pericardial effusion. Melanoma also metastasizes to the heart. Uremia and tuberculosis can also cause pericarditis. If no cause can be documented, idiopathic viral pericarditis is the most likely diagnosis, and treatment with nonsteroidal anti-inflammatory agents or high-dose aspirin usually resolves the condition.

- Causes of pericarditis: autoimmune and collagen diseases; postmyocardial infarction; radiation; neoplasm; breast, thyroid, and lung tumors; uremia; tuberculosis.

Pericardial Effusion

The response of the pericardium to inflammation is to exude fluid, fibrin, and blood cells, causing a pericardial effusion. The amount of effusion needed before it shows on the chest radiograph is 250 mL. If fluid accumulates slowly, the pericardial sac distends slowly with no cardiac compression. If fluid accumulates rapidly, such as with bleeding, tamponade can occur with relatively small amounts of fluid. Tamponade restricts the blood entering the ventricles and causes a decrease in ventricular volume. The raised intrapericardial pressure increases the ventricular end-diastolic pressure and mean atrial pressure, and the increased atrial pressure increases the venous pressure. The decreased ventricular volume and filling diminish cardiac output. Any of the previously listed causes of pericarditis can cause tamponade, but other acute causes of hemopericardium should be considered, such as ruptured myocardium after infarction, aortic dissection, ruptured aortic aneurysm, and sequelae of cardiac operation.

- Amount of pericardial effusion needed before it can be seen on chest radiograph is 250 mL.
- Tamponade can occur with small amounts of fluid.
- Tamponade restricts the blood entering the ventricles and decreases ventricular volume.

Clinical Features

Tamponade produces a continuum of features, depending on its severity. The blood pressure is low, the heart is small and quiet, jugular venous pressure is increased, and pulsus paradoxus develops (increased flow of blood into the right heart during inspiration, decreased flow into the left heart). An increase in inspiratory distention of the neck veins (Kussmaul's sign) is infrequent unless there is underlying constriction.

Treatment

Emergency pericardiocentesis is performed with echocardiography-directed guidance.

Constrictive Pericarditis

Diastolic filling of both ventricles is prevented by the pericardium. The smaller the ventricular volume, the higher the end-diastolic pressure. The most common causes are recurrent viral pericarditis, irradiation, previous open heart operation, tuberculosis, and neoplastic disease.

Symptoms

Dominantly right-sided failure, peripheral edema, ascites, and often dyspnea and fatigue are present.

- Symptoms of constrictive pericarditis: peripheral edema, ascites, dyspnea, and fatigue.

Physical Examination

The jugular venous pressure is elevated (remember to look at the patient when he or she is sitting or standing), and inspiratory distention of neck veins (Kussmaul's sign) is present. The jugular venous pressure may show rapid descents, and pericardial knock is present in fewer than 50% of cases (sound is probably due to sudden cessation of ventricular filling). Ascites and peripheral edema may be present. Chest radiography may show pericardial calcification, but no specific changes are found on electrocardiography.

- Signs of constrictive pericarditis: elevated jugular venous pressure, inspiratory distention of neck veins, rapid descents of jugular venous pressure, and pericardial knock in <50%.
- Chest radiograph may show pericardial calcification.
- No specific changes are found on electrocardiography.

Diagnosis

Echocardiography and Doppler may be helpful, particularly Doppler, which shows respiratory changes in mitral and tricuspid inflow velocities. Other methods such as computed tomography and magnetic resonance imaging help to delineate the thickness of the pericardium, although they do not prove physiologic significance. The major confounding diagnosis is restrictive cardiomyopathy, and the distinction can be very difficult. Diastolic expansion of both ventricles is affected equally; therefore, diastolic pressure is elevated and equal in all four chambers. Ventricular pressure curve shows characteristic "√" from rapid ventricular filling and equalization of pressures (also may be seen in restrictive cardiomyopathy). The "a" and v waves are usually equal and x and y descents are rapid. If pulmonary artery systolic pressure is >50 mm Hg, myocardial disease is likely. If the end-diastolic pulmonary artery pressure is <30% of systolic pressure, myocardial disease is likely. Both of these findings are nonspecific, however. The treatment of choice for constrictive pericarditis is exploratory operation to remove the pericardium.

- Constrictive pericarditis is diagnosed from respiratory changes in mitral and tricuspid inflow velocities.
- Major confounding diagnosis is restrictive cardiomyopathy.
- Diastolic pressure is elevated and equal in all four chambers.

EVALUATION OF THE PATIENT WITH CARDIAC DISEASE BEFORE NONCARDIAC OPERATION

Risks

The major risk for most patients with cardiac disease who undergo noncardiac operations arises from the presence of coronary artery disease. In patients without previous evidence of heart disease, the risk of perioperative myocardial infarction during a noncardiac procedure is 0.15%. In patients who have had myocardial infarction, the frequency of reinfarction during a major noncardiac operation is about 6%. The risk of perioperative reinfarction is inversely related to the interval between preoperative infarction and noncardiac operation (Table 3-3). With aggressive perioperative management and invasive hemodynamic monitoring, these rates may be significantly reduced. The mortality rate from a perioperative myocardial infarction is approximately 50%.

- In patients without previous heart disease, the risk of perioperative myocardial infarction during a noncardiac operation is 0.15%.
- In patients with previous myocardial infarction, the risk of reinfarction during a major noncardiac operation is 6%.
- The risk of perioperative infarction is inversely related to the time from previous infarction to noncardiac operation.
- The mortality rate from perioperative myocardial infarction is 50%.

Certain surgical procedures are associated with a threefold greater chance of myocardial infarction: major intrathoracic, upper abdominal, and great vessel surgical procedures. Other preoperative cardiac risks include age >70 years, S_3 gallop, jugular venous pressure >12 cm H_2O, and significant aortic stenosis. Electrocardiographic risk factors are a rhythm other than sinus, atrial ectopy, or >5 premature ventricular contractions per minute. Other factors to consider are general medical status (e.g., PaO_2 <60 or $PaCO_2$ >50 mm Hg, potassium <3 mEq/L, bicarbonate <20 mEq/L), blood urea nitrogen value >50 or creatinine value >3 mg/dL, chronic liver disease, general debilitation, and type of operation (e.g., emergency procedure or intraperitoneal, thoracic, or aortic procedure).

- Risk of myocardial infarction is threefold more with major intrathoracic, upper abdominal, and great vessel operations.

Because of a strong association between coronary disease and peripheral vascular disease, patients who are to undergo a

Table 3-3.--Risk of Perioperative Reinfarction, by Time From Initial Infarction

Time from MI to noncardiac operation, mo	Risk of perioperative MI, %
<3	27-37
3-6	11-16
>6	4-5

MI, myocardial infarction.

peripheral vascular operation are at high risk of having important coronary disease. In patients having routine coronary angiography before a vascular operation, approximately 60% with clinically suspected ischemic heart disease have severe multivessel or even inoperable coronary artery disease. Approximately 20% of patients with no prior history to suggest coronary artery disease have diffuse, severe coronary artery disease.

- There is a strong association between coronary disease and peripheral vascular disease.
- At routine angiography before a vascular operation, 60% of patients with clinically suspected ischemic heart disease have severe multivessel or inoperable coronary artery disease.
- Of patients without a history of coronary artery disease, 20% have diffuse, severe coronary artery disease.

Therefore, use of a cardiac risk index (e.g., Goldman) has limitations. Obviously, the risks are much higher, for example, in patients undergoing a vascular operation. Risk indices thus depend on referral patient population, nature of the operation, expertise of the surgeon and anesthesiologist, and uncommon problems or events (e.g., emergency procedure).

A low risk score index does not exclude a patient from having a perioperative event but rather indicates a low probability of a cardiac event. Preoperative cardiovascular assessment with a thorough cardiac history is important, corroborated by examination, chest radiography, and electrocardiography. The absence or presence and severity of angina pectoris and the efficacy of current medical therapy need to be considered. The history and time of the previous myocardial infarction are important. If operation is not urgent, waiting more than 6 months after myocardial infarction is probably appropriate.

- Low risk score index does not exclude a perioperative event but does indicate low probability of cardiac event.
- Preoperative cardiovascular assessment is important.
- History and time of previous infarction are important.

Mild Angina

Most patients who can perform vigorous activity of daily living and are functional class I or II tolerate the stress of most noncardiac operations. However, if they are to undergo one of the more risky procedures (intrathoracic, upper abdominal, or vascular), preoperative stress testing should be considered. If functional limitation is not clear from the history, stress testing should be performed, if possible.

Class III or IV Angina

Significant limitation because of symptoms suggests the need for direct coronary angiography.

- Patients limited by class III or IV angina need direct coronary angiography.

Exercise Testing

Different end points have been used in stress testing. If during routine exercise treadmill testing the patient has no ischemic changes and achieves >75% of maximal predicted heart rate, the risk of a perioperative myocardial infarction is low. If ischemia develops on the electrocardiogram during treadmill exercise testing and the patient can only exercise <5 METs, the risk is twice that with a normal exercise electrocardiogram and exercise >5 METs. For various reasons, some patients are unable to exercise, and for them dipyridamole thallium scanning may be useful. This has a high sensitivity (particularly when used before vascular operation) but not a very high specificity. The negative predictive value, however, is high. In other words, a negative dipyridamole thallium scan suggests a low risk of operation.

- Dipyridamole thallium scanning has high sensitivity but not specificity.
- Negative dipyridamole thallium scan suggests a low risk of operation.

Before a series of tests are done, the risks and benefits of coronary revascularization before a major noncardiac operation should be considered. For example, the Coronary Artery Surgery Study (CASS) found that the operative mortality rate was 2.3% with coronary artery bypass grafting, 2.9% when the left ventricular ejection fraction was <50%, and 7.9% in patients >70 years old. Thus, the risk of bypass may be higher than the potential risk of noncardiac operation. Each case needs to be considered individually. Angina therapy needs to be optimized. If left ventricular dysfunction is present, noninvasive assessment of the left ventricular ejection fraction may be indicated and treatment optimized. If the left ventricular dysfunction is severe, hemodynamic monitoring should be performed perioperatively, especially when optimization of cardiac status is not possible preoperatively. Antianginal therapy should be maintained perioperatively.

- Risk of coronary artery bypass grafting may be higher than the potential risk of noncardiac operation.
- Therapy for angina needs to be optimized.
- Antianginal therapy should be maintained perioperatively.

Aortic or Mitral Stenosis

Assess stenosis with two-dimensional and Doppler echocardiography. If it is severe, patients should have cardiac operation before a noncardiac procedure. Percutaneous balloon valvuloplasty can occasionally be used to "get patients through" the operation. Asymptomatic patients with significant aortic stenosis can often tolerate a noncardiac operation safely with careful anesthesia and hemodynamic monitoring.

- If aortic or mitral stenosis is severe, cardiac operation should be done before noncardiac procedure.
- Asymptomatic patients with significant aortic stenosis can often tolerate a noncardiac operation safely.

Mechanical Valvular Prostheses

Management depends on the degree of operation being undertaken. Depending on the risk and degree of the procedure, anticoagulant therapy can be discontinued 1 to 3 days preoperatively and restarted 2 to 5 days postoperatively with a low risk of a thromboembolic event. The risk of bleeding complications may be higher, depending on the extent of the operation. For patients needing more extensive procedures, oral anticoagulation may be changed to heparin, continued 6 hours before operation with resumption 24 hours postoperatively, or days later if necessary.

THE HEART IN SYSTEMIC DISEASE

Hyperthyroidism

Effects

The cardiovascular effects include increased heart rate, stroke volume, and cardiac output; decreased peripheral resistance; and widened pulse pressure. All of these lead to increased myocardial work and may precipitate angina. Symptoms include palpitations, tachycardia, and exertional dyspnea.

- Cardiovascular effects of hyperthyroidism: increased heart rate, stroke volume, cardiac output; decreased peripheral resistance; and widened pulse pressure.
- Effects lead to increased myocardial work and perhaps angina.

Physical Examination

Common findings are tachycardia, bounding pulse, forceful apical impulse, systolic ejection murmur, and scratchy systolic murmur at the left sternal border resembling a pericardial friction rub. Cardiac arrhythmias are common, particularly supraventricular tachycardia or atrial fibrillation. Atrial fibrillation occurs in 10%-20% of patients. Always suspect thyrotoxicosis in a patient with unexplained atrial fibrillation. Arterial embolization is rare.

- Findings of hyperthyroidism: tachycardia, bounding pulse, forceful apical impulse, and systolic ejection murmur.
- Cardiac arrhythmias are common (supraventricular tachycardia and atrial fibrillation).

- Suspect thyrotoxicosis in a patient with unexplained atrial fibrillation.

Hypothyroidism

This disorder causes a decrease in metabolic rate and circulatory demand, bradycardia, decreased myocardial contractility and stroke volume, and increased peripheral resistance.

Physical Examination

There may be cardiac enlargement due to either intrinsic myocardial disease or pericardial effusion. Myocardial contractility is reduced. These changes usually resolve with thyroid hormone therapy. Pericardial effusion occurs in approximately one-third of patients with hypothyroidism. Heart failure is rare in the absence of associated cardiac disease. Coronary atherosclerosis occurs twice as often in patients with hypothyroidism as in age- and sex-matched controls.

- Physical findings in hypothyroidism: cardiac enlargement, reduced myocardial contractility, and pericardial effusion in one-third.
- Heart failure is rare in the absence of associated cardiac disease.
- Coronary atherosclerosis occurs twice as often as in controls.

Diabetes Mellitus

This condition is frequently associated with premature coronary atherosclerosis, and the prevalence is increased among females. Fatal myocardial infarctions occur at least twice as often in diabetic men and three times as often in diabetic women as in the nondiabetic population. The cause is uncertain. The prevalence of hypertension is increased among diabetic patients. Hyperlipidemia is common. Angina and myocardial infarction are often manifested by atypical symptoms. The incidence of silent myocardial infarction is high. Congestive heart failure may be the first manifestation of coronary disease.

- Fatal myocardial infarction occurs twice as often in diabetic men and three times as often in diabetic women as in nondiabetics.
- Prevalence of hypertension is increased in diabetics.
- Angina and myocardial infarction are often manifested by atypical symptoms.
- Incidence of silent myocardial infarction is high.

There is some evidence that diabetes may also be associated with cardiomyopathy unassociated with coronary artery disease. Some studies suggest that this may be due to small vessel disease, similar to that in the kidney.

Amyloidosis

Primary amyloidosis is characterized by accumulation of

protein ground substance in many organs, typically the kidneys and the heart but also the tongue, skin, nerves, and liver. Secondary amyloidosis occurs in association with chronic disease (rheumatoid arthritis, tuberculosis, chronic infection, neoplasia). Cardiac abnormality is not a prominent feature. In senile systemic amyloidosis the heart is the most involved organ. The prevalence increases from age 60 on. Familial amyloidosis is autosomal dominant. The characteristic amyloid protein is prealbumin. It can involve the heart.

- Primary amyloidosis is characterized by protein ground substance in many organs.
- In secondary amyloidosis, cardiac abnormality is not a prominent feature.
- In senile systemic amyloidosis, the heart is the most involved organ.
- Familial amyloidosis is autosomal dominant, and it can involve the heart.

Primary Amyloidosis

About 90% of patients with primary amyloidosis have clinical evidence of cardiac dysfunction. The heart is often enlarged, due mostly to thickened ventricular myocardium caused by the infiltration, and the atria tend to enlarge. Abnormalities of conduction may occur. Amyloid also deposits in the cardiac valves, and there is a high frequency of atrioventricular valve regurgitation.

- In primary amyloidosis, 90% of patients have cardiac dysfunction.
- Abnormalities of conduction may occur.
- Amyloid also deposits in the cardiac valves.

Clinical Features

The following can occur: congestive heart failure, arrhythmias, sudden death, angina-like chest pain, pericardial effusion, and murmurs of atrioventricular valve regurgitation. The natural history is usually intractable biventricular cardiac failure. Diastolic abnormalities are common, particularly features of "restrictive cardiomyopathy." Most patients have evidence of renal disease associated with serum and urine protein abnormalities.

- Clinical features of primary amyloidosis: arrhythmias, sudden death, "restrictive cardiomyopathy," and evidence of renal disease.

Diagnosis

Electrocardiography shows classic low-voltage QRS complex, which is nonspecific. In addition to the systemic abnormalities described, echocardiography is particularly useful. This typically demonstrates the increased ventricular wall thickness without cavity dilatation and a granular appearance of the ventricular myocardium. Atria are usually dilated. The cardiac valves may also show some thickening and reduction in motion associated with atrioventricular valve regurgitation. Various hemodynamic features have been shown in amyloidosis, and Doppler techniques have recently been useful for characterizing these. An early-stage finding is prolonged relaxation with an important contribution to filling from atrial contraction. In later stages, rapid, early filling suggestive of restrictive cardiomyopathy may be found.

- Echocardiographic findings in primary amyloidosis: increased ventricular wall thickness, granular appearance of ventricular myocardium, and dilated atria.
- An early-stage finding is prolonged relaxation.
- In later stages, rapid, early filling is found.

Hemochromatosis

This is an iron-storage disease, either a primary form or a secondary form related to exogenous iron (usually from repeated blood transfusions). Iron deposits within the cardiac cells. Cardiac hemochromatosis never occurs alone and is always accompanied by involvement of other organs. A clue to the diagnosis is the tetrad of diabetes, liver disease, brown skin pigmentation, and heart disease. The condition may present with cardiomegaly and congestive failure or cardiac arrhythmias. It may have features of dilated or restrictive cardiomyopathy. Therefore, it can present with abnormalities of either systolic or diastolic dysfunction. Once clinical symptoms of heart failure or arrhythmias develop, most patients will be dead within 1 year unless treatment is initiated either with phlebotomy or iron chelation.

- In hemochromatosis, iron deposits within the cardiac cells.
- Cardiac hemochromatosis never occurs alone.
- A clue to diagnosis is the tetrad of diabetes, liver disease, brown skin pigmentation, and heart disease.

Carcinoid Heart Disease

Metastatic malignant carcinoid tumors produce a serotonin-like substance that causes systemic flushing. In patients with hepatic metastasis, right-sided valves are involved. Therefore, changes occur in the tricuspid and pulmonary valves. The tricuspid leaflets become thickened with deposition on the underside of the valve. Leaflets become thickened, stiff, and relatively immobile, and the chordae may also be involved. The dominant lesion is tricuspid regurgitation. There may be some element of stenosis. The pulmonary valve is also involved, and the leaflets become thickened and rigid. Pulmonary regurgitation is common, and the valve is also often stenotic. Surgical therapy includes tricuspid valve replacement (with a mechanical valve because carcinoid may also affect bioprostheses).

Pulmonary valve resection may be necessary.

- Carcinoid tumors produce serotonin-like substance that causes systemic flushing.
- Changes occur in the tricuspid and pulmonary valves.
- Dominant lesion is tricuspid regurgitation.
- Pulmonary regurgitation is common.
- Pulmonary valve is often stenotic.

PROSTHETIC VALVES

Bioprostheses

These are made of animal or human tissue, which may be unmounted or mounted in a frame. Different types include 1) homograft (human tissue), either aortic or pulmonary; 2) heterograft (porcine valve), e.g., Hancock or Carpentier-Edwards; and 3) pericardial (bovine valve), e.g., Ionescu-Shiley. Tissue valves have the advantage that they are not as thrombogenic as mechanical valves; thus, most patients in sinus rhythm do not require anticoagulation. There is a risk of systemic embolism, however, with biologic prostheses in patients with atrial fibrillation, particularly with a mitral prosthesis. The disadvantage is that tissue values degenerate and calcify and thus patients will need reoperation. Approximately 50% of patients will need valve replacement at 10 years. In young patients (≤20 years old), these valves may calcify very rapidly. Tissue valves last a little longer in the tricuspid position than in positions on the left side of the heart. Aortic valves have a slightly better durability than mitral valves. Prosthesis failure can be detected by clinical evaluation and two-dimensional and Doppler echocardiography.

- Tissue valves are not as thrombogenic as mechanical valves.
- Most patients with tissue valves who are in sinus rhythm do not require anticoagulation.
- There is a risk of systemic embolism with biologic prostheses in patients with atrial fibrillation, particularly with a mitral prosthesis.
- Tissue valves degenerate and calcify.
- About 50% of patients will need valve replacement.

Mechanical Valves

An example of a *ball valve* is the Starr-Edwards. It has excellent longevity and is a so-called high-profile valve. A small size may be associated with a higher transvalvular pressure gradient. Types of *tilting disc valves* are the Björk-Shiley and St. Jude. All mechanical valves have a risk of thromboembolism. Reported rates vary. For example, in a Mayo Clinic series of patients with a Starr-Edwards prosthesis, 81% were free of embolism at 5 years when the valve was in the aortic position, and 93% were free of embolism when it was in the mitral position. Hemolysis often occurs with mechanical prostheses, especially with perivalvular leak. Anticoagulation can also be associated with hemorrhage and thrombosis. The rate of minor hemorrhages is approximately 2%-4% per year, and that of major hemorrhages is 1%-2% per year.

- All mechanical valves have a risk of thromboembolism.
- Hemolysis often occurs with mechanical prostheses, especially with perivalvular leak.
- Anticoagulation can be associated with hemorrhage and thrombosis.

TUMORS OF THE HEART

Most cardiac tumors are metastatic. The most common primary cardiac tumor is myxoma.

Cardiac Myxoma

Most cardiac myxomas are sporadic, but there have been some reports of familial occurrence. A syndrome of cardiac myxomas with lentiginosis (spotty pigmentation) and recurrent myxomas has been recognized. About 75% are in the left atrium, 18% are in the right atrium, and the rest are in the ventricles. Most of the atrial tumors arise from the atrial septum, usually adjacent to the fossa ovalis. About 95% are single. Most myxomas have a short stalk, are gelatinous and friable, and tend to embolize. They occasionally calcify, so they may be visible on a chest radiograph.

The main clinical features are obstruction to blood flow, embolization, and systemic effects. Left atrial tumors prolapse into the mitral valve orifice and produce mitral stenosis. They mimic mitral valvular stenosis with symptoms of dyspnea, orthopnea, cough, pulmonary edema, and hemoptysis. Classically, symptoms occur with a change in body position. Physical findings suggest mitral stenosis. Pulmonary hypertension may also occur. An early diastolic sound, the tumor "plop," may be heard. This has a lower frequency than an opening snap.

- Most cardiac tumors are metastatic.
- Most common primary cardiac tumor is myxoma.
- 75% of cardiac myxomas are in the left atrium and 18% are in the right atrium; rest are in the ventricles.
- Clinical features are obstruction to blood flow, embolization, and systemic effects.
- Symptoms occur with a change in body position.
- An early diastolic sound, tumor "plop," may be heard.

Embolization

Systemic emboli may occur in 30%-60% of patients with left-sided myxoma, frequently to the brain and lower extremities. Histologic examination of embolized material is important. Coronary embolization is rare, but it should be considered in a young patient with no known previous cardiac disease. Systemic effects are fatigue, fever, weight loss, and arthralgia. Systemic effects may be associated with an elevated sedimentation rate, leukocytosis, hypergammaglobulinemia, and anemia. Elevated immunoglobulins are usually of IgG class.

Echocardiography is the preferred approach to diagnosis. Transesophageal echocardiography helps delineate the precise site of origin and accurately assesses tumor size and degree of mobility. Operation is indicated when the diagnosis is made.

- Systemic emboli occur in 30%-60% of cases of left-sided myxoma, frequently to the brain and lower extremities.
- Coronary embolization is rare.
- Systemic effects: fatigue, fever, weight loss, and arthralgia.
- Systemic effects may be associated with elevated sedimentation rate, leukocytosis, hypergammaglobulinemia, and anemia.
- Elevated immunoglobulins are usually IgG class.
- Echocardiography is the preferred approach for diagnosis.
- Operation is indicated.

Primary Cardiac Neoplasm

Rhabdomyoma is most common in women and children. It can produce obstruction of cardiac valves simulating other abnormalities and can cause cardiac arrhythmias. Other tumors, such as Kaposi's sarcoma associated with acquired immunodeficiency syndrome (AIDS), do not usually cause cardiac symptoms.

Secondary tumors most often originate from bone, breast, lymphoma, leukemia, and thyroid. More than half of patients with malignant melanoma have metastases to the heart.

- Rhabdomyoma is most common in women and children.
- More than half of patients with malignant melanoma have metastases to heart.

DIAGNOSTIC TESTS

Echocardiography

Echocardiography uses an ultrasonic beam (frequency, >20,000 cps) produced by electric excitation of a piezoelectric crystal. The properties of this beam include linear transmission through a homogeneous medium, poor transmission through air, and reflective/refractive phenomena when the directed waves traverse an interface between two media of differing density (acoustic impedances). The greatest reflection of ultrasound occurs when the acoustic impedances of the neighboring structures are dissimilar and when the beam strikes this interface at a perpendicular angle. The reflected waves return to the ultrasound generator (transducer) with a time delay proportional to the distance of the interface from the transducer. Knowledge of the velocity of the ultrasound beam allows relative distances (and dimensions) of various structures to be determined. This forms the basis of M-mode echocardiography, which displays the distances as continuous lines of varying intensities on a moving strip of paper. This technique gives a "one-dimensional" look at a small portion of the heart. If instead of a single crystal a linear array of crystals is excited sequentially, a plane of ultrasound is generated, which when reflected and appropriately analyzed produces a tomographic or two-dimensional image of cardiac structure. An infinite variety of planes transecting the heart is possible; the examiner orients the ultrasound plane appropriately to transect desired structures.

Doppler Echocardiography

Doppler echocardiography is able to detect and measure abnormal blood velocities in the cardiac chambers and great vessels. It uses the Doppler principle, which states that a sound beam reflected off a moving object will change its frequency. This change in frequency, known as the Doppler shift, is proportional to the velocity of the moving object. Thus, by reflecting the Doppler beam off moving erythrocytes, one can measure blood velocities. From this information, it is possible to calculate gradients across stenotic valves, intracardiac pressures, and cardiac output. A semiquantitative estimate of the severity of valvular regurgitation and intracardiac shunts may also be obtained. Color flow imaging allows a real-time visualization of blood flow by superimposing different color maps (indicating direction and velocity of blood flow) on top of a moving two-dimensional echocardiogram.

- Doppler echocardiography detects and measures abnormal blood velocities in the cardiac chambers and great vessels.
- Allows calculation of gradients across stenotic valves, intracardiac pressures, and cardiac output.
- Color flow imaging allows real-time visualization of blood flow.

Practical Applications of Echocardiography

Chamber Size and Function

Echocardiography is an excellent method for determination of the size of all four cardiac chambers. In addition, left ventricular function (ejection fraction) can be easily and accurately determined in most patients. Based on left ventricular dimensions in systole and diastole measured on M-mode echocardiography, the equation for ejection fraction is

$$\frac{[(\text{diastolic dimension})^2 - (\text{systolic dimension})^2]}{(\text{diastolic dimension})^2}$$

This has been well validated when compared with ejection fractions obtained by cardiac catheterization or radionuclide angiography.

- Echocardiography is excellent method for determination of the size of all four cardiac chambers.
- Left ventricular function (ejection fraction) can be easily and accurately determined.

Regional Wall Abnormalities

Because of its ability to determine endocardial motion, as well as myocardial thickening, echocardiography is an ideal method for evaluation of regional wall abnormalities. This is a sensitive marker for either ongoing ischemia or myocardial infarction. Currently, a subjective visual analysis is used to determine wall motion abnormalities.

- Echocardiography is ideal for evaluation of regional wall abnormalities.
- This is a sensitive marker for ongoing ischemia or myocardial infarction.

Valvular Abnormalities

M-mode and two-dimensional echocardiography are sensitive methods for analysis of structural valvular lesions. Calcified stenotic valves are easily identified. Prolapsed and flail valves as a cause of valvular regurgitation may be detected. Doppler echocardiography adds hemodynamic information to allow an accurate estimate of the severity of stenosis and regurgitation.

- M-mode and two-dimensional echocardiography are sensitive for analysis of structural valvular lesions.

Intracardiac Shunts

Both atrial septal defects and ventricular septal defects can be visualized on two-dimensional echocardiography if they are more than 2-3 mm in diameter. Color flow imaging has allowed the detection of even smaller shunts.

Cardiac Output

Knowledge of 1) the cross-sectional area of a valvular orifice or great vessel utilizing M-mode and two-dimensional echocardiography and 2) the velocity of blood flow through the area of Doppler echocardiography allows a volumetric flow rate to be calculated. This provides a noninvasive instantaneous measurement of cardiac output which is accurate and reproducible.

Miscellaneous

Two-dimensional echocardiography is the method of choice in the evaluation of pericardial effusion. It has greatly enhanced the safety and feasibility of pericardiocentesis by directing the placement and angle of the puncture needle. Intracardiac masses (tumors, thrombus) are well visualized with two-dimensional echocardiography. Valvular vegetations are also able to be detected.

Because echocardiography is totally noninvasive and risk-free, sequential examinations are facilitated. Because transmission of ultrasound through the chest wall to the heart requires an "ultrasonic window" (i.e., an area without overlying lung and resultant air dispersion of sound waves), not all patients can have adequate imaging with this technique, and a 10%-20% failure rate is the largest single drawback. Transesophageal echocardiography overcomes several of these drawbacks and is especially useful for examining 1) valve pathology (ruptured chord, vegetations), 2) atrial septum (? patent foramen ovale/atrial septal defect), 3) anomalous pulmonary veins, and 4) left atrial appendage, in a search for thrombus.

PART II
Stephen C. Hammill, M.D.
Marshall S. Stanton, M.D.

MYOCARDIAL CELLULAR CONDUCTION

Cells in the sinus and atrioventricular (AV) nodes are slow-conducting and activated by the opening of calcium channels and blocked by calcium channel blockers such as verapamil. Cells in the atrium, His-Purkinje system, and ventricle are fast-conducting and activated by the opening of sodium channels and blocked by sodium channel blockers such as class I antiarrhythmic drugs (e.g., quinidine, lidocaine, and propafenone).

MECHANISMS OF ARRHYTHMIAS

Reentry

Three conditions are required for reentry to occur (Fig. 3-4 and 3-5): 1) two or more anatomically or functionally distinct pathways connected proximally and distally to form a closed circuit, 2) unidirectional block in one pathway, and 3) slowed conduction in the other pathway.

Fig. 3-4. Reentry within the AV node demonstrates the two limbs of reentrant circuit. Recent evidence suggests that a portion of the reentrant pathway is separate from the AV node.

Fig. 3-5. AV nodal reentrant tachycardia. An atrial premature complex (APC) blocks in fast pathway but conducts over slow pathways to ventricle. Impulse then returns to atria over recovered fast pathway and can reenter slow pathway and initiate tachycardia. A, atrium; AV, atrioventricular node; V, ventricle.

Reentry is the most common mechanism responsible for cardiac arrhythmias and can occur in a microreentrant circuit within the sinus node, AV node, or small area of injured myocardium bordering a myocardial infarction. Large reentrant circuits involve the atrium (as in atrial flutter) or the atrium, AV conduction system, ventricle, and accessory pathway (as in patients with Wolff-Parkinson-White syndrome).

● Reentry is the most common mechanism for cardiac arrhythmias.

Automaticity

Automatic rhythms occur when accelerated phase IV depolarization results in enhanced automaticity. The sinus node demonstrates normal physiologic automaticity. When other cells in the heart have increased automaticity, they may exceed the rate of sinus node automaticity and replace the sinus node as the cardiac pacemaker. The factors that enhance automaticity are listed in Table 3-4.

Automaticity may be the mechanism responsible for multifocal atrial tachycardia in patients with decompensated lung disease and patients with ventricular ectopy early after myocardial infarction. In both cases, automaticity is enhanced by increased sympathetic tone, hypoxia, acid-base and electrolyte disturbances, and atrial or ventricular stretch. Accelerated idioventricular rhythm may also be due to abnormal automaticity.

● Automaticity is enhanced by increased sympathetic tone, hypoxia, acid-base and electrolyte disturbances, and atrial or ventricular stretch.

Parasystole

Parasystole is a type of abnormal automaticity. It occurs when an ectopic focus in the atrium or ventricle is isolated from the dominant rhythm because of conduction block into the focus. Cells within this area undergo automatic depolarization and, because of entrance block, are not constantly reset by the dominant rhythm. These cells capture the regional myocardium unless the myocardium is refractory from a previously conducted beat. This mechanism causes 3% of premature ventricular complexes (PVCs) noted during routine monitoring and, in general, is benign.

● Parasystole is caused by an ectopic focus in the atrium or ventricle.

Table 3-4.--Factors That Enhance Automaticity

Autonomic changes
Increased sympathetic tone
Decreased parasympathetic tone
Metabolic/ischemic changes
Increased carbon dioxide
Decreased oxygen
Increased acidity
Mechanical factors
Increased stretch
Drugs
Isoproterenol
Electrolyte alterations
Decreased potassium
Increased calcium

- Parasystole causes 3% of PVCs during routine monitoring.
- Parasystole is benign.

Triggered Activity

This mechanism for arrhythmias is so-named because each complex in the rhythm is generated (triggered) by the preceding one. The arrhythmia cannot begin without an initiating beat. Two types of triggered activity exist: delayed afterdepolarizations and early afterdepolarizations. *Delayed afterdepolarizations* arise during the resting phase of the action potential (phase 4) and may be the mechanism for digitalis-induced arrhythmias. *Early afterdepolarizations* arise during the plateau (phase 2) or repolarization (phase 3) of the action potential and may be responsible for the polymorphic ventricular tachycardia (torsades de pointes) caused by antiarrhythmic drugs such as quinidine.

DIAGNOSTIC TECHNIQUES

Ambulatory Electrocardiographic Monitoring and Transtelephonic Event Recording

Ambulatory (Holter) monitoring is used to document symptomatic and asymptomatic rhythm disturbances if they occur frequently enough to be recorded during the 24- or 48-hour recording period. It is also used to determine the effect of treatment, such as control of the ventricular response during atrial fibrillation. Patients may have adequate control of heart rate in response to atrial fibrillation at rest in the physician's office but inappropriately rapid heart rates in response to mild exercise. Such inappropriate rates can be shown by 24-hour monitoring or exercise testing.

Ambulatory monitoring can assess pacemaker function and determine the relationship of arrhythmia to daily activity (e.g., exercise). Finally, ambulatory monitoring may be used to confirm episodes of myocardial ischemia, most of which are usually not associated with typical symptoms of angina.

- Ambulatory monitoring assesses pacemaker function, documents the relationship of arrhythmia to daily activity, and confirms episodes of myocardial ischemia.

Transtelephonic event recording documents heart rate and rhythm during symptoms that occur infrequently. Patients either wear a device continuously for several days or weeks or briefly attach it to themselves during symptoms. The device permanently stores the electrocardiogram (ECG) in memory when the activation button is depressed, and this ECG is later transmitted over the telephone for evaluation. This device documents the rhythm when a patient experiences typical symptoms. About 20% of transmissions document abnormal heart rhythm, although often the transmissions are helpful for

patient management even if normal rhythm is identified. Continuous loop event recorders store the ECG occurring 30 seconds to 4 minutes before depression of the activation button and are very useful for patients whose symptoms are brief or of sudden onset.

- Transtelephonic event recording documents heart rate during symptoms that occur infrequently.
- About 20% of transmissions document abnormal heart rhythm.
- Transtelephonic event recording is often helpful for patient management even if normal rhythm is identified.

Exercise Testing

Exercise testing is helpful when patients describe symptoms consistent with cardiac arrhythmia which occur during exercise. This allows for evaluation in a controlled setting with ECG monitoring to determine whether cardiac arrhythmia is causing the exercise-related symptoms. Exercise testing is also useful to determine whether the beneficial effect of a drug at rest is reversed with exercise. Patients with atrial fibrillation may have adequate control of heart rate at rest but poor control with moderate exercise. Those with ventricular tachycardia or complex ventricular ectopy may have adequate suppression of arrhythmia at rest in response to medical therapy only to have ventricular tachycardia with exercise. Proarrhythmic effects of antiarrhythmic drugs can sometimes be provoked by exercise testing. This is particularly true of the class IC drugs (flecainide and propafenone), probably because of use-dependence and their long unbinding times from the sodium channel.

- Exercise testing evaluates cardiac arrhythmia during exercise.
- Exercise testing determines whether the effect of a drug is reversed with exercise.

PVCs occur during exercise testing in 10% of patients without and in 60% of patients with coronary artery disease. The response of PVCs during exercise does not predict severity of coronary artery disease. Elimination of PVCs with exercise is not an indication that coronary artery disease is less severe.

- PVCs occur during exercise in 10% of patients without and in 60% of patients with coronary artery disease.
- Response of PVCs during exercise does not predict severity of coronary artery disease.
- Elimination of PVCs with exercise does not indicate less severe coronary artery disease.

Exercise testing is useful for assessing sinus node function to determine whether there is chronotropic incompetence in a patient who complains of dyspnea on exertion or fatigue. It is also used to assess AV block. AV block at the AV node is usually benign and does not require pacing. This type of block (Wenckebach [Mobitz I]) improves with exercise when increased catecholamines enhance AV node conduction. AV block due to failure of conduction in the His-Purkinje system (Mobitz II) has a worse prognosis; it has a high incidence of complete heart block and requires pacing. This type of block often worsens with exercise because the increase in catecholamines enhances AV node conduction and results in increased frequency of activation of the diseased His-Purkinje system with progressive block.

- Exercise testing assesses sinus node function in patients with dyspnea on exertion.
- Mobitz I block may improve with exercise.
- Mobitz II block may worsen with exercise.
- Mobitz II block has a worse prognosis and requires pacing.

Signal-Averaged ECG

Signal-averaged ECG is a noninvasive test used to detect low-level signals, termed "late potentials," that result from delayed conduction through diseased myocardium. These signals usually arise in the border zone adjacent to a myocardial infarction, where conducting myocardial cells are mixed in among scar tissue. This disrupted architecture results in delayed conduction and is the substrate for myocardial reentry. Signal-averaged ECG amplifies this low-level signal by several thousandfold and averages multiple QRS complexes to eliminate random noise. The low-level activity is then measured to determine whether a late potential is present. Late potentials have independent prognostic value for identifying patients at risk for ventricular tachycardia after myocardial infarction and inducible ventricular tachycardia at the time of electrophysiologic testing. Signal-averaged ECG has a positive predictive accuracy of 25%-50% and a negative predictive accuracy of 90%-95% for identifying patients at risk for ventricular tachycardia. The test is used primarily to stratify patients at risk for ventricular tachycardia or ventricular fibrillation. It is not useful in the setting of right bundle branch block or in patients without coronary artery disease.

- Signal-averaged ECG is noninvasive.
- Signal-averaged ECG identifies patients at risk for ventricular tachycardia.
- Positive predictive accuracy is 25%-50%; negative predictive accuracy is 90%-95%.

Heart Rate Variability

More recently, research has increased in assessing how much the heart rate varies as a predictor of future arrhythmic events. It has been shown that heart rate variability decreases when there is relatively more sympathetic versus parasympathetic tone; the converse is also true. Decreased heart rate variability after myocardial infarction identifies a group with increased risk of ventricular arrhythmias. Currently, this should be considered a research tool in most instances; it does not have widespread clinical applicability.

Electrophysiologic Testing

Electrophysiologic testing involves placement of electrode catheters in the heart to record and stimulate heart rhythm. In general, catheters are placed in the high right atrium, across the tricuspid valve in the region of the AV node and His bundle, in the right ventricular apex, and, in selected patients, in the coronary sinus to record from the left atrium and ventricle. This testing is indicated in patients with cardiogenic syncope of undetermined origin, for evaluation of mechanism of supraventricular tachycardia, for assessing symptomatic patients with Wolff-Parkinson-White syndrome, and for evaluating patients with sustained ventricular tachycardia and survivors of out-of-hospital cardiac arrest. Ablative therapy can be curative for almost all patients with AV node reentry or Wolff-Parkinson-White syndrome, most patients with atrial tachycardia or typical atrial flutter, and selected patients with ventricular tachycardia. The complication rate of the test is 0.5%-1%.

- Electrophysiologic testing is invasive.
- Electrophysiologic testing is indicated for cardiogenic syncope of undetermined origin.
- The complication rate is 0.5%-1%.

THERAPY

Pacing

Pacing uses a four-letter classification system (Table 3-5). The first letter is the chamber paced; the second letter, the chamber sensed; and the third letter, the mode of response. In practice, the fourth letter is used to designate whether the pacemaker will automatically increase its rate in response to activity detected by a sensor within the pacemaker pulse generator. Common pacing modes are VVI, which is ventricular paced, ventricular sensed, and inhibited in response to a ventricular event; VVIR, in which rate responsiveness (R) is added; DDD, which is atrial and ventricular paced and sensed and also triggered and inhibited in response to a sensed atrial or ventricular event; and DDDR, which adds rate response to the DDD mode.

Physiologic pacing attempts to maintain heart rate with normal AV synchrony and increase heart rate in response to physical activity. DDD pacing is used to track atrial activation in patients with normal sinus node activity but some type of AV block. As sinus activity increases in response to exercise or some other stress, the pacemaker tracks this response and paces

Table 3-5.--Code of Permanent Pacing

Chamber(s) paced	Chamber(s) sensed	Mode(s) of response	Programmable capabilities
V = Ventricle	V = Ventricle	T = Triggered	R = Rate modulated
A = Atrium	A = Atrium	I = Inhibited	
D = Dual (atrium and ventricle)	D = Dual (atrium and ventricle)	D = Dual (triggered and inhibited)	
	O = None	O = None	

the ventricle with normal AV conduction delay (P-R interval) at a rate following sinus rate. In patients who have chronic atrial fibrillation, rate-modulated pacing (the "R" in VVIR) is used to increase heart rate in response to physical demand. An external sensor that senses body motion, respiratory rate, and blood temperature, or some other sensor, is used to drive the pacemaker to keep up with increased metabolic demands. This type of pacemaker increases exercise endurance during treadmill testing. A patient with sinus node dysfunction and AV conduction system disease would benefit from DDDR pacing.

- Physiologic pacing maintains heart rate with normal AV synchrony and increases the rate during physical activity.
- Rate-modulated pacing increases exercise endurance during treadmill testing.

Pacemaker syndrome is a complication that occurs during ventricular pacing in patients who have intact retrograde conduction between the ventricle and the atrium (Fig. 3-6). When the ventricle is paced, the impulse conducts retrogradely to the atrium and simultaneous atrial and ventricular contractions result. The atria are then trying to contract against closed tricuspid and mitral valves, and as a result, the atrial contribution to ventricular filling is eliminated and the atria are distended. The increased atrial pressure distends the neck veins and can result in hypotension; symptoms include a full sensation in the neck, light-headedness, and fatigue. These are eliminated with dual-chamber pacing.

- Pacemaker syndrome is a complication of pacemakers.
- Atria contract against closed tricuspid and mitral valves.
- Increased atrial pressure distends neck veins and results in hypotension.
- Symptoms: full sensation in neck, light-headedness, and fatigue.
- Dual-chamber pacing eliminates symptoms.

Pacemaker-mediated tachycardia occurs with DDD pac-

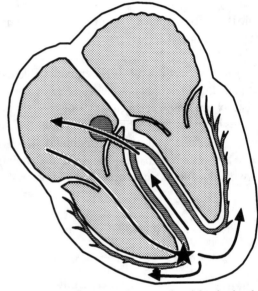

Fig. 3-6. Pacemaker syndrome with retrograde atrial activation during ventricular pacing (*star*), resulting in simultaneous atrial and ventricular contractions.

ing when there is intact retrograde conduction between the ventricle and atrium. In this type of tachycardia, the pacemaker generator acts as one limb of the reentrant circuit. Typically, a PVC occurs that conducts retrogradely to the atrium. The retrograde atrial activity is sensed by the pacemaker, which awaits the normal AV delay and then paces the ventricle. The ventricular activity then conducts retrogradely to the atrium and the reentrant circuit is completed. This abnormality is corrected through programming changes of the pacemaker generator.

- Pacemaker-mediated tachycardia occurs with DDD pacing when there is intact retrograde conduction between the ventricle and atrium.
- The abnormality is corrected by programming changes of the pacemaker generator.

Antiarrhythmic Drugs

Therapeutic range, half-life, and routes of metabolism of antiarrhythmic drugs are listed in Table 3-6. Table 3-7 lists the relative effectiveness of these drugs for treating PVCs, ventricular tachycardia, paroxysmal tachycardia using the AV node as part of the reentrant circuit, and atrial fibrillation.

Half-life is an important concept for use of antiarrhythmic drugs. It is the time required for 50% of the drug within the body to be eliminated. It takes 5 half-lives for a drug to reach steady state or to be eliminated. If a drug has a half-life of 90 minutes (e.g., lidocaine), a steady state will be reached in 6 hours; therefore, a loading dose is given to achieve a therapeutic level more promptly.

- Half-life is an important concept for use of antiarrhythmic drugs.
- Half-life is the time required for 50% of the drug within the body to be eliminated.

Proarrhythmic effect (Table 3-8), a common problem of all antiarrhythmic drugs, occurs when the drug creates an adverse rhythm disturbance (Fig. 3-7), including sinus node suppression and sinus bradycardia, AV block, or increased frequency of or new-onset atrial or ventricular arrhythmias. It was first described in association with quinidine and causes quinidine syncope, which occurs in an estimated 3% of patients who take this drug. In such patients, a rapid ventricular tachycardia with polymorphic morphology, termed "torsades de pointes," develops. The frequency of proarrhythmia is higher in patients who have decreased ventricular function and a history of sustained ventricular tachycardia or ventricular fibrillation. Unfortunately, it is these patients in whom antiarrhythmic drugs are most often required. Also, it can occur in structurally normal hearts.

- Proarrhythmic effect is a common problem of all antiarrhythmic drugs.
- Proarrhythmic effect occurs when a drug creates rhythm disturbance.
- Proarrhythmic effect causes quinidine syncope: a rapid ventricular tachycardia with polymorphic morphology (torsades de pointes).

The Cardiac Arrhythmia Suppression Trial (CAST) study indicated that patients with asymptomatic or mildly symptomatic ventricular ectopy after myocardial infarction had decreased survival rates with drug therapy, even though the drugs suppressed the spontaneous ectopy. These patients had approximately a threefold increase in death rate compared with the rate in patients taking placebo. The CAST study evaluated flecainide, encainide, and moricizine; however, similar results have been demonstrated for class IA drugs (quinidine,

Table 3-6.--Properties of Antiarrhythmic Drugs

Drug	Therapeutic range, µg/mL	Half-life, hours	Route of metabolism Hepatic, %	Renal, %
Class IA				
Quinidine	2-5	6-8	80	20
Procainamide	4-10	3-6	50	50
Disopyramide	2-5	4-8	50	50
Class IB				
Lidocaine	1.5-5	1-4	100	...
Mexiletine	1-2	8-16	100	...
Tocainide	5-12	9-20	60	40
Phenytoin	10-20	24	~100	...
Class IC				
Flecainide	0.2-1	12-27	75	25
Propafenone	Not helpful*	2-10	100	...
Class I				
Moricizine	0.8-2.0	2-6†	60	40
Class III				
Amiodarone	1-2.5	25-110 days	100	...
Sotalol	~2.5	7-18	...	100

*Therapeutic effects for propafenone are generally associated with a QRS width increase of 10% above baseline.

†Effects of moricizine persist for 14-24 hours; thus, an unmeasured metabolite is suggested.

From MKSAP IX: Part C Book 1, 1992. American College of Physicians. By permission.

Table 3-7.--Relative Effectiveness of Antiarrhythmic Drugs

Drug	Effectiveness*			
	PVCs	VT	PSVT	AF
Quinidine	2+	2+	2+	2+
Procainamide	2+	2+	2+	2+
Disopyramide	2+	2+	2+	2+
Lidocaine	2+	2+	0	0
Mexiletine	2+	2+	0	0
Tocainide	2+	1+	0	0
Flecainide	4+	2+	3+	2+
Propafenone	4+	2+	3+	2+
Moricizine	2+	2+	0-1+	0-1+
Amiodarone	4+	3+	3+	3+
Sotalol	3+	2-3+	3+	2+

*0, not effective; 1+, least effective; 4+, most effective.
AF, atrial fibrillation (prevention of paroxysmal AF); PSVT, paroxysmal tachycardia utilizing AV node as part of reentrant circuit; VT, ventricular tachycardia.

procainamide, and disopyramide) and the class IB drug mexiletine.

- CAST study indicated decreased survival rate with drug therapy in patients with asymptomatic ventricular ectopy after infarction.

Adenosine slows conduction in the AV node and is eliminated by uptake in endothelial cells and erythrocytes. Its half-life is 10 seconds. Adenosine is indicated in supraventricular reentrant tachycardia that uses the AV node as part of the reentrant circuit (i.e., AV nodal reentry or reentry using an accessory pathway). The drug does not terminate atrial fibrillation, flutter, or tachycardia, and it slows the ventricular rate for only a few seconds because of its short half-life. Both adenosine and verapamil have equal efficacy at the highest recommended doses (adenosine, 12 mg; verapamil, 10 mg). Because of adenosine's short half-life, approximately 10% of patients have recurrent supraventricular tachycardia after its administration, whereas recurrent supraventricular tachycardia is rare after termination by verapamil. In patients with a wide QRS tachycardia (ventricular tachycardia) or atrial fibrillation and associated Wolff-Parkinson-White syndrome, hemodynamic collapse is common when they are given verapamil. This problem is not associated with adenosine. The cost of adenosine is approximately twice that of verapamil.

- Adenosine slows conduction in the AV node.
- Adenosine is used for supraventricular reentrant tachycardia.

- Adenosine does not terminate atrial fibrillation, flutter, or tachycardia.
- Efficacy of 12 mg of adenosine is equal to that of 10 mg of verapamil.
- Cost of adenosine is twice that of verapamil.

Electrophysiology-Guided Serial Drug Testing

This technique is used to identify an effective drug for patients (before dismissal from the hospital) who have life-threatening arrhythmias and for whom outpatient management is unsafe. Arrhythmia is induced in the baseline state, an antiarrhythmic drug is then administered orally, and the electrophysiologic study is repeated. A drug that prevents induction of tachycardia is termed effective. In patients who have ventricular tachycardia occurring spontaneously, the chance of that tachycardia being induced in the laboratory is 95% if the patients have underlying coronary artery disease and 75% if they have dilated cardiomyopathy or valvular heart disease. In patients who present with out-of-hospital cardiac arrest and ventricular fibrillation, the chance of life-threatening ventricular arrhythmia being induced at testing is 70%. For patients with ventricular tachycardia, an effective drug is identified for approximately 40%, and each drug has a 25% chance of being effective with electrophysiology-guided serial drug testing. For patients who survive cardiac arrest and have inducible ventricular tachycardia, the survival rate at 1 year is 95% if an effective drug is identified. Alternatively, the 1-year survival rate is 65% if an effective drug cannot be identified and 85% if ventricular tachycardia is not inducible during baseline study and no therapy is given.

- Electrophysiology-guided serial drug testing, performed before hospital dismissal, identifies an effective drug for patients with life-threatening arrhythmias.
- With out-of-hospital cardiac arrest and ventricular fibrillation, the chance of inducing life-threatening arrhythmia during testing is 70%.
- Serial drug testing identifies an effective drug for 40% of patients with ventricular tachycardia.

Implantable Defibrillators

Because serial drug testing identifies only 40% of patients with life-threatening ventricular arrhythmias, alternative therapy has been developed to treat recurrences of tachycardia. The most effective therapy has been the implantable cardioverter-defibrillator. This device monitors the rhythm and treats a ventricular arrhythmia with an up to 34-joule shock or antitachycardia pacing as the initial therapy followed by low-energy cardioversion and high-energy defibrillation if needed. Current limitations of the device are a battery life of 3-5 years, large and cumbersome size, and presence of uncomfortable and potentially dangerous shocks during sinus rhythm or atrial fibrillation.

Table 3-8.--Toxicity and Side Effects of Antiarrhythmic Drugs

Drug	Frequency of side effects, %	Organ toxicity	% proarrhythmia during treatment for VT	Risk of congestive heart failure*		Side effects
				EF ≥ 30%	EF ≤ 30%	
Quinidine	30	Moderate	3	0	0	Nausea, abdominal pain, diarrhea, thrombo-cytopenia, hypo-tension, ↓ warfarin
Procainamide	30	High	2	0	1+	Lupus-like syndrome, rash, fever, headache, nausea, hallucinations, diarrhea
Disopyramide	30	Low	2	1+	4+	Dry mouth, urinary hesitancy, blurred vision, constipation, urinary retention
Lidocaine	40	Moderate	2	0	0	L-H, seizure, tremor, confusion, memory loss, nausea
Mexiletine	40	Low	2	0	0	L-H, tremor, ataxia, confusion, memory loss, altered liver function
Tocainide	40	High	2	0	0	L-H, tremor, ataxia, confusion, memory loss, blood dyscrasia, pulmonary fibrosis
Flecainide	30	Low	5	1+	3+	L-H, visual disturbance, headache, nausea
Propafenone	30	Low	5	0-1+	2+	L-H, headache, nausea, constipation, metallic taste, ↓ warfarin
Moricizine	30	Low	5	0	1+	L-H, nausea, headache, fatigue, dyspnea
Amiodarone	65	High	4	0	1+	Corneal deposits, photosensitivity, sleep disturbance, nausea, anorexia, tremor, ataxia, neuropathy, pulmonary fibrosis, thyroid disorders, hepatotoxicity, ↓ warfarin
Sotalol	30	Low	5	1+	3+	L-H, fatigue, dyspnea, nausea

*Congestive heart failure risk: 0, no risk; 4+, high risk.
EF, ejection fraction; L-H, light-headedness; PVC, premature ventricular complex; VT, sustained ventricular tachycardia.
Modified from MKSAP IX: Part C Book 1, 1992. American College of Physicians. By permission.

Fig. 3-7. Proarrhythmic response to quinidine. Quinidine resulted in prolongation of QT interval, and late-coupled PVC initiated polymorphic ventricular tachycardia, termed "torsades de pointes."

Implantable cardioverters-defibrillators have improved mortality in patients surviving sudden cardiac death when compared with historical controls. Historically, such patients had a 70% survival rate at 1 year with either no treatment or empiric antiarrhythmic drug therapy. Use of the device has improved the overall 1-year survival rate to 90%; recurrent sudden cardiac death occurs in 2% of patients at 1 year and in 4% of patients at 4 years.

Advances in technology have now made it possible to implant defibrillators in virtually all patients by using a nonthoracotomy approach. Also, the devices have been reduced in size so that most patients can have them implanted in the pectoral region, similar to a pacemaker.

- Limitations of implantable cardioverter-defibrillator: battery life of 3-5 years, large size, uncomfortable and potentially dangerous shocks during sinus rhythm or atrial fibrillation.
- Overall 1-year survival rate with the device is 90%.

Transcatheter Ablation

This technique involves placing an electrode catheter in a heart chamber. It is placed adjacent to a critical portion of a reentrant circuit, which might include one of the pathways participating in AV nodal reentrant tachycardia or an accessory pathway in patients with Wolff-Parkinson-White syndrome, an automatic atrial focus, or a portion of the reentrant circuit adjacent to a scar in the ventricle in patients with ventricular tachy-

cardia. Previously, direct current was then passed through the catheter; the current exited the catheter tip and produced a 1-cm scar that was 2-3 mm in depth. Most ablations are now performed with radio-frequency energy, which passes through the catheter tip and heats the adjacent tissue; the result is a smaller scar with a lesion size that is easier to control.

- Catheter ablation: AV nodal reentrant tachycardia, accessory pathway in Wolff-Parkinson-White syndrome, automatic atrial focus, atrial flutter, and some cases of ventricular tachycardia.
- Catheter ablation is performed with radio-frequency energy passed through a catheter.

Radio-frequency energy used to treat an accessory pathway (Wolff-Parkinson-White syndrome) or reentrant tachycardia within the AV node is successful in 95% of cases. About 1%-2% of patients have complications, including vascular injury where the catheters are placed, cardiac perforation, and infection. In addition, if the accessory pathway is close to the normal conduction system or if AV nodal reentrant tachycardia is ablated, there is a 5% risk of creating complete heart block that requires permanent pacing. Compared with previous surgical approaches for treatment of similar tachycardias, the technique has reduced the hospital stay from 7 days to 1-2 days and the time to return to work or school from 6-8 weeks to 3-5 days. The cost is approximately 40% of the surgical cost.

- Catheter ablation is successful in 95% of cases of accessory pathway or reentrant tachycardia in the AV node.
- The complication rate is 1%-2%.
- Catheter ablation reduces hospital stay to 1-2 days.
- The cost is 40% of the surgical cost.

Catheter ablation is also used to achieve complete heart block in patients with supraventricular tachycardias (usually atrial fibrillation or atrial flutter) that are refractory to medications and associated with rapid ventricular rates. Either direct-current or radio-frequency ablation results in heart block in >95% of patients, and permanent pacing is then required. Such patients have significant symptomatic improvement because the heart rate is regular and they respond normally to exercise because of rate-responsive pacing. This technique trades tachycardia-associated problems for problems associated with permanent pacemaker implantation and follow-up.

- Catheter ablation achieves complete heart block in supraventricular tachycardias that are refractory to medication and associated with rapid ventricular rates.
- Catheter ablation results in heart block in >95% of patients; permanent pacing is then required.
- Symptoms improve significantly.

Antitachycardia Surgery

Endocardial resection is a standard technique for treating ventricular tachycardia associated with aneurysm. The border zone adjacent to a myocardial scar (including aneurysm) is generally the location for the reentrant circuit. This border zone is located with mapping systems at the time of operation and is then removed with a technique called subendocardial resection. The operative mortality rate is approximately 10%; arrhythmia is cured in 85% of survivors.

- Endocardial resection is an option for treating ventricular tachycardia associated with aneurysm.
- Operative mortality rate is 10%.
- Arrhythmia is cured in 85% of survivors.

Endocardial resection is also a standard technique for treating an accessory pathway or AV nodal reentrant tachycardia. Either sharp dissection or cryoablation of the accessory pathway is used. Surgical success rates approach 95%. The surgical mortality rate is 1%, and the risk of heart block is 1%-2%.

For the most part, surgical techniques have been replaced by transcatheter radio-frequency ablation.

- Operation is standard for treating accessory pathway or AV nodal reentrant tachycardia.
- The success rate is 95%.

SPECIFIC ARRHYTHMIA PROBLEMS

Sinus Node Dysfunction

Sinus node dysfunction, also called "sick sinus syndrome," includes sinus bradycardia, sinus pauses, tachycardia-bradycardia syndrome (Fig. 3-8), and sinus arrest. It is usually associated with conduction system disease and lack of an appropriate junctional escape focus during sinus pause or sinus bradycardia. The diagnosis is made from the medical history and results of ECG and Holter monitoring, which are the most useful diagnostic tests. Electrophysiologic testing is used to evaluate patients with a history consistent with sinus node disease but in whom ECG or Holter monitoring has not shown the mechanism because of infrequent spells. Electrophysiologic testing has low sensitivity because patients may be in an increased adrenergic state in the laboratory and catecholamines prevent the sinus bradycardia or sinus pauses from being apparent. Prolonged monitoring with an event recorder is also useful for diagnosis.

- Sinus node dysfunction includes sinus bradycardia, sinus pauses, tachycardia-bradycardia syndrome, and sinus arrest.
- Sinus node dysfunction is associated with conduction system disease.
- The diagnosis is made from the history and the results of ECG and Holter monitoring.
- Electrophysiologic testing is used for patients in whom the mechanism of dysfunction is not shown by ECG or Holter monitoring.

Asymptomatic patients with sinus node dysfunction are followed without specific therapy. Symptomatic patients are usually treated with pacemakers. Often, patients with tachycardia-bradycardia have atrial fibrillation that at times presents with rapid ventricular rates and at other times with inappropriate, symptomatic bradycardia. Pacemakers are used to prevent the bradycardia, and drugs are used to slow conduction through

Fig. 3-8. Tachycardia-bradycardia with episode of atrial fibrillation terminating spontaneously; these are followed by a 4.5-second pause until sinus node recovers. (From MKSAP IX: Part C Book 1, 1992. American College of Physicians. By permission.)

the AV node and to prevent episodes of rapid ventricular rate.

- Asymptomatic patients with sinus node dysfunction: followed without specific therapy.
- Symptomatic patients with sinus node dysfunction: treated with pacemakers.

Conduction System Disorders

First-degree AV block results in a prolonged P-R interval and is usually due to conduction delay within the AV node. In patients with associated bundle branch block, the conduction delay may be distal to the AV node in the His-Purkinje system. Patients with *second-degree AV block of the Mobitz I* (Wenckebach) variety have a gradual prolongation of the P-R interval before the nonconducted P wave. The subsequent P-R interval is shorter than the P-R interval before the non-conducted P wave (Fig. 3-9 and 3-10). Also, the R-R interval that encompasses the nonconducted P wave is shorter than two R-R intervals between conducted beats. Wenckebach conduction often accompanies an inferior myocardial infarction, which results in ischemia of the AV node. This problem generally does not require pacing unless there are documented hemodynamic problems associated with the slow heart rate.

- First-degree AV block results in a prolonged P-R interval.
- Second-degree AV block of Mobitz I type results in a gradual prolongation of the P-R interval before the nonconducted P wave.
- Wenckebach conduction may accompany inferior myocardial infarction.
- Wenckebach conduction does not require pacing unless hemodynamic problems are associated with slow heart rate.

Second-degree AV block due to the Mobitz II mechanism is generally caused by conduction disease in the His-Purkinje system and is associated with bundle branch block (Fig. 3-11). This conduction abnormality is shown on the ECG as a sudden failure of a P wave to conduct to the ventricle with no change in the P-R interval either before or after the nonconducted P wave. This problem often heralds complete heart block, and strong consideration should be given to permanent pacing. *Complete heart block* is diagnosed when there is no relationship between the atrial rhythm and the ventricular rhythm and the atrial rhythm is faster than the ventricular escape rhythm (Fig. 3-12). The ventricular escape rhythm is either a junctional escape focus, with a conduction pattern similar to the conduction pattern seen during normal rhythm, or a ventricu-

Fig. 3-9. 3:2 Mobitz I (or Wenckebach) second-degree AV block in a patient with acute inferior myocardial infarction.

Fig. 3-10. Mobitz I second-degree AV block; note gradual P-R prolongation. P-R after nonconducted P wave is shorter than P-R preceding nonconducted P wave.

lar escape focus, with a wide QRS conduction pattern. Complete heart block is treated with permanent pacing in most cases.

- Second-degree AV block of Mobitz II type is usually due to conduction disease in His-Purkinje system.
- It often heralds complete heart block; consider permanent pacing.
- Complete heart block: no relationship between atrial rhythm and ventricular rhythm, and atrial rhythm is faster than ventricular escape rhythm.

Bifascicular block refers to left bundle branch block, right bundle branch block with left anterior fascicular block (marked left-axis deviation), or right bundle branch block with left posterior fascicular block (right-axis deviation). Bifascicular block is usually associated with underlying structural heart disease and has a 1% chance of progressing to complete heart block in asymptomatic persons. Patients presenting with syncope and bifascicular block may have intermittent complete heart block caused by their conduction system disease or ventricular tachycardia caused by the underlying myocardial disease. Permanent pacing can be used to treat syncope due to complete heart block, but syncope due to ventricular tachycardia requires antiarrhythmic medications, an implantable defibrillator, or surgery, depending on the clinical situation. Patients with syncope and bifascicular block should undergo electrophysiologic testing to determine whether they have ventricular tachycardia, because this rhythm occurs in 40% of such patients. If these patients receive only permanent pacing, the pacing, although it improves their syncope, does not decrease their risk of sudden death.

- Bifascicular block is usually associated with structural heart disease.

- Bifascicular block progresses to complete heart block in 1% of asymptomatic persons.
- Permanent pacing is used to treat syncope in complete heart block.
- Syncope due to ventricular tachycardia requires antiarrhythmic medications, implantable defibrillator, or surgery.
- Patients with syncope, bifascicular block, and ventricular tachycardia who receive only permanent pacing have improvement in syncope but no decrease in risk of sudden death.

High-degree AV block is diagnosed when there is a 2:1 or higher AV conduction block (Fig. 3-13). It might be caused by a Wenckebach or a Mobitz II mechanism. A Wenckebach mechanism is more likely if the QRS conduction is normal, and a Mobitz II-type mechanism is more likely if the QRS complex demonstrates additional conduction disease, such as bundle branch block.

During an electrophysiologic study, the *H-V interval* is measured. It is the conduction time after the impulse leaves the AV node to the time when the ventricles are activated (Fig. 3-14). The normal H-V interval is 35-55 ms. In asymptomatic persons, an H-V interval of 50-70 ms is associated with a 1% per year risk of complete heart block and does not require pacing, an H-V interval of 70-100 ms is associated with a 4% per year risk of complete heart block and treatment should be individualized, and an H-V interval >100 ms is associated with an 8% per year risk of complete heart block and should be treated with permanent pacing.

Indications for pacing include symptomatic Mobitz II heart block, complete heart block, and bifascicular block. Pacing should be considered in asymptomatic patients with Mobitz II and complete heart block.

- Indications for pacing: symptomatic Mobitz II heart block,

Fig. 3-11. Mobitz II second-degree AV block with no change in P-R interval before or after nonconducted P wave.

Fig. 3-12. Complete heart block with an atrial rate at 70 beats per minute and a ventricular escape rhythm at 30 beats per minute.

Fig. 3-13. High-grade 2:1 AV conduction block.

Fig. 3-14. Intracardiac recording of the AV node-His bundle area (HIS) with surface lead AVF. The A-H interval is conduction through AV node, and H-V interval is conduction through His-Purkinje system.

complete heart block, and bifascicular heart block.

- Pacing should be considered for asymptomatic persons with Mobitz II and complete heart block.

Carotid Sinus Syndrome

Carotid sinus massage is performed to identify carotid sinus hypersensitivity (Fig. 3-15). Approximately 40% of patients older than 65 years have a hyperactive carotid sinus reflex (3-second pause or decrease in blood pressure of 50 mm Hg), although most of these patients have no spontaneous syncope. Carotid sinus massage should be performed over the carotid bifurcation at the angle of the jaw in patients without evidence of carotid bruit on carotid auscultation or a history of cere-brovascular disease. Carotid sinus massage is performed with moderate pressure over the carotid bifurcation for 5 seconds while monitoring heart rate and blood pressure. Approximately 35% of patients with a hyperactive carotid sinus reflex have a pure cardioinhibitory component manifested only by a pause in ventricular activity exceeding 3 seconds. Fifteen percent of patients have a pure vasodepressor component, with a normal heart rate maintained but a decrease in blood pressure >50 mm Hg. Sixty percent of patients have a combined response, with both cardioinhibitory and vasodepressor components. In such patients, permanent pacing may prevent the cardioinhibitory response, but the vasodepressor response continues to produce symptoms.

Fig. 3-15. Carotid sinus massage resulting in sinus pause with junctional escape beats before sinus rhythm returns.

- Carotid sinus massage is used to identify carotid sinus hypersensitivity.
- About 40% of patients >65 years have a hyperactive carotid sinus reflex (3-second pause or decrease in blood pressure of 50 mm Hg).

Occasionally, associated neck abnormalities, including lymph node enlargement, previous neck surgery, and regional tumor, result in carotid sinus syndrome. Surgical techniques to treat this condition are usually unsuccessful, and the primary form of therapy is AV sequential pacing for the cardioinhibitory component and elastic stockings for the vasodepressor component. On occasion, patients respond to anticholinergic medications.

Atrial Flutter

Atrial flutter is identified by the characteristic sawtooth pattern of atrial activity at a rate of 240-320 beats per minute. Patients with normal conduction systems maintain 2:1 AV conduction; thus, the ventricular rate is often close to 150 beats per minute. Higher degrees of AV block (3:1 or higher) in the absence of drugs to slow AV node conduction (digoxin, β-adrenergic blocker, calcium antagonist) imply AV conduction disease (Fig. 3-16). Patients with 2:1 AV conduction and a heart rate of 150 beats per minute often have one of the flutter waves buried in the QRS complex. Carotid sinus massage results in increased AV block, revealing the flutter waves and establishing the diagnosis.

- Atrial flutter: atrial activity at 240-320 beats per minute.
- Ventricular rate is close to 150 beats per minute.

Treatment is aimed at preventing paroxysms and controlling the ventricular rate. Paroxysms of atrial flutter (or atrial fibrillation) can be prevented or decreased with class IA (quinidine, procainamide, disopyramide), class IC (propafenone, flecainide), and class III (amiodarone, sotalol) antiarrhythmic drugs. In general, these drugs control paroxysms of atrial flutter or atrial fibrillation in 30%-50% of patients during the first year of use. Side effects, including proarrhythmia, need to be weighed against symptoms during tachycardia to ensure that the potential benefits of therapy outweigh the risk.

- Antiarrhythmic drugs control atrial flutter (fibrillation) in 30%-50% of cases.

Atrial Fibrillation

Atrial fibrillation is diagnosed by the characteristic irregular baseline without clear-cut P waves and irregularly irregular ventricular response. A slow ventricular response in the absence of drugs to block the AV node implies associated AV conduction disease. Patients with this slow response may have prolonged sinus node recovery and so should be electrically cardioverted with temporal external pacing standby, because the combination of atrial fibrillation and a slow ventricular rate implies tachycardia-bradycardia syndrome or sinus node dysfunction.

Most patients with atrial fibrillation have a sympathetically mediated arrhythmia that may be made worse with sympathetic stimulation that occurs with activity, stress, smoking, and consumption of alcohol and caffeine. In about 5%-10% of patients with atrial fibrillation, the rhythm is due to increased parasympathetic activity that results in sinus bradycardia and dispersion of atrial refractoriness. An atrial premature complex then finds part of the atrium refractory, whereas other parts of the atrium are either partially refractory or fully recovered. This sets up the substrate for a reentrant arrhythmia and the development of atrial fibrillation. Typically, the arrhythmias occur during sleep or at rest. They are worse with drugs that slow sinus rate, such as digoxin and β-adrenergic blockers.

- Most patients with atrial fibrillation have a sympathetically mediated arrhythmia that may be worse with activity, stress, smoking, and alcohol and caffeine consumption.
- In 5%-10% of patients with atrial fibrillation, the rhythm is due to increased parasympathetic activity.

Acute atrial fibrillation or flutter should be treated with electrical cardioversion if there is hemodynamic compromise. In a patient who is adequately tolerating the new arrhythmia, initial therapy should be aimed at controlling the ventricular rate with digoxin, a β-adrenergic blocker, or a calcium antagonist. Attention then should be directed to reversing the underlying cause, which might include fever, anemia, thyrotoxicosis, myocardial infarction, pulmonary embolism, or worsening

Fig. 3-16. Atrial flutter with 3:1 conduction in a patient with AV conduction disease.

heart failure. A patient who has been in atrial fibrillation for >24-48 hours should undergo anticoagulation with warfarin for 3 weeks before and for 4 weeks after elective cardioversion. After 3 weeks of anticoagulation, chemical cardioversion can be tried with a class IA or IC antiarrhythmic agent. Treatment with these drugs should be initiated in the hospital during continuous monitoring to observe for proarrhythmia. If drugs are ineffective, electrical cardioversion can be performed; if sinus rhythm is obtained, treatment with the drug can be maintained for several weeks to help ensure maintenance of sinus rhythm. Continuation of drug therapy depends on the underlying heart disease and the propensity for relapse into atrial fibrillation or flutter. Use of the antiarrhythmic drug should be stopped if recurrent atrial fibrillation occurs, and it should not be used in patients with chronic atrial fibrillation.

- Acute atrial fibrillation or flutter is treated with electrical cardioversion if there is hemodynamic compromise.
- Initial therapy should be digoxin, β-adrenergic blocker, or calcium antagonist.
- The underlying cause should be reversed.
- If atrial fibrillation is present >24-48 hours, treat with warfarin for 3 weeks before elective cardioversion.
- If drugs are ineffective, perform electrical cardioversion.

Digoxin is not as effective as a β-adrenergic blocker or a calcium antagonist for controlling ventricular rate in response to exercise during atrial fibrillation. Patients with atrial fibrillation or flutter treated with digoxin may have adequate rate control at rest only to have inappropriately fast heart rates with exercise. Such patients benefit from the addition of either a β-adrenergic blocker or calcium antagonist to their drug regimen.

- Digoxin is not as effective as a β-adrenergic blocker for controlling ventricular rate in response to exercise during atrial fibrillation.
- Patients treated with digoxin may have control at rest but fast heart rates with exercise; a β-adrenergic blocker or calcium antagonist should be added to the drug regimen.

Anticoagulation with warfarin is indicated in patients with atrial fibrillation if there is associated heart disease or congestive heart failure. Anticoagulation is not indicated for lone atrial fibrillation (patients <60 years with no associated heart disease and no history of hypertension). Warfarin is better than aspirin and both are better than placebo for preventing stroke or major systemic embolization in patients with either chronic or paroxysmal atrial fibrillation. The optimal prothrombin time is 1.3-1.5 times normal (INR 2-3); in this range, the benefit of reducing stroke outweighs the risk of bleeding complications. Aspirin has not been helpful in patients >75 years, and hemorrhagic strokes with warfarin are increased in this age group.

- Anticoagulation is indicated if there is heart disease, congestive heart failure, or a previous transient ischemic attack/cerebrovascular accident.
- Anticoagulation not indicated for lone atrial fibrillation (patients <60 years, no heart disease, and no history of hypertension).
- Warfarin is better than aspirin for preventing stroke or major systemic embolization in patients with chronic or paroxysmal atrial fibrillation.

Supraventricular Tachycardia

Paroxysmal supraventricular tachycardia (PSVT) refers to cardiac arrhythmias of supraventricular origin using a reentrant mechanism with an abrupt onset and termination, a regular R-R interval, and a narrow QRS complex, unless there is rate-related or preexisting bundle branch block (Fig. 3-17). In patients with a normal QRS during sinus rhythm (lack of preexcitation), PSVT is due to reentry within the AV node in 60%, reentry utilizing a concealed accessory pathway in 30%, and reentry in the sinus node or atrium in the remaining 10% (Fig. 3-18). Episodes usually respond to vagal maneuvers; if these fail, intravenously administered adenosine or verapamil terminates the arrhythmia in 90% of patients.

- PSVT is arrhythmia with abrupt onset and termination.
- PSVT usually responds to vagal maneuvers; if not, adenosine or verapamil is effective in 90% of patients.

PSVT generally is not a life-threatening arrhythmia and only occasionally is associated with near-syncope or syncope. The rhythm is more serious when it is associated with significant heart disease, and cardiac decompensation results with the sudden increase in heart rate. This can occur in patients with congenital heart disease, cardiomyopathy, or ischemic heart disease. Patients with AV nodal reentrant tachycardia usually have simultaneous activation of the atrium and ventricle, in which case the atria contract against closed tricuspid and mitral valves (similar to pacemaker syndrome) and produce symptoms associated with atrial distention, including a fullness in the neck, hypotension, and polyuria. Hypotension and polyuria are due in part to release of atrial natriuretic peptide.

- PSVT generally is not a life-threatening arrhythmia.
- PSVT is more serious when associated with heart disease.

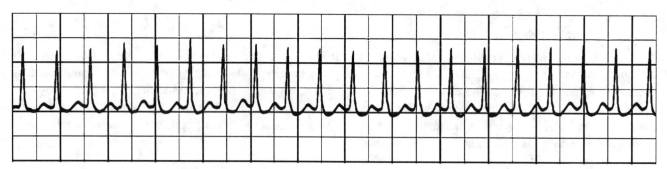

Fig. 3-17. Paroxysmal supraventricular tachycardia.

Fig. 3-18. Mechanisms of paroxysmal supraventricular tachycardia in patients with a normal ECG during sinus rhythm. SA, sinoatrial.

PSVT responds to most antiarrhythmic drugs, including drugs that suppress AV node conduction (digoxin, β-adrenergic blocker, and calcium antagonist), assuming that part of the reentrant circuit uses the AV node, and to drugs that slow conduction within the reentrant circuit, including class IA (quinidine, procainamide, disopyramide), IC (propafenone, flecainide), and III (amiodarone, sotalol) antiarrhythmic drugs.

● PSVT responds to most antiarrhythmic drugs.

Multifocal atrial tachycardia is an automatic atrial rhythm diagnosed when three or more distinct atrial foci (P waves of different morphology) are present and the rate exceeds 100 beats per minute (Fig. 3-19). The rhythm occurs primarily in patients with decompensated lung disease with associated hypoxia, increased catecholamines (exogenous and endogenous), atrial stretch, and local tissue acid-base and electrolyte disturbances. This rhythm is made worse by digoxin, which shortens atrial refractoriness, but does respond to improved oxygenation and slow channel blockade with verapamil or diltiazem.

● Digoxin worsens multifocal atrial tachycardia.

Distinguishing Supraventricular Tachycardia With Aberrancy From Ventricular Tachycardia

A wide QRS tachycardia may be due to supraventricular tachycardia with aberrancy or to ventricular tachycardia. Useful findings to identify ventricular tachycardia are listed in Table 3-9.

Approximately 85% of wide QRS tachycardias are ventricular in origin and are often well tolerated. The absence of hemodynamic compromise during tachycardia is not a clue that the tachycardia is supraventricular in origin. In patients with a wide QRS tachycardia and a history of ischemic heart disease (angina, myocardial infarction, Q wave on ECG), the tachycardia is ventricular in origin in 90%-95%. Therefore, the vast majority of wide QRS complex tachycardias are ventricular tachycardia (Fig. 3-20).

● About 85% of wide QRS tachycardias are ventricular in origin.
● In patients with wide QRS tachycardia and ischemic heart disease, tachycardia is ventricular in origin in 90%-95%.

Avoid intravenous administration of verapamil in patients with a wide QRS tachycardia unless the tachycardia is supraventricular in origin. Most patients with a wide QRS tachycardia have ventricular tachycardia, and verapamil causes hemodynamic deterioration that requires cardioversion in more than half of the patients. The use of verapamil results in peripheral vasodilatation, further increase in catecholamines, and decreased cardiac contractility, all of which contribute to adverse hemodynamics.

● Avoid intravenously administered verapamil for wide QRS tachycardia.
● Verapamil causes hemodynamic deterioration requiring cardioversion in ventricular tachycardia.

Table 3-9.--Findings That Identify Ventricular Tachycardia

Evidence of AV dissociation with P waves "marching through" the QRS complexes

A QRS width >0.14 second if the tachycardia has a right bundle branch block pattern and >0.16 second if the tachycardia has a left bundle branch block pattern

Northwest axis (axis between -90° and -180°)

A different QRS morphology in patients with a preexisting bundle branch block

A history of structural heart disease

Fig. 3-19. Simultaneous recordings from patient with multifocal atrial tachycardia, showing three or more P waves of different morphology. (*Lower panel*, From MKSAP IX: Part C Book 1, 1992. American College of Physicians. By permission.)

Wolff-Parkinson-White Syndrome

This abnormality is defined as 1) symptomatic tachycardia, 2) a short P-R interval (<0.12 second), 3) a delta wave, and 4) a prolonged QRS interval (>0.12 second).

In Wolff-Parkinson-White syndrome, normal activation of the ventricle is a fusion complex. Part of the activation is due to conduction over the accessory pathway, and the remaining activation is due to conduction through the normal His-Purkinje conduction system. Not all patients with preexcitation have a short P-R interval. Normal P-R conduction may occur if the accessory pathway is far removed from the AV node. In patients with a far left lateral accessory pathway, the heart is activated through the AV node before atrial activation reaches the accessory pathway. Thus, the P-R interval may be normal before the onset of the delta wave.

Ventricular activation is abnormal in patients with Wolff-Parkinson-White syndrome. Infarction, ventricular hypertrophy, and ST-T wave changes should not be interpreted after the diagnosis is established because these changes are usually due to the abnormal pattern of ventricular activation.

- In Wolff-Parkinson-White syndrome, the P-R interval may be normal before the onset of the delta wave.
- Ventricular activation is abnormal in Wolff-Parkinson-White syndrome.

Preexcitation occurs in about 2 of 1,000 patients; tachycardia subsequently develops in 70%. Of patients with tachycardia, 70% have PSVT and 30% have atrial fibrillation. The atrial fibrillation often occurs after a short episode of PSVT. Elimination of PSVT after surgery or catheter ablation generally eliminates problems with atrial fibrillation. The most serious rhythm disturbance is the onset of atrial fibrillation with rapid ventricular conduction over the accessory pathway resulting in ventricular fibrillation (Fig. 3-21). Most asymptomatic patients do not benefit from risk stratification with electrophysiologic testing, including induction of atrial fibrillation, unless they have a high-risk occupation. Patients who are asymptomatic have a negligible chance of sudden death, and in patients who are symptomatic, the incidence of sudden death is 0.0025 per patient-year.

- Preexcitation occurs in 2 of 1,000 patients; tachycardia develops in 70%.
- Of patients with tachycardia, 70% have PSVT and 30% have atrial fibrillation.
- Asymptomatic patients have a negligible chance of sudden death.
- In symptomatic patients, the incidence of sudden death is 0.0025 per patient-year.

Patients with Wolff-Parkinson-White syndrome may have either 1) a manifest accessory pathway resulting in preexcitation on the ECG (Fig. 3-22) due to antegrade conduction over the accessory pathway or 2) a concealed accessory pathway that is capable of conducting only in the retrograde direction, and, therefore, the surface ECG in sinus rhythm is normal. Both manifest and concealed accessory pathways have the

Fig. 3-20. Ventricular tachycardia with a wide QRS complex, northwest axis, and fusion complexes in a patient with normal blood pressure.

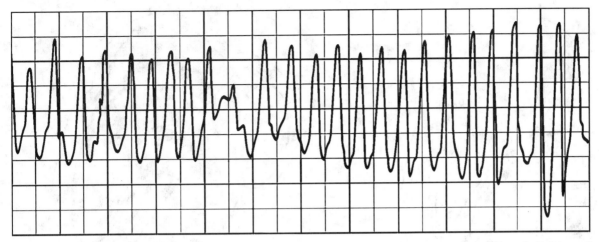

Fig. 3-21. Atrial fibrillation in a patient with Wolff-Parkinson-White syndrome shows wide QRS complex and irregular R-R intervals.

same mechanism of reentrant tachycardia, in which antegrade conduction over the normal conduction system results in a normal QRS complex (unless there is rate-related bundle branch block) and conduction continues through the ventricle, returns retrogradely over the accessory pathway, and continues through the atrium to complete the reentrant circuit, termed "orthodromic AV reentry" (Fig. 3-23). Five percent of patients may have reentrant tachycardia that goes in the reverse direction (antidromic AV reentry), in which ventricular activation over the accessory pathway activates the ventricle from an ectopic location; the result is a wide QRS complex tachycardia that is often confused with ventricular tachycardia (Fig. 3-24).

Electrophysiologic testing should be performed in patients with symptomatic Wolff-Parkinson-White syndrome. This testing identifies the pathway location, confirms that the pathway is an integral part of the reentrant circuit and not an inno-

cent bystander (i.e., the arrhythmia is AV nodal reentry), and evaluates for a second accessory pathway that occurs in approximately 15% of patients.

During acute atrial fibrillation, intravenously administered digoxin and verapamil should be avoided because they accelerate the ventricular rate. Digoxin may shorten the refractoriness of the accessory pathway, and verapamil results in vasodilatation with reflex increase in catecholamines and more rapid conduction over the accessory pathway. Both drugs have been associated with ventricular fibrillation when used to treat atrial fibrillation in the presence of Wolff-Parkinson-White syndrome. If the rate is rapid or there is hemodynamic compromise, cardioversion should be performed. Intravenously administered procainamide can be used to slow conduction over the accessory pathway and to attempt to convert the atrium to sinus rhythm if immediate cardioversion is not indicated.

- Avoid intravenously administered digoxin and verapamil during acute atrial fibrillation.
- If heart rate is rapid and there is hemodynamic compromise, perform cardioversion.
- Use intravenously administered procainamide to slow conduction and to convert the atrium to sinus rhythm.

PSVT in patients with an accessory pathway often ends with vagal maneuvers or intravenously administered adenosine or verapamil. Further episodes can be prevented with a β-adrenergic blocker, a calcium antagonist, and class IA (quinidine, procainamide, disopyramide), class IC (propafenone, flecainide), and class III (amiodarone, sotalol) antiarrhythmic drugs. Radio-frequency ablation is used to ablate the accessory pathway and to cure the tachycardia, thus eliminating the need for medical therapy.

- Further PSVT is prevented with a β-adrenergic blocker, a calcium antagonist, and class IA, IC, and III antiarrhythmic drugs.

Fig. 3-22. Conduction of sinus impulse in Wolff-Parkinson-White syndrome. Ventricles are activated over normal AV node–His-Purkinje system and accessory pathway; result is a fusion complex (QRS and delta wave).

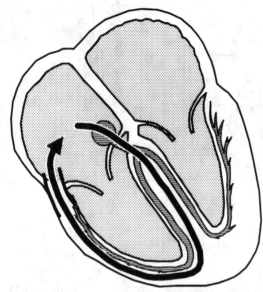

Fig. 3-23. Typical mechanism of supraventricular tachycardia in patients with Wolff-Parkinson-White syndrome; result is narrow QRS complex because ventricular activation is over the normal conduction system.

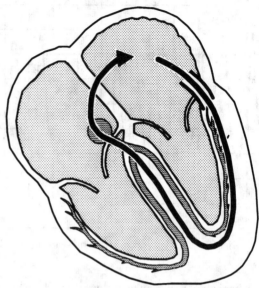

Fig. 3-24. Unusual mechanism of supraventricular tachycardia in patients with Wolff-Parkinson-White syndrome; result is a wide QRS complex because ventricular activation is over accessory pathway. This arrhythmia is difficult to distinguish from ventricular tachycardia.

- Radio-frequency ablation is used to cure tachycardia.

Tachycardia-Mediated Cardiomyopathy

Supraventricular tachycardia, atrial fibrillation with a rapid ventricular rate, and ventricular tachycardia have been associated with cardiomyopathy. Treatment of the tachycardia has allowed cardiac performance to return to near normal. When patients present with heart failure and tachycardia is identified, determine whether the heart failure is causing the tachycardia or the tachycardia has caused the heart failure. Control of ventricular rate often improves ventricular function. In a patient with heart failure who has a rhythm with an abnormal P-wave axis, tachycardia-mediated cardiomyopathy should be suspected.

Premature Ventricular Complexes

Complex PVCs are defined as >10 per hour, multiform morphology, PVC pairs, or runs of nonsustained ventricular tachycardia. Patients who are asymptomatic with a normal heart and complex PVCs have an excellent long-term prognosis, and the PVCs in general are considered benign. Management includes reassurance and antiarrhythmic drugs only if necessary for intolerable palpitations.

In patients with asymptomatic complex ventricular ectopy and associated heart disease, the risk for syncope or sudden death is 10%-20%. However, antiarrhythmic agents for all such patients are not warranted because 80%-90% will not have syncope or sudden death, and these agents would expose them to the risks of drug toxicity and proarrhythmia. Studies are now under way to identify the best test to stratify patients at highest risk for sudden death. These tests include the signal-averaged ECG, measuring of ventricular function, and electrophysiologic testing.

- In patients with asymptomatic complex ventricular ectopy and heart disease, the risk for syncope or sudden death is 10%-20%.
- Antiarrhythmic drugs are not warranted because 80%-90% of patients will not have syncope or sudden death.

Ventricular Tachycardia and Fibrillation

Patients who present with ventricular tachycardia or fibrillation or who survive sudden cardiac death have lethal ventricular arrhythmias and a significant risk of recurrence. Survivors of sudden cardiac death have a risk of death approaching 30% in 1 year after hospital dismissal. They should receive electrophysiology-guided therapy, which improves outcome. For about 40% of patients, an antiarrhythmic drug is identified that prevents induction of ventricular tachycardia or fibrillation, and these patients have approximately a 5% chance of death at 1 year if dismissed with that medication. Patients in whom the baseline electrophysiology study is negative or an antiarrhythmic drug cannot be identified to prevent tachycardia continue to have increased risk for sudden death and should be considered for antitachycardia surgery or an implantable cardioverter-defibrillator. This device has reduced the recurrence rate of sudden death to 2% at 1 year and to 4% at 4 years; the overall mortality rate is 10% at 1 year and 20% at 4 years.

- Patients with ventricular tachycardia or fibrillation who survive sudden cardiac death have significant risk of recurrence.

- Survivors of sudden cardiac death have a risk of death of 30% at 1 year after hospital dismissal.
- Electrophysiology-guided therapy improves outcome.
- For 40% of patients, an effective antiarrhythmic drug can be identified.

Torsades de Pointes

This is a form of ventricular tachycardia with a characteristic polymorphic morphology described as a "twisting of the points" (torsades de pointes) (Fig. 3-7). The QT interval is prolonged, and the tachycardia is initiated by a late-coupled PVC. The arrhythmia is usually due to a medication (quinidine, procainamide, disopyramide, sotalol, tricyclic antidepressants), electrolyte disturbance (hypokalemia), or bradycardia (especially after myocardial infarction). After the tachycardia has been converted to sinus rhythm (electrically or spontaneously), treatment should be aimed at shortening the QT interval until the offending drug can be metabolized or the electrolyte disturbance or bradycardia corrected. Treatment options include temporary overdrive pacing, isoproterenol infusion, or magnesium. Patients with QT prolongation in the absence of medications, electrolytes, or bradycardia have a congenital form of this problem and are usually treated with a β-adrenergic blocker.

- Torsades de pointes is a form of ventricular tachycardia involving a prolonged QT interval.
- Torsades de pointes is usually due to a medication, an electrolyte disturbance, or bradycardia.
- Treatment includes temporary overdrive pacing, isoproterenol, or magnesium.

Ventricular Arrhythmias During Acute Myocardial Infarction

Prevention of myocardial ischemia and the use of β-adrenergic blockers are essential after acute myocardial infarction to decrease the frequency of life-threatening ventricular arrhythmias. Asymptomatic complex ventricular ectopy, including nonsustained ventricular tachycardia, should not be treated empirically because the risk of proarrhythmia outweighs the potential benefit of therapy for reducing the incidence of sudden cardiac death after hospital dismissal. Studies are assessing the use of amiodarone or risk stratification with ejection fraction, signal-averaged ECG, and electrophysiologic testing after myocardial infarction in an attempt to decrease the incidence of sudden death.

Ventricular tachycardia and fibrillation occurring within 24 hours after myocardial infarction are independent risk factors for in-hospital mortality at the time of the acute myocardial infarction but are not risk factors for subsequent total mortality or mortality due to an arrhythmic event after hospital dismissal and do not require antiarrhythmic therapy.

Ventricular tachycardia and fibrillation occurring 24 hours or longer after an acute myocardial infarction in the absence of reinfarction are independent risk factors for increased total mortality and death due to an arrhythmic event after hospital dismissal. Patients should be assessed with electrophysiologic testing, and treatment options include serial-guided antiarrhythmic drug testing, implantable cardioverter-defibrillator, and endocardial resection.

Episodes of refractory ventricular tachycardia and fibrillation during acute myocardial infarction should be treated with intravenously administered lidocaine, procainamide, or bretylium, and patients should have adequate oxygenation and normal electrolyte values. If these drugs are ineffective, alternative therapies to prevent recurrences of tachycardia include overdrive pacing if the tachycardia follows a bradycardia event, high-dose amiodarone, interaortic balloon pump, and coronary revascularization.

- Refractory ventricular tachycardia and fibrillation during acute myocardial infarction should be treated with intravenously administered lidocaine, procainamide, or bretylium.
- Alternative therapies are overdrive pacing, high-dose amiodarone, and coronary revascularization.

Role of Pacing in Acute Myocardial Infarction

Among patients with an acute inferior myocardial infarction, 5%-10% have Mobitz I second-degree or third-degree block in the absence of bundle branch block, and the site is usually in the AV node. This is usually transient, tends not to recur, and requires pacing only if there are symptoms as a result of bradycardia.

Bundle branch block occurs in 10%-20% of patients with acute myocardial infarction; in half of these patients, it is present at initial presentation, often representing preexisting conduction system disease. Approximately 40% of patients with right bundle branch block and either left-axis or right-axis deviation (fascicular block) will have transient complete heart block in the first few days after myocardial infarction. In 20% of patients with new left bundle branch block or bundle branch block of uncertain duration, complete heart block develops. The appearance of new bundle branch block is an indication for prophylactic temporary pacing.

- Bundle branch block occurs in 10%-20% of patients with acute myocardial infarction.
- In 20% of patients with new left bundle branch block or bundle branch block of uncertain duration, complete heart block develops.

Death in patients with myocardial infarction and bundle branch block is usually due to advanced heart failure and ventricular arrhythmias rather than to development of complete heart block. Patients in whom transient complete heart block develops in association with bundle branch block are at risk for recurrent complete heart block and should undergo permanent pacing. New bundle branch block that never progresses to complete heart block is not an indication for permanent pacing.

- Death in patients with myocardial infarction and bundle branch block is due to advanced heart failure.
- New bundle branch block that never progresses to complete heart block is not an indication for permanent pacing.

PART III
Rick A. Nishimura, M.D.

Coronary artery disease, principally myocardial infarction, accounts for approximately one of three deaths in the U.S., or nearly 600,000 deaths annually. The substantial reductions in the death rate from acute myocardial infarction that have occurred in the last 2 decades (Fig. 3-25) are attributed to efforts in primary prevention and new interventions in the treatment of myocardial infarction. The variable presentation of myocardial infarction includes asymptomatic patients; ones with angina, silent ischemia, unstable angina, or myocardial infarction; and sudden death.

- About 1/3 of deaths annually in the U.S. are due to myocardial infarction.
- The substantial decrease in the last 2 decades in death from acute myocardial infarction is due to primary prevention and new treatments of myocardial infarction.

PRIMARY PREVENTION OF CORONARY ARTERY DISEASE IN MYOCARDIAL INFARCTION

The known risk factors for coronary artery disease are tobacco abuse, serum cholesterol level, a lower serum HDL cholesterol level, serum LDL cholesterol level, hypertension, physical activity, obesity, diabetes mellitus, estrogens, and alcohol. Primary prevention includes modification of the following risk factors (N Engl J Med 326:1406-1416, 1992):

- Smoking more than doubles the incidence of coronary artery disease and increases mortality by 70%.
- The relative risk of smokers who have quit smoking decreases rapidly, approaching the levels of nonsmokers within 2-3 years.
- A 1% decrease in total serum cholesterol yields a 2%-3% decrease in the risk of coronary artery disease.
- The estimated decreased risk of myocardial infarction is 2%-3% for each 1-mm Hg decrease in diastolic blood pressure.

- The estimated decrease in the risk of myocardial infarction with the maintenance of an active compared with sedentary lifestyle is 35%-55%.
- The adjusted mortality rates for coronary artery disease are two to three times higher in men with diabetes mellitus and three to seven times higher in women with diabetes mellitus.
- In postmenopausal women, the decrease in risk of coronary artery disease attributable to estrogen therapy is 44%.
- Although heavy alcohol use increases the risk of cardiovascular disease, moderate consumption decreases the risk of heart disease.

MECHANISM OF ATHEROSCLEROSIS

The "response to injury" hypothesis is the most prevalent explanation of atherosclerosis (N Engl J Med 326:242-250, 1992). According to this hypothesis, chronic minimal injury to the arterial endothelium is caused mainly by a disturbance in the pattern of blood flow (type I injury), potentiated by high cholesterol levels, infections, and tobacco smoke. Type I injury leads to accumulation of lipids and macrophages. Release of toxic products by macrophages produces type II injury, which is characterized by the adhesion of platelets. Macrophages and platelets with endothelial-release growth factors cause migration and proliferation of smooth muscle cells, which form a fibrointimal lesion or lipid lesion. Disruption of a lipid lesion with a thin capsule causes type III damage, with thrombus formation. The thrombus may organize and contribute to the growth of the atherosclerotic lesion or become totally occluded, culminating in unstable angina or myocardial infarction (Fig. 3-26).

- The most prevalent explanation for atherosclerosis is the "response to injury" hypothesis.
- Type II injury is characterized by the adhesion of platelets.
- Type III damage is disruption of a lipid lesion leading to thrombus formation.
- Lipid-laden coronary artery lesions with less severe angio-

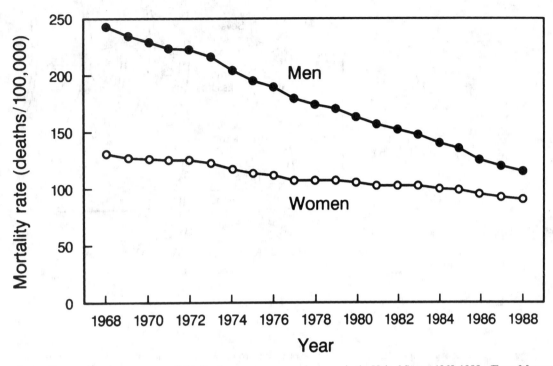

Fig. 3-25. Annual mortality rates from acute myocardial infarction among men and women in the United States, 1968-1988. (From Manson JE, Tosteson H, Ridker PM, Satterfield S, Hebert P, O'Connor GT, Buring JE, Hennekens CH: The primary prevention of myocardial infarction. N Engl J Med 326:1406-1416, 1992. By permission of the journal.)

graphic stenosis are more prone to rapid progression due to atherosclerotic plaque disruption.

- In up to two-thirds of cases of unstable angina or myocardial infarction, the lesion is a vessel with <50% stenosis.

CHRONIC STABLE ANGINA

Pathophysiology

In chronic stable angina, myocardial ischemia is caused chiefly by increased myocardial oxygen demand of the heart. Less important factors are perfusion pressure (aortic-to-right-atrial gradient), autoregulation (maintenance of coronary blood flow through a physiologic range of perfusion pressures), autonomic tone, and compressive effect (high left ventricular end-diastolic pressure decreases subendocardial flow). Normally, coronary blood flow can increase up to five times to meet myocardial oxygen demands of the heart. Ischemia occurs when flow reserve is inadequate, usually the result of fixed coronary artery disease. Resting blood flow does not cause ischemia unless vessel stenosis is >95%. However, a decrease in flow reserve begins to occur with about 60% stenosis, which is the mechanism for ischemia with exercise. The four factors that determine myocardial oxygen consumption are heart rate, afterload, contractility, and wall tension [wall tension = (left ventricular radius) x (left ventricular pressure)]. With a dilated, poorly contractile left ventricle, the contribution of wall tension to myocardial oxygen consumption outweighs

the other factors. The temporal sequence of events includes ischemia → diastolic dysfunction → regional wall motion abnormalities → electrocardiographic changes → pain.

- In chronic stable angina, myocardial ischemia is caused by increased myocardial oxygen demand.
- Normally, coronary blood flow can increase up to five times to meet myocardial oxygen demands.
- Resting blood flow does not cause ischemia unless stenosis is >95%.
- Four factors of myocardial oxygen consumption: heart rate, afterload, contractility, and wall tension.
- The temporal sequence of events: ischemia → diastolic dysfunction → regional wall motion abnormalities → electrocardiographic changes → pain.

Symptomatic Chronic Coronary Artery Disease

Many patients have symptoms of angina pectoris during physical activity. The pain is described variously as "pressure," "burning," "stabbing," "ache," "hurt," or "shortness of breath." It can be substernal or epigastric and can radiate to the neck, jaw, shoulder, elbow, or wrist. In chronic stable angina, the pain lasts 2-30 minutes and is usually relieved by rest. It is generally precipitated by any activity that increases myocardial oxygen consumption. The physical signs occurring with the pain include onset of a fourth heart sound and mitral regurgitant murmur due to papillary muscle dysfunction. ST-segment depression may be found on the electrocardiogram

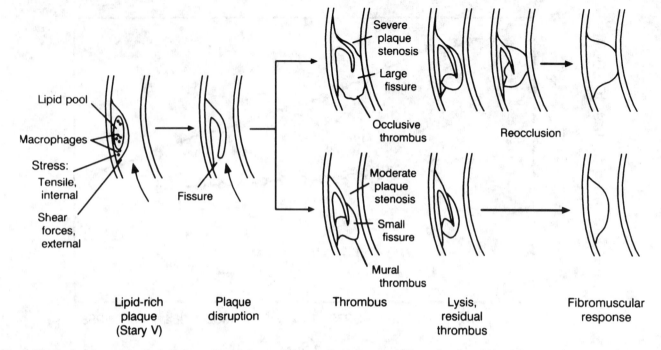

Fig. 3-26.--Typical dynamic evolution of complicated disrupted plaque. Curved arrows indicate direction of blood flow. (From Fuster V, Badimon L, Badimon JJ, Chesebro JH: The pathogenesis of coronary artery disease and the acute coronary syndromes [First of two parts]. N Engl J Med 326:242-250, 1992. By permission of the journal.)

(ECG), indicating subendocardial ischemia. The double product [(heart rate) x (systolic blood pressure)] is useful for defining myocardial oxygen demand. Nocturnal angina can be caused by unstable angina and also by increased wall tension with left ventricular dysfunction.

- The pain of angina pectoris during physical exercise is described in various ways.
- Physical signs occurring with the pain are a fourth heart sound and mitral regurgitant murmur due to papillary muscle dysfunction.
- The double product [(heart rate) x (systolic blood pressure)] is useful for defining myocardial oxygen demand.

Silent Ischemia

Silent ischemia is common in patients with symptomatic stable coronary artery disease, unstable angina, or after myocardial infarction. It is diagnosed by the presence of ST-segment depression in the absence of symptoms. Silent ischemia can occur either with an increase in myocardial oxygen consumption or at rest. The treatment is similar to that for chronic unstable angina; nitrates, β-blockers, and calcium channel blockers are effective agents. Whether percutaneous transluminal coronary angioplasty or coronary artery bypass grafting should be performed for silent ischemia alone is debated. The prognosis for this condition is the same as for symptomatic ischemia.

- Silent ischemia is common in patients with symptomatic stable coronary artery disease, unstable angina, or after

myocardial infarction.
- Silent ischemia is diagnosed by the presence of ST-segment depression in the absence of symptoms.
- Treatment is similar to that for chronic unstable angina.
- Nitrates, β-blockers, and calcium channel blockers are effective therapeutic agents in silent ischemia.
- Whether coronary angioplasty or bypass grafting should be performed for silent ischemia is debated.
- The prognosis is the same for silent ischemia and symptomatic ischemia.

Ancillary Testing

Ancillary tests for coronary artery disease include measurement of left ventricular function, stress testing, and coronary angiography. Left ventricular function is the most important predictor of prognosis and should be measured in all patients by two-dimensional echocardiography, radionuclide angiography, or left ventricular angiography. Exercise testing is performed with the treadmill or bicycle exertion test in conjunction with ECG monitoring, thallium scanning (perfusion of myocardium), radionuclide angiography (left ventricular function), or echocardiography (left ventricular function) to check for ischemia. During a standard treadmill test (i.e., exercise with stepped increases in workload every 2-3 minutes), heart rate, blood pressure, and the onset of subjective symptoms are monitored. Continuous monitoring of cardiac rhythm and 12-lead ECG at 1-minute intervals are performed. The ECG is positive for ischemia if a flat ST-segment depression is ≥1 mm. The ECG response is uninterpretable on the treadmill exertion test when there are resting T-wave abnormalities, left bundle branch block, left ventricular hypertrophy, paced rhythm, digoxin therapy, or mitral valve prolapse. For interpreting the results of this test, Bayes' theorem is important. According to this theorem, the predictive value of a test depends on the prevalence of the disease in the population studied.

- The most important predictor of prognosis is left ventricular function.
- The ECG is positive for ischemia if a flat ST-segment depression is ≥1 mm.
- T-wave abnormalities, left bundle branch block, left ventricular hypertrophy, paced rhythm, digoxin therapy, or mitral valve prolapse make the ECG response to the treadmill exertion test uninterpretable.
- Bayes' theorem--the predictive value of a test depends on the prevalence of the disease in the population studied.

As indicated in Figure 3-27, the sensitivity and specificity of ECG treadmill exertion testing are about 70% and 75%, respectively. Thus, a young patient with atypical chest pain and no risk factors (A in Fig. 3-27) has a low pretest probability (5%) of coronary artery disease. If the test results are negative, the probability decreases to 3%. However, if the results are positive, the probability is <15%. In comparison, an older man (B in Fig. 3-27) with typical chest pain and multiple risk factors has a high pretest probability (90%) of coronary artery disease, and even with negative test results, the probability is >70%. The treadmill exertion test should not be used to make the *diagnosis* of coronary artery disease.

Several different types of cardiac imaging modalities add to the sensitivity and specificity of ECG treadmill exertion testing. In thallium imaging, thallium-201 injected at peak exercise labels areas of perfusion; "cold spots" are nonperfused regions. Scanning is repeated 3 to 24 hours later. Persistent cold spots indicate previous infarction, and reperfused areas indicate ischemia. Single photon emission computed tomography (SPECT) thallium scanning (use of multiple tomographic planes) is more accurate than planar thallium scanning. In patients with left bundle branch block and severe left ventricular hypertrophy, thallium scanning gives false-positive results. In radionuclide angiography (multiple-gated acquisition scanning, MUGA), erythrocytes are labeled with technetium-99m and the left ventricular cavity is imaged during the cardiac cycle to measure, at rest and at peak exercise, left ventricular volume, ejection fraction, and regional wall motion abnormalities. MUGA is positive if the ejection fraction decreases (>5%-7%) and/or new regional wall motion abnormalities appear. Because multiple cycles are gated, MUGA cannot be used with irregular rhythms. In exercise echocardiography, two-dimensional echocardiography is performed at rest and at peak exercise. Digital acquisition allows side-by-side comparisons of images from the same view. The test is positive for ischemia if global systolic function decreases and/or new regional wall motion abnormalities appear.

- The sensitivity and specificity of ECG treadmill exertion testing are about 70% and 75%, respectively.
- The treadmill exertion test should not be used to make the diagnosis of coronary artery disease.
- Thallium scanning gives false-positive results in patients with left bundle branch block and severe left ventricular hypertrophy.
- MUGA is positive if the ejection fraction decreases (>5%-7%) and/or new regional wall motion abnormalities appear.
- Two-dimensional echocardiography is positive for ischemia if global systolic function decreases and/or new regional wall motion abnormalities appear.

All these imaging modalities are more expensive than the ECG treadmill exertion test. Because Bayes' theorem applies, imaging modalities should not be used for diagnosis of coronary artery disease over ECG treadmill testing except in cases of an uninterpretable ECG, or false-positive ECG results, or for localizing specific regions of ischemia (for future revascularization procedures).

Pharmacologic stress tests that provoke ischemia have been developed for patients who cannot exercise. These tests include the use of dipyridamole thallium, which redistributes flow away from ischemic myocardium. Adenosine thallium works in the same way as dipyridamole. In dobutamine echocardiography, the myocardial oxygen demand is increased. Pacing echocardiography increases heart rate.

Treadmill exertion testing identifies high-risk patients. High-risk patients are identified if the following are obtained on

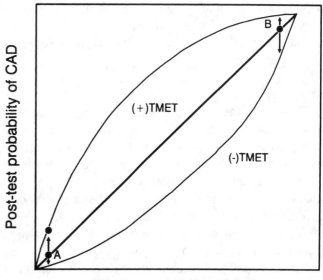

Fig. 3-27. The effect of Bayes' theorem on the ability of treadmill exertion testing (TMET) to diagnose coronary artery disease (CAD). Representative patients A and B are described in the text.

testing: less than stage I of the Bruce protocol, heart rate of <120 beats per minute, ST-segment depression >2 mm, ST-segment depression greater than 6 minutes' duration after stopping, decreased blood pressure, multiple perfusion defects, and an ejection fraction decrease >20%. In patients with poor prognostic factors, it is reasonable to proceed with coronary angiography to define the anatomy of the coronary arteries and the need for intervention. However, in patients who achieve a good work load without significant ST-segment depression and have appropriate blood pressure and heart rate responses, medical management is indicated because of the excellent prognosis.

- The major usefulness of stress testing is to identify high-risk patients, not to diagnose coronary artery disease.
- The treadmill exertion test should not be performed on patients with either unstable angina or severe aortic stenosis.

Coronary Angiography

Although coronary angiography has many limitations, it is the standard method for defining the severity of coronary artery disease. Subjective visual estimation of the percentage of stenosis may grossly underestimate the severity of the disease, especially if it is diffuse, because angiography outlines only the vessel lumen. The risk of serious complications of coronary angiography is about 1%; they include vascular complications (1.0%), myocardial infarction (0.5%), stroke (0.5%), ventricular fibrillation (0.5%), and death (0.1%). Risk is greater in older patients or in those with severe left ventricular dysfunction, left main coronary artery disease, or other coexistent medical diseases.

- Coronary angiography is the standard method for defining the severity of coronary artery disease.
- Visual estimation of the percentage of stenosis may grossly underestimate disease severity.
- The risk of serious complications in coronary angiography is about 1%.

Medical Therapy

The medical treatment for chronic stable angina should be given in a step-wise manner according to symptoms. Initial therapy is sublingual nitroglycerin as needed. Long-acting nitrates, calcium channel blockers, or β-blockers should be added sequentially if symptoms continue. A first-line drug should be increased to the optimal dosage before a second or third drug is added. Nitrates relieve angina mainly by producing venodilatation, which decreases wall tension. Calcium channel blockers relieve angina by decreasing afterload, heart rate, and contractility. Different calcium channel blockers have different relative effects (Table 3-10). β-Blockers relieve angina mainly by decreasing heart rate, reducing contractility, and decreasing (long-term) blood pressure (renin effect). β-Blockers are the most effective drugs for reducing the double product

(heart rate x blood pressure) with exercise.

Nitrate tolerance can occur with continuous exposure (use nitrate-free interval with dosing three times daily). Isosorbide dinitrate, at least 20-30 mg three times a day, needs to be used. β-Blockers should not be used if the patient has significant bronchospastic disease, congestive heart failure, or bradycardia. β-Blockers should be given at a dosage that keeps the resting heart rate <70 beats per minute. Always look for treatable underlying factors contributing to ischemia (anemia, thyroid abnormalities, hypoxia). In patients with left ventricular dysfunction and nocturnal angina, diuretics and angiotensin converting enzyme (ACE) inhibitors may be helpful in reducing wall tension.

- The initial therapy for chronic stable angina is sublingual nitroglycerin as needed.
- Add long-acting nitrates, calcium channel blockers, or β-blockers sequentially if symptoms continue.
- Nitrates relieve angina by producing venodilatation, which decreases wall tension.
- Calcium channel blockers relieve angina by decreasing afterload, heart rate, and contractility.
- β-Blockers relieve angina by decreasing heart rate, reducing contractility, and decreasing blood pressure.
- β-Blockers are the most effective drugs for reducing the double product.
- Nitrate tolerance can occur with continuous exposure.
- Do not use β-blockers if the patient has significant bronchospastic disease, congestive heart failure, or bradycardia.
- β-Blockers should be given at a dosage to keep the resting heart rate <70 beats per minute.
- Look for treatable underlying factors contributing to ischemia.
- Diuretics and ACE inhibitors may be helpful in patients with left ventricular dysfunction and nocturnal angina.

Antiplatelet agents may be helpful in patients with chronic stable angina pectoris. A low dose of aspirin probably does not prevent progression of atherosclerosis, but it may prevent acute myocardial infarction in patients with known coronary artery disease. In two large primary prevention trials, aspirin produced a 33% decrease in the risk for first, nonfatal myocardial infarction in men (no convincing data exist about the use of aspirin in women). The role of aspirin in primary prevention of stroke or overall cardiovascular mortality is uncertain.

- A low dose of aspirin probably does not prevent progression of atherosclerosis but may prevent acute myocardial infarction in patients with known coronary artery disease.
- No convincing data exist about the use of aspirin in women.
- The role of aspirin in primary prevention of stroke or overall cardiovascular mortality is uncertain.

Table 3-10.--Relative Effects of Calcium Channel Blockers

	Verapamil	Nifedipine	Diltiazem
Decrease heart rate	+++	±	+
Decrease blood pressure	++	+++	++
Decrease contractility	+++	+	++
Side effects	Constipation	Edema	Least
	AV block	Hypotension	
Lowest effective dose	360 mg/day	90 mg/day	300 mg/day

+, effective; ++, more effective; +++, most effective; ±, little effect.
AV, atrioventricular.

Catheter-Based Treatment

Percutaneous transluminal coronary angioplasty (PTCA) is the most common catheter-based intervention. PTCA is a combination of "splitting" the atheroma and stretching the noninvolved segment of artery. In experienced laboratories, the success rate is usually >90%. However, there is a risk of emergency coronary artery bypass (1%-2%), myocardial infarction (2%-4%), and death (1%). These risks are increased in long, tubular, eccentric, and calcified lesions and also in older women. Restenosis is a major problem (30%-45% restenosis at 6 months). Antiplatelet agents given before PTCA may reduce the rate of acute closure but do not prevent restenosis. Other catheter-based therapies (atherectomy, Rotoblator laser) have high restenosis rates similar to those of PTCA. These other catheter-based therapies are used in an attempt to prevent acute complications of balloon dilatation or to achieve a better result with balloon dilatation. Preliminary trials suggest that stent placement may reduce the rate of restenosis, but long-term follow-up is needed. No medical therapy has proved effective in preventing restenosis after PTCA or other catheter-based therapies.

- PTCA is a combination of splitting the atheroma and stretching the noninvolved segment of artery.
- The initial success rate is usually >90%.
- Restenosis is a major problem (30%-45% restenosis at 6 months).
- Antiplatelet agents do not prevent restenosis.
- No medical therapy is effective in preventing restenosis after PTCA.

Surgical Treatment

The surgical treatment for severely symptomatic patients with chronic stable angina is coronary artery bypass grafting (CABG) with either saphenous vein or internal mammary artery grafts. CABG provides excellent relief from symptoms (partial relief in >90% of patients and complete relief in >70%).

In-hospital mortality after CABG varies widely from 2% to 30%. Mortality increases with age, poor ventricular function, female sex, left main coronary artery disease, unstable angina, and diabetes mellitus. Complications of CABG include sternal wound infection (especially in patients with diabetes mellitus), severe left ventricular dysfunction (from inadequate cardioprotection), and late constrictive pericarditis. The procedure is not without latent problems. Closure rates of saphenous vein grafts are 20% and 50% at 1 year and 5 years, respectively. The patency rate is higher in internal mammary arteries, possibly up to 90% patency at 5 years.

- CABG provides excellent relief from symptoms.
- CABG gives partial relief in >90% of patients and complete relief in >70%.
- In-hospital mortality after CABG varies widely from 2% to 30%.
- Mortality increases with age, poor ventricular function, female sex, left main coronary artery disease, unstable angina, and diabetes mellitus.
- Closure rates of saphenous vein grafts are 20% and 50% at 1 year and 5 years, respectively.
- CABG does not prevent myocardial infarction.
- CABG does not uniformly improve left ventricular function.
- CABG does not decrease ventricular arrhythmias.
- CABG only improves survival in patients with 1) left main coronary artery disease, 2) three-vessel disease and moderately depressed left ventricular function, 3) three-vessel disease and severe symptoms of ischemia at a low workload, and 4) multivessel disease with involvement of the proximal left anterior descending artery. In all other subsets of patients, CABG should not be performed to improve survival.
- The indications for CABG versus medical therapy are 1) relief of symptoms in patients who have limiting symptoms unresponsive to medical management and 2) prolonging life in subsets of patients listed above.

Medical Versus Catheter-Based Versus Surgical Therapy

The decision about which therapy to use for a patient with chronic, stable angina is an individual one and must be based on the patient's age, lifestyle, and personal preference. However, randomized trials have compared the medical, catheter-based, and surgical therapies, and their results help in guiding decisions on which therapy to use for a selected subset of patients. The following summarizes the results of these trials.

1. Medical therapy versus PTCA (one-vessel disease):

- PTCA has a higher incidence of myocardial infarction and emergency CABG.
- PTCA does not decrease the future risk of myocardial infarction.
- PTCA does not improve resting left ventricular function.
- PTCA does not increase survival.

2. PTCA versus surgical therapy (multivessel disease--excluding left main coronary artery disease and totally occluded vessels):

- The incidences of death or myocardial infarction are similar.
- The rates of procedure-related mortality are similar (1%-2%).
- There are more procedure-related Q-wave infarctions with CABG versus PTCA (8%-10% versus 2%-3%), but events are well tolerated.
- The duration of initial hospitalization is longer for CABG versus PTCA.
- Patients undergoing CABG have less angina, require less antianginal medication, and are less likely to need a revascularization procedure than those undergoing PTCA.

Postcardiotomy Syndrome

Postcardiotomy syndrome occurs 2 weeks to 2 years postoperatively and consists of fever, pericarditis, and increased sedimentation rate. Rarely, it can present as pericardial tamponade. It is probably an autoimmune process (associated with antimyocardial antibodies); treatment is with aspirin and nonsteroidal anti-inflammatory drugs. Postperfusion syndrome is also characterized by fever and pericarditis but is associated with increased values on liver function tests and atypical lymphocytes, presumably due to cytomegalovirus syndrome. In patients with fever and pleuritic chest pain postoperatively, measure the sedimentation rate and perform a special blood smear to check for postperfusion or postcardiotomy syndrome.

- Postcardiotomy syndrome occurs 2 weeks to 2 years postoperatively.

- It consists of fever, pericarditis, and increased sedimentation rate.
- It is probably an autoimmune process (associated with antimyocardial antibodies).
- Treatment--aspirin and nonsteroidal anti-inflammatory drugs.
- Postperfusion syndrome: fever, pericarditis, increased values on liver function tests, and atypical lymphocytes.
- Measure the sedimentation rate and perform a special blood smear in patients with fever and pleuritic chest pain postoperatively to check for postcardiotomy or postperfusion syndrome.

UNSTABLE ANGINA

The definition of unstable angina is 1) accelerating pattern of angina, 2) rest pain or prolonged episodes of pain, 3) new onset of rapidly progressive angina, or 4) nocturnal angina. The mechanism is probably plaque rupture, with platelet aggregation and subsequent thrombus formation. Coronary artery spasm may have a role. The vasomotor response of coronary arteries is regulated by endothelial-relaxing and endothelial-constricting factors, which are activated partly by platelets. The diagnosis of unstable angina is made on the basis of the medical history, ST-segment changes on ECG, and the absence of increased creatine kinase-MB fraction. It is important to diagnose unstable angina because it may be the prelude to acute myocardial infarction.

- Unstable angina is 1) accelerating pattern of angina, 2) rest pain or prolonged episodes of pain, 3) new onset of rapidly progressive angina, or 4) nocturnal angina.
- The mechanism is probably plaque rupture, with platelet aggregation and subsequent thrombus formation.
- Coronary artery vasomotor response is regulated by endothelial-relaxing and endothelial-constricting factors.
- The diagnosis is made on the basis of the medical history, ST-segment changes, and the absence of increased creatine kinase-MB fraction.

Treatment of unstable angina consists of immediate hospitalization with ECG monitoring. It is important to decrease the myocardial oxygen demand. First and foremost, unstable angina is treated with sedation (to decrease anxiety and catecholamine stimulation of the heart). β-Blockers, nitrates, and calcium channel blockers are effective in decreasing myocardial oxygen demand (see Chronic Stable Angina, page 77). Antiplatelet agents, such as aspirin, are effective in decreasing the incidence of progression to myocardial infarction and should be used in all patients. Heparin given intravenously also reduces the incidence of progression to myocardial infarction and should be used in all patients without any contraindication.

- For unstable angina, immediate hospitalization with ECG monitoring.
- Decrease myocardial oxygen demand with β-blockers, nitrates, and calcium channel blockers.
- Antiplatelet agents are effective in decreasing the incidence of progression to myocardial infarction and should be used in all patients.
- Heparin given intravenously should be used in all patients without any contraindication.

The work-up for unstable angina is controversial. However, most cardiologists usually recommend coronary angiography to define coronary anatomy. Exercise testing is usually not performed because it may cause myocardial infarction. PTCA or CABG has not been shown to prevent myocardial infarction or to prolong longevity. However, even with optimal medical therapy, there is a high crossover to revascularization therapy in the following 6 months. Therefore, in certain clinical situations, it is reasonable to proceed with revascularization in patients with unstable angina and suitable coronary artery anatomy.

- Most cardiologists usually recommend coronary angiography for patients with unstable angina.
- Exercise testing usually is not performed.
- PTCA or CABG has not been shown to prevent myocardial infarction or to prolong longevity in patients with unstable angina but both are highly effective in relieving pain.

CORONARY ARTERY SPASM

The vasomotor tone of coronary arteries is important in the pathogenesis of coronary artery disease. Coronary artery vasoconstriction can be seen as a response to arterial injury. The endothelium affects vascular tone by releasing relaxing factors, e.g., prostacyclin and endothelium-derived relaxing factor, that prevent vasoconstriction and platelet deposition. With dysfunctional endothelium, these factors are absent and the coronary arteries may be more prone to spasm. Most clinical episodes of coronary artery spasm occur superimposed on atherosclerotic plaques. However, patients may have primary coronary artery spasm and angiographically normal coronary arteries.

- Endothelium affects vascular tone by releasing relaxing factors, e.g., prostacyclin and endothelium-derived relaxing factor.
- With dysfunctional endothelium, coronary arteries may be more prone to spasm.
- Most episodes of spasm occur superimposed on atherosclerotic plaques.
- Patients may have primary coronary artery spasm and angiographically normal coronary arteries.

The typical presentation of coronary artery spasm consists of recurrent episodes of rest pain in association with ST-segment elevation, which reverses with administration of nitrates. Coronary angiography with ergonovine challenge has been used to diagnose these patients, but its sensitivity and specificity are unknown. The use of acetylcholine to provoke spasm may be more useful. ST-segment elevation on the resting 12-lead ECG during an episode of rest pain is the standard criterion for diagnosing coronary artery spasm. Coronary artery spasm is treated with long-acting nitrates and/or calcium channel blockers.

- The typical presentation of coronary artery spasm is recurrent episodes of rest pain and ST-segment elevation that is reversed with nitrates.
- The standard criterion for diagnosis: spontaneous ST-segment elevation on resting 12-lead ECG during rest pain.

MYOCARDIAL INFARCTION

Background

Myocardial infarction accounts for a large percentage of morbidity and mortality in the U.S. in the 1990s. More than 500,000 people are admitted annually to a hospital because of myocardial infarction. However, >50% of people with myocardial infarction die before reaching the hospital. With the advent of coronary care units 3 decades ago, mortality from myocardial infarction was trimmed from 30% to 15% by treating ventricular arrhythmias. Beta-blockade has further decreased in-hospital and post-hospital mortality by 30%-40%. In the late 1980s, reperfusion therapy was shown to further improve survival and has become standard care for selected patients with myocardial infarction. Currently, overall in-hospital mortality is 5%-10%. After myocardial infarction, another 2%-10% die in the ensuing year.

- More than 50% of people with myocardial infarction die before reaching the hospital.
- By treating ventricular arrhythmias, mortality was trimmed from 30% to 15%.
- β-Blockade has reduced in-hospital and post-hospital mortality by 30%-40%.
- Thrombolytic therapy has reduced overall mortality to 5%-10%.

Pathogenesis

Acute transmural myocardial infarction is usually caused by sudden complete occlusion of a coronary artery. The mechanism of myocardial infarction is usually plaque rupture, leading to platelet aggregation and thrombus formation. Without collateral circulation, 90% of the myocardium supplied by an occluded artery is infarcted within 3 hours.

- The usual cause of acute transmural myocardial infarction is sudden complete occlusion of a coronary artery.
- The usual mechanism is plaque rupture, leading to platelet aggregation and thrombus formation.

Currently, two categories of myocardial infarction used clinically are based on the ECG. "Q-wave myocardial infarction" is diagnosed on the basis of chest pain with ST-segment elevation and subsequent development of Q waves. (This term replaces "transmural myocardial infarction," because not all myocardial layers are necessarily involved.) The likelihood of occlusive coronary artery thrombus at early coronary angiography is high (>85%). "Non-Q-wave myocardial infarction" is diagnosed by two of the following three criteria: 1) prolonged chest pain, 2) persistent ST-segment changes >24 hours, and 3) increased creatine kinase-MB fraction. (This term replaces "subendocardial myocardial infarction.") The likelihood of an occlusive coronary artery thrombus is about 30%-40%. In patients with non-Q-wave myocardial infarction, multivessel disease is likely, because long-standing multivessel disease provides collaterals that prevent transmural injury.

- Q-wave myocardial infarction is diagnosed on the basis of chest pain with ST-segment elevation and subsequent Q waves.
- Q-wave myocardial infarctions are associated with larger infarctions and higher in-hospital mortality than non-Q-wave myocardial infarctions.
- Non-Q-wave myocardial infarctions have a higher risk for reinfarction, continued angina, and even posthospital death.
- Some advocate predismissal coronary angiography for all patients with non-Q-wave myocardial infarction.

Several new concepts have been developed in the past decade for examining patients with myocardial infarction. "Stunned myocardium" occurs when a coronary artery is completely occluded and then opened. If reperfusion occurs early enough, systolic contraction of the affected myocardium may remain reduced after the event, although the myocardium remains viable. Systolic contraction then returns hours to days later. Currently, no clinical test differentiates "stunned myocardium" from infarcted, dead myocardium. "Ischemia at a distance" occurs when infarction is in the distribution of one coronary vessel and ischemia with subsequent hypokinesis occurs in the distribution of a second vessel in which there is a high-grade stenosis. When this is seen on echocardiography, the prognosis is poor because of recurrent myocardial infarction and increased mortality. "Infarct remodeling" occurs mainly after large anteroapical myocardial infarctions. An area of infarction may undergo thinning, dilatation, and dyskinesis. This is associated with a higher incidence of congestive heart failure and posthospital mortality. ACE inhibitors may help prevent infarct remodeling.

- Stunned myocardium--a coronary artery is completely occluded and then opened and transient akinesis of the myocardium occurs.
- Ischemia at a distance--infarction is in the distribution of one coronary artery, and ischemia and subsequent hypokinesis are in the distribution of a second vessel in which there is a high-grade stenosis.
- Infarct remodeling--occurs after large anteroapical myocardial infarctions.
- ACE inhibitors may help prevent infarct remodeling.

Presentation and Diagnosis

The typical presentation of myocardial infarction is anginal-sounding pain lasting >30-45 minutes associated with ECG changes and elevated creatine kinase-MB fraction. However, >25%-30% of infarctions are silent and present later as new ECG abnormalities or regional wall motion abnormalities. Silent myocardial infarctions occur especially in patients with diabetes mellitus and in the elderly. Increased incidence of myocardial infarction in the early morning is perhaps related to increased platelet aggregation. The pain of myocardial infarction mimics that of other diseases, e.g., gastrointestinal or pericardial disease or musculoskeletal pain. Remember that myocardial infarction may occur without ECG changes. Thus, all patients with ischemic-sounding pain should be hospitalized despite lack of ECG changes. In these patients, echocardiography or radionuclide angiography showing regional wall motion abnormalities may help confirm the clinical diagnosis of myocardial infarction.

- More than 25%-30% of infarctions are silent.
- Silent infarctions occur especially in patients with diabetes mellitus and in the elderly.
- Increased incidence of myocardial infarction in the early morning perhaps is related to increased platelet aggregation.
- The pain of myocardial infarction mimics that of other diseases.
- Myocardial infarction may occur without ECG changes.
- All patients with ischemic-sounding pain should be hospitalized.

An increased creatine kinase-MB fraction, indicative of myocardial necrosis, confirms the clinical diagnosis of myocardial infarction. The peak values are at 12-20 hours. Thus, negative creatine kinase-MB fraction at admission does not rule out myocardial infarction. Any creatine kinase-MB peak occurring earlier than 12 hours may indicate reperfusion. (SGOT and LDH levels, used in the past, have later peaks but are usually not required for diagnosis of myocardial infarction.)

- An increased creatine kinase-MB fraction indicates myocar-

dial necrosis.
- Negative creatine kinase-MB fraction at admission does not rule out myocardial infarction.

Basic and Drug Treatments

Bed rest and sedation are essential and are beneficial in the acute stage of myocardial infarction for decreasing myocardial oxygen demand. Analgesics, particularly morphine, are beneficial for recurrent pain. Currently, prolonged bed rest is not recommended, and the effort to shorten hospitalization is increasing. Many physicians recommend a gradual increase in activity level over 3-6 days for an uncomplicated myocardial infarction. During the acute 3-4-day period, ECG monitoring is recommended for both tachyarrhythmias and bradyarrhythmias. Oxygen has no benefit unless hypoxia is present. However, modest hypoxemia is not uncommon, even with uncomplicated myocardial infarction, and is due to ventilation/perfusion lung mismatch.

- Prolonged bed rest is not recommended.
- Oxygen has no benefit unless hypoxia is present.

Heparin is important in treating acute myocardial infarction. It prevents 1) recurrent infarction, especially after thrombolytic therapy, 2) deep venous thrombosis, and 3) intracardiac thrombus formation. Intracardiac thrombus formation occurs in 40% of patients with anterior myocardial infarction, and almost 50% of these patients have a systemic embolic event. Thus, heparin therapy is especially indicated in these patients. The benefits of subcutaneous versus intravenous heparin are unsettled. Aspirin reduces recurrent infarction by 49% in patients not receiving thrombolytic therapy. It also reduces mortality when given in addition to thrombolytic therapy.

- Heparin is important in treating acute myocardial infarction.
- Heparin prevents recurrent infarction, deep venous thrombosis, and intracardiac thrombus formation.
- Intracardiac thrombus formation occurs in 40% of patients with anterior myocardial infarction.
- Aspirin reduces recurrent infarction by 49% in patients not receiving thrombolytic therapy.

Nitroglycerin is useful for a subset of patients with myocardial infarction--for those with heart failure (by decreasing wall tension) and for those with continued pain. In the early stages of myocardial infarction, nitroglycerin given intravenously should be used instead of long-acting nitrates given orally to prevent acute decreases in blood pressure. Intravenous nitroglycerin may reduce infarct size by decreasing wall tension and affecting "remodeling." Also, it may decrease susceptibility to ventricular fibrillation. If mean blood pressure is >80 mm Hg, intravenous nitroglycerin may reduce mortality by 10%-

25%, specifically in patients with anterior myocardial infarction and poor left ventricular function. However, in patients with low blood pressure and those with inferior and right ventricular infarctions, nitroglycerin may decrease blood pressure too much and may cause increased mortality. The dosage of intravenous nitroglycerin is a 15-μg bolus and an initial infusion of 10 μg/min. Intravenous infusion should be increased every 5-10 minutes until the blood pressure decreases 10%-15%, up to a maximum of 150-200 μg/min. Mean blood pressure should be kept at >80 mm Hg. Nitrate intolerance occurs with infusions lasting >24 hours. Do not use intravenous nitroglycerin in patients with low blood pressure or right ventricular infarction. Intravenous nitroglycerin may improve mortality in patients with large anterior myocardial infarctions and congestive heart failure.

- Nitroglycerin is useful for patients with heart failure and those with continued pain.
- Intravenous nitroglycerin may reduce infarct size by decreasing wall tension and affecting remodeling.
- Nitroglycerin may decrease susceptibility to ventricular fibrillation.
- Nitrate intolerance occurs with infusions >24 hours.
- Do not use intravenous nitroglycerin in patients with low blood pressure or right ventricular infarction.
- Intravenous nitroglycerin may improve mortality in patients with large anterior myocardial infarctions and congestive heart failure.

β-Blockers are useful both in acute myocardial infarction and postmyocardial infarction setting. If given early, they decrease infarction size and in-hospital mortality. If given after myocardial infarction is completed, β-blockers can reduce posthospital reinfarction and mortality. In an acute setting, the typical dosage of metoprolol is 5 mg given intravenously three times, 5 minutes apart, followed by 100 mg given orally twice daily. β-Blockers will also decrease the incidence of ventricular fibrillation and decrease pain. The beneficial effects are probably multifactorial but include 1) decreased myocardial oxygen demand, 2) increased threshold for ventricular fibrillation, 3) decreased platelet aggregability, and 4) decreased sympathetic effects on myocardium. β-Blockers are most beneficial in patients with large infarctions, i.e., those at higher risk of complications. Acute intravenous β-blockers are also beneficial in those patients undergoing thrombolytic therapy. β-Blockers are especially useful for patients with hyperdynamic circulation and continued postinfarction pain and should be given to patients presenting with <12 hours of pain who do not have contraindications, especially those with anterior myocardial infarction.

- Acute intravenous β-blockers decrease infarction size and in-hospital mortality.

- Acute intravenous β-blockers decrease the incidence of ventricular fibrillation.
- Contraindications to β-blockers are bradycardia, atrioventricular block, hypotension, severe heart failure, and inferior myocardial infarction with high vagal tone.

Calcium channel blockers have been used to treat myocardial infarction, but their routine use has *no* proven benefit. Routine use of verapamil and nifedipine has no benefit and may increase mortality. Diltiazem, 60-90 mg given every 6 hours within 72 hours of myocardial infarction, may prevent later reinfarction and recurrent angina in patients with non-Q-wave myocardial infarction; however, it probably increases mortality in patients with Q-wave myocardial infarction and depressed left ventricular function. Because most patients with non-Q-wave myocardial infarction at risk for later events will probably be identified and have a revascularization procedure performed, routine use of calcium channel blockers is not indicated. However, by producing coronary vasodilatation and decreasing myocardial oxygen demand, calcium channel blockers may be beneficial in treating postinfarction angina.

- Routine use of calcium channel blockers for myocardial infarction has no proven benefit.
- Routine use of verapamil and nifedipine may increase mortality.
- Calcium channel blockers may be beneficial for patients with postinfarction angina and those with non-Q-wave myocardial infarction.

Treatment--Reperfusion Therapy

Early reperfusion therapy has had tremendous impact on the treatment of acute myocardial infarction. Overall, mortality is decreased 27% ± 3% when reperfusion is given early. In >50,000 patients in ISIS-3 and GISSI-2 studies, the 35-day in-hospital mortality was only 10% with thrombolytic therapy. Time is of the essence when giving reperfusion therapy. The faster the reperfusion, the better the extent of myocardial salvage and the better the effect on mortality. Without collaterals, 90% of the myocardium at risk is infarcted within 3 hours after occlusion. Very early reperfusion has a major effect on direct myocardial salvage. In a study in which thrombolysis was given <90 minutes after pain onset, the mortality was 1%. In most U.S. studies, the average time from pain onset to artery opening is 3.7 hours. The delay is in patient presentation (22%), transport (21%), in-hospital institution of the drug (35%), and reperfusion drug time (19%). Reperfusion at 2-6 hours salvages the peri-infarction zone, depending on the degree of collateral circulation. Thus, there is a lesser effect on myocardial salvage but an important effect on survival. The "open artery concept" describes a benefit in improvement in posthospital mortality in the presence of an open artery after thrombolytic therapy, which is not reflected in improved ventricular function. The reason for this is unclear but may be related to improved electrical stability or prevention of ventricular remodeling.

- Overall, mortality is decreased 27% ± 3% when reperfusion is given early.
- In >50,000 patients, 35-day in-hospital mortality was 10% with thrombolytic therapy.
- The faster the reperfusion, the better the extent of myocardial salvage.
- Without collaterals, 90% of the myocardium at risk is infarcted within 3 hours after occlusion.

Controversy exists about the effectiveness of intravenous thrombolytic therapy versus emergency PTCA in patients with acute myocardial infarction. After administration of thrombolytic therapy, emergency PTCA is not indicated in the absence of ongoing pain, because of a higher incidence of complications than in patients not undergoing emergency PTCA. The controversy is now about whether intravenous thrombolytic therapy should be given versus emergency-direct PTCA. Intravenous thrombolysis may not be as effective (65%-70%) in opening arteries as PTCA (90%). However, this is counterbalanced by faster administration of intravenous thrombolysis and wider availability of the intravenous drug. Less than 10% of all hospitals have the capability for emergency PTCA. Late patency (>24 hours) is 70%-80% for both methods. Thus, with the lack of available resources, intravenous thrombolytic therapy is still the treatment of choice in patients with acute myocardial infarction. Emergency PTCA may be used in patients with 1) contraindication for intravenous thrombolysis, 2) cardiogenic shock, or 3) continued ischemia after thrombolytic therapy.

- The effectiveness of intravenous thrombolytic therapy versus emergency PTCA in patients with acute myocardial infarction is controversial.
- After giving thrombolytic therapy, emergency PTCA is not indicated in the absence of ongoing pain.
- Intravenous thrombolysis may not be as effective (65%-70%) in opening arteries as PTCA (90%).
- Less than 10% of hospitals have the capability for emergency PTCA.
- Intravenous thrombolytic therapy is still the treatment of choice in stable patients with acute myocardial infarction with no contraindications.

Thrombolytic therapy definitely is indicated for patients presenting within 6 hours after the onset of pain who have ST-segment elevation and no contraindication. It should be considered for patients up to 12 hours after onset of symptoms with continued pain. Whether thrombolytic therapy should be given to patients later than 6 hours after pain onset who have no evidence of continued ischemia is unclear. It should also be considered for patients presenting within 6 hours of pain onset and left bundle branch block. Thrombolytic therapy is not clearly indicated for patients with pain and other ECG abnormalities (ST-segment depression).

- Thrombolytic therapy definitely is indicated for patients presenting within 6 hours after the onset of pain who have ST-segment elevation and no contraindication.
- Whether thrombolytic therapy should be given to patients later than 6 hours after pain onset who have no evidence of continued ischemia is unclear.
- Thrombolytic therapy is not clearly indicated for patients with pain and other ECG abnormalities (ST-segment depression).

Contraindications to thrombolytic therapy include a history of bleeding, severe hypertension, recent stroke, diabetic hemorrhagic retinopathy, recent cardiopulmonary resuscitation, previous allergy to streptokinase, recent surgical procedure, suspected aortic dissection or pericarditis, and pregnancy. Major complications of intravenous thrombolysis include major bleeding (5%-6%), intracranial bleeding (0.5%), major allergic reaction (0.1%-1.7%), and hypotension (2%-10%). A higher incidence of myocardial rupture may occur in patients given thrombolytic therapy late (>12 hours after pain onset).

- Major complications of intravenous thrombolysis are major bleeding (5%-6%), intracranial bleeding (0.5%), major allergic reaction (0.1%-1.7%), and hypotension (2%-10%).
- A higher incidence of myocardial rupture may occur in patients given thrombolytic therapy late (>12 hours after pain onset).

Three agents are available for intravenous thrombolysis (Table 3-11). Streptokinase, a nonselective thrombolytic agent, combines with circulating plasminogen to split circulating and thrombus-bound plasminogen into plasmin, which splits fibrin. It lyses circulating fibrinogen and thus has systemic effects. The dosage is a 250,000-U bolus and 1.5×10^6 U in 1 hour. TPA (tissue plasminogen activator) binds to preformed fibrin preferentially and lyses it without activating plasminogen in the general circulation. Thus, it has less effect on circulating fibrinogen and is "fibrin-specific." It has the fastest onset of action. The dosage is 100 mg over 90 minutes. Anistreplase (APSAC) is composed of anisoylated plasminogen and streptokinase bound together and inactivated by plasminogen. It requires spontaneous deacylation, which occurs in the plasma before the active streptokinase-plasminogen complex is generated, splitting plasminogen to plasmin. Thus, anistreplase is a more stable agent and may be given as a single intravenous bolus. The dosage is 30 U over 5 minutes.

In the large European trials, there was no proven benefit of one thrombolytic therapy over the others. In the GUSTO trial, there was a lower mortality rate when an accelerated dose of TPA was given with intravenous heparin as compared with streptokinase. TPA is more costly than streptokinase and has a slightly increased risk of cerebral hemorrhage, especially in the elderly. It is thus reasonable to preferentially give TPA in the younger patient who presents very early with a large myocardial infarction.

After intravenous thrombolysis, a high-grade residual lesion is usually present. Reocclusion or ischemia occurs in 15%-20% of patients and reinfarction occurs in 2%-3%. In the U.S., both heparin and aspirin are given after intravenous thrombolysis to prevent reinfarction. The benefit with aspirin is clear but is less clear with heparin. The indication for coronary angiography or PTCA after intravenous thrombolysis is continued pain or ischemia documented on functional testing. There is no benefit from routine intervention in all patients.

- After intravenous thrombolysis, reocclusion or ischemia occurs in 15%-20% of patients and reinfarction occurs in 2%-3%.

Table 3-11.--Thrombolytic Agents

	Clot specific	Half-life	Allergic reaction	Dosage	Cost
Streptokinase	+	++	++	1.5×10^6 U/hr	+
TPA (tissue plasminogen activator)	+++	+	-	10 mg i.v. bolus with 90 mg i.v. over 90 min	+++
APSAC (anisoylated plasminogen-streptokinase activator complex)	+	+++	+	30 U/5 min	++

-, none; +, some; ++, more; +++, most.

- Both aspirin and heparin are given after intravenous thrombolysis to prevent reinfarction.
- The benefit is clear with aspirin but not with heparin.
- Streptokinase is the least expensive thrombolytic therapy.
- TPA is the most clot-specific thrombolytic therapy.
- The least amount of antigenicity is with TPA.

Acute Mechanical Complications of Myocardial Infarction

Cardiogenic shock after myocardial infarction has a high mortality, approaching 90%. However, it is important to determine the cause of cardiogenic shock. Although most cases are due to extensive left ventricular dysfunction, there are other causes, e.g., right ventricular infarction and mechanical complications of myocardial infarction. Swan-Ganz catheterization and two-dimensional echocardiography may help in determining its cause (Table 3-12).

- Cardiogenic shock after myocardial infarction approaches 90% mortality.
- Most cases of cardiogenic shock are due to extensive left ventricular dysfunction.
- Swan-Ganz catheterization and two-dimensional echocardiography may help determine other causes of cardiogenic shock.

Right ventricular infarction occurs in up to 40% of patients with inferior myocardial infarction and is diagnosed by elevated jugular venous pressure in the presence of clear lung fields. ST-segment elevation in a V_{4R} lead is diagnostic of a large right ventricular infarction and portends a high mortality rate. In extreme circumstances, right ventricular infarction can cause cardiogenic shock, because the right ventricle is not able to pump effectively enough blood to fill the left ventricle. Treatment includes large amounts of fluids given intravenously and infusion of dobutamine. If right ventricular infarction is recognized early, reperfusion therapy is indicated.

- Right ventricular infarction occurs in up to 40% of patients with inferior myocardial infarction.

Myocardial free wall rupture may occur and cause abrupt decompensation. Free wall rupture occurs in 85% of all ruptures. It occurs suddenly, usually 2-14 days after transmural myocardial infarction, most commonly in elderly hypertensive women. It presents as electromechanical dissociation or death. If rupture is contained in the pericardium, tamponade may occur. If the diagnosis can be made by emergency echocardiography, surgery should be performed. If the rupture is sealed off, pseudoaneurysm may occur; operation is required because of the high incidence of further rupture.

- Free wall rupture occurs in 85% of all ruptures.
- It occurs suddenly, usually 2-14 days after transmural myocardial infarction.

Papillary muscle rupture occurs in 5% of all ruptures and usually 2-10 days after myocardial infarction. It is associated with inferior myocardial infarction, because of the single blood supply to the posteromedial papillary muscle. Papillary muscle rupture is heralded by the sudden onset of dyspnea and hypotension. Although a murmur may be present, it is not audible because of equalization of left atrial and left ventricular pressures. The diagnosis is made with echocardiography or Swan-Ganz catheterization, which demonstrates a large "V" wave on pulmonary capillary wedge pressure. The treatment is intra-aortic balloon pumping and emergency operation.

- Papillary muscle rupture occurs in 5% of all ruptures.
- It usually occurs 2-10 days after myocardial infarction.
- It is associated with inferior myocardial infarction.
- It is heralded by sudden dyspnea and hypotension.
- It is diagnosed with echocardiography and Swan-Ganz catheterization.

Table 3-12.--Diagnosis of Cause of Cardiogenic Shock

	Swan-Ganz catheterization				2-Dimensional echocardiography
	RA	PCWP	CO		
Left ventricular dysfunction	↑	↑↑	↓↓		Poor left ventricle
Right ventricular infarction	↑↑	↓	↓↓		Dilated right ventricle
Tamponade	↑↑	↑↑	↓↓	End-equalization	Pericardial tamponade
PM rupture	↑	↑↑	↓↓	Large "V"	Severe MR
VSD	↑	↑↑	↑	Step-up	Defect seen
PE	↑↑	=	↓	PADP > PCWP	Dilated right ventricle

CO, cardiac output; MR, mitral regurgitation; PADP, pulmonary artery diastolic pressure; PCWP, pulmonary capillary wedge pressure; PE, pulmonary emboli; PM, papillary muscle; RA, right atrial pressure; VSD, ventricular septal defect.

Ventricular septal defects occur in 10% of all ruptures, usually 1-20 days after myocardial infarction. It is equally frequent in inferior and anterior myocardial infarctions. Ventricular septal defects associated with inferior myocardial infarctions have a poorer prognosis because of the serpiginous nature of the rupture and associated ventricular infarction. They are indicated by the sudden onset of dyspnea and hypotension. A loud murmur and systolic thrill are always present. The diagnosis is made with echocardiography or Swan-Ganz catheterization, which demonstrates a step-up in oxygen saturation from the right atrium to the pulmonary artery. Treatment is intra-aortic balloon pump and emergency operation.

- Ventricular septal defects occur in 10% of all ruptures.
- They are equally frequent in inferior and anterior myocardial infarctions.
- They are indicated by the sudden onset of dyspnea and hypotension.
- A ventricular septal defect almost always has a thrill and loud murmur.

Prehospital Dismissal Evaluation

To properly evaluate a patient with myocardial infarction before dismissal from the hospital, determine the predictors of mortality. These include status of the left ventricle, ventricular arrhythmias, and presence of continued myocardial ischemia.

Rehabilitation treadmill exertion testing should be performed in most patients after myocardial infarction to detect continued ischemia. It is a low-risk test in properly selected patients and is performed 8-10 days after the infarction. It is usually a limited workload to 5 metabolic equivalents (METs) or 70% of the maximum heart rate. High-risk patients identified by treadmill exertion testing have >1-mm ST-segment depression, decrease in blood pressure, or inability to achieve 4 METs on the exercise test. Imaging exercise tests may identify additional high-risk patients by demonstrating multiple areas of ischemia. Pharmacologic stress tests (dobutamine echocardiography, dipyridamole thallium scanning, or adenosine thallium scanning) may be useful in patients unable to exercise. The role of stress testing in patients after thrombolytic therapy is less clear.

- After myocardial infarction, most patients should undergo rehabilitation treadmill testing.
- It is a low-risk test in properly selected patients and is performed 8-10 days after the infarction.

ACE inhibitors should be given to all patients with large anterior myocardial infarctions to prevent infarct remodeling and expansion. In patients with ejection fractions <40%, the administration of ACE inhibitors will prevent future congestive heart failure and improve mortality. The time to start ACE inhibitors is not settled. Acute, intravenous administration of ACE inhibitors within 24 hours of an infarction may be detrimental. However, oral ACE inhibitors given at least 2-3 days after the onset of myocardial infarction are beneficial.

Coronary angiography is indicated after myocardial infarction if the results of a rehabilitation treadmill exertion test are positive or postinfarction angina occurs. Some cardiologists recommend coronary angiography in all patients with non-Q-wave myocardial infarction.

- Coronary angiography is indicated if the results of a rehabilitation treadmill exertion test are positive or postinfarction angina occurs.

No randomized trials have examined the benefit of PTCA or bypass grafting after myocardial infarction. However, in high-risk patients (i.e., those with continued ischemia or positive results on the treadmill exertion test), it is reasonable to proceed with intervention. PTCA can be undertaken if there is a single-vessel high-grade lesion amenable to the procedure. CABG should be performed if there is left main or proximal three-vessel disease or two- or three-vessel disease that supplies a large portion of the myocardium, especially when associated with moderate depression in left ventricular function.

The following apply to patients who survive acute myocardial infarction:

- Aspirin decreases recurrent myocardial infarction by 31% and late mortality by 15%, more so in cases of non-Q-wave myocardial infarction.
- Warfarin may cause a similar decrease in mortality and reinfarction, but it is not routinely used in the U.S.
- Diltiazem may be beneficial after non-Q-wave myocardial infarction to prevent reinfarction.
- β-Blockers improve survival after myocardial infarction.
- β-Blockers are most effective in high-risk patients (i.e., decreased left ventricular function and ventricular arrhythmias) and may not be required in low-risk patients.
- High dosages of β-blockers, equivalent to 200 mg of metoprolol per day, need to be administered.
- β-Blockers are also effective after thrombolytic therapy.
- Because antiarrhythmic agents are associated with increased mortality, they should not be used to suppress ventricular ectopy.
- ACE inhibitors decrease mortality after anterior myocardial infarction and depressed left ventricular function, presumably by inhibiting infarct remodeling.
- A rehabilitation program is essential for the patient's well-being and cardiovascular fitness.

PART IV
Rick A. Nishimura, M.D.
Barry L. Karon, M.D.

DEFINITION

Heart failure is the inability of the heart to meet the metabolic demands of the body while maintaining normal ventricular filling pressures. Although the commonest cause is left ventricular dysfunction (as in dilated cardiomyopathy), other causes must be considered. To treat heart failure properly, the cause and precipitating factors must be identified. Backward heart failure is caused by elevated filling pressure, which affects the pulmonary circulation and causes shortness of breath and paroxysmal nocturnal dyspnea. Elevated filling pressure can also affect the systemic circulation and cause edema and ascites. Forward heart failure is caused by low cardiac output, which produces symptoms of fatigue and lethargy. Most patients will have a combination of the symptoms of backward and forward heart failure.

- Heart failure is the inability of the heart to meet the metabolic demands of the body.
- Its commonest cause is left ventricular dysfunction.
- Cause of backward heart failure is elevated filling pressure.
- Cause of forward heart failure is low cardiac output.

Myocardial dysfunction that causes heart failure may be due to systolic dysfunction, which is depression in contractile force of the myocardium leading to low stroke volume. The compensatory mechanism for improving stroke volume is ventricular dilatation. Ventricular dilatation results in increased end-diastolic pressures, which in turn cause symptoms of shortness of breath. Diastolic dysfunction is as important as systolic dysfunction in causing signs and symptoms of heart failure. As many as one-third of patients who present with heart failure have normal systolic function; diastolic dysfunction is predominantly the cause of their heart failure. Diastolic dysfunction is an abnormality of filling of the left ventricle so that there is a greater increase in pressure per unit volume.

- Myocardial dysfunction that causes heart failure may be due to systolic dysfunction.
- Systolic dysfunction is depression in contractile force of the myocardium.
- Diastolic dysfunction is as important as systolic dysfunction in causing signs and symptoms of heart failure.
- One-third of patients with heart failure have normal systolic function.
- Diastolic dysfunction is an abnormality of filling of the left ventricle.

Diastolic function is a complex process. Three of its major components are relaxation, passive filling, and atrial contribution. Relaxation is an active process in which calcium is removed from the actin myosin filaments, causing contracted muscle to return to its original length. After relaxation, filling of the ventricle continues, with an increase in pressure (passive filling). This is defined in terms of compliance, which is change in volume over change in pressure. Thus, abnormally low compliance produces high end-diastolic pressure. The contribution from atrial contraction further increases ventricular volume by as much as 15%-20% in normal subjects and 45%-50% in those with abnormality. In most disease states, a combination of systolic and diastolic abnormalities causes the signs and symptoms of heart failure.

- Three major components of diastolic function are relaxation, passive filling, and atrial contribution.
- In relaxation, calcium is removed from the actin myosin filaments.
- Reduced ventricular compliance means higher pressures are needed to produce volume changes.
- In most disease states, there is a combination of systolic and diastolic abnormalities.
- Atrial contraction takes on greater importance in patients with reduced ventricular compliance.

ETIOLOGY

The cause of heart failure must be defined to properly define therapy. Several different types of categories can be used. A simple one is given in Table 3-13.

Clinically, the commonest cause of heart failure is a myocardial process in which there is left ventricular contractile dysfunction. The treatment and prognosis are markedly different for other causes. Thus, the diagnosis is essential and is made on the basis of physical examination and noninvasive testing, e.g., echocardiography and radionuclide angiography.

PRECIPITATING FACTORS

It is necessary to define an underlying cause in patients with heart failure. However, one or more precipitating factors are usually responsible for "tipping" a patient into congestive heart failure. If the precipitating factors are not identified and corrected, the severe symptoms of heart failure frequently return after initial therapy. In every patient, the following categories must be investigated to determine a precipitating factor (Table 3-14).

In evaluating each patient with heart failure, take the fol-

Table 3-13.--Causes of Heart Failure and Treatment

Cause	Treatment
Myocardial	
Dilated cardiomyopathy	Angiotensin converting enzyme inhibitors, nitrates, hydralazine, digoxin, diuretics, heart transplant, coronary revascularization
Hypertrophic cardiomyopathy	β-Adrenergic blockers, calcium channel blockers, permanent pacing, surgery
Restrictive cardiomyopathy	Diuretics, heart transplant, treat underlying systemic disease
Pericardial	
Tamponade	Pericardiocentesis
Constrictive pericarditis	Pericardiectomy
Valvular	Valve repair or replacement
Hypertension (increased afterload)	Afterload reduction
Pulmonary hypertension	Heart-lung transplant, calcium channel blockers
High output	Correct underlying cause
Hyperthyroidism, Paget's disease	
Arteriovenous fistula	

Table 3-14.--Precipitating Factors of Heart Failure

Diet (increased sodium or fluid intake, alcohol)

Noncompliance with medication

Infection (infective endocarditis, urinary tract infection, upper respiratory tract infection)

Myocardial ischemia or infarction

Pulmonary embolus

Arrhythmia (atrial fibrillation, bradycardia)

Anemia

Metabolic (hyperthyroidism, hypothyroidism, chronic renal failure)

lowing steps: 1) medical history, including dietary history and history of medication compliance ("pill count"); 2) culture specimens of blood, urine, and sputum; 3) chest radiography and arterial blood gas studies should be performed to look for pneumonitis or pulmonary embolus; 4) electrocardiography (ECG) and creatine kinase-MB fraction blood test should be performed to rule out active ischemia. Other tests include hemoglobin, leukocyte count, sensitive thyroid-stimulating hormone, and creatinine. The heart rhythm should be documented.

- For different causes of heart failure, treatment and prognosis are different.
- For every patient with heart failure, precipitating factors must be sought and treated.

DEFINITION OF CARDIOMYOPATHIES

Cardiomyopathy is a disease of heart muscle without any known cause. Three major categories of cardiomyopathies are dilated, hypertrophic, and restrictive. Many other diseases have the same pathophysiology as true cardiomyopathies but have a known underlying cause. The different anatomical and pathophysiologic processes for each cardiomyopathy are listed in Table 3-15.

DILATED CARDIOMYOPATHY

The major abnormality in dilated cardiomyopathy is decreased systolic function (low ejection fraction) with enlargement of the left ventricular cavity and often increased left ventricular end-diastolic pressure due to coexistent diastolic dysfunction. The increased filling pressures and low cardiac output produce symptoms of shortness of breath and fatigue.

- In dilated cardiomyopathy, the major abnormality is decreased systolic function (low ejection fraction).

A true dilated cardiomyopathy is indicated by left ventricular dysfunction without any known cause. There appears to be a genetic link, with 20%-30% incidence of dilated cardiomyopathy in first-degree relatives. Some speculate that there is a viral cause, perhaps starting out with a viral myocarditis. Other causes of severe left ventricular dysfunction include severe coronary artery disease ("hibernating myocardium"), multiple areas of previous infarctions, ethanol abuse, hyperthyroidism or hypothyroidism, postpartum cardiomyopathy, toxins and drugs, tachycardia-induced cardiomyopathy, infil-

Table 3-15.--Anatomical and Pathophysiologic Processes for Each Cardiomyopathy

Type	Left ventricular cavity size	Left ventricular wall thickness	Systolic function	Diastolic function	Other
Dilated cardiomyopathy	↑	N/↑	↓	↓/N	
Hypertrophic cardiomyopathy	↓/N	↑	↑	↓	Left ventricular outflow obstruction
Restrictive cardiomyopathy	N/↑	N	N	↓	

↓, N, ↑, decreased, normal, increased, respectively.

trative cardiomyopathy (i.e., hemochromatosis, sarcoidosis, or amyloidosis), acquired immunodeficiency syndrome (AIDS), and pheochromocytoma.

- There seems to be a genetic link in dilated cardiomyopathy--20%-30% incidence in first-degree relatives.
- Other causes of severe left ventricular dysfunction: severe coronary artery disease ("hibernating myocardium"), multiple areas of previous infarction, ethanol abuse, hyperthyroidism or hypothyroidism, postpartum cardiomyopathy, toxins and drugs, tachycardia-induced cardiomyopathy, infiltrative cardiomyopathy (i.e., hemochromatosis, sarcoidosis, or amyloidosis), AIDS, and pheochromocytoma.

Clinical Presentation of Dilated Cardiomyopathy
The presentation of dilated cardiomyopathy is highly variable. The patient may be asymptomatic, in which case the diagnosis is made on basis of chest radiography, ECG, or echocardiography. Patients may have symptoms of mild to severe heart failure (New York Heart Association functional class II-IV). Other patients may present with the sudden onset of a systemic embolus. Atrial and ventricular arrhythmias are common in dilated cardiomyopathy. If heart failure is present, the following may be found on physical examination: jugular venous pressure is increased, up-stroke of carotid artery is low volume, left ventricular impulse is displaced and sustained with a rapid filling wave, third and fourth heart sounds are frequently audible, and apical systolic murmur of mitral regurgitation is present.

- Presentation of dilated cardiomyopathy is highly variable.
- Jugular venous pressure is increased, third heart sound is often audible, and the apex is displaced and sustained.

ECG frequently shows left ventricular hypertrophy, interventricular conduction delay, or left bundle branch block. Premature atrial contractions or atrial fibrillation occurs.

Premature ventricular contractions and short bursts of ventricular tachycardia are common. The chest radiograph often shows left ventricular enlargement. The diagnosis is made on the basis of reduced ejection fraction on analysis of left ventricular function (echocardiography, radionuclide angiography, or left ventriculography).

- ECG shows left ventricular hypertrophy, interventricular conduction delay, or left bundle branch block.
- Premature ventricular contractions and short bursts of ventricular tachycardia are common.
- Chest radiograph often shows left ventricular enlargement.

Evaluation of Dilated Cardiomyopathy
After the diagnosis of depressed left ventricular function is made, rule out treatable secondary causes of left ventricular dysfunction. Sensitive thyroid-stimulating hormone level should be determined to exclude hyperthyroidism or hypothyroidism. Iron and iron-binding capacities should be measured (or ferritin level) to rule out hemochromatosis. Serum angiotensin converting enzyme level should be measured. Metanephrine level should be measured if there is a history of severe labile hypertension or unusual spells. Ethanol or drug abuse must be documented. In severe coronary artery disease, reversible left ventricular dysfunction can be caused by hibernating myocardium. In this situation, long-standing diffuse ischemia depletes ATP stores in myocardial cells, which are thus functionally inactive. However, with revascularization, left ventricular function may gradually improve. Identifying affected patients is difficult. Currently, the standard method is positron emission tomography, which can demonstrate metabolic activity. Improvement in myocardial thickening after treatment with low doses of dobutamine or large areas of reperfusion on rest and delayed thallium scanning may help diagnose hibernating myocardium. Tachycardia-induced cardiomyopathy is a recently described entity. In patients with prolonged periods of tachycardia due

to either atrial fibrillation or atrial tachycardia, left ventricular systolic function may be depressed. The mechanism of this is unknown but may be related to abnormalities of neurohumoral mechanisms. This is an important cause to establish because systolic dysfunction can be completely reversed after the tachycardia is treated.

- After depressed left ventricular function is diagnosed, rule out treatable secondary causes of left ventricular dysfunction.
- Sensitive thyroid-stimulating hormone test can exclude hyperthyroidism and hypothyroidism as causes.
- Hibernating myocardium is a reversible cause of left ventricular dysfunction.
- Tachycardia-induced cardiomyopathy is reversible.

A certain number of patients have left ventricular dysfunction caused by acute myocarditis. The natural history of these patients is unknown. Many patients continue to have progressive left ventricular dysfunction that eventually may lead to dilated cardiomyopathy. A small percentage of patients may undergo spontaneous improvement with time. Thus, it is necessary to measure left ventricular function 3-6 months after making the diagnosis. Endomyocardial biopsy may help in diagnosing myocarditis (but may not be practical because there is no proven therapy for myocarditis). Myocarditis with concomitant skeletal myositis often responds to steroid therapy.

Pathophysiology

To treat heart failure associated with dilated cardiomyopathy, the pathophysiology of heart failure must be understood. The relationship of stroke volume to preload and afterload and the neurohumoral response to decreased myocardial contractility are important.

The relationship of stroke volume to preload is shown on the Starling curve in Figure 3-28.

The relationship of stroke volume to afterload is shown in Figure 3-29.

Figure 3-30 illustrates the neurohumoral response to decreased myocardial contractility. Decreased stroke volume produces a compensatory increase in left ventricular end-diastolic volume and end-diastolic pressure (Starling curve mechanism); this results in symptoms of pulmonary congestion. Decreased stroke volume activates baroreceptors and the sympathetic nervous system. Sympathetic nervous system stimulation causes an increased heart rate and contractility. Alpha-stimulation of the arterioles causes an increase in afterload. The renin-angiotensin system is activated by sympathetic stimulation, decreased renal blood flow, and decreased renal sodium. This system in turn activates aldosterone, causing increased renal retention of sodium and, thus, more pulmonary congestion. A low rate of renal blood flow results in renal retention of sodium. An increased level of angiotensin II causes vaso-

constriction and an increase in afterload. In congestive heart failure, there is an inappropriate increase in afterload, causing further decrease in stroke volume.

- Increase in preload causes increase in stroke volume.
- Increase in afterload causes decrease in stroke volume.
- Either increase in afterload or decrease in myocardial contractility can shift the Starling curve downward and to the right.
- Inappropriate increase in afterload in patients with heart failure causes further decrease in stroke volume.

Treatment of Dilated Cardiomyopathy

In treating dilated cardiomyopathy, it is important to diagnose and remove precipitating factors, as mentioned above. Treatment of congestive heart failure in patients with dilated cardiomyopathy should be based on the pathophysiologic mechanisms described above (Fig. 3-31).

- In treating dilated cardiomyopathy, diagnose and remove precipitating factors.

The mainstays of therapy in the 1990s are angiotensin converting enzyme (ACE) inhibitors. By blocking conversion of angiotensin I to angiotensin II, ACE inhibitors decrease afterload by inhibition of angiotensin II and decrease sodium retention by inhibition of aldosterone. Also, ACE inhibitors directly affect myocardial cells at the molecular level, which explains how ACE inhibitors prevent ventricular dilatation and improve

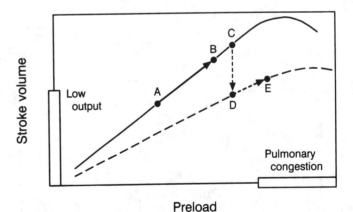

Fig. 3-28. Starling curve. Solid line is patient with normal contractility, and the dotted line is one with depressed systolic function. Normally, stroke volume depends on preload of the heart. Increasing preload increases stroke volume (A to B). Myocardial dysfunction causes a shift of the curve downward and to the right (C to D), causing a severe decrease in stroke volume, which leads to symptoms of fatigue and lethargy. The compensatory response to decrease in stroke volume is an increase in preload (D to E). Because the diastolic pressure-volume relationship is curvilinear, increased left ventricular volume produces increased left ventricular end-diastolic pressure, causing symptoms of pulmonary congestion. Note flat portion of the curve at its upper end; here, there is little increase in stroke volume for increase in preload.

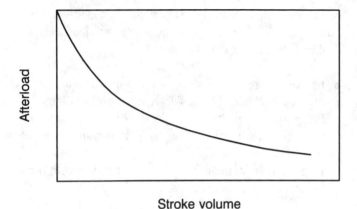

Fig. 3-29. As opposed to preload, increase in afterload produces a decrease in stroke volume. Therefore, a shift of the Starling curve up and to the left can be accomplished by either an increase in myocardial contractility or a decrease in afterload.

In asymptomatic or mildly symptomatic patients, ACE inhibitors prevent onset of heart failure and reduce the need for hospitalization. After anterior myocardial infarction, ACE inhibitors prevent progressive ventricular dilatation and reduce mortality. These agents need to be given initially as a small dose (comparable to 6.25 mg of captopril) because of a hypotensive effect. Dosage should be titrated up as tolerated, with a final dosage equivalent to 50 mg of captopril three times daily. To achieve this, diuretics should be withheld for several days before administering ACE inhibitors for equilibration of intravascular volume. Common side effects of ACE inhibitors include hypotension, hyperkalemia, dysgeusia, cough, acute renal failure (with markedly reduced renal blood flow, bilateral renal artery stenosis, or renal artery stenosis in a single kidney), and angioedema (mild or severe).

- In asymptomatic or mildly symptomatic patients, ACE inhibitors reduce the incidence of heart failure and reduce the need for hospitalization.
- After anterior myocardial infarction, ACE inhibitors prevent progressive ventricular dilatation and reduce mortality.
- ACE inhibitor side effects: hypotension, hyperkalemia, dysgeusia, cough, acute renal failure, and angioedema.

mortality. Overall, ACE inhibitors provide symptomatic improvement in patients with New York Heart Association functional class II-IV failure and improve mortality in patients with moderate and severe heart failure.

- ACE inhibitors are mainstays of therapy in the 1990s.
- ACE inhibitors decrease afterload by inhibition of angiotensin II and decrease sodium retention by inhibition of aldosterone.
- ACE inhibitors improve mortality in patients with moderate and severe heart failure.

Drugs that directly affect contractility include digoxin and phosphodiesterase inhibitors (milrinone and amrinone). Digoxin provides symptomatic relief if the ejection fraction is <40%, particularly in patients with a third heart sound or concomitant atrial fibrillation. Whether digoxin improves

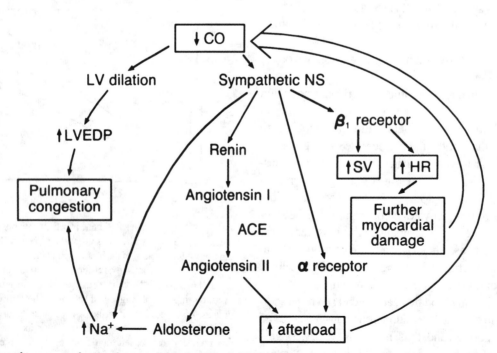

Fig. 3-30. Neurohumoral response to decreased myocardial contractility. ACE, angiotensin converting enzyme; CO, cardiac output; HR, heart rate; LV, left ventricle; LVEDP, left ventricular end-diastolic pressure; NS, nervous system; SV, stroke volume.

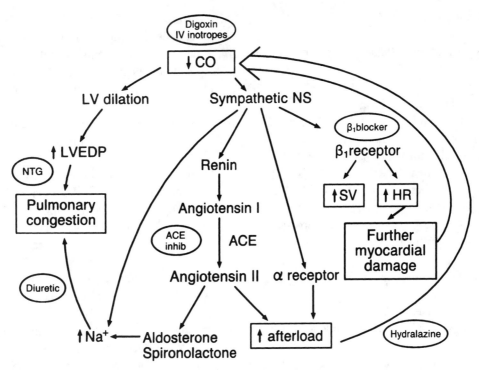

Fig. 3-31. The effect of various drugs used to treat heart failure on the neurohumoral responses in patients with dilated cardiomyopathy. IV, intravenous; NTG, nitroglycerin. Other abbreviations as in Figure 3-30.

mortality is unknown. Because digoxin is excreted by the kidneys, its dosage needs to be decreased with increased levels of creatinine and for older patients. The normal dosage is 0.25 mg/day but should be decreased to 0.125 mg/day if creatinine clearance is <70. In patients with chronic renal failure, digoxin can be given at a dosage of 0.125 mg three times weekly. Because of drug-to-drug interaction, digoxin dosage should be decreased with concomitant administration of quinidine, verapamil, and amiodarone. Although parenteral inotropic agents (milrinone and amrinone) may improve symptoms short-term, their overall effect is to increase mortality. Therefore, they should be used transiently only in severe cases of congestive heart failure.

- Digoxin and phosphodiesterase inhibitors (milrinone and amrinone) directly affect contractility.
- Because digoxin is excreted by the kidneys, its dosage needs to be decreased with increased levels of creatinine and for older patients.
- Digoxin dosage should be decreased with concomitant administration of quinidine, verapamil, and amiodarone.

Diuretics and nitrates reduce pulmonary congestion. Diuretics should be used in patients with symptoms of pulmonary congestion or physical evidence of fluid overload. The daily use of diuretics may cause neurohumoral and electrolyte imbalances. Mild fluid overload is initially treated with thiazide diuretics if renal function is normal. Loop diuretics are

needed if there is significant fluid overload, renal dysfunction, or fluid overload resistant to thiazides. Occasionally, a combination of thiazides and loop diuretics is needed for severe, tenacious fluid retention. Nitrates reduce preload through venodilatation. They should be given with a nitrate-free interval to prevent nitrate tolerance.

- Diuretics and nitrates reduce pulmonary congestion.
- Nitrates reduce preload through venodilatation.

With reduced afterload, stroke volume improves, as do symptoms. The combination of high-dose nitrates and hydralazine provides symptomatic improvement and improved mortality in patients with heart failure. However, the rate of intolerance to these doses of medications is high. When afterload reduction is used, diuretics are often useful concomitantly to prevent the compensatory increase in sodium retention.

- Stroke volume improves with reduced afterload.
- Combination of nitrates and hydralazine improves mortality and symptoms.

β-Adrenergic blockers may be helpful in the treatment of selected patients with dilated cardiomyopathy. β-Blockers are most useful in patients with resting tachycardia but need to be given carefully to prevent left ventricular decompensation. The benefit of beta-blockade may be achieved through prevention of sympathetic-induced myocardial necrosis.

- β-Blockade is most useful in patients with resting tachycardia.
- β-Blockade may prevent sympathetic-induced myocardial necrosis.

A 48-hour infusion of dobutamine gives symptomatic relief, but the effect is temporary (1-2 months) and mortality is increased. The infusion must be given with continuous ECG monitoring to look for arrhythmia. The usual dosage is 10-25 μg/kg per minute to get the resting heart rate 15-20 beats per minute above baseline. Dobutamine may replenish low catecholamine stores. This therapy is reserved for severely symptomatic patients who are unresponsive to other therapies; they may receive continuous outpatient infusions.

- 48-Hour infusion of dobutamine gives symptomatic relief.
- Effect is for 1-2 months.
- Dobutamine may cause increased mortality.
- Dobutamine may replenish low catecholamine stores.

Second-generation dihydropyridine calcium channel blockers may be beneficial for patients with dilated cardiomyopathy. Their major effect appears to be by lowering afterload.

First-generation calcium channel blockers (verapamil, dilitiazem, nifedipine) are relatively contraindicated because of their negative inotropic effects. Anticoagulation with warfarin is recommended for patients in atrial fibrillation and those with left ventricular thrombus or a history of systemic or pulmonary thromboembolism.

- Anticoagulation with warfarin is recommended in patients with atrial fibrillation, left ventricular thrombus, or a history of thromboembolism.

The prognosis for patients with dilated cardiomyopathy varies with functional class. Annual mortality ranges from 5%-10% for patients in New York Heart Assocation class II to as high as a 2-year mortality of 50% after symptoms are severe. Heart transplantation is the procedure of choice for patients with severe dilated cardiomyopathy and severe symptoms. With successful transplantation, the 1-year survival is 90%. The major contraindication for transplantation in an otherwise healthy patient is a high pulmonary arteriolar resistance (>4 Wood units/m^2). In the U.S., donor availability is the major limiting factor.

- After symptoms are severe, 2-year mortality is 50% for patients with dilated cardiomyopathy, even with optimal medical therapy.
- The procedure of choice for these patients is heart transplantation.
- With successful transplantation, 1-year survival is 90%.

Recapitulation of Drug Therapy of Heart Failure

- ACE inhibitors improve mortality in patients with symptomatic dilated cardiomyopathy.
- ACE inhibitors prevent deterioration and subsequent hospitalizations in patients with asymptomatic dilated cardiomyopathy.
- ACE inhibitors prevent ventricular dilatation and improve mortality in patients with anterior myocardial infarction.
- Combination of nitrates and hydralazines may improve symptoms to a greater degree than ACE inhibitors. These drugs improve mortality in symptomatic patients, but intolerance to these medications is high.
- Nitrates should be used with a nitrate-free interval to prevent nitrate tolerance.
- Digoxin is useful for symptomatic treatment of patients with dilated cardiomyopathy, particularly those in atrial fibrillation or with a third heart sound.
- Phosphodiesterase inhibitors and prolonged infusion of dobutamine directly increase contractility and may improve symptoms, but they probably increase mortality.

HYPERTROPHIC CARDIOMYOPATHY

Etiology

Hypertrophic cardiomyopathy is a disease in which massive hypertrophy of the myocardium occurs without any known cause. There is usually dynamic left ventricular outflow tract obstruction, but 20%-40% of patients have no obstruction. The diagnosis is based on the echocardiographic finding of severe hypertrophy of the myocardium in the absence of a secondary cause, such as hypertension, chronic renal failure, or infiltrative disease.

- Hypertrophic cardiomyopathy--massive hypertrophy of the myocardium without known cause.
- Dynamic left ventricular outflow tract obstruction occurs, but not in 20%-40% of patients.
- Diagnosis is based on the echocardiographic finding of severe myocardial hypertrophy.

The primary abnormality of patients with hypertrophic cardiomyopathy appears to be abnormal calcium metabolism at the cellular level. Hypertrophic cardiomyopathy is a hereditary disease (autosomal dominant), although sporadic cases are frequent. All patients with hypertrophic cardiomyopathy should have screening of first-degree relatives. Genetic counseling is advised for potential parents. A gene mutation is highly prevalent in certain families with hypertrophic cardiomyopathy. Patients with this gene mutation have a high incidence of sudden death.

- The primary abnormality apparently is abnormal calcium metabolism at the cellular level.
- It is a hereditary disease (autosomal dominant), but sporadic cases are frequent.
- Genetic counseling is advised.
- A gene mutation is highly prevalent in certain families with hypertrophic cardiomyopathy.
- Patients with this gene mutation have a high incidence of sudden death.

Symptoms

Hypertrophic cardiomyopathy has several different manifestations. There appears to be a bimodal age distribution of presentation. Young males (usually in the teens or early 20s) have a high propensity for syncope and sudden death. Older patients (in the 50s and 60s) present with symptoms of shortness of breath and angina and may have a better prognosis than young patients. The classic presentation of the younger group is a young male athlete undergoing a physical examination for participating in a sport who is found to have a heart murmur and left ventricular hypertrophy on ECG. The classic presentation of the older group is an elderly woman in whom pulmonary edema develops after noncardiac surgery and whose condition worsens, with diuresis, afterload reduction, and inotropic support (all of which worsen dynamic left ventricular outflow tract obstruction). The classic symptom triad is syncope, angina, and dyspnea. These symptoms are similar to those of patients with valvular aortic stenosis. Some patients have a small hyperdynamic left ventricle with hypertrophy due to hypertension and associated dynamic left ventricular outflow tract obstruction--"hypertensive-hypertrophic cardiomyopathy." Although they do not have true cardiomyopathy, the pathophysiology may be the same as for hypertrophic cardiomyopathy. These patients are not at increased risk for sudden death and ventricular fibrillation.

- The classic presentation of hypertrophic cardiomyopathy is the triad of angina, syncope, and dyspnea.
- Bimodal distribution of presentation: young males with high incidence of sudden death and older patients with dyspnea and angina.
- Prognosis for older patients may be better than for younger patients.
- Patients with hypertension may have hypertrophy and dynamic left ventricular outflow tract obstruction similar to those of patients with hypertrophic cardiomyopathy.

Pathophysiology

Signs and symptoms of hypertrophic cardiomyopathy are caused by four major abnormalities: diastolic dysfunction, left ventricular outflow tract obstruction, mitral regurgitation, and ventricular arrhythmias.

Diastolic dysfunction is caused by many mechanisms. Severe hypertrophy and increased muscle mass produce decreased compliance so that there is increased pressure per given volume entering the left ventricle during diastole. Marked abnormality in calcium metabolism causes abnormal ventricular relaxation. High afterload due to left ventricular tract obstruction also delays ventricular relaxation. All these events cause increased left ventricular diastolic pressure, which leads to angina and dyspnea.

In many patients, dynamic left ventricular tract obstruction is caused by the hypertrophied septum encroaching into the left ventricular outflow tract. This subsequently "sucks in" the anterior leaflet of the mitral valve (systolic anterior motion), creating left ventricular outflow tract obstruction. Because of this pathophysiologic process, a dynamic outflow tract obstruction increases dramatically with decreased preload or afterload or increased contractility.

Systolic anterior motion of the mitral valve distorts the mitral valve apparatus during systole and may cause significant mitral regurgitation. The degree of mitral regurgitation is also dynamic and depends on the degree of left ventricular outflow tract obstruction. Patients with severe mitral regurgitation usually have severe symptoms of dyspnea.

Because of cellular disarray in patients with hypertrophic cardiomyopathy, the electrical conduction system is dispersed, leading to a high propensity for ventricular arrhythmias. The frequent occurrence of ventricular arrhythmias may cause sudden death or syncope.

- The major pathophysiologic abnormality in patients with hypertrophic cardiomyopathy is diastolic dysfunction.
- Left ventricular outflow tract obstruction and mitral regurgitation are caused by distortion of the mitral valve apparatus (systolic anterior motion).
- The propensity for ventricular arrhythmias causing syncope and sudden death is high.

Examination

Hypertrophic cardiomyopathy can be diagnosed with the combination of carotid artery upstroke and left ventricular impulse. The carotid artery upstroke is very rapid compared with that of patients with aortic stenosis. If left ventricular outflow tract obstruction is significant, carotid artery upstroke has a bifid quality. The left ventricular impulse is always very sustained, indicating significant left ventricular hypertrophy. It frequently has a palpable "A" wave. Patients with significant left ventricular outflow tract obstruction have a triple impulse. The first heart sound is normal, and the second heart sound is paradoxically split. A loud systolic ejection murmur indicates left ventricular outflow tract obstruction. The murmur changes in intensity with changes in loading conditions (Table 3-16). A holosystolic murmur of mitral regurgitation may be present; it

Table 3-16.--Dynamic Left Ventricular Outflow Tract Obstruction

Increased obstruction
Decreased afterload
Amyl nitrite
Vasodilators
Angiotensin converting enzyme inhibitors
Increased contractility
Postpremature ventricular contraction beat
Digoxin
Dopamine
Decreased preload
Squat-to-stand
Nitrates
Diuretics
Valsalva maneuver
Decreased obstruction
Increased afterload
Handgrip
Decreased contractility
β-Blockers
Calcium channel blockers
Increased preload
Fluids

increases with increases in left ventricular outflow murmur. The changes in mitral regurgitation with different maneuvers are opposite the changes that occur with mitral regurgitation due to other causes. There is an increased intensity of the murmur on the beat after a premature ventricular contraction. Arterial pulse volume decreases because the obstruction is increased. This is due to increased contractility and decreased afterload and is called Brockenbrough's sign.

- Diagnosis of hypertrophic cardiomyopathy can be made by palpating sustained left ventricular impulse and rapid upstroke of the carotid artery.
- The murmur changes dramatically with changes in loading conditions of the heart.
- Mitral regurgitation murmur changes in same direction as that of left ventricular outflow tract obstruction under different loading conditions.
- First heart sound is normal, and the second heart sound is paradoxically split.

Diagnostic Testing in Patients With Hypertrophic Cardiomyopathy

Patients with hypertrophic cardiomyopathy almost always have an abnormal ECG, which shows significant left ventricular hypertrophy (Fig. 3-32). Apical hypertrophic cardiomyopathy is a variant of hypertrophic cardiomyopathy in which the hypertrophy is localized at the apex of the left ventricle. The ECG in these patients typically has large, diffuse, symmetrical T-wave inversions across the precordium (Fig. 3-33).

Hypertrophic cardiomyopathy is diagnosed with echocardiography, which shows severe hypertrophy of the myocardium (left ventricular wall thickness >16 mm in diastole) without any known cause. Although asymmetric septal hypertrophy was required for the diagnosis (septum-to-posterior-wall ratio >1.3), it is now recognized that hypertrophy can be in any part of the myocardium, e.g., lateral wall only or diffuse concentric hypertrophy. Therefore, the M-mode criterion of asymmetric septal hypertrophy is no longer valid. Doppler echocardiography is useful in diagnosing left ventricular outflow tract obstruction and measuring its severity. Mitral regurgitation can be detected with Doppler echocardiography.

Cardiac catheterization is no longer necessary for diagnosing dynamic left ventricular outflow tract obstruction because all diagnostic data can be obtained by two-dimensional and Doppler echocardiography. Because of a strong association with ventricular arrhythmias and sudden death, 48- to 72-hour Holter monitoring is recommended for all patients with hypertrophic cardiomyopathy.

- ECG usually shows evidence of left ventricular hypertrophy in cases of hypertrophic cardiomyopathy.
- Asymmetric septal hypertrophy is suspected by the presence of large inverted T-waves in precordial leads on ECG. It is confirmed by echocardiography, which demonstrates localized apical hypertrophy.
- Diagnosis of hypertrophic cardiomyopathy is made with echocardiography, which shows hypertrophy in absence of any known cause.
- Strong association with ventricular arrhythmias and sudden death.
- 48- to 72-Hour Holter monitoring recommended for all patients with hypertrophic cardiomyopathy.

Treatment

Treatment of Symptomatic Patients

For symptomatic patients with hypertrophic cardiomyopathy, treatment is with drugs that decrease contractility in an attempt to decrease left ventricular outflow tract obstruction (Fig. 3-34). The most effective medication is a high dose of β-blockers (>240 mg equivalent of propranolol/day). Although calcium channel blockers may be used if β-blockade fails, they

Fig. 3-32. Electrocardiogram in hypertrophic cardiomyopathy showing marked left ventricular hypertrophy.

Fig. 3-33. Electrocardiogram in apical hypertrophic cardiomyopathy with deep symmetric T-wave inversions in precordial leads.

may cause sudden hemodynamic deterioration in patients with high resting left ventricular outflow tract gradients because of their vasodilating properties. Disopyramide may give symptomatic improvement by decreasing left ventricular outflow tract obstruction, but anticholinergic side effects limit its use. All drugs that reduce afterload or preload and those that increase contractility must be avoided in patients with hypertrophic cardiomyopathy.

Surgical myectomy is reserved for patients who are severely symptomatic despite optimal medical therapy and produces dramatic symptomatic relief. Mortality associated with this procedure is 5%-10%. Its complications include complete heart block, aortic regurgitation, and ventricular septal defect. Myectomy is a highly operator-dependent procedure and should be performed only at medical centers that specialize in this procedure.

Dual-chamber pacing may prove to be an alternative to myectomy for patients with hypertrophic cardiomyopathy and severe left ventricular outflow tract obstruction. Its mechanism is unclear. Dual-chamber pacing can produce a modest improvement in gradient, and in the initial studies, symptomatic improvement may be achieved. More studies need to be completed before recommending dual-chamber pacing for all patients with symptomatic hypertrophic obstructive cardiomyopathy.

Sudden death is a problem in patients with hypertrophic cardiomyopathy. Predictors of sudden death include a family history of sudden death, young male, history of syncope, and nonsustained ventricular tachycardia on Holter monitoring. Genetic markers may identify patients with a strong propensity for sudden death. Whether to treat asymptomatic patients with nonsustained ventricular tachycardia is a controversial subject (Fig. 3-35). No conventional antiarrhythmic agent is effective and may make the arrhythmia worse. In selected patients with multiple risk factors for sudden death, a low dose of amiodarone or an automatic implantable cardiac defibrillator might be chosen. In patients who have already had an out-of-hospital arrest, treatment of choice is automatic implantable cardiac defibrillator.

- β-Blockade is treatment of choice for patients with symptomatic hypertrophic cardiomyopathy.
- Surgical myectomy is reserved for severely symptomatic patients unresponsive to medical therapy.
- Calcium channel blockers may cause sudden hemodynamic deterioration in patients with high resting left ventricular outflow tract obstruction.
- Predictors of sudden death: family history of sudden death, nonsustained ventricular tachycardia, young male, and history of syncope.
- No conventional antiarrhythmic agent is effective and may worsen the arrhythmia.
- Automatic implantable cardiac defibrillator is treatment of choice for patients with out-of-hospital arrest.

RESTRICTIVE CARDIOMYOPATHY

Definition
The primary abnormality in restrictive cardiomyopathy is diastolic dysfunction. As mentioned above, diastolic dysfunction causes abnormal left ventricular filling so that the increase in pressure per unit volume is greater. This is reflected back to the pulmonary and systemic circulations, causing symptoms of shortness of breath and edema. Also, because the ventricle cannot fill to meet its preload requirements (Starling mechanism), cardiac output is low, causing fatigue and lethargy. Systolic function is maintained in many patients with restrictive cardiomyopathy. However, at the end stage of the disease, there can be decompensation of systolic function as well.

- In restrictive cardiomyopathy, primary abnormality is diastolic dysfunction.
- Diastolic dysfunction causes abnormal left ventricular filling so that rise in pressure per unit volume is greater.
- Left ventricle cannot fill to meet its preload requirements.
- Low cardiac output causes fatigue and lethargy.

The cause of primary restrictive cardiomyopathy is unknown. There are two major categories: idiopathic restrictive cardiomyopathy and endomyocardial fibrosis. In idiopathic restrictive cardiomyopathy (seen mainly in the U.S.), there is progressive fibrosis of the myocardium. Endomyocardial fibrosis is probably an end stage of eosinophilic syndromes in which there is intracavitary thrombus filling of the left ventricle. This restricts filling and causes increased diastolic pressures. Secondary fibrosis may also involve the mitral valve, causing severe mitral regurgitation. There may be two different forms of endomyocardial fibrosis: active inflamma-

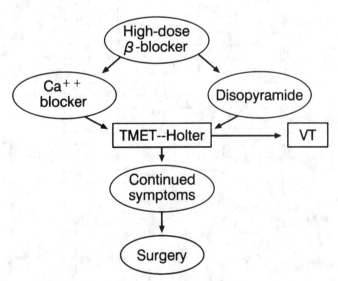

Fig. 3-34. Treatment of symptomatic patients. TMET, treadmill exertion test; VT, ventricular tachycardia.

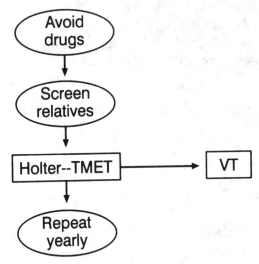

Fig. 3-35. Treatment of asymptomatic patients. Abbreviations as in Figure 3-34.

tory eosinophilic myocarditis in temperate zones and chronic endomyocardial fibrosis in tropic zones. Diseases that cause infiltration of the myocardium have a presentation and pathophysiology similar to those of primary restrictive cardiomyopathy. These diseases include amyloidosis and chronic renal failure. After radiation therapy and following heart transplantation, signs and symptoms similar to those of restrictive cardiomyopathy may also develop.

- Endomyocardial fibrosis is probably an end stage of eosinophilic syndromes.
- Secondary fibrosis may involve mitral valve, causing severe mitral regurgitation.
- Diseases causing infiltration of myocardium: amyloidosis and chronic renal failure.

Signs and Symptoms

Patients with restrictive cardiomyopathy usually present with edema, dyspnea, ascites, and low output symptoms. Atrial arrhythmias are frequently present, and the patient may present with atrial fibrillation. Jugular venous pressure is almost always elevated, with rapid X and Y descents. The precordium is quiet, and heart sounds are soft. There may be an apical systolic murmur of mitral regurgitation and a left sternal border murmur of tricuspid regurgitation. A third heart sound may be present. Dullness at the bases of the lungs is consistent with bilateral pleural effusions. ECG is usually low or normal voltage with atrial arrhythmias. Chest radiography shows pleural effusions with normal cardiac silhouette or atrial enlargement.

- Restrictive cardiomyopathy: severe right-sided failure, dyspnea, and low output symptoms.
- Atrial arrhythmias are frequently present.

- Jugular venous pressure is elevated, with rapid X and Y descents.

Diagnosis

Restrictive cardiomyopathy is diagnosed with echocardiography. Typical findings are normal left ventricular cavity size and function and marked enlargement of both atria. Echocardiography is usually nonspecific about the cause except in two instances. One, in endomyocardial fibrosis, the typical appearance of an echo density indicates thrombus in left ventricular apex. Two, amyloid heart disease has typical echocardiographic features of thickened myocardium with a scintillating appearance of the myocardium, pericardial effusion, and valvular regurgitation. Cardiac catheterization shows elevation and end-equalization of all end-diastolic pressures. A typical "square-root sign" or "dip and plateau" pattern consistent with early rapid filling is present. Endomyocardial biopsy usually is not helpful unless there is a systemic disease that has caused infiltration of the myocardium (i.e., amyloid).

- Restrictive cardiomyopathy is diagnosed with echocardiography.
- Typical findings: normal left ventricular cavity size and function and marked enlargement of both atria.
- Endomyocardial fibrosis: typical appearance of echo density indicating thrombus in left ventricular apex.
- Amyloid heart disease: typical echocardiographic features of thickened myocardium with scintillating appearance of myocardium, pericardial effusion, valvular regurgitation.

Treatment

There is no medical treatment for idiopathic restrictive cardiomyopathy. Diuretics decrease filling pressures and give symptomatic relief, but this may be at the expense of further decreasing cardiac output. Although calcium channel blockers have been proposed for treating diastolic dysfunction, they may be harmful and cause elevation of end-diastolic pressures. Digoxin usually is not helpful, because systolic contractility is maintained. Heart transplantation is the only proven therapy for patients with severe restrictive cardiomyopathy.

- There is no medical treatment for idiopathic restrictive cardiomyopathy.
- Diuretics decrease filling pressures.
- Digoxin usually is not helpful.
- Heart transplantation is only proven therapy.

It is important to differentiate restrictive cardiomyopathy from constrictive pericarditis. Both have similar presentations and findings on clinical examination and diagnostic studies. However, in constrictive pericarditis, pericardiectomy produces symptomatic improvement and, frequently, prolongation of longevity. Therefore, exploratory thoracotomy may be indicated in patients with normal left ventricular systolic function, large atria, and severe elevation of diastolic filling pressures if doubt remains after anatomic (fast computed tomography) and other tests (fast computed tomography, echocardiography).

- It is important to differentiate restrictive cardiomyopathy from constrictive pericarditis.
- In constrictive pericarditis, pericardiectomy produces symptomatic improvement and prolongation of longevity.

QUESTIONS

Multiple Choice (choose the one best answer)

1. Which statement is true of the bicuspid aortic valve?
   a. May cause isolated aortic regurgitation
   b. Produces an ejection click that becomes more delayed with increasing stenosis
   c. With increasing stenosis, the aortic closure sound moves earlier
   d. In a 20-year-old with severe stenosis, the ejection click has usually disappeared
   e. Is not subject to endocarditis if it functions completely normally

2. Which of the following is true of ventricular septal defects?
   a. Muscular defects never close spontaneously
   b. Small defects produce insignificant murmurs
   c. They do not need antibiotic prophylaxis unless there is associated valvular disease
   d. Large defects may produce an apical diastolic murmur
   e. When associated with Eisenmenger syndrome, they produce a loud systolic murmur

3. A 65-year-old man needs repair of an abdominal aortic aneurysm. He had an uncomplicated myocardial infarction 4 years ago and has angina after walking 25 yards. He takes atenolol (50 mg/day) and nitrates on a daily basis.
   a. Treadmill exercise test should be done before operation
   b. An exercise thallium test should be done
   c. The atenolol dose should be increased to 100 mg/day and operation should proceed
   d. Coronary angiography should be done before operation
   e. A dipyridamole thallium test should be done before operation

4. Which one of the following drugs is contraindicated in pregnancy?
   a. Propranolol
   b. Quinidine
   c. Digoxin
   d. Enalapril
   e. Verapamil

5. Which of the following is correct?
   a. Expiration increases the murmur of pulmonary stenosis
   b. Valsalva maneuver increases the murmur of mitral regurgitation
   c. Changing from supine to standing increases the murmur of pulmonary stenosis
   d. Handgrip increases the murmur of mitral regurgitation
   e. After a premature ventricular complex, the murmur of aortic stenosis increases

6. All of the following are common features of cardiac amyloid *except*:
   a. Atrioventricular valve regurgitation
   b. Valvular aortic stenosis
   c. Congestive heart failure
   d. Pericardial effusion
   e. Arrhythmias

7. Which of the following is true of mitral stenosis?
   a. It causes a diffuse apical impulse
   b. The more severe the stenosis, the shorter the diastolic murmur
   c. It causes a soft first heart sound
   d. The A_2-OS interval gets wider with increasing stenosis
   e. As the valve calcifies, the opening snap diminishes

8. Verapamil would be expected to cause the most depression on conduction through which of the following cardiac cells?
   a. Atrial
   b. Atrioventricular nodal
   c. Bundle of His
   d. Bundle branch
   e. Ventricular

9. A 52-year-old man is evaluated for recurrent palpitations

that are abrupt in onset, associated with light-headedness, occur once per month, and last 1-2 minutes. The most useful test for documenting the cause of this patient's arrhythmia is:

a. 12-lead electrocardiography
b. Signal-averaged electrocardiography
c. 24-hour ambulatory electrocardiography
d. Event recorder
e. Electrophysiologic study

10. Adenosine is usually effective in terminating which of the following arrhythmias?

a. Sinus tachycardia
b. Atrial flutter
c. Atrial fibrillation
d. Atioventricular nodal reentry
e. Ventricular tachycardia

11. Implantable cardioverter defibrillators are available with all of the following capabilities except:

a. Overdrive pacing for termination of ventricular tachycardia
b. Low-energy cardioversion shocks
c. Placement with transvenous leads so as to avoid thoracotomy
d. Single-chamber pacing
e. Dual-chamber pacing

12. Proarrhythmia from antiarrhythmic drugs:

a. Is invariably fatal
b. Usually occurs months after beginning treatment with class IA drugs such as quinidine
c. Only presents as torsades de pointes
d. Does not occur when treating atrial arrhythmias
e. Occurs more frequently in the setting of left ventricular dysfunction

13. Results of the Cardiac Arrhythmia Suppression Trial (CAST):

a. Are applicable to all antiarrhythmic drugs
b. Suggest that treatment of nonsustained ventricular tachycardia decreases mortality
c. Are no longer applicable because the drugs used in this trial are no longer manufactured
d. Show that flecainide is not safe for treating supraventricular arrhythmias
e. Show that no therapy may be safer than antiarrhythmic drug therapy for asymptomatic ventricular arrhythmias after myocardial infarction

14. A 28-year-old man comes to the emergency room complaining of palpitations and light-headedness. His blood pressure is 98/62 mm Hg. The accompanying electrocardiogram is obtained.

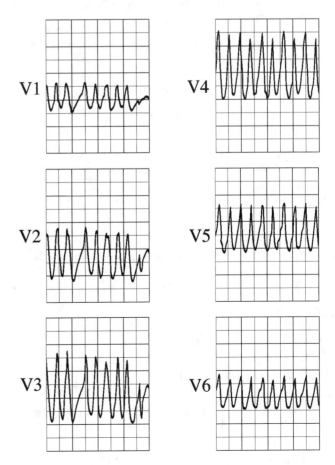

Of the following choices, the best intravenous medication to administer would be:
   a. Lidocaine
   b. Procainamide
   c. Digoxin
   d. Verapamil

e. Adenosine

15. A 48-year-old woman comes to your office complaining of shortness of breath. Her blood pressure is 114/70 mm Hg. The accompanying electrocardiogram is obtained.

The most appropriate acute treatment for her is:
   a. Adenosine
   b. Verapamil
   c. Lidocaine
   d. Bretylium
   e. Electrical cardioversion

16. A patient with Wolff-Parkinson-White syndrome presents with a regular, narrow QRS tachycardia. All of the following would be safe and effective acute therapy for this arrhythmia *except*:
   a. Adenosine
   b. Verapamil
   c. Procainamide
   d. Lidocaine
   e. Electrical cardioversion

17. All the following slow ventricular response *and* prevent recurrence of atrial fibrillation *except*:
   a. Digoxin

b. Flecainide
   c. Propafenone
   d. Sotalol
   e. Amiodarone

18. Which of the following is true about ventricular arrhythmias?
   a. Nonsustained ventricular tachycardia is a predictor of an increased risk of sudden death in the setting of a normal heart and warrants evaluation
   b. Frequent ventricular premature complexes (>30 per hour) indicate an increased risk of sudden death following myocardial infarction and require evaluation and treatment
   c. Out-of-hospital cardiac arrest is usually caused by an acute myocardial infarction
   d. Serial testing of antiarrhythmic drugs by electrophysiologic testing is accepted as a method of treating sustained ventricular tachycardia
   e. Sotalol is effective for treating supraventricular, but not ventricular, arrhythmias

19. The rhythm on the accompanying electrocardiogram is:

a. Sinus tachycardia
b. Atrial flutter
c. Atrial fibrillation
d. Atrioventricular nodal reentry
e. Ventricular tachycardia

20. Which of the following is not a risk factor for coronary artery disease?
    a. Low high-density lipoprotein (HDL)
    b. High low-density lipoprotein (LDL)
    c. Two beers per day
    d. Half a pack of cigarettes per day
    e. Diabetes mellitus

21. β-Blockers are associated with all the following *except*:
    a. Increased lipids
    b. Worsening claudication
    c. Depressed libido
    d. Lowering ventricular fibrillation threshold
    e. Improved survival after myocardial infarction

22. Which of the following is not a determinant of myocardial oxygen demand?
    a. Heart rate
    b. Contractility
    c. Wall tension
    d. Perfusion pressure
    e. Afterload

23. A 65-year-old man with multiple risk factors for coronary artery disease has had typical stable exertional angina for 2 years. A TMET is normal at 100% functional aortic capacity. Which of the following should be done?
    a. Esophageal manometry
    b. Coronary angiography
    c. Medical therapy
    d. Exercise thallium test
    e. Dobutamine echocardiography

24. Which of the following regimens is useful in the treatment of a patient with unstable angina?
    a. Streptokinase, heparin, and β-blockers
    b. Aspirin, heparin, and angiotensin converting enzyme (ACE) inhibitors
    c. Tissue plasminogen activator (TPA), heparin, and aspirin
    d. Aspirin, heparin, and β-blockers
    e. Calcium channel blockers, nitrates, and ACE inhibitors

25. Inferior myocardial infarction can be associated with all the following except:

a. Right ventricular infarction
b. Papillary muscle rupture
c. Ventricular septal defect
d. Apical thrombus
e. Bradycardia and hypotension

26. Which of the following is the most common cause of a Q-wave myocardial infarction?
   a. Plaque rupture with thrombus
   b. Coronary embolus
   c. Coronary artery spasm
   d. Increased myocardial oxygen demand
   e. Coronary artery dissection

27. A 19-year-old athlete has exertional chest pain and a systolic murmur. The electrocardiogram shows left ventricular hypertrophy. The most appropriate evaluation in this patient includes:
   a. A thallium exertion test
   b. Echocardiography
   c. Coronary angiography
   d. A dipyridamole thallium test
   e. Cardiac catheterization (right and left heart)

28. All of the following are common side effects of the angiotensin converting enzyme inhibitors except:
   a. Nonproductive cough
   b. Myositis
   c. Dysgeusia
   d. Hypotension
   e. Hyperkalemia

29. Dilated cardiomyopathy is diagnosed on the basis of:
   a. Cardiac catheterization showing a dip-and-plateau pattern
   b. Echocardiography showing a dilated and poorly contractile left ventricle
   c. A thallium scan with multiple perfusion defects
   d. A sustained left ventricular impulse on examination
   e. Chest radiograph showing an enlarged cardiac silhouette

30. Which of the following drugs would not be expected to cause hemodynamic deterioration in a patient with hypertrophic obstructive cardiomyopathy with a high gradient at rest?
   a. Digoxin
   b. Propranolol
   c. Furosemide
   d. Verapamil
   e. Nitroglycerin

31. Which of the following is *not* a feature of hypertrophic cardiomyopathy?

a. Dynamic left ventricular outflow tract obstruction
b. Mitral regurgitation
c. Low voltage on electrocardiogram
d. Severe left ventricular hypertrophy on echocardiography in the absence of known cause
e. Late peaking systolic ejection murmur with normal carotid upstrokes

32. Which of the following is *not* common in a patient with restrictive cardiomyopathy?
   a. Severe mitral regurgitation
   b. Enlarged atria
   c. Dip-and-plateau pattern on the left ventricular pressure curve
   d. Rapid X and Y descents in the jugular venous pulse
   e. End-equalization of diastolic pressures

33. A 57-year-old woman presents with severe shortness of breath and has an ejection fraction of 15%. Which of the following should not be given?
   a. Hydralazine
   b. Digoxin
   c. Enalapril
   d. Diltiazem
   e. Long-acting nitrates

True/False (indicate whether each answer is true or false)
34. Mitral valve prolapse
   a. Is more common in women
   b. Does not need bacterial endocarditis prophylaxis if unassociated with a murmur
   c. With Valsalva maneuver, the click moves later and the murmur becomes shorter
   d. Is associated with Marfan's syndrome
   e. Is the most common valve lesion associated with primum atrial septal defect
   f. Two-dimensional echocardiography can delineate which patients are at higher risk of stroke and chordal rupture

35. Which of the following is true/false about a woman with Marfan's syndrome?
   a. The risk of her child inheriting the disease is 1:4
   b. If her aortic root reaches 58 mm in size, it should be replaced
   c. If her aortic root has normal dimensions, she still has an increased risk of aortic dissection and rupture during pregnancy
   d. Angiotensin converting enzyme inhibitors have been proved to delay aortic dilatation
   e. If her aortic root is >4 cm diameter, she should be counseled against pregnancy
   f. If severe aortic regurgitation develops with an ejection fraction of 50%, the aortic valve should be replaced

36. A 65-year-old man presents with severe mitral regurgitation.
    a. The most common cause is rheumatic heart disease
    b. His ejection fraction will increase after valve replacement
    c. If the anterior leaflet is flail, the murmur will radiate to the aortic area
    d. The afterload of the left ventricle is increased
    e. If the cause is papillary muscle rupture, the most likely one to be affected is the posteromedial one
    f. The first heart sound is usually loud

37. A 55-year-old woman has chest pressure. Her rhythm is atrial fibrillation, with a ventricular response of 135 beats per minute while lying down. She states that she previously underwent cardiac catheterization. She has a 70% obstruction in her mid right coronary artery. She typically gets angina, similar to her present chest pain, only at high levels of exertion. The only treatment has been aspirin, 325 mg daily, for her coronary artery disease. The following would be effective for controlling the ventricular response during atrial fibrillation in this patient:
    a. Digoxin
    b. Verapamil
    c. Metoprolol
    d. Nifedipine
    e. Diltiazem
    f. Quinidine

38. The following are likely to prevent ventricular tachycardia or ventricular fibrillation after myocardial infarction:
    a. Aneurysmectomy
    b. Smoking cessation
    c. Participation in cardiac rehabilitation
    d. Empiric quinidine
    e. Empiric flecainide
    f. Implantable cardioverter defibrillator

39. Reentry is the underlying mechanism for the following arrhythmias:
    a. Sinus tachycardia
    b. Atrioventricular reciprocating tachycardia in Wolff-Parkinson-White syndrome
    c. Atrioventricular nodal tachycardia using slow and fast pathways
    d. Atrial flutter
    e. Nonparoxysmal junctional tachycardia
    f. Ventricular tachycardia late after myocardial infarction

40. The following are useful for documenting which arrhythmia is the cause of a patient's symptoms:
    a. History

b. 24-hour ambulatory ECG monitor
    c. Continuous loop-event recorder
    d. Signal-averaged ECG
    e. Heart rate variability
    f. Telephone transmitter

41. With regard to catheter-based interventions:
    a. They should be performed immediately after thrombolytic therapy
    b. Restenosis can be reduced with aspirin
    c. They have a high initial success rate of >90%
    d. They are useful in cardiogenic shock after myocardial infarction
    e. Lower restenosis rate with laser versus PTCA
    f. They have a better long-term outcome in multivessel disease than CABG does

42. With regard to CABG versus medical therapy, CABG:
    a. Improves survival in patients with multivessel disease and normal left ventricular function
    b. Prevents myocardial infarction in patients with high-grade proximal left anterior descending coronary artery disease
    c. Prevents ventricular fibrillation
    d. Improves left ventricular function in patients with 3-vessel disease and an ejection fraction of 20%
    e. Provides better relief of symptoms of angina
    f. Improves survival in patients with left main coronary artery disease

43. The following drug regimens are useful for a 50-year-old man with an acute anterior myocardial infarction of 3 hours' duration:
    a. Streptokinase, aspirin, β-blockers
    b. TPA, heparin, aspirin, β-blockers
    c. Streptokinase, aspirin, magnesium, lidocaine
    d. Emergency PTCA
    e. TPA, ACE inhibitor, calcium channel blocker
    f. Urokinase, magnesium, aspirin, calcium channel blocker

44. The following maneuvers will increase the left ventricular outflow murmur in a patient with hypertrophic cardiomyopathy:
    a. Squatting to standing position
    b. Administration of amyl nitrite
    c. Strain phase of the Valsalva maneuver
    d. Sublingual nitroglycerin
    e. Supine position with elevation of the feet

45. The following drugs will cause a significant increase of the digoxin level:
    a. Verapamil

b. Captopril
c. Quinidine
d. Amiodarone
e. Furosemide

46. In a 63-year-old man with class III symptoms of heart failure, an ejection fraction of 20%, and nonsustained ventricular tachycardia on Holter monitoring, the following drugs will improve survival:
    a. Quinidine
    b. Flecainide
    c. Enalapril
    d. Digoxin
    e. Nitrates/hydralazine

ANSWERS

1. Answer a.

The bicuspid aortic valve can cause isolated aortic regurgitation. With increasing stenosis, the ejection click moves *earlier* to the first sound because the high left ventricular pressure forces the valve open early. The aortic closure sound becomes more delayed with increasing stenosis and, when severe, may result in paradoxic splitting of the second sound. Bicuspid aortic valves frequently do not calcify until the third decade, and the valve may still be pliable even in the setting of severe stenosis. Thus, an ejection click is still frequently present in a 20-year-old despite severe stenosis. Even a normally functioning bicuspid aortic valve may be the substrate for infective endocarditis, and in such cases endocarditis prophylaxis is needed.

2. Answer d.

Ventricular septal defects, when small, usually produce a loud systolic murmur because they induce more turbulence, and therefore they may also be associated with a thrill. Muscular defects frequently close spontaneously, and all ventricular septal defects need antibiotic prophylaxis. When there is a large defect, there is an increased flow from the left to the right side of the heart. This results in increased return to the left side of the heart, producing a diastolic murmur across the mitral valve because of the increased flow (functional mitral stenosis). Large defects, which may be associated with Eisenmenger's syndrome, produce little or no murmur because right and left ventricular pressures are in equilibrium and there is no turbulence between the two ventricles.

3. Answer d.

This patient requires repair of an abdominal aortic aneurysm, which is one of the high-risk procedures associated with a strong likelihood of occurrence of a myocardial infarction peri-operatively. He has class III symptoms and needs to take nitrates every day. In the setting of his marked symptoms, he should have coronary angiography preoperatively. If he had class I or II symptoms, a stress test would be appropriate.

4. Answer d.

All angiotensin converting enzyme (ACE) inhibitors, including enalapril, are contraindicated in pregnancy. Digoxin is very safe and is not associated with any fetal problem during pregnancy. The β-adrenergic blockers, including propranolol, may be associated with impaired fetal growth, bradycardia, and hypoglycemia at the time of birth, but this is usually only when large doses are used, and they are not absolutely contraindicated in pregnancy. Similarly, quinidine and verapamil can be used if necessary and are not contraindicated.

5. Answer e.

Because of increased venous return to the right side of the heart during inspiration, inspiration increases all the murmurs on the right side of the heart, including pulmonary stenosis and tricuspid regurgitation. Changing from the supine to the standing position decreases venous return because the blood pools in the legs, and therefore the murmur of pulmonary stenosis gets softer on standing. Valsalva maneuver, by increasing the intrathoracic pressure, reduces preload, and therefore the murmur of mitral regurgitation gets softer. Indeed, most cardiac murmurs diminish in intensity during Valsalva maneuver except hypertrophic cardiomyopathy and mitral valve prolapse. In the latter case, the click may move earlier, and the murmur may get longer. After a premature ventricular complex, there is increased ventricular contractility, and so the murmur of aortic stenosis increases. This is one of the ways that aortic stenosis can be distinguished from mitral regurgitation at the bedside, because the murmur of mitral regurgitation is unchanged after a premature ventricular complex.

6. Answer b.

Cardiac amyloid deposits both in the myocardium and on the atrioventricular valves and can produce a thick-walled left ventricle with both systolic and diastolic dysfunction. Patients therefore can present with congestive heart failure, pericardial effusion, and arrhythmias. Atrial arrhythmias are particularly frequent. Because amyloid deposits on the atrioventricular valves, regurgitation of these valves is common. It does not deposit on the aortic valve particularly, and so it does not produce aortic stenosis.

7. Answer e.

Mitral stenosis causes a localized tapping apical impulse, which is actually the palpable fourth heart sound. As mitral stenosis increases in severity, the diastolic murmur becomes longer because the gradient persists throughout diastole. It causes a loud first heart sound, and the A_2-OS interval gets shorter with increasing stenosis, severe stenosis being associated with an A_2-OS interval of approximately 70 msec or less. The opening snap occurs only with a pliable valve, and so as the valve begins to calcify, the opening snap disappears.

8. Answer b.

The calcium channel blocking drugs verapamil and diltiazem affect slow conduction through the atrioventricular node. They have minimal effect on the other tissues listed. Slowing of the sinus node can also occur with these drugs.

9. Answer d.

This patient has symptoms that occur infrequently and last only a brief time. Thus, to document this patient's arrhythmia, he needs to be wearing a recording device at the time of his arrhythmia, and it should be one that he can activate but which already would have been recording the rhythm before the onset of symptoms. An event recorder would be most useful for this patient.

10. Answer d.

Adenosine can terminate atrioventricular nodal reentry in most cases by blocking the slow pathway. Sinus tachycardia may be slowed transiently but not terminated by adenosine. Atrial flutter and atrial fibrillation would not be directly affected, although the ventricular response would slow for a brief time. Most types of ventricular tachycardia would not be terminated by adenosine, although there are rare types that can be.

11. Answer e.

Currently, dual-chamber pacing is not available in implantable cardioverter defibrillators. This is being developed for future devices, but as of now, they have only single-chamber, fixed rate pacing.

12. Answer e.

Proarrhythmia can be fatal if not identified, but many patients can be saved, particularly if antiarrhythmic drug therapy is initiated in the hospital during continuous monitoring. Studies have shown that proarrhythmia typically is an early event, clustered within the first few days after beginning treatment with drugs such as class IA agents. Torsades de pointes is one form of proarrhythmia, but there are others, such as ventricular fibrillation and incessant ventricular tachycardia. Torsades de pointes is more typical of the proarrhythmia caused by drugs that prolong the QT interval, such as the class IA (quinidine, procainamide, and disopyramide) and class III (sotalol) drugs.

13. Answer e.

CAST was a trial of flecainide, encainide, and moricizine for suppression of premature ventricular complexes and nonsustained ventricular tachycardia after myocardial infarction. The trial showed that these drugs actually increased mortality even though they suppressed the ambient asymptomatic ventricular arrhythmia. The results can be applied only to those drugs. It showed that treatment of nonsustained ventricular tachycardia with these drugs increased mortality. Flecainide and morcizine are available, but encainide is no longer marketed. The study did not address flecainide in the treatment of supraventricular arrhythmias, and, in fact, flecainide is the only other drug aside from quinidine that is approved for treatment of supraventricular arrhythmias. Currently, no studies exist that are convincing enough to empirically use antiarrhythmic drugs for decreasing mortality after myocardial infarction. This does not include β-adrenergic blocking drugs, which have been shown to decrease mortality with empiric use after myocardial infarction.

14. Answer b.

The arrhythmia is atrial fibrillation with Wolff-Parkinson-White syndrome. This is diagnosed because the ventricular rhythm is grossly irregular, and this would be exceedingly rare to occur in monomorphic ventricular tachycardia. The QRS is wide and the rate is too fast to be conducting normally over the atrioventricular node. If the patient's condition is stable hemodynamically, the drug of choice is procainamide, which will block the accessory pathway and/or convert the patient form atrial fibrillation to normal sinus rhythm. Should the patient's condition be unstable, cardioversion would be the therapy of choice.

15. Answer c.

The arrhythmia is ventricular tachycardia: 2:1 ventriculoatrial conduction can be seen with P waves associated with every other QRS, best seen in lead V_1. The treatment of choice for hemodynamically stable ventricular tachycardia is lidocaine.

16. Answer d.

This regular narrow QRS tachycardia most likely is atrioventricular reentry going down the atrioventricular node and returning to the atrium, traveling up the accessory pathway. Lidocaine typically would not be effective in blocking the atrioventricular node or the accessory pathway. Adenosine and verapamil both would cause a block in the atrioventricular node, thus terminating the arrhythmia. Procainamide likely would block the accessory pathway. Electrical cardioversion would be used if the patient's condition were unstable.

17. Answer a.

Although digoxin can slow the atrioventricular node, and thus slow the ventricular response in atrial fibrillation, it has never been convincingly shown either to terminate acute atrial fibrillation or to prevent its recurrence. All the other antiarrhythmic drugs have been shown to prevent recurrent atrial fibrillation in some patients.

18. Answer d.

Serial drug testing is used frequently to identify the most effective therapy for sustained ventricular tachycardia. Nonsustained ventricular tachycardia is not an adverse prognosticator in the setting of a normal heart. Frequent premature ventricular complexes indicate an increased risk of sudden death after myocardial infarction; however, treatment of this arrhythmia has not been shown to decrease the incidence of sudden death, and it generally is not accepted that this needs to be evaluated further. Out-of-hospital cardiac arrest usually is not due to a reversible cause such as acute ischemia. Sotalol is effective for both supraventricular and ventricular arrhythmias.

19. Answer b.

The predominant ventricular response is 2:1, but in leads 2 and 3, there is a slightly higher atrioventricular block for a few atrial impulses and the atrial flutter waves can be identified.

20. Answer c.

Tobacco abuse is a definite risk factor for coronary artery disease. Diabetes mellitus is a definite risk factor for coronary artery disease. Hyperlipidemia is associated with an increased incidence of coronary artery disease. High low-density lipoprotein and high total cholesterol values are associated with an increased incidence of coronary artery disease. Conversely, low-density lipoprotein is a risk factor for coronary artery disease. Mild alcohol consumption (up to two beers per day) may actually be protective for coronary artery disease.

21. Answer d.

Side effects of β-blockers include a worsening claudication (due to unopposed α-receptor stimulation), depressed libido, and an increase in lipids. β-Blockers have been shown to improve survival after myocardial infarction. β-Blockers will actually increase ventricular fibrillation threshold rather than lower it.

22. Answer d.

Components of myocardial oxygen demand include heart rate, contractility, wall tension, and afterload. Perfusion pressure is the pressure between the aorta and right atrium. This is a determinant of myocardial oxygen supply, not demand.

23. Answer c.

The 65-year-old man has a high pretest probability of having coronary artery disease. Therefore, despite the "normal" treadmill exertion test, he still has a high probability of having coronary artery disease. With symptoms typical of angina pectoris, he does not need other diagnostic tests such as esophageal manometry. The fact that he was able to achieve 100% of his functional aerobic capacity indicates that he had a good prognosis. Therefore, he does not need coronary angiography. The exercise thallium test or dobutamine echocardiography will not add any more clinical information.

24. Answer d.

In the patient with unstable angina, both aspirin and heparin have been shown to prevent the progression to myocardial infarction. β-Blockers will decrease myocardial oxygen demand, and they also have been shown to prevent the progression to myocardial infarction. Thrombolytic agents have not been shown in any trial to be of benefit in patients with unstable angina. Angiotensin converting enzyme inhibitors have not been shown to be useful in patients with unstable angina.

25. Answer d.

Inferior myocardial infarction is associated with the mechanical complications of myocardial infarction, including papillary muscle rupture and ventricular septal defect. If there is a right dominant circulation, inferior myocardial infarction can frequently be associated with infarction of the right ventricle. An inferior myocardial infarction is frequently associated with bradycardia and hypotension due to ischemia to the sinoatrial node as well as activation of the Bezold-Jarisch reflex. An inferior myocardial infarction will not result in an apical thrombus, because the apex is most frequently supplied by blood in the anterior distribution.

26. Answer a.

A Q-wave myocardial infarction is usually caused by plaque rupture with thrombus formation. This results in 100% occlusion of the coronary artery. Myocardial infarction is rarely caused by coronary artery spasm or coronary artery dissection. Coronary artery embolus is a rare cause of myocardial infarction. In patients with severe coronary artery disease, non-Q-wave myocardial infarction can be caused by increased myocardial oxygen demand. However, a Q-wave infarction is almost always caused by complete occlusion of a coronary artery.

27. Answer b.

The finding of left ventricular hypertrophy on the electrocardiogram raises the differential diagnosis of athletic heart versus hypertrophic cardiomyopathy. This morphologic distinction should be make with echocardiography. Stress perfusion testing or coronary angiography would not define ventricular status. Cardiac catheterization could identify hyperdynamic ventricular function and even possibly obstruction but would not make the morphologic diagnosis of inappropriate hypertrophy, which would indicate hypertrophic cardiomyopathy.

28. Answer b.

Angiotensin converting enzyme inhibitors cause nonproductive cough, altered taste sensation (dysgeusia), hypotension, or hyperkalemia. Myositis is not a common side effect of these drugs.

29. Answer b.

The diagnosis of dilated cardiomyopathy is based on a finding of ventricular enlargement with poor contractile function. This is most easily obtained by either echocardiography or radionuclide imaging. Although a dip-and-plateau pattern might be seen in end-stage cardiomyopathy, its presence or absence neither confirms nor refutes the diagnosis because it is more common in other diseases such as restrictive cardiomyopathy. Perfusion defects on a thallium scan do not define contractile function. A sustained ventricular impulse is present in dilated cardiomyopathy but also present in hypertension, aortic stenosis, or hypertrophic cardiomyopathy. An enlarged cardiac silhouette on chest radiography is nonspecific.

30. Answer b.

Drugs that decrease left ventricular volume, increase left ventricular contractility, or decrease left ventricular afterload cause hemodynamic deterioration in patients with hypertrophic cardiomyopathy. Such drugs include digoxin, furosemide, and nitroglycerin. Verapamil decreases contractility but also decreases afterload; in patients with resting obstruction, the putative effect of the latter may overshadow the beneficial effect of the former, and it is therefore contraindicated. Propranolol would not be expected to be hemodynamically harmful in patients with hypertrophic cardiomyopathy with high resting gradients.

31. Answer c.

Hypertrophic cardiomyopathy is a diagnosis based on a finding of marked ventricular hypertrophy without cause. Dynamic outflow tract obstruction is usually present, as is mitral regurgitation. Physical examination reveals a late-peaking ejection murmur with normal carotid upstrokes, thus helping distinguish it from aortic stenosis. Typically the electrocardiogram shows high voltage. A finding of low voltage in combination with marked ventricular hypertrophy on echocardiography raises the thought of an infiltrative process such as amyloidosis.

32. Answer a.

Patients with restrictive cardiomyopathy have near normal ventricular size and function but markedly enlarged atria due to the chronically high ventricular filling pressures. Physical findings include elevated jugular venous pressures with rapid X and Y descents. Hemodynamics in this condition show high, equalized diastolic pressures with a dip-and-plateau pattern on the ventricular pressure curves. These high equalized pressures and the characteristic appearance can also be seen in constrictive pericarditis, and this important distinction needs to be made.

33. Answer d.

Patients with severe ventricular systolic dysfunction can safely receive hydralazine, digoxin, enalapril, and nitrates. The combination of nitrates and hydralazine as well as angiotensin converting enzyme inhibitors has been shown to improve symptom status and mortality. Digoxin improves symptom status in patients with severe symptoms. Diltiazem and the other first-generation calcium channel blockers are negatively inotropic and typically should not be given to patients with significant systolic dysfunction.

34. a, true; b, true; c, false; d, true; e, false; f, true.

Mitral valve prolapse is more common in women, and patients who do not have associated mitral regurgitation do not need to have endocarditis prophylaxis. The Valsalva maneuver reduces venous return so the left ventricle has a smaller volume within it. This distorts the ventricular geometry, causing the valve to prolapse earlier, and thus mitral regurgitation begins earlier, making the murmur longer. Mitral valve prolapse is one of the common associations of Marfan's syndrome. Patients with primum atrial septal defect have a cleft mitral valve, and this is a different anomaly from mitral valve prolapse. Two-dimensional echocardiography can delineate patients at higher risk of stroke and chordal rupture, because these are patients who have a thicker, more redundant mitral valve. Patients who have normal leaflet thickening and no redundancy have a very low risk of cardiovascular complications.

35. a, false; b, true; c, true; d, false; e, true; f, true.

Marfan's syndrome has autosomal dominant inheritance, and so the chance of a woman with Marfan's syndrome having a child with the same syndrome is approximately 50%. In general, if the aortic root reaches 55 mm in size, patients are at increased risk for dissection and rupture, and at that point it should be replaced. Nonetheless, the aorta in patients with Marfan's syndrome is not normal, even if it has normal dimensions. Because of the softening that takes place in the vascular tissues during pregnancy, patients are still at risk of dissection and rupture. In two reported series, β-adrenergic blockers were shown to delay aortic dilatation. Angiotensin converting enzyme inhibitors have not been shown yet to do this. Patients who have an aortic root >4 cm in diameter appear to be at more risk of aortic complications during pregnancy, and so they should be counseled against pregnancy. Patients with severe aortic regurgitation should have a hyperdynamic left ventricle, and if the ejection fraction has decreased to 50%, at least modest ventricular dysfunction is implied. The aortic valve should be replaced, preferably before ventricular dysfunction has developed.

36. a, false; b, false; c, false; d, true; e, true; f, false.

In a 65-year-old man with severe mitral regurgitation in the United States, rheumatic heart disease is not the most common cause; much more likely would be mitral valve prolapse or ischemic heart disease. Because mitral regurgitation "offloads" the left ventricle, replacing the valve removes this afterload reduction. As a result, the ejection fraction does not usually improve after valve replacement but either stays the same or may even decrease. The posteromedial papillary muscle rupture is the one most likely to be affected by ischemia because of its single blood supply. The first heart sound is usually soft with severe mitral regurgitation.

37. a, true; b, true; c, true; d, false; e, true; f, false.

Digoxin, β-adrenergic blocking drugs (metoprolol), and calcium channel blocking drugs (verapamil and diltiazem) slow the ventricular response in atrial fibrillation by slowing conduction through the atrioventricular node. Other calcium channel blocking drugs (nifedipine) do not clinically affect the atrioventricular node in vivo. Quinidine can enhance conduction through the node through its vagolytic effect and may actually increase the ventricular response during atrial fibrillation.

38. a, false; b, false; c, false; d, false; e, false; f, false.

Aneursymectomy does not remove the portion of the heart involved in the arrhythmia. To prevent recurrent ventricular tachycardia, the operation must include a subendocardial resection. Empiric antiarrhythmic drugs such as quinidine and flecainide have never been shown to decrease the rate of recurrence of ventricular tachycardia or ventricular fibrillation. Although implantable cardioverter defibrillators are effective in the treatment of ventricular tachycardia or ventricular fibrillation, they do not prevent their recurrence.

39. a, false; b, true; c, true; d, true; e, false; f, true.

Sinus tachycardia is due to automaticity. Atrioventricular reciprocating tachycardia and atrioventricular node tachycardia with dual physiology (i.e., slow and fast pathways) are well-defined reentrant rhythms that can be cured by ablation of a portion of the reentrant circuit. Classic atrial flutter has been shown to be due to reentry within the right atrium, with the waveform proceeding down the freewall and then up the atrial septum. Nonparoxysmal junctional tachycardia is thought to be due to triggered activity when caused by digitalis intoxication. It is not thought to be due to reentry under any circumstance. With mapping techniques, ventricular tachycardia occurring after chronic myocardial infarction has been shown to be due to reentry.

40. a, false; b, true; c, true; d, false; e, false; f, true.

To document which arrhythmia is the cause of a patient's symptoms, it is necessary to document the cardiac rhythm during the patient's symptoms. This can be done only with devices such as 24-hour Holter monitors if the arrhythmia occurs during the time the patient is wearing the monitor. Continuous loop event recorders are more useful for patients who have less frequent arrhythmias, because this device can be worn for a period of months. A telephone transmitter is useful for a patient whose symptoms last long enough that they can hook up this equipment and call in to a center to transmit their rhythm real-time. A history may give clues about the cause of a person's arrhythmia, but it will not document the arrhythmia. Signal-averaged ECG and heart rate variability are tools used to identify patients at increased risk of having ventricular arrhythmias, particularly after myocardial infarction. These tools do not show what the arrhythmia is that a patient has.

41. a, false; b, false ; c, true; d, true; e, false; f, false.

A catheter-based intervention can now be performed with a high initial success rate of >90%. However, there is a high restenosis rate approaching 50% at 6 months' time. The restenosis rate has not been shown to be decreased by any medications. Other types of catheter-based intervention aside from PTCA (laser angioplasty, atherectomy Rotoblator) have not been shown to decrease the incidence of restenosis. In acute myocardial infarction, PTCA should not be performed after thrombolytic therapy. However, PTCA is useful in the patient who presents with cardiogenic shock. The long-term outcome in multivessel disease is not better with PTCA than CABG.

42. a, false; b, false; c, false; d, false; e, true; f, true.

CABG has been evaluated in several randomized trials. As opposed to medical therapy, CABG will not prevent myocardial infarction, will not prevent ventricular fibrillation, and will not improve ventricular function. It improves survival only in certain subgroups of patients, including those with left main coronary artery disease and patients with three-vessel disease and depressed left ventricular function. CABG does provide better relief of symptoms of angina than medical therapy.

43. a, true; b, true; c, false; d, true; e, false; f, false.

In the patient who presents with a large anterior myocardial infarction, thrombolytic therapy with either tissue plasminogen activator (TPA) or streptokinase has been shown to be of benefit in decreasing mortality. Concomitant use of aspirin will also lower mortality. β-Blockade given acutely decreases mortality. Intravenous heparin should be given concomitantly with TPA. Neither calcium channel blockers nor magnesium have conclusively been shown to decrease mortality in patients with myocardial infarction. Emergency PTCA can be performed and will reduce mortality in patients with acute myocardial infarction, especially those with large anterior myocardial infarctions.

44. a, true; b, true; c, true; d, true; e, false.

The left ventricular obstruction in patients with hypertrophic cardiomyopathy is aggravated by conditions that reduce ventricular preload, decrease ventricular afterload, or increase myocardial contractility. Standing causes transient volume depletion, amyl nitrite causes a transient decrease in preload and afterload, the strain phase of the Valsalva maneuver decreases venous return and therefore decreases preload, and sublingual nitroglycerin acutely decreases preload. Therefore, all four of these maneuvers increase the degree of dynamic outflow tract obstruction, which in turn increases the severity of an outflow tract murmur.

45. a, true; b, false; c, true; d, true; e, false.

Significant drug-drug interactions occur between digoxin and verapamil, quinidine, and amiodarone. If these drugs are added to the regimen of someone taking digoxin, the digoxin dose should be empirically halved. Captopril and furosemide do not have such an interaction.

46. a, false; b, false; c, true; d, false; e, true.

Patients with class III heart failure due to impaired ventricular systolic function benefit in survival terms from angiotensin converting enzyme inhibitors, including enalapril and a combination of nitrates and hydralazine. Although digoxin might improve symptom status, it has not been proved to enhance survival. No drug therapy for ventricular dysrhythmias has been shown to enhance survival in these patients and, in fact, flecainide is strongly contraindicated in patients with ventricular systolic dysfunction.

NOTES

CHAPTER 4
CLINICAL PHARMACOLOGY AND TOXICOLOGY

Thomas F. Bugliosi, M.D.

EPIDEMIOLOGY

Most exposures to poison (69%) reported to the American Association of Poison Control Centers in 1993 occurred in persons younger than 19 years. Overall, accidental poisoning outnumbers intentional poisoning in all age groups. However, if only fatal cases are considered (626 in 1993), most occurred in adults, and suicide was the cause in 54%. It is important to remember that the vast majority of all poisonings are not deadly, and most patients do well with good supportive care (Am J Emerg Med 12:546-584, 1994).

- Most exposures to poison are in persons <19 years.
- Accidental poisoning outnumbers intentional poisoning.
- Vast majority of poisonings are not deadly.

DIAGNOSIS

Clinical

Any patient who presents with an altered mental status should be considered to have taken an overdose. The history provided by the patient is often unreliable, and every effort should be made to interrogate family, friends, paramedics, and law enforcement officers present at the scene. Ask them to bring in pill remnants and containers.

- Patient with altered mental status should be considered to have taken overdose.
- History given by patient is often unreliable.

The next step is a thorough general examination. Many of the most frequent poisonings produce classic physical signs and symptoms, and you should be familiar with these. The findings associated with various agents are listed below.

- Many poisonings produce classic physical signs and symptoms.

Anticholinergic syndrome (atropine, belladonna alkaloid, tricyclic antidepressants, antipsychotics, medications for Parkinson's disease, and antihistamines):
- Dry skin and mucous membranes
- Hyperthermia
- Flushing
- Tachycardia
- Hypertension
- Mydriasis
- ↓ Salivation
- ↓ Sweating
- Ileus
- Urinary retention
- Anxiety/confusion
- Seizures

Mnemonic: "Red as a beet, hot as a hare, dry as a bone, blind as a bat, and mad as a hatter"

Cholinergic syndrome (organophosphate poisoning):
- Sweating
- Salivation
- Lacrimation
- Miosis
- Bradycardia
- Vomiting
- Diarrhea
- Wheezing
- Muscle cramps/fasciculations
- Altered mental status
- Acronym is "SLUDGE":
- *S*alivation, *L*acrimation, *U*rination, *D*efecation, *G*astrointestinal upset, *E*mesis

Opiates (e.g., morphine, codeine, heroin, methadone):
- Miosis
- Respiratory depression
- Drowsiness
- Nausea/vomiting

115

Pulmonary edema
Seizures

Classic triad is depressed mental status, depressed respiration, miosis.

Barbiturates (e.g., pentobarbital, phenobarbital):
Central nervous system depression
Respiratory depression
Bradycardia
Hypotension
Hypothermia
Areflexia
Pulmonary edema
Blisters
Pupils variable

Stimulants (amphetamines, cocaine, aminophylline):
Central nervous system excitation/agitation
Seizures
Hypertension
Tachycardia
Hallucinations
Arrhythmias/cardiovascular collapse
Mydriasis

Substance withdrawal:
Agitation
Confusion
Mydriasis
Tachycardia
Hypertension
Nausea
Vomiting
Abdominal pain
Seizures

Laboratory Evaluation

Toxicologic Screening

Many misconceptions exist regarding the utility of the standard drug screen. Many commonly encountered drugs cannot be easily detected. The predictive value of a negative toxicologic test is only 40%. Of the drugs that can be detected, quantitative results can be obtained in only 5%-10% of cases. When quantitative results can be measured, they often correlate poorly with clinical signs and symptoms. Most qualitative tests require urine samples, and most quantitative tests require serum samples.

- Predictive value of negative toxicologic test is only 40%.
- Quantitative results reliable in only 5%-10% of cases.
- Most qualitative tests require urine samples; most quantitative tests require serum samples.
- Treat the patient on the basis of symptoms and signs, not results of toxicologic screening.

Quantitative drug levels have important therapeutic implications in only a handful of cases:
Acetaminophen
Salicylates
Theophylline
Methanol
Ethylene glycol
Iron
Lithium
Seizure medications (for seizure prophylaxis)
Carbon monoxide
Methemoglobin

Arterial Blood Gases

Perhaps the most useful ancillary blood test that can be performed is the arterial blood gas analysis. This not only will give critical acid-base information but also can diagnose specific poisonings such as carbon monoxide and methemoglobin.

- Arterial blood gas analysis is very useful test.

Osmolar Gap

This is calculated as the difference between the osmolarity as measured by freezing point depression and the calculated osmolarity.

- Calculated osmolarity = $2\,[Na^+] + \dfrac{BUN}{2.8} + \dfrac{Glucose}{18}$ (BUN, blood urea nitrogen).
- Osmolar gap = measured osmolarity - calculated osmolarity.
- If osmolar gap >10, consider acetone, ethanol, methanol, ethylene glycol, isopropanol, and diuretics (mannitol, glycerol, or sorbitol).

Anion Gap

The anion gap can be extremely useful in patients with suspected overdose.

Anion gap = $Na^+ - (Cl^- + HCO_3^-)$; normal gap is 8-12 mEq.

A decreased anion gap can occur in patients with hypermagnesemia, bromide or lithium ingestion, or hypoalbuminemia. An increased anion gap can occur in patients who have ingested methanol, ethylene glycol, propylene glycol, salicylates, strychnine, isoniazid, paraldehyde, phenformin, carbon monoxide, cyanide, or iron. Nontoxicologic causes of an increased anion gap include uremia, diabetic ketoacidosis, and lactic acidosis.

- Iron ingestion is a cause of increased anion gap that is often forgotten.
- Acetaminophen, narcotics, hallucinogens, and stimulants generally do not cause an increased anion gap.

ESSENTIALS OF CARE

Care of the poisoned patient can be divided into 1) supportive care, 2) prevention of further absorption, 3) enhancement of excretion, and 4) administration of a specific antidote.

Supportive Care

Any patient who presents with an altered mental status or confusing symptom complex should be evaluated for drug overdose. Secure airway, breathing, and circulation (ABCs). Most patients will do well with careful attention to the ABCs, including endotracheal intubation if necessary. Intravenous access and cardiac monitoring should be initiated. Confused, agitated, or violent patients require close observation and possibly physical restraints.

- Any patient with altered mental status should be evaluated for drug overdose.
- Secure airway, breathing, circulation (ABCs).
- Establish intravenous access and cardiac monitoring.

Dextrose (D_{50}) was once considered "standard" care of patients with altered mental status. A growing body of evidence, however, suggests that elevated glucose concentrations during cerebral ischemia worsen brain injury and decrease functional recovery. Therefore, every patient with altered mental status should have a quick fingerstick blood glucose determination. Dextrose should be administered to patients with documented hypoglycemia. In addition, administer 100 mg thiamine intramuscularly to alcoholic patients.

- Elevated glucose concentrations during cerebral ischemia may worsen brain injury and decrease functional recovery.
- Every patient with altered mental status should have quick fingerstick blood glucose determination.
- Alcoholic patients should be treated with 100 mg thiamine intramuscularly.

Naloxone (Narcan) was also considered standard care of patients with altered mental status. Naloxone has been reported to cause pulmonary edema in a few anecdotal case reports. Patients with hypoventilation, miosis, or other signs of narcotic abuse who present with altered mental status should be given 2 mg naloxone by intravenous push. Naloxone can also be given subcutaneously or intramuscularly or by endotracheal tube. Remember that many narcotics have longer half-lives than naloxone, so all patients require prolonged monitoring for resedation.

- Naloxone has been reported to rarely cause pulmonary edema.
- Naloxone 2 mg intravenously should be given in patients with hypoventilation, miosis, or signs of narcotic abuse.
- All patients require prolonged monitoring for resedation.

Prevention of Further Absorption

Many toxins can be absorbed through the skin, and decontamination of the skin is mandatory in such cases. Gastric emptying can be accomplished with induced emesis or gastric lavage utilizing a large-bore (32- to 40-French) tube. In general, there has been a significant trend away from these treatments for several reasons:

- No studies prove that these efforts positively influence outcome.
- Recent studies have shown that activated charcoal alone may be superior to either induced emesis or gastric lavage, and it seems to cause fewer complications.
- Gastric emptying is time-consuming in a busy emergency department.
- Either method of gastric emptying removes only about 30% of ingested material.

Induced Emesis

Syrup of ipecac is the only acceptable emetic. It acts centrally (medulla) and peripherally. Vomiting usually occurs within 20 minutes. The usual adult dose is 30 mL, which may be given again in 30 minutes if vomiting has not occurred.

An indication for ipecac is ingestion of a potentially toxic substance in the home setting in persons older than 6 months. Contraindications are nontoxic ingestions, caustic ingestions, hydrocarbon ingestions, age younger than 6 months, altered mental status, poor gag reflex, seizures, and substance likely to alter mental status rapidly (e.g., tricyclics). Complications are prolonged vomiting, Mallory-Weiss tear, aspiration pneumonia, intracranial hemorrhage, and delayed charcoal administration.

- Ipecac is the only acceptable emetic.
- Usual adult dose is 30 mL; may be repeated in 30 minutes.
- Aspiration is major concern with ipecac.
- Patient must be alert and likely to stay that way.

Gastric Lavage

This is accomplished with the patient in the left lateral decubitus position; a large-bore orogastric tube is used. A cuffed endotracheal tube should be placed before procedure if patient has altered mental status, depressed gag reflex, or seizures. Indications are recent (<1 hour) ingestion of a potentially toxic substance, substances not well bound by charcoal, or toxic substances that delay gastric emptying. Contraindications are nontoxic ingestions, caustic ingestions, and patients who present >1 hour after ingestion, except in cases of potentially delayed gastric emptying. Complications are aspiration pneumonia, perforation of esophagus or stomach, and inadvertent tracheal intubation.

- Before gastric lavage, cuffed endotracheal tube should be placed if patient has altered mental status, depressed gag reflex, or seizures.

Activated Charcoal

Activated charcoal is emerging as the treatment of choice for most poisonings. It is an inert compound that binds to most substances. The dose is generally 1 g/kg body weight. This may be given as a slurry down an orogastric tube or nasogastric tube, or the patient can drink it. Charcoal is generally ineffective for absorbing small ionic compounds such as lithium, magnesium, arsenic, and alcohols. In addition, charcoal should not be given in cases of caustic ingestions because the caustic substances are poorly bound by activated charcoal, and the subsequent endoscopic view will be obscured. Pulse charcoal in which 50 g of charcoal is given every 2 to 4 hours has theoretical value in overdoses involving drugs that undergo enterohepatic circulation (e.g., barbiturates, meprobamate, carbamazepine, theophylline, phenytoin, tricyclics). Data are not conclusive, however, and the complication rate may be increased. Administration of cathartics after charcoal administration has not been proved to be effective.

- Activated charcoal emerging as treatment of choice for most poisonings.
- Dose is 1 g/kg body weight.
- Charcoal generally ineffective for absorbing small ionic compounds such as lithium, magnesium, arsenic, alcohols.
- Charcoal should not be given for caustic ingestion.

Enhancement of Excretion

Several methods may enhance excretion: forced diuresis, alkaline or acid diuresis, hemodialysis, and hemoperfusion. A brief review of volume of distribution is necessary to understand the limited role enhancement of excretion plays in most overdoses.

The volume of distribution (V_d) is defined as that volume of fluid into which a drug seems to distribute with the concentration equal to that in plasma. It is a hypothetical volume only. It does not refer to any physiologic space. When V_d is large (>1 liter/kg), the tissue concentration is large (and vice versa).

$$V_d = \frac{A \text{ (amount ingested)}}{C \text{ (plasma concentration)}}$$

The V_d can be used to predict the serum level of a drug if the amount ingested is known. For example, if a 70-kg patient ingested 50 100-mg tablets of phenytoin ($V_d = 0.75$ liter/kg), the plasma level can be predicted:

$$V_d = \frac{A}{C} \qquad V_d = 0.75 \text{ liter/kg} \times 70 \text{ kg} = 52.5 \text{ liters}$$

$$52.5 \text{ liters} = \frac{5,000 \text{ mg}}{C} = 95 \text{ mg/liter}$$

Drugs are eliminated by first order, zero order, or combination kinetics. First-order elimination is how the kidney handles toxins. A constant fraction of the drug is eliminated per unit time. The higher the plasma concentration, the greater the amount of drug excreted per unit time. Zero-order elimination is how the liver handles toxins. This type of elimination involves saturable enzymes that, when saturated, allow only for a constant amount of drug to be eliminated. Once enzymes are saturated, serum levels can increase dramatically. Examples include phenytoin, salicylates, and ethanol. Combination elimination occurs with salicylates, phenytoin, and ethanol. These drugs switch their elimination from first-order to zero-order elimination.

- First-order elimination is how kidney handles toxins.
- Zero-order elimination is how liver handles toxins.
- Combination elimination occurs with salicylates, phenytoin, ethanol in the therapeutic range.

Forced Diuresis

Most attempts at increasing drug elimination by forced diuresis (thereby increasing urine flow) are not successful. In general, for many drugs, elimination by renal excretion is not dependent on urine flow rates. In addition, drugs that are highly protein-bound or have a large volume of distribution (V_d) are not affected by forced diuresis.

- Most attempts at forced diuresis are not successful.
- Drugs that are highly protein-bound are not affected by forced diuresis.

Urine Alkalinization

Weak acids such as salicylates, phenobarbital, and isoniazid are ionized in a more alkaline medium. Promoting an alkaline urine by alkalinizing a patient slows reabsorption of weakly acidic compounds because they will exist as anions that do not readily cross lipid membranes. As a result, urinary clearance is increased. An alkaline diuresis is accomplished by adding 1 ampule of $NaHCO_3$ to 1 liter of 0.45 normal saline and monitoring urine pH.

Urine Acidification

Although several drugs (e.g., amphetamines and phencyclidine) may have their elimination enhanced by acidifying the urine, this is not recommended because of the possibility of acute renal tubular necrosis caused by rhabdomyolysis.

- Urine acidification not recommended because of possibility of acute renal tubular necrosis.

Hemodialysis

Hemodialysis has very limited application in drug overdoses. Suitable substances should be of small molecular weight and soluble, have limited protein and lipid binding, and have a small volume of distribution (V_d). The driving force is the concentration gradient of unbound, ultrafiltrable solute.

Hemodialysis is indicated in some cases of the following overdoses (depending on patient's condition): ethylene glycol, methanol, lithium, salicylates, bromide. Hemodialysis is not indicated for overdoses of tricyclic antidepressants, antihistamines, benzodiazepines, digitalis, phenothiazines, opiates, or ethchlorvynol.

Hemoperfusion

Hemoperfusion is accomplished by pumping a patient's blood through an extracorporeal cartridge containing adsorbent particles (activated charcoal, carbon, or polystyrene resin). The factors that limit toxin removal in hemodialysis are not as important in hemoperfusion.

Hemoperfusion is indicated in some cases of ingestions of phenobarbital, other barbiturates, diphenylhydantoin, and theophylline. The major rate-limiting factors are the affinity of the adsorbent for the toxin and the rate of blood flow through the circuit. Complications include thrombocytopenia, leukopenia, hypoglycemia, and hypocalcemia. Most overdoses can be managed without hemodialysis or hemoperfusion. Applications must be considered on an individual basis.

- In hemoperfusion, major rate-limiting factors are affinity of adsorbent for toxin and rate of blood flow through circuit.
- Complications include thrombocytopenia, leukopenia, hypoglycemia, hypocalcemia.
- Most overdoses can be managed without hemodialysis or hemoperfusion.

Administration of an Antidote

There are specific antidotes for only a few agents involved in overdoses. Even when a specific antidote is available, it is often not needed, and supportive care is all that is necessary. A partial list of antidotes is included in Table 4-1.

CYCLIC ANTIDEPRESSANTS

Overdose with cyclic antidepressants (e.g., imipramine, amitriptyline, desipramine, doxepin) is one of the most serious types of overdose; it causes approximately 25% of all deaths due to poisoning. They are rapidly absorbed and readily distribute to body tissues and fat. In fact, tissue levels may be much higher than plasma levels. Cyclic antidepressants have a high degree of protein binding (85%-99%) and a huge volume of distribution (V_d) (i.e., not removed by hemodialysis or hemoperfusion). Increasing pH increases protein binding; thus, less free drug is available to exert its effect.

- Overdose with cyclic antidepressants one of most serious types of overdose.
- Causes about 25% of all deaths due to poisoning.
- Cyclic antidepressants are rapidly absorbed and readily

Table 4-1.--Antidotes for Agents Associated With Overdose

Drug/toxin	Antidote
Acetaminophen	*N*-Acetylcysteine
Anticholinergics	Physostigmine
Benzodiazepines	Flumazenil
Carbon monoxide	Oxygen
Cyanide	Amyl nitrite, sodium nitrite, sodium thiosulfate
Ethylene glycol	Ethanol
Iron	Deferoxamine
Isoniazid	Pyridoxine
Methanol	Ethanol
Narcotics	Naloxone
Nitrites	Methylene blue
Organophosphates	Atropine Pralidoxime
Tricyclics	Sodium bicarbonate

From Bryson PD: Comprehensive Review in Toxicology. Second edition. New York, Raven Press, 1989, p 11. By permission of publisher.

distribute to body tissues and fat.
- They have high degree of protein binding.

Tricyclics (most cyclic antidepressants have three rings) have four main actions (Table 4-2):
1. Class IA antiarrhythmic effects (quinidine-like)
3. Anticholinergic activity
3. Block reuptake of norepinephrine in central nervous system
4. Antihistamine (H1 and H2 antagonist)

Toxic effects vary, but rapid deterioration is common. Ventricular arrhythmias, seizures, hypotension, and respiratory depression are some of the more dangerous side effects to anticipate. Maprotiline (Ludiomil) is a tetracyclic antidepressant that causes more seizures but fewer cardiovascular side effects. Remember, cardiotoxicity is the main cause of death associated with cyclic antidepressants.

- Toxic effects vary, but rapid deterioration is common with overdose of cyclic antidepressants.

Treatment of patients who have overdosed on cyclic antidepressants first includes securing the ABCs. Because seizures or rapid deterioration is common, many patients require endotracheal intubation. Do not induce vomiting. After ABCs are secured, gastric lavage is indicated even if several hours have elapsed since ingestion because the anticholinergic effects cause delayed gastric emptying. Activated charcoal is recommended and, because of enterohepatic circulation, pulse charcoal may be of benefit. Cardiac monitoring is needed for

Table 4-2.--Effects of Tricyclic Antidepressants

Action	Clinical findings
1. Quinidine-like effect	↓ Myocardial contractility
	↑ Myocardial conduction
	Increased P-R and Q-T intervals
	Widened QRS
	Ventricular arrhythmia
	Hypotension
2. Anticholinergic	Supraventricular tachycardia, hyperthermia, mydriasis, anxiety, hallucinations, seizures, coma, death
3. Block reuptake of norepinephrine	↓ Myocardial contractility
	Hypotension
	Bradycardia
4. Antihistamine	

all patients for a minimum of 24 hours.

- Seizures or rapid deterioration is common with overdose of cyclic antidepressants.
- Do not induce vomiting.
- Activated charcoal is recommended.

Treatment of specific complications is outlined below:

1. Cardiotoxicity: Alkalinization causes more cyclic antidepressant to be protein-bound, leaving less free drug to exert its effect. It may be the best treatment of most forms of cardiovascular toxicity and can narrow widened QRS complexes, abolish arrhythmias, and improve perfusion. The goal is a serum pH of about 7.5. Dysrhythmias should be treated with alkalinization. Lidocaine and phenytoin are both reasonable choices for ventricular arrhythmias. Bretylium has an effect similar to that of the tricyclics and should be avoided. Class IA agents (quinidine, procainamide, and disopyramide) should be avoided.

2. Seizures: After alkalinization, diazepam and phenytoin are used, as for other patients with seizures. Refractory seizures should be treated with phenobarbital or general anesthesia.

3. Hypotension: After fluid challenge and alkalinization, you may need catecholamine pressors such as epinephrine, norepinephrine, or phenylephrine. Isoproterenol, dobutamine, and low-dose dopamine should be avoided because they may worsen hypotension through unopposed β-adrenergic effect. (Cyclic antidepressants produce strong α-adrenergic blockade.)

4. Anticholinergic toxicity: Physostigmine can reverse the anticholinergic effects of cyclic antidepressants, but its use is controversial. It has a low therapeutic:toxic ratio and can produce cholinergic crises. Its use should be limited to patients with severe hypertension, seizures, or dysrhythmias not responsive to other forms of therapy.

- Lidocaine and phenytoin are reasonable choices for ventricular arrhythmias.

- Refractory seizures should be treated with phenobarbital or general anesthesia.
- For hypotension, avoid isoproterenol, dobutamine, and low-dose dopamine.
- Physostigmine can reverse anticholinergic effects of cyclic antidepressants; it has low therapeutic:toxic ratio and can produce cholinergic crises.

ACETAMINOPHEN

Acetaminophen is the active metabolite of phenacetin and is a common over-the-counter antipyretic analgesic available in many forms. It is rapidly absorbed. Toxicity is from a minor metabolite formed via the cytochrome P450 system. Actually, most of an acetaminophen dose is conjugated with glucuronic acid and sulfate and then excreted by the kidneys. Only a very small amount is metabolized by the cytochrome P450 system. In cases of overdose, however, the sulfate and glucuronide conjugating systems are saturated, so more metabolism occurs through the cytochrome P450 system. Under normal circumstances, the metabolite of this system is conjugated with hepatic glutathione and excreted. In the case of overdose, however, hepatic glutathione is rapidly depleted and the metabolite binds to hepatocytes, producing cell death.

- Acetaminophen is active metabolite of phenacetin.
- It is rapidly absorbed.
- In acetaminophen overdose, sulfate and glucuronide conjugating systems are saturated, so more metabolism occurs through cytochrome P450 system.
- In overdose, metabolite binds to hepatocytes, producing cell death.

Hepatotoxicity, the main complication of acetaminophen overdose, can be predicted accurately with a nomogram (Fig. 4-1). This is based on the estimate that 15 g of acetaminophen in a single ingestion causes hepatotoxicity in an adult. For safety, and because patients with chronic liver disease have less glutathione stores, 7.5 g is used for the nomogram. Remember that patients taking phenobarbital and alcohol have stimulated cytochrome P450 systems and are more likely to experience toxicity at any given dose.

- Hepatotoxicity is main complication of acetaminophen overdose.

Treatment of acetaminophen overdose requires precise determination of the time of ingestion and quantified serum levels of acetaminophen. For patients who are in the "toxic" range on the nomogram, treatment with N-acetylcysteine is indicated. N-Acetylcysteine provides a -SH group for the toxic intermediary to bind to, thus sparing the hepatocytes. N-Acetylcysteine is given orally in the United States, but it has been used intravenously in other countries for years, and it should be given within 24 hours of ingestion. The loading dose of 140 mg/kg is followed by 70 mg/kg every 4 hours for 17 doses. The odor is offensive, and it may be best to give it through a nasogastric tube.

- For patients in toxic range of acetaminophen overdose, treatment with N-acetylcysteine is indicated.
- Treatment should be given within 24 hours of ingestion.

There is some debate regarding the initial treatment of acetaminophen overdose. There is theoretical concern that if activated charcoal is given initially, it may also bind the antidote (N-acetylcysteine). In practice, however, this is not a major concern, and because activated charcoal binds acetaminophen well, most investigators recommend it. Induced emesis should be avoided because prolonged vomiting may delay giving N-acetylcysteine if it is found to be indicated.

SALICYLATES

Salicylates are weak acids that are rapidly absorbed and have a small volume of distribution (V_d, 0.2 liter/kg). Although the half-life is short (15 minutes) under normal conditions, in case of overdose the half-life may be prolonged to 20 hours. Overall, the number of accidental ingestions has decreased, and most toxicity is now related to chronic salicylate use. A 50% increase in the daily dose of aspirin

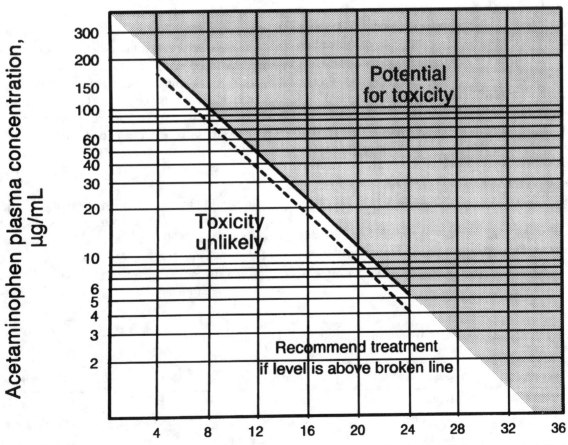

Fig. 4-1. Plasma or serum acetaminophen concentration vs. time after ingestion. Graph relates only to levels after a single acute overdose. Broken line represents 25% allowance below solid line; it is included to allow for possible errors in acetaminophen assays and estimated time from ingestion of overdose. (From Chiang WK, Wang RY: Evaluation and management of acute acetaminophen toxicity. Emerg Med Reports 14:83-90, 1993 and from McNeil Consumer Products Co., as adapted from Rumack BH, Matthews H. Acetaminophen poisoning and toxicity. Pediatrics 55:871-876, 1975. By permission of American Health Consultants, McNeil Consumer Products Co., and Pediatrics.)

can result in a 300% increase in plasma level. As salicylate levels increase, a typical pattern of acid-base disturbances occurs:

Respiratory → Respiratory → Metabolic acidosis
alkalosis   alkalosis   (anion gap)
                    +
               Metabolic acidosis
                  (anion gap)

This pattern may be accelerated in children. About the only abnormality that does not occur is metabolic alkalosis.

- In salicylate overdose, half-life may be prolonged to 20 hours.
- Most toxicity related to chronic salicylate use.
- 50% increase in daily dose of aspirin can result in 300% increase in plasma level.

Other symptoms and signs of salicylate overdose are listed in Table 4-3.

An elderly patient who is confused and has a high anion gap metabolic acidosis or unexplained respiratory alkalosis may have salicylate toxicity. This is a common presentation. Salicylate intoxication can cause noncardiogenic pulmonary edema.

Treatment includes usual supportive care and activated charcoal. Consider gastric lavage if the duration since ingestion is <1 hour. Fluids should be given to correct losses and to promote diuresis. Potassium levels need to be monitored carefully. Alkalinization increases urinary excretion of salicylates dramatically and may prevent salicylates from crossing the blood-brain barrier (ion trapping). Hemodialysis is used in certain cases, such as renal failure, noncardiogenic pulmonary edema, persistent or progressive central nervous system manifestations, and deterioration despite adequate supportive care and alkaline diuresis.

- Treatment of salicylate overdose: activated charcoal, fluids to correct losses and promote diuresis, monitoring of potassium levels, alkalinization to increase urinary excretion, hemodialysis in some cases.

THEOPHYLLINE

Theophylline is approximately 50% protein-bound, and about 90% of excretion occurs through liver metabolism. Metabolism is increased with cigarette smoking and use of phenobarbital or phenytoin. Metabolism is decreased with erythromycin, cimetidine, propranolol, ciprofloxacin, and heart failure or liver disease. The clinical presentation of theophylline toxicity depends not only on the amount of drug ingested but also on whether the patient is chronically maintained on theophylline. Patients who chronically take theophylline have more toxicity, in general, than their counterparts at the same serum level.

- Theophylline is 50% protein-bound; 90% of excretion is through liver metabolism.
- Patients who chronically take theophylline have more toxicity than their counterparts at same serum level.

Symptoms of theophylline toxicity are nausea and vomiting, agitation, tachypnea, cardiac arrhythmia (atrial fibrillation, multifocal atrial tachycardia, ventricular tachycardia, ventricular fibrillation), and seizures. Seizures increase mortality and may be first manifestation. Hypokalemia, hypophosphatemia, and hyperglycemia also occur.

Treatment includes routine supportive decontamination procedures. Pulse charcoal may be beneficial. Hemoperfusion is indicated for patients with increasing serum levels or seizures from sustained-release products and for patients whose condition is deteriorating despite appropriate initial management. Although levels do not correlate well with toxicity, if the plasma level is >40 μg/mL in chronic overdose or >80 μg/mL in acute overdose, consider hemoperfusion.

IRON

Iron poisoning is a common cause of pediatric ingestion emergencies. It is much less common in adults. Toxicity may occur at doses of 20-60 mg/kg. Lethal dose is 60-80 mg/kg of elemental iron.

Clinically, several phases are encountered in overdose:
Phase I (gastrointestinal symptoms 1/2 to 6 hours)--nausea,

Table 4-3.--Clinical and Laboratory Abnormalities in Salicylate Overdose

Central nervous system	Gastrointestinal	Pulmonary	Renal	Miscellaneous
Tinnitus	Nausea	Tachypnea	Tubular	Hyperpyrexia
Delirium	Vomiting	Noncardiogenic	necrosis	Hypokalemia
Stupor	Gastritis	pulmonary edema		Hypoglycemia
Coma				Platelet dysfunction
Seizures				Acid-base
				disturbances

vomiting, hematemesis, abdominal pain, diarrhea

Phase II (6-24 hours): latent period, patient seems to improve. Anion gap metabolic acidosis

Phase III (systemic toxicity): altered mental status, seizures, hepatic/renal failure, coagulopathy, death

Phase IV (late complications): gastrointestinal obstruction

Initial treatment includes standard supportive care and gastric emptying. Some authors recommend gastric lavage be performed with $NaHCO_3$, which converts iron to a less absorbable salt. This practice is controversial and not thoroughly investigated. Activated charcoal may be given but is of questionable value. Overall, iron is fairly resistant to various stomach decontamination regimes.

Patients suffering from significant iron overdose should have adequate crystalloid fluid resuscitation. Deferoxamine is a chelating agent that enhances iron elimination by producing a water-soluble substance (ferrioxamine) that can be excreted by the kidneys. It is administered intravenously at a rate of 15 mg/kg per hour. Deferoxamine should be given in any moderately or severely symptomatic patient regardless of iron levels, if serum iron level is >350 µg/dL, or in any patient whose serum iron level is greater than total iron-binding capacity.

A word of caution is in order in regard to treating patients for iron overdose. First, although iron tablets often are seen on abdominal radiograph, their absence is not a guarantee that a significant iron overdose has not occurred. Second, a patient who presents to the emergency department in phase II (latent period) may appear well despite having taken a serious overdose. Finally, do not withhold chelation therapy in moderately or severely symptomatic patients while waiting for determination of serum iron levels.

- Deferoxamine is a specific chelating agent for iron.
- Serum iron levels should not be solely relied on in determining need for deferoxamine therapy.
- A normal abdominal radiograph does not exclude severe iron overdose.

LITHIUM

In general, lithium has a low therapeutic index. In acute intoxication, serum levels may not accurately reflect the severity of overdose. Early signs of toxicity are nausea and vomiting, dysarthria, and hand tremor. Later signs are ataxia, fasciculations, hyperreflexia, confusion, seizures, coma, and cardiotoxicity (rare).

Charcoal is not used for treatment because it does not absorb lithium. Rehydration with normal saline is helpful (lithium can cause nephrogenic diabetes insipidus). Alkalinization of the urine can increase renal excretion of lithium. Hemodialysis should be considered for patients with renal failure, for patients with deterioration after appropriate treatment, or if serum lithium levels exceed 4 mEq/L.

β-ADRENERGIC BLOCKERS

Extremely small doses of β-adrenergic blockers can produce life-threatening reactions. Blood levels are not helpful. Clinical findings include bradycardia (many rhythm types), hypotension, peripheral cyanosis, pulmonary edema, altered mental status, and many electrocardiographic abnormalities.

The treatment of β-adrenergic blocker overdose includes gastric lavage rather than emesis induction because β-adrenergic blockers taken in large quantity exert their effects quickly. Activated charcoal should also be administered. The hypotension and bradycardia are often refractory to usual therapies, including dopamine, epinephrine, and atropine. Intravenous glucagon seems to be the most consistent agent for reversing the toxic effects of β-adrenergic blocker overdose. Glucagon is given as an intravenous bolus (0.05-0.15 mg/kg) followed by a continuous infusion at 2-5 mg/hour.

- Glucagon is most consistent agent for reversing β-adrenergic blocker toxicity.

DIGITALIS

Clinical manifestations of digitalis toxicity include both cardiac and noncardiac symptoms. Toxic effects of digitalis in patients receiving chronic therapy can occur at any serum level. Acute overdoses of digitalis are rare but usually severe.

Noncardiac signs and symptoms are nausea, vomiting, abdominal pain, confusion, hallucinations, occasionally seizures, visual disturbances (many), and hyperkalemia. Cardiac symptoms are junctional tachycardia, ventricular premature contractions, ventricular tachycardia, ventricular fibrillation, atrial flutter, atrial fibrillation, and all types of atrioventricular block. Although hypokalemia increases the risk of toxicity in patients chronically taking digitalis, hyperkalemia is a complication of acute digitalis overdose.

Treatment includes supportive care with cardiac monitoring, and gastric emptying if ingestion was recent. Treat dangerous hyperkalemia with intravenous glucose, insulin, and bicarbonate. AVOID calcium in cases of digitalis toxicity. Atropine may be effective for bradycardias, as may external pacemakers. Treat stable ventricular arrhythmias with lidocaine or phenytoin. Magnesium sulfate may be beneficial. Digoxin immune Fab (ovine) (Digibind) is digoxin-specific antibody fragments that have been induced in sheep. It acts by binding digoxin molecules, making them incapable of binding at their receptor, the Na^+K^+-ATPase. Its use should be reserved for severe intoxication. It is given intravenously, and its dose is titrated to clinical effect. Many vials are often required. Because serum digoxin levels reflect both bound and unbound drug, they may actually increase over several hours.

- Avoid calcium in digitalis toxicity.
- Atropine may be effective for bradycardias.
- Lidocaine or phenytoin is preferred agent for ventricular irritability.
- Digoxin-specific Fab fragments reserved for severe intoxication.

CYANIDE

Cyanide binds to iron in cytochrome oxidase, and the result is cellular hypoxia. It does not combine with the iron in hemoglobin. Cyanide is used in many industries, and the natural environment contains various cyanogenic glycosides that, when broken down and ingested, can release cyanide.

- Cyanide binds to iron in cytochrome oxidase.
- It does not combine with the iron in hemoglobin.

Clinical symptoms with inhalation (symptoms within seconds) are dry, burning throat, air hunger, hyperpnea, apnea, seizures, and death. Symptoms with ingestion (symptoms delayed) are nausea, vomiting, confusion, vertigo, giddiness, seizures, and cardiac dysrhythmias.

The diagnosis of cyanide overdose must initially be made clinically because rapid deterioration leading to death can occur well before any laboratory confirmation can be obtained. The history may provide clues to occupational cyanide exposure (electroplating, metallurgy, etc.), intentional cyanide exposure (suicide attempt), or accidental ingestion (apricot, plum, or peach pits). The odor of bitter almonds or peach pits is diagnostic of cyanide poisoning. Finally, altered mental status and tachypnea but no cyanosis suggest cyanide overdose.

Treatment includes supplemental high-flow 100% oxygen. If cyanide is ingested, consider gastric lavage and charcoal. Nitrite-thiosulfate is the therapy of choice in cyanide overdose. The nitrite causes creation of methemoglobin, which allows cyanide to bind to this rather than the cytochromic system. Thiosulfate then converts this to thiocyanate, which can be excreted by the kidney.

OPIOIDS

Opioids include many drugs that often are abused in society (e.g., morphine, heroin, methadone, codeine, propoxyphene, opium, fentanyl, meperidine). Morphine, opium, and codeine are the only natural (opium-derived) opioids. All other opioids require minor or major chemical alterations to produce.

Clinical features of opioid overdose are drowsiness, lethargy, respiratory depression, coma, nausea, vomiting, miosis, ileus, urinary retention, and pulmonary edema.

- Morphine, opium, and codeine are natural opioids.
- Heroin and methadone cause pulmonary edema.

- Classic opioid triad: respiratory depression, pinpoint pupils, coma.

Opioid ingestions are associated with other drugs in 90% of cases, and 95% of all emergency room visits by opioid abusers are for infections or trauma (not overdose). Thiamine, 100 mg intramuscularly, is given. If the blood glucose level is <80 mg/dL, 50 mL of dextrose (D_{50}, push) is given. Naloxone (Narcan), 2 mg by intravenous bolus, is given and repeated as necessary. A continuous infusion is occasionally required. Naloxone can be given intravenously, intramuscularly, or subcutaneously or by endotracheal tube. Many opioids have a longer half-life than naloxone, so prolonged monitoring for resedation is necessary.

- 90% of opioid ingestions are associated with other drugs.
- Patients successfully treated with naloxone require prolonged monitoring.

COCAINE

Although legally classified as a narcotic, cocaine is the only naturally occurring local anesthetic. When abused, it may be injected intravenously or subcutaneously, swallowed, smoked, or applied to oral or genital mucous membranes. Cocaine is cut with many substances, some of which have toxicity of their own.

Clinical features of cocaine use are excitement, euphoria, restlessness, nausea, vomiting, headache, seizures, tachycardia or hypertension, hypoventilation, psychosis, and mydriasis. Serious effects are malignant hyperthermia, seizures, and ventricular tachycardia.

The treatment of cocaine overdose is generally supportive. Seizures may be treated with diazepam and phenytoin. Propranolol can be used for severe hypertension or tachycardia, although some authors prefer labetalol (an α- and β-adrenergic blocker), which would not cause unopposed α-stimulation. Haloperidol can be used for hallucinations, although some authors prefer benzodiazepines.

In an attempt to smuggle cocaine, some patients have swallowed balloons or condoms filled with it ("body packers"). If an abdominal radiograph demonstrates this, consideration should be given to endoscopic or surgical removal.

AMPHETAMINES

Amphetamines are noncatechol sympathomimetic adrenergic agents that have more central nervous system stimulant activity than catecholamines. Symptoms of intoxication include tachycardia, headache, hypertension, euphoria, mydriasis, anxiety, hypothermia, seizures, diaphoresis, hallucinations, and arrhythmias. The hypertension and cardiac arrhythmias may be severe.

In general, emesis or lavage is not helpful for treatment. Phentolamine (α-adrenergic blocker) can be used to treat hypertensive crisis. Haloperidol is used for psychosis and agitation.

BENZODIAZEPINES

Benzodiazepines are a frequent cause of overdose (accidental, intentional, and iatrogenic) in adults. The associated morbidity and mortality are directly related to respiratory and central nervous system depression. In the past several years, an antagonist (flumazenil, Romazicon) has become available in the United States.

Flumazenil is a relatively pure antagonist with limited agonist or inverse agonist properties. It effectively antagonizes the neurologic, behavioral, and respiratory depressant effects of benzodiazepines. The initial dosage is 0.2 mg intravenously over 30 seconds. Subsequent dosages of 0.3-0.5 mg intravenously over 30 seconds can be given until desired effects are achieved or cumulative dose of 3 mg is given. Adverse reactions, including nausea, vomiting, dizziness, and, rarely, seizures, can occur, especially if cyclic antidepressants were also ingested. Two other problems can occur: 1) the precipitation of a withdrawal-type syndrome if the patient chronically uses benzodiazepines, and 2) resedation is very common, so prolonged monitoring is required.

Endotracheal intubation and ventilation is the treatment of choice for hypoventilatory patients. The exact role of flumazenil in benzodiazepine overdose has yet to be determined.

- For benzodiazepine overdose, endotracheal intubation and ventilation is used in hypoventilatory patients.
- Flumazenil can effectively reverse benzodiazepine-induced central nervous system and respiratory depression, but its role in overdose situations is unclear.

ALCOHOLS AND GLYCOLS

Ethanol, isopropyl alcohol (rubbing alcohol), methanol (wood alcohol), and ethylene glycol all produce an osmolar gap (see page 116). Methanol and ethylene glycol produce a large anion gap metabolic acidosis (serum bicarbonate level usually <10 mEq/L). Ethylene glycol produces calcium oxalate crystalluria. Isopropyl alcohol produces ketones but no acidosis.

Ethanol

Ethanol is the most abused drug. It is metabolized by liver alcohol dehydrogenase through zero-order kinetics (i.e., enzymes that are saturable). Blood alcohol levels are a poor predictor of level of impairment and anticipated morbidity. Clinical findings are slurred speech, ataxia, nystagmus, dulled sensory perception, tachycardia, hypoventilation, hypothermia, and coma.

Because alcoholics also experience trauma, hypoglycemia, and life-threatening infections, part of treatment is to be vigilant. Observation until the patient is sober is a good general rule. Thiamine, 100 mg intramuscularly, can be given. If blood glucose value is <80 mg/dL, 50 mL of dextrose is given.

Naloxone, 2 mg intravenously, should be given if any signs of narcotic overdose are present. Severe intoxication occasionally requires endotracheal intubation and gastric lavage (especially if multiple drugs are ingested).

- Alcoholics also experience trauma, hypoglycemia, life-threatening infection.
- General rule, observe patient until he or she is sober.
- If blood glucose value <80 mg/dL, give 50 mL dextrose.

Isopropyl Alcohol

Isopropyl alcohol is rubbing alcohol. It can cause toxicity by ingestion or inhalation, but it is not absorbed through the skin. On an equal-dose basis, it is more toxic than ethyl alcohol, causing more central nervous system depression. It is also metabolized by alcohol dehydrogenase, the end products being acetone, CO_2, and H_2O. Thus, it produces an osmolar gap and ketosis without significant metabolic acidosis.

- Isopropyl alcohol is rubbing alcohol.
- More toxic than ethyl alcohol.
- Produces osmolar gap and ketosis without significant metabolic acidosis.

Clinical effects are the same as those of ethanol; other effects are hemorrhagic gastritis, hypotension, rhabdomyolysis, hepatocellular toxicity, and breath with a sweet odor.

Treatment is generally supportive, as for ethanol. Only in extremely rare cases is hemodialysis considered (e.g., severe coma or isopropyl alcohol level >400 mg/dL).

Methanol

Methanol (wood alcohol) is metabolized by liver alcohol dehydrogenase to formaldehyde and formic acid (toxicity). Thus, it produces an osmolar gap and an impressively elevated anion gap metabolic acidosis. In fact, serum bicarbonate levels may reach 3 mEq/L. There is a latent period of 8-72 hours, and then visual symptoms (blurred vision, photophobia, papilledema), central nervous system effects (confusion, lethargy, coma), abdominal pain, nausea, and vomiting develop.

- Methanol produces osmolar gap and elevated anion gap metabolic acidosis.

Gastric lavage and activated charcoal are used for treatment. Ethanol has a greater affinity for alcohol dehydrogenase and, thus, helps prevent the formation of toxic metabolites. The goal is to achieve an ethanol level of 100 mg/dL. There are many dosing regimens. Hemodialysis works well and should be considered if methanol level is >50 mg/dL or if patient has deteriorated on ethanol therapy. Thiamine, other vitamins, magnesium, and glucose are given as needed. Bicarbonate therapy is controversial and should be guided by blood gas values.

- For methanol intoxication, gastric lavage and activated charcoal are used for treatment.
- Hemodialysis works well.
- Bicarbonate therapy controversial.

Ethylene Glycol

Ethylene glycol is commonly found in antifreeze and many other products. It is also metabolized by liver alcohol dehydrogenase to its toxic metabolites. Clinically, ethylene glycol overdose affects the central nervous system (ataxia, nystagmus, seizures, coma, papilledema), kidney (calcium oxalate crystals, acute tubular necrosis), and gastrointestinal tract (abdominal pain, nausea, vomiting). Late effects are pulmonary edema and cardiac failure. Similar to methanol, ethylene glycol produces an osmolar gap and an impressive anion gap metabolic acidosis.

- Ethylene glycol found in antifreeze.
- Produces an osmolar gap and impressive anion gap metabolic acidosis.
- Produces calcium oxalate crystalluria.

Treatment is similar to that for methanol toxicity, i.e., ethanol and hemodialysis if the ethylene glycol level is >50 mg/dL or there is clinical deterioration on ethanol therapy.

ORGANOPHOSPHATES

The inhibition of acetylcholinesterase by organophosphates results in increased cholinergic activity. Carbamates are also inhibitors of acetylcholinesterase, but they cause less toxicity because their binding is reversible. Clinical findings of pesticide overdose are bradycardia, lacrimation, salivation, sweating, urinary incontinence, wheezing, fecal incontinence, and miosis. Delayed effects are fasciculations, tachycardia, mydriasis, and hypertension.

Evaluation of patients includes determination of both serum (easier) and red blood cell (more accurate) cholinesterase levels.

- Organophosphates inhibit acetylcholinesterase.

Treatment includes establishment of an airway. Atropine, 2-4 mg, is given as needed. The stabilized patient is fully decontaminated by removing clothing and irrigating. Charcoal is used depending on route of contamination. Pralidoxime (Protopam, 2-PAM) reactivates cholinesterase and reverses cholinergic and nicotine effects. Dosage in adults is 1 g over 15 minutes.

- Treatment of pesticide toxicity includes atropine, 2-4 mg as needed.
- Pralidoxime also used.

CARBON MONOXIDE POISONING

Carbon monoxide is the leading cause of toxin-related death. It is a colorless, odorless, nonirritating gas that reversibly displaces oxygen in hemoglobin to produce carboxyhemoglobin (COHb). Symptoms are often vague and misdiagnosed.

Although at time of exposure COHb level can correlate with symptoms, the COHb level after initiation of treatment with 100% oxygen can be deceptively low (Table 4-4). Diagnosis is established from the history (especially if 100% oxygen administered) and from COHb levels.

- In carbon monoxide poisoning, carboxyhemoglobin level at exposure can correlate with symptoms, but after treatment with 100% oxygen, level can be deceptively low.

Treatment is administration of 100% oxygen (decreases half-life of COHb by 400%). The use of hyperbaric oxygen is very controversial. It may prevent delayed neurologic sequelae, but controlled studies are lacking. Consider it for patients in coma, those with neurologic deficits, chest pain, or acidosis, or in pregnant patients. COHb value >30% may also be an indication, but the decision should be based on the clinical picture.

METHEMOGLOBINEMIA

Methemoglobinemia is an abnormal, nonfunctioning ferric hemoglobin ($HbFe^{3+}$) that cannot bind oxygen. It is caused by hereditary diseases (rare) but also by drugs of abuse such as amyl nitrite and isobutyl nitrite. These are used for short-term "rush" effect and as orgasm enhancers.

Diagnosis is based on the finding of chocolate-brown cyanosis unrelieved by oxygenation and arterial blood

Table 4-4.--Relationship of Carboxyhemoglobin Levels to Clinical Presentation

COHb, %	Signs and symptoms
0	None
10	Headache
20	Headache, dyspnea
30	Nausea, dizziness, impaired judgment
40	Confusion, syncope
50	Coma, seizures
60	Hypotension, respiratory failure
70	Death

gases with low saturation but normal arterial oxygen partial pressure.

Treatment includes supplemental oxygen. Methylene blue acts as a cofactor in methemoglobinemia reductase system. Its use is reserved for patients with hypoxic symptoms or methemoglobin levels >30%. It may cause hemolysis in high doses.

QUESTIONS

Multiple Choice (choose the one best answer)

1. Which of the following substances would not be well bound by charcoal?
   a. Acetaminophen
   b. Theophylline
   c. Iron
   d. Phenobarbital
   e. Digoxin

2. A 16-year-old boy is brought to the emergency department by friends after taking an unknown number of diazepam (5 mg) pills and a large amount of ethanol. Initial examination reveals a blood pressure of 90/60 mm Hg, pulse 100, temperature of 37° C, respirations 8 and shallow. The patient is comatose, responding to pain only. Your initial management should include:
   a. Establishing intravenous access and administering 0.2 mg of flumazenil intravenously
   b. Establishing intravenous access and administering 0.5 mg of flumazenil intravenously
   c. Performing gastric lavage with a large-bore orogastric tube
   d. Administering 50 g of activated charcoal through a nasogastric tube
   e. Obtaining an emergency computed tomography scan of the patient's head to rule out an intracranial hemorrhage

3. All of the following can commonly increase the blood level of theophylline in a patient *except*:
   a. Phenobarbital
   b. Erythromycin
   c. Cimetidine
   d. Ciprofloxacin
   e. Conversion to a longer-acting preparation

4. Which of the following statements regarding overdose is true?
   a. Most overdoses occur in the elderly
   b. Most overdoses will require the administration of a specific antidote
   c. Accidental overdoses tend to occur in adults and are often fatal
   d. Most *fatal* overdoses occur in adults and were intentional (i.e., suicide attempt).
   e. Children rarely overdose

5. Pulmonary edema might occur in all of the following overdoses *except*:
   a. Acetaminophen
   b. Aspirin
   c. Heroin
   d. Methadone
   e. Ethylene glycol

6. Acidification of the urine and subsequent forced diuresis are indicated in:
   a. Cocaine overdose
   b. Phencyclidine overdose
   c. Amphetamine overdose
   d. Tricyclic overdose
   e. Such management is never indicated

7. Which of the following statements regarding gastric lavage is true?
   a. It should be performed in every overdose of a potentially toxic substance
   b. It should be reserved for patients with potentially toxic overdoses who are seen within 1-2 hours from time of ingestion
   c. It should never be performed because of the potential to cause aspiration pneumonia and other complications
   d. When performed by an experienced physician, it can remove 90% of an ingested substance
   e. It may be performed on an unconscious patient before endotracheal or nasotracheal intubation

True/False (indicate whether each answer is true or false)

8. The following commonly cause miosis in patients who have overdosed:
   a. Amphetamines
   b. Organophosphate

c. Opioids
d. Caffeine
e. Tricyclic antidepressants
f. Acetaminophen

9. Hemoperfusion is a consideration in the following overdoses:
a. Phenobarbital
b. Theophylline
c. Phenytoin
d. Lithium

e. Methanol
f. Digitalis

10. Common symptoms of organophosphate overdose include the following:
a. Excessive salivation
b. Excessive lacrimation
c. Miosis
d. Tachycardia
e. Dry, hot skin
f. Mydriasis

ANSWERS

1. Answer c.

Although activated charcoal binds many commonly encountered toxins well, it is generally ineffective for absorbing small ionic compounds, heavy metals, and the alcohols. It should also be avoided in cases of caustic ingestion.

2. Answer d.

The cornerstone of management of patients with overdose is excellent supportive care. An adequate airway must be assured in the unconscious patient who is at risk for aspiration. This should include endotracheal or nasotracheal intubation *before* gastric lavage. Flumazenil is a specific benzodiazepine antagonist, but its role in the management of overdose has not yet been established

3. Answer a.

The metabolism of theophylline is decreased with simultaneous use of erythromycin, cimetidine, propranolol, or ciprofloxacin, leading to a higher blood level. Changing to a longer-acting preparation may also increase blood levels of theophylline. Metabolism is increased (blood levels are therefore lowered) with phenobarbital or phenytoin.

4. Answer d.

Overall, most overdoses are accidental and occur in the pediatric age group. Fatal overdoses, however, more commonly occur in adults and were intentional.

5. Answer a.

Opioids, aspirin, and ethylene glycol all can produce

pulmonary edema. It would not be expected in acetaminophen overdose.

6. Answer e.

Although alkalinization is indicated in certain cases of overdose (barbiturates, aspirin, isoniazid, and lithium), acidification is no longer recommended.

7. Answer b.

Gastric lavage should be reserved for patients who have taken an overdose of a potentially toxic substance within 1 to 2 hours of presentation. Unconscious patients or those with a depressed gag reflex or seizures should have an endotracheal tube placed before lavage. Only 30%-40% of an ingested substance is successfully removed this way.

8. a, false; b, true; c, true; d, false; e, false; f, false.

Organophosphates and opioids commonly cause miosis in cases of overdose. Amphetamines, caffeine, and anticholinergic medications commonly cause mydriasis.

9. a, true; b, true; c, true; d, false; e, false; f, false.

Hemoperfusion is a consideration in some cases of overdose with phenobarbital, theophylline, or phenytoin. Hemodialysis may be indicated in some overdoses of aspirin, lithium, bromide, ethylene glycol, or methanol.

10. a, true; b, true; c, true; d, false; e, false; f, false.

The signs and symptoms of organophosphate poisoning can be remembered by the acronym "SLUDGE" (salivation, lacrimation, urination, defecation, gastrointestinal upset, emesis). In addition, patients may present with miosis, bradycardia, wheezing, and altered mental status.

CHAPTER 5

CRITICAL CARE MEDICINE

Steve G. Peters, M.D.

Critical Care Medicine encompasses multidisciplinary aspects of the management of severely ill patients. All areas of medicine may have relevance for critically ill patients, but this review focuses on aspects of cardiopulmonary monitoring and life support, technological interventions, and disease states typically managed in the intensive care unit (ICU).

A few general tips for preparing for the board examination: 1) Stress the acute care of common life-threatening conditions. Review a general manual or text of medical therapeutics. 2) Try to identify important areas with which you are less familiar or experienced. Also, review situations encountered in major hospitals of large U.S. cities, e.g., complications of alcohol, drug overdose, and trauma. 3) Common things are commonly tested, but be aware of unusual causes or features of common conditions, e.g., adult respiratory distress syndrome (ARDS) secondary to thrombotic thrombocytopenic purpura. 4) In reviewing drugs, stress common agents that have serious toxic effects, e.g., antihypertensive agents, theophylline, antibiotics, immunosuppressive agents, and antidepressants. 5) Know the indications for (and complications of) common invasive procedures, e.g., pulmonary angiography, cardiac catheterization, and hemodialysis.

- Stress acute care of common life-threatening conditions.
- Identify important areas with which you are less familiar or experienced.
- Be aware of unusual causes or features of common conditions.
- Know indications for (and complications of) invasive procedures.

RESPIRATORY FAILURE

Effective functioning of the respiratory system requires normal central nervous system control, neuromuscular transmission and bellows function, and gas exchange at the alveolar-capillary level. Respiratory failure may result from disease at any of these levels.

Physiologic Definitions and Relationships

Lung Volumes

TLC = total lung capacity--total volume of gas in the chest at the end of a maximal inspiration. VC = vital capacity--volume of a maximal breath (expired or inspired). V_T = tidal volume--volume of a normal breath. FRC = functional residual capacity--lung volume at the end of a normal expiration. It reflects the relaxation point of the respiratory system or the point at which outward recoil of the chest wall is balanced by inward recoil of the lungs. Compliance of the lungs or respiratory system is defined by the change in volume (ΔV) for a given change in pressure (ΔP).

$$C_{STATIC} = \frac{\Delta V}{\Delta P}$$

where ΔV is measured in liters (L) and ΔP in cm H_2O. Emphysema causes loss of recoil and, thus, increased compliance. Most other disease states, particularly interstitial diseases, fibrosis, pulmonary edema, and ARDS, cause decreased compliance (i.e., "stiff" lungs, or increased transpulmonary pressure for given volume change).

- Normal compliance = 0.2 L/cm H_2O.
- Emphysema causes loss of recoil and increased compliance.
- Interstitial diseases, fibrosis, pulmonary edema, and ARDS cause decreased compliance.

Resistance (R) to air flow is defined by the change in pressure (ΔP) for a given change in flow ($\Delta \dot{V}$)

$$R = \frac{\Delta P}{\Delta \dot{V}}$$

where ΔP is measured in cm H_2O and $\Delta \dot{V}$ in L/sec. Common causes of increased airway resistance include bronchospasm and airway secretions.

- Causes of increased airway resistance: bronchospasm and airway secretions.

The total pressure required to inflate the respiratory system (spontaneously or with a mechanical ventilator) is the pressure required to overcome elastic recoil plus the pressure to overcome flow resistance:

$$P_{inflation} = \frac{\Delta V}{C_{ST}} + R \times \Delta \dot{V}$$
$$\text{(Elastic)} \quad \text{(Resistive)}$$

Gas exchange requires alveolar ventilation for elimination of carbon dioxide, oxygen uptake across alveolar-capillary membrane, and delivery of O_2 to tissues. Hypoxemia may result from a decrease in the inspired partial pressure of O_2 (e.g., high altitude), hypoventilation, ventilation-perfusion ($\dot{V}/Q$) mismatch, shunting, or diffusion barrier. Estimation of the alveolar-arterial gradient (A-a) for oxygen is essential in analyzing the cause of hypoxemia. Important relationships include the following:

The partial pressure of carbon dioxide (P_{aCO_2}) in the blood is directly proportional to the amount of CO_2 produced ($\dot{V}_{CO_2}$), and inversely proportional to alveolar ventilation ($\dot{V}_A$):

$$P_{aCO_2} = k \frac{\dot{V}_{CO_2}}{\dot{V}_A}$$

Alveolar ventilation is equal to total ventilation ($\dot{V}_E$) minus dead space ventilation (V_D). Thus, physiologic dead space is defined by the portion of a breath that does not participate in gas exchange. Dead space may be anatomical (conducting airways) or alveolar (areas of ventilation that receive no perfusion):

$$\dot{V}_A = \dot{V}_E - V_D \times f$$

where f = breaths/min.

$$\frac{V_D}{V_T} \text{ normally is } <0.25 - 0.30$$

$$\frac{V_D}{V_T} = \frac{P_{aCO_2} - P_{E}CO_2}{P_{aCO_2}}$$

where $P_{E}CO_2$ is the partial pressure of expired CO_2. The dead space-to-tidal volume ratio is calculated by measuring the partial pressure of carbon dioxide in an arterial blood (P_{aCO_2}) gas sample and an expired gas sample ($P_{E}CO_2$). The greater the dead space, the greater the difference between P_{aCO_2} and $P_{E}CO_2$.

- Physiologic dead space is defined by the portion of breath not participating in gas exchange.
- Dead space may be anatomical or alveolar.

Alveolar gas consists of inspired gases saturated with water vapor. The alveolus also contains CO_2 delivered from the blood. The sum of the partial pressures of all gases present equals the ambient barometric pressure. The alveolar air equation defines this relationship:

$$P_{AO_2} = F_{IO_2} (P_B - P_{H_2O}) - \frac{P_{aCO_2}}{R}$$

where P_A is alveolar partial pressure, P_B is barometric pressure (about 760 mm Hg at sea level), P_{H_2O} is water vapor pressure (47 mm Hg), and R is the respiratory quotient ($\dot{V}_{CO_2} / \dot{V}_{O_2}$, normally about 0.8). The simplified equation is:

$$P_{AO_2} = F_{IO_2} (P_B - 47) - \frac{P_{aCO_2}}{0.8}$$

Breathing room air ($F_{IO_2} = 0.21$) at sea level:

$$P_{AO_2} = 0.21 (760-47) - \frac{40}{0.8}$$

or normal P_{AO_2} is approximately equal to 100 mm Hg.

The A-a O_2 difference is defined by P_{AO_2} minus P_{aO_2}, which is normally <10-20 mm Hg when breathing room air. The A-a gradient normally increases to approximately 50-100 mm Hg as the F_{IO_2} increases from 0.21 to 1.0. Hypoxemia due to hypoventilation is characterized by increased P_{aCO_2} and decreased P_{aO_2} but by a relatively normal A-a gradient. Hypoxemia due to ventilation-perfusion mismatch shows an elevated A-a gradient. A shunt is defined by perfusion in the absence of ventilation (i.e., V/Q = 0). With a pure shunt, P_{aO_2} does not increase even though F_{IO_2} is increased to 100%. Normal shunt fraction is <3%-5% of total cardiac output. The shunt fraction is measured on 100% O_2 and is expressed as:

$$\frac{Q_s}{Q_t} = \frac{Cc'_{O_2} - Ca_{O_2}}{Cc'_{O_2} - C\bar{v}_{O_2}} = \frac{P(A-a)_{O_2} \times 0.003}{P(A-a)_{O_2} \times 0.003 + (Ca-C\bar{v})_{O_2}}$$

The content of O_2 in the blood is the total amount of O_2 bound to hemoglobin plus the amount dissolved.

$$O_2 \text{ content: } C_xO_2 = 1.34 \times Hgb \times S_xO_2 + 0.003 \times P_xO_2$$
$$\text{(Bound)} \qquad \text{(Dissolved)}$$

where x may equal arterial, venous, capillary, etc.

Under steady state conditions, the amount of O_2 used by the tissues equals the amount taken up by the lungs. The O_2

uptake, $\dot{V}O_2$, can be defined by amount of O_2 leaving the lungs in pulmonary venous blood minus the amount of O_2 coming into the lungs in the pulmonary arteries. This should be familiar as the Fick equation:

$$\dot{V}O_2 = Q\,(Ca\text{-}C\bar{v})O_2$$

where Q is cardiac output.

- Hypoxemia due to hypoventilation: increased Pa_{CO_2}, decreased Pa_{O_2}, normal A-a gradient.
- Shunt is defined by perfusion in absence of ventilation, i.e., V/Q = O.
- Normal shunt fraction is <3%-5% of total cardiac output.
- A shunt leads to hypoxemia that shows little improvement after supplemental O_2.

Many applications of the Fick equation are important in managing critically ill patients. One application involves continuous monitoring of mixed venous O_2 saturation by recently developed pulmonary artery catheters. Expressing O_2 content in terms of saturation and rearranging the Fick equation to solve the $S\bar{v}O_2$ yields the following:

$$S\bar{v}O_2 = Sa_{O_2} - \frac{\dot{V}O_2}{Q \times Hgb \times 1.34}$$

Note that decreased mixed venous O_2 saturation may be due to decreased arterial saturation, increased O_2 consumption, decreased cardiac output, or decreased hemoglobin. Certain disease states, particularly early sepsis, may be characterized by normal or increased mixed venous O_2 saturation, because cardiac output initially increases, along with impaired O_2 uptake by the tissues. Later in sepsis, mixed venous $S\bar{v}O_2$ typically decreases due to decreased O_2 delivery.

- Decreased mixed venous O_2 may be due to: decreased arterial saturation, increased O_2 consumption, decreased cardiac output, or decreased hemoglobin.
- Early sepsis: normal or increased mixed venous O_2 saturation.

Under normal circumstances, O_2 demand by the tissues is met by the supply. O_2 delivery is defined by cardiac output times arterial O_2 content, i.e.,

$$O_2 \text{ delivery} = Q \times Ca_{O_2}$$

Although cardiac output may decrease, $\dot{V}O_2$ of the tissues may be maintained by increased O_2 extraction. Supply dependence of O_2 consumption refers to disease states in which O_2 delivery falls below a certain point where O_2 extraction cannot maintain the required $\dot{V}O_2$. Below such a threshold of O_2 delivery, O_2 consumption varies directly with the available supply. Such conditions usually imply coexisting anaerobic metabolism and accumulation of lactic acid.

- O_2 delivery = cardiac output x arterial O_2 content.
- Supply dependence of O_2 consumption may occur at very low levels of O_2 delivery.

ACID-BASE BALANCE AND ARTERIAL BLOOD GASES

The production of acid byproducts is the normal result of cellular metabolism. An acid is defined as a hydrogen ion, $[H^+]$, or proton donor. A base accepts protons. The dissociation constant (K) for an acid (HA) may be defined as

$$K = \frac{[H^+][A^-]}{[HA]}$$

Buffer systems minimize the changes in pH associated with the addition of acid or base. For carbonic acid:

$$H_2O + CO_2 \leftrightarrow H_2CO_3 \overset{K}{\leftrightarrow} H^+ + HCO_3^-$$

$$\text{and } K = \frac{[H^+][HCO_3^-]}{[H_2CO_3]}$$

The Henderson-Hasselbalch equation:

$$pH = pK + \log \frac{[HCO_3^-]}{[H_2CO_3]}$$

where $pH = -\log[H^+]$ and $pK = -\log K$. The pK for carbonic acid is 6.1. $[H_2CO_3]$ is often measured by taking $0.03 \times Pa_{CO_2}$ (i.e., dissolved CO_2). So the Henderson-Hasselbalch equation can be rewritten as

$$pH = 6.1 + \log \frac{[HCO_3^-]}{0.03 \times Pa_{CO_2}}$$

Hydrogen ions are buffered by several mechanisms in different body fluid compartments. In plasma and interstitial fluid, bicarbonate is the major buffer, with proteins and phosphate compounds contributing to a lesser extent. In erythrocytes, hemoglobin is the major buffer, but bicarbonate contributes approximately 30% and phosphate 10% of the buffering capacity. The kidney eliminates organic acid and also contributes by 1) reabsorption of bicarbonate from tubular fluids, 2) formation of titratable acid, and 3) elimination of $[H^+]$ as ammonium ions.

- Bicarbonate is the major buffer in plasma and interstitial fluid.
- In erythrocytes, hemoglobin is the major buffer.

- Kidney eliminates organic acid and reabsorbs bicarbonate from tubular fluids.

Given the importance of the carbonic acid-bicarbonate system, most acid-base problems involve some method for solving variables of the Henderson-Hasselbalch equation. Because pK is constant, given two of the three values for pH, P_{CO_2}, and $[HCO_3^-]$, the missing variable can be calculated. Graphic displays are commonly used; two of the variables are plotted at constant values (isopleths) for the third variable (the Davenport diagram is an example).

Patterns of Acid-Base Disorder

Respiratory Acidosis

Acute respiratory acidosis is defined by rapid development of CO_2 retention (P_{ACO_2} > 45 mm Hg) with a concomitant decrease in pH (<7.35). Common causes include respiratory depression by drugs such as narcotics, central nervous system injury, acute diaphragm or neuromuscular weakness, severe parenchymal respiratory failure, and cardiac failure. Because CO_2 diffuses quickly into cells and the cerebrospinal fluid, the physiologic effects of the acidosis may occur rapidly. Confusion, obtundation, and signs of cerebral edema are commonly observed. Chronic respiratory acidosis is typically seen in patients with severe chronic obstructive lung disease (particularly chronic bronchitis or bronchiectasis) and in other states associated with chronic alveolar hypoventilation. Chronic respiratory acidosis may be compensated partly by renal mechanisms, i.e., increased reabsorption of bicarbonate and excretion of acid in the urine.

- Acute respiratory acidosis: rapid onset of CO_2 retention with concomitant decrease in pH.
- Chronic respiratory acidosis is typically seen in patients with severe chronic obstructive lung disease or other states associated with chronic alveolar hypoventilation.

Respiratory Alkalosis

Acute respiratory acidosis is the result of a rapid decrease in P_{ACO_2} due to hyperventilation. Hyperventilation is usually associated with anxiety or pain. Other important causes are early shock states, pulmonary embolism, other causes of hypoxemia, hyperthermia, salicylate intoxication, liver failure, and disorders of the central nervous system. Patients with unexplained hypocapnia should be evaluated for these disorders. In mechanically ventilated patients, respiratory alkalosis may result from inadvertent over-ventilation, i.e., excessive tidal volume and/or respiratory rate, especially in an assist-control ventilator mode.

- Respiratory alkalosis is the result of alveolar hyperventilation.
- Common causes include anxiety, pain, shock, pulmonary

embolism, hypoxemia, fever, salicylate overdose, liver failure, and mechanical over-ventilation.

Metabolic Acidosis

Metabolic acidosis results from the accumulation of organic acids such as lactate, pyruvate, or keto acids. Acidosis may develop by increased acid production or decreased renal excretion of acid. Conditions causing metabolic acidosis are further characterized by the anion gap, i.e.:

$$[Na^+] - ([Cl^-] + [HCO_3])$$

with a normal value of 8-14 mEq/L.

A normal anion gap or non-anion gap acidosis is characterized by an increase in chloride balancing the loss of bicarbonate. Causes include gastrointestinal losses of bicarbonate, i.e., diarrhea, urinary diversion procedures, or intestinal fistulas. Renal losses of bicarbonate (renal tubular acidosis) are also associated with a normal anion gap. Causes of acidosis associated with other anions--increased anion gap disorders-- are diabetic ketoacidosis, lactic acidosis, uremia, and toxins (ethylene glycol, methanol, paraldehyde, and salicylate).

- Metabolic acidosis: result of accumulation of organic acids, e.g., lactate, pyruvate, keto acids.
- Normal anion gap or non-anion gap acidosis is characterized by increase in chloride balancing loss of bicarbonate.
- Increased anion gap disorders: diabetic ketoacidosis, lactic acidosis, uremia, toxins (ethylene glycol, methanol, paraldehyde, salicylate).

Metabolic Alkalosis

Metabolic alkalosis is characterized by increased bicarbonate and pH. Hypokalemia and hypochloremia are commonly associated and further perpetuate the alkalosis. Common causes are volume contraction states, particularly those associated with further loss of chloride and hydrogen ion (vomiting and nasogastric suctioning). Diuretic therapy and mineralocorticoids are also common contributing factors. Although respiratory compensation (hypoventilation) for metabolic alkalosis might seem counterproductive, it can occur and may contribute to hypoxemia. As with other acid-base disorders, therapy is directed at the underlying cause, but support with volume and potassium and chloride replacement are important.

- Metabolic alkalosis is characterized by increased bicarbonate and pH.
- Hypokalemia and hypochloremia are commonly associated and further perpetuate alkalosis.
- Common causes are volume contraction states, particularly those associated with further loss of chloride and hydrogen ion (vomiting, nasogastric suctioning).

Mixed Acid-Base Disorders

Mixed disorders are characterized by a combination of the primary abnormalities described above or by a primary disorder and compensatory changes in $Paco_2$ or bicarbonate. For example, combined respiratory and metabolic acidosis may occur in patients with depressed respiration and tissue hypoperfusion, as would occur with severe shock, after cardiorespiratory arrest, or with status epilepticus. In these situations, pH is severely depressed and immediate therapy is necessary. Treatment includes assisted ventilation plus measures to improve cardiac output and organ perfusion. Sodium bicarbonate might be given for severe acidemia (pH <7.0-7.1) but treatment must be directed at the underlying cause of the primary disorder.

- Combined respiratory and metabolic acidosis leads to severe acidemia.
- Treatment should be directed at the underlying disorder.

Respiratory acidosis and metabolic alkalosis typically occur in patients with chronic obstructive pulmonary disease (COPD) or chronic alveolar hypoventilation. Secondary bicarbonate retention may be augmented by concomitant corticosteroid therapy or diuretics. Because a given blood gas measurement showing increased $Paco_2$ and increased bicarbonate (with pH near 7.4) could occur by many mechanisms, the clinical history is essential for determining the most likely pathophysiology. If patients with chronic hypercarbia are mechanically ventilated, there is a risk of severe alkalosis if ventilator settings are adjusted to "normalize," the $Paco_2$ at approximately 40 mm Hg, without recognizing the chronic increase in bicarbonate.

- Respiratory acidosis plus metabolic alkalosis is seen most commonly in patients with chronic respiratory insufficiency plus bicarbonate retention.

Metabolic acidosis and respiratory alkalosis may occur in patients with tissue hypoperfusion and respiratory stimulation, as is commonly seen with early shock states, sepsis, and hepatic or renal failure. This pattern is also typical of salicylate intoxication.

- Metabolic acidosis and respiratory alkalosis are commonly seen with shock states, sepsis, or salicylate overdose.

Metabolic and respiratory alkalosis rarely occurs in spontaneously breathing patients but can develop quickly with mechanical ventilation. This is usually the result of a disorder causing respiratory alkalosis, as described above, combined with a metabolic alkalosis induced by volume contraction, gastric suctioning, hypokalemia, diuretics, or corticosteriods. Seizures and/or cardiac arrhythmias may result from severe alkalemia. Treatment usually requires replacement of volume, potassium, and chloride.

CLINICAL APPROACH TO ARTERIAL BLOOD GASES

There are many ways to assess problems of acid-base balance and gas exchange. When interpreting arterial blood gases, the following approach is useful:

1. Consider the pH. Are conditions normal (pH 7.35-7.45), acidemic (<7.35), or alkalemic (>7.45)?
2. Assess $Paco_2$. Does the $Paco_2$ change (from 40 mm Hg) account for the pH change (from 7.40)? Evaluation of this relationship requires calculation, graphic display, or a rule of thumb, such as: an acute change in $Paco_2$ of 10 mm Hg should be associated with a pH change in the opposite direction of approximately 0.08 unit. If an abnormal pH can be accounted for by the change in $Paco_2$, a simple respiratory disturbance is present. If not, a mixed acid-base disorder is defined.
3. The change in bicarbonate, i.e., base deficit or excess, should confirm the conditions already defined by pH and $Paco_2$.
4. Consider Pao_2. If hypoxemia is present, estimate the A-a gradient. If this is normal and $Paco_2$ is increased, hypoventilation alone should account for the hypoxemia. The A-a gradient should be increased in conditions of ventilation-perfusion mismatching, shunting, or diffusion barrier.
5. Compare the Pao_2 and the arterial saturation, Sao_2. The Sao_2 should correspond to the expected values for a normal O_2-Hgb dissociation curve. If saturation is lower than expected, consider the presence of other hemoglobin forms, e.g., carboxyhemoglobin or methemoglobin.

As examples, use the algorithm above to match the following arterial blood gases with the clinical scenarios listed below.

	pH	$Paco_2$	HCO_3^-	Pao_2(room air)	Sao_2
A.	7.35	60	32	50	85%
B.	7.50	46	34	85	94%
C.	7.24	70	28	55	89%
D.	7.28	33	15	110	99%
E.	7.38	30	18	105	75%

1. 20-year-old woman with diabetic ketoacidosis
2. 20-year-old man with acute narcotic overdose
3. 60-year-old man 1 week after an abdominal operation, with continuous nasogastric suction and diuretic therapy
4. 60-year-old woman with severe emphysema
5. 60-year-old man with carbon monoxide intoxication

(Answers: 1. D, 2. C, 3. B, 4. A, 5. E)

- Consider the pH.
- Assess $PaCO_2$.
- Change in bicarbonate should confirm the conditions already defined by pH and $PaCO_2$.
- Consider PaO_2 and A-a gradient.

Airway Management

Endotracheal intubation allows control of the airway, ability to deliver specific inspired O_2 and positive pressure ventilation, and protection from aspiration. Indications for intubation include: airway protection in cases of obstruction or loss of normal gag and cough reflexes, central nervous system injury or sedation with loss of normal controls of ventilation, and any cause of respiratory failure requiring positive pressure-assisted ventilation. Oral-tracheal intubation is usually achieved via direct visualization with a laryngoscope. In experienced hands, this procedure should be relatively quick and safe. Complications may include vomiting and aspiration, hypoxemia during the procedure, and inadvertent intubation of the esophagus. The major contraindication for laryngoscopic intubation is an unstable cervical spine (due to trauma or degenerative conditions such as rheumatoid arthritis). In such cases, fiberoptic intubation (passing a tube over a bronchoscope) or tracheostomy may be necessary. In semiconscious and spontaneously breathing patients, nasotracheal intubation may be accomplished "blindly" and may be more comfortable for patients. Complications include bleeding, obstruction of sinus drainage with sinusitis, and damage to nasal structures.

- Endotracheal intubation allows control of the airway.
- Contraindication: unstable cervical spine (trauma or rheumatoid arthritis).
- In semiconscious, spontaneously breathing patients, nasotracheal intubation may be an alternative.

In emergency situations in which airway control is required, cricothyrotomy may be lifesaving. This procedure involves identification and puncture of the cricothyroid membrane. In patients requiring prolonged mechanical ventilation or airway support, the timing of tracheostomy is controversial. Newer high-volume low-pressure endotracheal tube cuffs have decreased the frequency of tracheal injury and stenosis caused by prolonged intubation. Tracheostomy has the advantages of decreased laryngeal injury, increased patient comfort, ease of suctioning, and, in certain patients, allowance for oral ingestion and speech. Complications may include tracheal injury and stenosis, bleeding, tracheoesophageal fistula, and possibly increased bronchial or pulmonary infections. Tracheostomy is commonly considered in patients who have needed or are expected to need intubation and mechanical ventilation for >2-4 weeks.

- In emergency situations, cricothyrotomy may be lifesaving.
- High-volume low-pressure endotracheal tube cuffs have decreased frequency of tracheal injury and stenosis.
- Tracheostomy is for patients who have needed or are expected to need intubation and mechanical ventilation for >2-4 weeks.

Mechanical Ventilation

Mechanical ventilation may be valuable in various conditions of respiratory failure, including loss of respiratory controls, neuromuscular or respiratory pump failure, and disorders of gas exchange. Many specific variables have been suggested as criteria for ventilator support and are listed in Table 5-1.

Complications of Mechanical Ventilation

Complications of mechanical ventilation may relate to airway access, physiologic responses to positive pressure, and complications related to other organ systems. Examples are given in Table 5-2.

Other complications, such as pulmonary embolism or malnutrition, may also reflect the underlying disease state. Management of these complications requires ongoing surveillance and recognition. Diagnosis of pneumonia may be difficult in patients receiving mechanical ventilation because pulmonary infiltrates are frequently present, tracheal secretions may be colonized by bacteria, and signs such as fever and leukocytosis are frequently blunted. Prophylaxis is commonly given to reduce stress-related gastritis and ulceration. H_2-Blockers may increase colonization of the respiratory tract by gram-negative bacteria. Sucralfate or frequent use of antacids is an alternative. The hemodynamic complications of increased intrathoracic pressure may be overcome by fluid administration; however, there is often a coexisting condition of capillary leak and pulmonary edema that may worsen.

Table 5-1.--Criteria for Ventilator Support

Respiratory rate >30/min
Minute ventilation >10 L/min
Maximal inspiratory pressure <-20 cm H_2O
Vital capacity <10 mL/kg
PaO_2 <60 mm Hg with FIO_2 >0.60
PaO_2/FIO_2 <100-150
$P(A-a)O_2$ >300 mm Hg on FIO_2 1.0
VD/VT >0.60
$PaCO_2$ >50 mm Hg

Table 5-2.--Complications of Mechanical Ventilation

Airway injury, bleeding, infection
Ventilator malfunction--leaks, power loss, incorrect settings,
  or alarm failures
Barotrauma; pneumothorax; interstitial, subcutaneous, or
  mediastinal air
Decreased right ventricular filling, increased right ventricular
  afterload, decreased cardiac output, hypotension
Gastrointestinal bleeding, stress gastritis, ulceration
Decreased urine output
Alteration in intracranial pressure

- Diagnosis of pneumonia may be difficult in patients receiving mechanical ventilation.
- Prophylaxis is commonly given to reduce stress-related gastritis and ulceration.
- H_2-Blockers may increase colonization of respiratory tract by gram-negative bacteria.
- Sucralfate or frequent use of antacids is an alternative.

An important and occasionally subtle complication of positive pressure ventilation is called intrinsic positive end-expiratory pressure (PEEP), auto-PEEP, breath stacking, or dynamic hyperinflation. This refers to a phenomenon of inadequate time during the expiratory phase of the respiratory cycle, so that a mechanically assisted breath is delivered before passive expiration of the lungs is complete. Thus, a new machine breath is delivered before the previous breath is completely exhaled. This may worsen hyperinflation, increase intrathoracic pressure, and worsen the associated complications, especially in patients with airway obstruction. Intrinsic PEEP may exist in spontaneously breathing patients with obstructive airway disease, but the effect is most significant in mechanically ventilated patients. Treatment typically involves optimizing bronchodilator therapy and altering the ventilator cycle to allow maximal expiratory time.

"Modes of mechanical ventilation" refers to the pattern of cycling of the machine breath and its relation to the spontaneous breaths of the patient. Assist-control mode is defined by a machine-assisted breath for every inspiratory effort by the patient. If no spontaneous breaths occur during a preset time interval, a controlled breath of predetermined tidal volume will be delivered by the ventilator. The backup rate should determine the minimum minute ventilation the patient will receive. The advantage of the assist-control mode is that it should allow maximal rest for the patient and maximal control of ventilation. The disadvantage is that hyperventilation and/or air trapping can occur in patients making rapid inspiratory efforts. Intermittent mandatory ventilation (IMV) allows a preset number of machine-assisted breaths of a given tidal volume. Between machine breaths, patients may breathe spontaneously. The advantage of IMV is that the number of

machine breaths can be decreased gradually during weaning efforts, providing that the patient is able to maintain satisfactory spontaneous ventilation. This is common clinical practice but it has not been proved superior to other weaning techniques, e.g., T-piece trials alternated with full ventilator support.

- Assist-control mode: machine-assisted breath for every inspiratory effort by the patient.
- Assist-control mode advantage: allows maximal rest for patient and maximal control of ventilation.
- Assist-control mode disadvantage: hyperventilation and/or air trapping in patients making rapid inspiratory efforts.
- IMV: allows preset number of machine-assisted breaths of a given tidal volume.
- Between machine breaths, patients may breathe spontaneously.
- IMV advantage: number of machine breaths can be decreased gradually during weaning efforts.
- IMV not proved superior to other weaning techniques (T-piece trials).

Pressure support may be used to assist spontaneously breathing patients, with or without IMV breaths. In this technique, for each inspiratory effort of the patient, the ventilator delivers a high rate of flow of inspired gas, up to a preset pressure limit. This pressure support lasts only during the spontaneous inspiratory effort, so that the rate and pattern of respiration are determined by the patient. Initial ventilator settings require specification of the mode of ventilation, tidal volume, respiratory rate, inspiratory and expiratory ratio (I:E) for the respiratory cycle, FIO_2, level of pressure support, and PEEP.

- With pressure support ventilation, for each inspiratory effort of the patient, the ventilator delivers a high flow of inspired gas, up to preset pressure limit.

PEEP is intended to increase functional residual capacity, recruit partially collapsed alveoli, improve lung compliance, and improve $\dot{V}/Q$ matching. An adverse effect of PEEP is an excessive increase in intrathoracic pressure with decreased cardiac output. Overdistention of lung units may also worsen $\dot{V}/Q$ mismatch. At levels of PEEP >10-15 cm H_2O, barotrauma is of particular concern. Optimal, or best, PEEP may be defined as lowest level of PEEP needed to achieve satisfactory oxygenation at a nontoxic FIO_2.

- PEEP: to increase functional residual capacity, recruit partially collapsed alveoli, improve lung compliance, improve $\dot{V}/Q$ matching.
- Adverse effect of PEEP: excessive increase in intrathoracic pressure with decreased cardiac output.
- Overdistention of lung units may also worsen $\dot{V}/Q$ mismatch.

- Optimal, or best, PEEP: lowest level of PEEP needed to achieve satisfactory oxygenation at a nontoxic FIO_2.

Pulmonary O_2 toxicity appears to be the result of direct exposure to high tensions of inspired O_2 or alveolar O_2. For adults, O_2 toxicity is not believed to be a major clinical concern below an FIO_2 of 0.40-0.50. Higher levels of inspired O_2 may be associated with acute tracheobronchitis (most likely an irritant effect). After several days of exposure, a syndrome of diffuse alveolar damage and lung injury may develop. The pathologic picture may resemble that of ARDS.

- Pulmonary O_2 toxicity: result of direct exposure to high tensions of inspired O_2 or alveolar O_2.
- Syndrome of diffuse alveolar damage and lung injury may develop.

ADULT RESPIRATORY DISTRESS SYNDROME

Diffuse lung injury with acute hypoxic respiratory failure may result from various injuries. Acute lung injury is a frequent primary cause of critical illness and may occur as a complication or a coexisting feature of multisystem disease. Mortality from all causes averages about 50%. Existing therapies do not significantly alter overall mortality in established ARDS. Recent emphasis is on identification of patients at high risk for acute lung injury and on possible early interventions. ARDS is commonly defined as diffuse acute lung injury that has the following major features: diffuse pulmonary infiltrates, severe hypoxemia due to shunting and ventilation-perfusion mismatch, and normal or low pulmonary capillary wedge pressure (i.e., noncardiogenic pulmonary edema). Criteria for the diagnosis of ARDS are listed in Table 5-3.

Table 5-3.--Criteria for Diagnosis of Adult Respiratory Distress Syndrome

Appropriate setting
Pulmonary injury, shock, trauma
Acute event
Clinical respiratory distress, tachypnea
Diffuse pulmonary infiltrates on chest radiograph
Interstitial and/or alveolar pattern
Hypoxemia
PaO_2/FIO_2 ratio <150
Decreased compliance of respiratory system
<50 mL/cm H_2O
Exclude
Chronic pulmonary disease accounting for clinical picture
Left ventricular failure (most series require pulmonary artery wedge measurement <18 mm Hg)

- Diffuse lung injury with hypoxic respiratory failure may result from various injuries.
- Mortality from all causes averages about 50%.
- Existing therapies do not significantly alter overall mortality in established ARDS.

ARDS was initially described as a post-traumatic or shock-induced injury, but it occurs with various states, as outlined in Table 5-4.

Relative risks of developing ARDS have been estimated from studies of predisposed groups. The greatest frequency is among patients with sepsis (approximately 40%), gastric aspiration (30%), multiple transfusions (25%), pulmonary contusion (20%), disseminated intravascular coagulation (20%), pneumonia requiring ICU management (12%), and trauma with long-bone or pelvic fractures (5%).

The pathophysiology of ARDS depends on damage to the alveolar-capillary unit. The earliest histologic changes are endothelial swelling, followed by edema and inflammation. Mononuclear inflammation, loss of alveolar type I cells, and protein deposition in the form of hyaline membranes may occur within 2-3 days. Fibrosis may develop after days or weeks of the process. Damage to type II alveolar epithelial cells leads to loss of surfactant. The surfactant that is produced may also be inactivated by proteins present in the airways. Alveolar filling and collapse cause intrapulmonary shunting and V̇/Q̇ mismatch with hypoxemia.

Death from ARDS usually is not due to isolated hypoxemic respiratory failure. The most frequent causes of mortality are complications of infection, sepsis syndrome, and failure of other organ systems. In addition to clinical risk factors listed

Table 5-4.--Disorders Associated With Adult Respiratory Distress Syndrome

Shock	Any cause
Sepsis	Lung infections, other bacteremic or endotoxic states
Trauma	Head injury, lung contusion, fat embolism
Aspiration	Gastric, near-drowning, tube feedings
Hematologic	Transfusions, leukoagglutinin, intravascular coagulation, thrombotic thrombocytopenic purpura
Metabolic	Pancreatitis, uremia
Drugs	Narcotics, barbiturates, aspirin
Toxic	Inhaled--O_2, smoke
	Irritant gases--NO_2, Cl_2, SO_2, NH_3
	Chemicals--paraquat
Miscellaneous	Radiation, air embolism, altitude

above, specific variables associated with mortality include <10% band forms on peripheral blood smear, persistent acidemia, bicarbonate <20 mEq/L, and blood urea nitrogen >65 mg/dL. Therefore, the systemic effects associated with ARDS may be important to outcome.

- Death from ARDS is not usually due to isolated hypoxemic respiratory failure.
- Infection, sepsis syndrome, and failure of other organ systems are the usual causes of mortality.
- Variables associated with mortality: <10% band forms on peripheral blood smear, persistent acidemia, bicarbonate <20 mEq/L, blood urea nitrogen >65 mg/dL.

Traditional therapy of ARDS involves optimization of physiologic variables and supportive management of associated complications. Measures include optimization of gas exchange and hemodynamics, nutrition, ambulation, and control of infections. Hypoxemia is typically corrected with positive pressure ventilation with supplemental O_2 and PEEP. PEEP provides potential benefits of increased lung volume and lung compliance and improvement in ventilation-perfusion relationships. Beyond an optimal level of PEEP, increase in intrathoracic pressure may be associated with decreased venous return, increased pulmonary vascular resistance, decreased left ventricular filling, and corresponding decrease in cardiac output. Supportive management of associated complications includes screening for underlying infections and early antibiotic therapy. Selective bowel decontamination by oral or nasogastric administration of a combination of nonabsorbable antibiotics may decrease colonization of airway by gram-negative organisms (reported to decrease the incidence of pneumonia in patients receiving mechanical ventilation).

- Hypoxemia is typically corrected with positive pressure ventilation with supplemental O_2 and PEEP.
- Screen for underlying infections and early antibiotic therapy.
- Selective bowel decontamination may decrease colonization of airway by gram-negative organisms.

Because increased capillary permeability allows greater intravascular fluid leak at any given hydrostatic pressure, attempt to limit intravascular volume to that necessary for systemic perfusion. However, associated shock states may demand volume expansion or increased inotropic support. Crystalloids can provide adequate filling pressures in patients with shock states, but large volumes may be required. Specific applications for colloids in ARDS include blood products (e.g., for coagulopathies or anemia). Supplemental nutrition is typically provided throughout the course of critical illness. Many patients with ARDS have associated multiorgan injury and may have ileus and/or gastrointestinal dysfunction

precluding enteral feedings. Such feedings are recommended if tolerated. Consequences of malnutrition may include impairment of respiratory muscle function, depressed ventilatory drive, and limitation of host defenses. Mobilization, ambulation, and ventilator weaning are carried out as early as practical.

- Crystalloids can provide adequate filling pressures in patients with shock states.
- Many patients with ARDS have associated multiorgan injury.

Pharmacologic therapies have been directed against proposed biochemical and cellular mechanisms of ARDS. The presumed pathogenesis of acute lung injury is centered on the role of polymorphonuclear leukocytes. Activation of complement by many stimuli associated with lung injury may lead to recruitment and activation of neutrophils, which may injure endothelium by releasing proteolytic enzymes and liberating toxic O_2 species (e.g., hydrogen peroxide, hydroxyl radical, singlet oxygen, superoxide). Broncho-alveolar lavage fluid from patients with established ARDS and from high-risk patients may show increased numbers of cells, predominantly neutrophils. (Normal lavage fluid contains about 93% alveolar macrophages, with 5%-7% lymphocytes and few neutrophils.) The percentage of neutrophils is correlated with abnormalities of gas exchange and alveolar protein content. However, experimental lung injury may occur in the absence of neutrophils, and typical ARDS is seen in severely neutropenic patients. Thus, other mechanisms presumably have a role. Arachidonic acid metabolites are implicated in many biochemical events associated with acute lung injury. Arachidonic acid is released from cell membranes by phospholipases. Arachidonate may then be metabolized via the lipoxygenase pathway to leukotriene compounds or via the cyclooxygenase pathway to prostaglandins or thromboxane. These compounds are potentially crucial in the pathogenesis of acute lung injury. Thromboxane A_2, a potent vasoconstrictor, induces platelet aggregation. Prostacyclin, or PGI_2, has the opposite effects on smooth muscle and platelet aggregation and is a potential therapeutic agent for ARDS. PGE_1, a prostaglandin, relaxes vascular and bronchial smooth muscle and inhibits neutrophil chemotaxis.

- Acute lung injury: presumed pathogenesis centers on polymorphonuclear leukocytes.
- Neutrophils may injure endothelium by releasing proteolytic enzymes and liberating toxic O_2 species.
- Experimental lung injury may still occur in the absence of neutrophils.
- Arachidonic acid metabolites are implicated in many biochemical events associated with acute lung injury.

- Thromboxane A_2: potent vasoconstrictor, induces platelet aggregation.
- PGE_1: relaxes vascular and bronchial smooth muscle, inhibits neutrophil chemotaxis.

Potential therapeutic and prophylactic agents have been directed against steps in arachidonate pathways. Corticosteroids decrease cell membrane disruption and have other anti-inflammatory properties. However, in ARDS and sepsis syndrome, steroids are potentially harmful and have no known benefit. Specifically, no differences in mortality have been observed in prospective, randomized studies of ARDS patients receiving methylprednisolone or placebo. Trials of corticosteroids in sepsis have also shown no difference in overall mortality. Steroids may delay resolution of secondary infections; a greater number of deaths related to secondary infection after steroids has been observed.

- Corticosteroids decrease cell membrane disruption and have other anti-inflammatory properties.
- However, in ARDS and sepsis syndrome, corticosteroids are potentially harmful and have no proven benefit.
- In sepsis, no difference in overall mortality with corticosteroids.

Nonsteroidal anti-inflammatory drugs (NSAIDs), e.g., ibuprofen and indomethacin, block cyclooxygenase and thromboxane formation. In animal models of acute lung injury and septic shock, NSAIDs have beneficial effects if used prophylactically. However, no benefit is known for established ARDS. Other mediators, particularly those associated with sepsis, may be important factors in the pathogenesis of acute lung injury. Endotoxin, a complex lipopolysaccharide, may activate complement; it has been associated with neutrophilic alveolitis. Monoclonal antiendotoxin antibodies are reported to have beneficial effects in some septic patients.

The prognosis for recovery of lung function in patients who survive ARDS is good. Studies of survivors have shown nearly normal lung volumes and airflow 6-12 months after the illness, with mild impairment in gas exchange--decreased diffusing capacity, desaturation with exercise, or widened A-a gradient. Therefore, the incentive is strong to continue aggressive measures in those patients with otherwise reversible organ dysfunction.

- Prognosis for the recovery of lung function in patients surviving ARDS is good.

CARDIOPULMONARY RESUSCITATION

General clinical algorithms for standardized responses to cardiac dysrhythmias or arrest should be reviewed. Ideally, in ICUs, cardiorespiratory problems should be prevented or anticipated and recognized quickly.

Basic Life Support

Airway Control

Relieve obstruction. Remove any foreign bodies. If not dislodged or obstructing, dentures may improve the seal of a face mask. However, dentures are usually removed before endotracheal intubation.

Suction (saliva, emesis, blood). A rigid suction catheter is most useful. Use head-tilt, chin-lift, or forward thrust of the jaw to open the posterior pharynx. The oropharyngeal or nasopharyngeal airway may help maintain patency and facilitate suctioning and mask ventilation.

Supply a high rate of flow of supplemental O_2. Ventilation is usually begun with a bag-valve-mask technique. Because a combined respiratory and metabolic acidosis is common, hyperventilation should be carried out to the extent possible.

Endotracheal intubation provides better control of the airway for ventilation, oxygenation, and suctioning and should be performed as soon as practical during resuscitation effort. However, the best possible ventilation and oxygenation should be provided before any attempt at intubation, and efforts should be limited to 15-30 seconds before resuming mask ventilation.

For chest compressions, a 5:1 compression-to-ventilation ratio is recommended for two-person resuscitation. Check femoral pulse for effectiveness of compressions. Monitoring of expired CO_2 (capnometry) by various devices is used to assess adequacy of ventilation and confirm endotracheal (versus esophageal) intubation. Under conditions of controlled ventilation and cardiac resuscitation, expired CO_2 may be an indicator of effective chest compressions (i.e., by Fick equation for CO_2--$\dot{V}CO_2 = Q \times (C\bar{v}\text{-}Ca)$ CO_2- and CO_2 delivery to lungs depends on adequate cardiac output).

- Relieve obstruction.
- Oropharyngeal or nasopharyngeal airway may help maintain patency.
- Supply a high rate of flow of supplemental O_2.
- Endotracheal intubation: better control of the airway for ventilation.

Electrical Therapy

Ventricular fibrillation is the most common rhythm in sudden cardiac arrest. The time to defibrillation is the most important factor determining successful resuscitation. In monitored patients in ICUs, defibrillation should typically be the first treatment, with other life support efforts initiated only after immediate attempts at electrical conversion. Electrical pacing may be useful in some cases of bradycardia and heart block.

- Ventricular fibrillation is the common rhythm in sudden cardiac arrest.

- Time to defibrillation is the most important factor determining successful resuscitation.
- In monitored patients in ICUs, defibrillation should typically be the first treatment.

Drug Therapy

Several recent trends and changes in recommendations about drug use are noteworthy. Electrical defibrillation is the treatment of choice for ventricular fibrillation. As additional therapy, lidocaine and bretylium have similar results in clinical outcome. Because bretylium may have adverse hemodynamic effects (hypotension), lidocaine is the recommended first-line therapy.

Sodium bicarbonate is still often used despite potential adverse effects and lack of documented efficacy. A rapid bolus of sodium bicarbonate may induce osmotic and ionic shifts and, by generating CO_2, may transiently worsen intracellular acidosis. Currently, bicarbonate is recommended only after another initial treatment has been established and if persistent metabolic acidosis and/or hyperkalemia is documented.

- Bicarbonate is recommended only after another initial treatment has been established.

Calcium may provide positive inotropic effects and vasoconstriction, but benefits in cardiac arrest have not been confirmed. Current indications for calcium include calcium channel blocker toxicity, acute hyperkalemia, or hypocalcemia.

- Indications for calcium: calcium channel blocker toxicity, acute hyperkalemia, hypocalcemia.

Epinephrine is administered during resuscitation from cardiac arrest for documented effects of peripheral vasoconstriction and improved coronary artery and cerebral blood flow during cardiopulmonary resuscitation. Epinephrine should also increase contractility in the beating heart. However, myocardial O_2 consumption may also increase, and automaticity and arrhythmias may be promoted. The optimal dose of epinephrine is debated. Blood flow may increase to a greater extent at doses higher than the standard 1 mg recommended for adult humans. A high dose of epinephrine (about 0.2 mg/kg) increases coronary artery perfusion in humans. Outcome and complications between standard and high doses of epinephrine: no additional toxicity but no improvement in survival. Standard doses and interval should remain the routine.

- High dose of epinephrine (about 0.2 mg/kg) increases coronary artery perfusion in humans.

VASCULAR ACCESS AND HEMODYNAMIC MONITORING

Central Venous Catheterization

The first choice for access in stable patients requiring intravenous therapy is the peripheral veins. However, in ICUs, central venous catheterization is often necessary for the following indications: lack of adequate peripheral veins, need for hypertonic or phlebitic medications or solutions, need for long-term access, measurement of central pressures, and access for procedures (hemodialysis, cardiac pacing). Relative contraindications include inexperience of the practitioner, coagulopathy, inability to identify landmarks, infection or burn at entry site, and thrombosis of proposed central venous site. Central venous catheters are usually placed over a guide wire (modified Seldinger technique). Complications of central venous catheterization include infections, cardiac arrhythmias, pneumothorax, air embolism, catheter or guide wire embolism, catheter knotting, bleeding, and other potential complications of needle or catheter misplacement.

- Central venous catheterization is often necessary.
- Contraindications: inexperienced practitioner, coagulopathy, inability to identify landmarks, infection or burn at entry site, thrombosis of proposed central venous site.
- Complications: infections, cardiac arrhythmias, pneumothorax, air embolism, catheter or guide wire embolism, catheter knotting, bleeding.

Catheter-related infections are usually attributed to migration of bacteria from skin along catheter tract. Catheter-related infection is usually defined by >15 colonies (CFU/mL) on semiquantitative culture of catheter tip. Catheter-related bacteremia is defined by similar growth and blood cultures positive for the same organism. Risk factors include infected catheter site or cutaneous breakdown, multiple manipulations, number of catheter lumens, and duration of use of the same site (particularly after 3-4 days). Treatment should include catheter removal and replacement at another site if necessary.

- Catheter-related infections usually are attributed to migration of bacteria from skin along catheter tract.
- Risk factors: infected catheter site or cutaneous breakdown, multiple manipulations, number of catheter lumens, duration of use of same site.

Pulmonary Artery Catheterization

Although common use (or overuse) of pulmonary artery catheterization is criticized, data from pulmonary artery catheterization may aid diagnosis and therapy in many disorders encountered in ICUs. Physiologic data that may be obtained are listed in Table 5-5.

Table 5-5.--Hemodynamic Data Obtained With Pulmonary Artery Catheterization

Variable	Normal value
Right atrial pressure (RAP)	2-8 mm Hg
Pulmonary arterial pressure (PAP)	16-24/5-12 mm Hg
Pulmonary capillary wedge pressure (PCWP)	5-12 mm Hg
Cardiac output (Q)	4-6 L/min
Cardiac index (CI = Q/body surface area)	2.5-3 L/min per m^2
Stroke volume (SV = Q/heart rate)	50-100 mL/beat
Stroke volume index (SVI = SV/body surface area)	35-50 mL/m^2
Systemic vascular resistance [SVR = (blood pressure - RAP)/Q]	10-15 mm Hg/L per min (x80 to convert to 800-1,200 dyne • s/cm^5)
Pulmonary vascular resistance [PVR = (PAP - PCWP)/Q]	1.5-2.5 mm Hg/L per min (100-200 dyne • s/cm^5)

Clinical conditions for which hemodynamic data may be useful include shock states, pulmonary edema, oliguric renal failure, indeterminate pulmonary hypertension, and myocardial and valvular disorders. Intravascular volume may be assessed more accurately, and effects of therapeutic interventions (volume, vasodilator therapy, or inotropes) may be evaluated. Mixed venous oxygen saturation may also be measured, as indicated above. This may be particularly useful in assessing the effects of PEEP on O_2 delivery (i.e., improving arterial saturation but potentially decreasing cardiac output).

Complications of pulmonary artery catheterization include arrhythmias, right bundle-branch block, complete heart block in patients with preexisting left bundle-branch block, vascular or right ventricular perforation, thrombosis and embolism, catheter knotting, infection, and pulmonary infarction or rupture due to persistent wedging or overdistention of the balloon.

- Complications of pulmonary artery catheterization: arrhythmias, right bundle-branch block, complete heart block in patients with preexisting left bundle-branch block, vascular or right ventricular perforation, thrombosis and embolism, catheter knotting, infection, pulmonary infarction or rupture due to persistent wedging or overdistention of balloon.

Use of pulmonary capillary wedge pressure (PCWP) as indicator of left ventricular end-diastolic pressure assumes a continuous hydrostatic column from pulmonary capillary to left atrium. Although digital displays of PCWP are usually available, the pressure wave should be examined for potential artifacts and for degree of respiratory variation. Because varying intrathoracic pressure may be sensed by the pulmonary artery catheter, recorded PCWP should be obtained at end expiration. Even with these measures, PCWP may be influenced by airway pressure--thus, not accurately reflecting ventricular filling pressure--especially with high levels of PEEP.

- PCWP is indicator of left ventricular end-diastolic pressure.
- PCWP may be influenced by airway pressure, especially with high levels of PEEP.

SHOCK STATES

Shock is defined by evidence of end-organ hypoperfusion, usually (but not necessarily) associated with hypotension. A common classification is cardiogenic (decreased cardiac output), hypovolemic (decreased blood volume), and septic (variable cardiac output, decreased systemic vascular resistance). All forms of shock may be characterized by hypotension, tachycardia, tachypnea, altered mental status, decreased urine output, and lactic acidosis. The clinical history often helps determine the diagnosis, e.g., blood loss, trauma, myocardial infarction, systemic infection. Compared with other causes, septic shock is often characterized by relatively warm extremities and normal or increased cardiac output.

- Shock is defined by evidence of end-organ hypoperfusion, usually associated with hypotension.
- Common classification: cardiogenic, hypovolemic, septic.
- Shock is characterized by hypotension, tachycardia, tachypnea, altered mental status, decreased urine output, and lactic acidosis.
- Septic shock is often characterized by relatively warm extremities and normal or increased cardiac output.

Sepsis syndrome is typically defined by a known or presumed source of infection associated with fever (or hypothermia) and leukocytosis (or leukopenia) *and* evidence of systemic effects, including hypotension, decreased urine output, or metabolic acidosis. After rapid initial assessment, treatment is directed at the presumed source, e.g., volume (blood loss, hypovolemia), vasodilator, or inotropic therapy (cardiogenic) or fluids, antibiotics, and drainage of any infected space (sepsis). If the response to initial therapy is inadequate, and especially if intravascular volume status is uncertain clinically, pulmonary artery catheterization may be useful. For example, if the wedge pressure remains <12-15 mm Hg, further volume support and/or erythrocytes should be administered. If the wedge pressure is >18-20 mm Hg and there is evidence of cardiac dysfunction, a vasodilator (nitroprusside) and diuretic therapy might be considered. If "hyperdynamic" indices are observed, i.e., increased cardiac output and low peripheral resistance, fluids should first be given to achieve a high-normal wedge pressure. Low doses of dopamine, 2-5 μg/kg per minute, may improve renal perfusion. *After* volume support has been given and tissue perfusion is still inadequate, careful administration of vasoconstrictors (norepinephrine) may improve organ perfusion. Septic shock is commonly associated with multiorgan injury. Multisystem organ failure is typically defined as acute dysfunction of two or more organ systems lasting >2 days. Sepsis is the most common cause. The pathogenesis is attributed to the hemodynamic and immunologic effects of endotoxin, cytokines (tumor necrosis factor [TNF-α]), interleukins (IL-1, IL-2, IL-6), platelet activating factor, arachidonic acid metabolites, polymorphonuclear leukocyte-derived toxic products, and myocardial depressant factors. Corticosteroids have no known benefit and potential adverse effects in patients with sepsis syndrome, with or without ARDS.

- Sepsis syndrome is typically defined by known or presumed source of infection associated with fever (or hypothermia) and leukocytosis (or leukopenia) and evidence of systemic effects (hypotension, decreased urine output, metabolic acidosis).
- Treatment is directed at the presumed source.
- Septic shock is commonly associated with multiorgan injury.
- Multisystem organ failure: acute dysfunction of two or more organ systems lasting >2 days.
- Pathogenesis is attributed to hemodynamic and immunologic effects of endotoxin, cytokines (TNF-α), IL-1, IL-2, IL-6, platelet activating factor, arachidonic acid metabolites, polymorphonuclear leukocyte-derived toxic products, and myocardial depressant factors.
- Corticosteroids have no known benefit.

Mortality in patients with sepsis and multiorgan failure may be >70%-90%. Adverse risk factors include age >65 years, continued systemic signs of sepsis, persistent deficit in O_2 delivery, and preexisting renal or liver failure. Physiologic scoring systems (e.g., APACHE) may predict outcome more accurately for patient subgroups.

- Mortality in patients with sepsis and multiorgan failure may be >70%-90%.

ETHICS IN THE ICU

The principles listed in Table 5-6 provide a framework for assessing ethical issues in the ICU. However, the potential for conflict frequently arises because patients are often unable to participate in their own care, multiple family members may be involved, and medical staff may disagree about prognosis and proposed interventions.

Recent legal opinions have supported the concept that a competent person may refuse life-sustaining therapy. Decision making for incompetent patients is more controversial, and living-will legislation has been designed partly to address such conflicts.

- A competent person may refuse life-sustaining therapy.
- Decision making for incompetent patients is more controversial; living-will legislation has been designed partly to address such conflicts.

"Do Not Resuscitate" orders have become increasingly common and important in recent years. Guidelines of the American Medical Association include:

1. Consent to cardiopulmonary resuscitation is presumed unless the patient (or patient's surrogate) has expressed in advance the wish not to be resuscitated or if, in the judgment of the treating physician, an attempt to resuscitate the patient would be futile. Resuscitation efforts should be considered futile if they cannot be expected either to restore cardiac or respiratory function or to achieve the expressed goals of the patient.

Table 5-6.--Principles for Assessing Ethical Issues in Intensive Care Units

---

Beneficence--acting in the patient's benefit by sustaining life, treating illness, and relieving pain

Nonmaleficence--do no harm

Autonomy--fundamental right to self-determination

Informed consent--providing factual and adequate information for competent patients to make decisions about their care

Substituted judgment--ability of a family member, guardian, or other surrogate to make decisions on behalf of the patient on the basis of what he or she believes the patient would have chosen if competent

Social justice--allocation of medical resources according to need (note that this concept implies overt health care rationing and may conflict with perceived individual rights)

Advance directives--living will: designed for persons to express their wishes regarding life-sustaining treatment at such time when they are deemed terminally ill and no longer able to participate in such decisions; typically there is provision or request for denial of specific life-support measures and designation of a surrogate decision maker.

2. The appropriateness of cardiopulmonary resuscitation should be discussed with those patients at risk of cardiopulmonary arrest, preferably in the outpatient setting or early during hospitalization, and resuscitation status should be reassessed periodically.

3. The physician is ethically obligated to honor resuscitation preferences of the patient or surrogate except when this would mandate use of futile therapeutic efforts (potential conflicts may arise in the application of this principle).

4. "Do Not Resuscitate" orders should be entered in the medical record.

5. "Do Not Resuscitate" orders affect administration of cardiopulmonary resuscitation only; other therapeutic interventions should not be influenced by the order.

Withholding Life Support Versus Withdrawal of Existing Support

Recent deliberations and court rulings have supported the concept that withholding and withdrawing of life support are essentially equivalent. In general, an irreversible or terminal illness is considered a prerequisite for withdrawal of support, but interpretation may vary widely.

QUESTIONS

Multiple Choice (choose the one best answer)

1. Which one of the following is true regarding the alveolar-to-arterial oxygen gradient, $P(A-a)O_2$?
   a. Decreases with increasing FIO_2
   b. Normal if hypoxemia is due to hypoventilation
   c. Increases if hypoxemia is due to altitude
   d. Increases with anemia
   e. Normal if hypoxemia is due to pulmonary embolism

2. Signs of air trapping with hypotension, agitation, and increasing $PaCO_2$ develop in a patient with severe asthma who requires mechanical ventilation. Which one of the following ventilator setting changes is most appropriate?
   a. Increase PEEP
   b. Increase I:E ratio
   c. Increase tidal volume
   d. Increase respiratory rate
   e. Increase expiratory time

3. The most appropriate definition of "best PEEP" is the pressure that provides which one of the following?
   a. Best compliance
   b. Best PaO_2
   c. Satisfactory O_2 delivery at a non-toxic FIO_2
   d. Best SaO_2
   e. Lowest mixed venous oxygen saturation

4. Which one of the following findings in a patient with shock would suggest sepsis rather than other causes?
   a. Altered mental status
   b. Hypotension
   c. Oliguria
   d. Lactic acidosis
   e. Increased cardiac output

5. A 60-year-old man with severe chronic obstructive pulmonary disease is intubated and mechanically ventilated for pneumonia. He receives treatment with antibiotics, bronchodilators, corticosteroids, and diuretics. After 3

days, ABGs on F_{IO_2} 0.30, IMV 6/min show Pa_{O_2}, 70 mm Hg; Pa_{CO_2}, 60 mm Hg, pH 7.45; HCO_3^-, 40 mEq/L; K+ = 3.0 mEq/L; Cl^- = 88 mEq/L. Which one of the following interventions is most appropriate?

a. Increase KC1 replacement
b. Increase ventilator rate
c. Increase F_{IO_2}
d. Increase diuretic
e. Increase steroid dose

6. A 25-year-old man is brought to the emergency room by a friend who found him unconscious. No further history is available. An arterial blood gas on room air revealed the following: pH 7.24; Pa_{CO_2}, 60 mm Hg; HCO_3^-, 26 mEq/L; Pa_{O_2}, 70 mm Hg; Sa_{O_2}, 93%. Which one of the following diagnoses is most likely?

a. Carbon monoxide poisoning
b. Diabetic ketoacidosis
c. Acute hepatic failure
d. Narcotic ingestion
e. Pneumonia

7. Which one of the following measurements in an intubated 80-kg patient is most indicative of a need for continued mechanical ventilation?

a. V_D/V_T = 0.25
b. Spontaneous tidal volume, 200 mL
c. Maximal inspiratory pressure, -80 cm H_2O
d. Respiratory rate, 15/min
e. Minute ventilation, 8 L

True/False (indicate whether each answer is true or false)
8. A pulmonary artery catheter is placed in a patient with progressive dyspnea. Measurements include: right atrial pressure, 8 mm Hg; pulmonary artery pressure, 50/20 mm Hg; pulmonary capillary wedge pressure, 10 mm Hg; cardiac output, 4 L/min. The following diagnoses are consistent with these findings:

a. Severe chronic obstructive pulmonary disease
b. Cardiac tamponade
c. Mitral regurgitation
d. Primary pulmonary hypertension
e. Chronic pulmonary thromboembolism
f. Left ventricular failure

9. The following are characteristic of the adult respiratory distress syndrome (ARDS):

a. Decreased lung compliance
b. Evidence of intrapulmonary shunting
c. Dynamic hyperinflation
d. Improved survival with early steroid treatment
e. Pulmonary capillary wedge pressure >18 mm Hg
f. Neutrophilic alveolitis

10. A 70-year-old man was brought to the intensive care unit after an abdominal operation. He was intubated and was breathing spontaneously on a T-piece with F_{IO_2} 0.50. Arterial blood gas values were as follows: pH 7.42; Pa_{O_2}, 60 mm Hg; Pa_{CO_2}, 38 mm Hg; Sa_{O_2}, 90%; HCO_3^-, 24 mEq/L; Hgb, 13.9 g/dL. The following could account for the blood gas findings:

a. Narcotics and postoperative sedation
b. Right mainstem intubation
c. Mesenteric ischemia
d. Aspiration pneumonia
e. Pulmonary embolism
f. Methemoglobinemia

ANSWERS

1. Answer b.

The alveolar-arterial (A-a) O_2 gradient is normally <10 mm Hg breathing room air and may increase to approximately 50 mm Hg on 100% O_2. The A-a gradient will increase in any condition causing ventilation/perfusion mismatch, but it remains normal if inspired O_2 decreases (altitude) or if alveolar P_{CO_2} increases (hypoventilation).

2. Answer e.

Air trapping, hyperinflation, or intrinsic PEEP result in increased intrathoracic pressure, decreased venous return, and decreased cardiac output. Treatment is directed at decreasing airway obstruction and allowing maximal time for passive expiration.

3. Answer c.

Various methods have been proposed to determine optimal

levels of PEEP. No single physiologic measurement has been shown to be most useful, and "best PEEP" may be defined as the lowest PEEP yielding acceptable oxygen delivery (O_2 content x cardiac output) at a nontoxic F_{IO_2} (<60%-70%).

4. Answer e.

Shock from any cause results in signs of hypoperfusion. Hypovolemia and cardiogenic shock are associated with decreased cardiac output, whereas early sepsis is typically a hyperdynamic state.

5. Answer a.

The arterial blood gas and electrolyte values indicate a chornic respiratory acidosis and metabolic alkalosis, likely compensatory but worsened by hypokalemia and hypochloremia. Increasing the ventilator support is not necessary because oxgenation is satisfactory and pH is >7.4

6. Answer d.

The arterial blood gas value shows a pure respiratory acidosis with a normal alveolar-arterial gradient. Hypoventilation, as could occur after narcotic ingestion, accounts for these findings.

7. Answer b.

Rapid, shallow breathing is the most sensitive and specific indicator of failure to wean from the ventilator. Tidal volume should be about 5 mL/kg.

8. a, true; b, false; c, false; d, true; e, true; f, false.

The hemodynamics indicate pulmonary hypertension with normal filling pressures. The features are consistent with primary pulmonary hypertension or secondary causes.

9. a, true; b, true; c, false; d, false; e, false; f, true.

ARDS is characterized by noncardiogenic pulmonary edema with shunting, decreased compliance, and influx of neutrophils. Dynamic hyperinflation or air-trapping typically occurs in conditions with airway obstruction. Early steroid treatment has not been shown to be of benefit.

10. a, false; b, true; c, false; d, true; e, true; f, false.

The arterial blood gas values show marked hypoxemia given the F_{IO_2} of 50%. Alveolar ventilation is normal. The findings are consistent with any cause for ventilation perfusion mismatch or shunting.

CHAPTER 6
DERMATOLOGY

Marian T. McEvoy, M.D.

GENERAL DERMATOLOGY

Skin Cancer

Non-melanoma skin cancers (basal cell, squamous cell) are the most common malignancy in the United States population; more than 600,000 cases occur each year. Basal cell carcinomas outnumber squamous cell carcinomas by a ratio of 4:1. The incidence of non-melanoma skin cancer is increasing rapidly, and an additional 12 million new cases of non-melanoma skin cancer are expected during the next 50 years. The increasing incidence of non-melanoma skin cancer has been attributed to a combination of increased exposure to ultraviolet light, changes in clothing style, increased longevity, and ozone depletion.

Both basal cell and squamous cell carcinomas tend to occur on sun-exposed areas. Basal cell carcinomas are commonly slow growing and locally invasive. They often invade vital structures and can cause significant disfigurement. Basal cell carcinomas tend not to metastasize to regional lymph nodes. Squamous cell carcinomas, alternatively, can metastasize to regional lymph nodes, and approximately 2% of all squamous cell carcinomas lead to death. Fortunately, non-melanoma skin cancers are highly curable; the cure rate is 90% if they are detected and treated early.

- Basal cell carcinoma and squamous cell carcinoma occur on sun-exposed skin.
- Cure rate is 90% with early detection and treatment.

Malignant Melanoma

An estimated 32,000 new cases of malignant melanoma and 8,000 new cases of melanoma in situ were diagnosed in the United States in 1994. The incidence of malignant melanoma is increasing rapidly in the United States. At the current rate, malignant melanomas will develop during the lifetime of 1 of every 105 Americans born in 1993 (approximately 1%). In contrast, the risk in 1980 was 1 in 250, and the risk in 1936 was only 1 in 1,500. If the incidence of malignant melanoma continues to increase at the current rate, by the year 2000 the lifetime risk for development of melanoma will increase to 1 in 75.

Risk factors for the development of malignant melanoma include fair skin, blond hair, freckling, intermittent sunlight exposure with blistering sunburns during childhood or adolescence, and genetic predisposition. The "familial atypical mole-melanoma syndrome" is transmitted by an autosomal dominant gene. This is characterized by a predisposition to dysplastic nevi and cutaneous melanomas. Patients with non-familial dysplastic nevi also have an increased risk for development of malignant melanoma. Other risk factors that have been identified include a personal or family history of melanoma, a personal or family history of non-melanoma skin cancer, a large number of benign pigmented nevi, giant pigmented congenital nevus, immunosuppression, human immunodeficiency virus (HIV) positivity, and the use of tanning beds. Many primary melanomas occur on non-sun-exposed sites such as the back, scalp, and nails.

The key to improved survival with malignant melanoma has been early diagnosis. The most important prognostic feature of malignant melanoma is tumor thickness; this is defined as the measurement from the stratum granulosum to the deepest tumor cell in the histologic section and is referred to as Breslow's thickness. The 5-year survival rate approaches 100% in patients with lesions <0.75 mm thick, approximately 94% for lesions 0.76-1.50 mm, 84% for lesions 1.5-2.25 mm, 77% for lesions 2.26-3.00 mm, and 46% for lesions >3 mm. The 5-year survival rate is approximately 36% in patients with lymph node metastasis and 5% in patients with extranodal metastasis. Clark's levels of invasion (level 1, intraepidermal tumor only; level 2, tumor extending into papillary dermis; level 3, tumor pushing on papillary dermal-reticular dermal junction; level 4, lesion has invaded reticular dermis; level 5, invasion into subcutaneous fat) are not used for prognostic classification. Other factors such as sex and anatomic site have sometimes been cited as criteria of independent prognostic significance.

- Key to improved survival rate with malignant melanoma is early diagnosis.
- Most important prognostic feature is tumor thickness (Breslow thickness).

Stage I malignant melanoma consists of the cutaneous lesion without lymph node involvement, stage II consists of the primary skin lesion plus lymph node involvement, and stage III represents distant metastasis. The recommended management of stage I malignant melanoma is surgical. The previous recommendation of a 5-cm margin of excision for all types of malignant melanoma has been revised. Although "wide" excision of malignant melanoma is still the standard of treatment, excision margins >3 cm are no longer advocated. For excision of a thin melanoma (<1 mm thick), a 1-cm margin is generally recommended, and a 2- to 3-cm margin is advised for thicker lesions. Elective lymph node dissection does not improve outcome in patients with stage I disease. For stage II disease, excision of the primary skin lesion and regional lymph node dissection are usually recommended. Again, early diagnosis is the key to management, as no form of adjuvant therapy has been shown to improve survival in patients with advanced disease.

- Surgical management of stage I malignant melanoma consists of excision with tumor-free margins of 1-3 cm.

Prevention of Melanoma and Non-Melanoma Skin Cancer

Dermatologists encourage regular use of sunscreens with a sun protection factor (SPF) of at least 15. Sunlight exposure during the first 18 years of life accounts for up to 80% of cumulative lifetime sun exposure. Therefore, sunscreen use is particularly important in children and adolescents. Persons with light skin types and outdoor workers need to be particularly vigilant with sun protection. Because the prognosis with melanoma and non-melanoma skin cancer improves with early diagnosis, these lesions need to be recognized by health care workers and the general public alike.

Cutaneous T-Cell Lymphoma

Forms of cutaneous T-cell lymphoma are mycosis fungoides and Sézary syndrome. Mycosis fungoides generally manifests as discrete or coalescing patches, plaques, or nodules on the skin. Mycosis fungoides may progress to involve lymph nodes and viscera. From the time of extracutaneous involvement, the median duration of survival has been estimated at 2.5 years. The course of patients with patch- or plaque-stage cutaneous lesions, without extracutaneous disease, is less predictable, but the median duration of survival is approximately 12 years. Sézary syndrome is characterized by generalized erythroderma, keratoderma of the palms and soles, and a Sézary cell count of >1,000/mm^3 in the peripheral blood. Most patients have severe pruritus.

- Mycosis fungoides and Sézary syndrome are forms of cutaneous T-cell lymphoma.
- Mycosis fungoides may progress to involve lymph nodes and viscera.
- Median survival for patients with mycosis fungoides is 12 years; from time of extracutaneous involvement, it is 2.5 years.

Both mycosis fungoides and Sézary syndrome are characterized by the presence of Sézary cells (lymphocytes with hyperchromatic and convoluted nuclei) involving the epidermis (epidermotrophism) and dermis. Immunohistochemical stains of cutaneous lesions demonstrate that these neoplastic T cells usually express CD3 and CD4 antigens, and molecular genetic studies reveal clonal rearrangement of the T-cell receptor gene in lymphocyte populations from skin biopsy, lymph node, and peripheral blood specimens of patients with cutaneous T-cell lymphoma.

- Mycosis fungoides and Sézary syndrome are T-cell lymphomas characterized by presence of Sézary cells in skin and peripheral blood.

Treatment of cutaneous T-cell lymphoma includes topical nitrogen mustard, psoralen with ultraviolet-A light (PUVA), radiotherapy (electron beam, orthovoltage), and systemic chemotherapy. Interferon, retinoids, and other agents have also been used. Most recently, extracorporeal photopheresis has become popular in the treatment of cutaneous T-cell lymphoma. After ingestion of 8-methoxypsoralen, the patient's leukocytes are exposed to ultraviolet light A and then reinfused.

Psoriasis

Psoriasis occurs in approximately 1%-2% of the population of the United States. Onset of lesions is usually in the third decade of life, and about a third of patients have a family history of psoriasis. The cutaneous disease is usually chronic, and the most common presentation is with papules and plaques covered with a silvery scale. Removal of the scale results in pinpoint bleeding from a phenomenon referred to as Auspitz sign. Patterns of psoriasis include psoriasis vulgaris with large plaque-like lesions on the trunk and limbs and classic involvement of the elbows and knees. Guttate psoriasis is an acute form of psoriasis which often follows streptococcal throat infection and presents with small lesions (5-10 mm in diameter) of psoriasis on the trunk and limbs. Other, less common forms of psoriasis include pustular psoriasis, which may be localized to the hands and feet or may be generalized. Approximately 50% of patients have nail abnormalities, most commonly onycholysis, pitting, and oil spots. Lesions of psoriasis are characterized by koebnerization, which is a term used to describe the induction of lesions at sites of trauma.

- Onset of psoriasis lesions is in third decade of life.
- One-third of patients have family history.
- 50% of patients have nail abnormalities.

The treatment of psoriasis includes topical steroids, topical tar preparations, and phototherapy. A newer form of treatment of localized psoriasis is a topical synthetic vitamin D analogue, calcipotriene.

Ultraviolet Light

Natural sunlight may be divided into ultraviolet-B (UVB, 280-320 nm), ultraviolet-A (320-400 nm), and visible light. UVB radiation is responsible for the sunburn reaction. In treating inflammatory dermatoses, UVB has been used most commonly in combination with tar, as in the Goeckerman therapy of psoriasis. UVB may also benefit atopic dermatitis, lichen planus, and certain other inflammatory dermatoses.

PUVA

PUVA consists of ingestion of psoralen followed by exposure of the skin to ultraviolet-A light. PUVA has most commonly been used for therapy of generalized psoriasis, but it is also effective in the treatment of various dermatoses, including lichen planus, mycosis fungoides, urticaria pigmentosa, and vitiligo. PUVA therapy is associated with minimal or no systemic side effects. The main side effect of PUVA therapy is an increased risk (>12 times) of cutaneous squamous cell carcinoma in patients who have received long-term therapy.

- PUVA commonly used for therapy of generalized psoriasis.
- Associated with minimal or no systemic side effects.
- Main side effect is increased risk of cutaneous squamous cell carcinoma.

Atopic Dermatitis

The atopic diathesis is manifested by one or more of the following: atopic dermatitis, asthma, and allergic rhinitis or conjunctivitis. Atopic dermatitis often presents in the neonatal period with scaling and erythema of the scalp and face with later spreading to the trunk. The distribution is often extensor in the older infant, and by the age of approximately 3 years the more classic flexural distribution is observed. In adolescence, facial involvement (perioral, eyelid, and forehead) is not uncommon. Generalized flares of eczema can occur at any age.

Disturbances in cell-mediated immunity lead to an increased incidence of bacterial and viral infections. Secondary infection with *Staphylococcus aureus* is not uncommon and presents as a weeping, crusting dermatitis (impetiginization). Eczema herpeticum is the term used to describe a secondary infection with the herpes simplex virus, which may be generalized. Infections with the human papilloma virus and molluscum

contagiosum are also more common and the lesions are more numerous in patients with atopic dermatitis.

- Eczema herpeticum, a generalized herpes simplex virus infection, may occur in patients with atopic dermatitis.

Allergic Contact Dermatitis

Allergic contact dermatitis is a form of localized or generalized dermatitis that results from exposure to an antigen. This is a type 4 hypersensitivity reaction (delayed, cell-mediated). Recognition of antigens by T-lymphocytes requires participation of Langerhans cells, which are the "antigen-presenting" cells of the epidermis. Langerhans cells are dendritic cells of the epidermis, which express CD1 (OKT6) antigen and contain Birbeck granules. During investigation of the cause of allergic contact dermatitis, one must consider the anatomical location of the cutaneous lesions and environmental exposure to allergens, including occupational, household, and recreational contactants.

- Allergic contact dermatitis is type 4 hypersensitivity reaction (delayed, cell-mediated).
- Langerhans cells are "antigen-presenting" cells of epidermis.

Patch testing consists of application of various substances to the patient's back; each substance is under a small aluminum disk covered with adhesive tape. These are left on the patient's back for 48 hours, and the results are interpreted at 48 and 96 hours. Positive reactions occur most often to the following antigens: nickel sulfate, potassium dichromate, thimerosal, paraphenylenediamine, ethylenediamine, neomycin sulfate, benzocaine, thiuram, and formalin.

Nickel sulfate allergies are mainly associated with jewelry. Paraphenylenediamine is present in hair dyes and other cosmetics; *para*-aminobenzoic acid (PABA) in sunscreens is immunologically related to paraphenylenediamine. Potassium dichromate sensitivity is one of the most common types of occupational allergic contact dermatitis and occurs in construction workers exposed to cement, leathers, and certain paints. Formaldehyde is a common preservative in cosmetics and shampoos. Neomycin sulfate and benzocaine are components of many topical antimicrobial and analgesic preparations. Thimerosal is a commonly used preservative in contact lens solutions and in some intramuscular injections. Thiuram is a rubber accelerator and fungicide and therefore may correlate with occupational dermatitis or dermatitis related to wearing shoes containing rubber.

- Nickel sulfate allergies are associated with jewelry.
- Potassium dichromate sensitivity occurs in construction workers exposed to cement, leathers, certain paints.
- Formaldehyde is common preservative in cosmetics and shampoos.

Acne Vulgaris

Acne vulgaris is one of the most common problems seen in clinical dermatology. Acne occurs physiologically at puberty with varying degrees of severity. In some persons, acne persists into the second and third decades of life. The pathogenesis of acne is multifactorial; inheritance, increase in sebaceous gland activity, hormonal influences, disturbances of keratinization, and bacterial infection have all been implicated. The primary lesions of acne are noninflammatory and include microcomedones, closed comedones (whiteheads), and open comedones (blackheads). The secondary or inflammatory lesions include papules and pustules, nodules, and cysts. Acne may be divided into grades 1, 2, and 3 based on the clinical findings. Comedonal acne (grade 1) is treated with agents that cause dryness and peeling and help to eliminate comedones. Such agents include topical tretinoin (Retin A) and benzoyl peroxide. Treatment of papular or pustular acne (grade 2) is the same with the addition of topical or systemic antibiotics. Cystic acne (grade 3) is treated with systemic antibiotics; when it is severe and extensive or unresponsive to conventional therapy, isotretinoin (Accutane) is the treatment of choice.

Systemic Retinoids

Isotretinoin (13-*cis*-retinoic acid) is a synthetic vitamin A derivative used primarily for the treatment of severe nodulocystic acne vulgaris. The mechanism of action of 13-*cis*-retinoic acid in acne is probably multifactorial, including improvement in keratinization, decrease in sebum production, and decrease in inflammation. A 4- to 5-month course at a dosage of approximately 1 mg/kg per day is the standard regimen.

- Isotretinoin used for treatment of severe acne vulgaris.

The greatest risk associated with use of systemic retinoids is teratogenicity. Before isotretinoin is prescribed, female patients must be counseled on this side effect and follow contraception during therapy and for at least 1 month after use of the drug is discontinued.

- Greatest risk with use of systemic retinoids is teratogenicity.

The systemic retinoids are associated with various side effects, including xerosis, dermatitis, cheilitis, sticky skin, peeling skin, epistaxis, conjunctivitis, hair loss, and nail dystrophy. Symptoms of arthralgias and myalgias may also occur. Most patients develop some degree of hyperlipidemia, including hypertriglyceridemia and hypercholesterolemia. Other laboratory abnormalities include elevation of liver function measurements and leukopenia. Skeletal hyperostosis occurs particularly in association with long-term use.

- Side effects of systemic retinoids include xerosis, dermatitis, cheilitis, sticky skin, peeling skin, epistaxis, conjunctivitis, hair loss, nail dystrophy.

Etretinate has been used effectively for treatment of pustular psoriasis, erythrodermic psoriasis, and generalized chronic plaque-type psoriasis. It has been used successfully as a single agent or in combination with PUVA therapy. Because of its long half-life (at least 3 months) and deposition in subcutaneous fat, etretinate is not recommended for treatment of females of childbearing potential.

Autoimmune Bullous Diseases

Bullous pemphigoid is the most common autoimmune bullous disease. The disease predominantly occurs in elderly patients and usually presents with large, tense bullae on erythematous bases with a predilection for flexural areas (color plate 6-1). Lesions are often generalized but may be localized. The most common histologic pattern is a subepidermal bulla with eosinophils, although there is a subset of patients with neutrophil-rich lesions, noninflammatory lesions, or eosinophilic spongiosis without evidence of blisters histologically.

- Bullous pemphigoid is most common autoimmune bullous disease.
- Occurs predominantly in elderly patients.
- Presents as large, tense bullae with predilection for flexural areas.

Immunofluorescence testing is important for diagnosis of bullous pemphigoid. Direct immunofluorescence testing of perilesional skin shows deposition of C3 in a linear pattern at the basement membrane zone in almost all cases and of IgG in >90%. A minority (usually <20%) of biopsy specimens also have IgA or IgM in a linear pattern at the basement membrane zone. Indirect immunofluorescence testing of serum demonstrates IgG anti-basement-membrane zone antibodies in approximately 70% of cases. Routine indirect immunofluorescence testing of serum in patients suspected to have autoimmune bullous diseases is usually performed with monkey esophagus as substrate. The sensitivity of detection of anti-basement-membrane zone antibodies is increased by use of sodium chloride (NaCl)-split human skin as substrate. In addition, use of NaCl-split skin as substrate for indirect immunofluorescence testing is useful in distinguishing between bullous pemphigoid and epidermolysis bullosa acquisita, a rare blistering disease with a similar clinical presentation. On NaCl-split skin substrate, basement membrane zone antibodies from patients with bullous pemphigoid localize to the epidermal side (roof) of the substrate, or occasionally to both the roof and the floor of the substrate, whereas basement membrane zone antibodies from patients with epidermolysis bullosa acquisita localize to the dermal side (floor) of the substrate. This procedure often obviates immunoelectron microscopy to distinguish between bullous pemphigoid and epidermolysis bullosa acquisita.

- Immunofluorescence testing important for diagnosis of bullous pemphigoid.
- Almost all cases have deposition of C3 and IgG in linear pattern at basement membrane zone.

Immunoelectron microscopy of bullous pemphigoid lesions demonstrates deposition of IgG at the lamina lucida and hemidesmosomes. Immunoblotting and immunoprecipitation studies have demonstrated that bullous pemphigoid antigens are a heterogeneous group of noncollagenous glycoproteins, predominantly consisting of two proteins of 230 kd and 180 kd.

Treatment of bullous pemphigoid includes systemic corticosteroids, dapsone, azathioprine, and cyclophosphamide. In general, bullous pemphigoid requires less immunosuppressive therapy than does pemphigus. Also in contrast to pemphigus, the titer of circulating antibodies does not correlate with disease activity.

Epidermolysis bullosa acquisita is another subepidermal bullous disease. It is characterized clinically by blisters or erosions induced by trauma, which predominantly occur on acral locations. A small subset of patients have generalized lesions, which clinically may be difficult to distinguish from bullous pemphigoid. The histologic pattern is a subepidermal bulla, with or without eosinophils or neutrophils.

- Epidermolysis bullosa acquisita characterized by blisters or erosions induced by trauma.
- Occurs predominantly on acral sites.

Direct immunofluorescence testing reveals a pattern similar to that in bullous pemphigoid, namely, deposition of IgG and C3 in a linear pattern at the basement membrane zone. In contrast to bullous pemphigoid, C3 may be absent or IgG may be the dominant immunoreactant. Indirect immunofluorescence testing of serum on monkey esophagus substrate demonstrates IgG anti-basement-membrane zone antibodies in 25%-50% of patients; these antibodies localize to the dermal side (floor) of NaCl-separated human skin substrate. In patients who lack circulating antibodies, the NaCl-split skin technique may be applied to skin biopsy tissue from the patient. Immunoelectron microscopy demonstrates IgG deposits below and at the lamina densa. The epidermolysis bullosa acquisita antigen is a 290-kd collagenous glycoprotein, representing the globular carboxyl terminus of type VII procollagen. Epidermolysis bullosa acquisita tends to be resistant to immunosuppressive therapy.

- On direct immunofluorescence, epidermolysis bullosa acquisita shows deposition of IgG and C3 in linear pattern at basement membrane zone.
- Tends to be resistant to immunosuppressive therapy.

Cicatricial pemphigoid is characterized by mucosal lesions, with limited or no cutaneous lesions. The disease predominantly affects oral and ocular mucous membranes, and less frequently the genital, pharyngeal, or upper respiratory mucosa. This disease is also known as benign mucous membrane pemphigoid, which is often a misnomer because untreated ocular involvement may lead to blindness. Patients may present with oral erosions or diffuse gingivitis.

- Cicatricial pemphigoid affects oral and ocular mucous membranes, and less frequently genital, pharyngeal, or upper respiratory mucosa.

Direct immunofluorescence testing of mucosal tissue shows deposition of C3 and IgG in a linear pattern at the basement membrane zone, as in bullous pemphigoid. There may be IgA deposition, in addition to IgG and C3, in approximately 20% of patients. The diagnostic yield of oral mucosal tissue is better than that of conjunctiva. Serum rarely contains IgG anti-basement-membrane zone antibodies demonstrable on monkey esophagus substrate. Use of NaCl-split human skin or oral mucosa as substrate increases the sensitivity of detection of circulating anti-basement-membrane zone antibodies. Immunoelectron microscopy demonstrates deposition of IgG somewhat lower in the lamina lucida in cicatricial pemphigoid than in bullous pemphigoid. Immunoblotting and immunoprecipitation studies demonstrate that cicatricial pemphigoid antigens appear to be similar to bullous pemphigoid antigens by molecular weight, suggesting that the different disease expression is related to a different location of target antigens.

- In cicatricial pemphigoid, direct immunofluorescence shows deposition of C3 and IgG in linear pattern at basement membrane zone.

Treatment of cicatricial pemphigoid is similar to that of bullous pemphigoid, with systemic corticosteroids, dapsone, azathioprine, or cyclophosphamide. Cyclophosphamide has been used particularly in patients with ocular involvement.

Herpes gestationis, also referred to as pemphigoid gestationis, consists of intensely pruritic urticarial papules, plaques, or blisters usually occurring in last half of pregnancy. The lesions are histologically characterized by a subepidermal bulla with eosinophils.

- Herpes gestationis consists of intensely pruritic urticarial papules, plaques, or blisters.

Direct immunofluorescence testing of perilesional skin demonstrates deposition of C3 in a linear pattern at the basement membrane zone. In contrast to bullous pemphigoid, IgG is deposited at the basement membrane zone in only 30%-40% of cases. Direct immunofluorescence testing is particularly useful because the other dermatoses of pregnancy (such as pruritic urticarial papules and plaques of pregnancy, PUPP) are negative by immunofluorescence testing. The serum from approximately half of patients with herpes gestationis contains the "HG factor," which is a complement-fixing IgG anti-basement-membrane zone antibody. IgG1 is the major subclass in serum and tissue from patients with herpes gestationis, whereas it is IgG4 in patients with bullous pemphigoid. Immunoelectron microscopy of a skin lesion from herpes gestationis demonstrates deposition of C3 throughout the lamina lucida. The herpes gestationis antigen appears to be a 180-kd molecule, although a higher-molecular-weight antigen may also exist.

- In herpes gestationis, direct immunofluorescence shows deposition of C3 in linear pattern at basement membrane zone.

Linear IgA bullous dermatosis is characterized by vesicles or blisters on erythematous bases in a generalized distribution with a high rate of mucosal involvement. There is no association with gluten-sensitive enteropathy. *Chronic bullous disease of childhood* seems to be immunologically identical to linear IgA bullous dermatosis of adults. Both diseases have clinical and histologic features in common with dermatitis herpetiformis and bullous pemphigoid. The histologic pattern is a subepidermal bulla with features of dermatitis herpetiformis or pemphigoid.

The diseases are characterized by the direct immunofluorescence finding of IgA deposition in a linear pattern at the basement membrane zone, with or without C3 or IgG deposition. Circulating IgA anti-basement-membrane zone antibodies, usually in low titer, are better demonstrated with use of NaCl-split skin as substrate than with monkey esophagus as substrate. Immunoelectron microscopy demonstrates deposits of IgA in the lamina lucida, sublamina densa, or both locations. Treatment of linear IgA bullous dermatosis and chronic bullous disease of childhood includes systemic corticosteroids, dapsone, and sulfapyridine.

- In linear IgA bullous dermatosis and chronic bullous disease of childhood, direct immunofluorescence shows IgA deposition in linear pattern at basement membrane zone.

Dermatitis herpetiformis (color plate 6-2) is characterized by extremely pruritic, grouped vesicles occurring predominantly over the elbows, knees, buttocks, back of the neck and scalp, and low back, usually beginning in the third or fourth decade of life. The characteristic histologic pattern in skin biopsy tissue consists of papillary stuffing with neutrophils underlying a microvesicle. Virtually all patients have some degree of gluten-sensitive enteropathy, although it is usually low-grade and subclinical. This association is important in terms of management of dermatitis herpetiformis. Dermatitis herpetiformis is also associated with thyroid disease.

- In dermatitis herpetiformis, virtually all patients have some degree of gluten-sensitive enteropathy.

The hallmark of the diagnosis of dermatitis herpetiformis is the direct immunofluorescence finding of IgA deposits in a stippled, granular, or clumped pattern, concentrated in papillary bodies and along the basement membrane zone. It is recommended that skin biopsy specimens be obtained from an area 0.5 to 1 cm away from an active lesion. IgA deposits tend to persist in the skin over time. A small percentage of patients who strictly adhere to a gluten-free diet may show diminution in IgA deposits after many years, but IgA deposits in the skin are unaffected by pharmacologic therapy. The serum of patients with dermatitis herpetiformis may contain IgA anti-reticulin and IgA anti-endomysial antibodies. IgA anti-endomysial antibodies and IgA anti-reticulin antibodies are found in approximately 70% of patients with dermatitis herpetiformis or celiac disease and in close to 100% of such patients who have grade III or IV gluten-sensitive enteropathy. Testing for IgA anti-endomysial antibodies is useful for both diagnosis and management of dermatitis herpetiformis, although these antibodies correlate with the degree of gluten-sensitive enteropathy rather than the skin lesion per se.

- In dermatitis herpetiformis, direct immunofluorescence shows IgA deposits in stippled, granular, or clumped pattern.
- Testing for IgA anti-endomysial antibodies useful for diagnosis and management.

The mainstay of treatment of dermatitis herpetiformis consists of dapsone and a gluten-free diet. Patients who strictly adhere to a gluten-free diet may have a decreased need for dapsone. Patients must adhere to the diet for at least 8 months before its efficacy is assessed. The titer of IgA anti-endomysial antibodies decreases during strict adherence to a gluten-free diet. Systemic corticosteroids are generally not helpful in the treatment of dermatitis herpetiformis.

- Treatment of dermatitis herpetiformis: dapsone and gluten-free diet.

Bullous eruption of systemic lupus erythematosus shares clinical and histologic features with dermatitis herpetiformis. The blisters were therefore originally thought to represent the coexistence of dermatitis herpetiformis and lupus erythematosus, but they are now established as a distinct subset of lupus.

Direct immunofluorescence testing demonstrates deposition of IgG, IgM, IgA, or C3 in a linear or granular pattern at the basement membrane zone, similar to the classic "lupus band." Indirect immunofluorescence testing of serum may show IgG anti-basement-membrane zone antibodies; testing on NaCl-split skin substrate reveals a pattern identical to that of serum from patients with epidermolysis bullosa acquisita--staining of the floor (dermal side) of separated skin. The antigen of bullous lupus erythematosus appears to be the same as the epidermolysis bullosa acquisita antigen (a 290-kd glycoprotein).

- In bullous eruption of systemic lupus erythematosus, direct immunofluorescence shows deposition of IgG, IgM, IgA, or C3 in a linear or granular pattern at basement membrane zone.
- Antigen is same as that of epidermolysis bullosa acquisita.

The clinical variants of *pemphigus* include pemphigus vulgaris and pemphigus foliaceus (with subsets pemphigus erythematosus and fogo selvagem, the latter being an endemic form of pemphigus that occurs in South America). There is also a drug-induced variant of pemphigus, particularly associated with D-penicillamine, captopril, or other thiol-containing medications.

- A drug-induced variant of pemphigus is associated with D-penicillamine.

More than 50% of patients with pemphigus vulgaris present with oral lesions, and >90% have oral mucosal involvement at some point in the course of the disease. Pemphigus vulgaris is characterized by coalescing blisters and erosions, often with generalized involvement. In contrast, pemphigus foliaceus, considered to represent the "superficial" variant of pemphigus, may present with superficial scaling-crusting lesions of the head and neck area (in a seborrheic dermatitis-like pattern) or generalized distribution (color plate 6-3). The histologic hallmark of pemphigus is the presence of acantholysis (detachment of intercellular adhesion resulting in rounded keratinocytes). Pemphigus vulgaris is characterized by an intraepidermal bulla in a suprabasilar location. Pemphigus foliaceus involves acantholysis at the granular layer.

- Histologic hallmark of pemphigus is presence of acantholysis.

All types of pemphigus are characterized by the deposition of IgG and C3 at the intercellular space (epidermal cell surface) on direct immunofluorescence testing (intercellular substance antibody, ICS). Indirect immunofluorescence testing demonstrates IgG anti-ICS antibodies in approximately 90% of cases. The titer of IgG anti-ICS antibodies is useful in both diagnosis and management of pemphigus. IgG in pemphigus is predominantly IgG4.

- All types of pemphigus are characterized by direct immunofluorescence finding of IgG and C3 deposition at the epidermal cell surface.
- Titer of IgG anti-ICS antibodies is useful in diagnosis and management.

Pemphigus antibodies are pathogenic in that they have been demonstrated to induce acantholysis in vitro and in animal models. Immunoelectron microscopy shows that IgG and C3 are localized to cell membranes, not intracellularly. The pemphigus vulgaris antigen complex consists of a 130-kd glycoprotein (the binding site for pemphigus vulgaris antibodies) linked to plakoglobin. The pemphigus foliaceus antigen complex is composed of a 160-kd protein (which is desmoglein 1--the binding site for pemphigus foliaceus antibodies) linked to plakoglobin.

- Pemphigus antibodies induce acantholysis.

High-dose corticosteroids are generally required to control pemphigus. Various "steroid-sparing" immunosuppressive agents have been used, including azathioprine, cyclophosphamide, gold, and dapsone.

- High-dose corticosteroids generally are required to control pemphigus.

Erythema Multiforme

This is an acute, usually self-limited eruption of maculopapular, urticarial, occasionally bullous lesions characterized by "iris" or "target" morphology (color plate 6-4). A subset of patients with erythema multiforme may have recurrent lesions. When erythema multiforme presents with extensive cutaneous and mucosal lesions, it is referred to as Stevens-Johnson syndrome. Various etiologic factors have been implicated in erythema multiforme. The most commonly cited precipitating factor is viral infection, particularly herpes simplex virus. This is responsible for a significant percentage of recurrent erythema multiforme. Other infectious agents that have been noted to cause erythema multiforme include *Mycoplasma pneumoniae* and *Yersinia enterocolitica*. Drugs have been reported to induce erythema multiforme, particularly sulfonamides, but also barbiturates and anticonvulsants. Erythema multiforme may be associated with underlying connective tissue disease or malignancy. A small subset of patients with erythema multiforme have disease of the oral mucosa. Erythema multiforme tends to involve the lips, buccal mucosa, and tongue, in contrast to pemphigus vulgaris, which typically involves the pharynx, buccal mucosa, and tongue, and pemphigoid, which most often involves gingivae. Neither pemphigus nor pemphigoid tends to involve the lips.

- Most commonly cited precipitating factor is viral infection, particularly herpes simplex.
- Other agents: *Mycoplasma pneumoniae* and *Yersinia enterocolitica*.
- Drugs are reported to induce erythema multiforme: sulfonamides, barbiturates, anticonvulsants.

Erythema Nodosum

Erythema nodosum typically presents as tender, erythematous, subcutaneous nodules localized to the pretibial areas. The lesions may be acute and self-limited or chronic, lasting for months up to years. The most common cause is streptococcal pharyngitis. Other infectious agents that have been implicated in the development of erythema multiforme include *Yersinia enterocolitica*, *Coccidioides*, and *Histoplasmosis*. Drug-induced erythema nodosum is most often associated with oral contraceptives and sulfonamides. Other associations with erythema nodosum include sarcoidosis, inflammatory bowel disease, and Behçet's syndrome.

- Most common cause of erythema nodosum is streptococcal pharyngitis.
- Drug-induced erythema nodosum most often associated with oral contraceptives and sulfonamides.
- Other associations: sarcoidosis, inflammatory bowel disease, Behçet's syndrome.

Drug Reactions

The morphologic spectrum of reactions that may be induced by medications is broad, and hundreds of drugs may produce a cutaneous reaction. Types of cutaneous lesions induced by drugs include morbilliform maculopapular eruptions, acnefolliculitis, necrotizing vasculitis, vesiculobullous lesions, erythema multiforme, erythema nodosum, fixed drug eruptions, lichenoid reactions, photosensitivity reactions, and hair loss.

Approximately 2% of hospitalized patients have cutaneous drug reactions, and penicillin, sulfonamides, and blood products are responsible for approximately two-thirds of such reactions. The most common types of clinical presentations (in descending order of frequency) are exanthematous or morbilliform eruptions, urticaria or angioedema, fixed drug eruption, and erythema multiforme. Stevens-Johnson syndrome, exfoliative erythroderma, and photosensitive eruptions are less common. Urticarial drug reactions are most often related to aspirin, penicillin, or blood products. Photoallergic reactions are most often associated with sulfonamides, thiazides, griseofulvin, or phenothiazines. Phototoxic (sunburn-like, nonimmunologic) reactions may be induced by tetracyclines.

Chronic use of chlorpromazine may be associated with slate-gray discoloration of sun-exposed skin, and amiodarone has been associated with slate-blue discoloration of sun-exposed areas, particularly the face. Antimalarial drugs induce yellow pigmentation or blue-gray pigmentation, depending on the compound used.

- 2% of hospitalized patients have cutaneous drug reactions.
- Penicillin, sulfonamides, blood products responsible for about two-thirds of drug reactions.
- Urticarial drug reactions most often related to aspirin, penicillin, blood products.
- Photoallergic reactions most often associated with sulfonamides, thiazides, griseofulvin, phenothiazines.
- Phototoxic reactions may be induced by tetracyclines.

Exanthematous or morbilliform eruptions are the most common type of cutaneous drug reaction. This type of eruption usually begins within a week of onset of therapy, but it may occur >2 weeks after initiation of the drug or up to 2 weeks after use of the drug has been discontinued. Ampicillin, penicillin, and cephalosporins are commonly associated with morbilliform eruptions. A fixed drug eruption is one or several lesions that recur at the same anatomic location on rechallenge with the medication. The genital and facial areas are common sites of involvement. Phenolphthalein, barbiturates, salicylates, and oral contraceptives have been implicated in the cause of fixed drug eruptions.

- Exanthematous or morbilliform eruptions are most common cutaneous drug reaction.
- Fixed drug eruption is one or several lesions that recur at same location on rechallenge.
- Phenolphthalein, barbiturates, salicylates, oral contraceptives implicated in fixed drug eruptions.

Lichenoid drug eruptions are morphologically similar to lichen planus (with violaceous papules of the skin) and have most often been associated with gold and antimalarial drugs, although various medications may induce this type of reaction.

CUTANEOUS SIGNS OF UNDERLYING MALIGNANCY

Cutaneous metastasis occurs in 1%-5% of patients with metastatic neoplasms. The types of malignancy metastatic to the skin reflect the most common types of visceral carcinoma, in particular, lung, breast, kidney, gastrointestinal, melanoma, and ovary. Lesions usually present on the scalp, face, or trunk.

- Cutaneous metastasis occurs in 1%-5% of patients with metastatic neoplasms.
- Lesions usually present on scalp, face, trunk.

Paget's disease of the nipple is an erythematous, scaly, or weepy eczematous eruption of the areola. Virtually all patients with Paget's disease have an underlying ductal carcinoma of the breast. In contrast, *extramammary Paget's disease*, a morphologically similar eruption that usually occurs in the anogenital region, is associated with underlying carcinoma in only about 50% of cases. Extramammary Paget's disease may be associated with underlying cutaneous adnexal carcinoma or with underlying visceral carcinoma (particularly of the genitourinary or distal gastrointestinal tracts).

- Patients with Paget's disease have underlying ductal carcinoma of breast.
- Extramammary Paget's disease is associated with underlying carcinoma in only 50% of cases.

Acanthosis nigricans (color plate 6-5) consists of velvety hyperpigmentation of the intertriginous regions, particularly the axillae and groin. It has been associated with adenocarcinoma of the gastrointestinal tract, particularly the stomach, and insulin-resistant diabetes. Acanthosis nigricans may also be associated with obesity or certain medications (such as prednisone and nicotinic acid) or have an autosomal-dominant variant.

- Acanthosis nigricans associated with adenocarcinoma of gastrointestinal tract, particularly stomach, and insulin-resistant diabetes.
- May also be associated with obesity and certain medications.

Pyoderma gangrenosum (color plate 6-6) consists of ulcers with irregular, undermined, inflammatory, violaceous borders that heal with cribriform scarring. The lesions are most commonly associated with inflammatory bowel disease or rheumatoid arthritis. The bullous form of pyoderma gangrenosum is associated with malignancy of the hematopoietic system, particularly leukemia.

- Pyoderma gangrenosum most commonly associated with inflammatory bowel disease or rheumatoid arthritis.
- Bullous form is associated with leukemia.

The skin lesions of *glucagonoma syndrome (necrolytic migratory erythema)* (color plate 6-7) consist of erosions, crusting, and peeling, particularly involving the perineum and perioral areas, but may be generalized. The syndrome also includes stomatitis, glossitis (beefy tongue), anemia, diarrhea, and weight loss. It is associated with an islet cell (α) tumor of the pancreas.

- Glucagonoma syndrome consists of erosions, crusting, and peeling involving perineum and perioral areas.
- Associated with islet cell tumor of pancreas.

Leser-Trélat syndrome consists of sudden onset of numerous seborrheic keratoses, and it may be associated with underlying malignancy.

Torre's (Muir-Torre) syndrome consists of multiple sebaceous tumors of the skin associated with visceral carcinomas. These tumors are sebaceous adenomas, sebaceous epitheliomas, or sebaceous carcinomas. Patients may have one or numerous lesions. In addition, keratoacanthomas of the skin are also part of this syndrome. Of the underlying malignancies, carcinoma of the colon is the most common, although breast, hematologic, and other malignancies have been observed. There is a genetic predisposition and, in some cases, an association with the "cancer family syndrome."

- Torre's syndrome consists of multiple sebaceous tumors of skin associated with visceral carcinomas.
- Carcinoma of colon is most common underlying malignancy.

Cowden's syndrome has autosomal dominant inheritance. Cutaneous abnormalities include trichilemmomas, verrucous papules, and oral fibromas. The syndrome is associated with thyroid and breast carcinoma. There is an increased incidence of fibrocystic disease of breast and thyroid adenoma.

- Cowden's syndrome has autosomal dominant inheritance.
- Cutaneous abnormalities: trichilemmomas, verrucous papules, oral fibromas.

Gardner's syndrome is a hereditary (autosomal dominant) form of colonic polyposis. Clinical features include adenomatous polyps of the colon, osteomas of the skull and face, scoliosis, soft tissue tumors (including dermoids, lipomas, and fibromas), and sebaceous (epidermal inclusion) cysts of the face and scalp. There is a high incidence of colonic carcinoma. In approximately 60% of patients, adenocarcinoma of the colon develops by age 40 years, and malignancies of other sites have been associated with this syndrome, including adrenal, ovarian, and thyroid.

- Gardner's syndrome is a hereditary (autosomal dominant) form of colonic polyposis.
- Clinical features: soft tissue tumors, sebaceous cysts of face.
- There is a high incidence of colonic carcinoma.

Acquired ichthyosis has most often been associated with Hodgkin's disease, but it has been reported with other types of lymphoma, multiple myeloma, and various carcinomas.

- Acquired ichthyosis associated with Hodgkin's disease.

Paraneoplastic acrokeratosis of Bazex consists of psoriasiform lesions of the hands, feet, ears, and nose, onychodystrophy, and carcinoma of the upper respiratory system, pharynx, or esophagus.

- Paraneoplastic acrokeratosis of Bazex consists of psoriasiform lesions and carcinoma of the upper respiratory system.

Hirsutism may reflect androgen excess due to an adrenal or ovarian tumor.

Hypertrichosis represents increase in hair unrelated to androgen excess, such as hypertrichosis lanuginosa acquisita (growth of soft downy hairs). It has been associated with carcinoid tumor, adenocarcinoma of the breast, lymphoma, gastrointestinal malignancy, and other types of neoplasms.

Erythema gyratum repens presents with a striking pattern of concentric erythematous bands in a "wood grain" pattern almost universally associated with underlying malignancy. The classic association is with breast carcinoma, but other types of malignancy have been reported.

- Erythema gyratum repens classically associated with breast carcinoma.

Sweet's syndrome (acute febrile neutrophilic dermatosis) has skin lesions that consist of erythematous plaques and nodules, most commonly located on the extremities and face. The association is with leukemia, particularly acute myelocytic or acute myelomonocytic leukemia.

- Sweet's syndrome is associated with leukemia.

Generalized pruritus is the presentation for many cutaneous and systemic disorders. Pruritus may be the presenting symptom in lymphoma.

- Pruritus may be presenting symptom in lymphoma.

In *dermatomyositis*, the pathognomonic skin lesions are Gottron's papules (color plate 6-8) involving the skin over the joints of the fingers, elbows, and knees. Poikilodermatous lesions or erythematous macular-papular eruptions may diffusely involve the face, particularly the periorbital area ("heliotrope rash" [color plate 6-9]), and the trunk and extremities. The cutaneous lesions are photosensitive. The disease is characterized by proximal myositis. Although creatine phosphokinase levels are usually elevated in patients with myositis, it is important to verify the diagnosis by obtaining a muscle biopsy specimen. Dermatomyositis is associated with an increased incidence of underlying malignancy.

- Dermatomyositis may involve periorbital area ("heliotrope rash") or dorsal aspect of hands (Gottron's papules).
- Lesions are photosensitive.
- Characterized by proximal myositis.

Multiple mucosal neuromas syndrome is associated with autosomal dominant inheritance. The main features include neuromas of the skin or mucosa (anterior tongue, lips, eyelids, conjunctiva), medullary carcinoma of the thyroid, pheochromocytoma, and parathyroid adenoma.

- Multiple mucosal neuromas syndrome: medullary carcinoma of thyroid, pheochromocytoma, parathyroid adenoma.

Cutaneous *amyloidosis* may present clinically as macroglossia (color plate 6-10), waxy papules on the eyelids or nasolabial folds, pinch-purpura, and postproctoscopic purpura (color plate 6-11). Multiple myeloma may be associated with amyloid.

- Amyloidosis may be associated with multiple myeloma.

Tylosis is a rare disorder characterized by palmar-plantar keratoderma associated with esophageal carcinoma. It has autosomal dominant inheritance.

- Tylosis is associated with esophageal carcinoma.

The *autoimmune bullous diseases* are a heterogeneous group of disorders characterized by antibody deposition at the basement membrane zone or epidermis. An association with malignancy has been demonstrated in several of these disorders.

- Pemphigus is associated with thymoma with or without myasthenia gravis.
- Paraneoplastic pemphigus presents with clinical and histologic features of pemphigus and erythema multiforme and is associated with lymphomas and leukemia.
- Patients with dermatitis herpetiformis rarely develop intestinal lymphoma.
- Epidermolysis bullosa acquisita is associated with amyloidosis and multiple myeloma.
- Bullous pemphigoid has not been associated with an increased risk of underlying malignancy.

DERMATOLOGY: AN INTERNIST'S PERSPECTIVE

Respiratory

The skin is involved in 15%-35% of patients with *sarcoidosis*. Lesions may present as 1) lupus pernio (erythematous swelling of the nose), 2) translucent papules around the eyes and nasolabial folds, 3) annular lesions with central atrophy, 4) nodules on the trunk and extremities, and 5) scar sarcoid. Acute sarcoidosis may present with a combination of erythema nodosum, bilateral hilar lymphadenopathy, fever, and arthralgias (Löfgren's syndrome).

- Skin involved in 15%-35% of patients with sarcoidosis.

- Lesions may present as lupus pernio (erythematous swelling of nose).

Erythema nodosum (color plate 6-12) is a reactive condition that may be associated with acute sarcoidosis. Erythema nodosum typically presents as tender, erythematous, subcutaneous nodules localized to pretibial areas. The lesions may be acute and self-limited or chronic, lasting for months up to years.

- Erythema nodosum may be associated with acute sarcoidosis.

In *Wegener's granulomatosis*, cutaneous involvement occurs in >50% of patients and is manifested by cutaneous infarction, ulceration, hemorrhagic bullae, purpuric papules, or urticaria. A skin biopsy may show hypersensitivity vasculitis or granulomatous vasculitis.

- In Wegener's granulomatosis, cutaneous involvement occurs in >50% of patients.
- Manifestations: ulceration, hemorrhagic bullae, purpuric papules, urticaria.

Churg-Strauss granulomatosis/allergic granulomatosis syndrome is characterized by combination of adult-onset asthma, peripheral eosinophilia, and pulmonary involvement with recurrent pneumonia or transient infiltrates. Skin lesions have been reported in up to 60% of patients and consist of palpable purpura, cutaneous infarcts, and subcutaneous nodules.

- Skin lesions of Churg-Strauss granulomatosis occur in up to 60% of patients.
- Skin lesions include palpable purpura, cutaneous infarct, subcutaneous nodules.

In *relapsing polychondritis*, there is episodic destructive inflammation of cartilage of the ears, nose, and upper airways. There may be associated arthritis and ocular involvement. In the acute stage, the ears may be red, swollen, and tender. Later, they become soft and flabby. Nasal chondritis may lead to saddle-nose deformities. Relapsing polychondritis is mediated by antibodies to type II collagen.

- Relapsing polychondritis: episodic destructive inflammation of cartilage of ears, nose, upper airways.
- Nasal chondritis may lead to saddle-nose deformities.

Cardiovascular

In several syndromes, lentigines have been associated with cardiac abnormalities. These include the *LEOPARD*, *NAME*, and *LAMB* syndromes.

- LEOPARD syndrome (Moynahan's syndrome): *l*entigines, *e*lectrocardiographic changes, *o*cular hypertelorism, *p*ulmonary stenosis, *a*bnormal genitalia, *r*etardation of growth, *d*eafness.
- NAME syndrome: *n*evi, *a*trial myxoma, *m*yxoid neurofibromas, *e*philides.
- LAMB syndrome: *l*entigines, *a*trial myxoma, *m*ucocutaneous myxomas, *b*lue nevi.

Pseudoxanthoma elasticum may be transmitted by autosomal dominant or autosomal recessive inheritance. Yellow xanthoma-like papules are seen on the neck (plucked-chicken skin), axillae, groin, and abdomen. Angioid streaks may be seen in the fundus. Skin biopsy shows degeneration of elastic fibers. Systemic associations include stroke, myocardial infarction, peripheral vascular disease, and gastrointestinal hemorrhage.

- Pseudoxanthoma elasticum associated with stroke, myocardial infarction, peripheral vascular disease, and gastrointestinal hemorrhage.

Ehlers-Danlos syndrome includes 10 subgroups that vary in severity and systemic associations. Cutaneous findings are skin hyperextensibility with hypermobile joints and fish-mouth scars. Angina, peripheral vascular disease, and gastrointestinal bleeding may be associated.

- Ehlers-Danlos syndrome associated with angina, peripheral vascular disease, gastrointestinal bleeding.

Erythema marginatum is one of the diagnostic criteria for acute rheumatic fever. This uncommon eruption occurs on the trunk and is characterized by erythematous plaques with rapidly mobile serpiginous borders.

- Erythema marginatum is one of diagnostic criteria for acute rheumatic fever.

Gastrointestinal

Osler-Weber-Rendu syndrome (hereditary hemorrhagic telangiectasia), with autosomal dominant inheritance, is manifested by cutaneous and mucosal telangiectasias. Frequent nosebleeds and gastrointestinal bleeds may be a presenting feature. Pulmonary arteriovenous malformations and central nervous system angiomas are also features of this syndrome.

- Osler-Weber-Rendu syndrome has autosomal dominant inheritance.
- Features: nosebleeds, gastrointestinal bleeds, pulmonary arteriovenous malformations, central nervous system angiomas.

Acrodermatitis enteropathica is an inherited (autosomal recessive) or acquired disease characterized by zinc deficiency (failure of absorption or failure to supplement). The clinical features include angular cheilitis, a seborrheic dermatitis-like eruption, erosions, blisters, and pustules, with skin lesions particularly involving the face, hands, feet, and perineum. Alopecia and diarrhea are other features of this syndrome.

- Acrodermatitis enteropathica: inherited (autosomal recessive) or acquired disease.
- Characterized by zinc deficiency (failure of absorption or failure to supplement).
- Alopecia and diarrhea are other features.

Peutz-Jeghers syndrome is an inherited (autosomal dominant) syndrome of intestinal polyposis. Patients have hamartomas, mostly involving the small bowel, without an increased risk of developing carcinoma. Cutaneous lesions include macular pigmentation (freckles) of the lips, periungual skin, fingers, and toes and pigmentation of the oral mucosa.

- Peutz-Jeghers syndrome is inherited (autosomal dominant) syndrome of intestinal polyposis.
- No increase in risk of developing carcinoma.

Dermatitis herpetiformis (color plate 6-2) is an immune-mediated bullous disease that presents with intensely itchy vesicles on extensor surfaces (elbows, knees, buttocks, scapula). Gluten-sensitive enteropathy occurs in up to 70% of patients.

- Dermatitis herpetiformis is immune-mediated bullous disease.
- Gluten-sensitive enteropathy occurs in up to 70% of patients.

Extensive *aphthous ulceration* may be associated with Crohn's disease or gluten-sensitive enteropathy.

- Aphthous ulceration may be associated with Crohn's disease or gluten-sensitive enteropathy.

Pyoderma gangrenosum (color plate 6-6) presents with ulceration, predominantly on the lower extremities, with inflammatory undermined borders. The lesions heal with cribriform scarring. The phenomenon whereby lesions occur at sites of trauma is known as pathergy--the occurrence of the disease at sites of trauma is classic. Systemic disease associations include inflammatory bowel disease (ulcerative colitis more commonly than Crohn's disease), rheumatoid arthritis, and paraproteinemia.

- Pyoderma gangrenosum occurs at sites of trauma.
- Associated diseases are inflammatory bowel disease (ulcerative colitis more than Crohn's disease), rheumatoid arthritis, paraproteinemia.

Cutaneous Crohn's disease may present as skin nodules with granulomatous histology. Other manifestations include pyostomatitis vegetans (granulomatous inflammation of the gingivae), granulomatous cheilitis, oral aphthous ulceration, perianal skin tags, and perianal fistulae.

- Manifestation of Crohn's disease: pyostomatitis vegetans (granulomatous inflammation of gingivae).

Bowel bypass syndrome presents with a flu-like illness with fever, malaise, arthralgias, myalgias, and inflammatory papules and pustules on the extremities and upper trunk. The disease is recurrent and episodic and occurs in up to 20% of patients after jejunoileal bypass. The condition responds to antibiotics or to reversal of the bypass procedure.

- Bowel bypass syndrome: flu-like illness, inflammatory papules and pustules.
- Occurs in up to 20% of patients after jejunoileal bypass.

Gardner's syndrome and *glucagonoma syndrome* are described on page 153.

Nephrology
Partial lipodystrophy is associated with C3 deficiency and the nephrotic syndrome.

Neurocutaneous
Fabry's disease is an X-linked recessive disorder due to deficiency of the enzyme α-galactosidase A. The skin changes consist of numerous vascular tumors (angiokeratomas) that develop during childhood and adolescence. Corneal opacities are present in 90% of patients. Systemic manifestations include paresthesias and pain due to involved peripheral nerves, renal insufficiency, and vascular insufficiency of the coronary and central nervous system.

- Fabry's disease is recessive disorder due to deficiency of α-galactosidase A.
- Systemic manifestations: paresthesias, renal insufficiency, vascular insufficiency.

The clinical features of *ataxia-telangiectasia* include cutaneous and ocular telangiectasia, cerebellar ataxia, choreoathetosis, IgA deficiency, and recurrent pulmonary infections.

Tuberous sclerosis may be inherited in an autosomal dominant pattern (25%) or may occur sporadically (new mutation). Predominant cutaneous lesions include hypopigmented macules, adenoma sebaceum, subungual or periungual fibromas, and shagreen patch (connective tissue nevus) (color plate 6-13). This syndrome is associated with epilepsy (80%) and mental retardation (60%). Rhabdomyomas may occur in the heart in childhood. Angiomyolipomas occur in the kidneys in up to 80% of adults with this syndrome.

- Tuberous sclerosis may be inherited in autosomal dominant pattern or be sporadic.
- Associated with epilepsy (80%) and mental retardation (60%).
- Angiomyolipomas occur in kidneys in up to 80% of affected adults.

Neurofibromatosis (von Recklinghausen's disease) (color plate 6-14) occurs in 1 in 3,000 births. Inheritance is autosomal dominant, and approximately 50% of cases are new mutations. The major signs of the disease are café-au-lait spots, axillary freckling (Crowe's sign), neurofibromas, and Lisch nodules of the iris.

- Neurofibromatosis is autosomal dominant.
- Major signs: café-au-lait spots, axillary freckling, neurofibromas.

Neurofibromatosis has various clinical manifestations, as reflected in Ricardi's classification:

1. Classic: Neurofibromas, café-au-lait spots, Lisch nodules of iris, chromosome 17, positive family history.
2. Central: Bilateral acoustic neuromas, few neurofibromas, few café-au-lait spots, *no Lisch nodules*, chromosome 22, positive family history.
3. Mixed: Features of no. 1 and no. 2, central nervous system tumors, positive family history.
4. Variant: Variable family history, diffuse café-au-lait spots, neurofibromas, with or without central nervous system tumors.
5. Segmental or dermatomal: Neurofibromas or café-au-lait spots, skin involvement only, negative family history.
6. Multiple café-au-lait spots: Skin involvement only, negative family history, no neurofibromas.
7. Late onset: Cutaneous disease for >30 years.
8. Other: Clinical syndromes not fitting the above classifications.

The associated central nervous system tumors include acoustic neuromas, optic gliomas, and meningiomas. Other associated tumors include pheochromocytoma, neuroblastoma, and Wilms' tumor. Café-au-lait spots and neurofibromas frequently occur in the absence of neurofibromatosis. The diagnostic criteria for neurofibromatosis include two or more of the following:

1. Six or more café-au-lait macules > 0.5 cm in greatest diameter in prepubertal patients, or >1.5 cm in diameter in adults.
2. Two or more neurofibromas of any type, or one plexiform neurofibroma.
3. Freckling of skin in axillary or inguinal regions.
4. Optic gliomas.

5. Lisch nodules.
6. An osseous lesion such as sphenoid dysplasia or thinning of long bone cortex with or without pseudarthrosis.
7. A first-degree relative with neurofibromatosis that meets the above diagnostic criteria.

Sturge-Weber-Dimitri syndrome is characterized by capillary angioma (port-wine stain) in the distribution of the upper or middle branch of the trigeminal nerve. There may be associated meningeal angioma in the same distribution. Intracranial tramline calcification, mental retardation, epilepsy, contralateral hemiparesis, and visual impairment may be associated.

- Sturge-Weber-Dimitri syndrome characterized by capillary angioma in distribution of upper or middle branch of trigeminal nerve.
- Associated features: intracranial calcification, mental retardation, epilepsy, contralateral hemiparesis, visual impairment.

Klippel-Trenaunay-Weber syndrome is the constellation of hemangiomas in a dermatomal distribution with associated arteriovenous malformation.

Cobb's syndrome is a noninherited disorder in which port-wine stain or angiokeratoma occurs in a dermatomal distribution associated with spinal cord angioma within one or two segments of the cutaneous lesions.

Sneddon's syndrome involves extensive livedo reticularis and cerebrovascular accidents, possibly as manifestation of the antiphospholipid syndrome.

Cerebral granulomatous angiitis is a sequela of ophthalmic herpes zoster and is responsible for the combination of ophthalmic zoster followed by a delayed contralateral hemiplegia (weeks to months; average, 8 weeks).

Rheumatology: Cutaneous Associations of Arthritis

Psoriatic arthritis occurs in 4%-5% of patients with psoriasis. It is characterized by involvement of the distal interphalangeal joints, but also with involvement of the proximal interphalangeal joints. Most patients have asymmetric involvement of few joints of the fingers or toes. A small percentage of patients have symmetric polyarthritis resembling rheumatoid arthritis. The most severe form of psoriatic arthritis, arthritis mutilans, is associated with osteolysis resulting in "telescoping" of digits and dissolution of distal phalanges. Approximately 5% of patients with psoriatic arthritis have ankylosing spondylitis.

- Psoriatic arthritis occurs in 4%-5% of patients with psoriasis.
- Characterized by involvement of distal interphalangeal joints.
- 5% of patients have ankylosing spondylitis.

Reiter's syndrome consists of the triad of urethritis, conjunctivitis, and arthritis. The disease usually affects young men. Two-thirds of patients have skin lesions, namely, circinate balinitis, consisting of erythematous plaques of the penis, and keratoderma blennorrhagicum, a pustular psoriasiform eruption of the palms and soles. Most patients are HLA-B27 positive.

- Reiter's syndrome triad: urethritis, conjunctivitis, arthritis.
- Most patients are HLA-B27 positive.

Multicentric reticulohistiocytosis may affect the skin, mucosa, joints, bones, and viscera. Most patients have skin lesions and arthritis. Skin lesions consist of red-brown papules and nodules, most commonly located on the dorsal aspects of hands and face. Approximately half of all patients have mucosal lesions, particularly of the lips, buccal mucosa, tongue, gingiva, or nose. The arthritis consists of severely destructive and mutilating involvement, particularly of the interphalangeal joints of the hands ("opera glass hand" or "telescope fingers"), knees, wrists, hips, ankles, feet, elbows, and spine. Multicentric reticulohistiocytosis has also been associated with underlying malignancy.

- Multicentric reticulohistiocytosis involves skin lesions and arthritis.
- May be associated with underlying malignancy.

Erythema chronicum migrans is an annular, sometimes urticarial, erythematous lesion presenting as a manifestation of Lyme disease. The lesion develops subsequent to, and surrounding the site of, a tick bite. Lesions are single in 75% of patients and multiple in 25%. Other acute features of Lyme disease include fever, headaches, myalgias, arthralgias, and lymphadenopathy. The tick, *Ixodes dammini*, contains a spirochete, *Borrelia burgdorferi*, that is responsible for the syndrome. Arthritis is a late complication of Lyme disease. Weeks or months after the initial illness, patients may develop meningoencephalitis, peripheral neuropathy, myocarditis, atrioventricular node block, or destructive erosive arthritis.

- Erythema chronicum migrans presents as manifestation of Lyme disease.
- Lesion develops subsequent to and surrounding site of tick bite.
- Lesions are single in 75% of patients and multiple in 25%.

In *rheumatoid arthritis,* nodules occur over the extensor surfaces of joints, most commonly on the dorsal hands and elbows. Rheumatoid vasculitis with ulceration may occur in the setting of rheumatoid arthritis with a high circulating rheumatoid factor.

During the late stages of *gout*, tophi (urate deposits with surrounding inflammation) occur in the subcutaneous tissues.

Improved methods of treatment account for the decrease in the incidence of tophaceous gout in recent years.

- With gout, tophi occur in subcutaneous tissues.

In *lupus erythematosus* (LE), cutaneous abnormalities occur in approximately 80% of patients. LE has been classified into chronic cutaneous LE (localized discoid LE and generalized discoid LE), subacute cutaneous LE, and acute cutaneous LE (malar rash, generalized macular-papular erythema, or bullous LE).

- In LE, cutaneous abnormalities occur in 80% of patients.

Discoid LE (color plate 6-15) is characterized by erythematous papules and plaques with follicular hyperkeratosis and scaling. Localized discoid LE is usually not associated with systemic LE. Generalized discoid LE or disseminated discoid LE refers to lesions involving the head and neck area or the trunk and extremities. Discoid LE most commonly affects the face, scalp, and ears. Although most patients with discoid LE lack manifestations of systemic LE, approximately 25% of patients with systemic LE have had cutaneous lesions of discoid LE at some point during the course of their illness.

- Discoid LE characterized by erythematous papules and plaques with follicular hyperkeratosis and scaling.
- Discoid LE most commonly affects face, scalp, ears.
- 25% of patients with systemic LE have had cutaneous manifestations of discoid LE.

Subacute cutaneous LE (color plate 6-16) usually presents with generalized annular or polycyclic papules and plaques. The lesions may appear papulosquamous or vesiculobullous. Subacute cutaneous LE is characterized by the presence of anti-Ro (anti-SSA) antibodies in serum and photosensitivity.

- Subacute cutaneous LE presents with annular or polycyclic papules and plaques.
- Characterized by presence of anti-Ro (anti-SSA) antibodies and photosensitivity.

The "lupus band test" consists of the finding of immunoglobulin and complement at the basement membrane zone of skin biopsy tissue as determined by direct immunofluorescence testing. In biopsy of lesional tissue from discoid LE or systemic LE, immunoglobulin and complement are demonstrable at the basement membrane zone in >90% of patients. Only 50%-60% of patients with subacute cutaneous LE have a positive lupus band test of lesional skin. The lupus band test is positive in nonlesional skin (normal-appearing, non-sun-exposed skin, typically buttock) from 50% of patients with systemic LE and in nonlesional sun-exposed skin of the forearm from 75% of patients with systemic LE, and it is generally negative in nonlesional skin of patients with discoid LE. Therefore, direct immunofluorescence testing of nonlesional, non-sun-exposed skin is specific, but not highly sensitive, for LE.

- Only 50%-60% of patients with subacute cutaneous LE have positive lupus band test of lesional skin.
- Direct immunofluorescence testing of nonlesional, non-sun-exposed skin is specific, but not sensitive, for LE.

Circulating antinuclear antibodies are demonstrable in most patients with systemic LE and subacute cutaneous erythematosus, but they are present in only a small percentage of patients with discoid LE. A homogeneous antinuclear antibody pattern tends to correlate with the diagnosis of systemic LE, peripheral (rim) pattern correlates with lupus nephritis, speckled anticentromere pattern is associated with the CREST variant of scleroderma (CREST: *c*alcinosis cutis, *R*aynaud's phenomenon, *e*sophageal dysmotility, *s*clerodactyly, and *t*elangiectasia), nucleolar pattern usually correlates with the diagnosis of scleroderma and uncommonly with lupus, and the particulate pattern is associated with various connective tissue diseases, including LE. In addition to association with subacute cutaneous LE, anti-Ro (anti-SSA) antibodies are associated with Sjögren's syndrome, LE with C2 deficiency, and neonatal LE.

Scleroderma encompasses a spectrum of diseases, including progressive systemic sclerosis, localized scleroderma/localized morphea, generalized morphea, linear scleroderma (including en coup de sabre), facial hemiatrophy, CREST syndrome, and eosinophilic fasciitis.

Morphea manifests as discrete sclerotic plaques with white shiny center and erythematous or violaceous periphery. Localized or linear scleroderma may have various presentations depending on extent, location, and depth of sclerosis. Most lesions are characterized by sclerosis and atrophy associated with depression or "delling" of the soft tissue; underlying bone may be affected in linear scleroderma.

- Morphea manifests as discrete sclerotic plaques with white shiny center.
- Underlying bone may be affected in linear scleroderma.

Systemic scleroderma consists of diffuse sclerosis associated with smoothness and hardening of the skin, with mask-like face and microstomia. Sclerodactyly, periungual telangiectasia, hyperpigmentation, and cutaneous calcification may be observed. Esophageal, pulmonary, renal, and cardiac involvement may be associated with systemic scleroderma. The CREST syndrome (color plate 6-17) is associated with circulating anticentromere antibodies.

- Systemic scleroderma may include sclerodactyly, periungual telangiectasia, hyperpigmentation, and cutaneous calcification.

Eosinophilic fasciitis manifests as tightly bound thickening of the skin and underlying soft tissue of the extremities. Other features include arthralgias, hypergammaglobulinemia, and peripheral blood eosinophilia.

- Eosinophilic fasciitis manifests as tightly bound thickening of skin and underlying soft tissue of extremities.

Hematologic

Graft-versus-host disease (GVHD) most commonly occurs after bone marrow transplantation and represents the constellation of skin lesions, diarrhea, and liver function abnormalities. GVHD occurs in 60%-80% of patients who undergo allogeneic bone marrow transplantation.

- GVHD commonly occurs after bone marrow transplantation.
- Includes skin lesions, diarrhea, liver function abnormalities.

GVHD generally occurs in two phases. Acute GVHD begins 7-21 days after transplantation, and chronic GVHD begins within months to 1 year after transplantation. One or both phases may occur in the same patient. Acute GVHD results from attack of donor immunocompetent T lymphocytes and null lymphocytes against host histocompatibility antigens. Chronic GVHD results from immunocompetent lymphocytes that develop in the recipient.

The cutaneous abnormalities of acute GVHD include pruritus, numbness or pain of the palms and soles, an erythematous macular-papular eruption of the trunk, palms, and soles, and blisters that, when extensive, resemble toxic epidermal necrolysis. Acute GVHD also includes intestinal abnormalities resulting in diarrhea and liver function changes.

- Cutaneous abnormalities of GVHD: pruritus, numbness or pain of palms and soles, erythematous macular-papular eruption of trunk, palms, and soles.

Chronic GVHD mainly affects skin and liver. Early chronic GVHD is characterized by a lichenoid reaction consisting of cutaneous and oral lesions that resemble lichen planus, with coalescing violaceous papules, but also pigmentary changes. Late chronic GVHD is characterized by cutaneous sclerosis, poikilodermatous-reticulated lesions, and scarring alopecia. The histologic pattern of GVHD includes lymphocytes in proximity to dyskeratotic keratinocytes, so-called satellite cell necrosis. The cutaneous infiltrate is composed predominantly of suppressor/cytotoxic T cells.

- Chronic GVHD: lichenoid reaction consisting of cutaneous and oral lesions.

Mastocytosis (mast cell disease) can be divided into four groups, depending on the age at onset and the presence or absence of systemic involvement: 1) urticaria pigmentosa arising in infancy or adolescence without significant systemic involvement, 2) urticaria pigmentosa in adults without significant systemic involvement, 3) systemic mast cell disease, and 4) mast cell leukemia.

The cutaneous lesions may be brown to red macules, papules, nodules, or plaques that urticate on stroking. Less commonly, the lesions may be bullous, erythrodermic, or telangiectatic. The systemic manifestations are due to histamine release and consist of flushing, tachycardia, and diarrhea.

- Cutaneous lesions of mastocytosis: brown to red macules, papules, nodules, or plaques that urticate on stroking.
- Systemic manifestations--flushing, tachycardia, diarrhea--due to histamine release.

Necrobiotic xanthogranuloma--indurated plaques with associated atrophy and telangiectasia with or without ulceration--may occur on the trunk or periorbital areas. Serum electrophoresis shows an IgG κ paraproteinemia or multiple myeloma.

Endocrine

Diabetes Mellitus

Several dermatologic disorders have been described in diabetes.

Necrobiosis lipoidica diabeticorum (color plate 6-18) classically occurs on the shins and presents as yellow-brown atrophic telangiectatic plaques that occasionally ulcerate. Two-thirds of patients have diabetes.

- Necrobiosis lipoidica diabeticorum occurs on shins.
- Two-thirds of patients have diabetes.

Granuloma annulare is an asymptomatic eruption consisting of small, firm, flesh-colored or red papules in an annular configuration (color plate 6-19) (less commonly nodular or generalized). The association with diabetes is disputed.

- Granuloma annulare consists of small, firm, flesh-colored or red papules in annular configuration.

Rarely, patients with poorly controlled diabetes present with spontaneously occurring *subepidermal blisters* (bullosa diabeticorum) on the dorsal aspects of the hands and feet.

The *stiff hand syndrome* has been reported in juvenile-onset insulin-dependent diabetes. Patients have limited joint mobility and tight waxy skin on the hands. There is an increased risk of subsequent renal and retinal microvascular disease.

- Stiff hand syndrome: increased risk of subsequent renal and retinal microvascular disease.

In *scleredema,* there is an insidious onset of thickening and stiffness of the skin on the upper back and posterior neck. The condition is more common in middle-aged men with diabetes. The diabetes is often long-standing and poorly controlled.

- Scleredema is more common in middle-aged men with diabetes.
- Diabetes is often long-standing and poorly controlled.

Thyroid

Pretibial myxedema and thyroid acropachy are cutaneous associations of Graves' disease.

Metabolic

The *porphyrias* are a group of inherited or acquired abnormalities of heme synthesis. Each type is associated with deficient activity of a particular enzyme. The porphyrias are usually divided into three types: erythropoietic, hepatic, and mixed.

Erythropoietic porphyria (Günther's disease) is a hereditary form (autosomal recessive) characterized by marked photosensitivity, blisters, scarring alopecia, hirsutism, red-stained teeth, hemolytic anemia, and splenomegaly. The skin lesions are severely mutilating. Onset is in infancy or early childhood.

- Erythropoietic porphyria is autosomal recessive.
- Skin lesions are severely mutilating.

Erythropoietic protoporphyria is an autosomal dominant syndrome that usually begins during childhood. It is characterized by variable degrees of photosensitivity and a marked itching, burning, or stinging sensation that occurs within minutes after sun exposure. It is associated with deficiency of ferrochelatase.

- Erythropoietic protoporphyria is autosomal dominant.
- It is associated with deficiency of ferrochelatase.

Porphyria cutanea tarda, one of the hepatic porphyrias, is an acquired or hereditary (autosomal dominant) disease associated with a defect in uroporphyrinogen decarboxylase. The disease may be precipitated by exposure to toxins (such as chlorinated phenols or hexachlorobenzene), alcohol, estrogens, iron overload, and infection with hepatitis C. Porphyria cutanea tarda usually presents in the third or fourth decade of life. Clinical manifestations include photosensitivity, skin fragility, erosions and blisters (particularly on dorsal surfaces of the hands) (color plate 6-20), hyperpigmentation, milia, hypertrichosis, and facial suffusion. Some patients develop sclerodermoid skin changes. The diagnosis is confirmed by the finding of elevated porphyrin levels in the urine. Treatment includes phlebotomy and low-dose chloroquine.

- Porphyria cutanea tarda is acquired or hereditary (autosomal dominant).
- Associated with defect in uroporphyrinogen decarboxylase.
- May be precipitated by exposure to toxins or infection with hepatitis C.

Pseudoporphyria is a porphyria cutanea tarda-like clinical syndrome induced by drugs, including tetracycline, furosemide, and nalidixic acid, or by hemodialysis. The clinical features resemble those of porphyria cutanea tarda, but there is usually no demonstrable biochemical abnormality of porphyrin metabolism.

- Pseudoporphyria is induced by drugs (tetracycline, furosemide, nalidixic acid) or by hemodialysis.

Acute intermittent porphyria ("Swedish porphyria") lacks skin lesions and is characterized by acute attacks of abdominal pain or neurologic symptoms.

- Acute intermittent porphyria lacks skin lesions.
- Involves acute attacks of abdominal pain or neurologic symptoms.

Variegate porphyria (mixed porphyria) also follows autosomal dominant inheritance. Variegate porphyria is characterized by cutaneous abnormalities that are similar to those of porphyria cutanea tarda and by acute abdominal episodes, as in acute intermittent porphyria. Variegate porphyria tends to be precipitated by drugs, such as barbiturates and sulfonamides.

- Variegate porphyria is autosomal dominant.
- Tends to be precipitated by drugs, such as barbiturates and sulfonamides.

NAIL CLUES TO SYSTEMIC DISEASE

Onycholysis consists of distal and lateral separation of the nail plate from the nail bed. Onycholysis may be due to psoriasis, infection (such as *Candida* or *Pseudomonas*), a reaction to nail cosmetics, or a drug reaction. Drugs that have been noted to induce onycholysis include tetracycline and chlorpromazine. Association with thyroid disease (hyperthyroidism more than hypothyroidism) has also been observed.

- Onycholysis may be due to psoriasis, infection (*Candida* or *Pseudomonas*), nail cosmetics, or drug reaction.

Pitting is a common feature of psoriatic nails. Pits have also been associated with alopecia areata.

Twenty-nail dystrophy is most often associated with lichen planus or alopecia areata.

Terry's nails consist of whitening of the proximal or entire nail as a result of changes in the nail bed. This abnormality is associated with cirrhosis.

- Terry's nail associated with cirrhosis.

Muehrcke's lines consist of white parallel bands associated with hypoalbuminemia.

- Muehrcke's lines associated with hypoalbuminemia.

"Half-and-half" nails (Lindsay's nails) are nails in which the proximal half is white and the distal half is red. This abnormality may be associated with renal failure.

- "Half-and-half" nails may be associated with renal failure.

Yellow nails are associated with chronic edema, pulmonary disease, pleural effusion, chronic bronchitis, bronchiectasis, and lung carcinoma.

Beau's lines are transverse grooves in the nail associated with high fever, systemic disease, and drugs.

Koilonychia (spoon nails) is associated with iron-deficiency anemia, but it may also be idiopathic, familial, or related to trauma.

- Koilonychia associated with iron-deficiency anemia.

Blue-colored lunula is associated with hepatolenticular degeneration (Wilson's disease) and argyria.

Mees' lines are white bands associated with arsenic.

- Mees' lines associated with arsenic.

CUTANEOUS MANIFESTATIONS OF AIDS

Epidemic Kaposi's sarcoma usually presents as oval papules or plaques oriented along skin lines of the trunk, extremities, face, and mucosa. This presentation is in contrast to that of classic Kaposi's sarcoma seen in elderly patients, which occurs predominantly on the distal lower extremities. Although epidemic Kaposi's sarcoma is most commonly associated with human immunodeficiency virus (HIV) infection, the finding of a small percentage of homosexual men with Kaposi's sarcoma who are HIV negative has suggested that Kaposi's sarcoma may be related to another sexually transmitted infectious disease.

- Epidemic Kaposi's sarcoma: oval papules or plaques along skin lines of trunk, extremities, face, mucosa.
- Most commonly associated with HIV infection.

Severe herpes simplex virus infection, manifested as chronic progressive erosions or ulcers, has been associated with HIV infection.

Herpes zoster infection is considered a sign of underlying HIV infection and occurs 7 times more often in homosexual men with HIV than in HIV-negative controls.

Oral hairy leukoplakia is caused by Epstein-Barr virus infection of the oral mucosa and usually occurs in patients with advanced HIV infection.

Molluscum contagiosum, a common viral infection of otherwise healthy children, has been observed in 10%-20% of patients with HIV infection.

- Molluscum contagiosum observed in 10%-20% of patients with HIV infection.

Bacillary angiomatosis consists of one or more vascular papules or nodules caused by a *Rickettsia*-like organism related to *Rochalimaea quintana*.

Syphilis, which is severe and often resistant to therapy, is commonly associated with HIV disease.

There is a marked increase in the incidence of *Reiter's syndrome* in HIV infection.

Eosinophilic pustular folliculitis is associated with HIV disease.

Color plate 6-1. Bullous pemphigoid.

Color plate 6-2. Dermatitis herpetiformis.

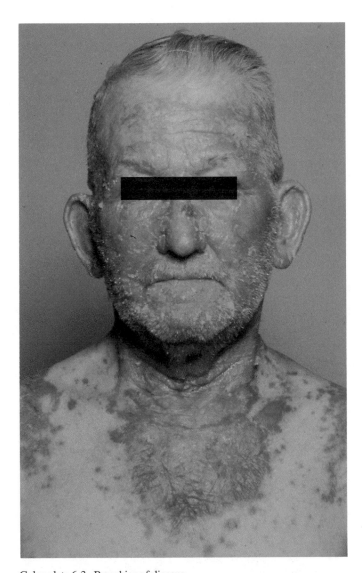

Color plate 6-3. Pemphigus foliaceus.

Color plate 6-4. Erythema multiforme.

Color plate 6-5. Acanthosis nigricans.

Color plate 6-6. Pyoderma gangrenosum.

Color plate 6-7. Glucagonoma syndrome (necrolytic migratory erythema).

Color plate 6-8. Dermatomyositis: Gottron's papules.

Color plate 6-9. Dermatomyositis: heliotrope discoloration.

Color plate 6-10. Amyloidosis: macroglossia.

Color plate 6-11. Amyloidosis: postproctoscopic purpura.

Color plate 6-12. Erythema nodosum.

Color plate 6-13. Tuberous sclerosis: adenoma sebaceum and forehead plaque.

Color plate 6-14. Neurofibromatosis: plexiform neurofibroma.

Color plate 6-15. Discoid lupus erythematosus.

Color plate 6-16. Subacute cutaneous lupus erythematosus.

Color plate 6-17. Scleroderma: CREST syndrome.

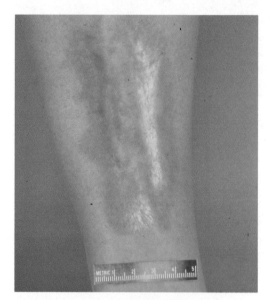

Color plate 6-18. Necrobiosis lipoidica diabeticorum.

Color plate 6-19. Granuloma annulare.

Color plate 6-20. Porphyria cutanea tarda.

Multiple Choice (choose the one best answer)
1. The following are features of dermatomyositis *except*:
   a. Photosensitivity
   b. Proximal myopathy
   c. Erosive arthritis
   d. Heliotrope discoloration of the eyelids
   e. Gottron's papules

2. Erythema nodosum may occur with each of the following *except*:
   a. Streptococcal throat infection
   b. Sarcoidosis
   c. *Yersinia enterocolitica*
   d. Ankylosing spondylitis
   e. Behçet's syndrome

3. Hereditary hemorrhagic telangiectasia is associated with each of the following *except*:
   a. Telangiectasia on the mucosal surface
   b. Frequent nosebleeds
   c. Pulmonary arteriovenous malformations
   d. Autosomal recessive inheritance
   e. Central nervous system angiomas

4. Dermatitis herpetiformis--the following are true *except*:
   a. Associated gluten sensitivity
   b. Blistering on the elbows and knees
   c. Rapid response to gluten elimination
   d. IgA deposition seen on direct immunofluorescence studies of the skin
   e. Pruritus

5. Erythema chronica migrans--the following are true *except*:
   a. Occurs at the site of a tick bite
   b. Resolves spontaneously
   c. Is a cutaneous manifestation of Lyme disease
   d. Early treatment will prevent the development of later sequelae of Lyme disease
   e. Resolves with scarring

6. Circulating antibodies have been identified in each of the following diseases *except*:
   a. Bullous pemphigoid
   b. Porphyria cutanea tarda
   c. Pemphigus
   d. Epidermolysis bullosa acquisita
   e. Herpes gestationis

7. Porphyria cutanea tarda may present with all the following *except:*
   a. Abdominal pain
   b. Increased facial hair
   c. Skin fragility
   d. Photosensitivity
   e. Milia formation

True/False (indicate whether each answer is true or false)
8. Pyoderma gangrenosum may be associated with:
   a. Rheumatoid arthritis
   b. Sarcoidosis
   c. Ulcerative colitis
   d. Hematologic malignancy
   e. Osteoarthritis
   f. Streptococcal throat infection

9. The following are recognized *topical* therapies for psoriasis:
   a. Corticosteroids
   b. Anthralin
   c. Calcipotriene (Dovonex)
   d. Cyclosporine
   e. Crude coal tar
   f. Sulfur

10. Subacute cutaneous lupus erythematosus (SCLE) is associated with:
   a. Renal involvement
   b. Photosensitivity
   c. Positive anti-Ro/anti-SSA antibodies
   d. Congenital heart block in children born to mothers with SCLE
   e. Neonatal lupus erythematosus
   f. Panniculitis

ANSWERS

1. Answer c.
Clinical features of dermatomyositis are photosensitivity, heliotrope discoloration of the eyelids, and the finding of Gottron's papules on the knuckles in association with a proximal myopathy. Erosive arthritis is not a feature of this disorder.

2. Answer d.
Erythema nodosum is a reactive phenomenon and may occur in association with several disorders, including streptococcal throat infection, sarcoidosis, and *Yersinia* infection and as a component of Behçet's syndrome. Ankylosing spondylitis is not associated with erythema nodosum.

3. Answer d.
Hereditary hemorrhagic telangiectasia is autosomal dominant in inheritance. Telangiectasias, frequent nosebleeds, pulmonary arteriovenous malformations, and central nervous system angiomas are features of this syndrome.

4. Answer c.
Dermatitis herpetiformis presents with a pruritic, blistering eruption of the elbows and knees which on direct immunofluorescence shows IgA deposition. There may be associated gluten-sensitive enteropathy. The response to gluten elimination is slow and may take many months.

5. Answer e.
Erythema chronica migrans occurs at the site of a tick bite and resolves spontaneously without treatment. This is an early manifestation of Lyme disease, and treatment will prevent the development of later sequelae of Lyme disease. The lesions heal without scarring.

6. Answer b.
All of the diseases listed are blistering diseases and all are immunologically mediated with identifiable circulating antibodies with the exception of porphyria cutanea tarda. Direct immunofluorescence studies in porphyria cutanea tarda show no evidence of antibody deposition in the basement membrane zone.

7. Answer a.
Acute abdominal pain is not a feature of porphyria cutanea tarda. The other features listed are classic clinical findings in porphyria cutanea tarda.

8. a, true; b, false; c, true; d, true; e, true; f, false.
Rheumatoid arthritis, ulcerative colitis, and hematologic malignancy are classic associations of pyoderma gangrenosum. Sarcoidosis and streptococcal throat infection are associated with erythema nodosum but not pyoderma gangrenosum.

9. a, true; b, true; c, true; d, false; e, true; f, false.
Topical corticosteroids, anthralin, crude coal tar, and calcipotriene (Dovonex) are recommended topical therapies for psoriasis. Cyclosporine is not used topically in the treatment of psoriasis but has been used systemically in the treatment of psoriasis in patients who have failed other therapies. Topical sulfur is a drying agent occasionally used for treating acne or rosacea.

10. a, false; b, true; c, true; d, true; e, true; f, false.
Subacute cutaneous lupus erythematosus is associated with photosensitivity and the finding of a positive anti-Ro/anti-SSA antibody. A congenital heart block and neonatal lupus erythematosus have been described in children born to mothers with this disorder. Renal involvement is not associated with this subtype of lupus erythematosus. Similarly, panniculitis may occur in patients with systemic lupus erythematosus but not in those with subacute cutaneous lupus erythematosus.

CHAPTER 7
ENDOCRINOLOGY

Charles F. Abboud, M.D.

HYPOTHALAMIC-PITUITARY DISORDERS

The Pituitary Gland

The pituitary gland has two distinct parts: the adenohypophysis (or anterior pituitary) and the neurohypophysis (or posterior pituitary). The adenohypophysis is composed of the anterior lobe, intermediate lobe, and pars tuberalis. It is an endocrine gland with at least five types of cells that produce at least eight hormones (Table 7-1). The neurohypophysis is composed of the supraoptic and paraventricular hypothalamic nuclei, their axons, the pituitary stalk, and the posterior lobe. The posterior lobe is not an endocrine gland; rather, it is a storehouse for hormones of the supraoptic and paraventricular nuclei, i.e., arginine vasopressin (AVP) and oxytocin. You should know well the anatomical relationships of the pituitary gland (Fig. 7-1). Blood supply—The adenohypophysis does not have a direct arterial supply; the long portal venous system from superior hypophyseal arteries and the short portal system from inferior hypophyseal arteries form its arterial blood supply; its venous return is via the cavernous and the inferior petrosal sinuses.

Table 7-1.--Anterior Pituitary Hormones and Their Hypothalamic Regulators

Anterior pituitary cell type	Pituitary hormone	Hypothalamic regulatory hormone
Somatotrope	Somatotropin or growth hormone (GH)	(-) Growth hormone release-inhibiting hormone (somatostatin)
		(+) Growth hormone-releasing hormone (GHRH), dominant
Lactotrope	Lactotropin or prolactin (PRL)	(-) Prolactin-inhibiting hormone (dopamine), dominant
		(+) Vasoactive intestinal peptide (VIP)
Thyrotrope	Thyrotropin or thyroid-stimulating hormone (TSH)	(+) Thyrotropin-releasing hormone (TRH), dominant
		(-) Somatostatin
Gonadotrope	Follicle-stimulating hormone (FSH) Luteinizing hormone (LH)	(+) Gonadotropin-releasing hormone (GnRH)
Corticotrope	Corticotropin or adrenocorticotropic hormone (ACTH) Lipotropin (β-LPH) Endorphin (β-END)	(+) Corticotropin-releasing hormone (CRH)

(+), stimulatory effect; (-), inhibitory effect.

169

Fig. 7-1. Anatomical relationships of the pituitary gland. A, sagittal and, B, frontal views. (From Netter FH: The CIBA Collection of Medical Illustrations. Vol 4. Endocrine System and Selected Metabolic Diseases. Summit, New Jersey, CIBA, 1965, pp 6-7. By permission of CIBA Pharmaceutical Company.)

Adenohypophysis: an endocrine gland with at least five types of cells producing at least eight hormones.
Posterior lobe: not an endocrine gland but a storehouse for hormones (AVP and oxytocin) of the supraoptic and paraventricular nuclei.

Anterior Pituitary Gland

Gonadotropins (LH, FSH), corticotropin (ACTH), and thyrotropin (TSH) are discussed in the sections dealing with their respective target glands.

1. Growth Hormone. Growth hormone (GH) is secreted by the somatotroph-cells in bursts. Its biologic effects are 1) a generalized protein-anabolic effect, 2) generation of insulin-like growth factors (IGF) by the peripheral tissues (IGFs mediate the growth-promoting effect), and 3) control of intermediary metabolism. IGF-I (somatomedin-C [SM-C]) is a peptide that resembles proinsulin and is produced by GH-responsive peripheral tissues. It acts in autocrine, paracrine, and endocrine ways. Circulating IGF-I is derived principally from the liver and circulates bound to six binding proteins (IGF-BPs). IGF-BP3 is regulated by GH and may become an

important tool in the assessment of GH secretion.

Cell differentiation and growth require both GH and IGF-I. GH secretion is under the control of neural influences, is sleep-entrained, and is subject to feedback by IGF-I and intermediary metabolites such as glucose, amino acids, and fatty acids (Fig. 7-2). GH-releasing hormone (GHRH) is the dominant hypothalamic control and is stimulatory; somatostatin is the inhibitory hypothalamic hormone.

- Biologic effects of GH: anabolic effect, generation of IGF-I by peripheral tissues, and control of intermediary metabolism.
- IGF-I mediates the growth-promoting effect.
- IGF-I acts in autocrine, paracrine, and endocrine ways.
- Cell differentiation and growth require both GH and IGF-I.
- GH secretion is under feedback control by IGF-I and intermediary metabolites.
- GHRH is the dominant hypothalamic control and is stimulatory; somatostatin is inhibitory

2. Prolactin. Prolactin (PRL) is also secreted in bursts. Its main biologic effects are on breast development and lactogenesis. Its physiologic role in the fetus, children, and adult males is not known. PRL levels begin to increase early in pregnancy and continue to increase through the third trimester, reaching a level about 10x normal. PRL levels are high in the postpartum state and decrease to normal within a few weeks in nonlactating females. PRL secretion is under neural influence and is sleep-entrained; it is stimulated by suckling and stress and inhibited by PRL itself (Fig. 7-3). Dopamine (DA) is the dominant hypothalamic control and is inhibitory.

- PRL: main biologic effects are on breast development and lactogenesis.
- PRL levels increase early in pregnancy and continue to rise through third trimester.
- DA is the dominant hypothalamic control and is inhibitory.

Manifestations of Hypothalamic Disease

Anatomical effects are produced by mass lesions (e.g., craniopharyngioma, germinoma, or metastases) and include obstructive hydrocephalus and chiasmal syndrome.

- Anatomical effects are produced by mass lesions.

Functional effects are related to disordered hypothalamic vegetative or endocrine functions. These include 1) vegetative dysfunction such as disorders of thirst, appetite, or temperature regulation and 2) endocrine disorders affecting AVP and/or hypophysiotropic functions; these may include diabetes insipidus, syndrome of inappropriate antidiuretic hormone (ADH), hypopituitarism, or hyperpituitarism.

- Functional effects are related to disordered hypothalamic vegetative or endocrine functions.

Hypopituitarism

Disorders of the anterior pituitary gland can affect one, more than one, or all of its hormones. When more than one hormone is affected, the disorder can affect the hormones concurrently or in succession. In multitropic failure, a common sequence of hormone loss is GH, LH/FSH, TSH, ACTH, and PRL. However, failure can occur in any sequence.

- Disorders of the anterior pituitary gland can affect one, more

Fig. 7-2. Hypothalamic-pituitary-growth hormone axis. CNS, central nervous system; GHRH, growth hormone-releasing hormone.

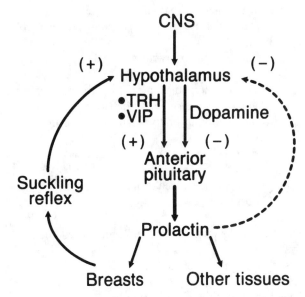

Fig. 7-3. Hypothalamic-pituitary-prolactin axis. CNS, central nervous system; TRH, thyrotropin-releasing hormone; VIP, vasoactive intestinal peptide.

than one, or all of its hormones concurrently or in succession.

The causes of hypopituitarism are outlined in Table 7-2, and the usual presentations of hypopituitarism are described in Table 7-3. The usual presentation is one of gradual onset and slow progression. However, hypopituitarism can present acutely: 1) acute adrenocortical crisis may be precipitated by acute medical/surgical illness or by thyroid hormone replacement in a patient with associated unrecognized ACTH deficiency, 2) hypoglycemia (lack of ACTH and GH), 3) hyponatremia (lack of ACTH and TSH), and 4) sedative/anesthetic "sensitivity" (lack of ACTH and TSH).

● Hypopituitarism usually presents as a slowly evolving disease, but it can present acutely: 1) acute adrenocortical crisis, 2) hypoglycemia, 3) hyponatremia, and 4) sedative/anesthetic "sensitivity."

Diagnostic Approach

Endocrine Evaluation

1. GH. Low serum level of GH unresponsive to stimulation. a) Definitive provocative options: insulin-hypoglycemia, L-dopa, arginine, propranolol-glucagon, or clonidine. Insulin hypoglycemia is the standard test;

Table 7-2.--Causes of Hypopituitarism

Primary pituitary disease
   Congenital--idiopathic
   Traumatic--neurosurgical (pituitary tumors, breast carcinoma, diabetic retinopathy); radiotherapeutic (to sella, nasopharynx, or intracranial contents)
   Inflammatory or infiltrative--infections (tuberculosis, syphilis, fungal), sarcoidosis, hemochromatosis, autoimmune hypophysitis
   Vascular
      Ischemic necrosis--postpartum pituitary necrosis (Sheehan's syndrome), diabetes mellitus, temporal arteritis, sickle-cell disease and trait, eclampsia
      Pituitary apoplexy
   Neoplastic
      Primary--pituitary tumors, craniopharyngioma
      Metastatic
   Miscellaneous--primary empty sella syndrome, idiopathic
Secondary pituitary disease: hypothalamic
   Destruction of pituitary stalk--trauma, neurosurgical, compression by tumor or aneurysm
   Hypothalamic or other central nervous system disease
      Functional
         Stress--psychogenic
         Nutritional--starvation, obesity
         Anorexia nervosa/bulimia syndrome
         Systemic disease--renal, hepatic failure, uncontrolled diabetes mellitus
         Drugs--vincristine
         Hormones--glucocorticoids, gonadal steroids, thyroid hormones
      Organic
         Congenital--hypothalamic hormone genetic defects, GnRH (Kallman's syndrome)
         Traumatic--neurosurgery, irradiation
         Inflammatory/infiltrative--sarcoidosis, histiocytosis X
         Neoplastic
            Primary--gliomas, ectopic pinealoma, craniopharyngioma
            Metastatic
            Lymphoma and leukemia
         Idiopathic
Extrasellar disease
   Parasellar--meningioma, optic nerve glioma, chordoma
   Cysts--arachnoid
   Nasopharyngeal carcinoma
   Sphenoid sinus mucocele
   Aneurysm of internal carotid artery
   Cavernous sinus thrombosis

Table 7-3.--Manifestations of Hypopituitarism

Hormone lack	Childhood-adolescence	Adulthood
Growth hormone	Shortness of stature Hypoglycemia	Hypoglycemia(?) Asthenia
Prolactin	None	Failure of postpartum lactation in women None in men
Gonadotropin	Failure of sexual maturation in adolescents	Failure of gametogenesis in both sexes and of maintenance of secondary sex characteristics and of other sex steroid hormone-dependent functions
Thyrotropin	Impairment of central nervous system development in newborn infants Slowing of emotional, mental, and physical functions Failure of sexual maturation in adolescents	Slowing of emotional, mental, and physical functions
Corticotropin	Ill health, anorexia, weight loss, gastrointestinal disturbances, weakness, orthostatic hypotension, hypoglycemia, inability to excrete a water load, pallor, inability to tan, and propensity to adrenocortical crises	Same as in childhood and adolescence

other tests are used if insulin hypoglycemia is not safe, e.g., in the elderly or in those with central nervous system (CNS) or ischemic myocardial disorder. b) Screening provocative options: sleep or exercise. c) Low IGF-I levels can be seen in GH deficiency or in nutritional disorders. Measurement of IGF-I and IGF-BP3 has been used as a screen for GH deficiency. (In GH-deficiency, both IGF-I and IGF-BP3 are low; in nutritional deficiency, IGF-I is low but IGF-BP3 is normal.) Currently, GH provocative tests are not indicated in adults with suspected hypopituitarism, pending future knowledge regarding the implications of GH deficiency syndrome and delineation of risks/benefits of GH therapy in adults. d) The role of GHRH testing has not been delineated.

- Low serum level of GH unresponsive to stimulation; low serum levels of IGF-I and IGF-BP3.
- GH provocative tests are not needed in adults with suspected hypopituitarism.

2. PRL. Low serum level of PRL is unresponsive to stimulation. Options: TRH, chlorpromazine, metoclopramide, or insulin-hypoglycemia. Provocative tests for PRL are rarely needed in clinical practice.

- Low serum level of PRL unresponsive to stimulation (clinically not indicated).

3. Gonadotropins. Males: low sperm count, low serum level of testosterone and free testosterone, and inappropriately low serum levels of LH and FSH. Females: low serum levels of estradiol and inappropriately low serum

levels of LH and FSH. Provocative tests for LH and FSH are not indicated clinically.

- Males: low sperm count, low serum level of testosterone, and inappropriately low serum levels of LH and FSH.
- Females: low serum level of estradiol and inappropriately low serum levels of LH and FSH.

4. ACTH. Low serum levels of cortisol and inappropriately low serum level of ACTH. The cosyntropin (Cortrosyn) test usually shows no response unless ACTH lack is partial or of recent onset. Prolonged exogenous ACTH tests show a stepwise response. Other provocative tests, including insulin-hypoglycemia and metyrapone tests, document pituitary ACTH-adrenal unresponsiveness.

- Low serum level of cortisol and inappropriately low serum level of ACTH.
- Cosyntropin test usually shows no response.
- Prolonged exogenous ACTH tests show stepwise response.

5. TSH. Low serum levels of T_4 and free T_4 (or free thyroxine index [FTI]) and an inappropriately normal or low serum level of TSH.

- Low serum levels of T_4 and free T_4 or FTI and an inappropriately low serum level of TSH.

"Anatomical" Evaluation

Computed tomography (CT) or magnetic resonance imaging (MRI) and ophthalmic evaluation to assess visual fields, visual acuity, and optic disks.

- Anatomical evaluation: CT or MRI and ophthalmic evaluation.

In diagnosing hypopituitarism, the physician must document the presence of hypopituitarism and delineate its cause. For tropic hormone deficiencies, the diagnosis rests on the evaluation of the function of the target gland. If target gland failure is present, tropic hormone levels are required to distinguish between primary target gland failure and target gland failure due to hypothalamic-pituitary disease.

- In diagnosing hypopituitarism, the presence of hypopituitarism must be documented and its cause delineated.
- Diagnosis of tropic hormone deficiencies rests on the evaluation of target gland function.
- If target gland failure is present, additional studies are needed to distinguish between primary target gland failure and failure due to hypothalamic-pituitary disease.

In hypothyroid patients, a high serum level of TSH or the presence of goiter points to primary hypothyroidism, and an inappropriately low serum level of TSH confirms the diagnosis of TSH deficiency.

- In hypothyroid patients, an inappropriately low serum level of TSH confirms the diagnosis of TSH deficiency.

In suspected hypogonadism, high serum levels of LH and FSH point to primary gonadal failure. In hypogonadism due to hypothalamic-pituitary disease, serum levels of LH and FSH are inappropriately low.

- In hypogonadism due to hypothalamic-pituitary disease, serum levels of LH and FSH are inappropriately low.

If a hypocortisol state is present, a diagnosis of primary adrenocortical failure is supported by the presence of hyperpigmentation and mineralocorticoid deficiency It is documented by increased serum levels of ACTH or lack of adrenocortical responsiveness to exogenous ACTH stimulation. In adrenocortical failure due to hypothalamic-pituitary disease, there is pallor, loss of tanning ability, no mineralocorticoid deficiency, inappropriately low serum levels of ACTH, and adrenal responsiveness to prolonged exogenous ACTH stimulation.

- Adrenocortical failure due to hypothalamic-pituitary disease: pallor, loss of tanning ability, no mineralocorticoid deficiency, inappropriately low serum levels of ACTH, and adrenal responsiveness to prolonged exogenous ACTH stimulation.

For the nontropic hormones, GH and PRL, a high-normal or high basal value excludes deficiency; otherwise, a provocative test is needed to assess hormone reserve. Clinically, such provocative tests are needed to document GH deficiency only in children with hypopituitarism.

- GH and PRL (nontropic hormones): high-normal or high basal value excludes deficiency.
- Otherwise, a provocative test is needed to assess hormone reserve.

In determining the cause of hypopituitarism, suspected functional causes (Table 7-2) must be removed or corrected. Normalization of pituitary function lends support to "functional" hypopituitarism. If functional causes are excluded or if hypopituitarism persists despite removal or correction of a functional cause, then evaluate for organic hypothalamic-pituitary disease. This evaluation is based on the clinical setting and appropriate endocrine and anatomical studies.

- In determining the cause of hypopituitarism, suspected functional causes must be removed or corrected.
- Next, evaluate for organic hypothalamic-pituitary disease based on the clinical setting and appropriate laboratory and radiologic studies.

Diagnostic Pitfalls

1) Failure to determine the extent and degree of hypopituitarism. It is important to evaluate all pituitary functions in patients with suspected hypopituitarism. 2) Failure to rule out functional causes. These are important causes of hypopituitarism because they are common and potentially reversible. 3) Failure to look for an organic cause and to follow up closely those patients with hypopituitarism in whom no organic cause is found. Hypopituitarism may precede by a long time the clinical appearance of its cause.

- Do not fail to determine the extent and degree of hypopituitarism.
- Do not fail to rule out functional causes.
- Do not fail to look for organic cause and to follow up those patients with hypopituitarism in whom no organic cause is found.

Therapy of Hypopituitarism

Therapy includes treating the cause and, when applicable, administering pituitary hormones or hormones of the target gland.

- Therapy: treat cause and, if needed, administer pituitary hormones or those of the target glands.

1. Glucocorticoids. Hydrocortisone, 20 mg in early a.m. and 10 mg in early p.m. for adults (or equivalent dosage of prednisone). Instruct patients in dose modification during acute illness (see Adrenal Cortex). In patients with combined ACTH-TSH lack, initiate glucocorticoid therapy before thyroid hormone therapy to avoid thyroid hormone-induced increased need for cortisol and precipitation of acute adrenocortical crisis.

- Instruct patients in dose modification during acute illness.
- In patients with combined ACTH-TSH lack, initiate glucocorticoid therapy before thyroid hormone therapy.

2. Thyroid hormones. T_4 is the drug of choice. Initiate therapy with a low dose and gradually increase it over a period of weeks. Assess the adequacy of therapy by feeling of well-being and serum levels of free T_4 (see Thyroid). Do not use sTSH levels to monitor the adequacy of T_4 dosage, because they are characteristically low in untreated persons.

- T_4 is the drug of choice.
- Initiate therapy with a low dose and gradually increase it over a period of weeks.
- Do not use sTSH levels to monitor the adequacy of therapy. Use the patient's clinical state and a measurement of free thyroxine or FTI.

3. Gonadal hormone replacement. 1) In females, conjugated estrogens, 0.6-1.25 mg (or equivalent) daily. Use progestational agents for women with a uterus: medroxyprogesterone acetate, 10 mg daily for days 1-12 of each month (see Female Gonadal Disorders). 2) In males, long-acting testosterone parenteral preparation (testosterone enanthate or cypionate), 100-200 mg every 2-3 weeks. The goal is to restore full androgenicity (see Male Gonadal Disorders). Assess the prostate status in middle-aged and elderly men before therapy and follow annually.

For restoration of fertility, FSH/LH (or gonadotropin-releasing hormone [GnRH] therapy in patients with hypothalamic disorders) may be indicated. Delay therapy in puberty to avoid premature closure of epiphyses and to allow maximal linear growth. Evaluate psychosexual needs and patient's lifestyle to assess the impact of the therapy.

- In hypogonadal females, use estrogen therapy, e.g., conjugated estrogens; use supplemental progestational agents for women with a uterus.
- In hypogonadal males, use long-acting parenteral testosterone esters.
- In adolescents, delay sex hormone therapy as long as possible to avoid premature closure of the epiphyses.

4. GH. In children, GH is used to treat impaired linear growth due to GH deficiency. Recombinant GH is given parenterally until an acceptable height is attained (goal, 5'4"). Careful attention is given to concomitant thyroid and cortisol replacement in order to avoid under- or overtreatment. To avoid premature closure of the epiphyses, delay using sex steroid therapy. In GH-deficient adults, GH therapy improves lean body mass and muscle strength and decreases fat mass. Currently, because no long-term studies are available, this use of GH is considered experimental.

- GH: used in children to treat impaired linear growth due to GH deficiency.

Pituitary Tumors

Pituitary tumors are "microadenomas" (<10 mm) or "macroadenomas" (>10 mm) in size, "sellar" or "sellar/extrasellar" in extent, and "functioning" or "nonfunctioning." In functioning tumors, the incidence is: PRL, 50%; GH, 15%; ACTH, 15%; LH/FSH, 5%; TSH, α-glycoprotein subunit, 5%; and "nonfunctioning," 10%. Pituitary tumors can be "isolated" or part of multiple endocrine neoplasia type I (MEN I) (see below).

- Tumor size: microadenoma (<10 mm) or macroadenoma (>10 mm).
- Tumor extent: sellar or sellar/extrasellar.
- Tumor may be functioning or nonfunctioning.
- Pituitary tumor may be isolated or part of MEN I.

Clinical Manifestations

Chronic

Mass effects include headaches and evidence of tumor extension beyond the confines of the sella. 1) Superior extension of the tumor may cause: a) chiasmal syndrome with impaired visual acuity and visual field defects; b) hypothalamic syndrome with vegetative disturbance in thirst, appetite, satiety, sleep, and temperature regulation and with endocrine disorder of diabetes insipidus or syndrome of inappropriate ADH; c) obstructive hydrocephalus; and d) frontal lobe dysfunction. 2) Lateral extension of the tumor may cause impairment of cranial nerves III, IV, V, and VI, with diplopia, facial pain, and temporal lobe dysfunction. 3) Inferior extension of the tumor may lead to a nasopharyngeal mass or cerebrospinal fluid (CSF) rhinorrhea.

- Mass effects: headaches and evidence that the tumor extends beyond the sella.

Endocrine effects result from either 1) hypersecretory states or 2) hypopituitarism caused by destruction of the pituitary gland by tumor growth. Hyperpituitarism can cause gigantism/acromegaly (GH excess), hyperprolactinemic syndrome (PRL excess), Cushing's disease and Nelson/Salassa syndrome (ACTH excess), and thyrotoxicosis (TSH excess). Generally, LH/FSH and α-subunit excess are clinically silent. Hypopituitarism can be expressed in several ways. Endocrine associations of pituitary tumors include MEN I, i.e., parathyroid tumor or hyperplasia (primary hyperparathyroidism), endocrine pancreas tumor or hyperplasia (various endocrine pancreatic syndromes), and other endocrine gland tumors (thyroid, adrenal) and lipomas.

- Endocrine effects: due to hypersecretory states or to hypopituitarism.
- Endocrine associations of pituitary tumors: MEN I.

Acute

Pituitary apoplexy (see below) may occur in patients with known pituitary tumor. Occasionally, it may be the first indication of an underlying tumor.

- Pituitary apoplexy may occur in patients with known pituitary tumor.
- It may be the first clinical expression of the underlying tumor.

Diagnosis

The presence of a pituitary tumor is suggested by the clinical features and by the results of CT or MRI of the pituitary region. Neuro-ophthalmologic evaluation, including assessing visual acuity, visual fields, and optic disks, is important, particularly if a suprasellar extension is present. Endocrine evaluation includes evaluation for hormonal excess (see below under the various functioning pituitary tumor syndromes) or hormonal lack and for the presence of any associated MEN I. A diagnosis of a pituitary tumor is made if the sellar mass is associated with anterior pituitary hormone excess (except for mild hyperprolactinemia, which can occur with other masses in the area and "stalk-effect"). Otherwise, the diagnosis is confirmed at surgical exploration.

- Pituitary tumor: presence is suggested by clinical assessment and CT and MRI findings.
- Neuro-ophthalmologic evaluation is important, particularly with suprasellar extension.
- Endocrine evaluation should assess for hormonal excess or lack and the presence of any associated MEN I.

The differential diagnosis includes 1) other hypothalamic or pituitary masses (outlined below), and 2) pituitary hyperplasia of pregnancy, target gland primary failure (e.g., primary hypothyroidism), and hypothalamic regulatory hormone disorder (eutopic or ectopic excess production).

Treatment

Pituitary tumors usually are treated with surgical ablation or irradiation. Drug therapy is available for PRL-, GH-, or TSH-producing tumors; it can be a useful adjunct to ablative therapy. Treat associated hypopituitarism.

- Treatment: surgical ablation or irradiation.
- Drug therapy is an option for PRL-, GH-, or TSH-producing tumors and can be a useful adjunct to ablation.

1. Surgery. Transsphenoidal surgery is the operation of choice for most tumors; transfrontal operation is reserved for tumors with large suprasellar extension. Surgical morbidity and mortality as well as available neurosurgical expertise should be considered.
2. Radiotherapy. Issues to be considered are 1) long latent period (few months to years), 2) postradiation hypopituitarism (30%-40% of patients), and 3) potential for CNS damage (rare) or development of CNS tumors (very rare).
3. Drug therapy. Dopamine agonists (bromocriptine in the U.S.) for management of prolactinoma or GH-producing tumors. Somatostatin analog (octreotide) for GH- or TSH-producing tumors. Consider the efficacy, long-term safety, and cost.
4. No therapy. This can be an option if the tumor is small and has no effect on quality/quantity of life.

Follow-up is essential for all therapeutic options to monitor for persistence, recurrence, and development of other aspects of MEN I.

- Observation can be an option if the tumor is small and not associated with "anatomical" or functional effects.
- Follow-up is essential for any therapeutic option to monitor for persistence, recurrence, and development of other aspects of MEN I.

Hyperprolactinemic Syndrome and Prolactinomas

Pituitary tumors associated with hyperprolactinemia may be prolactinomas, "mixed" tumors (e.g., GH- and PRL-producing tumors), or any tumor or mass lesion with suprasellar extension and "stalk effect." (In the "stalk effect" type, the serum level of PRL is usually <200 ng/mL; bromocriptine can control the hyperprolactinemia but does not cause regression of tumor size.) The causes of hyperprolactinemia are outlined in Table 7-4.

- Pituitary tumors associated with hyperprolactinemia: prolactinomas, mixed tumors, or any tumor/mass lesion with suprasellar extension and stalk effect.

Table 7-4.--Causes of Hyperprolactinemia

Physiologic
    Newborn, pregnancy, lactation, stress
Pathologic
    Eutopic pituitary disorder
        Primary pituitary disease
            Pituitary tumors
            Hypophysitis
            Empty sella syndrome
        Secondary pituitary disorder
            Hypothalamic/stalk disease
                Functional
                    Drugs
                    Primary hypothyroidism
                    Chest wall disease
                    Chronic renal or hepatic failure
                Organic
                    Traumatic
                    Inflammatory/infiltrative
                    Vascular
                    Neoplastic, primary or secondary
    Ectopic tumors--lung, kidney, ovary

Clinical Manifestations

Prolactinomas usually present with manifestations of hyperprolactinemia and, occasionally, with pituitary mass effects. The characteristic presentation is amenorrhea/galactorrhea in women, decreased libido and potency in men, and delayed sexual maturation in adolescents.

- Prolactinomas: usually present with manifestations of hyperprolactinemia and, occasionally, with mass effects.
- Characteristic presentation: amenorrhea/galactorrhea in women, decreased libido and potency in men, and delayed sexual maturation in adolescents.

Endocrine effects include: 1) effects of hyperprolactinemia: a) in women, galactorrhea, ovulatory and menstrual dysfunction (short luteal phase or anovulation leading to infertility); oligo/amenorrhea and hypogonadism; hyperandrogenic manifestations (hirsutism or acne), and decreased libido; b) in men, libido and potency impairment, oligospermia (infertility), and, very rarely, galactorrhea or gynecomastia; and c) in adolescents, delayed puberty; 2) associated pituitary dysfunction (hypopituitarism); and 3) associated MEN I.

- Endocrine effects: hyperprolactinemia, associated pituitary dysfunction, and associated MEN I.

Neurologic effects are caused by the mass effects of pituitary tumors.

- Neurologic effects: mass effects.

In men, the recognition of hyperprolactinemia frequently is delayed because decreased libido and impaired potency may be dismissed by the patient and physician as a result of psychiatric factors. In those harboring a pituitary tumor, marked hyperprolactinemia and a macroprolactinoma are usual at the time of presentation.

- In males, recognition of hyperprolactinemia is frequently delayed; a macroprolactinoma is usually present at diagnosis.

Diagnostic Approach

1. Rule out physiologic causes. A pregnancy test is an essential part of the work-up of any female of reproductive age.

- Rule out physiologic cause: pregnancy test is essential.

2. Check serum level of PRL. a) If the serum level is >10x normal (>250 ng/mL), it establishes the diagnosis of prolactinoma. However, prolactinomas may be associated with lower levels. b) If the serum level is <10x normal (<250 ng/mL), rule out functional causes, e.g., exclude drugs, irritative lesion of the chest wall, primary hypothyroidism, and chronic renal failure. i) If a functional cause is present, remove or treat if possible. If hyperprolactinemia does not resolve in about 3 months, evaluate for hypothalamic-pituitary disease. ii) If no functional cause is present, rule out organic hypothalamic-pituitary disease by CT or MRI and by evaluating other pituitary functions and the visual fields if necessary. Diagnostic possibilities include pituitary tumor, other organic hypothalamic-pituitary disease, or "idiopathic" hyperprolactinemia.

- Check the serum level of PRL.
- Level >250 ng/mL: establishes the diagnosis of prolactinoma (but prolactinomas may be associated with lower levels).
- Level <250 ng/mL: first, rule out functional cause, e.g., exclude drugs, irritative lesion of the chest wall, primary hypothyroidism, and chronic renal failure.
- If no functional cause is present, rule out organic hypothalamic-pituitary disease by CT or MRI.

Comments

1. If the patient is taking a drug that can cause hyperprolactinemia, decide whether use of the drug can be discontinued. If use of the drug is discontinued, the serum level of PRL is checked again in a few weeks. If the repeat serum level of PRL is normal, the diagnosis is drug-related hyperprolactinemia. If use of the drug cannot be discontinued or if the hyperprolactinemia persists

despite discontinued use, the work-up is continued to rule out organic disease.

2. A careful history and physical examination and appropriate laboratory and radiologic studies are usually sufficient to rule out a chest wall lesion, renal or hepatic failure, systemic disease, or metastatic disease. The next step is to rule out primary hypothyroidism. An sTSH should be performed in all hyperprolactinemia patients because many patients with primary hypothyroidism are asymptomatic and the findings may be subtle.

3. If a functional cause has been excluded, the next step is to rule out a pituitary tumor or other hypothalamic-pituitary mass lesion. The diagnosis of pituitary tumor is based on considering the serum level of PRL and CT or MRI findings on scans of the pituitary area. Most patients with a serum level of PRL >100 ng/mL and almost all patients with PRL levels >250 ng/mL harbor a prolactinoma. A substantial portion of patients with serum levels of PRL between 25 and 100 ng/mL have pituitary tumors; therefore, marginally increased values do not rule out a tumor. Radiologic studies, especially CT or MRI, are crucial for the diagnosis. Pituitary tumors associated with hyperprolactinemia may be prolactinomas, "mixed" tumors (e.g., GH- and PRL-producing tumors), or any tumor or mass lesion with suprasellar extension and "stalk effect." (In the "stalk effect" type caused by a non-PRL-producing tumor, the serum level of PRL is usually <200 ng/mL. In a prolactinoma of a comparable size, the serum level of PRL is between 500 and 20,000 ng/mL.)

4. If, after a thorough evaluation, a discernible cause is not found, the hyperprolactinemia is considered to be of indeterminate origin. Follow-up evaluation is critical in these patients because some of them may harbor microadenomas or other hypothalamic-pituitary space-occupying lesions that are below the limit of radiologic detection, and follow-up examinations may show evidence of a mass. The serum level of PRL should be checked every 6-12 months and a CT or MRI scan should be repeated in 1-2 years or earlier if deemed necessary by the development of new symptoms.

Treatment of Microprolactinoma or Idiopathic Hyperprolactinemia

Treatment is indicated for management of infertility, hypogonadism, significant galactorrhea, and hirsutism or to meet the patient's desire. Treatment options include bromocriptine or transsphenoidal surgery for microprolactinoma. Otherwise, observe, check the serum level of PRL annually, and perform CT or MRI every 2-3 years.

Treatment of Macroprolactinoma

1. Surgical excision is usually incomplete; for persistent disease, the options are a) postoperative radiotherapy with or without interim bromocriptine or b) bromocriptine. 2. Radiotherapeutic ablation with a) interim bromocriptine while awaiting the effects of radiotherapy or b) surgical excision for persistent or progressive disease. 3. Pharmacologic—In the U.S., the dopamine agonist bromocriptine is the mainstay of medical treatment; surgical excision or radiotherapy is reserved for persistent or progressive disease or for drug intolerance.

Bromocriptine

Bromocriptine is a dopamine agonist. It suppresses hyperprolactinemia and restores gonadal function (80%-90% of patients), and it may decrease tumor size (<50%). Its effect may be dramatic. The drug is not antimitotic. It is costly and can have side effects that are usually minimal and include nausea, fatigue, nasal stuffiness, and postural hypotension. Its long-term safety is unknown. The usual dose in cases of prolactinoma is 5.0-7.5 mg/day. To prevent or minimize the side effects, bromocriptine treatment is started with a small dose (1.25-2.5 mg) with food and at bedtime; the dose is increased in steps every 3-5 days. Bromocriptine is a temporizing therapy and discontinuation of its use leads to resumption of tumor growth and endocrine dysfunction.

- Bromocriptine is a dopamine agonist.
- It suppresses hyperprolactinemia and restores gonadal function.
- It may decrease tumor size.
- Discontinuation of its use: resumption of tumor growth and endocrine dysfunction.

Bromocriptine and Pregnancy

Restoration of gonadal function and fertility is the major goal of drug therapy. The use of bromocriptine should be stopped at the earliest sign of pregnancy. In pregnancy, the risk of tumor growth for microprolactinoma is <5% and for macroprolactinoma, 20%-40%. Observe patients closely, especially if they have macroprolactinomas, and periodically perform clinical and visual field evaluations. If significant tumor growth complicates pregnancy, consider surgical excision or reinstituting bromocriptine therapy.

- Use of bromocriptine should be stopped at earliest sign of pregnancy.
- During pregnancy, the risk of tumor growth for microprolactinoma is <5% and for macroprolactinoma, 20%-40%.
- If significant tumor growth complicates pregnancy, consider surgical excision or reinstituting bromocriptine therapy.

Surgical Treatment for Prolactinomas

The surgical cure rates for microadenomas and macroadenomas are 60%-80% and 0%-30%, respectively. The recurrence rate for hyperprolactinemia is 10%-50% and for pituitary tumors, 5%-10%. Morbidity is <1%-5%, and mortality is 0%-1%.

GH-Producing Tumors

Etiology

1) Pituitary disorder: >99% are due to GH-producing pituitary tumors. 2) Very rarely, acromegaly may be caused by ectopic GH-producing tumors or hypothalamic or extrahypothalamic GHRH-producing tumors.

Clinical Features

The clinical presentations are related to GH/IGF-I excess, to the pituitary tumor, and to the associations of acromegaly. 1) Excess GH/IGF-I leads to acromegalic features/gigantism, hyperhidrosis, heat intolerance, increased skin porosity and oiliness, carbohydrate intolerance (20% of patients; frank diabetes mellitus is rare), hypercalciuria, hyperphosphatemia, acroparesthesias, nerve entrapment syndromes, myopathy, hypertension or cardiomyopathy, Raynaud's phenomenon, fibromas or acanthosis nigricans, and sleep apnea or narcolepsy. 2) Pituitary tumor manifestations include hypopituitarism, hyperprolactinemia (which may be caused by mixed tumor or stalk effect of extrasellar extension of a large GH-producing macroadenoma), and anatomical effects related to extrasellar extension. 3) The associations of acromegaly include diffuse or nodular goiter, thyrotoxicosis (which may be related to mixed GH/TSH tumor, associated Graves' disease, or multinodular toxic goiter), or MEN I.

- Clinical presentation of GH-producing tumors: related to GH/IGF-I excess, pituitary tumor, and to associations of acromegaly.

Diagnostic Approach

Assess the clinical features. A random serum level of GH may be helpful. Values <1 ng/mL exclude acromegaly, and those >50 ng/mL confirm acromegaly. Values in the range of 2 to 50 ng/mL are nondiagnostic. Perform an oral glucose tolerance test with GH responses; nonsuppressible GH during an oral glucose tolerance test is the reference standard test. GH levels will not suppress to <1 ng/mL in active acromegaly. Measure serum IGF-I (Som-C): increased levels confirm the diagnosis of acromegaly (if one excludes physiologic elevations of pregnancy and adolescence). If the results are borderline, check for paradoxical GH responses to TRH or L-dopa. (In about 60% of acromegalics, TRH may stimulate GH secretion, whereas L-dopa may suppress levels of GH.) When the diagnosis is documented biochemically, proceed with imaging of the sella (CT or MRI). If no tumor is found (a rare event), obtain serum GHRH levels to exclude a GHRH-producing tumor and search for evidence of a GH-producing tumor.

- Assess the clinical features.
- Random serum level of GH may be helpful.
- Perform an oral glucose tolerance test with GH responses: failure of GH to suppress to <1 ng/mL is diagnostic of acromegaly.
- Measure the serum level of IGF-I: increased serum level confirms the diagnosis.
- If the results are borderline, check for paradoxical GH responses to TRH or L-dopa.
- When acromegaly is documented biochemically, proceed with imaging of the sella. If no tumor is visible, obtain the serum level of GHRH and look for evidence of a GH-producing tumor.

Usually, there is no problem in the diagnosis of flagrant cases. The challenge is to make the diagnosis early, because untreated chronic disease can cause irreversible physical changes, increase patients' morbidity (by the effects of tumor, GH hypersecretion, and other endocrine dysfunction), and increase mortality (from hypertension, diabetes mellitus, and cardiovascular effects). The syndrome should be considered in the differential diagnosis of increased perspiration, oiliness of the skin, hyperpigmentation, menstrual irregularities, galactorrhea, hypertension, diabetes mellitus, premature and significant degenerative joint disease, carpal tunnel and other entrapment neuropathies, peripheral neuropathy, sellar enlargement, and chiasmal syndrome and in the setting of MEN I.

Treatment

Pituitary tumor. There are several options. Surgical excision is the treatment of choice. Transsphenoidal surgery is the usual approach; the transfrontal operation is reserved for tumors with a large suprasellar extension. For postoperatively persistent disease, consider radiotherapy plus interim pharmacologic therapy (either bromocriptine or somatostatin analogue or both). Radiotherapy—Interim pharmacologic therapy can be considered; for persistent or progressive disease, one can proceed with surgical therapy.

- Therapy of choice: surgical excision.
- Transsphenoidal approach is the usual one.
- For persistent disease: radiotherapy plus interim pharmacologic therapy.

Ectopic GH or GHRH tumor. Surgical resection is the therapy of choice. For persistent disease, consider somatostatin analogue.

Transsphenoidal surgery has a cure rate of 60%-80%; it may be complicated by hypopituitarism (5%-10%), diabetes insipidus (2%-3%), and mortality (<1%). Radiation therapy has a cure rate of 70% after 10 years; hypopituitarism can occur in up to 50% of patients in 10 years; other morbidity is rare. The major disadvantage of radiotherapy is its long latent period (months to years) before it controls disease activity. In bromocriptine therapy, the usual dose is 5-20 mg/day or higher; normal GH/Som C, <10%; tumor shrinkage, <10%. This is a temporizing therapy. Somatostatin analogue (octreotide) is an effective therapeutic option: the average dose is 100-200 μg/8 hours given subcutaneously; it can normalize GH/Som C in 80% of patients and can lead to tumor shrinkage in 30%-50%. The side effects of octreotide include nausea, flatulence, mild malabsorption, cholelithiasis (10% of patients), and impairment of glucose tolerance. This, too, is a temporizing therapy. Gallbladder ultrasonography is performed initially and repeated at intervals of 1-2 years.

In patients with acromegaly, there appears to be a two- to threefold increase in the development of malignant tumors, and a three- to eightfold excess risk of colon cancer and premalignant colon polyps. Currently, it seems prudent to use colonoscopy to screen all patients with acromegaly at diagnosis and then at 2-3-year intervals.

Gonadotropin-Producing Tumors

Gonadotropin-producing tumors are rare, accounting for 3%-4% of all pituitary tumors. They usually are macroadenomas. These tumors may be selective for gonadotropins or may be plurihormonal. There usually is hypersecretion of FSH, occasionally of FSH and LH, and rarely of LH only. Also, these tumors may secrete α-glycoprotein subunit. Clinically, the tumor may present at any age but usually in middle-aged or elderly persons, predominantly males. Extrasellar effects dominate the clinical picture, and some degree of hypopituitarism is usually present. Rarely, in children, sexual precocity may be the presenting feature. Laboratory findings are high levels of FSH (85% of patients), high levels of LH and FSH (10%-15% of patients), or high levels of LH only (rarely). In males, serum levels of testosterone are variable and semen analysis is normal or oligospermic. CT or MRI reveals the sellar mass with extrasellar extension. Chiasmal syndrome may be present. The treatment is usually surgical, with or without postoperative irradiation. Endocrine replacement therapy is given for management of hypopituitarism. Currently, no effective medical therapy is available.

- Gonadotropin-producing tumors: are rare; 3%-4% of all pituitary tumors.
- They usually occur in middle-aged or elderly persons, predominantly males.
- They are usually macroadenomas.
- "Extrasellar" effects usually dominate the clinical picture.
- High serum level of FSH in 85% of patients; high serum levels of LH and FSH in 10%-15% of patients.
- Treatment: surgical, with or without postoperative irradiation.

Thyrotropin-Producing Tumors

The clinical presentations of primary TSH tumors include diffuse goiter and hyperthyroidism. The major differential diagnosis is Graves' disease. In TSH-producing tumors, and in contrast to Graves' disease, one finds equal sex incidence, absence of ophthalmopathy/dermopathy, normal or high sTSH values in patients with hyperthyroidism, and absence of thyroid-stimulating immunoglobulins. Other presentations include extrasellar mass effects and hypopituitarism. Laboratory evaluation reveals that, in a thyrotoxic patient, the sTSH value is normal or high, α-glycoprotein subunit levels are high, and TSH responsiveness to thyrotropin-releasing hormone (TRH) is absent. CT or MRI shows a sellar mass with or without extrasellar extension. Treatment options include ablation (either surgically or with irradiation), pharmacologic therapy with somatostatin analogue, and ancillary measures for the management of thyrotoxicosis.

- Clinical presentation of primary TSH tumors: diffuse goiter and hyperthyroidism.
- Major differential diagnosis: Graves' disease.
- Normal or high sTSH values are the distinguishing feature from all other causes of the hyperthyroid state.
- Other presentations: mass effects and hypopituitarism.
- Treatment: ablative or pharmacologic (somatostatin analogue).

α-Glycoprotein Subunit-Producing Tumors

These rare tumors may be unihormonal, with selective hypersecretion of the α-subunit, or plurihormonal, with cosecretion of GH, PRL, LH/FSH, or TSH. α-Subunit excess is clinically silent. The dominant clinical presentations are mass effects with extrasellar manifestations and hypopituitarism. Also, there may be clinical features of the cosecreted hormone excess, such as acromegaly, hyperprolactinemia, or thyrotoxicosis. Laboratory evaluation documents the high serum level of the α-subunit. Radiologic imaging reveals a sellar mass with or without extrasellar extension. Therapy for selective α-subunit tumors is either surgical excision or irradiation. Radiotherapy is also indicated as a secondary treatment for surgical patients with postoperative persistence or recurrence of tumor.

- Dominant clinical presentations: mass effects and hypopituitarism.
- High serum levels of α-subunit.
- Therapy for selective α-subunit tumors: surgical excision or irradiation.

ACTH-Producing Tumors

These are discussed below in the section on the adrenal gland.

The Pituitary Incidentaloma

Autopsy studies suggest that 10%-20% of persons harbor small pituitary tumors. CT or MRI of the head performed for nonendocrine reasons shows mass lesions in the sella >3 mm in 4%-20% of cases. In the management of such a radiologic finding, you should determine the serum levels of PRL, IGF-I, thyroxine, sTSH, LH, FSH, α-glycoprotein subunit, and a.m. cortisol to look for evidence of a hyperfunctioning tumor. If the results of any of these tests are positive, perform the appropriate additional studies. If the results are negative and no extrasellar extension or effects are found, observe and repeat the imaging study in 6-12 months and then later at less frequent intervals. Increase in the size of the incidentaloma dictates surgical intervention.

Empty Sella Syndrome

Primary empty sella syndrome may be a normal variant that is commonly seen in obese females who are evaluated for headache. Many patients, however, have been found to have circulating antipituitary antibodies, indicating a possible autoimmune hypophysitis preceding pituitary atrophy. Some patients with empty sella syndrome who present with headaches have increased intracranial pressure. Visual changes are absent (unless primary empty sella syndrome is associated with increased intracranial pressure). Clinical hypopituitarism is rare, although decreased pituitary reserve by laboratory testing is seen in up to 40% of patients. Primary empty sella syndrome can occur in association with other pituitary disorders, e.g., pituitary microadenomas.

- Primary empty sella syndrome may be a normal variant commonly found in obese females.
- Visual changes are absent.
- Clinical hypopituitarism is rare.
- Primary empty sella syndrome can occur in association with other pituitary disorders.

Secondary empty sella syndrome occurs in the setting of previous pituitary surgery/irradiation or apoplexy, Sheehan's syndrome, hypophysitis, or in idiopathic hypopituitarism. Its presentation includes headaches and visual defects due to traction on the optic pathways. The major diagnostic challenge is to differentiate it from recurrent pituitary tumor.

- Secondary empty sella syndrome: occurs in the setting of previous pituitary surgery/irradiation or apoplexy, Sheehan's syndrome, hypophysitis, or in idiopathic hypopituitarism.
- Presentation: headaches and visual defects.
- Major diagnostic challenge: differentiation from recurrent pituitary tumor.

Radiology of empty sella. A lateral skull film may show the characteristic ballooned or cupped enlarged sella. A radiographic clue may be the presence of myelographic dye in the sella in patients who have had previous myelographic studies. CT or MRI reveals a sella filled with CSF; the stalk is midline and extends down to the compressed pituitary gland in the floor of the sella (Fig. 7-4). The major radiologic diagnostic feature in the differentiation from a cystic pituitary tumor is that in cystic tumors the pituitary stalk is displaced or obscured.

- CT/MRI: sella filled with CSF; stalk is in the midline and extends down to the compressed pituitary gland in the floor of the sella.

Craniopharyngioma

Craniopharyngioma is a slow-growing encapsulated squamous cell tumor originating from remnants of Rathke's pouch. It is the most common pituitary region tumor in childhood but can occur at any age. Two-thirds of the tumors are suprasellar, and one-third originate in or extend into the sella. Most are cystic, and some are solid or mixed. These tumors have a propensity to calcification. The clinical presentation includes obstructive hydrocephalus, hypothalamic syndrome (diabetes insipidus/hyperprolactinemia), chiasmal defects, hypopituitarism, or calcification in or around the sella, as seen incidentally on radiography. Radiography shows calcification in intrasellar or suprasellar regions (75% of children; 25% of adults). CT or MRI reveals a mass or cysts, calcification on CT, and low attenuation values (cholesterol content).

Fig. 7-4.--Magnetic resonance image of case of empty sella syndrome.

- Craniopharyngioma: a slow-growing encapsulated squamous cell tumor.
- The most common pituitary region tumor in children, but these tumors can occur at any age.
- Propensity to calcification.
- Clinical presentation: obstructive hydrocephalus, hypothalamic syndrome, chiasmal defects, hypopituitarism, or calcification in or around sella.

Treatment—Surgery: biopsy for diagnosis; excision is possible for only small craniopharyngiomas. Decompression for large craniopharyngiomas includes cyst puncture and evacuation or subtotal solid mass excision. A ventriculoperitoneal shunt is used for obstructive hydrocephalus. Other treatments include postoperative radiotherapy and management of endocrine dysfunction.

- Treatment: surgical, postoperative radiotherapy, and management of endocrine dysfunction.

Pituitary Apoplexy

Pituitary apoplexy refers to hemorrhagic infarction of the pituitary gland with or without underlying disease. The usual clinical setting is that of a pituitary tumor, irradiated pituitary tumor, pregnancy, anticoagulation, increased intracranial pressure, vascular disease (e.g., diabetes mellitus), or vasculitis (e.g., temporal arteritis). Clinical presentation: 1) asymptomatic if small or gradual bleeding; 2) acute if sudden or large hemorrhage—severe headache, ophthalmoplegia, visual defects, meningismus, depressed sensorium, and acute adrenocortical crisis. Death may occur. The diagnosis is made on the basis of the characteristic clinical, radiologic, and surgical findings. Treatment includes neurosurgical decompression and hormonal support. Late sequelae may include hypopituitarism, secondary empty sella syndrome, or regression of hypersecretory syndrome in infarcted functioning pituitary tumor.

- Pituitary apoplexy: hemorrhagic infarction of pituitary gland with or without underlying disease.
- Acute if sudden or large hemorrhage.
- Severe headache, ophthalmoplegia, visual defects, meningismus, depressed sensorium, and acute adrenocortical crisis.
- Death may occur.
- Characteristic clinical, radiologic, and surgical findings.
- Treatment: neurosurgical decompression and hormonal support.

Lymphocytic Hypophysitis

Lymphocytic hypophysitis is presumed to be of autoimmune origin. It usually occurs in association with other autoimmune endocrinopathies, and it affects adults, predominantly women, especially during pregnancy and the postpartum state.

The clinical presentation may include hypopituitarism or the presence of a sellar mass associated with hyperprolactinemia. The major differential diagnoses are prolactinoma and Sheehan's syndrome. The diagnosis depends on the associations and the results of surgical exploration. No specific therapy is available. Hormonal replacement is given as needed.

- Lymphocytic hypophysitis: autoimmune origin.
- Affects adults, predominantly women, especially during pregnancy and postpartum state.
- Clinical presentation: hypopituitarism; sellar mass associated with hyperprolactinemia.

THE NEUROHYPOPHYSIS

The biologic effects of AVP (or ADH) and its regulatory influences are outlined in Figures 7-5 and 7-6.

Control of water balance. The input and output of water are regulated by changes in the volume of the liquid ingested, which is controlled by thirst, and in urine volume, which is controlled by AVP. Thirst and AVP secretion are regulated primarily by hypothalamic neurons in response to changes in plasma osmolality and volume. Increased plasma osmolality causes shrinkage and stimulation of the hypothalamic osmoreceptors, leading to increased AVP secretion and increased thirst. Osmoreceptors are extremely sensitive to changes in plasma osmolality, even to changes <1%. In extreme circumstances, decreased plasma volume sensed by volume receptors in the atria or pulmonary vessels, carotid sinuses, and aortic arch can also produce increased thirst and AVP secretion. Volume stimuli can override the effects of osmolality stimuli.

- Thirst and AVP secretion: regulated primarily by hypothalamic neurons in response to changes in plasma osmolality and volume.
- Osmoreceptors: extremely sensitive to changes in plasma osmolality, even changes <1%.
- Volume stimuli can override the effects of osmolality stimuli.

Vasopressin Deficiency: Diabetes Insipidus

Etiology

Diabetes insipidus can result from decreased production of AVP ("central diabetes insipidus"), unresponsiveness of renal tissue to AVP ("nephrogenic diabetes insipidus"), or functional suppression of AVP ("primary polydipsia"). The causes of diabetes insipidus are outlined in Table 7-5.

Polyuria (3-15 L/day) and polydipsia, often with preference for ice-cold water, are characteristic. Both of them are almost always accompanied by nocturia, except in psychogenic primary polydipsia. The abrupt onset of symptoms usually points to central diabetes insipidus. No other ill effects are

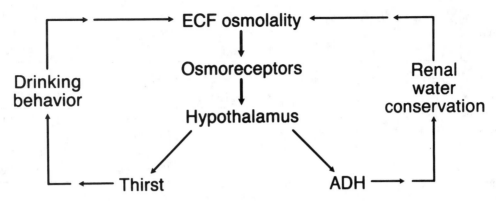

Fig. 7-5. Homeostatic control of extracellular fluid (ECF) osmolality. ADH, antidiuretic hormone.

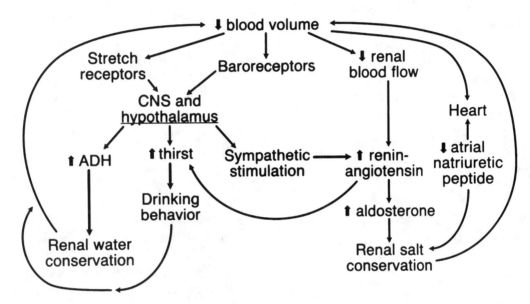

Fig. 7-6. Homeostatic control of blood volume. ADH, antidiuretic hormone; CNS, central nervous system.

seen unless patients do not have access to water. When access to water is restricted, hypertonic encephalopathy and circulatory collapse may ensue. In hypertonic encephalopathy, loss of cellular water leads to brain shrinkage and disturbances of consciousness that range from lethargy to coma. If it develops acutely, mortality is considerable. Those who survive may have permanent neurologic sequelae. If hyperosmolarity develops gradually, the brain adapts by accumulation of idiogenic osmoles and the incidence of encephalopathy is decreased. In childhood, dilatation of the bladder, ureters, and renal pelvis may occur.

- Diabetes insipidus characteristics: polyuria (3-15 L/day) and polydipsia, with preference for ice-cold water.
- Abrupt onset of symptoms usually points to central diabetes insipidus.
- When access to water is restricted, hypertonic encephalopathy and circulatory collapse may ensue.

Diagnostic Approach

The diagnosis consists of: 1) a careful and complete clinical evaluation to rule out solute diuresis (e.g., diabetes mellitus), electrolyte abnormalities (hypercalcemia, hypokalemia), associated diseases (e.g., sickle cell disease), and drugs. 2) Check random plasma and urine osmolality values and, if necessary, perform the water deprivation/exogenous AVP test. Plasma and urine osmolalities in different types of diabetes insipidus are shown in Table 7-6.

The responses of patients with different types of diabetes insipidus to water deprivation/exogenous AVP test are shown in Table 7-7.

Consider compulsive water drinking if urine volume is >18 L/24 hours, random plasma osmolality is <285 mOsm/kg, or if symptoms are intermittent or have varying intensity.

The water deprivation test: begin the night before the test in patients with mild polyuria, and start the morning of the test in patients with severe symptoms. Keep a careful watch on

Table 7-5.--Causes of Vasopressin Deficiency (Diabetes Insipidus)

AVP-deficient (neurogenic, hypothalamic, or central)
  Idiopathic
    Familial--autosomal dominant
    Sporadic--30%-40% of all cases
  Secondary
    Congenital
    Trauma--surgical, accident
    Inflammation
      Infections--meningitis, encephalitis, etc.
      Granulomatous--sarcoidosis, histiocytosis
    Vascular--Sheehan's syndrome, aneurysms, vasculitis, etc.
    Neoplasia
      Primary hypothalamic
      Extrahypothalamic--craniopharyngioma
      Metastatic
AVP-resistant (nephrogenic)
  Idiopathic
    Familial--X-linked recessive
    Sporadic
  Secondary
    Metabolic--hypercalcemia, hypokalemia
    Toxic--lithium, demeclocycline, methoxyflurane, colchicine
    Vascular--sickle cell disease or trait
    Inflammatory--pyelonephritis, sarcoidosis, Sjögren's syndrome
    Degenerative--amyloidosis
    Postobstructive
    Polycystic disease
Primary polydipsia
  Psychogenic
  Dipsogenic
    Idiopathic
    Secondary--sarcoidosis, vasculitis, etc.
    Drug-induced--thioridazine, chlorpromazine
AVP-resistant diabetes insipidus of pregnancy
  Presence of vasopressinase (rare)

Table 7-6.--Plasma and Urine Osmolality in Different Types of Diabetes Insipidus

Osmolality		
Plasma	Urine	Diagnosis
Decreased	Decreased	Primary polydipsia
Increased	Decreased	Central or nephrogenic diabetes insipidus
Normal	Decreased	Any type of diabetes insipidus

Table 7-7.--Water Deprivation/Exogenous Vasopressin Test

Water conservation	Response to vasopressin	Diagnosis
Normal	Absent	Primary polydipsia
Impaired	Present	Central diabetes insipidus
Impaired	Absent	Nephrogenic diabetes insipidus

the patient's state of hydration, weight, and blood pressure.

Give exogenous AVP when two sequential urine osmolalities vary by <30 mOsm/kg or when 3%-5% of body weight is lost.

A normal person, in the face of water deprivation, produces AVP and has maximal distal nephron responsiveness to it. Exogenous AVP adds <5% increase in urine osmolality. Patients with central diabetes insipidus do not respond to water deprivation; their AVP levels remain low (< 2 pg/mL). They have >50% increase in urine osmolality after administration of exogenous AVP. Patients with nephrogenic diabetes insipidus have maximal endogenous secretory response and AVP levels >10-20 pg/mL, but they do not respond to exogenous water deprivation or to exogenous AVP. Patients with primary polydipsia have a normal AVP axis, and their response to dehydration is limited only by the renal medullary concentration gradient, which may be reduced because of the "washout" of water diuresis; therefore, they concentrate the urine to a variable degree and do not show further response to exogenous AVP.

After diabetes insipidus and its type have been diagnosed, appropriate studies are needed to define the cause. In cases of central diabetes insipidus, perform CT or MRI, examine the visual fields, and assess anterior pituitary function. Imaging may reveal a mass lesion in the hypothalamic-pituitary region; thickening of the stalk may be an early sign of histiocytosis X or suprasellar germinoma. Diagnostic pitfalls include differentiating partial central diabetes insipidus, partial nephrogenic diabetes insipidus, and primary polydipsia with renal medullary washout. These are best differentiated by plotting plasma osmolality against plasma AVP values obtained during the water deprivation test and using standard nomograms

- After diagnosing diabetes insipidus and its type, determine the cause.
- In central diabetes insipidus, perform CT or MRI, examine the visual fields, and assess anterior pituitary function.

Therapy

There is no need for drug therapy for patients with mild diabetes insipidus (urine output, 2-5 L/day) and free access to water. For central diabetes insipidus, desmopressin acetate (DDAVP) is currently the drug of choice. It is administered by nasal instillation or spray in a dose of 5-10 μg once or twice daily. As yet, oral desmopressin is not approved in the U.S. Desmopressin is also available for parenteral use in a solution of 4 μg/mL; the usual dose is 0.5 to 2 μg. For patients with partial central diabetes insipidus, AVP agonists such as chlorpropamide (250-500 mg/day; carbamazepine is less desirable) or thiazides such as hydrochlorothiazide (50-100 mg daily) can be used. Note that the effect of thiazides, which is primarily due to volume contraction, is diminished by ample salt intake. For nephrogenic diabetes insipidus, thiazides are the only treatment available.

- No need for drug therapy in patients with mild diabetes insipidus and free access to water.
- For treating central diabetes insipidus, desmopressin acetate is the drug of choice.
- For treating partial central diabetes insipidus, use AVP agonists such as chlorpropamide, 250-500 mg/day.
- For nephrogenic diabetes insipidus, thiazides are the only treatment available.

The treatment of hypertonic encephalopathy includes the gradual replenishment of body water, which should be administered at a rate to decrease the serum concentration of sodium by 1 mEq/L every 2 hours. Caution: rapid repletion leads to translocation of water into brain cells and cerebral edema. If volume contraction is mild, use hypotonic saline. If volume contraction is significant, treat initially with normal saline to restore volume; 5% dextrose in water can be used in the absence of circulatory insufficiency; the rate should be less than that which induces glycosuria.

Vasopressin Hypersecretion: Syndrome of Inappropriate ADH

Pathophysiology

For the clinical expression of the syndrome, AVP excess and continued water intake should be present. Renal retention of water leads to hypo-osmolality of extracellular body fluids and hyponatremia, relative hyperosmolality of urine (usually >300 mOsm/kg), and increased extracellular fluid volume. Expansion of the extracellular fluid volume produces increased glomerular filtration rate, increased atrial natriuretic peptide secretion, and suppression of the renin-aldosterone system. Natriuresis follows. Syndrome of inappropriate ADH is also characterized by the absence of edema and low serum levels of creatinine and uric acid. This syndrome is often asymptomatic, particularly if the hyponatremia is mild or has

developed gradually over a few weeks to months. Otherwise, frequent symptoms are anorexia, nausea, or vomiting. If hyponatremia is severe or develops acutely, CNS dysfunction occurs, with symptoms of cerebral edema, irritability, confusion, or convulsions. Coma may occur.

- Syndrome of inappropriate ADH: basic events are AVP excess and continued water intake.
- Relative hypo-osmolality of body fluids, relative hyperosmolality of urine, and increased extracellular fluid volume.
- Natriuresis; absence of edema.
- Often asymptomatic, particularly if hyponatremia is mild or has developed gradually.
- Anorexia, nausea, or vomiting are frequent symptoms.
- In severe or acute hyponatremia, CNS dysfunction occurs.

The causes of hypersecretion of AVP are outlined in Table 7-8.

Diagnostic Approach

1) Is hyponatremia present? Check serum concentration of sodium. If it is normal, and syndrome of inappropriate ADH is still suspected, consider water loading. 2) Is it true hyponatremia? Check serum osmolality. Rule out factitial (hyperlipidemia, hyperproteinemia, or hyperglycemia) and hyperosmolar states (e.g., hyperglycemia). 3) Is it due to syndrome of inappropriate ADH? Rule out appropriate AVP excess, and exclude generalized edema, volume depletion, cortisol deficiency, and thyroid deficiency. 4) What is the cause of the syndrome? Look for a eutopic or ectopic disorder.

- Check the serum concentration of sodium; if normal, consider water loading.
- Is it true hyponatremia? Check serum osmolality.
- Is it due to syndrome of inappropriate ADH? Rule out appropriate AVP excess.
- What is the cause of syndrome of inappropriate ADH? Look for eutopic or ectopic disorder.

The major diagnostic challenge is to differentiate syndrome of inappropriate ADH from subclinical hypovolemia. Consider urine concentration of sodium, serum levels of creatinine and uric acid, and plasma renin activity.

- Major challenge: distinguishing syndrome of inappropriate ADH from subclinical hypovolemia.

Treatment

The treatment of syndrome of inappropriate ADH includes 1) water restriction to 800-1,000 mL daily. Follow patient's weight and serum concentration of sodium. 2) Use AVP antagonists if necessary: demeclocycline, 900-1,200 mg/day. Lithium is not recommended because of its potential serious

Table 7-8.--Causes of Hypersecretion of Vasopressin

Vasopressin hypersecretion
    Physiologic or appropriate ADH secretion
        Hyperosmolar states
        Decreased effective blood volume/pressure
            States with generalized edema
            States with volume depletion
    Pathologic or inappropriate ADH secretion
        Exogenous
            AVP or its analogues
            Oxytocin
        Ectopic
            Malignancy
                Cancer--bronchus, pancreas, ureter, prostate,
                    bladder
                Lymphoma, leukemia
                Thymoma, mesothelioma
        Benign pulmonary disorders
            Pneumonia, lung abscess, empyema,
                pneumothorax
            Tuberculosis, cystic fibrosis
            Asthma, positive pressure breathing
      Eutopic
        Central nervous system/hypothalamic disease of
           diverse causes
            Traumatic
            Inflammatory/degenerative
            Vascular
            Neoplastic
        Drugs that stimulate AVP secretion and/or
           action--vincristine, vinblastine, cyclophospha-
           mide, phenothiazines, monoamine oxidase
           inhibitors, tricyclic antidepressant agents,
           chlorpropamide, clofibrate, carbamazepine,
           nicotine
        Postoperative period
        Old age

side effects. 3) If acute neurologic sequelae are present, give hypertonic saline intravenously, 200-300 mL of 5% NaCl over 3-4 hours. Achieve a gradual increase in serum Na (do not exceed 0.5 mEq/hour or 12 mEq/24 hours); continue hypertonic saline until neurologic symptoms cease and a "safe" serum Na level of 120 mEq/L is reached. Rapid correction of hyponatremia can lead to central pontine myelinolysis, which is often fatal. 4) Identify and correct the cause.

- Treatment of syndrome of inappropriate ADH: water restriction.
- AVP antagonists, if necessary.
- For acute neurologic sequelae, hypertonic saline.
- Rapid correction of hyponatremia can lead to central pontine myelinolysis.
- Identify and correct the cause.

THYROID DISORDERS

Physiology

The normal hypothalamic-pituitary-thyroid axis is shown in Figure 7-7. Euthyroidism is maintained by a negative feedback system. TRH is the dominant hypothalamic regulator of TSH secretion. Thyroid hormones feed back principally at the pituitary level: triiodothyronine (T_3) directly and T_4 mainly by its intracellular monodeiodination to T_3. T_4 is produced exclusively by the thyroid gland. T_3 has two sources: 20% from the thyroid and 80% from peripheral deiodination of T_4. Peripheral deiodination of T_4 by deiodinase can lead to the formation of T_3, the bioactive hormone, or reverse T_3, which is bioinert. Thyroid hormones circulate in two forms: bound to binding proteins (thyroxine-binding globulin [TBG], thyroxine-binding prealbumin [TBPA], albumin) and free. (99.95% of T_4 and 99.50% of T_3 are bound, and 0.05% of T_4 and 0.50% of T_3 are free.) The free hormone is the physiologically active component responsible for thyroid function. The bound hormone is bioinert; its quantity depends on availability and affinity of binding proteins.

- Euthyroidism is maintained by a negative feedback system.
- TRH is the dominant hypothalamic regulator of TSH secretion.
- T_4 is produced exclusively by the thyroid gland.
- T_3 has two sources: 20% from the thyroid and 80% from peripheral deiodination of T_4.
- Thyroid hormones circulate in two forms: bound and free.
- T_4: 99.95% bound and 0.05% free.
- T_3: 99.50% bound and 0.50% free.

Assessment of the Thyroid Axis

1. Serum T_4. The two determinants are thyroid function and the quantity and quality of binding proteins. *Decreased* T_4: hypothyroidism, euthyroid patients with low concentration of binding proteins in the serum (androgen and anabolic steroid therapy, glucocorticoid excess, chronic liver disease, acromegaly, genetic TBG deficiency), and euthyroid sick syndrome. *Increased* T_4: thyrotoxicosis, euthyroid patients with increased TBG (estrogen use, pregnancy, acute hepatitis, acute intermittent porphyria, perphenazine use, and familial TBG excess), patients with genetic excess in albumin or prealbumin-binding protein, peripheral resistance to thyroid hormones, and euthyroid sick syndrome.

2. Serum T_3. Determinants: thyroid function, conversion of T_4 to T_3 in peripheral tissues, and binding proteins. *Decreased* T_3: hypothyroidism; euthyroid state in the neonate, elderly, euthyroid sick syndrome, and patients with caloric deprivation; use of drugs such as propranolol, glucocorticoids, certain iodinated contrast agents,

Fig. 7-7. The hypothalamic-pituitary-thyroid axis. CNS, central nervous system; TRH, thyrotropin-releasing hormone; TSH, thyroid-stimulating hormone; T_3, triiodothyronine; T_4, thyroxine.

and amiodarone that block T_4 to T_3 conversion; and states with decreased TBG levels. *Increased* T_3: thyrotoxicosis (including the T_3 toxicosis variety), euthyroid patients with TBG excess, and peripheral hormone resistance.

3. Free T_4. The determinant is thyroid function. *Decreased* free T_4: hypothyroidism and euthyroid sick syndrome. *Increased* free T_4: hyperthyroidism and euthyroid patients with euthyroid sick syndrome or peripheral hormone resistance.

4. FTI. Determinants: total T_4 and resin T_3 uptake (an indirect measure of TBG). FTI is equivalent to the free T_4. *Decreased* FTI: hypothyroidism and euthyroid sick syndrome. *Increased* FTI: hyperthyroidism; euthyroid patients with euthyroid sick syndrome, peripheral hormone resistance, genetic albumin and prealbumin-binding protein excess, and anti-T_4 antibodies.

5. Serum sTSH. With each successive generation of sTSH, sensitivity is increased tenfold. It clearly delineates low-normal from low values. Its major impact: a) diagnosis of hyperthyroidism: sTSH is low or undetectable in all types of thyrotoxicosis except that due to a TSH-producing tumor, and b) monitoring replacement or suppressive thyroid hormone therapy. Serum sTSH can be used alone as a thyroid function screening test in outpatients. A normal sTSH value implies absence of thyroid dysfunction, and no further studies are indicated. If sTSH is increased, determine FTI: in primary hypothyroidism, FTI is decreased, whereas it is increased in TSH-producing tumor. If sTSH is decreased, determine FTI: increased levels are found in thyrotoxicosis; decreased levels point to central hypothyroidism.

6. Thyroid scanning. The main indications for thyroid scanning are the documentation of thyroid agenesis/dysgenesis and ectopic thyroid and the evaluation of nodular goiter, retrosternal goiter, struma ovarii, or metastatic-functioning thyroid tumor.

7. Radioactive iodine (^{131}I) uptake. A 24-hour ^{131}I uptake is indicated for a) the differential diagnosis of thyrotoxicosis with diffuse goiter (Graves' disease [high uptake]; silent thyroiditis [low]), b) the diagnosis of silent or subacute thyroiditis (low), c) the diagnosis of exogenous or ectopic hyperthyroidism (low), d) pre-^{131}I treatment of thyrotoxicosis, and e) postoperative management and follow-up of differentiated thyroid malignancy.

8. Serum level of thyroglobulin. Although thyroglobulin levels can be increased in many benign or malignant thyroid disorders, their main clinical usefulness is as a tumor marker for follow-up of differentiated thyroid carcinoma and in distinguishing between silent thyroiditis (high serum level) and exogenous hyperthyroidism (low).

9. TSH receptor-stimulating immunoglobulins. These are markers for Graves' disease and are helpful in diagnosing euthyroid endocrine ophthalmopathy, predicting relapse of drug-treated Graves' disease, and predicting neonatal thyrotoxicosis in an infant born to a mother with present or past history of Graves' disease.

10. Antithyroglobulin and antimicrosomal antibodies. These usually are used to assess the presence of autoimmune thyroid disorder. The antimicrosomal antibodies are more specific as indicators of such a disorder. Highest titers occur in Hashimoto's thyroiditis (95%). Lower titers are found in primary atrophic hypothyroidism and Graves' disease, and modest or low titers can be found

in other autoimmune disorders (e.g., systemic lupus erythematosus and rheumatoid arthritis). Negative test results do not exclude the presence of autoimmune thyroid disease.

11. Thyroid ultrasonography. Potential indications include assessing thyroid size and configuration, assessing nodular goiter size and consistency of the nodule, and following up thyroid malignancy to demonstrate preclinical cervical metastatic nodes.

Hypothyroidism

The causes of hypothyroidism are outlined in Table 7-9.

Atypical Presentations: The Great Mimicker

- Neuropsychiatric: dementia, dysarthria, deafness, cerebellar ataxia, carpal tunnel syndrome, peripheral neuropathy, or psychoneurosis/psychoses.
- Cardiopulmonary: hypertension, cardiomegaly/failure, pericardial/pleural effusions, or respiratory depression.
- Gastrointestinal: constipation, ileus, or ascites.
- Genitourinary: potency impairment in males and menorrhagia, dysmenorrhea, or amenorrhea/galactorrhea in females.
- Musculoskeletal: arthritis or cramps/stiffness.
- Hematologic: normocytic, macrocytic, or microcytic anemia.
- Endocrine: growth retardation, abnormalities of sexual maturation, galactorrhea, associated autoimmune endocrinopathies, or syndrome of inappropriate ADH.
- Metabolic/laboratory findings: hyperlipidemia, hypercalcemia, hyperuricemia, or increased serum glutamic-oxaloacetic transaminase (SGOT)-lactic dehydrogenase (LDH)-creatine phosphokinase (CPK).

Diagnostic Approach

The diagnosis of hypothyroidism is based on the assessment of clinical features and the evaluation of the results of FTI and sTSH. The diagnostic process should delineate the presence of hypothyroidism, its type (whether primary or central), its cause, and whether it is reversible.

- Diagnosis of hypothyroidism: assessment of the clinical features and the results of FTI and sTSH.

Diagnostic clues: 1) normal FTI and sTSH exclude hypothyroidism; 2) normal FTI and high sTSH point to subclinical hypothyroidism; 3) low FTI and high sTSH point to primary hypothyroidism (rule out reversible causes and associated autoimmune disease); 4) low FTI and low sTSH point to hypothalamic-pituitary disease (check other pituitary functions and perform radiologic studies); 5) high FTI and high sTSH point to peripheral resistance to thyroid hormone.

Table 7-9.--Causes of Hypothyroidism

Primary thyroid failure (95% of cases)
Permanent--Hashimoto's thyroiditis, primary atrophic, postablative (surgery, radioiodide, radiation), others
Reversible--hypothyroid phase of subacute or silent thyroiditis, iodide deficiency, goitrogens (iodides, antithyroid agents, lithium)
Secondary/tertiary failure or central hypothyroidism (5% of cases)
Permanent--organic hypothalamic-pituitary disease, postpartum necrosis, tumors, others
Reversible--withdrawal of thyroid hormone therapy in euthyroid person
Tissue resistance to thyroid hormone (rare)

- Normal FTI, high sTSH: subclinical hypothyroidism.
- Low FTI, high sTSH: primary hypothyroidism.
- Low FTI, low sTSH: hypothalamic-pituitary disease.
- High FTI, high sTSH: peripheral resistance to thyroid hormone.

Hashimoto's thyroiditis is a common form of thyroiditis and is the most common cause of spontaneous primary hypothyroidism. It can affect any age or sex, but predominantly older women. It is familial and tends to occur in association with other autoimmune disorders. Two morphological types occur: goitrous and atrophic. It is commonly encountered in clinical practice: antimicrosomal antibodies occur in 10% of women and 3% of men; 10%-20% of patients have subclinical hypothyroidism.

- Hashimoto's thyroiditis affects predominantly older women.
- It is an autoimmune disorder and occurs in association with other autoimmune disorders.
- It is familial.
- 10%-20% of patients have subclinical hypothyroidism.

In Hashimoto's thyroiditis, the size of the goiter is variable and the texture is rubbery to firm. It usually is diffuse but may be nodular. The patient may be euthyroid or hypothyroid, and the hypothyroidism may be overt or subclinical. Occasionally, Hashimoto's thyroiditis may present with thyrotoxicosis, indistinguishable from Graves' disease. Postpartum thyroiditis is believed to be a variant of Hashimoto's thyroiditis (see Hyperthyroidism).

- Goiter: variable size, rubbery to firm, usually diffuse (may be nodular).
- Euthyroid or hypothyroid; hypothyroidism may be overt or subclinical.

• May present with postpartum thyroid dysfunction.

Laboratory evaluation in Hashimoto's thyroiditis. Antimicrosomal antibodies (antigen is thyroid peroxidase), 95% of patients; antithyroglobulin antibodies, 50%-60%. FTI and sTSH may reveal euthyroidism, subclinical primary hypothyroidism, or overt primary hypothyroidism. Radioiodide uptake is variable, and isotopic scan usually shows heterogeneous uptake; these tests are not indicated. Fine needle aspiration may be needed in the evaluation of "nodular goiter." In Hashimoto's thyroiditis, it shows the characteristic lymphocytic infiltration.

• Antimicrosomal antibodies (antigen in thyroid peroxidase), 95% of patients; antithyroglobulin antibodies, 50%-60%.
• FTI and sTSH may show euthyroidism, subclinical primary hypothyroidism, or overt primary hypothyroidism.

Radiation thyroiditis is another major cause of hypothyroidism in the U.S. It is a common and permanent result of radioiodine therapy for Graves' disease. It may also result from external neck irradiation exceeding 25 Gy, as used in the management of lymphoma and cancers of the head and neck. Hypothyroidism can develop within 3-6 months after therapy. Transient reversible hypothyroidism may occur in hypothyroid phases of subacute or silent thyroiditis and, in susceptible patients, with the use of goitrogens such as excess iodides or lithium.

Iodide deficiency is the most common cause of hypothyroidism on a worldwide basis.

Secondary, or central, hypothyroidism may result from any cause of hypothalamic-pituitary disease. The most common cause is a functioning or nonfunctioning pituitary adenoma. It is characterized by decreased TSH production and atrophy of the thyroid gland. It may be associated with other pituitary hormone(s) deficiency. It is important to remember that primary hypothyroidism may lead to hypothalamic-pituitary dysfunction. It may cause 1) hyperprolactinemia, sometimes with pituitary enlargement (due to thyrotroph hyperplasia), and may mimic a prolactinoma; the hyperprolactinemia resolves and enlargement regresses with T_4 therapy; 2) GH deficiency; 3) hypogonadotropism; and 4) inappropriate ADH secretion. Rarely, it can cause sexual precocity in children.

Therapy

Synthetic T_4 is the drug of choice: it is well absorbed from the gastrointestinal tract (>90%); its long half-life (>7 days) allows single daily dosing; and serum levels of T_4 and T_3 (derived from conversion of T_4 to T_3 by the peripheral tissues) are stable. Select and stay with a particular manufacturer's preparation. Some generic preparations may have variable standardization of drug potency and are preferably avoided. Dessicated thyroid extract or T_3-containing preparations are

not recommended (T_3 has a short half-life [<1 day], need for multiple daily dosing, leads to intermittently high serum levels of T_3, and the serum level of T_4 cannot be used to monitor therapy).

The usual replacement dose is 1.5 mg T_4/kg, and the average dose is 0.1 mg/day. Start low and increase the dose slowly every 3-4 weeks (except in young patients or if hypothyroidism is of recent onset). Monitor sTSH and clinical response in primary hypothyroidism: the therapeutic goal is a normal sTSH. After the proper dose is achieved, continue to monitor therapy every 6-12 months. In patients with primary hypothyroidism receiving previously documented adequate therapy, an increase in sTSH may indicate substandard medication, poor compliance, malabsorption (e.g., bile acid sequestrant therapy, use of ferrous sulphate or sucralfate), ongoing progressive thyroid disease, or increased hormone clearance (pregnancy or the use of phenytoin or rifampin). A decrease in sTSH may indicate reduced requirements of aging, patient's self-induced overmedication, regeneration of autonomous thyroid remnant, or decreased clearance. In central hypothyroidism, the therapeutic goal is the patient's well-being and a normal serum level of free T_4 or FTI.

• Synthetic T_4 is the drug of choice.
• Start low and increase slowly (except in young patients or if hypothyroidism is of recent onset).
• Monitor sTSH and clinical response in primary hypothyroidism.
• Monitor clinical response and serum level of free T_4 or FTI in central hypothyroidism.

With initiation of T_4 therapy, watch for a change in dosage needs of oral anticoagulants (decrease) and of insulin/oral antidiabetic agents (increase). Women with primary hypothyroidism who become pregnant may need higher T_4 dosage during pregnancy because of increased clearance to maintain euthyroidism. Check sTSH periodically, and adjust dosage if necessary, but avoid overreplacement. In the postpartum period, decrease the dosage of T_4 to prepregnancy levels.

Hypothyroidism does not contraindicate urgent surgery, but caution needs to be exerted with regard to dosing with anesthetics, sedatives, or narcotics and to the decreased ability to excrete a water load. In a hypothyroid patient with coronary heart disease, the dangers of thyroid hormone therapy are worsening of the ischemic pains, induction of arrhythmias, and myocardial infarction. Start treatment with T_4 at a low level (12.5-25 µg/day) and increase slowly by 12.5-25 µg every 3-4 weeks. If ischemic pain worsens, decrease the dose; 40% of patients with angina cannot tolerate a full T_4 replacement dose.

Replacement therapy for subclinical hypothyroidism is a matter of controversy. Of middle-aged and elderly patients, particularly women, 20%-40% may progress to overt hypothyroidism in few years. T_4 treatment is advised for those patients who have had ^{131}I therapy for Graves' disease or who are likely to have Hashimoto's thyroiditis (i.e., who have a goiter, antimicrosomal antibodies, or a personal/family history of autoimmune disorders).

Management of Hashimoto's thyroiditis. For euthyroid goiter, T_4 therapy may be considered to decrease goiter size (successful in 50% of patients) and to preempt development of hypothyroidism (5%-10%/year). For subclinical or overt hypothyroidism, T_4 therapy. For obstructive goiter, surgical decompression/excision if no response to T_4 treatment. For thyrotoxicosis, treat as for Graves' disease.

Hyperthyroidism

The causes of hyperthyroidism are outlined in Table 7-10.

Graves' Disease

Graves' disease is an autoimmune, multisystem disease characterized by the triad of hyperthyroidism, diffuse goiter, and mesenchymal extrathyroidal manifestations of ophthalmopathy, dermopathy, and thyroid acropachy. These manifestations can occur singly or in combination. Graves' disease is the most common cause of hyperthyroidism. Although it is seen most often in young females, it can occur at any age and in either sex. There is a strong familial predisposition. The immediate cause of the hyperthyroidism is the production of thyroid-stimulating autoantibodies that bind to the TSH receptor, activating it and causing cellular growth and increased hormonogenesis. Spontaneous remissions can occur. The goiter is usually 2x-3x normal size, diffuse, smooth, and somewhat firm. Twenty percent of the patients, especially the elderly, may not have a palpable goiter. The two types of ocular findings are infiltrative and noninfiltrative. The infiltrative findings (lid puffiness, chemosis, proptosis, extraocular muscle dysfunction, optic neuritis, or atrophy) are specific for Graves' disease. The noninfiltrative findings (lid lag and lid retraction) can occur with any type of thyrotoxicosis. Localized pretibial myxedema (raised thickened peau d'orange changes usually affecting the dorsum of the feet and legs) occurs in patients who either have or have had Graves' thyroid disease and ophthalmopathy. Thyroid acropachy may accompany the dermal changes.

- Graves' disease: an autoimmune multisystem disease.
- Characteristic triad: hyperthyroidism, diffuse goiter, and mesenchymal extrathyroidal effects (ophthalmopathy, dermopathy, and thyroid acropachy).
- It is the most common cause of hyperthyroidism.
- Strong familial predisposition.
- Immediate cause of hyperthyroidism: production of thyroid-stimulating antibodies.
- 20% of patients, especially elderly, may not have goiter.
- Two types of ocular findings: infiltrative and noninfiltrative.
- Infiltrative findings: specific for Graves' disease.
- Noninfiltrative findings: can occur with any type of thyrotoxicosis.

Table 7-10.--Causes of Hyperthyroidism

Exogenous
  Thyroid hormones
  Iodides
Endogenous
  Eutopic
    Primary thyroid disease
      Nodular goiter--single, multiple
      Thyroiditis--silent, subacute
      Follicular carcinoma
    Abnormal thyroid regulation
      Autoimmune
        Antibody-mediated--Graves' disease
      TSH--pituitary tumor
      hCG--hydatidiform mole
  Ectopic
    Struma ovarii

Toxic Multinodular Goiter

Toxic multinodular goiter is a disease of the elderly and occurs in patients who have had a long-standing simple nodular goiter with autonomy in one or more nodules. The hyperthyroidism is usually less severe than that of Graves' disease and may be characterized by the dominance of organ-specific manifestations. Cardiovascular effects (arrhythmias, congestive heart failure), weakness (and frequently muscle wasting), loss of appetite, and listlessness may dominate the picture—the so-called apathetic hyperthyroidism. The goiter is usually large, nodular, and asymmetrical; it may be difficult to palpate in some patients because of either a short neck or substernal extension.

- Toxic multinodular goiter: disease of the elderly.
- Occurs in patients with long-standing simple nodular goiter with autonomy in one or more nodules.
- Hyperthyroidism may be characterized by the dominance of organ-specific manifestations.
- The goiter may be difficult to palpate because of a short neck or substernal extension.

Toxic Adenoma

Toxic adenoma is caused by a hyperfunctioning autonomous follicular adenoma and is seen most often in middle-aged women. The solitary nodule is >3 cm in diameter, easily palpable, and firm. Radioisotopic scan shows intense uptake in the nodule, with no uptake in the rest of the gland.

- Solitary nodule: >3 cm in diameter, easily palpable, and firm.
- Radioisotopic scan: intense uptake in nodule but none elsewhere.

Thyroiditis

Thyrotoxicosis can occur in thyroiditis because of release of stored hormone from the inflamed, damaged thyroid follicles. It is transient and lasts a few weeks, until the hormone stores are depleted. A short period of hypothyroidism may ensue until the thyroid recovers. Thyroiditis-induced thyrotoxicosis can be caused by subacute thyroiditis and by painless lymphocytic thyroiditis (see below).

- Thyrotoxicosis can occur in thyroiditis through release of stored hormone from damaged thyroid follicles.
- It is transient, lasting a few weeks.
- A short period of hypothyroidism may occur until the thyroid recovers.
- It can be caused by subacute thyroiditis or painless lymphocytic thyroiditis.

Painless Lymphocytic Thyroiditis

Painless lymphocytic thyroiditis is probably a variant of Hashimoto's thyroiditis. It occurs most commonly in females, especially in the postpartum period. This type of hyperthyroidism may account for 5%-20% of all cases of hyperthyroidism. It is usually mild and transient, lasting for several weeks, and, in about one-third of patients, may be followed by transient hypothyroidism lasting several weeks. The small diffuse, painless, nontender goiter may be firm. Painless lymphocytic thyroiditis has a tendency to recur, especially in subsequent pregnancies. In the hyperthyroid phase, FTI is increased and sTSH is suppressed; uptake of ^{131}I is suppressed. Antithyroid antibodies are normal or modestly increased; leukocyte count is normal, and erythrocyte sedimentation rate is normal or slightly increased. There is no associated ophthalmopathy or dermopathy. The differential diagnosis includes Graves' disease and factitial hyperthyroidism. 1) Graves' disease with iodide exposure and low uptake of ^{131}I: history of iodide exposure and high urinary iodide. 2) Factitial hyperthyroidism: no goiter, ^{131}I uptake is low, and the serum thyroglobulin level is low (in contrast to painless thyroiditis, in which the serum thyroglobulin level is high).

Painless lymphocytic thyroiditis is self-limiting, and the thyroid dysfunction is transient. No treatment is required for most patients. Use β-blockers if hyperthyroidism is symptomatic. Symptomatic hypothyroidism may have to be treated with T_4 for a few months. If recurrences are significant, the gland may have to be ablated with ^{131}I in the euthyroid state to prevent recurrences. Annual follow-up of thyroid function is needed because of the increased risk of permanent hypothyroidism.

- Painless lymphocytic thyroiditis: most common in females, especially in the postpartum period (5%-10% incidence).
- This type of hyperthyroidism may account for 5%-20% of all cases of hyperthyroidism.

- It is usually mild and transient.
- It may be followed by transient hypothyroidism in about a third of patients.
- Tendency to recur.
- FTI is increased, sTSH is suppressed, low uptake of ^{131}I, and antithyroid antibodies are normal or modestly increased.
- No associated ophthalmopathy or dermopathy.
- Disease is self-limiting.
- No treatment is required in most patients.
- The major differential diagnosis is Graves' disease with expanded iodide pool and factitial hyperthyroidism.

Exogenous Hyperthyroidism

Exogenous hyperthyroidism can be caused by prescribed or factitiously ingested thyroid hormone(s), ingestion of iodides in susceptible persons (see below), or ingestion of ground meat contaminated with thyroid tissue. Factitial thyrotoxicosis should be suspected in thyrotoxic patients with no palpable goiter who have suppressed ^{131}I uptake and low serum levels of thyroglobulin.

- Causes of exogenous hyperthyroidism: prescribed or factitiously ingested thyroid hormone(s), ingestion of iodides, and ingestion of ground meat contaminated with thyroid tissue.
- Factitial thyrotoxicosis is suspected in thyrotoxic patients with no palpable goiter, suppressed ^{131}I uptake, and low serum levels of thyroglobulin.

Atypical Presentations of Hyperthyroidism

Cardiac: tachyarrhythmias, congestive heart failure, or systolic hypertension. Gastrointestinal: hyperdefecation, chronic diarrhea, or increased alkaline phosphatase and other liver enzymes. Reproductive: oligomenorrhea/amenorrhea or gynecomastia in men. Neurologic: myopathy or hypokalemic periodic paralyses, particularly in Asian males. Metabolic bone disease: osteoporosis.

Diagnostic Approach

- FTI and sTSH are the cornerstones of laboratory diagnoses.
- Serum T_3 assay may be needed in the 10%-20% of patients who present with T_3 toxicosis. ^{131}I uptake is needed in the differential diagnosis of hyperthyroidism with diffuse goiter, in the diagnosis of hyperthyroidism associated with thyroiditis or ectopic struma ovarii, and with the use of exogenous thyroid hormones.
- TRH test is needed rarely and has been replaced by the sTSH assay.
- Normal FTI and normal sTSH exclude hyperthyroidism.
- High FTI and low sTSH indicate euthyroid sick syndrome or thyrotoxicosis of any type except TSH tumor.

- Low FTI and low sTSH indicate the need for serum T_3 assay. Increased T_3 points to T_3 toxicosis; if T_3 is low, think of euthyroid sick syndrome or hypothalamic-pituitary disease.
- High FTI and high sTSH point to TSH-producing tumor or peripheral hormone resistance.
- Presence of mesenchymal manifestations of infiltrative ophthalmopathy in a hyperthyroid patient points to Graves' disease.
- Diffuse goiter; no mesenchymal manifestations: decreased sTSH and increased ^{131}I uptake = Graves' disease. Decreased sTSH and decreased ^{131}I uptake = silent thyroiditis. Normal or increased sTSH = TSH-producing tumor.
- Nodular goiter: single = toxic nodule, multinodular = toxic multinodular goiter, and metastasis = follicular carcinoma.
- Painful tender goiter = subacute thyroiditis (increased erythrocyte sedimentation rate and decreased radioiodine uptake).
- No goiter and presence of pelvic mass = struma ovarii; otherwise, exogenous or factitial thyrotoxicosis.

T_3 toxicosis: the serum level of T_4 is low (without deficiency of binding proteins) and the serum level of T_3 is increased. It occurs in about 20% of patients with thyrotoxicosis and may develop in any type of thyrotoxicosis. It may be the first manifestation of hyperthyroidism and may herald relapses and recurrences of the disease. It may also be caused by exogenous supraphysiologic T_3 therapy.

- T_3 toxicosis: low serum level of T_4 without deficiency of binding proteins and increased serum level of T_3.
- T_3 toxicosis: occurs in about 20% of patients with thyrotoxicosis.
- It may be the first manifestation of hyperthyroidism.
- It may herald relapses and recurrences.

T_4 toxicosis: the serum level of T_4 is increased, with a normal or low serum level of T_3. This may occur in the thyrotoxic elderly or sick. It usually is seen in the hospital setting. T_4 toxicosis is due to a decrease in the conversion of T_4 to T_3.

- T_4 toxicosis: the serum level of T_4 is increased, with a normal or low serum level of T_3.
- It may occur in the thyrotoxic elderly or sick and is usually seen in the hospital setting.

Familial dysalbuminic hyperthyroxinemia enters in the differential diagnosis of T_4 toxicosis. It is familial; an albumin variant is inherited which has increased affinity to T_4 but not T_3. T_4 levels are increased, but T_3 levels and T_3 resin uptake are normal. The serum level of free T_4 by equilibrium dialysis is normal, as is sTSH. Radiolabeled T_4 binding-electrophoresis shows increased tracer in the albumin peak.

Management

Available modalities include symptomatic (rest, β-blockers), ablative (surgery, radioiodide), and temporizing (block thyroid hormone formation, antithyroid drugs; block release of thyroid hormones, iodides [days]) therapies.

Antithyroid Drugs

Methimazole and propylthiouracil (PTU) block thyroid hormone formation and may decrease the production of thyroid-stimulating immunoglobulins. Also, PTU decreases the conversion of T_4 to T_3. The effect of these drugs is temporary and lasts only while the drugs are being given. They do not damage the thyroid and are given to control hyperthyroidism and, in Graves' disease, with the hope that the disease will enter a spontaneous remission during their use (<50% chance). Therapy is initiated with either methimazole, 20 mg daily as a single dose, or with PTU, 300-450 mg/day in divided doses. Improvement is evident in 1-2 weeks, and euthyroidism is usually achieved in 6-8 weeks. Maintenance doses are then given to maintain euthyroidism. In Graves' disease, therapy is continued for 6-12 months; the use of the drug is then discontinued and the patient is assessed periodically. Most recurrences develop in the first few months after discontinuing use of the drug. Side effects are uncommon (<5%). Remember the serious side effects of agranulocytosis, vasculitis, hepatitis, and aplastic anemia (<0.2%). Agranulocytosis can develop abruptly within a few hours. The risk of agranulocytosis increases with age, is independent of the dose of PTU, but is dose-dependent for methimazole. The onset usually occurs within 2 months, and rarely after 4 months, after initiation of therapy.

- Methimazole and PTU block thyroid hormone formation and may decrease the production of thyroid-stimulating immunoglobulins.
- PTU: decreases T_4 to T_3 conversion.
- These drugs are given to control hyperthyroidism (in Graves' disease, with the hope of spontaneous remission — <50% chance).
- In Graves' disease, treat for 6-12 months; discontinue therapy and assess the patient periodically.
- Serious side effects: agranulocytosis, vasculitis, hepatitis, and aplastic anemia (<0.2%).
- Agranulocytosis can develop abruptly within a few hours.

Radioiodine

Radioiodine therapy is safe and effective. Its major drawback is the almost certain eventual development of ^{131}I-induced hypothyroidism. It does not carry the risk of thyroid carcinogenesis, leukemogenic potential, or gonadal damage. [131]I can be given to the young and old, with the only absolute contraindication being pregnancy. However, in practice, most physicians avoid its use in very young patients. The usual dose is 150-200 mCi/g (estimated weight). Lower doses are less likely to relieve hyperthyroidism and do not obviate eventual hypothyroidism. The maximal effect from a given dose of ^{131}I is obtained in 2-3 months. Doses can be repeated if necessary. Radiation thyroiditis may appear in 7-10 days and is rarely severe. It is most likely to occur in the elderly. Because of the risk of aggravating thyrocardiac disease, it is best to render these patients euthyroid with antithyroid drug therapy before administering ^{131}I. Pretreatment ophthalmopathy may worsen with treatment of hyperthyroidism, and particularly with ^{131}I treatment, probably because of the higher incidence of post-treatment hypothyroidism.

- ^{131}I: safe and effective.
- The major drawback is the eventual development of ^{131}I-induced hypothyroidism.
- The only absolute contraindication is pregnancy.
- In practice, most physicians avoid using it in very young patients.
- The maximal effect is obtained in 2-3 months.
- Radiation thyroiditis may appear in 7-10 days and is most likely to occur in the elderly.

Treat post-^{131}I hypothyroidism promptly to avoid worsening of ophthalmopathy.

Surgery

As a therapeutic option, subtotal thyroidectomy is reserved for the management of toxic nodular goiter and for patients with Graves' disease who are young, pregnant, or with large obstructive-compressive goiters. It is customary to render the patient euthyroid and to give iodides for 7-10 days preoperatively to prevent thyrotoxic crisis and excessive bleeding from the overactive friable gland. Damage to the recurrent laryngeal nerves or parathyroid glands is rare occurrence for experienced surgeons.

- Subtotal thyroidectomy: reserved for toxic nodular goiter and patients with Graves' disease who are young, pregnant, or with large obstructive-compressive goiters.
- It is customary to render the patient euthyroid and to give iodides 7-10 days preoperatively.

Special Considerations

Inorganic iodides have a transient inhibitory effect on hormone release (7-10 days). Iodides can be used as adjunctive agents in patients being prepared for surgery, with severe thyrocardiac disease, or with an actual or impending crisis. Iodides are also a temporary expedient while awaiting the full effect in those patients given radioiodine treatment.

- Iodides: for patients being prepared for surgery or with actual or impending crisis.

- Temporary expedient while awaiting full effect of radioiodine therapy.

β-Blockers should be used only as adjunctive therapy. Propranolol is used most commonly in a dose of 40-120 mg/day. Such therapy only controls the adrenergic manifestations of hyperthyroidism and may also decrease the conversion of T_4 to T_3. The major uses of these drugs are in thyrotoxic crisis and while awaiting the effects of more definitive therapy. These drugs should not be used alone in the preoperative preparation of thyrotoxic patients, because they do not prevent thyrotoxic crisis.

- β-Blockers: use only as adjunctive therapy.
- Major uses: in thyrotoxic crisis and while awaiting effects of more definitive therapy.
- Should not be used alone in preoperative preparation of thyrotoxic patients.

Summary of Management of Hyperthyroidism

Graves' disease: radioiodine therapy (unless pregnant or very young, in which case use surgical excision or antithyroid drugs).

Severe hyperthyroidism: antithyroid drugs until euthyroid, then ^{131}I or surgical excision.

Toxic single nodule: surgical excision or ^{131}I.

Toxic multinodular: surgical excision or ^{131}I plus temporizing antithyroid drug therapy.

Silent thyroiditis: symptomatic supportive.

Subacute thyroiditis: symptomatic supportive plus steroids.

Tumor-induced, e.g., struma, hydatidiform, or pituitary: surgical excision.

Goiter

Diffuse Euthyroid Goiter

Causes: simple goiter, Hashimoto's thyroiditis, euthyroid Graves' disease, goitrogens, lymphoma, and Riedel's thyroiditis.

Diagnostic approach: the two most important issues in the clinical evaluation of diffuse goiter in a euthyroid patient are an assessment of the onset and course of development of the goiter and an inquiry into the use of or exposure to goitrogens.

1. Goitrogen: history, removal of goitrogen leads to resolution of goiter.
2. If there is gradual onset and slow progression: consider Hashimoto's thyroiditis (bosselated goiter, high antibody titer, presence of other autoimmune diseases), Graves' disease (ophthalmopathy/dermopathy and presence of thyroid-stimulating immunoglobulins), or simple goiter (adolescence, spontaneous resolution in 1-2 years).
3. If there is rapid onset and progression: consider Hashimoto's thyroiditis or lymphoma. Check thyroid antibodies. Tissue diagnosis is critical.

Multinodular Euthyroid Goiter

Causes. Benign: sporadic multinodular goiter or Hashimoto's thyroiditis. Malignant: primary carcinoma, metastatic carcinoma, or lymphoma.

Diagnostic approach. If any nodule is dominant: manage as a single nodule (see below). If any feature suggests malignancy: need for tissue diagnosis (fine needle aspiration) and surgical therapy. If gradual onset and slow progression: differential diagnosis is benign multinodular goiter versus Hashimoto's thyroiditis; check for other autoimmune disorders and thyroid antibodies.

Single or Dominant Thyroid Nodule

Etiology. Benign: adenoma, cyst, focal thyroiditis, benign multinodular goiter with dominant nodule, or remnant hyperplasia (postsurgical ablation). Malignant: 1) primary (thyroid follicle—differentiated [papillary or follicular] or undifferentiated [anaplastic]—or parafollicular C cell [medullary carcinoma]). 2) Secondary (metastatic or lymphoma).

Diagnostic approach. Identify any factors that increase suspicion of malignancy: young age, male, rapid growth, invasive characteristics, history of irradiation, family history of thyroid cancer, or appearance while patient is receiving suppressive doses of thyroid hormone.

- Identify any factors that increase suspicion of malignancy.

Obtain serum sTSH: A suppressed sTSH points to a hyperfunctioning nodule that in all likelihood is benign; an increased sTSH should prompt consideration of focal autoimmune thyroiditis as the cause of the nodule.

Fine needle aspiration is the most important diagnostic step. It is a safe and effective outpatient procedure (sensitivity for detection of thyroid malignancy is 95%-98%). Interpretation of the aspirated tissue by an experienced cytopathologist is critical for the usefulness of the procedure.

- "Benign aspirate": observe.
- "Suspicious" aspirate: request a thyroid isotopic scan. "Hot nodule," observe or ablate; "cold nodule," surgical excision.
- "Malignant" aspirate: surgical excision.
- "Nondiagnostic" aspirate (10%): repeat fine needle aspiration or make decisions based on clinical assessment.

Thyroid Cancer

Thyroid cancer may arise from the thyroid follicle or parafollicular C cells. Also, the thyroid gland may be affected by lymphoma or metastatic disease. Thyroid carcinoma may be differentiated (papillary or follicular) or undifferentiated (anaplastic). Medullary thyroid cancer arises from the parafollicular C cells.

- Thyroid cancer: may arise from thyroid follicle or parafollicular C cells.
- Thyroid may also be affected by lymphoma or metastatic disease.

Papillary cancer is the most common type (50%-60% of patients). Its incidence peaks in early and late adulthood. Papillary cancer spreads typically to lymph nodes and usually has the best prognosis. It can present with a thyroid mass or cervical lymphadenopathy or it can be found incidentally in surgically excised thyroid glands. Follicular carcinoma (20% of patients) spreads preferentially by the hematogenous route. Its follicles can form thyroid hormones. Its presentations are with a thyroid mass or metastatic deposits (can be stained with antithyroglobulin stains). Rarely, if the tumor burden is large, follicular carcinoma can lead to thyrotoxicosis. Anaplastic carcinoma usually presents in the elderly with a rapidly progressive thyroid mass. It has a poor prognosis and longevity is <6-9 months.

- Papillary cancer: the most common type (50%-60% of patients). It spreads to lymph nodes and has the best prognosis. Presentation: thyroid mass, cervical lymphadenopathy, found incidentally in excised thyroid glands.
- Follicular carcinoma (20% of patients): spreads preferentially by hematogenous route. Presentation: thyroid mass, metastatic deposits. It can lead to thyrotoxicosis (rare).
- Anaplastic carcinoma: usually presents in the elderly with rapidly progressive thyroid mass. Prognosis is very poor.

Treatment of Differentiated Thyroid Cancer

Surgical excision is the definitive therapy: either lobectomy with or without subtotal contralateral lobectomy or near total thyroidectomy. The affected lymph nodes are selectively excised, and postoperatively, the thyroid remnant may be ablated with ^{131}I. Suppressive doses of T_4 are used (monitored by sTSH). Follow-up on regular basis with physical examination, chest radiography, serum thyroglobulin, high-resolution ultrasonography of the thyroid and neck. A radioiodide study may be needed every 1-5 years depending on the aggressiveness of the differentiated thyroid cancer. Radioiodine therapy is given for functioning metastases. Radiotherapy is given for local bony painful metastasis. The treatment of anaplastic carcinoma is palliative.

- Surgical excision is the definitive therapy for differentiated thyroid cancer.
- Suppressive doses of T_4 are used (monitored by sTSH).
- Radioiodine therapy is given for functioning metastases.

Medullary Carcinoma of the Thyroid

Medullary carcinoma of the thyroid arises from C cells and

has the distinctive pathologic feature of amyloid deposits among sheets of cells. It secretes calcitonin and can occur sporadically or be familial. Familial medullary carcinoma of the thyroid may be isolated or part of an endocrine complex. In MEN IIA, it may be associated with primary hyperparathyroidism and pheochromocytoma, and in MEN IIB, it occurs in association with pheochromocytoma, mucosal neuroma syndrome, and a distinctive marfanoid habitus. Medullary cell hyperplasia may precede medullary carcinoma in some of the affected families. Medullary carcinoma of the thyroid can present with a thyroid nodule, cervical lymphadenopathy, or metastatic disease. It may be detected in an asymptomatic relative during a family screen. In addition, the tumor may secrete other hormones such as ACTH, AVP, serotonin, and histamine and present with "ectopic" humoral syndromes. A search for associated pheochromocytoma and hyperparathyroidism should be conducted in all patients. The diagnosis is confirmed by an increased serum level of calcitonin or an abnormal calcitonin response to a calcium and/or pentagastrin stimulation test. Treatment is surgical (after the exclusion of pheochromocytoma) and in all patients should include total thyroidectomy and central node dissection. Currently, no effective chemotherapy is available.

Recently, it has been shown that 98% of patients with familial medullary carcinoma of the thyroid, MEN IIA, or MEN IIB have point mutations in the *ret* oncogene. DNA testing has become an important tool in the diagnosis and screening for these disorders.

- Medullary carcinoma of the thyroid: arises from C cells. Calcitonin is the tumor marker.
- Feature: amyloid deposits.
- It can occur sporadically or be familial.
- The familial form may be isolated or part of an endocrine complex, e.g., MEN IIA or MEN IIB.
- In some families, medullary cell hyperplasia may precede medullary carcinoma of the thyroid.
- Presentation: thyroid nodule, cervical lymphadenopathy, or metastatic disease.
- Search for associated pheochromocytoma and hyperparathyroidism in all patients.
- Medullary carcinoma of thyroid may secrete other hormones and present with "ectopic" humoral syndromes.
- Diagnosis is confirmed by an increased serum level of calcitonin or abnormal calcitonin response to a calcium and/or pentagastrin stimulation test.
- Treatment: surgical.

"Painful" Goiter

Cause: inflammatory (subacute thyroiditis, acute suppurative thyroiditis, and, rarely, Hashimoto's thyroiditis), hemorrhage into cyst or adenoma, or neoplastic (anaplastic carcinoma or lymphoma). Diagnostic approach: clinical (onset, course, duration, systemic features, e.g., recent viral disease, pyogenic source), characteristics of goiter, and search for cervical lymphadenopathy. Laboratory studies: leukocyte count and differential, erythrocyte sedimentation rate, FTI, sTSH, ^{131}I uptake, other thyroid antibodies, and, when needed, fine needle aspiration.

Subacute Painful Thyroiditis (Granulomatous or de Quervain's)

Subacute painful thyroiditis, probably a viral illness, is the most common cause of a painful, tender thyroid. It occurs mostly in women in the 3rd-5th decades. The onset is gradual or abrupt, and the dominant symptom is a painful, tender thyroid area. Pain may radiate to the upper neck, jaws, throat, or ears. Many patients may have fever, malaise, myalgia, and a history of upper respiratory tract infection. The thyroid is tender and enlarged: involvement is usually diffuse but may be unilateral and involve the two lobes sequentially. Hyperthyroidism of a few weeks' duration may be present in 50% of patients; almost all patients have biochemical hyperthyroidism related to follicular destruction. It may be followed by transient hypothyroidism. The illness is self-limiting, usually subsiding in weeks to months. The disease is characterized by remissions and relapses, but it eventually resolves completely. Restoration of function is the rule, but permanent hypothyroidism occurs in <5% of patients. Marked increase in the erythrocyte sedimentation rate is characteristic. The leukocyte count is mildly increased. FTI is increased and sTSH is suppressed in the hyperthyroid phase; ^{131}I uptake is suppressed. In the ensuing hypothyroid phase, the FTI is decreased, but the sTSH may still be suppressed (it may take 8 weeks to recover). The antibody titers are low or minimally increased. The major differential diagnosis is with hemorrhage into a thyroid nodule. In hemorrhage into a thyroid nodule, there are no systemic features, the erythrocyte sedimentation rate is normal, ^{131}I uptake is normal, and resolution occurs in a few days. Other differential diagnoses include radiation thyroiditis and pyogenic thyroiditis. Therapy—The disease is self-limited. For mild disease, no treatment is needed. For moderate disease, use nonsteroidal anti-inflammatory drugs; for severe disease, prednisone (20-40 mg/day); prompt response (a therapeutic test), treat for 2-3 weeks and withdraw over 3 weeks. For the hyperthyroid phase, use β-blockers. For the hypothyroid phase, T_4 treatment for a few months may be needed.

- Subacute painful thyroiditis: probably a viral illness.
- Onset: gradual or abrupt.
- Many patients: fever, malaise, myalgia, and a history of an upper respiratory tract infection.
- Involvement: usually diffuse, may be unilateral.
- Hyperthyroidism of few weeks' duration may be present

in 50% of patients.

- May be followed by transient hypothyroidism.
- Illness is self-limited.
- The disease is characterized by remissions and relapses.
- Restoration of function is the rule.
- Marked increase in erythrocyte sedimentation rate is characteristic.
- FTI is increased and sTSH is suppressed in the hyperthyroid phase; ^{131}I uptake is suppressed.
- The major differential diagnosis is with hemorrhage into a thyroid nodule.
- For moderate disease, use nonsteroidal anti-inflammatory drugs.
- For severe disease, prednisone (20-40 mg/day); prompt response (therapeutic test).

Euthyroid Sick Syndrome: "Adaptive Hypothyroidism"

The following abnormalities in thyroid hormone(s) values can occur in acute and chronically sick hospitalized patients:

- Decreased serum T_3 and increased reverse-T_3 levels (decreased peripheral T_3 production from T_4).
- Decreased serum levels of T_4 and T_3 (decreased serum T_4 and T_3 binding).
- Increased serum level of T_4 (decreased hormone clearance).
- Decreased sTSH (central effect).

Note that the thyroid hormone abnormalities in the euthyroid sick syndrome can mimic 1) central hypothyroidism: decreased T_4 and T_3, normal or decreased sTSH; and 2) thyrotoxicosis: increased T_4 and decreased sTSH.

- In euthyroid sick syndrome, thyroid hormone abnormalities can mimic central hypothyroidism and thyrotoxicosis.

With recovery from the illness, thyroid function values return to normal within a few days.

sTSH cannot be used alone as a thyroid function screening test in hospitalized patients. Suppressed sTSH can be seen in medical/surgical illness (20% of patients) and in psychiatric illness (20% of patients). Drugs: glucocorticoids and dopamine. Increased sTSH may be seen during recovery from illness.

- sTSH cannot be used alone as a thyroid function screening test in hospitalized patients.

Iodide-Induced Thyroid Dysfunction

In susceptible persons, exposure to excess iodides may lead to thyroid dysfunction. Common causes of iodide-induced thyroid dysfunction are contrast agents, inorganic iodides, and amiodarone. Iodide-induced *hypothyroidism* may occur in Hashimoto's thyroiditis, in Graves' disease after radioiodine therapy or surgery, and in fetal and neonatal thyroid. Iodide-induced *hyperthyroidism* may occur in patients with autonomous nodular thyroid (jodbasedow) or Graves' disease. Infrequently, iodide-induced dysfunction can occur in patients without a discernible underlying thyroid disorder.

Pregnancy and the Thyroid

In women with primary hypothyroidism, optimize the therapy before pregnancy is contemplated. Untreated hypothyroidism may lead to early loss of pregnancy. Also, closely follow sTSH levels during pregnancy, because the dose of thyroid hormone may need to be increased. The dosage is returned to prepregnancy dosage after delivery.

- In women with hypothyroidism, optimize therapy before pregnancy is contemplated.
- Closely follow sTSH levels during pregnancy.
- The dose of thyroid hormone may need to be increased.
- After delivery, dosage is returned to prepregnancy dosage.

In women with a diffuse euthyroid goiter early in pregnancy, check antithyroid antibodies. Positive antimicrosomal antibodies may identify patients at increased risk for developing postpartum thyroid disease.

- If diffuse euthyroid goiter occurs early in pregnancy, check antithyroid antibodies.
- Positive antibodies: may identify patients at increased risk for postpartum thyroid disease.

Thyrotoxicosis in pregnancy—In normal pregnancy, T_4 and T_3 levels increase because of estrogen-induced increase in TBG. The resin T_3 uptake is decreased, and the FTI is normal. The sTSH may be decreased modestly, as low as 0.1 mU/mL (normal, 0.4-5 mU/mL). The thyroid may be slightly enlarged. An increase in FTI and an sTSH <0.1 mU/mL point to thyrotoxicosis. Obviously, a ^{131}I uptake test is absolutely contraindicated.

- In normal pregnancy, T_4 and T_3 levels increase, principally because of an increase in TBG.
- Resin T_3 uptake is decreased; FTI is normal.
- sTSH may be decreased modestly.
- Increase in free T_4 or FTI and an sTSH <0.1 mU/mL indicate thyrotoxicosis.
- [131]I uptake test is absolutely contraindicated.

For management of Graves' thyrotoxicosis in pregnancy, most physicians rely on antithyroid drug therapy. Surgical excision may be an option after the first trimester. Antithyroid drugs cross the placenta and have an effect on the fetal thyroid; however, maternal T_4 and T_3 do not cross the placenta. Therefore, antithyroid drugs should be given in the smallest doses necessary to control the disease, usually <200 mg/day of PTU. Radioiodine therapy is absolutely contraindicated. Also, β-blockers should not be given, because of fetal growth retardation and neonatal respiratory depression. Inorganic iodides should be avoided; they can cross the placenta and cause fetal goiter and hypothyroidism.

- For Graves' thyrotoxicosis in pregnancy, most physicians rely on antithyroid drug therapy.
- Surgical excision may be an option after the first trimester.
- Antithyroid drugs cross the placenta.
- Maternal T_4 and T_3 do not cross the placenta.
- Antithyroid drugs: give in the smallest dose necessary to control the disease.
- Radioiodine therapy is absolutely contraindicated.
- β-Blockers should not be given.

Thyrotoxic Crisis

Thyrotoxic crisis is a rare disorder seen in untreated or inadequately treated hyperthyroid patients undergoing surgical treatment or who have an acute nonthyroidal illness. It may be seen postoperatively in poorly prepared patients with thyrotoxicosis undergoing subtotal thyroidectomy. It is characterized by extreme irritability, delirium, hyperpyrexia, tachycardia, hypotension, vomiting, diarrhea, prostration, and coma. If untreated, it is fatal. Perform the appropriate diagnostic blood tests promptly, and start treatment without waiting for confirmation of the diagnosis. Give PTU to block thyroid hormone synthesis (150-250 mg/2-6 hours), followed 1 hour later by sodium iodide to inhibit release of thyroid hormones (1 g in slow intravenous infusion). Propranolol is given as a β-blocker and to decrease T_4 conversion to T_3 (20-60 mg/6 hours orally or 0.5-2 mg/4 hours intravenously). Support the patient with fluids given intravenously, vitamin B complex, dexamethasone (2 mg/6 hours), and with symptomatic therapy. After recovery, plan for definitive therapy.

- Thyrotoxic crisis: seen in untreated or inadequately treated hyperthyroid patients undergoing surgical treatment or who have acute nonthyroidal illness.
- Characteristics: extreme irritability, delirium, hyperpyrexia, tachycardia, hypotension, vomiting, diarrhea, prostration, and coma.
- If untreated, it is fatal.
- Start treatment without waiting for confirmation of diagnosis.
- Give PTU to block thyroid hormone synthesis.
- Give sodium iodide to inhibit the release of thyroid hormones.
- Propranolol is given as a β-blocker and to decrease T_4 con-

version to T_3.
- Support the patient.
- After recovery, plan for definitive therapy.

Myxedema Crisis

Myxedema crisis occurs in patients with severe hypothyroidism and is either spontaneous or precipitated by acute illness, exposure to cold, or use of sedatives or opiates. It carries a high mortality rate (20%-50%). The onset is gradual, with progressive stupor culminating in coma. Seizures may occur, and hypothermia, hypotension, hypoventilation, hyponatremia, and hypoglycemia may be present. Most often, the patients are elderly and have overt hypothyroidism. Treatment—Perform confirmatory blood tests and start treatment promptly. Do not wait for the laboratory results. Institute supportive therapy and aggressively give thyroid hormone therapy. Conserve body heat; do not warm externally. Conserve vital functions; consider tracheal intubation and ventilatory support if respiratory depression occurs. Cautiously maintain hydration and hemodynamic functions and watch out for hyponatremia (syndrome of inappropriate ADH). Give T_4, 2 mg/kg intravenously over 5-10 minutes and 100 mg/24 hours intravenously thereafter. Support the patient by giving glucocorticoids in high doses (hypothyroidism may have slowed down adrenal responsiveness and there may be associated Addison's disease).

- Myxedema crisis: occurs in severe hypothyroidism (either spontaneously or precipitated by acute illness), exposure to cold, or with the use of sedatives or opiates.
- It carries a high mortality (20%-50%).
- The onset is gradual, with progressive stupor culminating in coma.
- Hypothermia, hypotension, hypoventilation, hyponatremia, and hypoglycemia may occur.
- Perform confirmatory blood tests, and promptly start treatment.
- Institute supportive therapy and give aggressive thyroid hormone therapy.
- Support the patient by giving glucocorticoids in high doses.

THE PARATHYROID GLANDS AND METABOLIC BONE DISEASE

Physiology

Parathyroid Hormone

Parathyroid hormone (PTH) is critical for maintenance of eucalcemia. It acts on bone to mobilize calcium and phosphate (osteolytic osteolysis and osteoclastic bone resorption), an effect that needs the permissive action of calcitriol, 1-25(OH)$_2$D. Its renal effects include stimulation of calcium reabsorption by the distal tubule, inhibition of phosphate reabsorption and stimulation of 1-hydroxylation of 25(OH)D to 1-25(OH)$_2$D by the proximal tubule. PTH, indirectly via 1-25(OH)$_2$D, stimulates the absorption of calcium and phosphate from the gut. PTH acts via cell membrane receptors and activates adenylate cyclase; cyclic AMP is the second messenger. The serum level of calcium is the major determinant of PTH secretion: low serum levels of calcium stimulate and high serum levels suppress PTH secretion. Magnesium is necessary for the secretion and action of PTH. PTH is a single-chain polypeptide of 84 amino acids; its N-terminal (1-34) is biologically active and has a short half-life. The C-terminal is biologically inert, has a long half-life, and is excreted by the kidney. Standard assays use C-terminal, N-terminal, or mid-region antisera. C-terminal assay values are falsely increased in renal failure. New immunoradiometric assays measure the intact PTH molecule with high sensitivity and specificity and are the immunoassays of choice.

- PTH: critical for maintenance of eucalcemia.
- Bone effects: mobilization of calcium and phosphate.
- Renal effects: stimulation of calcium reabsorption by distal tubule, inhibition of phosphate reabsorption, and stimulation of 1-hydroxylation of 25(OH)D to 1-25(OH)$_2$D by proximal tubule.
- Intestinal effect: stimulation of absorption of calcium and phosphate indirectly via 1-25(OH)$_2$D.
- Serum calcium is the major determinant of PTH secretion.
- Magnesium is necessary for PTH secretion and action.
- PTH: single-chain polypeptide of 84 amino acids.
- N-terminal (1-34) is biologically active.
- C-terminal is biologically inert.
- New immunoradiometric assays: measure PTH molecule assays with high sensitivity and specificity and are the immunoassays of choice.

Vitamin D

The sources of vitamin D are the diet and the irradiation of vitamin D precursors in the skin. The bioactivation of vitamin D is shown in Figure 7-8.

1-25(OH)$_2$D, or calcitriol, is the active hormone. It stimulates active absorption of calcium and phosphate from the gut, has a permissive role in the PTH effect on bone, and optimizes calcium-phosphate product in the extracellular fluids to allow mineralization of new osteoid. It has other effects on the skin and immune system. 1-25(OH)$_2$D is a steroid and acts through specific intracellular cytoplasmic or nuclear receptors.

- Sources of vitamin D: diet and irradiation of vitamin D precursors in the skin.
- 1-25(OH)$_2$D is the active hormone.
- It stimulates active absorption of calcium and phosphate from the gut.
- It has a permissive role in the PTH effect on bone.

- It optimizes calcium-phosphate product in extracellular fluids to allow mineralization of new osteoid.

Calcium

Total body calcium is 1,000-1,200 g. Bone and teeth contain about 99%; cells, 1%; and extracellular fluid, 0.1% (about 1 g). The total serum calcium is ionized (50%); complexed to citrate, phosphate, and other anions (5%-10%); and bound to protein (40%), especially albumin. Ionized calcium is the biologically active component and the major determinant of PTH secretion. The average intake of calcium is 400-1,000 mg/day. Absorption occurs in the proximal small intestine and is enhanced by 1-25(OH)$_2$D. Calcium is filtered by the glomeruli; 98%-99% of the filtered calcium is reabsorbed by the renal tubules, mostly in the proximal tubule; distal tubular reabsorption is enhanced by PTH. In men, 24-hour urine excretion is <275 mg and in women, <250 mg.

- Total serum calcium: ionized (50%); complexed to citrate, phosphate, and other anions (5%-10%); and bound to protein (40%), especially albumin.
- Ionized calcium is the biologically active component and major determinant of PTH secretion.
- Gut absorption occurs in the proximal small intestine and is enhanced by 1-25(OH)$_2$D.
- Distal tubular reabsorption is enhanced by PTH.

Syndrome of Hypercalcemia

Clinical Presentation

Hypercalcemia may be asymptomatic or present with a single or multisystem disorder. Renal: polyuria, polydipsia due to nephrogenic diabetes insipidus; renal colic, nephrolithiasis; and chronic renal failure. Neuropsychiatric: fatigue, weakness,

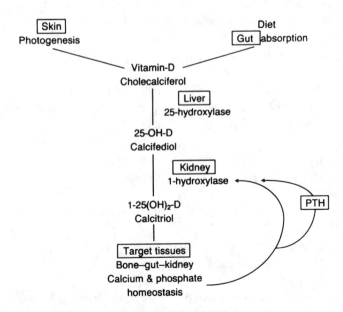

Fig. 7-8. The biosynthesis of calcitriol, 1-25(OH)$_2$D.

impairment of consciousness, confusion, depression, and hyporeflexia. Gastrointestinal: anorexia, nausea, vomiting, and constipation; hypercalcemia may be associated with peptic ulcer and pancreatitis. Cardiovascular: hypertension and arrhythmias; hypercalcemia potentiates the cardiac effects of digitalis; ECG may show shortened QT intervals. Metastatic calcification: band keratopathy or nephrocalcinosis.

- Hypercalcemia: may be asymptomatic or present with a single or multisystem disorder.

Etiology

The causes of hypercalcemia are outlined in Table 7-11. Fundamentally, hypercalcemia can result from increased bone resorption, increased intestinal absorption, or decreased urinary excretion of calcium. More than one mechanism may be involved in any given disorder. The causes can most usefully be categorized as either PTH-dependent or PTH-independent.

Parathyroid-Dependent Hypercalcemia

Primary hyperparathyroidism. Adenoma is the most common cause. It can be single (80% of patients) or multiple (3%); hyperplasia of all four glands occurs in 15% of patients; carcinoma is rare (2%). Adenoma may be ectopic in 6%-10% of patients and be found in the thyroid, thymus, or mediastinum. Primary hyperparathyroidism may be sporadic or familial. The familial form may be a part of MEN I (in association with tumors of the anterior pituitary and endocrine pancreas) or MEN IIA (in association with medullary carcinoma of the thyroid and pheochromocytoma). The usual parathyroid lesion in familial hyperparathyroidism is hyperplasia. Most patients with primary hyperparathyroidism are asymptomatic and identified by random blood screening; others may present with features of hypercalcemia (see above). Characteristic skeletal lesions include osteopenia, subperiosteal bone resorption, salt-and-pepper lesions in the skull, and ostitis fibrosis cystica. Primary hyperparathyroidism has known associations with chondrocalcinosis and pseudogout. Hypercalcemia may be mild and intermittent; serum levels of phosphate are usually low but may be normal; chloride is often increased and bicarbonate is often decreased. Urine calcium is usually normal or modestly increased, which helps to differentiate primary hyperparathyroidism from familial hypocalciuric hypercalcemia. The ECG may show a short QT interval or arrhythmia. The serum level of PTH is increased (90% of patients); it may be "normal" in 10% of patients, but it is always inappropriately increased for the degree of hypercalcemia. Immunoradiometric assay of PTH is most reliable, and in most patients, it distinguishes between primary hyperparathyroidism and humoral hypercalcemia of malignancy. Preoperative localization is not required except in the surgical management of postoperative persistent or recurrent disease (high-resolution ultrasonography

Table 7-11.--Causes of Hypercalcemia

Parathyroid hormone-dependent
Hyperparathyroidism--primary or tertiary
Familial benign hypocalciuric hypercalcemia
Drug-induced--thiazides, lithium
Ectopic hyperparathyroidism (rare)
Parathyroid hormone-independent
Malignancy
With bone metastasis
Hematologic--multiple myeloma, leukemia, lymphoma
Humoral hypercalcemia (PTH-rp and others)
Endocrine disorders
Thyroid dysfunction
Pheochromocytoma
Adrenal insufficiency
Acromegaly
Hypervitaminosis D
Exogenous vitamin D
Endogenous--granulomatous disorders, some lymphomas
Immobilization, especially in patients with high turnover of bone as in Paget's disease
Milk-alkali syndrome

for cervical adenomas and CT scan, thallium/technetium subtraction scan, or angiography for mediastinal tumors). Conservative therapy may be indicated in cases of mild uncomplicated disease, especially in the elderly; otherwise, adenomectomy for adenoma and subtotal parathyroidectomy (leaving 50 mg of parathyroid tissue) for hyperplasia. Medical therapy for chronic hypercalcemia is usually not effective; options include phosphate and estrogen given orally.

- Primary hyperparathyroidism: adenoma is the most common cause.
- It can be single (80% of patients) or multiple (3%).
- Hyperplasia of all four glands occurs in 15% of patients.
- Carcinoma is rare (2% of patients).
- It may be isolated or familial.
- Familial hyperparathyroidism: may be part of MEN I or MEN IIA.
- The usual parathyroid lesion in familial hyperparathyroidism: hyperplasia.
- Most patients with hyperparathyroidism are asymptomatic.
- Characteristic skeletal lesions: osteopenia, periosteal bone resorption, salt-and-pepper lesions in the skull, and ostitis fibrosis cystica.
- Primary hyperparathyroidism: known associations with chondrocalcinosis and pseudogout.
- Urine calcium: usually normal or moderately increased

(helps distinguish from familial hypocalciuric hypercalcemia).

- Serum PTH is increased (90% of patients), may be "normal" in 10%, but is always inappropriately increased for the degree of hypercalcemia.
- Immunoradiometric PTH is most reliable and in most patients distinguishes primary hyperparathyroidism from humoral hypercalcemia of malignancy.
- Preoperative localization is not necessary except in surgical management of postoperative persistent or recurrent disease.
- Conservative therapy may be indicated in mild uncomplicated disease (especially in the elderly).
- Adenomectomy for adenoma.
- Subtotal parathyroidectomy for hyperplasia.

Familial hypocalciuric hypercalcemia. This is characterized by hypercalcemia in a relatively young patient, normal or slightly increased PTH, low-to-normal phosphate, and decreased fractional excretion of calcium and magnesium. The measured calcium clearance-to-creatinine clearance ratio is <0.01. The parathyroid glands show chief cell hyperplasia. Familial hypocalciuric hypercalcemia is inherited in an autosomal dominant pattern; the hypercalcemia may be detected in affected family members before age 10. Recent data point to genetic mutations in the parathyroid-calcium receptor as the etiologic factor that increases the set point for PTH suppression in response to the ambient levels of calcium. Screening of family members is important. Hypercalcemia is usually asymptomatic and uncomplicated by end-organ effects. No medical or surgical therapy is indicated. Surgical therapy does not relieve hypercalcemia unless all parathyroid tissue is removed.

- Familial hypocalciuric hypercalcemia: hypercalcemia in a relatively young patient.
- PTH is normal or slightly increased.
- Decreased fractional excretion of calcium and magnesium: the calcium clearance-to-creatinine clearance ratio is <0.01.
- It is autosomal dominant.
- Hypercalcemia may be detected in affected family members before age 10.
- Hypercalcemia is usually asymptomatic and uncomplicated.

Thiazides. Thiazides may potentiate the effects of PTH on bone and kidney and may cause mild hypercalcemia. Unlike other diuretics, thiazides decrease urine calcium. The mild hypercalcemia should resolve within a few weeks after discontinuing use of the drug. Many patients have underlying mild primary hyperparathyroidism. Use thiazides with caution in patients with increased bone turnover and hypercalciuria, e.g., Paget's disease and thyrotoxicosis.

- Thiazides: may potentiate the effects of PTH on bone and kidney.
- Mild hypercalcemia should resolve in few weeks after use of the drug is discontinued.
- Use thiazides with caution in patients with increased bone turnover and hypercalciuria.

Lithium. Hypercalcemia occurs in 10% of patients who take lithium. Lithium increases the set-point of parathyroid secretion. The hypercalcemia is reversible if the use of lithium is discontinued.

- Hypercalcemia occurs in 10% of patients who take lithium.
- Lithium increases the set-point of parathyroid secretion.

Parathyroid-Independent Hypercalcemia

Humoral hypercalcemia. Hypercalcemia of malignancy is common, often develops acutely, and may be quite severe. It is the most common cause of hypercalcemia in hospitalized patients. Its causes include local bone destruction by metastasis or myeloma, increased synthesis of 1-25(OH)$_2$D by lymphoma, and elaboration of other mediators of bone resorption (e.g., PTH-related protein, tumor necrosis factor, transforming growth factor, and cytokines) by tumors such as of the lung and kidney and squamous cell carcinoma. Ectopic PTH is uncommon. PTH-related protein shares with PTH its renal and bone effects; levels are increased in most patients with humoral hypercalcemia of malignancy and are low or normal in patients with primary hyperparathyroidism. Most PTH antisera do not cross react with PTH-related protein. Most patients with humoral hypercalcemia of malignancy show suppressed PTH by radioimmunoassay.

- Hypercalcemia of malignancy: common, often develops acutely, and may be severe.
- It is the most common cause of hypercalcemia in hospitalized patients.
- Cause: local bone destruction by metastasis or myeloma, increased synthesis of 1-25(OH)$_2$D by lymphoma, or elaboration of other mediators of bone resorption.
- Increased levels of PTH-related protein are seen in most patients.
- Most patients show suppressed PTH on radioimmunoassay.

Vitamin D intoxication. Hypercalcemia, hypercalciuria, renal insufficiency, and soft tissue calcification follow prolonged ingestion of vitamin D in high dosages. The condition may persist for months after discontinuing use of vitamin D, because of fat storage of the vitamin. Levels of 1-25(OH)$_2$D are increased. The response to glucocorticoids is prompt.

- Vitamin D intoxication may persist for months after discontinued use of the vitamin.

- The response to glucocorticoids is prompt.

Sarcoidosis and other granulomatous disorders. Hypercalcemia occurs in 15% of patients (hypercalciuria is more common) and is caused by increased gut absorption and increased bone resorption. It is vitamin D-mediated. Levels of 25(OH)D are normal; the serum level of 1-25(OH)$_2$D is increased because granulomas have 1-hydroxylase and can generate 1-25(OH)$_2$D from circulating 25(OH)D. The condition is responsive to glucocorticoids.

- Hypercalcemia is vitamin D-mediated.
- Serum levels of 1-25(OH)$_2$D increase because granulomas have 1-hydroxylase.
- It is glucocorticoid responsive.

In Addison's disease, hypercalcemia is frequent and related to an increase in the protein-bound fraction; it is reversible with glucocorticoid therapy.

In thyrotoxicosis, enhanced bone resorption is greater than bone formation. Hypercalcemia occurs in 25% of patients; hypercalciuria, in 50%. Hypercalcemia resolves with treatment of thyrotoxicosis.

Immobilization may result in hypercalcemia in patients with rapid bone turnover, such as adolescents and patients with Paget's disease.

Milk-alkali syndrome is a combination of high calcium intake and absorbable alkali. Features: hypercalcemia, low urine calcium, alkalosis, renal failure, and soft tissue calcification. It is preventable.

Diagnostic Approach

Rule out laboratory error and factitial causes. Confirm the hypercalcemia with repeated measurements. If serum albumin abnormalities are present, correct for serum albumin levels or measure ionized calcium. A change of 1.0 g/dL in serum albumin changes serum calcium by about 0.8 mg/dL in the same direction.

- Rule out laboratory error and factitial causes.
- Correct for serum albumin or measure ionized calcium.

If drug-induced hypercalcemia is suspected, stop use of the drug and reassess the serum concentration of calcium in a few weeks (a few months in case of vitamin D). If hypercalcemia persists, proceed with evaluation.

- If drug-induced, stop use of the drug.
- Reassess the serum concentration of calcium.

Determine the serum level of PTH. This is a critical step in the diagnostic approach. The best assay is the two-site immuno-metric assay that measures intact PTH and is unaffected by renal function.

- Determine the serum level of PTH.
- Best assay: two-site immunometric assay.

A suppressed PTH points to parathyroid-independent hypercalcemia. Proceed with careful clinical, biochemical, and radiologic assessment to identify the cause. Increased PTH-related protein points to humoral hypercalcemia of malignancy, and an increased 1-25(OH)$_2$D suggests a granulomatous disorder or some type of lymphoma.

- Suppressed PTH: parathyroid-independent hypercalcemia.
- Increased PTH-related protein: humoral hypercalcemia of malignancy.
- Increased 1-25(OH)$_2$D: granulomatous disorder or some type of lymphoma.

A high serum level of PTH points to primary hyperparathyroidism. A "normal" or "minimally elevated" serum level of PTH may be due to thiazides, lithium, familial hypocalciuric hypercalcemia, or primary hyperparathyroidism. A family history, benign clinical course, and low urinary concentration of calcium point to familial hypocalciuric hypercalcemia. Note that the serum concentration of phosphate may be low in any hypercalcemic state. A high serum concentration of phosphate points to renal insufficiency or to non-PTH-dependent hypercalcemia. A low urinary level of calcium is seen in familial hypocalciuric hypercalcemia and with the use of thiazides. Significant hypercalciuria (>400 mg/24 hours) usually points to a nonparathyroid cause.

- High serum PTH level: primary hyperparathyroidism.
- "Normal" or "minimally elevated" serum level of PTH: thiazides, lithium, familial hypocalciuric hypercalcemia, or primary hyperparathyroidism.
- Family history, benign clinical course, low urinary concentration of calcium: familial hypocalciuric hypercalcemia.

Treatment

Specific treatment. Treatment of the primary cause, if feasible, is the most important therapeutic option. For example, parathyroid adenomectomy for primary hyperparathyroidism and medical management of thyrotoxicosis. Glucocorticoids are the drugs of choice for the hypercalcemia seen in Addison's disease and in vitamin D excess, either of exogenous or endogenous origin (sarcoidosis and other granulomatous disorders). They are also effective for specific antitumor effects in some malignancies, such as multiple myeloma, some lymphomas, and breast cancer with metastasis. Indomethacin or aspirin as antiprostaglandins are usually ineffective.

- Most important therapeutic option: treatment of primary cause.
- Glucocorticoids: drugs of choice for hypercalcemia in Addison's disease and in vitamin D excess (exogenous or endogenous origin).
- Glucocorticoids may be effective in some malignancies: multiple myeloma, some lymphomas, and breast cancer with metastasis.

Nonspecific treatment. Consider the rapidity of the onset, severity of the hypercalcemia, coexisting illness, and age of the patient. Nonspecific therapy is designed to decrease bone resorption and increase renal excretion.

- Nonspecific therapy: to decrease bone resorption and increase renal excretion.

Rehydration. Severe hypercalcemia leads to a decrease in renal concentrating ability, dehydration, decreased renal blood flow and glomerular filtration rate, and enhanced renal tubular absorption of calcium along with sodium. Rehydration is an essential first step in the treatment to correct these abnormalities. Forced saline diuresis can increase calcium urinary losses and reduce serum calcium level by 1-3 mg/dL. Furosemide, 40 mg/1-2 hours given intravenously, adds to the sodium/calcium renal losses. Replace volume and electrolytes. Do not initiate forced saline diuresis until volume repletion is achieved. Often, central venous pressure monitoring and bladder catheterization are necessary. Treatment is temporizing. The dangers include cardiac decompensation, life-threatening hypokalemia, hypomagnesemia, and hypophosphatemia.

- Rehydration is an essential first step in the treatment.
- Do not initiate forced saline diuresis until volume repletion is achieved. Watch for volume or electrolyte abnormalities.

Calcitonin. It has a direct antiresorptive effect on osteoclasts; also, it is hypercalciuric. Calcitonin is nontoxic and has a rapid onset of action (few hours). Give in a dose of 2-8 IU/kg intravenously, intramuscularly, or subcutaneously every 6 hours. Unfortunately, the effect is modest and variable, and tachyphylaxis often develops (concomitant administration of glucocorticoids may prolong its effect). Side effects include nausea, flushing, and skin rash.

- Calcitonin has a direct antiresorptive effect on the osteoclasts; it also is hypercalciuric.
- It has a rapid onset of action.
- The effect is modest and variable.
- Tachyphylaxis often develops.

Bisphosphonates. These are analogues of pyrophosphate, with a high affinity to hydroxyapatite of bone. They are taken up by osteoclasts and inhibit bone resorption. In addition, bisphosphonates inhibit the differentiation of progenitor cells to osteoclasts. Etidronate is a first-generation bisphosphonate. It is poorly absorbed when given orally; thus, to be effective in managing hypercalcemia, it has to be given intravenously. The dose is 7.5 mg/kg daily in 5% dextrose in water over 2 hours for 3 successive days. It causes a dramatic decrease in the serum concentration of calcium, but it normalizes calcium in only 30%-40% of patients. The improvement may last 5-7 days. The side effects include nausea, vomiting, and abdominal pain.

- Bisphosphonates: analogues of pyrophosphate.
- They inhibit bone resorption.
- Etidronate: a first-generation bisphosphonate.
- It has to be given intravenously.
- It causes a dramatic decrease in the serum concentration of calcium.
- It normalizes calcium in 30%-40% of patients.
- Improvement may last 5-7 days.

Pamidronate, a new generation bisphosphonate, is an extremely potent antiresorptive agent that recently was approved by the FDA for management of hypercalcemia. It is given as a single intravenous dose of 60-90 mg. Pamidronate is effective in 24-48 hours (in 70% to >90% of patients) and normalizes the serum concentration of calcium for weeks or months. The drug given orally is also effective. Unlike etidronate, chronic administration is not associated with mineralization defect. Side effects include low-grade fever (20% of patients), hypocalcemia (10%), hypophosphatemia, hypomagnesemia, and reversible hepatic injury.

- Pamidronate: a new generation bisphosphonate.
- It is an extremely potent antiresorptive agent.
- It is given as a single intravenous dose of 60-90 mg.
- It is effective in 24-48 hours in most patients.
- It normalizes the serum concentration of calcium for weeks or months.
- Unlike etidronate, chronic administration of pamidronate is not associated with mineralization defect.

Plicamycin (mithramycin). It inhibits osteoclastic resorption. A dose of 15-25 mg/kg is given over a period of 4-24 hours. The effect is rapid (24-48 hours); it normalizes calcium in 40%-60% of patients. The effect may last 5-7 days. Side effects include thrombocytopenia and qualitative platelet defects, renal insufficiency, and liver abnormalities. Bisphosphonates have replaced plicamycin as "first-line" therapy.

- Plicamycin: inhibits osteoclastic resorption.
- Its effect is rapid.

- It normalizes calcium in 40%-60% of patients.
- The effect may last 5-7 days.
- Bisphosphonates have replaced plicamycin as "first-line" therapy.

Gallium nitrate. It, too, inhibits osteoclastic bone resorption. A dose of 200 mg per square meter of body surface area in 1 L of fluid daily for 5 days. Therapy achieves eucalcemia in 75% of patients. This effect may last 7-10 days. Side effects include nausea, hypotension, and renal insufficiency.

- Gallium nitrate: inhibits osteoclastic bone resorption.
- Achieves eucalcemia in 75% of patients.
- The effect may last 7-10 days.

Phosphate. Phosphate given intravenously can have a dramatic effect in decreasing the serum level of calcium by precipitating calcium phosphate in the skeleton and in soft tissues, including the kidneys and heart. It is hazardous and can precipitate acute renal failure and hypotension. This treatment has been superseded by the other agents described above. Phosphate given orally is minimally effective, if at all.

- Phosphate given intravenously: hazardous; it can precipitate renal failure and hypotension.

Dialysis. Peritoneal dialysis and hemodialysis are reserved for patients with renal failure.

- Dialysis (peritoneal or hemodialysis): reserved for patients with renal failure.

Syndrome of Hypocalcemia

Clinical Presentation

Hypocalcemia may be asymptomatic and detected only by biochemical screening. The symptoms of hypocalcemia reflect not only the degree but also the rate of its development. Neuromuscular: paresthesias and muscle spasms, such as carpopedal spasms, laryngeal stridor, and convulsions. Apathy, lethargy, and depression may occur. Specific neurologic sequelae include basal ganglia calcification, extrapyramidal manifestations, and benign intracranial hypertension. Gastrointestinal: abdominal pain, nausea, vomiting, and malabsorption. Cardiovascular: prolonged QT interval and congestive heart failure resistant to standard therapy but responsive to normalization of the serum level of calcium. Other effects: premature cataracts, alopecia, and mucocutaneous candidiasis. Children may have enamel hypoplasia and failure of secondary dentition. The signs of Chvostek and Trousseau are characteristic of hypocalcemia, although they can rarely be elicited in normal persons.

- Symptoms of hypocalcemia reflect not only the degree but also the rate of its development.
- Carpopedal spasms, laryngeal stridor, and convulsions.
- Basal ganglia calcification, extrapyramidal manifestations, and benign intracranial hypertension.
- Cardiovascular effects: prolonged QT interval and congestive heart failure resistant to standard therapy but responsive to normalization of the serum level of calcium.
- Chvostek's and Trousseau's signs: characteristic of hypocalcemia.

Etiology

The causes of hypocalcemia are outlined in Table 7-12. Basically, hypocalcemia may result from decreased secretion of PTH or PTH resistance, from decreased production of vitamin D or vitamin D resistance, and from other miscellaneous disorders that decrease the mobilization of calcium from bone or increase calcium deposition in tissues.

Hypoparathyroidism may result from inadvertent surgical damage to the parathyroid glands during thyroidectomy, radical neck dissection, or surgical management of primary hyperparathyroidism. It may be transient or permanent, and it may appear shortly or in a few months or years after the surgical insult. Occasionally, hypoparathyroidism may result from other organic disorders: autoimmune, infiltrative (hemochromatosis or Wilson's disease), or congenital (DiGeorge syndrome). Idiopathic hypoparathyroidism often appears as a familial disorder, and may have an autoimmune basis. It occasionally accompanies other endocrine deficiency states.

Table 7-12.--Causes of Hypocalcemia

Decreased secretion of parathyroid hormone
Hypoparathyroidism
Functional--hypomagnesemia
Organic--postoperative
Autoimmune
Hypomagnesemia
Decreased action of parathyroid hormone
Pseudohypoparathyroidism
Vitamin D deficiency
Nutritional
Malabsorption
Chronic liver disease
Anticonvulsant agents
Renal failure
Vitamin D resistance--types I and II
Other
Phosphate excess
Increased bone avidity for calcium, e.g., osteoblastic metastases
Miscellaneous, e.g., acute pancreatitis

Hypomagnesemia is a cause of functional hypoparathyroidism; it decreases the secretion and action of PTH.

- Surgical hypoparathyroidism: may result from inadvertent damage to the parathyroid glands and may be transient or permanent.
- May occasionally result from organic disorders: autoimmune, infiltrative, or congenital.
- Idiopathic hypoparathyroidism: often appears as a familial disorder; it may have an autoimmune basis.
- Hypomagnesemia: an important cause of hypoparathyroidism.
- Hypomagnesemia decreases the secretion and action of PTH.

Pseudohypoparathyroidism is an inherited disorder characterized by end-organ resistance to PTH action. The resistance may affect bone and kidney differentially; thus, clinical manifestations may vary. In type IA pseudohypoparathyroidism, there is a 50% decrease in the activity of G-stimulatory protein, the stimulatory guanyl nucleotide-binding protein coupled to adenylate cyclase; other hormone actions (e.g., TSH and gonadotropins) may be affected. In type IB, there may be a problem with the PTH receptor. In type II, there is a postreceptor defect. The characteristic features of type IA are short stature, round face, obesity, short neck, short metacarpals and metatarsals, subcutaneous calcification, and mild mental retardation. A variant disorder called "pseudopseudohypoparathyroidism" presents with the same characteristic physical features but without the biochemical abnormalities.

- Pseudohypoparathyroidism: inherited and characterized by end-organ resistance to PTH action.
- Type IA: characteristic features are short stature, round face, obesity, short neck, short metacarpals and metatarsals, subcutaneous calcification, and mild mental retardation.
- Pseudopseudohypoparathyroidism: variant disorder with the same characteristic physical features but without the biochemical abnormalities.

In both hypoparathyroidism and pseudohypoparathyroidism, hypocalcemia of variable degree and hyperphosphatemia are present. The serum level of PTH is low in hypoparathyroidism and high in pseudohypoparathyroidism. Basal ganglia calcification may occur in either disorder.

- Hypoparathyroidism and pseudohypoparathyroidism: hypocalcemia (variable degree) and hyperphosphatemia.
- Serum level of PTH: low in hypoparathyroidism, high in pseudohypoparathyroidism.
- Basal ganglia calcification may occur in either disorder.

For vitamin D deficiency and resistance, see Osteomalacia.

Diagnostic Approach

Rule out laboratory error and factitial hypocalcemia. Adjust for serum albumin abnormalities (if present)—for every 1-g change in albumin, the serum concentration of calcium changes by 0.8 mg/dL in the same direction—or measure the serum concentration of ionized calcium. Confirm by repeated measurements. Rule out hypomagnesemia and renal insufficiency. If hypomagnesemia is present, treat; if hypocalcemia persists, proceed with evaluation. Check the serum level of PTH. A low or undetectable level of PTH points to hypoparathyroidism; a high level may be related to pseudohypoparathyroidism, vitamin D deficiency, or renal failure. The diagnosis of pseudohypoparathyroidism is based on clinical stigmata, family history, and unresponsiveness to exogenous PTH. Vitamin D deficiency is suggested by the clinical setting and is confirmed by assays of 25(OH)D or 1-25(OH)$_2$D.

- Rule out laboratory error and factitial hypocalcemia.
- Adjust for serum albumin abnormalities (if present).
- Rule out hypomagnesemia and renal insufficiency.
- Low/undetectable serum level of PTH: hypoparathyroidism.
- High serum level of PTH: pseudohypoparathyroidism, vitamin D deficiency, or renal failure.

Treatment

The treatment of hypocalcemia includes treating the cause when identifiable and feasible, e.g., replacement of magnesium. Calcium supplementation and/or vitamin D therapy are the mainstays of therapy. Overreplacement leads to hypercalcemia, hypercalciuria, nephrolithiasis, or nephrocalcinosis. Therefore, it is important to monitor the efficacy of the therapy and to maintain the serum concentration of calcium in the range of 8.0 to 8.5 mg/dL and the 24-hour urine concentration of calcium to <300 mg/24 hours.

- Hypocalcemia: treat the cause when identifiable and feasible.
- Mainstays of therapy: calcium supplementation and vitamin D therapy.
- It is important to monitor the efficacy of therapy.
- Serum level of calcium: maintain at 8.0-8.5 mg/dL.
- 24-hour urine concentration of calcium: maintain at <300 mg/24 hours.

If hypocalcemia is life-threatening, give calcium intravenously: calcium gluconate is administered slowly over a period of 5-10 minutes (10-20 mL; 93 mg of elemental calcium per 10 mL). It can be repeated if symptoms persist. Frequently monitor the serum level of calcium. Remember that calcium given intravenously may be hazardous in patients taking digitalis. For chronic therapy, give calcium orally. Vitamin D is usually needed in addition. Calcium carbonate (40% elemental calcium) is preferred, up to 2 g of elemental calcium daily. Ergocalciferol is started in a dose of 25,000 U/day (or dihydrotachysterol in a dose of 0.125 mg/day or calcitriol in a dose of 0.25 mg/day). Useful adjuncts in some patients include thiazides (to decrease urinary calcium excretion) and oral phosphate binders.

- If hypocalcemia is life-threatening, give calcium intravenously.
- Useful adjuncts in some patients: thiazides (to decrease urinary calcium excretion) and oral phosphate binders.

Osteoporosis

By definition, "osteoporosis" refers to a decrease in bone mass that compromises the mechanical support function of the skeleton. The remaining bone is morphologically normal. Calcium homeostasis is not affected.

Etiology

The causes of osteoporosis are outlined in Table 7-13.

Clinical Presentation

Fracture after minimal trauma (especially of the vertebrae, distal radius, or femoral neck), loss of height, dorsal kyphosis, and drooping of the rib cage should suggest osteoporosis.

Diagnostic Approach

Document osteopenia. Radiography of the spine or other affected bones is a relatively insensitive diagnostic test. On spine films, the vertebral bodies may show loss of transverse trabeculations, thinning and sharpening of cortical margins, wedging, or collapse. In radiologic studies, it is important to look for specific signs of other disorders, such as subperiosteal resorption of primary hyperparathyroidism or Looser's zones of osteomalacia. Bone densitometry is the diagnostic procedure of choice: single-photon absorptiometry of the forearm, dual-photon absorptiometry of the spine, or dual energy x-ray absorptiometry of the spine and hip. The Scientific Advisory Board of the National Osteoporosis Foundation has outlined the following indications for bone densitometry, all based on its potential impact on other diagnostic or therapeutic implications: 1) in estrogen-deficient women to determine who might benefit from estrogen replacement therapy and to enable the patient to make an enlighted decision; 2) in patients with radiologic evidence suggestive of osteopenia to determine if osteopenia is really present; 3) in glucocorticoid-treated patients to establish who might have osteopenia and who needs a change in therapeutic plans; 4) in patients with mild primary hyperparathyroidism to identify those with low bone mineral density who might benefit from parathyroidectomy. Bone densitometry may also be used to monitor the clinical response to a given therapeutic intervention.

- Document osteopenia.

- Radiography of the spine or other affected bones is a relatively insensitive diagnostic test.
- In radiologic studies, look for specific signs of other disorders, e.g., subperiosteal resorption of primary hyperparathyroidism and Looser's zones of osteomalacia.
- Bone densitometry is the diagnostic procedure of choice.
- Single-photon absorptiometry of forearm, dual-photon absorptiometry of spine, or dual energy x-ray absorptiometry of spine and hip.

Table 7-13.--Causes of Osteoporosis

Primary (idiopathic)
  Postmenopausal (type I)
  Senile (type II)
  Juvenile
Secondary
  Endocrine
    Cushing's syndrome
    Thyrotoxicosis
    Hyperparathyroidism
    Hypogonadism of any cause, including
      hyperprolactinemia
    Diabetes mellitus
  Malignancy
    Multiple myeloma
    Leukemia
    Lymphoma
    Systemic mastocytosis
  Immobilization
    Generalized
    Localized
  Genetic abnormalities in bone collagen synthesis
    Homocystinuria
    Ehlers-Danlos syndrome
    Osteogenesis imperfecta
  Drugs
    Corticosteroids
    Heparin therapy
    Methotrexate
    GnRH analogues
    Lithium
    Cyclosporine
  Nutritional
    Protein malnutrition
    Ascorbic acid deficiency
    Alcoholism
  Gastrointestinal
    Cirrhosis
    Malabsorption
    Postgastrectomy

Identify the cause of osteoporosis. Rule out secondary causes of osteoporosis by history, physical examination, and appropriate laboratory and radiologic tests. The endocrine tests that are required include serum level of calcium (and, if necessary, PTH), sTSH, screen for Cushing's syndrome with 1-mg overnight dexamethasone suppression test or 24-hour urinary free cortisol, and serum level of sex steroids (LH and FSH) to rule out hypogonadism. Tests to rule out myeloma and malabsorption are important. In idiopathic osteoporosis, the serum levels of calcium and phosphate are normal and the urine concentration of calcium is variable; alkaline phosphatase is normal unless there has been a recent fracture. Bone scans identify recent fractures but are otherwise negative. Localized increased uptake in the absence of fractures may indicate Paget's disease or neoplasm. Bone biopsy (after a double tetracycline label) is indicated in osteopenia in all men, black women, and premenopausal white women when the cause is undetermined to confirm the diagnosis and to rule out osteomalacia and other bone diseases.

- To identify the cause: first rule out secondary causes of osteoporosis.
- Required endocrine tests: serum level of calcium (and PTH if necessary), FTI, sTSH, screen for Cushing's syndrome, and assessment of gonadal status.
- Tests to rule out myeloma and malabsorption are important.
- Bone scan in idiopathic osteoporosis: identifies recent fractures, otherwise negative.
- Localized increased uptake, on bone scan, in the absence of fracture may indicate Paget's disease or neoplasm.
- Bone biopsy is indicated in osteopenia in all men, black women, and premenopausal white women when the cause is undetermined to confirm the diagnosis and to rule out osteomalacia or other bone disorders.

Differential Diagnosis

Osteomalacia. Presence of biochemical abnormalities: low serum levels of calcium and phosphate and increased serum level of alkaline phosphatase (these values are normal in uncomplicated osteoporosis). Pseudofractures are almost pathognomonic. The diagnosis is confirmed by bone biopsy. Remember that osteoporosis and osteomalacia can coexist.

- Presence of biochemical abnormalities, pseudofractures, or characteristic bone biopsy findings point to osteomalacia.
- Osteoporosis and osteomalacia can coexist.

Metastatic bone disease. It is strongly suspected if vertebral collapse occurs above vertebra T-9, if a primary tumor is present, if the lesion affects the posterior arches of the vertebra, or if hypercalcemia or hypercalciuria is present. Bone scan is positive. MRI should clarify the situation. Bone biopsy, if necessary, is diagnostic.

- Strongly suspect metastatic bone disease if vertebral collapse occurs above T-9, the lesion affects the posterior arches of the vertebrae, or hypercalcemia or hypercalciuria is present.
- Bone scan is positive.
- Bone scan, if necessary, is diagnostic.

Management of Postmenopausal Osteoporosis

Prevention: adequate calcium intake, 1,000 mg/day in premenopausal women and up to 1,500 mg/day in postmenopausal women of elemental calcium is recommended. Calcium carbonate is 40% elemental calcium and is the most inexpensive preparation. It should be taken with food (achlorhydric patients cannot absorb it well on an empty stomach). Calcium citrate (24% elemental calcium) is absorbed well in the presence of achlorhydria and has enhanced bioavailability. Also, adequate vitamin D of 400-800 U/day, adequate weight-bearing exercise program, and effective and rapid treatment of secondary causes of osteoporosis. If there are no known contraindications, initiate estrogen therapy as early as possible after the development of menopause and continue the therapy for life. A minimum dose of 0.625 mg of conjugated estrogens (or their equivalent) is necessary. The concomitant administration of progesterone is necessary only in women with an intact uterus to prevent endometrial hyperplasia and cancer.

- Adequate calcium intake.
- Adequate vitamin D.
- Adequate weight-bearing exercise program.
- Effective and rapid treatment of secondary causes of osteoporosis.
- For the management of menopause and in the absence of known contraindications, initiate estrogen therapy as soon as possible after menopause develops.
- Minimum dose necessary: 0.625 mg conjugated estrogens.
- Concomitant administration of progesterone: only if the uterus is intact.

Treatment: the goals are to decrease bone resorption and/or enhance bone formation. Estrogen, calcium, and calcitonin are the only drugs approved for reduction of bone resorption.

Estrogen replacement is the therapy of choice for prevention and treatment of established osteoporosis in women who do not have contraindications to its use. It decreases bone resorption and decreases the incidence of osteoporotic fractures by 50%. Estrogen is started as early as possible after the onset of the estrogen-deficient state and is continued for at least 10-15 years and, preferably, for life. It can be given orally, transdermally, topically, or by injection. Progestin is added if the patient has an intact uterus to reduce the risk of endometrial hyperplasia/endometrial carcinoma. Progestin can be added sequentially or continuously. Endometrial biopsy is indicated if the woman is overweight (greater incidence of endometrial hyperplasia), has irregular bleeding pretreatment, or unscheduled or severe bleeding develops with therapy. Yearly breast examination and mammography are indicated because of the possibility of small increase in the risk of breast cancer.

Calcitonin is an approved antiresorptive agent (this effect is greatest in patients with high bone turnover). It is given parenterally (nasal calcitonin is not available in the U.S.). Its long-term efficacy has not been established. The parenteral dose is 100 IU every other day subcutaneously. Side effects include nausea, flushing, and reactions at injection sites. In addition to its antiresorptive effect, calcitonin has a potent analgesic effect.

Bisphosphonates (analogues of pyrophosphate) are adsorbed on the hydroxyapatite crystals and are antiresorptive. They are not approved for use in osteoporosis in the U.S. They have a long skeletal life. Etidronate, the bisphosphonate of greatest use in the U.S., may impair bone mineralization. It is given cyclically for 2 weeks out of every 3 months with supplemental calcium. It decreases the incidence of fractures at 2 years in postmenopausal women but not at 3 years. Newer bisphosphonates with a more potent antiresorptive action but without mineralization impairment are being tested.

No therapy that is effective and safe for increasing bone formation is available. Fluoride can increase bone formation, but it is associated with inadequate mineralization and increased incidence of appendicular fractures; therefore, it is not recommended. Androgens in females may have unacceptable androgenic side effects.

- Treatment goals: decrease bone resorption and/or enhance bone formation.
- Only drugs approved for reduction of bone resorption: estrogen, calcium, and calcitonin.
- Bisphosphonates (etidronate): reduce bone resorption, have to be given cyclically (2 weeks every 3 months), are experimental.

Osteomalacia

Definition

Osteomalacia refers to failure of mineralization of bone osteoid resulting in an excess of unmineralized osteoid and deficiency of mature mineralized bone. In children, the disorder is known as "rickets" and is associated with failure of maturation of the growth plate and gross skeletal deformities.

Etiology

The causes of osteomalacia are outlined in Table 7-14. Basically, osteomalacia can result from vitamin D deficiency or resistance, phosphate deficiency, or abnormal bone cell, matrix, or crystal.

- Osteomalacia: failure of mineralization of bone osteoid.
- Result: excess of unmineralized osteoid.

Clinical Features

Bone pain and tenderness, fractures, deformity, proximal weakness, and waddling gait are clinical features of osteomalacia.

- Clinical features: bone pain and tenderness, fractures, deformity, proximal weakness, and waddling gait.

Diagnostic Approach

The diagnosis of osteomalacia depends on the 1) clinical picture; 2) biochemical abnormalities of serum levels of calcium, phosphate, creatinine, and alkaline phosphatase; and 3) radiologic osteopenia and characteristic Looser's zone or pseudofractures. Pseudofractures are areas of linear decalcification perpendicular to the periosteal surface and along the course of blood vessels. They usually are bilateral and symmetrical; occur in the scapula, pelvis, proximal long bones; and represent stress fractures. In children, the epiphyses are wide, cupped, and irregular. Occasionally, the skeletal findings of secondary hyperparathyroidism may be seen. Bone scan may

Table 7-14.--Causes of Osteomalacia

Disorders of vitamin D metabolism
Vitamin D deficiency
Nutritional
Malabsorption syndromes
Defects of 25(OH)D generation
Anticonvulsant agents
Severe hepatic disease
Defects of 1-25(OH)$_2$D generation
Renal failure
Hyperphosphatemia
Hereditary disorders
Vitamin D-resistant rickets, types I and II
Phosphate deficiency
Phosphate-binding antacids
Renal phosphate loss
X-linked hypophosphatemic rickets
Proximal tubular defects
Isolated
Generalized (Fanconi)
Renal tubular acidosis
Nonfamilial adulthood hypophosphatemia
Neoplasms--oncogenic osteomalacia
Abnormal bone cell, matrix, crystal
Familial hypophosphatasia
Fibrogenesis imperfecta ossium
Axial osteomalacia
Fluoride toxicity
Aluminum toxicity
Bisphosphonates

identify pseudofractures before skeletal radiographs show positive findings. 4) Definitive diagnosis of osteomalacia rests on bone biopsy findings after tetracycline labeling.

- Clinical diagnosis depends on: clinical picture; biochemical abnormalities of serum levels of calcium, phosphate, creatinine, and alkaline phosphatase; and radiologic osteopenia and characteristic Looser's zone or pseudofractures.
- Bone scan may identify pseudofractures before skeletal radiographs show positive findings.
- Definitive diagnosis of osteomalacia rests on bone biopsy findings after tetracycline labeling.

Delineation of the cause depends on the clinical picture and the results of laboratory/radiologic ancillary tests. Check the serum levels of calcium, phosphate, creatinine, alkaline phosphatase, and PTH to assess whether vitamin D deficiency is present.

Decreased or normal serum levels of calcium and high levels of PTH point to a vitamin D deficiency state: 1) high phosphorus and creatinine = renal osteodystrophy; 2) if phosphorus is low, check 25(OH)D; 3) low phosphorus and low 25(OH)D = vitamin D deficiency, liver disease, or use of anticonvulsant agents; and 4) if phosphorus, creatinine, and 25(OH)D are normal, check serum levels of 1-25(OH)$_2$D. Low 1-25(OH)$_2$D = vitamin D-dependent rickets; high 1-25(OH)$_2$D = vitamin D-resistant rickets.

Normal serum levels of calcium and PTH point to non-vitamin D-dependent osteomalacia/rickets: 1) low phosphate = phosphate depletion; 2) normal phosphate, low alkaline phosphatase = hypophosphatasia; and 3) normal phosphate, normal alkaline phosphatase = primary disorder of bone with abnormal matrix, bone cell, or bone crystal.

Renal osteodystrophy is related to phosphate retention, decreased 1-25(OH)$_2$D, and acidosis. Three major disorders are a part of the syndrome: predominant hyperparathyroid bone disease (osteitis fibrosa), predominant impaired mineralization of bone (osteomalacia), and a mixed hyperparathyroid/osteomalacic disorder. Another form of bone disease, amyloid arthropathy, is recognized with increasing frequency in patients receiving long-term hemodialysis and is attributable to an increased plasma level of β_2-microglobulin, a microglobulin deposited in tissues as amyloid fibrils.

- Renal osteodystrophy: related to phosphate retention, decreased 1-25(OH)$_2$D, and acidosis.
- Three major disorders are part of the syndrome: hyperparathyroid bone disease, predominant impaired mineralization of bone, and a mixed hyperparathyroid/osteomalacic disorder.

Oncogenic osteomalacia is characterized by renal phosphate leak that occurs in association with certain neoplasms, principally with benign mesenchymal tumors, fibrous dysplasia, prostate cancer, and, rarely, with other neoplasms (breast, lung, leukemia, or multiple myeloma). These patients typically present with muscle weakness and have hypophosphatemia, normocalcemia, and a normal PTH level. Serum levels of calcitriol and 1-25(OH)$_2$D are low. Removal of the tumor results in resolution of the oncogenic osteomalacia. The humoral cause in unknown.

Treatment

Correct the underlying disorder if possible. Also, replenish the necessary minerals. Vitamin D is the mainstay of therapy; doses may be as low as 2,000-4,000 U/day in nutritional deficiency and up to 25,000-100,000 U/day in severe malabsorption. Equivalent doses of more potent analogues may be reasonable alternatives in some forms of osteomalacia, e.g., 1-hydroxylated derivatives in osteomalacia of renal failure. Supplemental calcium is given in a dose of 1-3 g of elemental calcium per day. Oral phosphate is added in hypophosphatemic states. Bone disease may take several months to heal. Be careful to avoid the complications of vitamin D therapy, i.e., hypercalciuria, hypercalcemia, nephrolithiasis, or nephrocalcinosis.

- Correct the underlying disorder.
- Replenish necessary minerals.
- The mainstay of therapy: vitamin D.
- Doses from 2,000-4,000 U/day (in nutritional deficiency) to 25,000-100,000 U/day (in severe malabsorption).
- Supplemental elemental calcium is given in a dose of 1-3 g/day.
- Add oral phosphate in hypophosphatemic states.
- Be careful to avoid the complications of vitamin D therapy.

Paget's Disease

Paget's disease, a disorder of unknown cause, is characterized by disorganized bone remodeling, structurally weakened bone, skeletal pain, and deformities. Genetic factors and "slow virus" infection may have a role in its pathogenesis. Although this disease is rare in persons <40 years, it affects 3% of the population >45 years. Pagetoid bone is enlarged and characteristically evolves through three phases—the early "lytic phase" is followed by excessive bone formation and the "mosaic pattern" and finally by the "sclerotic phase." Paget's disease may be monostotic or polyostotic; it affects the axial skeleton more than the appendicular skeleton. Sites of predilection are the sacrum, spine, femur, tibia, skull, and pelvis.

- Paget's disease is characterized by: disorganized bone remodeling, structurally weakened bone, skeletal pain, and deformities.

- It affects 3% of the population >45 years old.
- Pagetoid bone is enlarged and evolves through three phases: lytic phase, mosaic pattern, sclerotic phase.
- It may be monostotic or polyostotic.
- Sites of predilection: sacrum, spine, femur, tibia, skull, and pelvis.

Clinical Presentation

The clinical presentation varies from asymptomatic to crippling disease. Common presentations include pain, deformity, fracture, deformity and bowing of long bones, enlargement of the skull, erythema and warmth of overlying skin, and dorsal kyphosis. Complications include compressive neurologic manifestations, high-output cardiac failure, malignant transformation (especially of lesions in the femur or humerus), and hypercalcemia with immobilization. Angioid streaks are seen in the optic fundus in 15% of patients.

- Pain, deformity, or fractures.
- Complications: compressive neurologic manifestations, high-output cardiac failure, malignant transformation (especially of tumors in the femur or humerus), and hypercalcemia with immobilization.

Evaluation

Laboratory evaluation. Increased serum level of alkaline phosphatase, which reflects increased osteoblastic activity, correlates with disease activity. It may be normal in monostotic disease. The serum levels of calcium are usually normal except with immobilization or coexistent primary hyperparathyroidism. Markers of bone turnover are usually increased, e.g., increased urinary hydroxyproline correlates with increased bone matrix resorption.

- Increased serum level of alkaline phosphatase correlates with disease activity.
- It may be normal in monostotic disease.
- Serum levels of calcium are usually normal except with immobilization or coexistent primary hyperparathyroidism.

Radiologic evaluation. This may show an early lytic lesion in the skull (osteoporosis circumscripta), in the ends of long bones (sharply defined V shape), or in the vertebra (picture frame). There may be mixed lesions in the skull (honeycomb or cotton wool), pelvis, and long bones or sclerotic lesions in the patella or vertebrae. Radioisotopic scans are more sensitive than radiography for detecting the lesions of Paget's disease. Active lesions appear hot. CT of the spine may be helpful in delineating arthritic from spinal compressive manifestations.

- Lytic lesion in the skull (osteoporosis circumscripta) and in the ends of long bone (sharply defined V shape).

- Mixed lesions in the skull, pelvis, and long bones.
- Radioisotopic scans: more sensitive than radiography for lesions of Paget's disease.
- CT: may help distinguish arthritic from spinal compressive manifestations.

Diagnostic Approach

Diagnosis is based on the clinical picture, increased serum level of alkaline phosphatase, and characteristic radiologic findings. Look for arthritic, neurologic, or cardiac complications, and keep in mind the possibility of malignant transformation. Note the differentiation from osteoblastic metastasis, especially in the pelvis: in Paget's disease, the external dimensions of the bone are increased. There is thickening of the pelvic brim and iliopectineal line (brim sign) and enlargement of the pubic and ischial bones.

- Diagnosis is based on the clinical picture, increased serum level of alkaline phosphatase, and characteristic radiologic findings.
- Look for arthritic, neurologic, or cardiac complications.
- Keep in mind the possibility of malignant transformation.
- Differentiate Paget's disease from osteoblastic metastasis, especially in the pelvis.

Treatment

The objectives of medical treatment are to decrease bone pain, to prevent or reverse complications in the CNS, heart, or weight-bearing joints, and to prepare patients for orthopedic surgery (to minimize surgical bleeding and prevent hypercalcemia of immobilization). Medical treatment is monitored with serial alkaline phosphatase determinations every 2-3 months and serial annual radiographs of lytic lesions. Calcitonin—This is the mainstay of treatment. Currently, it is given parenterally as salmon calcitonin, 50-100 MRC units/day subcutaneously. The effects are usually seen in 2-4 weeks. Maintenance doses are 50 MRC units 3 times weekly. Calcitonin can be given in courses of 6-12 months. Side effects include nausea, facial flushing, and rash. The beneficial effects may be limited by antibody formation (such patients may respond to human calcitonin). Bisphosphonates—Etidronate is the only bisphosphonate approved for such use in the U.S. at this time. It is given orally in a dose of 5-10 mg/kg daily for 6 months. Higher doses or more prolonged administration may lead to osteomalacia. Supplemental calcium is given. More potent bisphosphonates, with lesser risk of osteomalacia, are being tested. Plicamycin—It is an effective alternate therapy in refractory progressive cases. It is not approved by the FDA. Platelet, renal, and hepatic toxicity may be associated with its use. Surgical therapy—This is indicated for decompression of neurologic sequelae or to enable ambulation (total hip arthroplasty, tibial osteotomy).

- Objectives of medical treatment: to reduce bone pain; to prevent or reverse complications in CNS, heart, or weight-bearing joints; and to prepare patients for orthopedic surgery.
- Calcitonin: the mainstay of treatment.
- Calcitonin can be given in courses of 6-12 months.
- Beneficial effects may be limited by antibody formation.
- Etidronate is only bisphosphonate approved for such use in the U.S.
- Plicamycin: an effective alternative therapy in refractory progressive cases.
- Surgical therapy: for decompression of neurologic sequelae and to enable ambulation.

PANCREAS

Diabetes Mellitus

Diabetes mellitus is a metabolic disorder whose basic defect is an absolute or relative lack of insulin. In its complete form, it is manifested by hyperglycemia, accelerated atherosclerosis, microvascular disease (retina and kidney), and neuropathy. It affects about 5% of the population in the U.S.

- Diabetes mellitus: a metabolic disorder whose basic defect is an absolute or relative lack of insulin.
- The complete form is manifested by: hyperglycemia, accelerated atherosclerosis, microvascular disease (retina and kidney), and neuropathy.

Type I, insulin-dependent, ketosis-prone diabetes mellitus, juvenile-onset diabetes mellitus (IDDM) is characterized by severe absolute insulin deficiency, the patient's dependence on exogenous insulin therapy, and a high predisposition to ketosis. It affects 10%-20% of the diabetic population, usually appearing in patients <20 years old, but it can occur at any age. Both genetic and environmental factors are involved in its pathogenesis. There is concordance in twins in about 50% of cases, frequent association with certain histocompatibility antigen HLA types, and association with abnormal immune responses, including islet-cell antibodies. Five components are probably present in the pathogenetic process: genetic susceptibility, an initiating environmental event (viral or otherwise), an insulitis in the pancreas, an alteration in the beta cell that renders it "non-self," and an immune response: the end result is the destruction of the beta cells and the emergence of frank diabetes. A strong association exists between IDDM and certain HLA types encoded on chromosome 6. Associations exist between class I alleles (A,B,C), class II alleles (D), and IDDM. The D locus is considered to be of primary importance. DR3/x, DR4/x, DR3/DR4 enhance the risk; DR2 is protective. There may be an even closer association with class II DQ antigens. Candidate islet-cell antigens that initiate the autoimmune response include glutamic acid decarboxylase (GAD), insulin, and other beta-cell cytoplasmic proteins.

Some patients with IDDM may show a remission of up to several months after initial insulin therapy restores the metabolic balance. This "honeymoon" is transient and followed by recurrence of insulin deficiency and symptomatic diabetes mellitus.

- IDDM is characterized by: severe absolute insulin deficiency, patient's dependence on exogenous insulin therapy, and a high predisposition to ketosis.
- IDDM affects 10%-20% of the diabetic population.
- Genetic and environmental factors are involved in its pathogenesis.
- Concordance in twins: about 50% of cases.
- Frequent association with certain histocompatibility antigen HLA types.
- Association with abnormal immune responses.
- Some patients may have remission of up to several months after initial insulin therapy restores metabolic balance. This "honeymoon" is transient.

The risks of developing IDDM in the population at large are 1/500, in siblings 1/14, in monozygotic twins 1/3, in offspring of a female with IDDM 1/50, and in the offspring of a male with IDDM 1/20.

Type II, non-insulin-dependent, ketosis-resistant diabetes mellitus (NIDDM) is characterized by partial absolute or relative insulin deficiency (and, thus, not ketosis-prone), and, in most patients, by insulin resistance at target tissues (the bulk of the insulin resistance is postreceptor in site, particularly at the glycogen synthesis step). Deposits of amylin are found in the islets of affected patients. Amylin is a 37-amino-acid peptide normally produced and packaged with insulin by beta cells. The role of amylin in the insulin secretory defect or in insulin resistance is not known. Which of these defects is primary is not known, but both defects are required for the expression of NIDDM. In the evolution of NIDDM, three phases are recognized: 1) the phase of insulin resistance and hyperinsulinemia but with normal glucose tolerance; 2) the phase of worsened insulin resistance, continued hyperinsulinemia, and impaired glucose tolerance; and 3) the phase of decline in insulin secretion and the emergence of hyperglycemia and frank diabetes. NIDDM affects 80%-90% of the diabetic population and can occur at any age, but it usually appears in older obese patients. Genetic susceptibility is strong (the nature of the genetic influence is not known in most patients), and twin concordance is almost 100%. Environmental factors such as obesity have a definite role in the development of the disease.

- NIDDM is characterized by: partial absolute or relative insulin deficiency, resistance to development of ketosis, and (in most patients) insulin resistance at target tissues.
- It affects 80%-90% of the diabetic population.
- It usually appears in older obese patients.

- Genetic susceptibility is strong.
- Twin concordance is almost 100%.
- Environmental factors such as obesity have a definite role in the development of NIDDM.

Maturity-onset diabetes of the young is clearly linked to mutations in the glucokinase gene located on the short arm of chromosome 7. It is transmitted as an autosomal dominant trait and is expressed as mild hyperglycemia and resistance to ketosis in young persons.

Clinical Presentation

IDDM usually has a dramatic onset related to abrupt severe insulin deficiency. It usually presents with polyuria, polydipsia, polyphagia with associated weight loss, severe dehydration, ketoacidosis, and, eventually, coma. In very young children, nocturnal enuresis may signal the onset of disease.

- IDDM: usually has a dramatic onset related to abrupt severe insulin deficiency.
- Presentation: polyuria, polydipsia, polyphagia with associated weight loss, severe dehydration, and ketoacidosis.

NIDDM usually has an insidious onset. Initially, the patient may be asymptomatic, and the diagnosis is suggested by the presence of glycosuria or is made by the finding of fasting hyperglycemia. Patients may complain of blurring of vision and myopia, generalized pruritus, and episodes of recurrent infections, carbuncles, furuncles, urinary tract infections, monilial vaginitis in females, and balanitis in males. Occasionally, patients may present with evidence of chronic diabetic complications (neuropathy, nephropathy, or retinopathy) without symptoms relating to glucose intolerance. Polyuria, polydipsia, and polyphagia may develop under certain conditions when the insulin output is stressed, e.g., in pregnancy, with infection, and with the use of certain drugs such as glucocorticoids. Occasionally, patients can present with hyperosmolar nonketotic coma. Some patients may present with transient postprandial hypoglycemia. The diagnosis should be suspected in women who have delivered large babies (>9 pounds) or who have a history of hydramnios, preeclampsia, and unexplained fetal losses.

- NIDDM: usually of insidious onset.
- Initially, patients may be asymptomatic.
- Episodes of recurrent infections, carbuncles, furuncles, urinary tract infections, monilial vaginitis, or balanitis.
- Evidence of chronic diabetic complications.
- Under certain conditions when insulin output is stressed, polyuria, polydipsia, polyphagia may develop.
- Patients occasionally present with hyperosmolar nonketotic coma.
- Suspect the diagnosis in women who deliver large babies (>9 pounds) or who have a history of hydramnios, preeclampsia, or unexplained fetal losses.

Diagnosis

Confirm the Presence of Diabetes

1. Fasting plasma glucose. The normal fasting plasma glucose is <115 mg/dL. In adults (but not pregnant women), values ≥140 mg/dL on two or more separate occasions confirm the diagnosis of diabetes mellitus.
2. Oral glucose tolerance test. The main usefulness of this test is to establish or refute the diagnosis of diabetes mellitus in the following circumstances: when the fasting plasma glucose values are borderline (between 115 and 139 mg/dL), when the patient presents with symptoms related to diabetes mellitus or its known chronic complications and fasting plasma glucose is normal or borderline, and when a diagnosis of diabetes mellitus must be made during pregnancy.

- In adults (not pregnant women): fasting plasma glucose values ≥140 mg/dL on two or more separate occasions confirm the diagnosis of diabetes.
- The main usefulness of the oral glucose tolerance test: establish or refute the diagnosis of diabetes mellitus when fasting glucose values are borderline, when patient presents with symptoms related to diabetes mellitus or its known chronic complications and fasting plasma glucose is normal or borderline, and when the diagnosis of diabetes mellitus must be made during pregnancy.

3. A diagnosis of diabetes mellitus is made if on two separate occasions the fasting plasma glucose is ≥140 mg/dL and the 2-hour value and 1 additional value between 0.5 and 1.5 hour are ≥200 mg/dL. A 2-hour plasma glucose value <140 mg/dL effectively rules out the diagnosis of diabetes mellitus.
4. A diagnosis of impaired glucose tolerance is made if the fasting plasma glucose is <140 mg/dL, the 2-hour value is 140-200 mg/dL, and the intervening values are ≥200 mg/dL. Over time, patients with impaired glucose tolerance may decompensate to frank diabetes, may revert to normal glucose tolerance, or may remain unchanged. They should be reevaluated periodically or if clinical indications develop.

- Over time, patients with impaired glucose tolerance may decompensate to frank diabetes, revert to normal glucose tolerance, or remain unchanged.
- They should be reevaluated periodically.

5. Patients with previous abnormality of glucose tolerance have a history of documented hyperglycemia and have

subsequently returned to normal glucose homeostasis. They include those with gestational diabetes and those in whom hyperglycemia developed during the acute phase of myocardial infarction, during serious trauma or sepsis, or during ingestion of diabetogenic drugs.

- Patients with previous abnormality of glucose tolerance have a history of documented hyperglycemia and have subsequently returned to normal glucose homeostasis.

6. Patients with potential abnormality of glucose tolerance have normal glucose tolerance but compared with the general population are at increased risk for development of diabetes. They include monozygotic twins or other first-degree relatives of diabetic patients, obese persons, women who have delivered babies of >9 pounds, and certain racial/ethnic groups such as Native Americans and African and Hispanic Americans.

- Have normal glucose tolerance but are at increased risk for developing diabetes.
- They include: monozygotic twins or other first-degree relatives of diabetic patients, obese persons, women who delivered babies >9 pounds, and certain racial/ethnic groups.

7. Pregnancy. Early detection and optimal management of diabetes during pregnancy can prevent congenital malformations and decrease neonatal morbidity and mortality. Screening for glucose intolerance is advisable in all pregnancies. Give 50 g of glucose orally at 24-26 weeks of gestation. Measure the plasma level of glucose 1 hour later; if the value is >140 mg/dL, perform the oral glucose tolerance test. In the oral glucose tolerance test during pregnancy, 100 g of glucose is given orally. The diagnostic criteria are those of O'Sullivan and Maher. Two or more of the following plasma glucose values must be met or exceeded: fasting, 105 mg/dL; 1 hour, 190 mg/dL; 2 hours, 165 mg/dL; and 3 hours, 145 mg/dL. By these criteria, 2%-3% of all pregnancies in the U.S. are attended by gestational diabetes. The status of the carbohydrate intolerance should be reclassified in the postpartum period. Reclassification can fall into three categories: diabetes mellitus, impaired glucose tolerance, and normal with previous abnormality of glucose tolerance.

- Early detection and optimal management of diabetes during pregnancy can prevent congenital malformations and decrease neonatal morbidity and mortality.
- Screening for glucose intolerance is advisable in all pregnancies and is usually done at 24-26 weeks of gestation.
- Oral glucose tolerance test during pregnancy: give 100 g of glucose orally. Diagnostic criteria of O'Sullivan and Maher.

- Reclassify status of carbohydrate intolerance in the postpartum period.

Rule Out Secondary Diabetes

Diabetes mellitus may develop secondarily to destructive lesions or surgical removal of the pancreas or to hypersecretion of hormones with actions that are antagonistic to insulin or that interfere with insulin secretion.

- Diabetes mellitus may develop secondarily to: destructive lesions/surgical removal of pancreas and hypersecretion of hormones antagonistic to insulin or that interfere with insulin secretion.

1. Pancreatic diabetes may be caused by surgical removal of more than two-thirds of the pancreas or to chronic relapsing pancreatitis. Pancreatic diabetes differs from spontaneous IDDM by requiring (in most patients) no more than 20-40 units of insulin per day, by a greater tendency to insulin-induced hypoglycemia, by a lesser tendency to ketosis, and by its usual association with exocrine pancreatic insufficiency. Hemochromatosis is often associated with "bronze diabetes." Diabetes can be explained by increased insulin resistance resulting from cirrhosis, insulin deficiency caused by the effects of iron deposits in the pancreas, or associated genetic predisposition to diabetes. Pancreatic carcinoma should be considered in new onset of diabetes in elderly patients, particularly if associated with abdominal pain, weight loss, and depression.

- Pancreatic diabetes (unlike IDDM): requires no more than 20-40 units of insulin per day.
- Greater tendency to insulin-induced hypoglycemia.
- Lesser tendency to ketosis.
- Usually associated with exocrine pancreatic insufficiency.

2. Features common to virtually all forms of endocrinopathy-associated diabetes mellitus include reversibility of the hyperglycemia after the underlying endocrine disorder is cured and, in most patients, absence of ketosis, because of the ongoing availability of endogenous insulin. In acromegaly, the prevalence of glucose intolerance is as high as 60%, fasting hyperglycemia is observed in only 15%-30% of patients, and <10% of patients require insulin. In Cushing's syndrome, whether of an exogenous or endogenous cause, there is insulin antagonism and increased neoglucogenesis. Fasting hyperglycemia is present in 20%-25% of patients. In pheochromocytoma, excess catecholamines interfere with either insulin secretion or its action. The degree of hyperglycemia is usually mild. Carbohydrate intolerance and, rarely, frank diabetes may accompany the hypokalemia of primary

aldosteronism and is due to reversible inhibition of insulin secretion. Glucagon and somatostatin-secreting tumors of the pancreas (glucagonoma and somatostatinoma) are rare causes of the diabetic syndrome. In glucagonoma, there is weight loss, diarrhea, erythematous bullous skin eruption (necrolytic migratory erythema), anemia, hypokalemia, pancreatic tumor, and increased plasma levels of glucagon. In somatostatinoma, there is weight loss, abdominal discomfort, diarrhea, steatorrhea, hypochlorhydria, increased incidence of cholelithiasis, pancreatic tumor, and high plasma levels of somatostatin. Isolated growth hormone deficiency is associated fairly commonly with glucose intolerance. Diabetes mellitus may coexist with multiple autoimmune endocrine deficiency syndromes, including Addison's disease, Hashimoto's thyroiditis, Graves' disease, hypoparathyroidism, primary gonadal failure, and pernicious anemia.

- Features common to virtually all forms of endocrinopathy-associated diabetes mellitus: reversibility of hyperglycemia after correction of the underlying endocrine disorder and absence of ketosis.

3. Stress hyperglycemia occurs in association with acute illness (e.g., sepsis, myocardial infarction, burns, stroke, and severe trauma) and results from increased catecholamines and glucagon and decreased insulin release. It may unmask previous mild carbohydrate intolerance. Patients may not have evidence of diabetes before or after the episode. The tests of glucose tolerance should not be performed until several weeks or months after recovery and restoration of adequate nutrition and physical activity.
4. Uremia and liver cirrhosis, particularly when accompanied by portal hypertension, may be associated with glucose intolerance caused by insulin resistance and hyperglucagonemia.

In all these circumstances associated with secondary diabetes mellitus, the diagnosis is based on clinical suspicion, clinical setting, appropriate laboratory studies, and hormonal studies.

Chronic Complications

Diabetic Eye Disease

In IDDM, the prevalence of diabetic retinopathy is 50% by 10-15 years and 80% by 20 years. It is rare in those who have had diabetes mellitus for <5 years. In NIDDM, the prevalence is 50% by 15 years.

Simple background nonproliferative retinopathy can be manifested early with increased capillary permeability (detected with fluorescein angiography), occlusion and dilatation of capillaries (microaneurysms), and dilated veins. Intraretinal

hemorrhages—"dot" in the deep retinal layers and "blot" in the superficial layers—may occur. Exudates may develop—"cotton wool" from microinfarcts and "hard" from leakage of protein and lipids from the damaged capillaries. Retinal ischemia can lead to retinal and macular edema, which is the most common cause of decreased vision in diabetics, especially in older NIDDM patients. In most patients, simple retinopathy tends to remain stable. In 10 years, there is progression to proliferative retinopathy in 10%-15% of patients.

- Early manifestations of simple retinopathy: increased capillary permeability, microaneurysms, dilated veins.
- Intraretinal hemorrhages: "dot" and "blot."
- Exudates: cotton wool (microinfarcts) and hard exudates.
- In simple retinopathy, the most common cause of decreased vision is retinal and macular edema.
- In 10 years, 10%-15% of patients show progression to proliferative retinopathy.

Proliferative retinopathy consists of vascular lesions that extend from the retina and result from new vessel formation that occurs in response to the underlying retinal ischemia. It is heralded by advancing capillary and arteriolar closure with more widespread ischemia: an increase in the number of cotton wool infarcts and hemorrhages, larger intraretinal hemorrhages, venous beading, and a small network of weblike intraretinal vessels. New vessels may develop over any portion of the retina, but mostly they develop around the optic disk and penetrate into the vitreous. They present as small floating specks or cobwebs in the visual fields or as sudden and profound visual loss. Two complications may occur: 1) preretinal and vitreous hemorrhage and 2) retinal detachment due to the growth of fibrous tissue into the vitreous and the subsequent contraction of the fibrous tissue. Proliferative retinopathy is the leading cause of blindness in the 20- to 64-year-old age group in the U.S. (Proliferative retinopathy may also be caused by sickle cell anemia, retinal vein obstruction, and retrolental fibroplasia.) Pregnancy is associated with accelerated retinal lesions and poses an additional risk to vision.

- Proliferative retinopathy: due to new vessel formation that occurs in response to underlying retinal ischemia.
- Two complications: preretinal and vitreous hemorrhage and retinal detachment.
- It can present with sudden loss of vision in one eye.
- It is the leading cause of blindness in persons 20-64 years old in the U.S.

Other ophthalmic problems in diabetic patients include 1) temporary changes in the shape of the lens and marked fluctuation of visual acuity because of hyperglycemia; 2) increased frequency of cataract and glaucoma; 3) neoproliferation of vessels in the iris; and, occasionally, 4) isolated primary pupillary abnormalities such as anisocoria and Argyll Robertson pupil (i.e., decreased reactivity to light but normal reactivity in accommodation).

- Temporary changes in the shape of the lens.
- Increased frequency of cataract and glaucoma.
- Isolated primary pupillary abnormalities.

Dilated ophthalmic evaluation by an experienced ophthalmologist is critical for all diabetic patients, at least annually. In NIDDM, screen annually beginning at the time of diagnosis. In IDDM, screen postpubertally and annually beginning 5 years after the onset of IDDM. For pregnant women with IDDM, obtain an ophthalmologic consultation in the first trimester and follow closely during pregnancy. No screening is required for women with gestational diabetes. In all cases, the severity of diabetic retinopathy is worsened by increasing duration of the diabetes, poor control, and hypertension. Diabetes and hypertension should be controlled early and adequately. The Diabetes Control and Complications Trial (DCCT) has conclusively proven that intensive insulin management can reduce the risk of developing retinopathy (76%) and of progression of mild nonproliferative retinopathy (54%). Transient worsening of existing retinopathy occurs in 25% of patients in the first year of intensive treatment but there is no reduction in the long-term benefits of this therapy. Photocoagulation is used for the management of macular edema and proliferative retinopathy. Vitrectomy and repair of retinal tears are considered in the appropriate setting.

- Dilated ophthalmic evaluation is critical for all diabetic patients: in NIDDM, at diagnosis and then annually; for IDDM, after puberty and annually beginning 5 years after the diagnosis.
- In all cases, the severity of diabetic retinopathy is worsened by the duration of the diabetes, poor control, and hypertension.
- Intensive insulin therapy and improved control of diabetes can reduce the risk of the development and progression of the early stages of retinopathy.

Diabetic Renal Disease

Diabetic nephropathy is present in 15% of patients with IDDM after 15 years and in 30%-40% after 30 years. It affects about 10% of patients with NIDDM. Diabetic nephropathy is the leading cause of end-stage renal disease in the U.S. Important factors in its pathogenesis include: duration of diabetes, degree of control, hypertension or family history of hypertension, high protein intake, and genetic propensity. Early lesions are those of microvascular glomerular disease, with glomerular hypertrophy, hyperfiltration, and microalbuminuria. As the disease progresses, diffuse thickening of the basement membrane and increased mesangial volume occur. This

increased mesangial volume may lead to glomerular occlusion and diffuse or nodular (Kimmelstiel-Wilson) lesions. Microalbuminuria (30-250 mg/24 hours) precedes overt proteinuria and can identify patients at risk for nephropathy. It can be reversed with adequate control of diabetes and blood pressure. The development of persistent proteinuria in IDDM (>0.5 g/24 hours) heralds a relentless progression to end-stage renal disease. In patients with NIDDM, proteinuria occurs earlier, and its occurrence does not necessarily indicate such progression. Persistent proteinuria of >3.5 g/day may progress to classic nephrotic syndrome and usually means that renal failure will occur within 3-5 years. The rate of progression of late phases can be affected by several factors: hypertension, infection, obstruction, or use of contrast agents. Glycemic control is of no benefit in the later stages of nephropathy; protein restriction is under study. Hypertension is volume-dependent and can be treated with salt restriction, thiazide or loop diuretics, angiotensin converting enzyme (ACE) inhibitors, or calcium channel blockers. Studies suggest that the use of ACE inhibitors in the microalbuminuria stage and before the development of hypertension may decrease the risk of the development of nephropathy.

- Diabetic nephropathy: occurs in 15% of patients with IDDM after 15 years and in 40% after 30 years.
- Early lesions: glomerular hypertrophy, hyperfiltration, and microalbuminuria.
- With disease progression: diffuse thickening of the basement membrane. May lead to glomerular occlusion and diffuse or nodular (Kimmelstiel-Wilson) lesions.
- Microalbuminuria (30-250 mg/24 hours) precedes overt proteinuria and can identify patients at risk for nephropathy.
- Can be reversed with adequate control of diabetes and blood pressure.
- Persistent proteinuria in IDDM (>0.5 g/24 hours) heralds relentless progression to end-stage renal disease.
- Persistent proteinuria of >3.5 g/day may progress to classic nephrotic syndrome. It usually means renal failure within 3-5 years.
- The rate of progression of late phases is affected by hypertension, infection, obstruction, and the use of contrast agents.
- Use of ACE inhibitors in the microalbuminuria stage even before hypertension develops may decrease the risk of developing nephropathy.

The use of contrast dyes in diabetes mellitus may induce rapid deterioration of renal function and acute renal failure. This deterioration is manifested as oliguria and an increasing serum level of creatinine (which peaks in 2-4 days and resolves in 1-4 weeks) or as acute renal failure. Predisposing factors include old age, dehydration, preexisting renal impairment, and liver disease. Do not perform contrast studies unless they are clearly indicated and the benefits of the study outweigh the risks. Before and after the study, hydrate the patient well, monitor fluid balance, and check the serum level of creatinine every 12 hours until a pattern is established.

- Contrast dyes: may induce rapid deterioration of renal function and acute renal failure.
- Deterioration is manifested as oliguria and an increased serum level of creatinine or as acute renal failure.

Other manifestations of diabetic kidney disease include syndrome of hyporeninemic hypoaldosteronism (see below), renal tubular acidosis after diabetic ketoacidosis, necrotizing papillitis, and acute/chronic pyelonephritis.

- Syndrome of hyporeninemic hypoaldosteronism.
- Acute renal tubular acidosis after diabetic ketoacidosis.
- Necrotizing papillitis.
- Acute/chronic pyelonephritis.

Prevention. Most important are intensive treatment of hyperglycemia and adequate control of hypertension. Added benefits are derived from restriction of dietary protein and the avoidance of nephrotoxic dyes or drugs. The use of ACE inhibitors has been shown to delay the onset and progression of diabetic nephropathy in IDDM and to stabilize albuminuria and renal function in NIDDM. The renal protective effects are independent of the effects on systemic blood pressure.

Detection. Microalbuminuria, defined as excretion of 30-300 mg of albumin/day, is associated with renal morphologic and hemodynamic changes and predicts the impairment of renal function in IDDM. In NIDDM, microalbuminuria is not so predictive. In both types of diabetes, microalbuminuria is an independent risk factor for death due to cardiovascular disease.

Check for microalbuminuria: in IDDM, annually in postpubertal patients who have had the disease for 5 years or more; in NIDDM, annually. Use quantitative assays in a 24-hour collection or in a single-voided early morning urine and adjusted for creatinine. Do not test for microalbuminuria after exercise or during a urinary tract infection or diabetic ketoacidosis.

Treatment. Optimal control of diabetes in the early phases, antihypertensive therapy (see below), and protein restriction.

Diabetes and the Nervous System

Neuropathy may occur early in diabetes mellitus, but the frequency and severity increase in proportion to the duration and severity of the hyperglycemia. Neuropathy is clinically evident in about 30% of patients with diabetes of more than 10 years' duration.

- Neuropathy may occur early in diabetes mellitus.
- The frequency and severity of neuropathy increase proportionally to the duration and severity of hyperglycemia.

- Neuropathy is clinically evident in about 30% of patients with diabetes of more than 10 years' duration.

Prevention. Intensive treatment of hyperglycemia. DCCT has shown that better control of hyperglycemia decreases the occurrence of clinical neuropathy by 60%. The use of aldose reductase inhibitors is experimental.

Peripheral polyneuropathy is the most commonly encountered type. It is usually bilateral and symmetrical and affects the lower extremities more commonly than the upper extremities. It presents with numbness, paresthesias, or hyperesthesia or with deep-seated moderate-to-severe pain that is worse at night. The onset may be insidious or acute, often occurring during the loss of diabetic control because of infection or another stress. Peripheral polyneuropathy also presents with abnormalities of proprioceptive fibers, leading to gait abnormalities and development of Charcot's joints (painless progressive destruction of articular cartilage and joint architecture and function; radiography commonly reveals loss of the arch and multiple fractures of the tarsal bones). Neurotrophic ulcers may develop, particularly on the plantar aspect of the feet, and may be complicated by osteomyelitis. Examination shows absence of deep tendon reflexes and decreased vibration sense. Therapy—Optimize control of diabetes; use amitriptyline with or without fluphenazine or local capsaicin cream for pain relief.

- Peripheral polyneuropathy: the most common type encountered.

Mononeuropathy, probably of vascular origin, can affect any single nerve trunk and characteristically can present with sudden wristdrop, footdrop, or painful diplopia resulting from cranial nerve III, IV, or VI dysfunction. There is a high degree of spontaneous reversibility, usually over several weeks. In cranial nerve mononeuropathy, pain precedes the development of paralysis by 5-10 days. When cranial nerve III is involved, there is a characteristic sparing of the pupillary fibers in >80% of patients. Aneurysms or intracranial mass lesions generally involve both the pupillary fibers and the fibers to the extraocular muscles.

- Mononeuropathy: probably of vascular origin.
- Characteristic presentation: sudden wristdrop, footdrop, or painful diplopia resulting from cranial nerve III, IV, or VI dysfunction.
- High degree of spontaneous reversibility.
- When cranial nerve III is involved, characteristic sparing of pupillary fibers in >80% of patients.

Radiculopathy is a sensory syndrome that can present with pain in the distribution of one or more spinal nerves, usually in the chest wall, abdomen, and lower extremities. It is also usually self-limited.

- Radiculopathy: sensory syndrome with pain in the distribution of one or more spinal nerves.
- It is usually self-limited.

Autonomic neuropathy can involve virtually every organ system, but the gastrointestinal tract is the primary target. Although constipation is the most common manifestation of this autonomic neuropathy, it tends to be overshadowed by the common, distressing diabetic diarrhea, which consists of intermittent explosive diarrhea that is not preceded by cramps and is seemingly worse at night. Radiologic studies may demonstrate characteristic patterns of disordered small-bowel motility. Steatorrhea suggests coexisting celiac disease or other causes of malabsorption. Diabetic gastroparesis may present with early satiety and nausea or vomiting. Radiologic or electrophysiologic studies may reveal impaired peristalsis and delayed gastric emptying. This complication is important because, as a result of the inconsistency of food absorption, there may be unpredictable swings in plasma levels of glucose and in levels of diabetic control. Esophageal dysfunction and dysphagia may also occur. Treatment options for gastroparesis, which occasionally responds to drug therapy, include the use of erythromycin (750 mg/day), metoclopramide (10 mg three to four times daily), and cisapride (10 mg four times daily). Erythromycin is the drug of first choice. Diabetic diarrhea is treated with tetracycline (200-500 mg) at the beginning of the attack; if ineffective, treat with diphenoxylate with atropine.

- Autonomic neuropathy: can involve virtually every organ system.
- The gastrointestinal tract is the primary target.
- The most common manifestation: constipation.
- Diabetic diarrhea can be managed with the use of tetracycline at the beginning of the attack.
- Steatorrhea suggests coexisting celiac disease or other diseases of malabsorption.
- Diabetic gastroparesis: important because as a result of inconsistency of food absorption there may be unpredictable swings in the plasma level of glucose and in levels of diabetic control. Erythromycin is the drug of first choice.

Genitourinary involvement includes urinary bladder dysfunction, which occurs in >50% of patients with diabetes of more than 20 years' duration. It can present as hesitancy, delayed and incomplete emptying, and residual urine. A voiding cystometrogram may reveal decreased propulsive efforts and increased residual urine. Urinary bladder dysfunction may be complicated initially by bacteriuria and later by overt urinary tract infection. Therapy is bladder drainage, antibacterial therapy for infections, and encouraging voiding every 3 hours by manual pressure. Potency impairment occurs in >50% of men with long-standing diabetes and may be the initial presentation of the diabetic syndrome. Another cause of potency impairment in diabetic patients is penile vascular insufficiency caused by aortoiliac occlusive disease (Leriche's syndrome). Diabetic male patients may also have retrograde ejaculation.

- Urinary bladder dysfunction is common and may be complicated by bacteriuria and overt urinary tract infection.
- Potency impairment in diabetic males may be due to (among other causes) autonomic neuropathy or penile vascular insufficiency.

Features of cardiovascular autonomic neuropathy may include manifestations of persistent resting tachycardia, orthostatic hypotension, and neuropathic edema. For orthostatic hypotension, encourage slow changes in position, Jobst leg compression, and use of fludrocortisone for orthostatic hypotension. Irregularity of sweating and partial and total anhidrosis may be observed; a patchy distribution of sweating may be particularly evident in the face. An unusual variant of autonomic instability may be manifested in some diabetic patients by gustatory sweating after eating.

Diabetic neuromuscular disease presents with symmetrical painless atrophy and weakness of the intrinsic hand muscles that may be associated with sensory impairment. It occurs more commonly in elderly patients and in males. Diabetic amyotrophy refers to a progressive weakness and wasting that involves the muscles of the pelvic girdle and anterior thigh compartments, most commonly the quadriceps femoris. It is usually accompanied by severe pain and may be distributed asymmetrically. It characteristically occurs in elderly men and generally resolves in 6-12 months after the time of diagnosis. A similar but less painful variant occurs in the upper extremities.

- Diabetic amyotrophy: progressive weakness and wasting of muscles of pelvic girdle and anterior thigh compartment.
- It usually is accompanied by severe pain.
- It may be distributed asymmetrically.
- It occurs characteristically in elderly men.
- It resolves in 6-12 months after diagnosis.

In diabetic neuropathy, electromyography may show a decrease in motor and sensory nerve conduction velocity, evidence of denervation and fasciculation, and characteristic distribution of nerve dysfunction. Examination of the CSF may show a slight increase in protein content.

Macrovascular Disease

Arteriosclerosis, which appears earlier and is more extensive in diabetic patients than in the general population, can present clinically as peripheral vascular disease (with intermittent claudication, gangrene, and impotence), coronary artery disease (with angina and myocardial infarction), and cerebrovascular disease (e.g., stroke). Coronary artery disease accounts for 70% of the deaths in the diabetic population. It tends to involve the proximal and distal vessels in the right and left coronary arterial systems. Atypical manifestations may occur. Angina may present with epigastric distress, heartburn, and neck or jaw pain. Myocardial infarction may be silent (in 15% of patients) because of autonomic neuropathy. It should be suspected in those patients with sudden onset of left ventricular failure. Diabetes mellitus may also be associated with cardiomyopathy and heart failure (in 17% of patients) in the absence of other identifiable causes and with a normal coronary arterial system by angiography. Peripheral vascular disease has a higher frequency of distal involvement, particularly in the lower extremities. Arteriography should be used with caution if the patient has diminished renal function, because acute tubular necrosis may develop. Arteriography should be reserved for patients who are candidates for vascular surgery.

- Arteriosclerosis can present as: peripheral vascular disease, coronary artery disease, or cerebrovascular disease.
- Atypical manifestations may occur.
- Myocardial infarction may be silent.
- Suspect myocardial infarction in patients with sudden onset left ventricular failure.
- Peripheral vascular disease: higher frequency of distal involvement, particularly lower extremities.
- Arteriography: use cautiously; reserve for candidates for vascular surgery.

Diabetic foot ulcers result from the effects of neuropathy and vascular disease. Abnormal pressure distribution results in callus formation; ill-fitting shoes cause blisters; and foreign bodies lead to abrasions and punctures. The ulcers are painless and frequently complicated by infection and osteomyelitis. Therapy consists of prevention or relief of maldistribution of pressure, prompt treatment of infections, and documentation and correction of vascular insufficiency.

- Diabetic foot ulcers: painless; frequently complicated by infection and osteomyelitis.

Hypertension

ACE inhibitors are the first line of therapy in hypertensive diabetic patients with normal renal function. ACE inhibitors normalize intraglomerular pressure, reduce proteinuria, and have no adverse effects on glucose and lipid levels. *Caution*: they may cause acute deterioration of renal function in patients with renal artery stenoses; therefore, monitor the serum level of creatinine carefully at the initiation of therapy. ACE inhibitors may also worsen the hyperkalemia of hyporeninemic hypoaldosteronism. Calcium channel blockers are reasonable alternatives, especially for patients with coexistent coronary artery

disease. They may induce minimal impairment in glucose tolerance but have no adverse effects on lipids. Avoid nifedipine because it dilates the efferent and afferent glomerular arterioles and can increase glomerular pressure and microalbuminuria. Use nicardipine or diltiazem. A low dose of a combination of ACE inhibitors and calcium channel blockers is effective and associated with fewer side effects. Thiazides are no longer a first-line therapy, especially in NIDDM, because of their metabolic side effects. In addition to inducing hypokalemia, they impair glucose tolerance, partly due to hypokalemia, and increase low-density lipoprotein cholesterol (LDL-C) and triglycerides. If a decision to use thiazides is made, do not use >50 mg/day or its equivalent. β-Blockers are also undesirable because of their metabolic side effects: glucose intolerance, masking of hypoglycemia, and hyperlipidemia. α-Adrenergic antagonists are effective and can reduce microalbuminuria; they have minimal metabolic side effects.

- ACE inhibitors: first line of therapy in hypertensive diabetic patients with normal renal function. Monitor serum creatinine levels carefully at the initiation of therapy.
- Calcium channel blockers: reasonable alternatives, especially for patients with coexistent coronary artery disease. Avoid nifedipine.
- A low dose of a combination of ACE inhibitors and calcium channel blockers is effective and associated with fewer side effects.
- Thiazides: no longer first-line therapy, especially in NIDDM, because of their metabolic side effects.
- Avoid β-blockers if possible: can impair glucose tolerance, mask hypoglycemic manifestations, and induce an atherogenic lipid profile.
- Can use α-adrenergic antagonists.

Hyperlipidemia

Diabetes mellitus often leads to abnormalities in the three major classes of lipoproteins. In IDDM, lipid levels are usually normal if the diabetic state is well controlled and there is no renal impairment. Diabetic ketoacidosis is associated with increased very-low-density lipoprotein (VLDL) synthesis by the liver and decreased catabolism of VLDL and chylomicrons because of inhibition of lipoprotein lipase. Triglyceride levels may reach very high levels, and eruptive xanthomas may appear. In NIDDM, triglyceride-rich lipoproteins are increased because of overproduction of VLDL and decreased lipoprotein lipase activity. Both defects are corrected with better control of the diabetic state. High-density lipoprotein-cholesterol (HDL-C) levels are low; the increased triglycerides play a role here. The levels do improve but usually do not normalize with control of diabetes. LDL-C levels are usually not affected by the diabetic state but may be elevated in the presence of renal failure, genetic diseases, or other associated diseases such as hypothyroidism. However, compositional changes in LDL may occur (including glycosylation, increased susceptibility to oxidation, and small dense low-density lipoproteins). These compositional changes may increase the atherogenicity of LDL-C in patients with diabetes.

Infections

Although infections may not occur more frequently in diabetic than in nondiabetic patients, they tend to be more severe because of the presence of hyperglycemia (which impairs leukocyte function) and because of associated macro- and microvascular disease, which decreases regional blood flow. In diabetic patients, there is an increased frequency of cutaneous infections (*Staphylococcus* infections, furuncles, pyoderma, and carbuncles), urinary tract infections (cystitis, pyelonephritis, and papillary necrosis), lung infections (pneumonia), extremity infections (gram-negative and anaerobic infections), and genital tract infections (vulvovaginitis and balanitis). Three unusual conditions appear to have specific relationships with the diabetic syndrome: malignant external otitis, rhinocerebral mucormycosis, and emphysematous cholecystitis.

- Diabetic patients have an increased frequency of: cutaneous, urinary tract, lung, extremity, and genital tract infections.
- Three unusual conditions having specific relationships with the diabetic syndrome: malignant external otitis, rhinocerebral mucormycosis, and emphysematous cholecystitis.

Dermatologic Complications

Various cutaneous lesions may occur in diabetic patients. Necrobiosis lipoidica diabeticorum consists of plaque-like lesions with central yellowish areas surrounded by a brownish border, usually occurring over the anterior surfaces of the legs. Ulceration may occur. Diabetic dermopathy consists of small rounded plaques with a raised border and occurs over the anterior tibial surfaces. The plaques may ulcerate centrally and crust at the edges. As these lesions heal, there is a depressed scar and diffuse brown discoloration. Dupuytren's contractures occur in 5%-20% of diabetic patients. Diabetic cheirarthropathy occurs in IDDM and presents with finger stiffness, periarticular swelling, and waxy thickened skin, resembling scleroderma. Eruptive xanthomas caused by significant hypertriglyceridemia may occur in uncontrolled diabetes.

Management of Diabetes Mellitus

Goals of Therapy

"Practical" goals. These apply to all patients and include 1) the elimination of ketosis and symptomatic hyper- and hypoglycemia, 2) preservation of well-being in adults and normal growth and development in children, 3) achieving and maintaining ideal body weight, and 4) provision of accessible care that encourages self-care and periodic surveillance. Currently, the available standard therapeutic regimens can achieve these goals in most patients. Unfortunately, such regimens do not normalize the metabolic derangements in many patients and are associated with a high incidence of micro- and macrovascular complications, which develop with increasing duration of the disease.

Restoration of euglycemia. This goal, which is based on the assumption that normalization of hyperglycemia will prevent/delay the micro- and macrovascular complications of the disease, is difficult to achieve. In pregnancy-associated diabetes, current evidence mandates attempts at achieving and maintaining euglycemia before and certainly during pregnancy. The Diabetes Control and Complications Trial has shown that restoration of euglycemia in IDDM prevents or reverses early manifestations of microvascular complications.

- In pregnancy-associated diabetes: achieving and maintaining euglycemia before and during pregnancy are mandated.
- Restoration of euglycemia in IDDM prevents or reverses early manifestations of microvascular complications.

The Diabetes Control and Complications Trial (1993). Intensive insulin therapy in patients with uncomplicated or minimally complicated IDDM leads to unequivocal and significant reduction in retinopathy, microalbuminuria, albuminuria, and clinical neuropathy.

Clinically important progression in retinopathy was reduced by 62% (by 76% if no retinopathy was present at baseline, and by 54% if mild nonproliferative retinopathy was present at baseline). Clinically significant nephropathy was reduced by 56%, and sustained microalbuminuria was decreased by 46%. Clinically significant neuropathy was reduced by 66%. Whether these encouraging results will apply to IDDM patients with significant microvascular and macrovascular complications or to NIDDM patients is not known. It is important to note that intensive insulin therapy was fraught with some significant complications: increased incidence of hypoglycemia (threefold), hypoglycemia unawareness, and increase in weight.

The generally accepted biochemical indices of metabolic control are listed in Table 7-15.

The modalities currently available in the U.S. are diet, exercise, oral antidiabetic agents, insulin, and combination therapy. Metformin was recently introduced in the U.S. Diet therapy—This is the first step. Its main objective is to restore and maintain normal weight in all diabetics. In many patients with NIDDM, this can decrease insulin resistance, improve insulin secretion, and restore euglycemia. An optimal diet plan should address caloric content, distribution of nutrients, and, in those receiving insulin therapy, timing of meals and snacks. Nutrient distribution should be roughly 50%-60% complex carbohydrates (restrict glucose and sucrose and increase dietary fiber),

Table 7-15.--Biochemical Indices of Metabolic Control

	Ideal	Acceptable	Poor
Fasting plasma glucose, mg/dL	<115	116-140	>200
Postprandial plasma glucose, mg/dL	<140	141-200	>235
Hemoglobin A_{1c}, %	<6	6-8	<10
Serum cholesterol, mg/dL	<200	200-239	>240
Serum triglycerides, mg/dL	<150	150-249	>250
Serum HDL cholesterol, mg/dL	>40	---	---

15%-20% proteins, and 20%-30% fats (<10% saturated fat and <300 mg cholesterol). In insulin-requiring patients, the distribution of calories is important. Different distributions may be required for different lifestyles. Exercise—A regular exercise program is encouraged. Its benefits include reduction in cardiovascular risk factors, weight reduction, increased insulin sensitivity, and improved sense of well-being. The risks of exercise include hypoglycemia, arrhythmia, myocardial infarction or sudden death, increased blood pressure, vitreous hemorrhage, and injuries. If initial diabetic control is poor, exercise worsens glycemic control. The major problem with diet/exercise therapy is patient noncompliance.

- Treatment modalities available in U.S.: diet, exercise, oral antidiabetic agents, insulin, and combination therapy.
- Diet therapy is the first step.
- Objective: restore and maintain normal weight.
- Optimal diet plan should address: caloric content, distribution of nutrients, and the timing of meals and snacks (for patients receiving insulin therapy).
- A regular exercise program is encouraged.
- Major problem with diet/exercise therapy: patient noncompliance.

When patients fail to meet the above outlined goals by diet and exercise, the therapeutic program should be advanced. The patient's age, weight, duration of diabetes, environment, and general health are among the factors that need to be considered in selecting the appropriate therapy.

Oral Sulfonylureas (Oral Antidiabetic Agents)

Oral sulfonylureas act primarily by increasing the ability of the pancreatic islets to secrete insulin. The dose, effectiveness, and duration of the action of these drugs are listed in Table 7-16.

- Oral sulfonylureas: act primarily by increasing the ability of pancreatic islets to secrete insulin.

Indications: fasting plasma level of glucose <250 mg/dL, age at onset of NIDDM >40 years, duration of diabetes <5 years, normal or excessive weight, and no previous therapy with insulin or insulin dose <40 U/day. Contraindications: IDDM, pregnant or lactating diabetic women, hepatic/renal insufficiency, and sulfa allergy. Efficacy: the primary failure rate is about 20%. Secondary failure occurs in about 5%-10% of patients a year and is probably caused by continued deterioration of islet reserve and/or progression of insulin resistance. Remember that transient failures may be due to intercurrent acute medical/surgical illness, failure to adhere to the diet, and weight gain. Complications: few serious adverse effects. The most serious one is hypoglycemia, especially in elderly patients who are ill-nourished and have renal/hepatic failure. Other side effects are gastrointestinal, dermatologic, and hematopoietic. Side effects uniquely associated with chlorpropamide use include antabuse-like effect and syndrome of inappropriate ADH. Selection of agent: consider potency, duration of action, dosage range, metabolism, side effects, cost, convenience, and potential drug interactions. Also consider the known contraindications. Prescribe the lowest effective dose and increase it weekly until satisfactory control or the highest recommended dose is reached. Those patients who respond to oral antidiabetic agents should undergo periodic reassessment to find the lowest effective dose and to assess for secondary failure.

Table 7-16.--Oral Sulfonylureas

Name Generic	Brand	Daily dose, mg	Relative effectiveness	Duration of action, hr
Tolbutamide	Orinase	500-3,000	1	6-12
Chlorpropamide	Diabinese	100-500	5	60
Acetohexamide	Dymelor	250-1,500	2.5	12-18
Tolazamide	Tolinase	100-1,000	5	12-24
Glipizide	Glucotrol	5-40	20	12-24
Glyburide	DiaBeta, Micronase	2.5-20	40	16-24

- Indications: fasting plasma glucose <250 mg/dL, age at disease onset >40 years, duration of disease <5 years, normal or excessive weight, and no previous insulin therapy or insulin dose <40 U/day.
- Contraindications: IDDM, pregnant or lactating diabetics, hepatic/renal insufficiency, and sulfa allergy.
- Efficacy: primary failure rate, 20%; secondary failure, 5%-10% a year.
- Transient failure due to: intercurrent acute medical/surgical illness, failure to adhere to diet, and weight gain.
- Most serious complication: hypoglycemia, especially in the elderly who are ill-nourished and have hepatic/renal failure.
- Side effects specifically related to chlorpropamide include: antabuse-like effect and syndrome of inappropriate ADH.

Second-generation agents (glyburide, glipizide) are analogues of first-generation drugs and are considerably more potent (50x-100x). There is no difference in mechanism of action, efficacy, contraindications, or complications. Secondary failures may be less common. These drugs are nonionically bound to plasma proteins and so are not displaced by other ionically charged drugs such as warfarin and phenylbutazone. Concurrent use of the latter medications does not lead to variation in bioavailability of the second-generation oral antidiabetic agents.

- Second-generation agents: glyburide and glipizide.
- They are nonionically bound to plasma proteins and, thus, not displaced by other ionically charged drugs, e.g., warfarin and phenylbutazone.

Treatment of oral antidiabetic agent failure. When patients fail to meet treatment goals, therapy should be escalated. Various approaches have been evaluated, and it is clear that any treatment that improves glycemic control can potentially improve the response to oral antidiabetic agents. The options are 1) stress treatment with diet; this may correct the postreceptor defect and improve endogenous insulin response. 2) Try another oral agent; 10%-15% of patients failing to respond to one agent may respond to another. 3) Discontinue use of the oral agent and start treatment with insulin. 4) Add insulin to the oral agent if patient continues to show some response to the drug; combination therapy may lead to better control than with an oral antidiabetic agent alone. Similar control can be achieved with insulin alone, although generally larger doses are required. Administration of insulin at bedtime to control fasting hyperglycemia has some merit and may require lower doses and cause less perturbation of a patient's lifestyle.

- Stress treatment with diet.
- Try another oral agent.
- Discontinue using oral agent and start treating with insulin.

- Add insulin to the oral agent.

Biguanides (Metformin and Phenformin)

The use of phenformin has been discontinued in the U.S. because of its possible association with lactic acidosis. Metformin has been introduced recently. These drugs act by inhibiting neoglucogenesis and by enhancing insulin action (increased insulin receptor number and activity). Metformin therapy rarely causes lactic acidosis and is not complicated by hypoglycemia. It should not be given to patients with renal disease. Its use should be stopped if nausea, vomiting, diarrhea, or intercurrent disease develops.

Insulin Therapy

Because the types of insulin are well known, they will not be discussed here. Some important caveats are: 1. Peak effects and duration of action vary from patient to patient and depend on the dose given and the route of administration. 2. Insulin action is delayed in many patients who have been treated chronically with insulin, probably because of the presence of insulin antibodies. 3. Lente and NPH insulins are roughly equivalent; Lente insulin is slightly more immunogenic and mixes less well with regular insulin

Conventional Therapy

This involves the administration of one or two injections of intermediate-acting insulin such as Lente or NPH with or without the addition of small doses of regular insulin. 1) A single daily injection of insulin will provide adequate control only in patients who have some residual capacity to secrete insulin. 2) Patients with poorly controlled diabetes should receive a split insulin program: about two-thirds of the insulin dose is given in the morning before breakfast and one-third before supper. Many physicians routinely add regular insulin to each dose. 3) Commercial premixed insulins (70/30 intermediate/regular) are acceptable and convenient for many patients. 4) All patients should be taught insulin-dose modifications: increase the insulin dose by 2-3 units every 2-3 days for better control of hyperglycemia, and, in the management of hypoglycemia, decrease by 2 units the following day. 5) For patients willing to self-monitor blood glucose levels, an algorithm can be provided. 6) Self-monitoring of blood glucose is essential in all treatment schedules using variable insulin dosages. Measurement of urinary glucose is obsolete; however, measurement of urinary ketones continues to play an important part in the care of insulin-dependent diabetics. 7) The only demonstrable clinical advantage to using highly purified or human insulin is a decline in the incidence of local reactions, insulin allergy/immune resistance, and lipoatrophy.

Intensive Insulin Therapy

Simply stated, the goals of intensive insulin therapy are to achieve euglycemia and to avoid hypoglycemia. It attempts to duplicate the physiologic pattern of insulin release in nondiabetic persons and uses either an insulin pump or a multiple-dose insulin (MDI) program. It provides:

1. Basal rate of insulin. Pump—Constant delivery of 0.6 U/hour of CZI in a 50-kg patient. An increase in the basal rate may sometimes be required between 4 a.m. and 8 a.m. to meet increased insulin needs (dawn phenomenon). MDI—Usually a single dose of Ultralente (at times a split dose is required). The basal rate is about half of the total daily dose and must be individually adjusted.
2. Preprandial boluses of CZI are superimposed to control postprandial glucose excursions. The bolus is delivered 15-60 minutes before a meal.

● Intensive insulin therapy: to achieve euglycemia and to avoid hypoglycemia.
● It attempts to duplicate the physiologic pattern of insulin release.
● Use either an insulin pump or MDI program.

In addition, various schemes that use intermediate insulin have been proposed. They include two regimens. 1) A regimen with mixed crystalline zinc insulin and intermediate-acting insulin at breakfast, crystalline zinc insulin at dinner, and intermediate-acting insulin at bedtime. 2) A regimen with premeal crystalline zinc insulin and bedtime intermediate-acting insulin. In general, these regimens are less preferable for the following reasons: 1) the peak of intermediate insulin may vary from patient to patient and in any individual patient; 2) in the attempt to suppress overnight hepatic neoglucogenesis, the patient may be exposed to the risk of hypoglycemia during peak activity of the intermediate-acting insulin.

● Various schemes that use intermediate-acting insulin have been proposed.

Indications for intensive therapy: children with IDDM who are older than 7 years (younger age may be associated with more significant CNS damage from hypoglycemia); prepregnancy in IDDM to prevent congenital malformations; during pregnancy in IDDM to prevent fetal macrosomy, respiratory distress syndrome, and perinatal mortality; after renal transplantation.

Requirements for intensive therapy include careful patient selection (i.e., sophisticated, motivated patients), formal education and training program, intensive dietary and physical activity instruction, self-monitoring of blood glucose 4 times/day and at 3 a.m. at least once weekly, and frequent outpatient visits to review data and make adjustments. Avoid intensive therapy in patients with established diabetic complications and those at greater risk for hypoglycemia.

● Only firm indications for therapy: pregnancy and patients

with IDDM, particularly early in the disease.

Complications of intensive insulin therapy include:

1. Hypoglycemia. This is the major complication of intensive insulin therapy, and the risk is twofold to threefold. The goal of euglycemia brings patients closer to hypoglycemic levels. Insulin pumps do not turn themselves off when blood glucose levels are low. Intensive therapy lowers the threshold for hypoglycemia awareness and for the release of counterregulatory hormones (see below).
2. Diabetic ketoacidosis. "Pump-treated" patients are more prone to diabetic ketoacidosis because of limited insulin depot and frequent transient interruption of flow.
3. Catheter abscess. This occurs in about 10%-15% of patients. Skin care at insertion sites is important.

● Hypoglycemia: the major complication of intensive insulin therapy.
● Intensive therapy: lowers threshold for hypoglycemia awareness and for release of counterregulatory hormones. Many diabetic patients have impaired glucagon and epinephrine response to hypoglycemia.
● Diabetic ketoacidosis: "pump-treated" patients.
● Catheter abscess.

Insulin Therapy in NIDDM

Indications include 1) temporary use during pregnancy, major surgery, or serious infection. 2) Newly diagnosed NIDDM in a patient <40 years old of normal or below-normal weight and who has evidence of insulin lack, i.e., hyperglycemia >250 mg/dL, glycosuria, ketosis, and weight loss greater than can be accounted for by dehydration. Insulin therapy leads to rapid control of metabolic abnormalities. In these patients, oral antidiabetic agents are less likely to succeed and may take many weeks to achieve control. 3) Diet/exercise/oral agent failure: about 40% of patients with NIDDM require insulin therapy to achieve acceptable metabolic control.

● Temporary use during pregnancy, major surgery, and serious infection.
● Newly diagnosed NIDDM in patient: <40 years old, normal/below-normal weight, evidence of insulin lack (hypoglycemia >250 mg/dL, ketosis, weight loss greater than accounted for by dehydration).
● Diet/exercise/oral agent failure.

Special Considerations in the Management of Diabetes

Hypoglycemia in Diabetics

Treated diabetics (except those taking metformin) are vulnerable to hypoglycemia because of insulin excess and counterregulatory failure. Early in the course of diabetes, glucagon responses to hypoglycemia are lost and the patient becomes dependent on the early release of catecholamines, and later of cortisol and GH, for recovery from hypoglycemia. These counterregulators increase glycogenolysis, decrease neoglucogenesis, and decrease glucose utilization. The catecholamine responsiveness is critical for early and rapid recovery. Loss of this catecholamine responsiveness can lead to hypoglycemia unawareness and to impaired recovery from hypoglycemia. It can occur in autonomic neuropathy and with the use of β-blockers. The occurrence of hypoglycemia can impair catecholamine responsiveness for some time (hours to days) by lowering the glycemic set-point for release of catecholamines.

- Treated diabetics (except for metformin) are vulnerable to hypoglycemia because of insulin excess and counterregulatory failure.
- Glucagon secretion is lost early in the course of diabetes.
- Epinephrine is important for hypoglycemia awareness and for effective early recovery from hypoglycemia. Cortisol and GH contribute to the late phase of recovery.
- Loss of catecholamines can lead to hypoglycemia unawareness and impaired recovery from hypoglycemia.
- This can occur after hypoglycemia, in autonomic neuropathy, and with the use of β-blockers.

The symptoms of hypoglycemia are catecholaminergic and neuroglycopenic. In general, catecholaminergic symptoms appear first if the rate of decrease of plasma glucose is rapid. Neuroglycopenic symptoms predominate if the decrease in plasma glucose is slow, when the degree of hypoglycemia is severe, when the patient has hypoglycemia unawareness, in patients with autonomic neuropathy or those who are taking β-blockers, and particularly in patients receiving intensive insulin programs.

Possible causes of hypoglycemia include missing a meal, heavy exercise, insulin or oral agent overdose, recent hypoglycemia (lowers glycemic threshold for catecholamine release), intensive insulin therapy and hypoglycemia unawareness, autonomic neuropathy, loss of counterregulatory cortisol in adrenocortical failure, development of renal failure (increased half-life of insulin and impaired neoglucogenesis), primary hypothyroidism because of need for lower doses of insulin/oral agents for control, and, rarely, the presence of insulin antibodies and coexistence of insulinoma.

Hypoglycemia is life-threatening. It should be prevented if at all possible; if not, it should be treated promptly and effectively.

All patients, members of their immediate family, and close friends need to be made aware of hypoglycemic manifestations, their prevention, and treatment. An ampule of glucagon (1 mg) should be given intramuscularly if the patient is unable to have oral sugar (candy or beverage). Help should be summoned promptly when appropriate.

Hypoglycemia is less frequent with oral agents but can be severe and prolonged. Hospitalization is mandatory in all patients with sulfonylurea-induced hypoglycemia.

- Hypoglycemia associated with the use of oral sulfonylureas can be severe and prolonged. Hospitalization is necessary for adequate management.

Early Morning Hyperglycemia in Treated Diabetics

This may be due to posthypoglycemic hyperglycemia, the so-called Somogyi phenomenon. This refers to rebound hyperglycemia following hypoglycemia and is due to counterregulatory hormone-excess; it is probably rare in adults but more common in children. It should be suspected if wide swings occur over a short period of time (even if the patient is asymptomatic) and if excessive hunger and weight gain occur in the context of worsening hyperglycemia. Management requires a decrease in insulin dosage. Early morning hyperglycemia may also be due to the so-called dawn phenomenon, the early morning increase in plasma glucose. It probably is related to the nocturnal surge in GH secretion. Management requires an increase in insulin dosage.

Differentiation between the two causes is best made by measuring the blood glucose level at 3:00 a.m. In the Somogyi phenomenon, the level is low, but in the dawn phenomenon, the level is high. For the Somogyi phenomenon, treat by decreasing the insulin dose; for the dawn phenomenon, increase the insulin dosage.

- Early morning hyperglycemia in treated diabetics can be due to the Somogyi phenomenon or the dawn phenomenon. To distinguish between them, measure plasma glucose level at 3:00 a.m.

For Surgical Procedures

The use of oral agents is stopped; the dose of intermediate insulin is halved; glucose infusions are covered (1 unit / 3 g of glucose); frequent sampling for blood glucose; supplemental regular insulin as needed until the patient can start eating (when a gradual return to the preoperative program can be accomplished).

For Difficult to Control Situations

Consider increased caloric intake, inadequate dose, failure to take insulin properly, infection/acute illness, emotional stress, use of thiazides or corticosteroids, dawn and Somogyi phenomena, presence of gastroparesis, and insulin resistance.

- In difficult to control situations, consider: increased caloric intake, inadequate dose, failure to take insulin properly, infection/acute illness, emotional stress, use of thiazides or corticosteroids, dawn and Somogyi phenomena, diabetic gastroparesis, and insulin resistance.

Poorly Controlled Diabetes

In poorly controlled diabetes brought under good control with insulin, patients frequently experience a significant decrease in insulin requirements after several days or weeks (hyperglycemia aggravates insulin resistance and impairs the beta cell secretory responses, so-called glucose toxicity). Correction of the hyperglycemia leads to resolution of the glucose toxicity.

Acute Complications of Diabetes Mellitus

Diabetic Ketoacidosis

Definition. Diabetic ketoacidosis is characterized by severe insulin deficiency, significant hyperglycemia, hypertonic dehydration, and ketonemia. Its pathophysiology includes insulin deficiency and counterregulatory hormone excess; hyperglycemia, osmotic diuresis, dehydration, and hyperosmolar state; and lipolysis, ketogenesis, ketonemia, and metabolic acidosis.

- Diabetic ketoacidosis: severe insulin deficiency, significant hyperglycemia, hypertonic dehydration, and ketonemia.

Clinical presentation. The patient usually has insulin-dependent diabetes; in fact, diabetic ketoacidosis may be the initial presentation of this disorder. The features include gradual or abrupt onset of polyps, dehydration, anorexia, nausea and vomiting, abdominal pain, tachypnea, obtundation, and coma. Note that abdominal pain usually is not due to diabetic ketoacidosis if the patient is >40 years old or, if <40 years, the bicarbonate level is >10 mEq/L. It is important to know the precipitating factors: failure to take insulin, infection, other intercurrent illness such as myocardial infarction, pancreatitis, stroke, trauma, or emotional stress.

- Diabetic ketoacidosis: patient usually has IDDM.
- It may be the initial presentation of the disease.
- Abdominal pain is not due to diabetic ketoacidosis if the patient is >40 years or (if <40 years) the bicarbonate level is >10 mEq/L.
- Know precipitating factors: failure to take insulin, infection, and other intercurrent illness (myocardial infarction, pancreatitis, stroke, trauma, or emotional stress).

Diagnosis. Diagnosis is based on demonstrating significant hyperglycemia, ketonemia, and metabolic acidosis. Pitfalls: hyperglycemia may be of only moderate degree (plasma glucose level <500 mg/dL), particularly with pregnancy or alcohol use. Ketoacidosis may be present with negative findings on nitroprusside tests (Ketostix, Acetest). Such tests react mainly with acetoacetate, less so with acetone, and none at all with β-hydroxybutyrate. The ratio of β-hydroxybutyrate to acetoacetate is usually 3:1. At pH 7.1, it increases to 6:1 and may be >30:1 in the presence of alcohol excess or lactic acidosis (altered redox state). The diagnostic process is not complete without a thorough search for precipitating factors and assessment of complications.

- Diagnosis is based on demonstrating: significant hyperglycemia, ketonemia, and metabolic acidosis.
- Ketoacidosis may be present with negative finding on nitroprusside tests (Ketostix, Acetest).
- The diagnostic process is not complete without a thorough search for precipitating factors and assessment of complications.

Management. The goals of therapy are to correct the hyperglycemia, hyperketonemia and acidosis, hyperosmolar dehydration, and electrolyte depletion. These goals are achieved by insulin administration, replacement of fluid and electrolytes, treatment of precipitating factors, and avoidance of complications. Metabolic and volume correction have to be initiated rapidly. After improvement is established, one can proceed more cautiously.

- Goals: to correct hyperglycemia, hyperketonemia and acidosis, hyperosmolar dehydration, and electrolyte depletion.
- Achieve goals by: insulin administration, replacement of fluid and electrolytes, treatment of precipitating factors, and avoidance of complications.

1. Insulin. Regular insulin is the mainstay of therapy. Initially, give a priming dose of 10-20 U intravenously and then set up an insulin infusion at the rate of 10 U/hour. This provides a plasma level of about 200 mU/mL, adequate to inhibit lipolysis and hepatic glucose production and maximize glucose uptake. Insulin infusion is preferred over subcutaneous or intramuscular insulin regimens because it provides smoother control with less risk of hypoglycemia.

- Regular insulin: the mainstay of therapy.
- Insulin infusion is preferred over subcutaneous or intramuscular insulin regimens.

2. Fluids. The aim is to restore volume and to correct electrolyte and fluid losses and hyperosmolarity. The average fluid deficit in the adult is 5-8 L. Give 2 L of normal saline in the first hour, 1 L/hour in the second and third hours, and then 250-500 mL/hour until the vital signs stabilize. Next, switch to 0.45% saline and adjust as needed. As plasma glucose values approach 300 mg/dL, change to 0.45% saline in 5% dextrose in water. Maintain plasma glucose value between 200 and 250 mg/dL dur-

ing the first 12-24 hours to reverse ketosis, to avoid rapid decrease in osmolarity and cerebral edema, and to avoid hypoglycemia.

3. Electrolytes. The potassium deficit is about 300-500 mEq. Regardless of the initial serum level of potassium, the total body stores of potassium are low. With therapy and correction of acidosis and hyperglycemia, the serum level of potassium decreases. Potassium should be added to the intravenous fluids as soon as renal perfusion and urine flow are assured. Add 40 mEq of potassium to each liter of intravenous fluid as potassium chloride. In controlled trials, potassium phosphate is of no benefit. Phosphate repletion is indicated in the presence of phosphate levels <1 mg/dL. Give phosphate in the dose of 0.08 mM/kg intravenously over 6 hours. (Neutral potassium phosphate, 1 ampule contains 3 mM phosphate and 15 mEq of potassium.) Monitor the serum level of phosphate carefully because of the risk of hypocalcemia, seizures, and death. Bicarbonate: if pH is <7.1, give bicarbonate (44 mEq/L) until pH increases to about 7.1. Avoid excessive bicarbonate because it exacerbates hypokalemia and may result in paradoxical CSF fluid acidosis.

- With therapy and correction of acidosis and hyperglycemia, the serum level of potassium decreases.
- Add potassium to intravenous fluids as soon as renal perfusion and urine flow are assured.
- If the pH is <7.1, give bicarbonate (44 mEq/L) until pH is about 7.1.

Complications. The major complications of diabetic ketoacidosis result mostly from therapy failures. In most patients, persistent ketosis/acidosis, hypoglycemia, hypokalemia, paradoxical CSF acidosis, cerebral edema, and metabolic alkalosis can be prevented.

Prognosis. The mortality rate is 5%-15% (higher among the elderly). With myocardial infarction, mortality is 50%. After successful therapy, the goal is to avoid recurrence by properly managing the diabetic state and by patient education.

- Prognosis: 5%-15% mortality; higher rate among the elderly.
- After successful therapy, the goal is to avoid recurrence by properly managing the diabetic state and by patient education.

Hyperglycemic Hyperosmolar Nonketotic Coma

Hyperglycemic hyperosmolar nonketotic coma is characterized by significant hyperglycemia and dehydration without ketoacidosis. Its pathophysiology includes insulin deficiency, osmotic diuresis, dehydration, and decreased renal function; however, enough insulin is available to inhibit excess lipolysis and ketogenesis. It occurs predominantly in NIDDM.

It is often precipitated by acute illness such as myocardial infarction, pancreatitis, pneumonia or other infections, surgical stress, dialysis, hyperalimentation, and the use of such drugs as glucocorticoids, thiazides, and phenytoin. Hyperglycemic hyperosmolar nonketotic coma may be the first presentation of NIDDM.

- Characteristics: significant hyperglycemia and dehydration without ketoacidosis.
- Pathophysiology: insulin deficiency, osmotic diuresis, dehydration, and decreased renal function.
- Enough insulin is available to inhibit excess lipolysis and ketogenesis.
- Occurs predominantly in NIDDM.
- It is often precipitated by acute illness.
- It is precipitated by the use of: glucocorticoids, thiazides, or phenytoin.
- It may be the first presentation of NIDDM.

Diagnostic approach. The disorder should be suspected in any diabetic patient presenting with altered sensorium, obtundation or coma, and severe dehydration. Laboratory evaluation reveals significant hyperglycemia (plasma glucose level is often >600 mg/dL), absence of significant ketonemia, and plasma hyperosmolarity (>320 mOsm/L). Associated findings may include renal insufficiency and lactic acidosis. After the diagnosis is made, prompt management is indicated; at the same time, search for complications and the precipitating disorder.

- Suspect the disorder in any diabetic patient with: altered sensorium, obtundation/coma, and severe dehydration.
- Laboratory evaluation shows: significant hyperglycemia (plasma glucose level is often >600 mg/dL), no significant ketonemia, and plasma hyperosmolarity (>320 mOsm/L).
- Associated findings: renal insufficiency and lactic acidosis.
- Prompt management is indicated.
- Search for complications and precipitating disorder.

Management. The objectives are to restore volume and osmolarity and to manage the hyperglycemia. Supportive measures are initiated to manage shock, coma, and, in patients who have been or are receiving steroids, to provide increased dosages appropriate for an acute illness. Initial fluid therapy should be with normal saline to correct the volume deficit: 1 L normal saline per hour for 2-4 hours or more followed by 0.45% saline to correct the hyperosmolarity. As the level of blood glucose decreases with appropriate insulin therapy, 5% dextrose in water can be added. A dose of 20 U of regular insulin is given intravenously if the plasma glucose level is >600 mg/dL, then insulin infusion is begun. It is important to decrease the plasma glucose gradually to a level around 200 mg/dL. Next, stop the infusion, and start giving insulin subcutaneously. Potassium, phosphate, and magnesium replacements are as outlined above for diabetic ketoacidosis. Lactic acidosis usually responds to volume replacement; if the pH is <7.1, bicarbonate can be given. The patient's condition has to be monitored closely. Repeated neurologic evaluation is needed because focal deficits or seizures may become apparent during therapy.

- Objectives: restore volume and osmolarity and manage hyperglycemia.
- Initial fluid therapy: give normal saline to correct volume deficit.
- Next, 0.45% saline to correct hyperosmolarity.
- Regular insulin.
- Lactic acidosis: responds to volume replacement.
- If pH is <7.1, can give bicarbonate.
- Patient must be monitored closely.

Complications. The complications include vascular events such as myocardial infarction or cerebrovascular accident, hypoglycemia, cerebral edema, and hypokalemia. Mortality is 50%.

- Complications: vascular events (myocardial infarction or cerebrovascular event), hypoglycemia, cerebral edema, and hypokalemia.
- Mortality: 50%.

Diabetes and Pregnancy

Diabetes may be newly diagnosed in pregnancy ("gestational diabetes") or antedate pregnancy in young females with IDDM. The well-being of the fetus dictates tight glucose control. Inadequate control early in pregnancy increases the risk of congenital malformations, and inadequate control in the latter part of pregnancy increases the risk of macrosomia, neonatal hypoglycemia, hypocalcemia, polycythemia, hyperbilirubinemia, and respiratory distress. The normal gestational changes in fuel metabolism include 1) fetal siphoning of glucose and neoglucogenic precursors, resulting in a tendency to fasting maternal hypoglycemia and to starvation ketosis; and 2) anti-insulin action of placental hormones (human placental lactogen, estrogen, and progesterone) and increased cortisol secretion. Because of these stresses, gestational diabetes may develop in those with reduced beta-cell reserve. In those with established diabetes, there is worsening of control.

- The well-being of the fetus dictates tight glucose control.
- Inadequate control in early pregnancy: increased risk of congenital malformations.
- Inadequate control in latter part of pregnancy: increased risk of macrosomia, neonatal hypoglycemia, hypocalcemia, polycythemia, hyperbilirubinemia, and respiratory distress.

Gestational diabetes complicates 2%-3% of all pregnancies. An increased risk is seen in patients with diabetes in a first-degree relative, previous abnormality of glucose tolerance, obesity, advanced maternal age, and abnormal obstetric history, i.e., large babies, unexplained stillbirths, congenital anomalies, and polyhydramnios. All pregnant women should be screened at 24-28 weeks or, if at high risk, at the first visit. A 50-g oral glucose load is given and the plasma glucose level is measured 1 hour later. A plasma glucose level >140 mg/dL indicates the need for a complete oral glucose tolerance test (see above).

- Gestational diabetes complicates 2%-3% of all pregnancies.
- Increased risk in patients with: diabetes in a first-degree relative, previous abnormality of glucose tolerance, obesity, advanced maternal age, or abnormal obstetric history.
- Screen all pregnant women at 24-28 weeks; if at high risk, screen at first visit.
- 50-g oral glucose load; 1 hour later, plasma glucose level >140 mg/dL indicates need for complete oral glucose tolerance test.

The goals of therapy are 1) to ensure tight control of diabetes, with avoidance of hypoglycemia and fasting ketonemia (fasting and preprandial values of 70-100 mg/dL; 1 hour postprandial, <140 mg/dL; 2 hours postprandial, <120 mg/dL; normal glycohemoglobin; 2) to ensure adequate nutrition and optimal weight gain; and 3) home monitoring for blood glucose and urine ketones. Insulin therapy is essential for achieving these goals, and dosage should be adjusted appropriately. Regular office visits and monthly glycohemoglobin values are required. In patients with prepregnancy diabetes, insulin requirements may decrease early in pregnancy, but after mid pregnancy, requirements increase progressively. Immediately post partum, insulin requirements usually return to prepregnancy levels. Timing of the delivery is based on tests of fetal maturity. An uncomplicated pregnancy should be allowed to progress to at least 37 weeks.

- Goals of therapy: ensure tight control of diabetes (avoiding hypoglycemia and fasting ketonemia), ensure adequate nutrition and optimal weight gain, and home monitoring for blood glucose and urine ketones.
- Insulin therapy is essential.
- In patients with prenatal diabetes, insulin requirements may decrease early in pregnancy and increase progressively after mid pregnancy.
- Immediately post partum, insulin requirements usually return to prepregnancy levels.
- Timing of delivery: based on tests of fetal maturity.

Those with gestational diabetes who become euglycemic

in the postpartum state should be followed up periodically; the risk of developing NIDDM approaches 60% in 15 years.

- Periodic follow-up of patients with gestational diabetes who become euglycemic post partum.
- Risk of developing NIDDM is almost 60% at 15 years

In women with IDDM and significant chronic diabetic complications, pregnancy may exacerbate retinopathy. Nephropathy may lead to toxemia, and borderline cardiac status may be decompensated. Well-controlled patients with mild and early chronic complications have a good chance for a normal pregnancy, without harm to the mother or the fetus.

Hypoglycemic Syndrome

Etiology

The maintenance of euglycemia involves a balance between glucose production and glucose utilization. Hypoglycemia can result from decreased production and/or increased utilization of glucose. Factors involved in glucose production include glucose input from the gastrointestinal tract and from hepatic glycogenolysis and neoglucogenesis. Insulin and the counterregulatory hormones glucagon, epinephrine, cortisol, and GH exert major influences on glucose production and utilization. Insulin stimulates tissue utilization of glucose and inhibits hepatic production of glucose. The counterregulatory hormones inhibit utilization and increase hepatic glucose output. The causes of hypoglycemia are outlined in Table 7-17.

Postprandial hypoglycemia. It is due to asynchronous or excessive insulin secretion relative to prandial plasma glucose levels and is characterized by symptomatic hypoglycemia occurring 1-5 hours after food ingestion. Postprandial hypoglycemia can occur as a rare hereditary abnormality in children. In these patients, hypoglycemia may follow the ingestion of fructose, galactose, or leucine. Postprandial hypoglycemia does not occur in patients with frank diabetes mellitus. However, in some patients who have impaired glucose tolerance with normal fasting plasma levels of glucose, symptomatic hypoglycemia, or "diabetic" hypoglycemia, may develop 4-6 hours after glucose ingestion. It is attributed to an excessive and delayed insulin response to a glucose load.

- Postprandial hypoglycemia: due to asynchronous or excessive insulin secretion relative to prandial plasma glucose levels.
- Characteristic: symptomatic hypoglycemia occurring 1-5 hours after food ingestion.

"Alimentary" hypoglycemia most often follows gastrectomy, jejunostomy, or vagotomy and pyloroplasty. Symptomatic hypoglycemia in alimentary hypoglycemia occurs earlier (1-2 hours after a glucose meal) than in other forms of postprandial hypoglycemia. The mechanism is believed to be due to

Table 7-17.--Causes of Hypoglycemia

Postprandial or reactive hypoglycemia
  Reactive, functional, or idiopathic
  "Diabetic"
  Alimentary
Fasting hypoglycemia
  Hepatic
    Extensive surgical resection
    Acute fulminant hepatic necrosis--viral, toxic
    Cirrhosis
    Hereditary enzyme deficiencies
      Glycogen storage diseases
      Galactosemia
      Hereditary fructose intolerance
  Endocrine
    Insulin excess
      Insulinoma
      Insulin and oral hypoglycemia agents--therapeutic error, factitial
      Autoimmune
    Hypopituitarism
    Cortisol deficiency
  Alcohol
  Severe medical illness
    Chronic renal failure
    Severe malnutrition
    Infection and sepsis
  Extrapancreatic islet tumors
    Mesenchymal tumors
    Hepatoma
    Adrenocortical carcinoma
    Gastrointestinal tract, bronchial, or pancreatic carcinoma
  Drugs and poisons
    β-Blockers
    Salicylates
    Mushroom poisoning
    Akee fruit
    Hepatotoxins

the rapid entry of large amounts of glucose into the small bowel, causing a precipitous increase in the plasma glucose level and dramatic secretion of insulin. Alimentary hypoglycemia may also occur in patients with thyrotoxicosis or rapid gastric emptying of unknown cause.

Contrary to popular belief, idiopathic postprandial syndrome (reactive or functional) is distinctly rare. Normal subjects may have a low circulating level of glucose after an oral glucose load. Those who have hypoglycemia after oral glucose frequently have normal glucose levels after a mixed meal. Symptoms do not correlate with glucose levels. Also, patients frequently have psychiatric disorders.

- Contrary to popular belief, idiopathic postprandial syndrome (reactive or functional) is rare.

Fasting hypoglycemia. The causes of symptomatic fasting hypoglycemia include 1) significant extensive liver disease, such as severe cirrhosis or acute fulminant hepatic necrosis of viral or toxic origin, or after extensive surgical resection and 2) inborn defects of hepatic enzymes required for normal carbohydrate metabolism; these are rare and include glycogen storage diseases, galactosemia, and hereditary fructose intolerance.

Insulinomas are rare islet-cell pancreatic tumors that can occur in all ages, but they occur most frequently in patients in the 4th-7th decades, with a slight preponderance in females. Of the affected patients, 80% have a single benign tumor; 10% of the insulinomas are multiple, and another 10% are malignant. Of the insulinomas, 10% occur in the setting of MEN I.

- 80% of patients with insulinoma have a single benign tumor.
- 10% of the insulinomas are multiple.
- 10% are malignant.
- 10% occur in the setting of MEN I.

Autoimmune hypoglycemia is a rare entity that can occur in patients who have antibodies to insulin (without previous exposure to insulin) or in patients with autoantibodies to insulin receptors of indeterminate cause.

Drug-related hormonal causes are the most common causes of hypoglycemia. Insulin administration in a known diabetic can cause hypoglycemia. Surreptitious administration of insulin may also cause hypoglycemia, as may excessive dosage in oral antidiabetic therapy related to decreased degradation or excretion (e.g., in kidney failure), potentiation by other drugs (e.g., barbiturates, warfarin, phenylbutazone, salicylates, sulfonamides, thiazide, or monoamine oxidase inhibitors), or surreptitious administration.

Glucocorticoid deficiency, whether related to primary adrenal disease or secondary to hypothalamic-pituitary disease, can cause fasting or late postprandial hypoglycemia because of impaired hepatic neoglucogenesis. This deficiency can be corrected completely by adequate steroid replacement. In children, GH deficiency can cause clinical hypoglycemia because of enhanced peripheral glucose utilization related to unopposed insulin effects.

Hypoglycemia associated with severe medical illness can occur in chronic renal failure, in severely malnourished children or adults, and in infection and sepsis. Certain extrapancreatic tumors may be associated with hypoglycemia. Hypoglycemia can occur in patients with tumors of any histologic type but most frequently in those with mesenchymal tumors, massive fibroma or sarcoma (e.g., retroperitoneal or intrathoracic), hepatomas, adrenocortical carcinomas, and gastrointestinal, bronchial, and exocrine pancreatic carcinoma. The cause of the hypoglycemia is likely related to insulin-like growth factors. Hypoglycemia can be caused by other drugs and poisons: β-adrenergic blockers, salicylates, and, most commonly in children, drugs that interfere with glucose metabolism in the liver. Ingestion of certain poisonous plants, e.g., mushrooms and akee fruit, and hepatotoxins can cause fatal hypoglycemia. Alcohol-induced hypoglycemia is a common cause of fasting hypoglycemia. It occurs most commonly in chronically malnourished alcoholics who stopped food and alcohol intake 10-20 hours earlier. It can also occur in healthy adults or children after a short drinking spree. Hypoglycemia results mainly from inhibition of gluconeogenesis by the products of ethanol metabolism; NADH accumulates in the liver and prevents entry of substrates into the gluconeogenic pathway.

- Hypoglycemia associated with severe medical illness: most frequently in those with mesenchymal tumors.
- Can occur with large extrapancreatic tumors and is likely related to insulin-like growth factors.
- Hypoglycemia can be caused by other drugs and poisons.
- Alcohol-induced hypoglycemia is a common cause of fasting hypoglycemia.

Clinical Manifestations

Clinical manifestations are related to hypoglycemia and its cause. The degree of hypoglycemia required to produce symptoms and the clinical manifestations reported by different patients vary widely. However, a similar pattern of symptoms generally recurs in any one person. Hypoglycemic symptoms may be hyperepinephrinemic, resulting from sympathetic activation, or neuroglycopenic, resulting from impaired central nervous system function. Hyperepinephrinemic symptoms usually occur when the plasma glucose levels decrease rapidly. These symptoms include sweating, palpitation, tremor, nervousness, hunger, faintness, weakness, and acral and perioral numbness. They may be blunted or absent in patients receiving β-adrenergic blocking agents, e.g., propranolol. Neuroglycopenic symptoms usually predominate when the plasma glucose levels decline slowly and reach lower levels (≤40 mg/dL). These symptoms include headache, diplopia, confusion, inappropriate affect, motor incoordination, and, when hypoglycemia is severe, seizures, coma, and (ultimately) death. Hypoglycemic manifestations can mimic many neurologic and psychiatric abnormalities. In patients with cerebrovascular disease, hypoglycemic manifestations may occur at higher plasma glucose levels, and the localized neurologic findings may correlate with the underperfused regions of the brain. The manifestations of hypoglycemia are generally reversible, but permanent brain damage can result from a prolonged severe episode.

- Clinical manifestations are related to hypoglycemia and its cause.
- Hypoglycemic symptoms may be hyperepinephrinemic or neuroglycopenic.
- Hyperepinephrinemic symptoms occur when the plasma glucose levels decrease rapidly. Symptoms may be blunted or absent in patients receiving β-adrenergic blocking agents.
- Neuroglycopenic symptoms usually predominate when the plasma glucose levels decline slowly and reach lower levels (≤40 mg/dL).
- Hypoglycemic manifestations can mimic many neurologic and psychiatric abnormalities.
- Manifestations of hypoglycemia: usually reversible, but permanent brain damage can result from a prolonged severe episode.

Diagnostic Approach

Evaluation of patients for possible hypoglycemia has two diagnostic objectives: 1) to demonstrate that the clinical manifestations are due to hypoglycemia and 2) to identify the underlying cause. The most important step in the diagnostic approach to hypoglycemia is to document Whipple's triad, i.e., to show that typical symptoms and hypoglycemia occur during a spontaneous attack or a provocative test and that the symptoms are relieved promptly by the ingestion or infusion of glucose. The actual level of plasma glucose that defines hypoglycemia is a matter of controversy. A reasonable diagnostic criterion is a glucose level, <50 mg/dL in males and <40 mg/dL in females, that is associated with clinical symptoms. It is important to rule out artifactual hypoglycemia. Whole-blood glucose values may be spuriously low in polycythemia vera and in leukemia, but measurement of plasma glucose in these conditions should provide an accurate result. The possibility of laboratory error should be excluded by repeated measurements.

- Two diagnostic objectives in evaluating hypoglycemia: demonstrate that clinical manifestations are due to hypoglycemia and identify the underlying cause.
- The most important step in the diagnostic approach to hypoglycemia: documenting Whipple's triad.
- Actual level of plasma glucose that defines hypoglycemia: a controversial matter.
- A reasonable diagnostic criterion is a glucose level (<50 mg/dL in males and <40 mg/dL in females) that is associated with clinical symptoms.
- Exclude artifactual hypoglycemia and the possibility of laboratory error.

Fasting Hypoglycemia

In evaluating fasting hypoglycemia, the two critical laboratory determinations are measurement of plasma glucose (to document hypoglycemia) and serum insulin (to categorize its cause). They can be measured during a spontaneous attack, can be measured during a spontaneous attack, after an overnight fast, or after a provoked attack (during a 72-hour fast).

- Two critical laboratory determinations in evaluating fasting hypoglycemia: measuring plasma glucose (to document hypoglycemia) and serum insulin (to categorize cause).
- Measurements performed: during spontaneous attack, after overnight fast, after provoked attack (during 72-hour fast).

When fasting glucose levels are <50 mg/dL, normal insulin production by the beta pancreatic cells is suppressed and serum insulin levels decrease to <10 mU/mL. When plasma glucose values are <40 mg/dL, insulin values should be <5 mU/mL. During continued fasting in normal persons, plasma glucose and serum insulin levels decline together. As a result, the ratio of insulin to plasma glucose remains constant and <0.3. Hyperinsulinism is identified by plasma insulin levels >6 mU/mL in association with plasma glucose of <50 mg/dL in males and <40 mg/dL in females. In most patients with hyperinsulinism, the ratio of insulin to plasma glucose is >0.3.

- Hyperinsulinism: plasma insulin levels >6 mU/mL in association with plasma glucose of <50 mg/dL in males and <40 mg/dL in females.

If hyperinsulinism is present, the diagnostic considerations are insulinoma or the surreptitious administration of insulin or oral antidiabetic agents.

- If hyperinsulinism is present, consider insulinoma or surreptitious administration of insulin or oral antidiabetic agents.

Surreptitious administration of insulin or oral antidiabetic agents occurs most commonly in family members of insulin-dependent diabetics or in hospital personnel who have ready access to insulin, syringes, and oral agents. All patients should be examined carefully for injection marks, and if surreptitious administration of insulin is suspected, the hospital room may need to be searched for hidden insulin and syringes. Detection of insulin antibodies in the plasma of a nondiabetic patient supports the diagnosis (remember: insulin autoantibodies also occur in some persons who have not received exogenous insulin). The diagnosis is confirmed by the measurement of serum C peptide. In patients with hyperinsulinism, a high C-peptide level implies endogenous insulin secretion, whereas a low C-peptide level suggests an exogenous source. The diagnosis of surreptitious ingestion of oral antidiabetic agents as a cause of the hypoglycemic syndrome is confirmed by the measurement of either plasma drug levels or urinary metabolites.

- Measurement of C peptide is critical in evaluating hyperinsulinemic states.
- In hyperinsulinism: high C-peptide levels imply endogenous

insulin secretion and can result from insulinoma or the ingestion of sulfonylureas.

- Confirm the diagnosis of sulfonylurea-induced hypoglycemia by measuring plasma sulfonylurea levels or urinary metabolites.
- Low C-peptide levels suggest exogenous source.

The exclusion of surreptitious administration of drugs points to insulinoma as the cause of the hyperinsulinemic state. The diagnosis can be supported further by high serum levels of proinsulin. In >85% of patients with insulinoma, the percentage of proinsulin is >25%, and the more undifferentiated the tumor, the higher the percentage of proinsulin. The use of an exogenous insulin suppression test can help distinguish physiologically controlled pancreatic beta cell islet from autonomous nonsuppressible insulin production in insulinoma. Suppression is assessed by measuring serum C peptide after administering insulin to produce hypoglycemia. Provocative agents such as tolbutamide, glucagon, leucine, or calcium elicit more insulin secretion from insulinomas than from normal beta cells. These provocative tests can be helpful in selected patients.

- In hyperinsulinemic states, the exclusion of surreptitious administration of drugs points to insulinoma as the cause of the hyperinsulinemic state.

After the diagnosis of insulinoma is made, an attempt to anatomically delineate the tumor is pursued. Ultrasonography, CT or MRI of the pancreas can delineate tumors >1-2 cm. Angiography may be needed to detect smaller tumors. Transhepatic venous sampling after the administration of calcium to stimulate insulin secretion may be helpful. The use of intraoperative ultrasonography has contributed significantly to identification of small tumors. Serum levels of human chorionic gonadotropin (hCG) or its α or β subunits are increased in two-thirds of patients with malignant insulinomas but not in those with benign disease.

- After making the diagnosis of insulinoma: anatomical delineation of the tumor is necessary.

If hyperinsulinism is absent in patients with documented hypoglycemia, the differential diagnosis includes hypopituitarism, hypoadrenalism, liver disease, drug-induced hypoglycemia, and extrapancreatic tumor. If the clinical evidence suggests hypopituitarism or hypoadrenalism, appropriate endocrine tests are in order. Severe liver disease or ingestion of alcohol, drugs, or toxins can generally be distinguished by the medical history, physical examination, and liver function tests. With inborn hepatic enzyme defects, symptoms usually begin in infancy, and the diagnosis depends on the clinical setting and appropriate enzyme assays. The diagnosis of primary liver disease is usually obvious, but physicians should remember that if hypoglycemia is noted in the course of cirrhosis, the presence of hepatoma needs to be excluded. The presence of an extrapancreatic tumor that causes hypoglycemia is likely if the clinical findings and specific laboratory tests do not support one of the above conditions, especially if significant wasting or an abdominal mass is present.

- If hyperinsulinism is absent in patients with documented hypoglycemia, the differential diagnosis includes hypopituitarism, hypoadrenalism, liver disease, drug-induced hypoglycemia, and extrapancreatic tumor.
- For hypoglycemia noted in the course of cirrhosis, exclude hepatoma.
- The presence of extrapancreatic tumor causing hypoglycemia is likely if the clinical findings and specific laboratory tests do not support one of the above conditions, especially in the presence of wasting or an abdominal mass.

Remember that alcohol-induced hypoglycemia is a frequent cause of fasting hypoglycemia. Its manifestations are often mistakenly attributed to drunkenness. The plasma glucose level should be determined in all symptomatic patients with a history of significant alcohol intake. Diabetic patients taking insulin or oral agents are especially susceptible to ethanol-induced hypoglycemia. Also, bear in mind that blood alcohol levels may not be increased when a patient with hypoglycemia is examined.

- Remember: alcohol-induced hypoglycemia is a frequent cause of fasting hypoglycemia.
- Its manifestations are often mistakenly attributed to drunkenness.
- Diabetic patients taking insulin or oral agents are especially susceptible to ethanol-induced hypoglycemia.
- When a patient with alcohol-induced hypoglycemia is examined, blood alcohol levels may not be increased.

Postprandial Hypoglycemia

It is important to remember that 1) postprandial hypoglycemia is uncommon; 2) patients are inclined to attribute many types of symptoms to hypoglycemia; 3) the lack of energy, chronic anxiety, lethargy, mental dullness, and similar complaints rarely result from hypoglycemia, and 4) the physician's responsibility is to demonstrate that these symptoms have been incorrectly attributed to hypoglycemia. The patient is instructed in the use of glucose oxidase strip reagents (e.g., Chemstrip BG) and asked to measure the plasma glucose at the time of the symptoms. If the levels are >80 mg/dL, the diagnosis of hypoglycemia is ruled out. If the levels are <80 mg/dL, a glucose or mixed meal tolerance test is indicated. The patient should avoid drugs known to influence glucose tolerance and ingest at least 150 g of complex carbohydrates for 3 days before the test.

- Postprandial hypoglycemia is uncommon.
- Patients are inclined to attribute many symptoms to hypoglycemia.
- Physician's responsibility: demonstrate that the symptoms have been incorrectly attributed to hypoglycemia.
- Measure the plasma glucose level at the time of the symptoms.
- If the levels are <80 mg/dL, a glucose or mixed meal tolerance test is indicated.

ADRENAL CORTEX

Physiology

The steroidogenic pathway for the synthesis of aldosterone, cortisol, and testosterone in the adrenal cortex is shown in Figure 7-9. The hypothalamic-pituitary-adrenal axis is shown in Figure 7-10. Its three regulatory influences are diurnal rhythm, negative feedback, and stress. ACTH and cortisol are secreted episodically. ACTH is produced by the anterior pituitary corticotroph cell and is under the regulation of corticotropin-releasing hormone (CRH). Cortisol circulates in bound (96%-98%) and free (2%) forms. It is bound to transcortin, a specific binding protein, and to albumin. The free form is biologically active. Cortisol enters the target cells freely and is recognized by a specific cytoplasmic and nuclear receptor. It has a critical permissive role in intermediary metabolism, in optimizing cardiovascular function, in the ability of the kidney to excrete a water load, and in central nervous sys-

tem activity. It also has a role in the checks and balances of the inflammatory response and immune reaction.

- Three regulatory influences: diurnal rhythm, negative feedback, and stress.
- ACTH is produced by the anterior pituitary corticotroph cell under the regulation of CRH.
- Cortisol circulates in bound (96%-98%) and free (2%) forms.
- The free form is biologically active.
- Cortisol: critical permissive role in intermediary metabolism, optimizing cardiovascular function, kidney's ability to excrete water load, and central nervous system activity.
- Cortisol: a role in checks and balances of inflammatory response and immune reaction.

The renin-angiotensin-aldosterone system and its control are shown in Figure 7-11. The dominant physiologic effect of aldosterone is at the distal renal tubule, where it enhances sodium reabsorption and potassium excretion. Aldosterone has a crucial role in maintaining sodium balance, extracellular fluid volume, and potassium balance. Its major regulatory influences are blood volume (through its effects on renal perfusion, renin secretion, and atrial natriuretic hormone production), β-adrenergic influences, and serum potassium level. Decreased blood volume, increased β-adrenergic stimulation, and increased serum potassium levels stimulate aldosterone secretion. Increased blood volume, atrial natriuretic hormone,

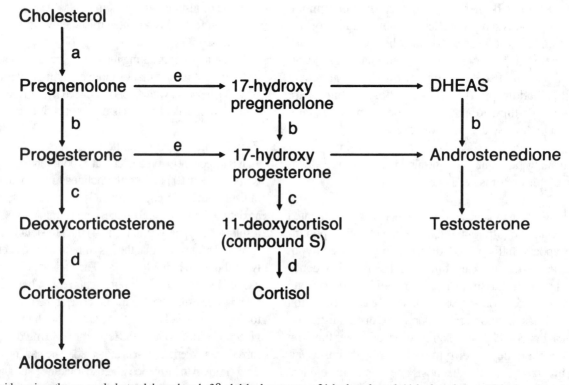

Fig. 7-9. Steroidogenic pathway. a, cholesterol desmolase; b, 3β-ol-dehydrogenase; c, 21-hydroxylase; d, 11-hydroxylase; e, 17-hydroxylase.

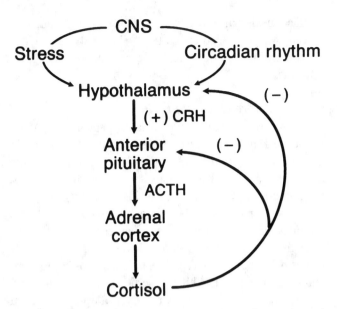

Fig. 7-10. Hypothalamic-pituitary-adrenal axis. ACTH, adrenocorticotropic hormone; CNS, central nervous system; CRH, corticotropin-releasing hormone.

and hypokalemia suppress its secretion. ACTH has a minor, permissive role in aldosterone secretion.

- Dominant physiologic effect of aldosterone: at the distal renal tubule.
- It enhances sodium reabsorption and potassium excretion.
- Aldosterone: crucial role in maintaining sodium balance, extracellular fluid volume, and potassium balance.
- Its major regulatory influences: blood volume, β-adrenergic influences, and serum potassium level.
- ACTH: minor, permissive role in aldosterone secretion.

Adrenocortical Failure

Clinical Features

The clinical features include weakness, fatigue, poor appetite, nausea, vomiting, weight loss, diarrhea, abdominal pain, salt craving, muscle cramps, and hypotension with orthostatism. A small heart is seen on chest radiography. Other features are hypoglycemia, hyponatremia, hyperkalemia, amenorrhea and loss of sexual hair in women, pigmentary disorder (hyperpigmentation or vitiligo), neutropenia, lymphocytosis, and eosinophilia. Adrenal calcification is seen on abdominal radiography. About 25% of patients present with adrenocortical crisis.

- Features: weakness, fatigue, poor appetite, hypotension with orthostatism, hypoglycemia, hyponatremia, and hyperkalemia.
- Pigmentary disorder.
- About 25% of patients present with adrenocortical crisis.

Etiology

The causes of adrenocortical failure are outlined in Table 7-18.

Primary Adrenocortical Failure

Autoimmune Addison's disease is the most common cause of adrenocortical failure in the U.S. (>80% of patients). Patients have circulating anti-adrenal antibodies (70%) with or without antibodies directed against other endocrine glands, e.g., antithyroid (80%). It may occur in association with other autoimmune endocrine disorders such as Graves' disease, Hashimoto's thyroiditis, hypoparathyroidism, IDDM, hypogonadism, pernicious anemia, and vitiligo. Forty percent of patients have a family history of associated endocrinopathies.

Fig. 7-11. Renin-angiotensin-aldosterone axis. ACTH, adrenocorticotropic hormone.

- Autoimmune Addison's disease: the most common cause of adrenocortical failure in the U.S. (>80%).
- May occur in association with other autoimmune endocrine disorders.
- 40% of patients have a family history of associated endocrinopathies.

Tuberculous Addison's disease is not associated with other endocrinopathies. Evidence of hematogenous dissemination and of adrenal calcification occurs in 50% of patients. Bilateral adrenal hemorrhage is probably the second most common cause of adrenocortical failure in the U.S. It may be the result of systemic infections (e.g., meningococcemia), trauma, or the use of anticoagulant agents. AIDS may cause adrenocortical failure in two ways: adrenalitis due to viral, bacterial, or fungal infections and hyporeninemic-hypoaldosteronism and hyperkalemia.

Table 7-18.--Causes of Adrenocortical Failure

Primary adrenocortical failure
  Glandular disease
    Autoimmune
    Bilateral adrenal hemorrhage
    Granulomatous
      Tuberculosis
      Histoplasmosis
      Coccidioidomycosis
      Toxoplasmosis
    Metastatic disease
    Systemic bacterial infections
      Meningococcal
      Staphylococcus
    Infiltrative disorder
      Sarcoidosis
      Amyloidosis
      Hemochromatosis
    Trauma
    Iatrogenic
      Anticoagulants
      Adrenolytic agents
      Blockers of steroidogenesis
    Adrenoleukodystrophy
    Intrinsic functional derangement
      Congenital adrenal hyperplasia
      Congenital adrenal hypoplasia
      Resistance of ACTH
Secondary adrenocortical failure (see the section on the Pituitary)
    Organic hypothalamic pituitary disease
    Functional: prior treatment with glucocorticoid
Peripheral resistance to glucocorticoids

- Bilateral adrenal hemorrhage: is probably the second most common cause of adrenocortical failure in the U.S. It may result from: systemic infections, trauma, or anticoagulant agents.

Secondary Adrenocortical Failure

In organic disease of the hypothalamic-pituitary unit, ACTH deficiency may be isolated or be part of hypopituitarism. The most common cause of ACTH deficiency is functional suppression by prolonged exogenous steroid therapy. It may also occur after removal of a tumor causing Cushing's syndrome. From 6 to 12 months may be needed for the hypothalamic-pituitary-ACTH axis to recover after cessation of therapy, hence the need for interim steroid coverage. In ACTH lack, there is pallor but no hyperpigmentation. Aldosterone secretion is usually normal. Although serum levels of sodium may be low because of the inability to excrete a water load due to cortisol or thyroid lack, the serum level of potassium is normal. Other features of hypothalamic-pituitary disease are usually present.

- The most common cause of ACTH deficiency: functional suppression by prolonged exogenous steroid therapy.
- May occur after removal of a tumor causing Cushing's syndrome.
- From 6 to 12 months may be needed for the hypothalamic-pituitary-ACTH axis to recover after cessation of therapy.

Aldosterone Deficiency

Aldosterone deficiency can result from decreased production or decreased tissue effect. Decreased production may be the result of:

1. Primary adrenocortical failure (decreased plasma aldosterone, increased plasma renin activity). This results from aldosterone and cortisol lack (from congenital adrenal hyperplasia or acquired adrenocortical failure, as in Addison's disease) or from isolated aldosterone lack due to 18-hydroxylase deficiency.
2. Abnormal regulation due to decreased renin (decreased plasma renin activity, decreased plasma aldosterone). This may result from acquired chronic renal disease or the use of drugs such as β-blockers and prostaglandin synthesis inhibitors. Abnormal regulation is also caused by decreased angiotensin II (decreased plasma aldosterone, increased PRA) due to the use of drugs such as ACE inhibitors.

- Aldosterone deficiency: results from decreased production or decreased tissue effect.
- Decreased production results from: primary adrenocortical failure, abnormal regulation due to decreased renin, or decreased angiotensin II.

Hyporeninemic hypoaldosteronism can occur in the elderly, especially those with diabetes mellitus and mild-to-moderate renal impairment. In the usual case, one can find hyperkalemia, mild metabolic acidosis, and hypertension related to associated renal disease. In such patients, drugs that can suppress the renin-angiotensin-aldosterone axis must be used with caution. These drugs include nonsteroidal anti-inflammatory agents, ACE inhibitors, β-blockers, calcium channel blockers, and chronic heparin therapy.

- Hyporeninemic hypoaldosteronism can occur in the elderly, especially in those with diabetes mellitus and mild-to-moderate renal impairment.
- In such patients, drugs that suppress the renin-angiotensin-aldosterone axis must be used with caution.

Diagnostic Approach

Plasma cortisol level and 24-hour urinary levels of free cortisol, 17-hydroxysteroids, 17-ketogenic steroids, and 17-ketosteroids are not usually helpful in diagnosing adrenocortical failure. Plasma cortisol levels can be normal in partial adrenocortical failure. Low values can be seen in eucortisol normal patients (because of the timing of the sampling relative to the diurnal rhythm or episodic secretion) and in patients with decreased cortisol-binding globulin (hypothyroidism, liver disease, nephrotic syndrome, and multiple myeloma). It is important to remember that "normal" values of plasma cortisol in a patient who is acutely sick are strong indications of adrenocortical failure.

- Not helpful in diagnosing adrenocortical failure: plasma cortisol level and 24-hour urinary levels of free cortisol, 17-hydroxysteroids, 17-ketogenic steroids, and 17-ketosteroids.
- "Normal" values of plasma cortisol in a patient who is acutely sick are strong indications of adrenocortical failure.

Assays for urinary free cortisol are not sensitive enough to differentiate between low-normal and low values. The urinary levels of cortisol metabolites are usually low in adrenocortical failure (except for adrenocortical failure due to some types of congenital adrenal hyperplasia); however, they can be low in eucortisol persons because of inadequate 24-hour collections, starvation, liver disease, use of drugs that alter cortisol degradation (e.g., phenytoin and phenobarbital), hypothyroidism, and renal failure.

For the diagnosis of adrenocortical failure, adrenocortical provocative tests are critical. The cosyntropin test, overnight metyrapone test, or insulin hypoglycemia test can be used singly or in combination.

- Diagnosis of adrenocortical failure: adrenocortical provocative tests are essential.

- Cosyntropin test, overnight metyrapone test, and insulin hypoglycemia test: use singly or in combination.

Is Adrenocortical Failure Present?

A cosyntropin test is performed. The normal response is a plasma cortisol increment >7 mg/dL, with peak cortisol >18 mg/dL. Subnormal cortisol responses establish the diagnosis of adrenocortical failure but cannot differentiate Addison's disease from secondary failure due to hypothalamic-pituitary disease. A normal cortisol response to cosyntropin excludes Addison's disease but does not rule out secondary adrenocortical failure that is partial or of recent onset.

- Perform the cosyntropin test.
- Subnormal cortisol response: establishes the diagnosis of adrenocortical failure. Cannot differentiate Addison's disease from failure due to hypothalamic-pituitary disease.
- Normal cortisol response: excludes Addison's disease. Does not rule out secondary adrenocortical failure that is partial or of recent onset.

One can elect to proceed initially with the overnight metyrapone test or the insulin hypoglycemia test. A normal response to the metyrapone test is a serum level of 11-deoxycortisol (immediate precursor of cortisol) >7 mg/dL. A normal response to insulin hypoglycemia is a cortisol level >18 mg/dL. A normal response to either test indicates a normal hypothalamic-pituitary-adrenal axis. An impaired response documents adrenocortical failure but does not localize the level of axis impairment.

- One may initially proceed with the overnight metyrapone test or the insulin hypoglycemia test.
- A normal response (either test) indicates a normal hypothalamic-pituitary-adrenal axis.
- An impaired response documents adrenocortical failure but does not localize the level of axis impairment.

What Is the Cause of the Adrenocortical Failure?

The serum level of ACTH is critical in distinguishing between Addison's disease (high levels, >200 pg/mL) and secondary adrenocortical failure (low values, <50 pg/mL). If ACTH assays are not available, perform the 3-day prolonged ACTH stimulation test. In Addison's disease, the adrenal glands remain unresponsive; however, a stepwise response is seen in patients with secondary failure. In patients who have normal cosyntropin responsiveness and in whom partial or recent secondary failure is still suspected, an impaired response to the metyrapone test or insulin hypoglycemia test confirms the diagnosis.

- Serum level of ACTH: critical for distinguishing between

Addison's disease and secondary adrenocortical failure.

- If ACTH assays are not available, perform the 3-day prolonged ACTH stimulation test.
- In patients who have normal cosyntropin responsiveness and still suspected to have partial or recent secondary failure, an impaired response to metyrapone or insulin hypoglycemia test confirms the diagnosis.

After the diagnosis is established, search for the cause. In secondary failure, proceed with the work-up outlined above in the section on Hypopituitarism. In Addison's disease, a search for the cause includes clinical assessment and a search for other autoimmune disorders, infections, and neoplasms.

- After the diagnosis is established, search for the cause.

Treatment

Chronic. Primary adrenocortical failure requires glucocorticoid therapy and usually mineralocorticoid therapy. In most patients, secondary failure requires only glucocorticoid therapy. The patient needs to be educated about the disease, its replacement therapy, how to handle dosage during acute illness, and how to inject steroids when needed. Therapy in primary adrenocortical failure usually consists of the following: 1) hydrocortisone (20 mg in a.m. and 10 mg in early p.m.) or prednisone (5 mg in a.m. and 2.5 mg in early p.m.). Monitor the clinical symptoms; ACTH levels are not reliable for monitoring the adequacy of therapy because they do not always decrease and are not widely available or reliable. 2) Mineralocorticoid therapy in the form of fludrocortisone, 0.05-0.2 mg orally; liberal salt intake. Monitor the supine and standing blood pressure, presence of edema, serum potassium level, and, if needed, plasma renin activity.

- Primary adrenocortical failure requires glucocorticoid and usually mineralocorticoid therapy.
- Secondary failure (in most patients) requires only glucocorticoid therapy.
- Therapy for primary adrenocortical failure: hydrocortisone, 20 mg in a.m. and 10 mg in early p.m., or equivalent.
- Mineralocorticoid therapy: fludrocortisone, 0.05-0.2 mg orally; liberal salt intake.

Acute illness coverage. In mild-to-moderate acute illness, increase the glucocorticoid dosage x3 for the duration of the illness. In the presence of severe illness or if vomiting is present, the patient needs to use parenteral dexamethasone (4 mg intramuscularly) and seek prompt medical help. The patient should wear an identification necklace or bracelet. For minor procedures performed under local anesthesia and most radiologic procedures, no special preparation is required. For moderately stressful procedures such as endoscopy, hydrocortisone (100 mg intravenously) should be given just before the pro-

cedure. For major surgery, give 100 mg hydrocortisone intravenously before induction of anesthesia and continue with 100 mg every 6-8 hours for the first 24 hours and taper dose rapidly (decrease by 50% per day) to maintenance level.

Management of adrenal crisis. Suspect a crisis in the presence of dehydration, hypotension, or shock out of proportion to severity of current illness, nausea, vomiting with a history of anorexia and weight loss, abdominal pain (may mimic acute abdomen), unexplained fever, hyponatremia, hyperkalemia, azotemia, hypercalcemia, eosinophilia, and hypoglycemia.

Prompt management is critical. Establish intravenous access: draw blood for measuring electrolytes, glucose, plasma cortisol level, and serum ACTH level. Do not wait for the results, but institute management as soon as the diagnosis is suspected. Promptly infuse saline/dextrose to restore blood and extracellular fluid volume; give dexamethasone, 4 mg intravenously (hydrocortisone, 100 mg every 6 hours, may be used but will interfere with measurements of cortisol during the cosyntropin test). Mineralocorticoids are not necessary at this time. Use other supportive measures as needed.

- Prompt management is critical.
- Draw blood for measuring electrolytes, glucose, plasma cortisol level, and serum ACTH level.
- Do not wait for results.
- Institute management as soon as the diagnosis is suspected.

After the patient's condition is stabilized, continue infusions but at a lower rate. Search for and treat possible infections and precipitating causes. Perform the cosyntropin stimulation test and determine the type and cause of adrenocortical failure. Taper glucocorticoids to maintenance, and begin mineralocorticoid replacement, if needed, after saline infusion is stopped.

- After stabilization, continue infusions at a lower rate.
- Search for and treat possible infections and precipitating causes.
- Perform the cosyntropin stimulation test.

Cushing's Syndrome

Clinical Features

1) Obesity with cushingoid characteristics. 2) Evidence of protein wasting such as thin skin, easy bruising, striae, muscle weakness and atrophy, or osteoporosis. 3) Diabetes mellitus. 4) Hypertension with or without hypokalemia. 5) Hyperandrogenicity with acne/hirsutism, menstrual disorders, and, rarely, virilization. 6) Psychiatric problems with depression or psychosis. 7) Hyperpigmentation (related to excess ACTH). 8) Growth failure in children. 9) Discovery of a pituitary, ectopic, or adrenal mass.

- Obesity with cushingoid characteristics.
- Evidence of protein wasting.
- Diabetes mellitus.
- Hypertension with or without hypokalemia.
- Hyperandrogenicity
- Psychiatric problems.
- Growth failure in children.
- Pituitary, ectopic, or adrenal mass.

Etiology

The causes of Cushing's syndrome are outlined in Table 7-19.

Cushing's disease is caused by an ACTH-producing pituitary tumor (>90% of patients) or hyperplasia (<10%). It usually presents with the classic clinical cushingoid picture of gradual onset and slow progression and affects predominantly women between 20 and 40 years old. Hyperpigmentation and hypokalemic metabolic alkalosis are rare. Laboratory evaluation shows a normal-to-modestly increased serum level of ACTH (40-200 pg/mL), mild-to-moderate cortisol excess, and mild proportionate increase in adrenal androgen production. The hypothalamic-pituitary-ACTH axis is impaired but responsive (cortisol hypersecretion is high-dose dexamethasone suppressible in >70% of patients). An ACTH-producing tumor is shown radiologically in about 50% of patients. Currently, MRI is the procedure of choice.

- Cushing's disease is caused by an ACTH-producing pituitary tumor (>90% of patients) or hyperplasia (<10%).
- Usual presentation: classic clinical picture of gradual onset and slow progression.
- Affects predominantly women 20-40 years old.
- Hyperpigmentation and hypokalemic metabolic alkalosis are seen only rarely.
- ACTH levels are normal or modestly elevated.
- The hypothalamic-pituitary-ACTH axis usually responds to high-dose dexamethasone suppression.
- Sellar imaging reveals the tumor in about 50% of cases.

Most ectopic ACTH-producing tumors occur in men 50-70 years old. The ectopic tumor is evident, such as lung carcinoma, thymoma, pancreatic carcinoma, medullary carcinoma of the thyroid, pheochromocytoma, and others. The hypercortisol state has a rapid onset and progression and is severe. The presentation includes weakness, debility, weight loss, hypertension, hypokalemic alkalosis, edema, diabetes mellitus, and hyperpigmentation. Cushingoid features are absent because of the short duration of the illness. There is an associated proportionate increase in mineralocorticoid and androgen production; ACTH is moderately to significantly increased, with 65% of patients having ACTH levels >200 pg/mL. The ACTH ectopic tumor is autonomous, and the hypothalamic-pituitary-ACTH axis is suppressed. Thus, cortisol secretion is non-high-

Table 7-19.--Causes of Cushing's Syndrome

Exogenous (most common)
Glucocorticoid therapy
ACTH therapy (rare)
Endogenous
Bilateral adrenal hyperplasia
ACTH-dependent
Cushing's disease (70%)
CRH-producing tumors (very rare)
Ectopic ACTH tumors (20%)
Non-ACTH dependent
Bilateral nodular hyperplasia (rare)
Adrenal tumors (10%)
Adenoma
Carcinoma

dose dexamethasone-suppressible. (For bronchial carcinoid, see below.)

- Most ectopic ACTH-producing tumors occur in men 50-70 years old.
- The ectopic tumor is usually evident, such as lung carcinoma, thymoma, pancreatic carcinoma, medullary carcinoma of thyroid, pheochromocytoma, and others.
- The hypercortisol state has a rapid onset and progression and is severe.
- Cushingoid features are absent because of the short duration of the illness.
- Plasma ACTH levels are high; hypokalemic alkalosis, hyperglycemia, and edema may occur.

Iatrogenic Cushing's syndrome is the most common cause of the syndrome. It is more likely to be associated with benign intracranial hypertension, glaucoma, cataracts, pancreatitis, or avascular necrosis of the femur head. Cessation of therapy may be followed by clinical evidence of hypothalamic-pituitary-adrenal axis suppression and may need glucocorticoid replacement until recovery of the hypothalamic-pituitary-ACTH axis. To assess recovery of the axis, use the cosyntropin test; a basal serum cortisol level >11 mg/dL and a post-ACTH level >20 mg/dL indicate recovery.

- Iatrogenic Cushing's syndrome is the most common cause of the syndrome.
- More likely associated with: benign intracranial hypertension, glaucoma, cataracts, pancreatitis, or avascular necrosis of the femur head.
- Cessation of therapy may be followed by clinical evidence of hypothalamic-pituitary-adrenal axis suppression.
- Glucocorticoid replacement may be needed until the hypothalamic-pituitary-ACTH axis recovers.

Adrenal tumors may be benign or malignant. Benign tumors are well differentiated and produce cortisol predominantly (pure syndrome). Malignant tumors are dedifferentiated and inefficient in steroidogenesis; they produce mineralocorticoids, glucocorticoids, and principally sex steroids in excess (mixed syndrome). ACTH levels are suppressed. CT or MRI of the adrenals confirms the presence of the tumor.

- Adrenal tumors may be benign or malignant
- Benign adenomas are differentiated and produce "pure" glucocorticoid excess.
- Adrenocortical cancer is undifferentiated and produces a "mixed" syndrome.
- Plasma ACTH is suppressed.
- Imaging shows the adrenal tumor.

Diagnostic Approach

Is Cushing's Syndrome Present?

Diagnosis depends on the clinical picture and the biochemical demonstration of a pituitary-adrenal axis that does not suppress normally. The best screening tests are the 1-mg overnight dexamethasone suppression test or the 24-hour urinary free cortisol. The definitive test is the low-dose (2 mg/day for 2 days) dexamethasone suppression test. The demonstration of abnormal dexamethasone suppressibility or a significantly increased urinary free cortisol point to a diagnosis of Cushing's syndrome, but only after alcoholism, depression, and acute illness have been excluded.

- Diagnosis depends on the clinical picture and the biochemical demonstration of a pituitary-adrenal axis that does not suppress normally.
- Best screening test: 1-mg overnight dexamethasone suppression test or 24-hour urinary free cortisol.
- Definitive test: low-dose (2 mg/day for 2 days) dexamethasone suppression test.
- Exclude alcoholism, depression, and acute illness.

The 1-mg dexamethasone suppression test is a reliable screening test. The normal response is a plasma cortisol value <5 mg/dL. Patients with Cushing's syndrome usually have values >10 mg/dL. False-positive test results occur in 13% of patients with simple obesity and in 25% of chronically ill patients. Other causes of false-positive responses include acute illness, depression, estrogen use, pregnancy, and the use of drugs that can accelerate dexamethasone metabolism (phenytoin and barbiturates).

Urinary free cortisol is increased in >97% of patients with Cushing's syndrome. However, it can also be increased in acute illness, trauma, surgery, alcoholism, and depression. Importantly, it can be modestly increased in simple obesity.

The 2-mg low-dose dexamethasone suppression test is the standard test for the diagnosis of Cushing's syndrome. False-positive results can be seen in patients with acute illness, severe stress, alcoholism, or depression and with the use of drugs known to accelerate dexamethasone metabolism (phenytoin and barbiturates).

What Is the Cause of Cushing's Syndrome?

In searching for the cause, the most important diagnostic tools are serum ACTH level, high-dose (8 mg) dexamethasone suppression test, and radiologic studies for pituitary, ectopic, or adrenal tumors.

- In searching for the cause, the most important diagnostic tools are serum ACTH level, high-dose (8 mg) dexamethasone suppression test, and radiologic studies for pituitary, ectopic, or adrenal tumors.

If Cushing's syndrome is caused by an adrenal tumor, one will find a low or undetectable level of ACTH, nonsuppressible hypercortisol state, and an adrenal mass on abdominal CT. Adrenal adenomas show "pure" glucocorticoid excess of a gradual progressive nature, and the tumor is usually <3 cm in size. However, in adrenal carcinoma, the hypercortisol state develops rapidly and is "mixed" with mineralocorticoid and androgen overproduction; the tumor is usually >6 cm in size.

- Cushing's syndrome caused by adrenal tumor: low/undetectable ACTH level, nonsuppressible hypercortisol state, and an adrenal mass found on abdominal CT.

Cushing's syndrome caused by an ectopic ACTH tumor is characterized in most patients by an evident ectopic tumor, rapid clinical course, very high ACTH levels (>200 pg/mL), and nonsuppressibility.

- Cushing's syndrome caused by ectopic ACTH tumor: evident ectopic tumor, rapid clinical course, very high ACTH levels (>200 pg/mL), and nonsuppressibility.

In Cushing's disease, ACTH values are "normal" or moderately increased (<200 pg/mL), the hypercortisol state is dexamethasone-suppressible in >66% of patients, and CT or MRI of the sella may show a pituitary tumor. However, about 50% of patients have normal sellar radiographic features, and 33% have nonsuppressibility. Also, patients with bronchial carcinoids may be clinically and biochemically indistinguishable from patients with Cushing's disease. If CT or MRI of the sella and CT of the chest do not show any abnormality, resort to petrosal sinus selective venous sampling with CRH provocative testing. A central-to-peripheral ACTH gradient ≥2:1 points to Cushing's disease. Petrosal sinus sampling is very helpful in localizing the side that harbors the pituitary state, but only in the unoperated person.

- Cushing's disease: ACTH values are normal/moderately increased (<200 pg/mL), hypercortisol state is dexamethasone suppressible in >66% of patients, and CT/MRI of the sella may show a pituitary tumor.
- About 50% of patients have normal sellar radiographic features, and about 33% have nonsuppressibility.
- Patients with bronchial carcinoids: clinically and biochemically may be indistinguishable from patients with Cushing's disease.
- If CT/MRI of the sella and CT of the chest show no abnormality, resort to petrosal sinus selective venous sampling with CRH provocative testing.

Differential Diagnosis

False-positive biochemical evaluation. 1) Simple obesity: urinary free cortisol, urinary ketogenic and ketosteroids, and other urinary steroids may be mildly increased. Overnight dexamethasone suppression may be abnormal in 10%-20% of obese patients, but the low-dose 2-mg dexamethasone suppression test shows normal suppressibility. 2) Estrogen, oral contraceptives, and pregnancy: high cortisol-binding globulin and increase in plasma cortisol. Overnight 1-mg dexamethasone suppression test may give abnormal results, but urinary free cortisol is normal. Results of a low-dose 2-mg dexamethasone suppression test are normal. 3) Pseudo-Cushing's syndrome in alcoholics: exclude this in every patient with suspected Cushing's syndrome. Clinical and biochemical similarities to Cushing's syndrome. Increased cortisol production and a nonsuppressible low-dose 2-mg dexamethasone suppression test. Abnormalities return to normal in a few weeks to a few months after abstention from alcohol. 4) Depression: biochemical similarities to Cushing's syndrome include increased cortisol production and a nonsuppressible low-dose dexamethasone test. Typical features of Cushing's syndrome are absent. These patients maintain normal cortisol responses to the insulin provocative test (patients with true Cushing's syndrome have blunted cortisol responses to hypoglycemia). The hypercortisol state is reversible with recovery from depression. 5) Acute and chronic illness in a hospital setting: steroid values may be increased and dexamethasone suppression may be impaired. Repeat the steroid evaluation after the illness resolves.

- False-positive evaluation occurs with: simple obesity; estrogen, oral contraceptives, pregnancy; pseudo-Cushing's syndrome in alcoholics; depression; and acute and chronic illness in a hospital setting.

False-negative evaluation. This occurs in patients with delayed dexamethasone clearance or with periodic hormono-genesis. Periodic hormonogenesis can occur with any cause of endogenous Cushing's syndrome. The hypercortisol state is periodic or cyclic, lasting a few weeks to a few months; between cycles of activity, cortisol secretion and dexamethasone suppressibility are normal. Repeated evaluations at intervals of a few weeks to a few months are required to establish the cyclic nature of the disorder.

- False-negative evaluation occurs in patients with delayed dexamethasone clearance or with periodic hormonogenesis.

Treatment

Cushing's disease. Transsphenoidal adenomectomy is the treatment of choice. The tumor can be identified in >90% of patients, surgical cure can be achieved in >80%, and for experienced surgeons, mortality and morbidity should be <1%. Alternatively, heavy particle irradiation or conventional radiotherapy can be given (only one medical center in the U.S. can deliver heavy particle irradiation). Radiotherapy, although effective in children with Cushing's disease, is effective in only 15%-25% of adults. If therapy fails, consider bilateral adrenalectomy and, in addition, in those in whom transsphenoidal surgery failed, postoperative pituitary irradiation. Drug therapy, such as cyproheptadine or valproic acid, to inhibit ACTH secretion is rarely successful. However, drugs that inhibit cortisol secretion, such as ketoconazole, metyrapone, aminoglutethimide, or the antimitotic op'DDD, can be used as adjunctive therapy or when therapy has failed. These drugs are expensive, have frequent side effects, and may produce a hypocortisol state.

- Cushing's disease: transsphenoidal adenomectomy is the treatment of choice.
- Radiotherapy is effective in children but in only 15%-25% of adults.
- If therapy fails: bilateral adrenalectomy plus (in those in whom transsphenoidal surgery failed) postoperative pituitary irradiation.

Ectopic ACTH. Surgical excision of the tumor is possible in only a small number of patients. If cortisol excess (rather than the primary tumor) is life-threatening, consider bilateral adrenalectomy. Otherwise, drug therapy is used (see above).

Adrenal tumor. For adrenal adenoma, surgical excision is curative. In adrenal carcinoma, surgical excision or debulking is undertaken with generally poor results; op'DDD and/or other drug therapy is given for residual disease.

It is important to remember that in Cushing's syndrome of whatever cause, the normal hypothalamic-pituitary-adrenal axis is suppressed. After tumor ablation, the axis may take up to 1-2 years to recover. During this time, glucocorticoid replacement therapy should be given.

Aldosteronism

Clinical Features

The most important clinical clues are hypertension and hypokalemia. Symptoms related to potassium deficiency include fatigue, muscle weakness, polyuria/polydipsia (due to either nephrogenic diabetes insipidus or diabetes mellitus), orthostatic hypotension, and paresthesias/tetany.

- Most important clinical clues: hypertension and hypokalemia.

Etiology

The causes of aldosterone excess are outlined in Table 7-20.

Diagnostic Approach

Document hypokalemia. If unprovoked hypokalemia is present, continue with the work-up. If the patient has a normal serum level of potassium and has been taking a potassium-sparing diuretic, discontinue use of the drug and reassess in a few weeks. If the patient has a normal serum level of potassium and has been on a low salt diet, salt load and measure the serum level of potassium in a few days. Of patients with mild primary aldosteronism, 20%-30% have normokalemia. In these patients measure the plasma aldosterone-to-plasma renin activity ratio: a ratio >25 confirms the diagnosis.

- Document hypokalemia.
- If the patient has a normal serum level of potassium and takes a potassium-sparing diuretic, discontinue use of drug and reassess in a few weeks.
- If the patient has a normal serum level of potassium and has been on a low sodium diet, salt load and measure the serum level of potassium in a few weeks.
- 20%-30% of patients, particularly those with mild disease, have normokalemia. If suspicion is still strong, measure the plasma aldosterone-to-plasma renin activity ratio.

If the patient has hypokalemia and has been taking a potassium-wasting diuretic, two options are available: 1) you can stop use of the diuretic, replenish the potassium, and repeat the serum level of potassium in about 2 weeks. If hypokalemia persists, proceed with the study. 2) Alternatively, you can check the plasma renin activity. If it is suppressed in a patient receiving diuretic therapy, it points to mineralocorticoid excess. Then, proceed with the study.

- If the patient has hypokalemia and has been taking a potassium-wasting diuretic, stop the use of the diuretic, replenish potassium, and repeat the serum level of potassium in about 2 weeks.

Document kaliuresis. Check the urinary potassium level. In

Table 7-20.--Causes of Aldosteronism

Primary aldosteronism
Adenoma (70% of patients)
Hyperplasia (25%-30% of patients)
Carcinoma (3% of patients)
Glucocorticoid remediable (rare)
Secondary aldosteronism
With hypertension
Increased renin
Renal artery stenosis
Malignant hypertension
Primary reninism
Renal renin tumor
Ectopic renin tumor
Increased angiotensinogen
Estrogen
Without hypertension
Increased renin
Decreased renal perfusion
Volume depletion
Congestive heart failure
Nephrosis
Cirrhosis-ascites
Increased angiotensinogen
Pregnancy
Excessive potassium intake
Bartter's syndrome

mineralocorticoid excess, urinary potassium in hypokalemic patients is >30 mEq/L.

- Document kaliuresis. Check the urinary potassium level.

Document aldosterone overproduction. Check the plasma or urinary aldosterone level. Note that because potassium is an aldosterone secretagogue and because significant hypokalemia may decrease aldosterone secretion in primary aldosteronism, potassium should be replenished before aldosterone measurements are made. If aldosterone levels are high, proceed with the work-up. If aldosterone levels are low, consider other causes of hypertension and hypokalemia.

- Document aldosterone overproduction. Check the plasma or urinary aldosterone levels.
- Replenish potassium before measuring aldosterone.

Document the type of aldosterone overproduction. Check the plasma renin activity. If low, it points to primary aldosteronism; high values imply that the aldosteronism is secondary.

- Document the type of aldosterone overproduction. Check the plasma renin activity.

Identify the cause of primary aldosteronism. Distinguishing between adenoma and hyperplasia in most patients is impossible on clinical and biochemical grounds and is best achieved by radiographic study. Abdominal CT is the imaging procedure of choice. If findings are negative, one can proceed with selective bilateral adrenal venous sampling. Aldosterone levels are 2x-3x higher on the side harboring the adenoma. The selective sampling procedure is technically difficult and laborious. Alternatively, one may elect to proceed with medical treatment for hyperaldosteronism and repeat the CT study in 1-2 years.

- Identify the cause of primary aldosteronism.
- Distinguishing between adenoma and hyperplasia in most patients is impossible on clinical and biochemical grounds.
- Distinguishing between the two is achieved with radiography.
- Abdominal CT is the imaging procedure of choice.

Many patients with adenoma have an anomalous postural decrease in the plasma level of aldosterone and increased 18-hydroxycorticosterone levels; unfortunately, in individual patients, these tests usually are of limited value.

Differential diagnosis—1) Hypertension, hypokalemia, low aldosterone level, and suppressed renin: other mineralocorticoid excess such as deoxycorticosterone-secreting tumor, 11- and 17-hydroxylase deficiency, licorice ingestion, and 11-β-hydroxysteroid dehydrogenase deficiency. 2) Hypertension, hypokalemia, high aldosterone level, suppressed renin: familial glucocorticoid-remediable aldosteronism; correction of clinical abnormalities occurs after few weeks of dexamethasone therapy at 1-2 mg/day.

Special Considerations

The syndrome of apparent mineralocorticoid excess is characterized by hypertension, hypokalemia, suppressed renin, and suppressed aldosterone. The defect is in 11-β-hydroxysteroid dehydrogenase, which catalyzes the conversion of the active cortisol to the inactive cortisone in the peripheral tissues. Thus, tissue cortisol levels increase and the cortisol binds to the mineralocorticoid receptor. The diagnosis is made by measuring metabolites of cortisol and cortisone in the urine. Licorice-induced mineralocorticoid excess syndrome occurs because licorice inhibits 11-β-hydroxysteroid dehydrogenase.

- Syndrome of apparent mineralocorticoid excess: hypertension, hypokalemia, suppressed renin, and suppressed aldosterone.
- Defect: 11-β-hydroxysteroid dehydrogenase.
- Diagnosis: measure the metabolites of cortisol and cortisone in the urine.
- Licorice-induced mineralocorticoid excess syndrome: due to licorice inhibition of 11-β-hydroxysteroid dehydrogenase.

Glucocorticoid-remediable aldosteronism is a rare syndrome, familial and autosomal dominant, that primarily affects young males. Hyperaldosteronism is dexamethasone suppressible; cortisol and ACTH secretion are normal.

Treatment

Surgical excision is the treatment of choice for aldosteronoma unless the patient is a poor surgical risk. For such patients and those with hyperplasia, medical treatment is indicated. This consists of dietary salt restriction and the use of potassium-sparing diuretics. Spironolactone, an aldosterone antagonist, is given in a dose of 25-100 mg/8 hours. It restores normokalemia and normalizes blood pressure in most patients. In men, it is associated with gynecomastia and impaired libido and potency. For such patients, use amiloride or triamterene. Surgical treatment in hyperplasia requires bilateral adrenalectomy; it normalizes potassium but rarely restores blood pressure to normal levels. For this reason, surgical treatment is not indicated in the management of hyperplasia. In glucocorticoid-remediable hyperaldosteronism, one may give dexamethasone in the dose of 1 mg/day.

- Surgical excision: the treatment of choice for aldosteronoma (unless the patient is a poor surgical risk).
- For patients who are poor surgical risks and for those with hyperplasia, give medical treatment.
- Medical treatment: dietary salt restriction and potassium-sparing diuretics.
- In glucocorticoid-remediable hyperaldosteronism: dexamethasone at 1 mg/day.

THE ADRENAL MEDULLA

The sympathochromaffin system consists of the sympathetic nervous system and the chromaffin tissues of the adrenal medulla. The catecholamines norepinephrine, epinephrine, and dopamine are the hormones and neurotransmitters of this system. The biosynthesis and biodegradation of these hormones are outlined in Figure 7-12. Tyrosine hydroxylase is the rate-limiting enzyme. Epinephrine is a hormone of the adrenal medulla. Norepinephrine is the neurotransmitter of sympathetic ganglionic neurons. Dopamine is principally a neurotransmitter in the CNS. The catecholamines exert their biologic actions by binding to cell membrane α and β receptors in the target tissues. Their principal endocrine role is to provide an integrated homeostatic stress response.

- Sympathochromaffin system: the sympathetic nervous system plus the chromaffin tissues of the adrenal medulla.
- Catecholamines: norepinephrine, epinephrine, and dopamine.
- They are hormones and neurotransmitters of the sympathochromaffin system.

Fig. 7-12. Catecholamine synthesis and degradation.

- Epinephrine: the hormone of the adrenal medulla.
- Norepinephrine: neurotransmitter of sympathetic ganglionic neurons.
- Principal endocrine role of catecholamines: integrated homeostatic stress response.

Pheochromocytoma

Pheochromocytomas are rare chromaffin tumors. They are important because they 1) may be potentially malignant; 2) present with a distinctive hypertensive syndrome (although rare — <1% of all hypertensive disorders—it can be cured, and if untreated, it can be potentially lethal); and 3) they may be familial. More than 90% of the tumors are sporadic, adrenal, unilateral, and benign. Familial pheochromocytomas are more likely to be intra-adrenal, bilateral, and malignant. Extra-adrenal tumors are usually located in the abdomen. Less than 1% of pheochromocytomas are in the chest or neck. Pheochromocytomas generally secrete both epinephrine and norepinephrine. Epinephrine-secreting tumors are located in either the adrenals or the organs of Zuckerkandl. Pheochromocytomas can secrete catecholamines persistently or episodically.

- Pheochromocytomas are important because they are potentially malignant and may present with a distinctive hypertensive syndrome.
- They may be familial.
- More than 90% of the tumors are sporadic, adrenal, unilateral, and benign.
- Extra-adrenal tumors are usually in the abdomen.
- Less than 1% are in the chest or neck.
- They generally secrete epinephrine and norepinephrine.
- Epinephrine-secreting tumors: either in the adrenals or the organs of Zuckerkandl.
- Pheochromocytomas can secrete catecholamines persistently or episodically.

Clinical Presentations

Pheochromocytomas are great mimickers. They can be asymptomatic and discovered incidentally on abdominal imaging. More commonly, they are suspected because of the presence of: 1) hypertension, particularly if it is labile, intermittent, or refractory to treatment; 2) paroxysmal symptoms of headaches, palpitations, sweating, anxiety with a feeling of impending doom, and pallor; 3) heat intolerance, sweating, and weight loss; 4) unexplained abdominal or chest pain; 5) orthostatic hypotension or unexplained shock after trauma, surgery, or parturition; and 6) family history of pheochromocytoma, MEN IIA (Sipple's syndrome) or MEN IIB (mucosal neuroma syndrome), or von Hippel-Lindau disease or neurofibromatosis. In most patients, the paroxysmal symptoms are stereotyped and vary only in severity or frequency. The common symptoms are headaches, palpitations, and sweating; absence of all three in a hypertensive patient strongly points away from pheochromocytoma.

- Pheochromocytomas: great mimickers.
- They can be asymptomatic; discovered incidentally on abdominal imaging.
- More commonly, they are suspected because of hypertension.
- Paroxysmal symptoms.
- Heat intolerance, sweating, and weight loss.
- Unexplained abdominal or chest pain.
- Orthostatic hypotension.
- Unexplained shock.
- Family history of pheochromocytoma, MEN IIA, or MEN IIB.
- In most patients, paroxysmal symptoms are stereotyped and vary only in severity or frequency.
- Common symptoms: headache, palpitations, and sweating.
- Absence of all three symptoms in a hypertensive patient: strongly points away from pheochromocytoma.

Diagnostic Approach

Document Catecholamine Hypersecretion

1. Check the levels of urinary catecholamines or metabolites. Diagnosis is based principally on urinary measurements of free catecholamines and their urinary metabolites, metanephrines, and vanillylmandelic acid. No one measurement is clearly superior to the others, and, in practice, the three measurements are made on the same 24-hour urine collection. Demonstration of increased values in hypertensive patients establishes the diagnosis if such conditions as severe stress, intercurrent illness, and acute myocardial ischemia are excluded. Normal values in hypertensive or otherwise symptomatic patients are adequate to exclude the diagnosis. In borderline cases, the urinary studies can be repeated. In patients who have

paroxysmal symptoms, the diagnostic yield can be significantly increased by initiating collection during or shortly after a paroxysm. In all urine collections, assay for creatinine to ensure the adequacy of the sample. Among the drugs that can interfere with the usefulness of the assay are α-methyldopa, labetalol, monoamine oxidase inhibitors, and β-adrenergic blockers.

- Document catecholamine hypersecretion.
- Check urinary catecholamines or metabolites.
- Increased values in hypertensive patients establish diagnosis (if severe stress, intercurrent illness, and acute myocardial ischemia are excluded).
- In patients with paroxysmal symptoms, diagnostic yield is increased significantly by initiating collection during or shortly after a paroxysm.

2. Plasma catecholamines are used as adjuncts to urinary studies. They must be obtained under strict conditions: basal state, supine position, and special collection tools. They represent secretion over a short period of time and are most useful if obtained during a paroxysm or in conjunction with provocative or suppression tests.

- Plasma catecholamines: adjuncts to urinary studies.
- Most useful if obtained during a paroxysm or in conjunction with provocative or suppression tests.

3. Provocative testing with glucagon or histamine is potentially hazardous and has no place in routine evaluation. Very occasionally, it may be useful for normotensive patients with a history of paroxysmal symptoms suggestive of pheochromocytoma. In these patients, the provocative test needs to be done under strictly monitored circumstances and only after α-blockade has been instituted to prevent adverse cardiovascular effects. Plasma catecholamine levels >2,000 pg/mL within 3-5 min after administering 1 mg of glucagon IV point to the presence of pheochromocytoma. The clonidine suppression test is of limited usefulness. A 50% decrease in plasma catecholamines within 3 hours after administering 0.3 mg of clonidine points away from pheochromocytoma.

- Provocative testing with glucagon or histamine is potentially hazardous; has no place in routine evaluation.
- Clonidine suppression test has limited usefulness.

Localize the Pheochromocytoma

CT or MRI of the abdomen (if findings are negative, image the pelvis and thorax) is the mainstay of radiologic localization procedures. They have a >90% sensitivity and specificity. CT has better spatial resolution. MR is better at characterizing the mass, with pheochromocytomas showing high-signal intensity on T2-weighted images. Labelled ^{123}I-metaiodobenzylguanidine (^{123}I-MiBG) is taken up by the chromaffin tissue and can be used as an adjunct to CT or MRI. Its advantages are that it can be used for whole-body scanning and is better at delineating extra-adrenal tumors and metastases. It may even be helpful in delineating the preclinical adrenal medullary hyperplasia. The disadvantages include a higher false-negative rate and the requirement of several days for completion.

- Localize the pheochromocytoma.
- CT or MRI of the abdomen (if negative findings, image the pelvis and thorax): the mainstays of radiologic localization.
- CT: better for spatial resolution.
- MR: better characterization of the mass.
- Labelled ^{123}I-MiBG is taken up by chromaffin tissue; used as adjunct to CT or MRI.

Treatment

Surgical excision of the tumor is curative. Medical treatment is used in preoperative preparation to diminish perioperative morbidity and mortality and on a chronic basis in surgical failures. α-Adrenergic blockade is the cornerstone of medical therapy and should be instituted as soon as the diagnosis is made. Phenoxybenzamine is the drug of choice to control the hypertension and to restore plasma volume. Start with a dose of 10 mg twice daily and increase every few days until the desired effect is obtained. Its major side effect is postural hypotension. Alternate drugs include prazosin, terazosin, labetalol, nifedipine, and ACE inhibitors. β-Blockade may be necessary to control tachyarrhythmias. These drugs should be used only after adequate α-blockade. Propranolol 10 mg 3-4 times daily is usually adequate. For hypertensive emergencies, phentolamine, an α-blocker, is the drug of choice and can be given in 5-10-mg doses every 5-15 minutes as needed. Alternatively, nitroprusside or labetalol can be used. Long-term follow-up is important to assess for persistence, recurrence, or development of other manifestations of MEN IIA or IIB. If hypertension persists postoperatively, consider missed or metastatic pheochromocytoma, surgically induced renal ischemia, or underlying essential hypertension. For an inoperable pheochromocytoma, add metatyrosine, a competitive inhibitor of tyrosine hydroxylase, to the treatment.

- Surgical excision of the tumor is curative.
- Medical treatment: use preoperatively to diminish perioperative morbidity and mortality and on a chronic basis in surgical failures.
- α-Adrenergic blockade: the cornerstone of medical therapy. It should be instituted as soon as the diagnosis is made.
- β-Blockade: may be necessary to control tachyarrhyth-

mias; use only after adequate α-blockade.

- For hypertensive emergencies: phentolamine (α-blocker) is the drug of choice.
- Long-term follow-up: important to assess for persistence, recurrence, and development of other manifestations of MEN IIA or IIB.
- If hypertension persists postoperatively, consider missed or metastatic pheochromocytoma, surgically induced renal ischemia, or underlying essential hypertension.

Incidentally Discovered Adrenal Mass

Small (1-6 cm) adrenal masses are found in up to 9% of unselected autopsies and in 0.7% of all abdominal CT scans. Most of these are nonfunctioning adenomas; a few are functioning adenomas or carcinomas of the adrenal cortex or medulla. Metastatic disease to the adrenal glands is frequent.

The challenges posed by operations on unsuspected functioning adrenal neoplasms include 1) unsuspected pheochromocytoma and the risk of anesthetic/surgical acute catecholamine excess and 2) unsuspected cortisol-producing adenoma: ACTH is suppressed and the contralateral adrenal cortex is atrophic. After adrenalectomy, postoperative acute adrenal crisis may occur. Such patients need cortisol replacement until recovery of the ACTH-adrenal axis, which may require 1-3 years.

The diagnostic approach should include:

1. Screening for pheochromocytoma. Measure 24-hour urinary metanephrines, vanillylmandelic acid, and fractionated catecholamines.
2. Screening for Cushing's syndrome. Use 1-mg overnight dexamethasone suppression test or a 24-hour urinary free cortisol.
3. Screening for primary aldosteronism. Use serum level of potassium in patients not taking diuretics and receiving >200 mEq of sodium per day; measure plasma renin activity.
4. For androgen-producing tumors, check serum dehydroepiandrosterone sulfate (DHEAS).
5. In addition, chest radiography to screen for carcinoma, tuberculosis, and fungal infection.
6. Assess size and nature of the mass on abdominal CT or MRI.

- Screen for pheochromocytoma.
- Screen for Cushing's syndrome.
- Screen for primary aldosteronism.
- Check for androgen-producing tumors.
- Chest radiography.
- Assess size and nature of mass on abdominal CT or MRI.

The only place for CT-guided adrenal needle biopsy in the evaluation of incidentalomas is in patients who have primary tumors with the potential of metastasis to the adrenals. Biopsy should not be done until pheochromocytoma has been excluded by appropriate urinary studies.

Management: surgical excision is indicated for functioning adrenal masses, large solid or solid-cystic masses (>6 cm in size), and cystic masses that have bloody contents on CT-guided needle aspiration. Otherwise, observation is indicated. The imaging study should be repeated in 3, 6, 12, and 24 months; an increase in size indicates the need for surgical treatment.

- Surgical excision is indicated for: functioning adrenal masses, large solid or solid-cystic masses (>6-cm size), and cystic masses with blood contents on CT-guided needle aspiration.
- Otherwise, observation is indicated.

MALE GONADAL DISORDERS

Physiology

The male gonadal axis is shown in Figure 7-13. The testis has two physiologic compartments: 1) the Leydig cells are endocrine cells whose main function is to secrete testosterone, and 2) the seminiferous tubules contain Sertoli cells and gametes. The full cycle of spermatogenesis takes 70-90 days. Sertoli cells also secrete inhibin.

- Two physiologic compartments of the testis: Leydig cells and seminiferous tubules (Sertoli cells and gametes).
- Full cycle of spermatogenesis: 70-90 days.

Testosterone has two functions: 1) an endocrine function that includes the development, growth, and maintenance of internal and external genitalia, secondary sex characteristics, libido and potency, pubertal growth spurt, and muscular development; and 2) a paracrine function, in which testosterone enters the adjoining seminiferous tubules and stimulates the early stages of spermatogenesis. Testosterone is a steroid that circulates in two forms: bound to a specific sex hormone-binding globulin (SHBG) and albumin (98%) and in a free form (2%). Testosterone acts intracellularly by binding to cytoplasmic- or nuclear-specific receptors. It also may function as a prohormone. Testosterone may undergo target-tissue transformation to dihydrotestosterone (DHT) by 5α-reductase (this occurs in such tissues as the genitalia, prostate gland, and hair follicles) or to estradiol (E_2) by aromatase (as in the hypothalamus).

- Two functions of testosterone: endocrine and paracrine.
- Testosterone: a steroid that circulates in bound (98%) and free (2%) forms.
- It also functions as a prohormone.
- It undergoes transformation to DHT by 5α-reductase in target tissue.

● Transformation to E_2 by aromatase.

A specific anterior pituitary cell, the gonadotrope, secretes the two pituitary hormones LH and FSH. These are glycoproteins consisting of α and β subunits. The α subunits are identical in the two hormones (and in TSH and hCG). The β subunit is hormone-specific and is responsible for its biologic effect. The male gonadal axis is regulated by one hypothalamic hormone, GnRH. GnRH is a decapeptide that is secreted in bursts every 70-90 minutes and stimulates the production of LH and FSH by gonadotropes. The hypothalamic-pituitary-gonadal system in the male is regulated by negative feedback, as shown in Figure 7-13. Inhibin has recently been isolated and characterized; it is a protein consisting of α and β polypeptide subunits and is synthesized by the Sertoli cells. Inhibin blocks GnRH-stimulated release of FSH. Activin, a newly described testicular peptide consisting of a dimer of the β-chains of inhibin, stimulates FSH secretion in vitro. The role of inhibin and activin in human physiology and disease states is not clear.

● Gonadotrope: specific anterior pituitary cell that secretes LH and FSH.
● The male gonadal axis is regulated by one hypothalamic hormone, GnRH, and by negative feedback from testosterone and inhibin.
● Inhibin is synthesized by Sertoli cells and blocks GnRH-stimulated release of FSH. Testosterone is the negative feedback regulator of LH secretion.

Sexual Development in Males

Testosterone is critical for the development of the male phenotype. Sex development in the male fetus proceeds in three phases: development of chromosomal sex, gonadal sex, and phenotypic sex. The chromosomal sex is 46,XY. In the presence of certain Y chromosome genes, the bipotential gonad develops into a testis. The fetus has bipotential internal and external genitalia; the internal genitalia are the wolffian and müllerian ducts. The fetal testes produce two hormones: testosterone and müllerian inhibitory factor (MIF). Testosterone is necessary for the development of the wolffian ducts into the male internal genitalia; MIF inhibits the development of the müllerian ducts. Testosterone is transformed by 5α-reductase in the bipotential external genitalia to DHT, which leads to the development of the male external genitalia.

● Three phases of sex development: development of chromosomal sex, gonadal sex, and phenotypic sex.
● Chromosomal sex: 46,XY.
● In the presence of certain Y chromosome genes, bipotential gonad develops into testis.
● Fetal testis produces two hormones: testosterone and MIF.
● Testosterone: necessary for the development of the wolffian duct; MIF inhibits the development of the müllerian duct.
● Testosterone is transformed by 5α-reductase in bipotential genitalia to DHT. DHT leads to the development of male external genitalia.

Laboratory Tests in Assessment of Male Gonadal Function

Semen analysis: normal volume, 2-5 mL; sperm count varies considerably but usually is >20 million/mL; motility, >60% at 2 hours; morphology, >60% normal forms. A normal semen analysis, with rare exceptions, rules out hypogonadism.

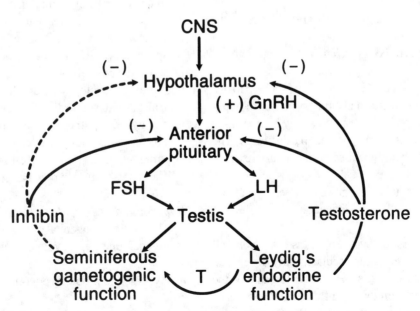

Fig. 7-13. Hypothalamic-pituitary-gonadal axis in males. CNS, central nervous system; FSH, follicle-stimulating hormone; GnRH, gonadotropin-releasing hormone; LH, luteinizing hormone; T, testosterone.

- Normal semen analysis, with rare exceptions, rules out hypogonadism.

Serum level of testosterone: measures bound (98%) and free (2%) testosterone. Its determinants are normal Leydig cell function and levels of SHBG. Low values indicate male hypogonadism. The serum level of testosterone may be low in eugonadal men with decreased SHBG, as in hypothyroidism, obesity, and acromegaly.

- Serum testosterone: determinants are normal Leydig cell function and levels of SHBG.

Serum level of free testosterone: measures the free biologically active fraction. It is not affected by conditions that modify SHBG levels.

Serum level of E_2: Low-normal or minimally increased levels may occur in primary testicular failure. Low levels occur in hypogonadotropism due to hypothalamic-pituitary disease. Increased levels occur in hypogonadotropism due to estrogen-producing tumor.

Serum levels of LH and FSH: LH and FSH levels are increased in patients with primary testicular failure and are "normal" or low in hypogonadotropism. Because of assay sensitivity limitations, values may be low in some eugonadal males. Always evaluate the serum level of LH in relation to the serum level of testosterone and evaluate the serum level of FSH in relation to semen analysis. LH, and less so FSH, is secreted in a pulsatile pattern. Thus, for optimal evaluation, obtain 3 samples at 30- to 60-minute intervals and assay hormones in pooled sample.

- LH and FSH: increased in primary testicular failure.
- Normal or low in hypogonadotropism.
- Always evaluate the serum level of LH in relation to the serum level of testosterone.
- Evaluate serum level of FSH in relation to semen analysis.

GnRH stimulation test: the GnRH test does not help to distinguish between hypothalamic and pituitary causes of hypogonadotropism. Unexpectedly, responses may be normal in pituitary disorders and absent in hypothalamic disorders. The test may sometimes be helpful in assessing pituitary reserve.

- GnRH test: does not help distinguish between hypothalamic and pituitary causes of hypogonadotropism.

hCG stimulation test: a provocative test to assess Leydig cell reserve; 4,000 IU are given intramuscularly daily for 4 days. The serum level of testosterone is measured before and on the 4th day of the test. It is useful in the differential diagnosis of cryptorchidism (normal response) from anorchia (no response).

Buccal smear: useful in the etiologic diagnosis of primary

testicular failure. The presence of Barr bodies in >15% of mucosal cells in a male confirms the presence of an extra X chromosome (Klinefelter's syndrome and its variants), but the test results may be negative in Klinefelter's mosaics.

- Buccal smear: useful in the etiologic diagnosis of primary testicular failure.

Karyotype: identifies sex chromosomal abnormalities, including mosaicism. However, it may not reveal mosaicism if this is present only in tissues other than those examined.

- Karyotype: identifies sex chromosomal abnormalities including mosaicism.

Testicular biopsy: useful in the diagnosis of severe oligospermia or azoospermia in males with normal testicular size and normal levels of testosterone and FSH. Such findings may be present in patients with spermatogenic arrest or ductal obstruction. Testicular biopsy and vasograms are needed for such differentiation.

Male Hypogonadism

Clinical Presentation

In adult males, hypogonadism can present as decreased libido, impaired potency, decreased ejaculate volume, or infertility. Also, decreased energy and stamina, decreased sexual hair growth, and classic hypogonadal facies, with pallor and fine wrinkling around the mouth and eyes. There is also altered fat distribution, testicular atrophy, decrease in prostate size, osteoporosis, and gynecomastia. If hypogonadism develops acutely, hot flashes may occur.

In adolescents, hypogonadism presents as failure of sexual and physical maturation and sexual infantilism. There is absence of pubertal growth spurt, eunuchoid habitus, i.e., ratio of upper (crown to pubis)-to-lower (pubis to floor) segment is <1 and the ratio of span-to-height is >1, high-pitched voice, poor muscle development, and female pattern of fat distribution, also, small soft testes <2 cm in length and <2 mL in volume or gynecomastia. Note that small firm testes should suggest the presence of Klinefelter's syndrome and an associated anosmia/hyposmia points to Kallmann's syndrome.

The causes of male hypogonadism are outlined in Table 7-21.

Hypergonadotropic Hypogonadism

This may be congenital or acquired, and it may affect spermatogenic function, Leydig cell function, or both.

- Hypergonadotropic hypogonadism: may be congenital or acquired.
- It may affect spermatogenic function and/or Leydig cell function.

Table 7-21.--Causes of Male Hypogonadism

Primary--testicular diseases (hypergonadotropic
hypogonadism)
  Genetic and developmental
    Klinefelter's syndrome
    Male Turner's syndrome
    Noonan's syndrome
    46,XX male
    47,XYY male
    Functional prepubertal castrate
    Myotonia dystrophica
    Sertoli-cell-only syndrome
  Acquired
    Postpubertal testicular failure
    Cirrhosis
    Castration--trauma, surgery
    Irradiation
    Chemotherapy
  Male pseudohermaphroditism
    Complete
    Incomplete
      Androgen receptor defect
      5α-reductase deficiency
      Enzyme defect in testicular biosynthesis
      Lack of müllerian inhibitory factor
Secondary--hypothalamic-pituitary diseases
(hypogonadotropic hypogonadism)
  Functional
    Systemic disease
    Malnutrition
    Anorexia nervosa
    Drugs
    Hyperprolactinemia
    Estrogen-producing tumors
    Thyroid disorders
    Adrenal disorders
  Organic
    Developmental
      Gonadotropin deficiency
        Isolated (Kallmann's syndrome, fertile eunuch
          syndrome)
        In association with deficiency of other pituitary
          hormones
    Traumatic
    Inflammatory
      Sarcoidosis
      Histiocytosis
      Granulomatous disease--tuberculosis
    Degenerative--hemochromatosis
    Vascular--carotid aneurysm
    Neoplastic
      Pituitary tumors
      Craniopharyngioma
      Glioma
      Other primary and metastatic malignancies

Klinefelter's syndrome: The basic defect in this common sex-chromosome anomaly (1:400-500) is the presence of one or more extra X chromosomes. The classic karyotype is 47,XXY. Variants include XXYY, poly X plus Y, and mosaicism. Pathologically, it is characterized by the development at puberty of seminiferous tubule hyalinization and clumping and varying levels of Leydig cell dysfunction. Clinically, it is characterized by small firm testes, gynecomastia, varying degree of testosterone deficiency and eunuchoidism, azoospermia, increased gonadotropin levels, and a positive buccal smear. Confirmation is by karyotyping of blood lymphocytes or testicular tissue. Patients with Klinefelter's syndrome have a slightly increased incidence of diabetes mellitus, chronic obstructive pulmonary disease, autoimmune disorders, varicose veins, malignancy of the breast, lymphoma, and germ cell neoplasm. The clinical picture may differ in variants and mosaics. If more than one X chromosome is present, the incidence of mental retardation and somatic abnormalities is increased. In mosaics, the clinical manifestations are less severe; if an XY line is present, fertility may be present. Infertility in classic Klinefelter's syndrome is irreversible. Testosterone therapy is given for androgen deficiency, and reduction mammoplasty is performed if the gynecomastia is a source of emotional distress.

- Klinefelter's syndrome: the basic defect is one or more extra X chromosomes.
- Classic karyotype is 47,XXY.
- Characterized pathologically by: seminiferous tubule hyalinization and clumping and varying levels of Leydig cell dysfunction.
- Characterized clinically by: small firm testes, gynecomastia, varying degree of testosterone deficiency and eunuchoidism, azoospermia, increased gonadotropin levels, and positive buccal smear.
- Confirmation: karyotyping of blood lymphocytes or testicular tissue.
- Clinical picture may differ in variants and mosaics.
- In classic Klinefelter's syndrome, infertility is irreversible.
- Testosterone therapy is given for androgen deficiency.

Noonan's syndrome (Bonnevie-Ulrich): autosomal recessive, presence of Turner's stigmata in a patient with normal male karyotype, and primary testicular failure.

Acquired testicular disorders: first and foremost, impair spermatogenic function. Leydig cell failure occurs only in severe cases. Such disorders may include mumps orchitis in postpubertal males, chronic liver disease, and chronic renal failure. Testicular damage may result from irradiation: >6 Gy damage the seminiferous tubules and >8 Gy lead to Leydig cell damage. Cytotoxic agents, especially alkylating agents, damage spermatogenic function (consider sperm banking before therapy if fertility is an issue).

- Acquired testicular disorders: first and foremost, impaired spermatogenecity.
- Only if severe, lead to Leydig cell dysfunction.

Sertoli-cell-only syndrome: azoospermia, testicular size somewhat reduced, normal or increased serum level of FSH, normal serum level of testosterone, no chromosome abnormality, no gynecomastia. Diagnosis is made by testicular biopsy. No treatment is available.

Myotonic dystrophy: 90% of men with this disorder have testicular failure that is usually hypergonadotropic but may be hypogonadotropic in nature. Therapy consists only of testosterone therapy for Leydig cell failure.

Cryptorchidism: may be unilateral or bilateral; undescended testis may be intra-abdominal, inguinal, prescrotal, or ectopic. Associated indirect inguinal hernia (50%-90% of patients). Infertility is often present, even in unilateral cases; Leydig cell function is usually normal. Increased incidence of testicular cancer that is not reduced by surgical transposition. Correction should be performed by age 12 months; options include orchiopexy, endocrine therapy with GnRH or hCG (or both), or orchiectomy.

Aging in normal men: modest decrease in total and free testosterone; decreased spermatogenesis; modest increase in LH and FSH; increased incidence of sexual dysfunction; decreased muscle and bone mass. In summary, modest primary gonadal failure with reduction in spermatogenic and Leydig cell functions; fertility may not be affected.

Hypogonadotropic Hypogonadism

A hypothalamic-pituitary disorder may lead to decreased gonadotropin secretion and thus to decreased spermatogenesis and testosterone production. Rarely, it may be associated with isolated LH or FSH deficiency. It may be functional or organic and may or may not be associated with other primary function abnormalities (see section on Hypopituitarism).

- Hypogonadotropic hypogonadism: hypothalamic-pituitary disorder may lead to decreased gonadotropin secretion and thus decreased spermatogenesis and testosterone production.
- May be functional or organic.
- May or may not be associated with other pituitary function abnormalities.

Kallmann's syndrome. This syndrome is characterized by isolated hypogonadotropism plus anosmia/hyposmia. It is a congenital disorder, often familial, that is related to maldevelopment of the olfactory lobes and the GnRH-producing cells. Studies have shown that GnRH neurons, as well as the olfactory bulbs, develop originally in the epithelium of the olfactory placode and then migrate to their ultimate anatomical location in the hypothalamus and anterior cranial fossa, respectively. This neural migration is facilitated by migration-facili-tating proteins. Gene defects recently have been found in these proteins leading to anosmia and hypogonadotropic hypogonadism characteristic of Kallmann's syndrome. Clinically, the patient presents with delayed puberty. Sexual infantilism, eunuchoidism, and, occasionally, a micropenis are present. Anosmia/hyposmia is present in 80% of patients. Other midline defects such as cleft lip or palate, color blindness, cryptorchidism, and skeletal abnormalities may also be present. Laboratory evaluation reveals hypogonadotropic hypogonadism. Other pituitary functions are normal. There may be unresponsiveness to a first single dose of GnRH; however, repeated GnRH stimulation leads to normal LH and FSH response. Therapy includes androgen replacement for sexual development and maintenance of sexual functions and secondary sex characteristics. Also, GnRH or gonadotropin therapy is warranted for fertility (is less effective if cryptorchidism is present).

- Kallmann's syndrome: isolated hypogonadotropism plus anosmia/hyposmia.
- It is a congenital disorder, often familial, and related to maldevelopment of olfactory lobes and GnRH-producing cells.
- Clinically, patients present with delayed puberty.
- Anosmia/hyposmia is present in 80% of patients.
- Laboratory evaluation: hypogonadotropic hypogonadism; other pituitary functions are normal.
- Therapy: androgen replacement and GnRH or gonadotropin for fertility.

Acquired hypogonadotropism. It may be isolated or part of a more generalized hypopituitarism. The evaluation and management of hypogonadotropic hypogonadism are outlined above (see above, Hypopituitarism). Remember hyperprolactinemia, which suppresses GnRH and presents with hypogonadotropism. Search for its cause. Therapy is with the dopamine agonist bromocriptine with or without androgen replacement.

- Acquired hypogonadotropism: Evaluate for organic and functional hypothalamic-pituitary disorders. Remember hyperprolactinemia, which suppresses GnRH and presents with hypogonadotropism.

Diagnostic Approach

Adult Male Hypogonadism

Diagnosis depends on assessing the clinical features, a semen analysis if feasible, and the serum level of testosterone. For practical purposes, a normal semen analysis excludes hypogonadism. A low serum level of testosterone, total and free, points to hypogonadism (see below). Serum levels of LH and FSH determine whether the hypogonadism is primary testicular (hypergonadotropic) or secondary to hypothalamic-pituitary disease (hypogonadotropic). The cause of hypergonadotropism is usually obvious from the clinical setting. A karyotype is required to confirm sex chromosome abnormalities. If the hypogonadism is hypogonadotropic, assess other pituitary functions and check the clinical setting for clues to functional disease (see Hypopituitarism). Among the functional disorders, the endocrine disorders of hyperprolactinemic syndrome, estrogen-producing tumors, and primary thyroid and adrenal disorders need to be considered. Perform CT or MRI of the hypothalamic-pituitary region and check visual fields if necessary.

- Diagnosis depends on: assessing clinical features, semen analysis if feasible, and serum level of testosterone.
- Normal semen analysis (for practical purposes) excludes hypogonadism.
- Low serum levels of testosterone may reflect hypogonadism or SHBG abnormalities. Check free testosterone. Low free testosterone defines hypogonadism
- Serum levels of LH and FSH: determine whether hypogonadism is primary testicular (hypergonadotropic) or secondary to hypothalamic-pituitary disease (hypogonadotropic).
- Cause of hypergonadotropism is usually obvious from the clinical setting.
- If hypogonadism is hypogonadotropic, assess other pituitary functions and check clinical setting for clues to functional disease.
- If functional hypogonadotropism is excluded, image (CT/MRI) the hypothalamic-pituitary region and check visual fields if necessary.

Adolescent Male

The clinical setting and assessment of testicular volume are critical for the evaluation. If testicular volume is >4 mL, puberty has begun; observation and reassurance are indicated. If the volume is <4 mL, check the serum levels of testosterone, LH, and FSH to document the disorder and to evaluate the axis level of dysfunction.

- Clinical setting and assessment of testicular volume are critical for evaluation.
- If testicular volume is >4 mL, puberty has begun and you can observe the patient for pubertal progression.
- If the volume is <4 mL, check serum levels of testosterone, LH, and FSH.

If hypogonadism is hypergonadotropic, diagnosis depends on the clinical setting and karyotype. If it is hypogonadotropic, evaluate the sense of smell. The presence of anosmia/hyposmia, other midline congenital defects, and positive family history point to Kallmann's syndrome. If smell sensation is normal, check other pituitary functions and perform CT or MRI of the pituitary area. All the following point to constitutional delay of puberty: absence of other pituitary function abnormalities, no abnormality seen on imaging study, and a positive family history of delayed but eventually normal puberty. Full pubertal development appears on follow-up examination.

The presence of other pituitary function abnormalities and abnormal CT or MRI findings point to organic hypothalamic-pituitary disorder (see above, Hypopituitarism).

- If hypergonadotropic, diagnosis depends on the clinical setting and karyotype.
- If hypogonadotropic, evaluate the sense of smell.
- If smell sensation is normal, check other pituitary functions and image (CT/MRI) the pituitary area.

Treatment of Male Hypogonadism

Androgen Therapy

In adults, androgen therapy is aimed at restoring and maintaining androgenic functions. In the hypogonadal pubertal male, it is designed to initiate and induce full pubertal development. It is important to remember that systemic testosterone cannot produce the high intratesticular levels of testosterone required to stimulate spermatogenesis. The drugs of choice for androgen replacement are testosterone enanthate or cypionate, long-acting 17-hydroxyl esters of testosterone. They are effective and safe. The usual dose is 200 mg intramuscularly every 10-20 days. Transdermal testosterone has recently become available but experience with it is still limited in the U.S. Aggressive testosterone therapy in pubertal patients may lead to premature closure of the epiphyses and compromise adult height. The dose is 50-100 mg/2 weeks given intramuscularly and is generally increased to full replacement. Oral preparations available in the U.S. are all 17α-alkylated derivatives of testosterone. They are less effective, more costly, and can be associated with the potentially serious side effects of hepatotoxicity, induction of peliosis hepatis, and hepatic tumors. Methyltestosterone is given in a dose of 25-50 mg daily by mouth or 10-25 mg daily buccally. Fluoxymesterone is given orally in a dose of 5-10 mg daily. Absolute contraindications for testosterone therapy are androgen-dependent tumors of the prostate and male breast. Relative contraindications include mental retardation, psychopathy, and elderly men with prostatism. Side effects include acne, mild weight gain, edema, increased erythropoiesis, and induction or worsening of obstructive sleep apnea.

- In adults, the aims of androgen therapy: restore and maintain androgenic function.
- In hypogonadal pubertal males: to initiate and induce full pubertal development.
- Drugs of choice for androgen replacement: testosterone enanthate or cypionate.
- Aggressive testosterone therapy in pubertal patients may

lead to premature closure of epiphyses and compromise adult height.

- Oral preparations: all 17α-alkylated derivatives of testosterone. They can have potentially serious side effects.
- Absolute contraindications for testosterone therapy are androgen-dependent tumors of the prostate and male breast.

Gonadotropin or GnRH Therapy

The aim of gonadotropin or GnRH therapy is to induce spermatogenesis and to establish fertility in hypogonadotropic patients. Therapy is expensive and requires multiple injections for gonadotropin therapy and pump administration for GnRH. For gonadotropin therapy, treatment is initiated with hCG alone in the dose of 2,000 IU subcutaneously or intramuscularly 3 times/week for 6-12 months. The aim is to increase intratesticular testosterone to induce maturation of the Sertoli cells and spermatogenesis. This is followed by the addition of human menopausal gonadotropin (hMG) in the dose of 75 IU intramuscularly or subcutaneously 3 times/week; spermatogenesis is completed and sperm may appear in the semen in 6-24 months. Although sperm counts are usually low in response to this therapy, fertility is restored in a substantial number of patients. After spermatogenesis is initiated, it may be maintained by hCG alone. In postpubertal patients with acquired hypogonadotropism, hCG alone may be sufficient to restore spermatogenesis. Pulsatile GnRH has been used successfully in patients with GnRH deficiency, such as Kallmann's syndrome. It requires a portable infusion pump with doses of GnRH given subcutaneously every 2 hours (to maintain gonadotrope responsiveness).

- Aim of therapy: to induce spermatogenesis and establish fertility in hypogonadotropic patients.
- Therapy is expensive.
- Requires multiple injections for gonadotropin therapy and pump administration for GnRH.
- For gonadotropin therapy: initiate treatment with hCG alone for 6-12 months.
- This is followed by the addition of hMG.
- In postpubertal patients with acquired hypogonadotropism, hCG alone may be sufficient to restore spermatogenesis.
- Pulsatile GnRH: has been successful in patients with GnRH deficiency such as Kallmann's syndrome; requires a portable infusion pump.

Anabolic Steroids and Athletes

Androgens have been and continue to be used to increase strength and performance in athletes. Because the potential risks outweigh the benefits, such androgen use should strongly be discouraged. Among the undesirable sequelae are hepatotoxicity, decreased spermatogenesis, and induction of hepatic tumors. Virilization effects are seen in prepubertal boys and

girls and in women. Other side effects include lowering of HDL-C, gynecomastia, and hypertension; there is also the risk of syringe-sharing when anabolic steroids are given parenterally. The long-term effects of use of anabolic steroids are unknown.

- Such androgen use should be strongly discouraged.
- Among the undesirable sequelae are hepatotoxicity, decreased spermatogenesis, and induction of hepatic tumors.
- Virilization can occur in prepubertal children and in women.

Male Infertility

Male infertility may result from 1) abnormal sperm count and quality; although this most commonly is "idiopathic" and related to impaired spermatogenesis, it occasionally may be related to a well-defined disorder affecting the hypothalamic-pituitary-gonadal axis. 2) Ductal obstruction, which may be caused by congenital defects, vasectomy, postinfection obstruction, or cystic fibrosis. 3) Disorders of the accessory sex organs, ejaculation, or coital techniques. The major challenge in the etiologic diagnosis of azoospermia is to differentiate spermatogenic defects from ductal obstruction. An increased level of FSH points to a spermatogenic defect. However, FSH levels may be normal in both conditions. Diagnosis then depends on testicular biopsy and vasographic study.

- Male infertility may result from: abnormal sperm count and quality (is usually "idiopathic"); ductal obstruction; or disorders of accessory sex organs, ejaculation, or coital technique.
- The major challenge in etiologic diagnosis of azoospermia: differentiating spermatogenic defects from ductal obstruction. Determination of serum FSH level and, in some cases, testicular biopsy are needed to make the differentiation.

Varicocele is a common disorder that affects 10% of the general population. Its incidence in infertile men is 30%. It is usually left-sided (90% of men) and may be associated with infertility, decreased sperm count and motility, and abnormal morphology. Serum levels of testosterone, LH, and FSH are normal. Surgical repair improves fertility. Note that if the varicocele is right-sided, venous obstruction by malignancy and situs inversus should be ruled out.

- Varicocele is common, affecting 10% of the general population.
- It is usually left-sided (90%).
- It may be associated with infertility.
- The serum levels of testosterone, LH, and FSH are normal.
- Surgical repair improves fertility.

Impotence

The causes of potency impairment are outlined in Table 7-22.

Table 7-22.--Causes of Impotence

Psychogenic, <50%
Vasculogenic--arterial, venous
Neurogenic--disorders of brain, spinal cord, or peripheral or
    autonomic nervous system
Endocrine
    Diabetes mellitus
    Neurogenic, vasculogenic, psychogenic, or mixed
Other endocrine disorders
    Gonadal disorders
    Hyperprolactinemia
    Thyroid disorders
    Adrenal disorders
Systemic disease
    Renal failure
    Liver disorder
    Chronic bronchopulmonary disorders
    Neoplastic disorders
Penile disorders--trauma, Peyronie's disease
Pharmacologic
    Alcohol
    Amphetamines, antidepressant agents, tranquilizers
    Some antihypertensive drugs
    Antiandrogens--cimetidine, spironolactone
    Estrogens
    Drugs associated with hyperprolactinemia

Diagnostic Approach

1) A complete medical history, physical examination, and selected appropriate laboratory studies can exclude or confirm many causes. The onset, clinical course, and effects on morning erections help differentiate psychogenic from organic causes. Any occurrence of erection, even if rare, suggests a psychogenic cause. Check for evidence of diabetes mellitus, alcohol abuse, aortoiliac disease, and other endocrinopathies. Review all medications and inquire into substance abuse. Tumescence study serves to confirm loss of erectile function. The "postage stamp" test is simple, inexpensive, and effective as a screen. 2) Endocrine evaluation includes measuring serum levels of testosterone, E_2, LH and FSH, PRL, T_4 and TSH, and cortisol. 3) The screening test for vasculogenic impotence consists of Doppler ultrasonography both in the flaccid state and after the intracavernous injection of a vasoactive drug such as papaverine, phentolamine, or prostaglandin E_1. Failure to achieve a normal response documents a vasculogenic disorder but does not distinguish between arterial and venous abnormalities. Additional vascular studies include penile arteriography (for arterial insufficiency) and cavernosometry and cav-

ernosography (for venous incompetence). 4) Evaluation for neurogenic impotence: the presence of neurogenic bladder suggests the diagnosis. Evaluate bulbocavernous reflex latency with electromyography, and study the somatosensory evoked response of the dorsal nerve to assess peripheral and sacral spinal cord function.

- A complete medical history, physical examination, and selected appropriate laboratory studies.
- Endocrine evaluation: measure serum levels of testosterone, E_2, LH and FSH, PRL, T_4 and TSH, and cortisol.
- Screening test for vasculogenic impotence.
- Evaluation for neurogenic impotence.

Management

If possible, treatment is directed to the cause, such as removing the offending drug or alcohol. Institute bromocriptine therapy for hyperprolactinemic disorders and testosterone therapy for hypogonadism. Recommend psychiatric counseling if appropriate. Other available modalities include: 1) intracavernous pharmacotherapy; the risks include priapism (1% of patients), corporal fibrosis (25%) with repeated injections, and hepatic dysfunction in those receiving papaverine; 2) external vacuum device or penile prosthesis; and 3) penile vascular surgery.

Gynecomastia

The causes of gynecomastia are outlined in Table 7-23. The basic mechanism of gynecomastia is relative estradiol excess which can result from 1) decreased androgen effect caused by a decrease in androgen production (aging, primary or central testicular failure, or use of inhibitors of testosterone biosynthesis such as ketoconazole), an increase in androgen-binding (hyperthyroidism or liver failure) or androgen-receptor blocker (use of spironolactone, cimetidine, or flutamide); 2) absolute increase in E_2 production (Klinefelter's syndrome, adrenal cancer, Leydig cell tumor, or hCG-producing tumor); 3) increased estrogen precursor availability (androgen-secreting tumors, exogenous androgen use, or hyperthyroidism); 4) exogenous estrogen effect (digitalis or synthetic estrogens); and 5) displacement of estrogen from SHBG and increased free estradiol (ketoconazole and spironolactone).

In healthy young pubertal males, the most likely cause is transient physiologic gynecomastia. Anabolic steroid use and Klinefelter's syndrome may account for a small number of cases. All other causes are rare in this age group.

In adults, the two most common causes are drugs and alcohol-related liver disease. Less common causes include recovery from malnutrition or other serious chronic illness. Rarely encountered are ectopic hCG-producing tumors, feminizing adrenal and testicular tumors, and pituitary tumors. In about 10% of cases, the cause of gynecomastia is indeterminate.

Diagnostic Approach

If bilateral, rule out pseudogynecomastia (fatty enlargement). If unilateral, rule out tumors, especially carcinoma. Gynecomastia is identified by its firmness, fine nodularity, a central location posterior to the areola from which it spreads radially, and a well-defined outer border. Signs that should arouse suspicion of malignancy include eccentric location relative to the areola, unusual firmness, fixation, ulceration, bloody discharge from the nipple, and the presence of axillary lymphadenopathy. Mammography and excisional biopsy may be necessary for definitive diagnosis. A complete medical history, physical examination, and appropriate laboratory studies should rule out physiologic, pharmacologic, alcohol-related, and refeeding types of gynecomastia. Endocrine tests should include measurement of testosterone, E_2, LH and FSH, βhCG, sTSH, DHEAS, and PRL. If needed, karyotyping should be performed.

Table 7-23.--Causes of Gynecomastia

Physiologic
  Newborn
  Adolescence
  Aging
Pathologic
  Decreased testosterone production
    Primary testicular failure
    Hypothalamic-pituitary testicular failure
  Decreased testosterone action
    Congenital
    Acquired
      Spironolactone, cimetidine
  Increased estradiol production
    hCG-producing tumors
    Estrogen-producing tumors
    Increased conversion of androgen to estrogen
      Liver disease/alcohol
      Thyrotoxicosis
      Marked obesity
      Hepatoma
  Exogenous
    Estrogenic drugs, alcohol
  Refeeding gynecomastia
  Hyperprolactinemic states
  Uncertain causes
    Methyltestosterone
    Cytotoxic drugs
    Amphetamine
    Marihuana
  Idiopathic

- If gynecomastia is bilateral, rule out pseudogynecomastia.
- If unilateral, rule out tumors.
- Signs that arouse suspicion of malignancy: eccentric location relative to the areola, unusual firmness, fixation, ulceration, bloody discharge from the nipple, and axillary lymphadenopathy.
- Complete medical history, physical examination, appropriate laboratory studies to rule out: physiologic, pharmacologic, alcohol-related, and refeeding types of gynecomastia.
- Endocrine tests: testosterone, E_2, LH and FSH, βhCG, sTSH, DHEAS, and PRL. (Karyotype is added when appropriate.)

One can start with measurements of the serum levels of LH and FSH: 1) High serum levels of LH and FSH point to primary testicular failure, including Klinefelter's syndrome. 2) Isolated high LH usually points to an hCG-secreting tumor, because of the crossreaction between LH and hCG. Check serum βhCG subunit level. 3) Low levels of LH and FSH should prompt consideration of androgen- or estrogen-producing tumor, exogenous sex steroid use, and hypogonadotropism including that associated with hyperprolactinemia. Inquire about use of sex steroids. If negative, check free testosterone and E_2 levels and proceed as indicated. A low level of free testosterone implies hypogonadotropism and should prompt a complete hypothalamic-pituitary evaluation. A high level of estradiol should prompt evaluation for feminizing adrenal or testicular tumors. 4) If serum levels of LH, FSH, and sex steroids are normal, an underlying endocrinopathy is unlikely. These patients can be observed and reevaluated periodically.

- First check LH and FSH measurements.
- High LH and FSH: primary testicular failure.
- High LH and normal FSH: check βhCG.
- Low LH and FSH: endogenous or exogenous sex steroid excess.
- Normal LH and FSH: an endocrinopathy is unlikely.

Management

Therapy may include reassurance, correction of underlying disorders, and tamoxifen (usually not helpful), or cosmetic surgery.

FEMALE GONADAL DISORDERS

Physiology

The female gonadal axis is shown in Figure 7-14. The function of the female gonadal system is characterized by cyclicity. Its dominant aspects are the ovarian cycle and the endometrial menstrual cycle. The ovarian cycle is responsible for ovulation and the secretion of sex steroids and is under the control of the hypothalamic-pituitary-gonadal axis.

- Cyclicity characterizes the function of the female gonadal axis during reproductive life.
- Ovarian cycle: responsible for ovulation and secretion of sex steroids.
- It is under the control of the hypothalamic-pituitary-gonadotropin axis.

The ovarian cycle consists of three phases: 1) the follicular phase, primary follicle to mature graafian follicle; 2) ovulation; and 3) the luteal phase, dominated by the corpus luteum. If pregnancy does not occur, the corpus luteum regresses in 14 days and another ovarian cycle is started. The hormone of the follicular phase is E_2; luteal phase hormones are E_2 and progesterone. These hormones are responsible for the endometrial menstrual cycle. In the follicular phase, E_2 leads to proliferative endometrium. In the luteal phase, E_2 and progesterone lead to a secretory endometrium. With regression of the corpus luteum, steroid levels decrease, the endometrium is sloughed, and menstrual flow ensues.

- Three phases of the ovarian cycle: follicular phase, ovulation, and luteal phase.
- E_2: hormone of follicular phase.
- E_2 and progesterone: hormones of luteal phase.

The hypothalamic-pituitary unit controls the ovarian cycle. The hypothalamic decapeptide GnRH is secreted in bursts every 70-90 minutes. The anterior pituitary gonadotroph secretes the glycoproteins LH and FSH. Secretion of GnRH, LH, and FSH is cyclic. In the follicular phase, both gonadotropins are needed for follicular maturation and hormone secretion; LH leads to the synthesis of androgens by the thecal cells, and FSH promotes the growth of the granulosa cells and the aromatization of androgens to estrogens by these cells. A mid-cycle LH peak causes ovulation. LH is needed for corpus luteum function. The female gonadal axis functions under negative and positive feedback. In general, steady or decreasing estrogen levels exert negative effects, increasing estrogen levels have positive effects, and the presence of both estrogen and progesterone has a negative effect. Documentation of ovulation is by 1) biphasic temperature curve (progesterone is thermogenic), 2) serial changes in cervical mucous and vaginal cell smear, 3) the presence of secretory endometrium on endometrial sampling, and 4) the increase in the serum level of progesterone in the luteal phase.

- GnRH (a hypothalamic decapeptide) is secreted in bursts every 70-90 minutes.
- GnRH, LH, and FSH: secretion is cyclic.
- In the follicular phase, both gonadotropins are needed for follicular maturation and hormone secretion.
- Mid-cycle LH peak causes ovulation.
- LH: needed for luteal function.
- The female gonadal axis functions under negative and positive feedback.
- Document ovulation: biphasic temperature curve; presence of secretory endometrium on endometrial sampling; and increase in serum levels of progesterone in the luteal phase.

E_2 is secreted by the ovarian follicle and corpus luteum. It is responsible for the initiation of female pubertal changes, development and maintenance of the genitalia and secondary sex characteristics, pubertal growth spurt and epiphyseal fusion, proliferative endometrium and receptive cervical mucus, breast duct development, negative and positive hypothalamic-pituitary feedback effect, and anabolic functions. Progesterone is secreted by the corpus luteum and is responsible for the secretory endometrium, hostile cervical mucus, breast and alveolar growth, hypothalamic-pituitary-gonadotropic axis feedback, and thermogenic effect. Androgens in females are responsible for libido, sexual hair growth, and anabolic functions.

Female sexual development has three phases: 1) chromosomal sex (46,XX in normal females); 2) gonadal sex, i.e., an ovary (absence of the Y chromosome and the presence of XX chromosomal constitution is necessary for full gonadal development); and 3) phenotypic sex. The ovary does not produce testosterone or MIF; therefore, the wolffian duct regresses and the müllerian duct develops into the female internal genitalia (fallopian tubes, uterus, and upper 2/3 of the vagina). In the

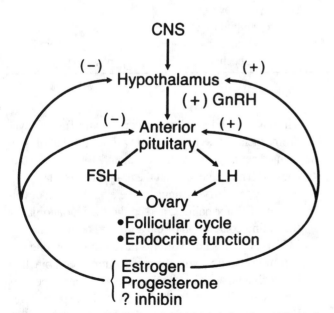

Fig. 7-14. Hypothalamic-pituitary-gonadal axis in females. Abbreviations same as in Fig. 7-13.

absence of testosterone, no DHT is formed in the bipotential external genitalia and these structures develop into the female external genitalia.

- Three phases of female sexual development: chromosomal sex (46,XX), gonadal sex (ovary), and phenotypic sex.
- The ovary does not produce testosterone or MIF. The Wolffian duct regresses, and the müllerian duct forms the female internal genitalia.
- Without testosterone, no DHT is formed in bipotential external genitalia, resulting in female external genitalia.

Amenorrhea

Etiology

The causes of amenorrhea are outlined in Table 7-24. Clinically, amenorrhea is best categorized as "primary amenorrhea," which refers to absence of menarche in a phenotypic female who is at least 17 years old, and "secondary amenorrhea," which refers to cessation of menstruation for at least 3 months in a woman with previously established menstrual function. Amenorrhea can result from impaired function of any component of the hypothalamic-pituitary-gonadal axis or from an anatomical abnormality of the genital tract.

- Amenorrhea is categorized clinically as "primary" and "secondary" amenorrhea.
- It can result from impaired function of any component of the hypothalamic-pituitary-gonadal axis or from an anatomical abnormality of the genital tract.

Outflow tract abnormalities are uncommon causes of primary or secondary amenorrhea. Developmental anomalies include imperforate hymen, isolated absence of the uterus, and vaginal aplasia or atresia. Acquired disorders include postabortive or postpartum endometritis, overzealous dilatation and curettage with destruction of the endometrial basal layer, and formation of adhesions and obliteration of the endometrial cavity (Asherman's syndrome and endometrial atrophy related to prolonged use of progestational agents or after treatment of endometriosis).

- Outflow tract abnormalities: uncommon causes of primary or secondary amenorrhea.

Ovarian disorders, including developmental and acquired disorders, account for most of the causes of primary amenorrhea:

1. Turner's 45/XO gonadal dysgenesis is the most common cause of primary amenorrhea. It is estimated to affect 1 in 3,000 newborn females and is characterized by fibrous gonadal streaks, female phenotype, short stature, skeletal and developmental anomalies, and, in adolescent patients, primary ovarian failure and sexual infantilism.

Table 7-24.--Causes of Amenorrhea

Physiologic
   Premenarchal
   Pregnancy
   Postpartum state
   Postmenopausal
Pathologic
   Outflow tract disorders--genital tract aplasia, atresia, acquired destructive processes (e.g., Asherman's syndrome)
   Gonadal disorders
      Gonadal dysgenesis and its variants
      Other developmental disorders
      Autoimmune oophoritis and other destructive processes
      Polycystic ovaries
      Ovarian tumors
   Hypothalamic-pituitary disorders
      Functional
         Stress, diet, exercise
         Postpill
         Drugs
         Systemic disease
         Other endocrine disease
            Thyroid
            Adrenal
            Hyperprolactinemia
            Diabetes mellitus
         Delayed puberty
      Organic
         Isolated hypogonadotropism (e.g., Kallmann's syndrome)
         Hypopituitarism
            Various organic diseases--pituitary tumors, Sheehan's syndrome, hypophysitis

The physical abnormalities associated with Turner's syndrome include a webbed neck, low-set ears, multiple pigmented nevi, micrognathia, epicanthal folds, shield-like chest with microthelia, short metacarpals and metatarsals, an increased carrying angle at the elbows, renal developmental abnormalities, and cardiovascular anomalies (including coarctation of the aorta and aortic stenosis). In Turner's mosaics, patients have more than one sex chromosomal line, with the most common combination being 45/XO, 46/XX; the degree of ovarian dysgenesis varies depending on the ratio of XO to XX germ cells. Patients may present with primary or secondary amenorrhea. In cases of Turner's mosaics, the patients are not invariably short and may have few or many of the physical stigmata of Turner's syndrome, depending on which tissues get the XO chromosomal line.

- Ovarian disorders are the most common cause of primary amenorrhea.
- Turner's 45/XO gonadal dysgenesis: the most common cause of primary amenorrhea.
- Characterized by: fibrous gonadal streaks, female phenotype, short stature, skeletal and developmental anomalies, and, in adolescent patients, primary ovarian failure and sexual infantilism.
- Physical abnormalities associated with Turner's syndrome: renal developmental abnormalities and cardiovascular anomalies.
- Turner's mosaics: patients have more than one sex chromosomal line.
- The degree of ovarian dysgenesis varies depending on the ratio of XO to XX germ cells.
- Turner's mosaics: patients may present with primary or secondary amenorrhea.

2. 46/XX gonadal dysgenesis is characterized by a normal female karyotype, gonadal fibrous streaks, phenotypic female, and, in adolescent females, primary ovarian failure with failure of sexual maturation and primary amenorrhea. The patient has eunuchoidal features and does not have the physical stigmata of Turner's syndrome.

3. 46/XY gonadal dysgenesis is characterized by fibrous streaks with a variable amount of testicular tissue, a female phenotype, and, in adolescent females, failure of normal sexual maturation and primary amenorrhea. Often, there is postpubertal virilization as a result of androgen secretion by the dysgenetic gonad. Such gonads are at an increased risk of neoplastic transformation; hence, gonadectomy is advisable as soon as the diagnosis is made.

4. True hermaphroditism is defined by the presence of both ovarian and testicular tissues in either the same or opposite gonads. The karyotype can be 46/XX or 46/XY, although some patients have mosaicism. The external genitalia are often ambiguous but can be distinctly female or male. The uterus is present in virtually all patients. At puberty, significant breast development occurs in most and menstruation in more than half of the patients. Some patients present with primary amenorrhea.

5. Testicular feminization is a hereditary disorder transmitted as an X-linked recessive trait that affects genetic males. It is characterized by peripheral tissue unresponsiveness to androgen (testosterone and dihydrotestosterone) because of androgen receptor or post-receptor abnormality. The vagina is often shallow, ending in a blind pouch. The testes may be inguinal and simulate an "inguinal hernia" or may be intra-abdominal. These male pseudoher-

maphrodites are raised as females. In adolescence, with the gonadotropin pubertal surge and increased estrogen production by the testes, normal breast and female secondary sexual maturation occurs except for the absence of sexual hair (which is androgen-dependent) and for primary amenorrhea. Gonadectomy is required after completion of pubertal development to forestall the development of neoplastic changes.

- Testicular feminization: affects genetic males.
- Characterized by peripheral tissue unresponsiveness to androgen (testosterone and dihydrotestosterone) because of androgen receptor abnormality.
- In adolescence, normal breast and female secondary sexual maturation occurs except for absence of sexual hair and for primary amenorrhea.
- Gonadectomy required after completion of pubertal development.

Ovarian disorders are common causes of secondary amenorrhea. The most common disorder is polycystic ovary syndrome (see Hirsutism). Ovarian destructive processes are an uncommon cause of secondary amenorrhea and premature menopause. These processes include autoimmune oophoritis as part of polyendocrine autoimmune disease, various forms of mosaic gonadal dysgenesis that lead to premature exhaustion of the complement of ovarian follicles, abdominal irradiation, chemotherapy with such agents as cyclophosphamide and vincristine, and ovarian tumors that cause secondary amenorrhea by hormonal abnormalities (hypersecretion of estrogen, androgen, or hCG) or, if bilateral, by destruction of the ovarian tissue.

- Ovarian disorders: common causes of secondary amenorrhea.
- The most common disorder: polycystic ovary syndrome.
- Ovarian destructive processes: uncommon cause of secondary amenorrhea and premature menopause.

Hypothalamic-pituitary disease can cause gonadotropin deficiency and amenorrhea by 1) destruction of pituitary gonadotrophs or the hypothalamic GnRH cell population by organic diseases of various origins or 2) functional suppression of these cells, commonly by a hyperprolactinemic state, nutritional disorder, or anorexia nervosa (see above, Hypopituitarism).

Hypothalamic disorders are the least frequent causes of primary amenorrhea. 1) Isolated deficiency of GnRH occurs in females but much less than in males. In some patients, it is associated with anosmia or hyposmia caused by hypoplasia or aplasia of the olfactory lobe (Kallmann's syndrome). This syndrome is familial and may be associated with midline craniofacial defects and other skeletal abnormalities. 2) Constitutional delay in puberty can occur in females but less frequently than in males. It may be genetic, and a parent or a sibling may have experienced a similar delay. The patients have evidence of delayed growth throughout childhood and delayed bone age, but they ultimately progress through the normal stages of puberty. 3) Organic hypothalamic-pituitary disease due to various causes is an uncommon cause of primary amenorrhea. In young adults, craniopharyngioma is the most common space-occupying lesion; prolactinomas occur in this age group but are rare. 4) Functional hypothalamic disorders account for a small percentage of cases of primary amenorrhea.

- Hypothalamic-pituitary disease can cause gonadotropin deficiency and amenorrhea by destruction of pituitary gonadotropin or the hypothalamic GnRH cell population.
- Or, by functional suppression of these cells (by hyperprolactinemic state, nutritional disorder, or anorexia nervosa).
- Hypothalamic disorders: the least frequent causes of primary amenorrhea.
- In young adults, craniopharyngioma is the most common space-occupying lesion.

Hypothalamic-pituitary disorders are the most common pathologic causes of secondary amenorrhea and may be either functional or organic. Functional hypogonadotropism results from hypothalamic dysfunction caused by a defect in the cyclic center, inhibition of the mid-cycle surge of GnRH and LH, and the failure of ovulation. Mild disorders of GnRH release may be triggered by situational stresses or mild weight loss: FSH secretion is low-normal, E_2 production continues, the endometrium is proliferative, and exogenous progesterone leads to withdrawal bleeding. Moderate or severe disorders of GnRH release may occur with severe weight loss, severe emotional stresses, competitive athletics, systemic disease, thyroid disorders, uncontrolled diabetes mellitus, or a hyperandrogenic state caused by an adrenal or ovarian disorder. Under these circumstances, estrogen levels are low, the endometrium is atrophic, and exogenous progesterone does not lead to withdrawal bleeding. Postpill amenorrhea is common and occurs in about 2% of women who take birth control pills and who may or may not have had prepill menstrual irregularity. Generally, spontaneous recovery occurs in one to a few months. Of patients with postpill amenorrhea, a minority have hyperprolactinemia and some of these may have underlying pituitary adenoma. Psychotropic drugs, especially the phenothiazine family, can cause hypogonadotropism by a direct effect at the hypothalamic level or secondary to hyperprolactinemia from the antidopaminergic effect of these drugs.

- Hypothalamic-pituitary disorders: the most common pathologic cause of secondary amenorrhea.
- It may be functional or organic; functional hypogonadotropism is common.

Anorexia nervosa, a syndrome seen almost exclusively in young females, is manifested predominantly by weight loss, amenorrhea, and behavioral disorder. The age at onset is usually <25 years. Weight loss can be extreme and accompanied by a distorted and implacable attitude toward eating and weight. The patients deny their illness and fail to recognize their nutritional needs. Some may manifest unusual hoarding and handling of food. Bulimia (excessive food intake) and vomiting are seen in 50% of the patients. Amenorrhea occurs in all young female patients with anorexia nervosa, and in 25% of them, it precedes the weight loss. Other features include bradycardia, hypotension, constipation, impaired temperature regulation (inability to shiver and maintain body temperature in face of hypothermia or hyperthermia), lanugo hair growth, hypercarotenemia, and, in severe cases, dependent edema. Endocrine findings include hypogonadotropism, normal or increased serum levels of GH and low IGF-I, normal serum levels of T_4 and TSH but decreased levels of T_3 and increased reversed T_3 levels, serum cortisol levels are generally increased and show normal suppressibility with dexamethasone, decreased 24-hour urinary 17-ketogenic and 17-ketosteroids, and a normal serum level of PRL.

- Anorexia nervosa: is seen almost exclusively in young females.
- Predominant manifestations: weight loss, amenorrhea, and behavioral disorder.
- Amenorrhea occurs in all the young female patients, and in 25%, it precedes the weight loss.
- Endocrine findings: hypogonadotropism, normal/increased GH serum level, low IGF-I, normal T_4 and TSH levels, decreased T_3 and increased reversed T_3 levels, increased serum cortisol levels (normal suppressibility with dexamethasone), and normal serum level of PRL.

Primary hypothyroidism can lead to amenorrhea via three mechanisms: 1) anovulation (in mild cases may lead to breakthrough bleeding and menorrhagia; in severe cases, to amenorrhea); 2) hyperprolactinemia (can occur in 20%-30% of patients with primary hypothyroidism, can cause functional suppression of the hypothalamic-pituitary-gonadotropin axis); and 3) associated autoimmune primary ovarian failure and consequent amenorrhea. Adrenal disorders can lead to amenorrhea through a hyperandrogenic state (congenital adrenal hyperplasia, Cushing's syndrome, adrenal tumors), through chronic adrenocortical insufficiency (by its effects on general health and nutrition), or by its association with autoimmune primary ovarian failure.

- Primary hypothyroidism can lead to amenorrhea.
- Three mechanisms: anovulation, hyperprolactinemia, and associated autoimmune primary ovarian failure.

Hypogonadotropism can be the only manifestation of hypothalamic-pituitary organic disease or it can occur in association with other pituitary function abnormalities (see above, Hypopituitarism). Hyperprolactinemia is a common cause of secondary amenorrhea, accounting for 25%-40% of all cases. Postpartum pituitary necrosis (Sheehan's syndrome), previously a common cause, has declined in incidence with improvement in obstetric care.

- Hypogonadotropism can occur as the only manifestation of hypothalamic-pituitary disease or in association with other pituitary function abnormalities.
- Hyperprolactinemia: a common cause of secondary amenorrhea (25%-40% of all cases).

Diagnostic Approach to Amenorrhea

Endocrine Tests

Serum level of E_2: low values occur in hypogonadism of any cause. Because normal values may be found in anovulatory states, they may not be indicative of a normal gonadal axis.

- Low values of E_2: occur in hypogonadism of any cause.

Serum levels of LH and FSH: these gonadotropins are secreted in a cyclic, pulsatile fashion; thus, normal values vary depending on the phase of the ovulatory cycle. LH and FSH should always be evaluated in relation to menstrual function or serum levels of E_2. In hypogonadal females, high values indicate primary ovarian failure, but "normal" or low values indicate hypogonadism of hypothalamic-pituitary origin. A high LH/FSH ratio (>2) is common in polycystic ovarian syndrome.

- LH and FSH: always evaluate in relation to menstrual function or serum E_2 levels.
- Hypogonadal females: high values indicate primary ovarian failure; normal/low values indicate hypogonadism of hypothalamic-pituitary origin.

Progestin withdrawal test: oral medroxyprogesterone acetate is given 10 mg/day for 5 days; alternatively, progesterone is given in a dose of 100 mg intramuscularly. Typically, this is the first test performed after pregnancy has been excluded and serves as a bioassay for LH, FSH, and E_2 secretion and for uterine responsiveness. Withdrawal bleeding indicates estrogen-endometrial priming and points to an anovulatory state resulting from very mild hypothalamic dysfunction or polycystic ovaries. Absence of withdrawal bleeding in a nonpregnant female indicates estrogen deficiency and more serious hypothalamic dysfunction, pituitary disease, or ovarian failure.

- Progestin withdrawal test can serve as a bioassay for gonadal-axis endocrine function.
- Withdrawal bleeding points to an anovulatory disorder.
- Absence of withdrawal bleeding, with pregnancy excluded, points to estrogen deficiency and a significant hypothalamic-pituitary-ovarian disorder.

Serum level of PRL: this should always be assessed in the evaluation of amenorrhea. Hyperprolactinemia is a common cause of hypogonadotropism and points to a hypothalamic-pituitary disorder. Remember that the most common cause of amenorrhea and hyperprolactinemia is pregnancy.

- Serum prolactin level: always assess it in evaluating amenorrhea.
- The most common cause of amenorrhea and hyperprolactinemia: pregnancy.

The GnRH test: usually is not helpful in distinguishing between hypothalamic and pituitary causes of hypogonadotropism. The gonadotropin responses may be exaggerated, normal, or decreased in disorders of either the hypothalamus or the pituitary.

- GnRH test: usually not helpful in distinguishing between hypothalamic and pituitary causes of hypogonadotropism.

Secondary Amenorrhea

The usual causes are hypothalamic dysfunction (30% of patients); polycystic ovaries (30%); pituitary disorder, principally prolactinoma (15%); primary ovarian failure (10%); and uterine problems (5%).

1) Rule out physiologic amenorrhea: clinical setting and pregnancy test. 2) Rule out genital tract outflow disorders: evaluate clinical setting; in outflow disorders, progesterone test and estrogen/progesterone test results are negative. 3) Rule out hyperandrogenic state (see Hirsutism). 4) Measure the serum levels of E_2, LH, and (particularly) FSH to distinguish ovarian from hypothalamic-pituitary disorders.

- Rule out: physiologic amenorrhea, genital tract outflow disorders, and hyperandrogenic state.
- Measure serum levels of E_2, LH, and FSH to distinguish ovarian from hypothalamic-pituitary disease.

Low serum levels of E_2 and increased levels of FSH and LH point to primary ovarian failure (a karyotype is necessary in patients <35 years old). In the absence of any readily apparent cause for ovarian failure such as trauma, chemotherapy, or radiotherapy, one should consider an autoimmune disorder. Appropriate tests for other evidence of autoimmune endocrinopathy such as sTSH, antimicrosomal antithyroid antibodies, and cosyntropin stimulation tests are indicated.

- Low serum levels of E_2 and increased levels of FSH and LH: primary ovarian failure.

Low serum levels of E_2 and inappropriately low levels of LH and FSH point to a hypothalamic-pituitary disorder. Rule out a functional disorder; if present, correct it; if periods resume, the diagnosis is functional disorder. If functional disorder is not present or if its correction does not lead to the resumption of menstrual function, proceed with tests to rule out organic hypothalamic-pituitary disease. These include determining the serum level of PRL and other pituitary hormones, CT or MR imaging of the sella, and testing visual fields, if necessary. If an identifiable organic disease is found, treat it appropriately, but if no such organic disease is found, consider the amenorrhea to be of indeterminate cause and pursue long-term follow-up; an identifiable cause may become apparent in months or years.

- Low serum levels of E_2 and inappropriately low levels of FSH and LH: hypothalamic-pituitary disorder.
- If hypogonadotropic, rule out functional disorder.
- If no functional disorder, perform tests to rule out organic hypothalamic-pituitary disease.
- If no organic disease, consider amenorrhea to be of indeterminate cause and pursue long-term follow-up.

Primary Amenorrhea

Evaluate the secondary sex characteristics: 1) If the sex characteristics are those of an adult female and pregnancy test results are negative, consider outflow obstruction (imperforate hymen), genital tract anomalies (such as absent uterus), or testicular feminization. Diagnosis depends on the clinical picture, pelvic examination, and use of pelvic ultrasonography. 2) If hyperandrogenic manifestations are present, proceed with work-up (as for hirsutism). 3) If sexually infantile, check serum levels of E_2, LH, and FSH and proceed as described under secondary amenorrhea work-up.

- Evaluate secondary sex characteristics.
- If adult female sex characteristics and negative results with pregnancy test: consider outflow obstruction, genital tract anomalies, and testicular feminization.
- If sexually infantile: check serum levels of E_2, LH, and FSH and proceed as for secondary amenorrhea.

Management of Hypogonadal Females

It is important to identify and treat the cause. Reversing the cause of functional amenorrhea—e.g., restoring lost weight, reducing excessive physical exercise, surgical treatment for pituitary tumors, bromocriptine therapy for hyperprolactinemic disorders—usually restores normal menstrual function. If successful treatment of the cause is not possible, estrogen replacement is indicated.

- It is important to identify and treat the cause.
- If successful treatment of the cause is not possible, estrogen replacement is indicated.

The goals of estrogen therapy include controlling vasomotor instability, preventing genitourinary atrophy, preserving secondary sex characteristics, preventing osteoporosis, reducing the risk of coronary artery disease (probable), and restoring a sense of well-being. Absolute contraindications to estrogen therapy include known or suspected estrogen-dependent neoplasm (breast or uterus), cholestatic hepatic dysfunction, active thromboembolic disorder, history of thromboembolic disorder associated with previous estrogen use, neuro-ophthalmologic vascular disease, and undiagnosed vaginal bleeding.

The complications of estrogen replacement include: 1) increased risk of endometrial cancer, which is dose- and duration-dependent (4x-8x); such cancer is usually stage I with no excess mortality. This risk is prevented by progestin supplementation. 2) Possible risk of breast cancer; the weight of present evidence indicates no such increased risk. Pretreatment breast examination and mammography (and annually thereafter) are essential. 3) Increased risk of surgical gallbladder disease.

- Complications of estrogen treatment: increased risk of endometrial cancer (prevented by progestin supplementation), possible risk of breast cancer, and increased risk of surgical gallbladder disease.

Estrogen therapy can be administered orally, parenterally, topically, or transdermally. In women with a uterus and who need supplemental progestin, the therapy can be given sequentially or in combination. In sequential therapy, estrogen may be given as conjugated equine estrogen (or equivalent) in a dose of 0.625 mg daily in patients >45 years (or 0.9-1.25 mg in those <45 years) on days 1-25 of each month and supplemented with a progestin, such as medroxyprogesterone acetate in a dose of 10 mg/day, days 14-25 of each month. Such sequential therapy results in predictable cyclic withdrawal bleeding in 50%-60% of patients. For unpredictable bleeding, endometrial biopsy is indicated.

- Sequential therapy results in predictable cyclic withdrawal in 50%-60% of patients.
- For unpredictable bleeding: endometrial biopsy.

Combination therapy mimics oral contraceptive combinations. Its goal is to induce endometrial atrophy and amenorrhea in those who find cyclic withdrawal bleeding inconvenient or unacceptable. Conjugated equine estrogen is given in the same doses daily and medroxyprogesterone acetate in a dose of 2.5 mg daily. Most patients become amenorrheic in 4-6 months and can expect irregular spotting during that time.

- Combination therapy mimics oral contraceptive combinations.
- Goal: induce endometrial atrophy and amenorrhea in those who find cyclic withdrawal bleeding inconvenient or unacceptable.

Estrogen replacement therapy must be individualized and be given only after a thorough discussion with the patient about the pros and cons of the therapy. Start therapy as soon as possible after the diagnosis of estrogen deficiency and continue it indefinitely or until the cause has been reversed. No estrogen preparation is superior to the other, and the cardioprotective effect of transdermal estradiol is unproved. Supplemental progestin is indicated only for women who have a uterus; medroxyprogesterone acetate is preferred rather than 19-nortestosterone derivatives, because it is less likely to lower HDL-C levels. Before estrogen therapy is initiated, it is advisable to give medroxyprogesterone acetate, 10 mg daily for 10-14 days. If no withdrawal bleeding occurs, an atrophic endometrium is present (after ruling out pregnancy in appropriate setting) and estrogen therapy can be initiated. However, if withdrawal bleeding occurs, the endometrium is estrogen-primed and consideration should be given to performing endometrial biopsy to rule out endometrial hyperplasia before initiating estrogen replacement therapy.

- Estrogen replacement therapy: must be individualized.
- Give it only after thoroughly discussing the pros and cons.

Ovulation Induction

Hypogonadal women who desire fertility can receive treatment with clomiphene citrate, gonadotropin, or GnRH. The drug of choice for hyperprolactinemic infertility is the dopamine-agonist bromocriptine (see Hyperprolactinemic Syndrome and Prolactinomas).

Clomiphene citrate acts like an antiestrogen at the hypothalamic level and stimulates endogenous gonadotropin secretion. Its main use is in patients with chronic anovulation related to functional hypothalamic disorder and in patients with polycystic ovarian disease. It is given in a dose of 50 mg/day for 5 days; the dose can be increased by increments of 50 mg/day in successive cycles to a maximum of 250 mg/day for 5 days. An ovulatory surge occurs 5-12 days after completion of clomiphene and can be documented by basal body temperature or serum progesterone level. If needed, hCG can be given 7 days after the last dose of clomiphene. Ovulation occurs in about 80% of patients, and 40%-50% achieve pregnancy. Multiple pregnancy rate (twins in most cases) occurs in <10% of patients. Side effects occur in <5% of patients and include vasomotor flushes, nausea or vomiting, abdominal discomfort, and visual symptoms. Symptomatic ovarian enlargement is rare.

- Clomiphene citrate: acts like an antiestrogen at the hypothalamic level.
- It stimulates endogenous gonadotropin secretion.
- Main use: patients with chronic anovulation related to functional hypothalamic disorder and patients with polycystic ovarian disease.

Gonadotropin therapy is indicated for patients with organic pituitary disease and for those in whom a trial of clomiphene was unsuccessful. Gonadotropin therapy should be initiated and followed by an experienced reproductive endocrinologist: hMG, consisting of FSH and LH, or human FSH is given to achieve follicular development; hCG is then given to simulate the LH surge. This therapy is expensive and may have significant complications, including a 30% incidence of multiple pregnancies and ovarian hyperstimulation syndrome. The latter is the major side effect and consists of ovarian enlargement, with multiple follicular cysts and edema, ascites, hypovolemia, and hemoconcentration. Gonadotropin therapy is monitored by measuring E_2 levels and pelvic ultrasonography. When hyperstimulation syndrome is present, conservative treatment is indicated; avoid pelvic examination because of the danger of ovarian rupture. The condition resolves slowly over 7 days.

- Gonadotropin therapy: indicated for patients with organic pituitary disease and for those in whom a trial of clomiphene was unsuccessful.
- Therapy should be initiated and followed by an experienced reproductive endocrinologist.

GnRH therapy may be used for patients with a hypothalamic syndrome and intact pituitary gland. It is most effective in hypothalamic anovulation. Administer 5-20 mg (intravenously, subcutaneously, or by pump) every 90 minutes or so. Hyperstimulation is extremely unlikely. Its major disadvantage is the need for an elaborate setup.

- GnRH therapy: for patients with hypothalamic syndrome and intact pituitary gland.

Oral Contraceptives

Oral contraceptives are widely used and are of two types: 1) a combination of estrogen and progestin and 2) a progestin-only pill. The estrogen component is either mestranol or ethinyl estradiol, and the progestin component is one of six derivatives of 19-nortestosterone. Oral contraceptives inhibit GnRH secretion and the mid-cycle LH surge. They also render the cervical mucus scanty, thick, and viscid and decrease fallopian tube motility, among other effects. Endometrial atrophy ensues (decreased vaginal menstrual flow), and vaginal epithelial maturation is decreased (increased incidence of candidial vaginitis). The failure rate is 0.1% in the first year.

- Two types of oral contraceptives: combination of estrogen and progestin and progestin-only.
- Oral contraceptives inhibit GnRH secretion and mid-cycle LH surge.
- Failure rate in the first year: 0.1%.

The metabolic effects of oral contraceptives include insulin resistance and impaired glucose tolerance, increased VLDL and triglycerides, increased HDL-C (estrogen effect), and increased LDL-C (progestin effect), increased hepatic production of α_2-globulins (including angiotensinogen), and increase in blood coagulation factors and carrier proteins (e.g., TBG or transcortin). In young women with dyslipidemia, it may be prudent to use a pill with minimal lipid-worsening effect (pills with the newer progestin desogestrel or with low doses of norethindrone). The complications of oral contraceptives are related principally to the estrogen component and include: increased risk (4x-10x) of thromboembolism, increased risk of coronary artery disease (2x-10x for myocardial infarction) and strokes (4x-9x for thrombotic strokes and 2x for hemorrhagic stroke—advanced maternal age and smoking are major risk factors), increased frequency and severity of migraine headaches, hypertension (which is usually reversible), increased risk of development of hepatic adenoma (which may rupture and can be fatal), and cholestatic jaundice. The beneficial effects of oral contraceptives, in addition to contraception, include a decreased risk of benign breast disease, endometrial and ovarian cancer, and pelvic inflammatory disease. The relation of oral contraceptives to cervical cancer, pituitary tumors, and melanoma is unclear. No increased incidence of pituitary tumors has been observed.

- Metabolic effects of oral contraceptives: insulin resistance and impaired glucose tolerance, increased VLDL and triglycerides, increased hepatic production of α_2-globulins, and an increase in blood coagulation factors and carrier proteins.
- Complications: related principally to estrogen component.
- Complications include: increased risk of thromboembolism; coronary artery disease and strokes; increased frequency and severity of migraine headaches; hypertension; increased risk of hepatic adenoma; and postpill amenorrhea.

The absolute contraindications to the use of oral contraceptives include thrombophlebitis and thromboembolic disorders, cardiovascular disease, impaired liver function, known or suspected estrogen-dependent tumors of the breast or uterus, pregnancy, and familial hypertriglyceridemia (for fear of precipitating pancreatitis). Oral contraceptives should be used very cautiously in women who smoke, are obese, or have varicose veins. If elective surgery is planned for a patient taking oral contraceptives, use of the medication is stopped 2 weeks preoperatively and resumed 2 weeks postoperatively.

Amenorrhea during pill use: Is the patient taking the pill regularly? If not, check pregnancy test; if yes, consider decreasing the dose of progestin or, if the patient is taking a pill with only 35 μg of ethinyl estradiol, consider increasing the estrogen dose.

Postpill amenorrhea: typically resumption of ovulatory cycles occurs within 3 months; 95%-98% occurs within 1 year. Consider pregnancy, return to prepill menstrual disorder, or development of a new gonadal disorder while on the pill (which had been masked while using the pill), e.g., prolactinoma.

Progestins as Contraceptives

Levonorgestrel implants use six slender Silastic tubes containing levonorgestrel. The tubes are implanted subdermally. Levonorgestrel, which is released slowly and continuously for 5 years, suppresses ovulation. The pregnancy rates over 5 years are 0.6%-4%. The advantages of levonorgestrel implants are convenience and the absence of clinically significant metabolic effects. The disadvantages are cost and irregular bleeding (60% of patients), which may last for months.

Intramuscular medroxyprogesterone acetate is approved for use as a contraceptive and is given as 150 mg every 3 months. If the drug is used correctly, the pregnancy rate is <1%. Disadvantages include inconvenience and irregular bleeding.

Hyperandrogenic Syndrome: Hirsutism/Virilization

Sources of Circulating Androgens in Females

The sources of circulating androgens in females are shown in Figure 7-15. Total serum testosterone includes free (1%-2%) and bound (98%-99%) components. Testosterone is bound to SHBG and albumin. Only the free fraction is biologically active. In hyperandrogenic females, a high level of testosterone and a high level of dehydroepiandrosterone (DHEAS) point to an adrenal origin, whereas a high level of testosterone and normal or slightly increased level of DHEAS point to ovarian origin of the hyperandrogenic state.

- Total serum testosterone: free (1%-2%), bound (98%-99%). The free fraction is biologically active.
- In hyperandrogenic females: a normal or high level of testosterone and a high level DHEAS point to adrenal origin.
- A high level of testosterone and a normal/slightly increased level of DHEAS point to ovarian origin.

In hair follicles, testosterone is converted to dihydrotestosterone through the activity of 5α-reductase. Dihydrotestosterone is the active androgen in hair follicles. It is metabolized within the pilosebaceous unit to 3α-androstenediol glucuronide.

- In hair follicles, testosterone is converted to dihydrotestosterone via 5α-reductase.
- Dihydrotestosterone: active androgen in hair follicles.

Clinical Presentations

In order of increasing severity, the hyperandrogenic state may present with acne, hirsutism, menstrual and ovulatory disorders, defeminization, and masculinization (temporal hair recession, deepening voice, increased muscle mass, and clitorimegaly).

- Clinical presentation in order of increasing severity: acne, hirsutism, menstrual and ovulatory disorders, defeminization, and masculinization,

The causes of hyperandrogenicity are outlined in Table 7-25. The source of increased androgen may be either exogenous or endogenous. Endogenous production may originate from the ovary, the adrenal cortex, or both and, in either case, may be benign or malignant. Hyperinsulinism resulting from insulin resistance triggers excessive ovarian androgen production. Obesity is associated with hyperinsulinism and with reduction in concentration of SHBG.

Idiopathic hirsutism. There is a modest increase in androgen production (mostly ovarian), with increased peripheral androgen production and increased sensitivity of the hair follicle. The hyperadrenogenicity is mild and LH-dependent. Also, the onset is at puberty and the disease has very slow progression. Menstrual cycles are ovulatory, and the results of pelvic examination are normal. The serum levels of testosterone and DHEAS and the LH:FSH ratio are normal. Pelvic ultrasonographic findings are normal.

- Idiopathic hirsutism: modest increase in androgen production (mostly ovarian).
- Other features: LH-dependent, onset at puberty, slow progression, menstrual cycles are ovulatory, normal serum levels of testosterone and DHEAS, and normal LH:FSH.

Polycystic ovarian syndrome. This is the most common cause of nonvirilizing hyperandrogenicity, but its pathogenesis is poorly understood; gonadotropin dynamics are abnormal with loss of the LH surge, increased LH levels, and increased LH/FSH ratio. The ovaries are usually enlarged (70% of patients) but may be normal in size and characteristically have multiple cysts and stromal thickening. Hyperandrogenicity is mild to moderate and is LH-dependent. In many patients there is associated obesity and hyperinsulinism, further contributing to the androgen excess. Disease onset is at puberty and shows slow progression; hirsutism (70% of patients), menstrual abnormality (88%), infertility and anovulation (75%), and obesity (50%) are usually present. The serum level of testosterone is normal or modestly increased (70% of patients) and is nearly always <200 ng/mL. DHEAS levels are normal or mildly increased in 25% of patients, and the LH:FSH ratio is >2 in 75%. Changes seen on pelvic ultrasonography are characteristic (70%); hyperprolactinemia may be present in 25%-30% of patients. Serum levels of E_2 are normal; estrone levels are increased, and the risk of endometrial hyperplasia is increased.

- Polycystic ovarian syndrome: the most common cause of hyperandrogenicity.

Table 7-25.--Causes of Hyperandrogenism

Exogenous--drugs
    Androgens
    Anabolic steroids
    Androgen-related progestin
    Metyrapone
Endogenous
    Neoplastic--autonomous production of androgens
        Ovarian tumors
        Adrenal tumors--benign, malignant
    Non-neoplastic--trophic hormone-dependent production
      of androgens
        Ovarian--LH-dependent
            Idiopathic hirsutism
            Polycystic ovaries
            Others/rare
        Adrenals--ACTH-dependent
            Late-onset congenital adrenal hyperplasia
                21-hydroxylase deficiency
                11-hydroxylase deficiency
                3β-ol-dehydrogenase deficiency
        Cushing's syndrome
        Hyperprolactinemic disorders

Fig. 7-15. Sources of circulating androgens in females. DHEA, dehydroepiandrosterone; DHEAS, dehydroepiandrosterone sulfate.

- Hyperandrogenicity: mild to moderate and LH-dependent.
- Features: onset at puberty, slow progression, hirsutism (70% of patients), menstrual abnormality (88%), infertility and anovulation (75%), and obesity (50%).
- Serum level of testosterone: normal or modestly increased (70%).
- Serum level of DHEAS: normal or mildly increased.
- LH:FSH ratio is >2 in 75% of patients.
- Hyperprolactinemia in 25%-30% of patients.

Ovarian hyperthecosis may be seen in association with acanthosis nigricans and insulin resistance.

Virilizing ovarian tumors include arrhenoblastomas and hilus cell tumors.

Late-onset congenital adrenal hyperplasia may be of the "classic" type, with severe enzyme deficiency and neonatal and postnatal presentation. It may also be "nonclassic" or "cryptic," in which the enzyme deficiency is mild and the presentation is pubertal or "late onset." It is inherited as an autosomal recessive trait closely linked to the HLA gene region Steroidogenic block may be of the 21-hydroxylase type (most common), 11β-hydroxylase, or 3β-ol-dehydrogenase block. As a result of the steroidogenic block, cortisol secretion is decreased, ACTH is increased, and cortisol precursor build-up occurs with shunting toward androgen pathways. The presentation is usually at puberty. Serum levels of testosterone are increased except in 3β-ol-dehydrogenase. Serum levels of DHEAS are increased and 17-hydroxyprogesterone is increased in 21- and 11β-hydroxylase deficiency; 17-hydroxypregnenolone is increased in 3β-ol-dehydrogenase deficiency. All androgen abnormalities are ACTH-dependent and, hence, dexamethasone suppressible. 21-Hydroxylase deficiency, the most common congenital adrenal hyperplasia, shows increased basal levels of 17-hydroxyprogesterone to >300 ng/dL; if normal, cosyntropin test is indicated; 30 minutes after the administration of ACTH, a value >1,200 ng/dL is diagnostic. Clinically significant cortisol lack does not occur. Late-onset congenital adrenal hyperplasia may occur in 5%-20% of patients with features of polycystic ovaries.

- Nonclassic or cryptic type: enzyme deficiency is mild; presentation at puberty or late onset.
- Steroidogenic block: may be 21-hydroxylase (most common type), 11-hydroxylase, or 3β-ol-dehydrogenase block.
- All androgen abnormalities are ACTH-dependent, hence dexamethasone suppressible.
- 21-Hydroxylase deficiency (most common congenital adrenal hyperplasia): increased basal levels of 17-hydroxyprogesterone to >300 ng/dL. If normal, cosyntropin test is indicated; 30 minutes after giving ACTH, a value >1,200 ng/dL is diagnostic.

For hyperprolactinemic syndromes, see the Pituitary.

Hyperprolactinemia stimulates excessive production of DHEA by the adrenal cortex. For Cushing's syndrome and adrenal tumors, see the Adrenal Cortex. Virilizing tumors of the ovary and adrenal can occur at any age; they produce a hyperandrogenic state that is severe and of rapid onset and progression. Adrenal tumors characteristically are associated with high levels of DHEAS, whereas ovarian tumors produce high levels of testosterone. Diagnosis requires anatomical delineation: abdominal CT for adrenal tumors and pelvic ultrasonography or CT for ovarian tumors. Rarely, one needs to resort to selective venous sampling for localization.

Drugs can cause hirsutism. Most potent are the anabolic steroids such as oxandrolone, which may be used surruptiously by some young women involved in competitive body building or athletics. Other drugs include danazol (used in the management of endometriosis), and oral contraceptives containing androgenic progestins. Phenytoin, glucocorticoids, cyclosporine, diazoxide, and minoxidil can cause hirsutism by nonadrenergic mechanisms.

Diagnostic Approach

The usual causes of hirsutism are polycystic ovaries (75%), idiopathic hirsutism (15%), and late onset congenital adrenal hyperplasia (3%); the rest of the cases are accounted for by Cushing's syndrome, hyperprolactinemia, drugs, and ovarian or adrenal tumors.

The most important clinical diagnostic clues relate to evaluation of the time at onset, tempo of progression, and severity of the hyperandrogenic state. Also, search for pelvic or abdominal masses, features of Cushing's syndrome, and galactorrhea. A benign disorder is suggested by disease onset at puberty and a mild, slowly progressive course. The rapid onset of disease at any age and a severe, rapidly progressive course point to a malignant disorder.

- The most important diagnostic clues relate to evaluating the time at onset, tempo of progression, and severity of hyperandrogenic state.
- A benign disorder is suggested by onset at puberty and a mild, slowly progressive course.
- A malignant disorder is suggested by a rapid onset at any age and a severe, rapidly progressive course.

A detailed drug and family history is important. A positive family history may be seen in familial/racial hirsutism, polycystic ovarian syndrome, and late-onset congenital adrenal hyperplasia. A young woman whose hirsutism is mild and pubertal in onset or who has southern European ancestry, whose menstrual function is normal, and who is free of underlying significant disorder need not undergo detailed endocrine testing. If the onset of hirsutism is pubertal and associated with menstrual irregularity (oligomenorrhea or amenorrhea) but without virilization, the differential diagnosis includes polycystic ovaries, late-onset congenital adrenal hyperplasia, and hyperprolactinemia. Severe hirsutism developing at any age and progressing rapidly to other manifestations of virilization points to a malignant androgen-producing tumor of the ovary or adrenal.

The serum levels of testosterone and DHEAS are essential for diagnostic laboratory evaluation. Also, a screen for Cushing's syndrome (overnight 1-mg dexamethasone suppression test or 24-hour urinary free cortisol) and the serum level of PRL are also required. In selected patients and as guided by the clinical history and findings, determining the serum level of 17-hydroxyprogesterone, with or without the cosyntropin test for confirmation of congenital adrenal hyperplasia, and determining the serum LH:FSH ratio for support of the diagnosis of polycystic ovarian syndrome might be needed. Also, in selected patients suspected of having neoplasm, pelvic ultrasonography and abdominal CT are necessary.

- Serum levels of testosterone and DHEAS: essential for diagnostic laboratory evaluation.
- Screen for Cushing's syndrome.
- Serum level of PRL is required.

If plasma DHEAS is >7 ng/dL, the differential diagnosis is between adrenal tumor and late-onset congenital adrenal hyperplasia. Proceed with CT scan of the abdomen; if the findings are negative, proceed with serum 17-hydroxyprogesterone and cosyntropin test. Also, test for dexamethasone suppressibility of DHEAS.

- If the plasma level of DHEAS is >7 ng/dL, the differential diagnosis is between adrenal tumor and late-onset congenital adrenal hyperplasia.

Plasma levels of DHEAS that are <7 ng/dL exclude adrenal tumor and congenital adrenal hyperplasia. Proceed with measuring the serum level of testosterone; levels >200 ng/dL should raise the suspicion of ovarian tumor; pelvic ultrasonography and CT are required and, if necessary, laparoscopy and exploration. A serum level of testosterone <200 ng/dL points to polycystic ovarian syndrome.

- If the plasma level of DHEAS is <7 ng/dL, measure the serum level of testosterone.
- If the serum level of testosterone is >200 ng/dL, suspect ovarian tumor.
- If the serum level of testosterone is <200 ng/dL, polycystic ovarian syndrome.

Endocrine Therapy

Endocrine therapy is temporizing and may need 6-12 months to show a clinical effect. The goal is to decrease androgen production or to inhibit the androgen effect of hair follicles.

Oral contraceptives are indicated for managing idiopathic hirsutism and polycystic ovaries. This therapy suppresses LH, increases SHBG, and inhibits DHT binding to its receptor. It is important to avoid the progestin norgestrel because of its androgenic effect. The primary role of glucocorticoid therapy is in the management of late-onset congenital adrenal hyperplasia, but it may also be used in polycystic ovaries if DHEAS levels are increased. Dexamethasone, 0.25-0.75 mg, or prednisone, 5-7.5 mg, is given at bedtime. The well-known risks of exogenous Cushing's syndrome and hypothalamic-pituitary-adrenal axis suppression may occur. In congenital adrenal hyperplasia, the efficacy of glucocorticoid therapy can be monitored by measuring the level of 17-hydroxyprogesterone. Spironolactone, the well-known aldosterone antagonist, is also an androgen receptor blocker and inhibitor of androgen action. It also decreases androgen production by its effect on steroidogenesis. The usual dose is 50-200 mg daily; spironolactone should be used only in conjunction with effective contraception. Cimetidine is an alternate androgen receptor blocker but is less effective than spironolactone. Newer promising approaches include use of flutamide (an androgen-receptor blocker) and finasteride (a 5α-reductase blocker). Cyproterone acetate is an antiandrogen that decreases dihydrotestosterone production and action. It also decreases LH release. It is given with topical or oral estrogen and is not available in the U.S.

- Endocrine therapy is temporizing.
- It may need 6-12 months to show an effect.
- Goal: decrease androgen production or inhibit androgen effect of hair follicles.
- Oral contraceptives: for managing idiopathic hirsutism and polycystic ovaries.
- Glucocorticoid therapy: primary role in managing late-onset congenital adrenal hyperplasia.
- Spironolactone: blocks androgen receptor and inhibits androgen action.

SOME FAMILIAL ENDOCRINE DISORDERS

Multiple Endocrine Neoplasia (MEN)

MEN Type I (MEN I)

MEN I, or Wermer's syndrome, refers to the association of neoplasms of the parathyroid, endocrine pancreas, and anterior pituitary. It is familial and inherited as an autosomal dominant trait with essentially 100% penetrance. The MEN I locus has been mapped to a specific region on chromosome 11; the gene itself has not been identified but is believed to belong to the category of tumor suppressor genes. Each affected person carries one mutated gene transmitted as an autosomal dominant trait; if the normal copy from the unaffected parent is mutated, the syndrome results.

Primary hyperparathyroidism. This is the most common manifestation; it shows nearly 100% penetrance by age 40-50 and usually is caused by parathyroid hyperplasia and, occasionally, by single or multiple adenomata. Hypercalcemia is commonly expressed by age 40, and it is similar in presentations and complications to sporadic hyperparathyroidism. Diagnosis is by the presence of hypercalcemia and increased intact PTH. The differential diagnosis includes other familial syndromes associated with hypercalcemia: 1) familial hyperparathyroidism: differentiation is based on family history and long-term observation to determine whether other features of MEN I develop and 2) familial hypocalciuric hypercalcemia: hypercalcemia is present at birth, hypocalciuria, usually not associated with complications of hypercalcemia. Therapy: two options are 1) removal of 3½ parathyroids or 2) total parathyroidectomy and transplantation of parathyroid tissue into the forearm; the rate of recurrence of hyperparathyroidism is high.

Islet cell neoplasia. This is the second most common neoplasm in MEN I and is probably the most important manifestation because of its malignant potential. Hypersecretory syndromes include hypersecretion of pancreatic polypeptide (75%-85% of patients), gastrin (60%), insulin (25%-35%), VIP (3%-5%), glucagon (5%-10%), and somatostatin (1%-5%). Islet cell tumors may hypersecrete other peptides, including ACTH, CRH, and GHRH. Distinctively, one third of the tumors are malignant. Diagnosis—depends on the clinical recognition of characteristic syndromes, measurement of hormones with or without provocative stimulation, and radiologic techniques. Gastrinoma, or Zollinger-Ellison syndrome: clinical features of increased gastric acid production, recurrent multiple peptic ulcers, diarrhea, and esophagitis. Diagnosis—increased gastric acid secretion, increased basal gastrin, and an exaggerated gastrin response to secretin or calcium. Insulinoma: characterized by fasting hypoglycemia and hyperinsulinism in the absence of exogenous insulin or oral sulfonylureas. Diagnosis—measure the plasma level of glucose, serum level of insulin, and C peptide during either a spontaneous or a provoked attack (e.g., 72-hour fast). In insulinoma: Whipple's triad, hyperinsulinism, and increased C peptide plus absence of oral sulfonylurea metabolites in the blood and urine. Localization studies: MR or CT imaging has suboptimal sensitivity; better results are obtained with transhepatic venous catheterization, with basal and calcium-stimulated insulin levels in the portal circulation, and intraoperative ultrasonography.

Pituitary tumors. More than 15% of gene carriers express pituitary tumors; the tumors are usually multicentric. The most common tumor is a prolactinoma. Acromegaly in MEN I may be caused by a pituitary GH tumor or by an ectopic GHRH tumor. Cushing's syndrome in MEN I may be caused by ACTH-pituitary tumor or by an ectopic ACTH or CRH tumor. (For diagnosis, see Pituitary and Adrenal Cortex.)

Other manifestations of MEN I include 1) carcinoid tumors, mostly of the foregut, which may produce serotonin, calcitonin, or CRH; 2) thyroid and adrenal adenomas; and 3) subcutaneous or visceral lipomas.

Screening for MEN I. Currently, there is no compelling evidence that early detection decreases mortality and morbidity. If a decision is made to screen asymptomatic family members, this is best done with serum levels of calcium (albumin-adjusted or ionized) and intact PTH. Laboratory evaluation and/or imaging studies for pancreatic or pituitary tumors are not indicated in the absence of relevant symptoms. Specific genetic testing for MEN I awaits identification of the single responsible gene and its key mutation(s).

MEN Type II (MEN II)

MEN II includes two major syndromes: MEN IIA (medullary carcinoma of the thyroid, pheochromocytoma, and primary hyperparathyroidism) and MEN IIB (medullary carcinoma of the thyroid, pheochromocytoma, mucosal neuromas, intestinal ganglioneuromatosis, and marfanoid features). These two familial syndromes are inherited in an autosomal dominant pattern with high penetrance.

MEN IIA

1) Medullary carcinoma of the thyroid (see Thyroid) is the most common manifestation (>90% of patients) of MEN IIA; it develops in childhood and usually begins as C-cell hyperplasia. Measurement of calcitonin after provocation with pentagastrin or calcium allows for early diagnosis. 2) Pheochromocytomas occur in about 50% of patients and about 50% of the tumors are bilateral. These tumors have an increased incidence of malignancy (20%-40%) and of epinephrine-producing tumors. In the 50% with apparently unilateral disease, unilateral adrenalectomy is followed in about 50% of patients by development of a contralateral tumor in 8-10 years. 3) Hyperparathyroidism develops in 15%-20% of affected patients.

MEN IIA has two subtypes: familial medullary carcinoma of the thyroid and MEN IIA with cutaneous lichen amyloidosis.

MEN IIB

The endocrine manifestations differ from those of MEN IIA 1) in the absence of hyperparathyroidism and 2) medullary carcinoma of the thyroid develops earlier in life and appears to be more virulent. The occurrence of hypercalcemia should make one think about osseous metastases. Mucosal true neuromas are the most distinctive features of MEN IIB. They may occur at the tip of the tongue, on the eyelids or lips, and along the gastrointestinal tract. Intestinal neuromas may cause intermittent obstruction or diarrhea.

Genetics of MEN II

The genetic locus is in the pericentromeric region of chromosome 10; abnormal mutation in the *RET* gene is present in 95%-98% of affected persons. Other chromosomal abnormalities may aid in the progression of the disease.

Screening for MEN II

Medullary carcinoma of the thyroid is potentially fatal, but it can be cured or prevented by early thyroidectomy. This provides the strongest rationale for screening. Screening includes DNA analysis for *RET* mutations; basal and provoked calcitonin; urinary fractionated catecholamines, metanephrines, and vanillylmandelic acid; and serum levels of calcium and PTH. Begin screening in early childhood, preferably before age 5.

There are other genetic tumor syndromes that do not fit neatly into either the MEN I or MEN II pattern, e.g., mixed syndromes such as familial pheochromocytoma and islet cell tumors.

Polyglandular Autoimmune Disorder (PGA)

Three syndromes have been delineated: PGA type I, PGA type II, and PGA type III.

PGA Type I—Autoimmune Polyendocrinopathy-Candidiasis-Ectodermal Dystrophy (APECED)

This syndrome, which is usually recognized in the first decade of life, is inherited as an autosomal recessive trait and has no HLA associations. It consists primarily of the triad of hypoparathyroidism, mucocutaneous candidiasis, and adrenal failure. Other features include dystrophy of the teeth and nails, vitiligo, gonadal failure, primary hypothyroidism, and pernicious anemia. IDDM is less common than in PGA type II. Because these endocrine features may not develop until the fourth decade, patients and their families should have long-term follow-up.

PGA Type II

This syndrome is inherited as an autosomal dominant trait and is usually associated with DR3 or DR4 haplotype or both. Twin concordance is about 50%. The syndrome tends to develop later in life and includes: 1) IDDM, the most common manifestation (50% of patients); 2) autoimmune thyroid disease (Hashimoto's or Graves' disease); 3) adrenal failure; 4) primary hypogonadism; 5) dermatologic conditions such as vitiligo, alopecia totalis, and alopecia areata are common; and 6) transient hypoparathyroidism develops in a few patients because of parathyroid blocking antibodies. Mucocutaneous candidiasis does not occur. PGA II is present in >25% of patients with myasthenia gravis, especially when thymoma is present.

PGA Type III

This syndrome has the same genetic pattern as PGA type II. PGA type III is characterized by the occurrence of only two endocrinopathies: either IDDM and autoimmune thyroid disease or autoimmune thyroid disease and adrenal failure.

Screen for PGA

Screen affected families every 1-2 years up to about age 50 in families with PGA type II or III and until age 40 in families with type I. Endocrine screening includes ionized calcium and, if necessary, PTH for hypoparathyroidism; antimicrosomal antibodies and sTSH for autoimmune thyroid disorder; fasting plasma glucose for IDDM; cosyntropin test for adrenocortical failure; sex steroids, LH, and FSH for gonadal failure.

QUESTIONS

Multiple Choice (choose the one best answer)

1. The presence of hypopituitarism should be considered in all of the following clinical presentations except:
   a. Acute adrenocortical crisis
   b. Fasting hypoglycemia
   c. Hyponatremia
   d. Failure of lactation in a postpartum woman
   e. Hyperkalemia

2. Hyperprolactinemia may be caused by all the following except:
   a. Use of dopaminergic drugs
   b. Primary hypothyroidism
   c. Chronic renal failure
   d. Metastatic tumors to the median eminence
   e. A nonfunctioning pituitary tumor with a significant suprasellar extension

3. In familial multiple endocrine neoplasia type I (MEN I), pituitary tumors may be associated with:
   a. Pheochromocytoma
   b. Pseudohypoparathyroidism
   c. Hyperplasia or adenomas of the parathyroid glands and tumors of the endocrine pancreas
   d. Tumors of the C cells (or parafollicular cells) of the thyroid
   e. Hyporeninemic hypoaldosteronism

4. A patient who complains of diffuse bone pain and weakness and who has the radiologic finding of pseudofractures of the pelvis (Looser's zones) may have:
   a. High serum level of calcium, low serum level of phosphorus, and high serum level of immunoreactive parathyroid hormone
   b. Low serum level of calcium, high serum level of phosphorus, and low serum level of immunoreactive parathyroid hormone
   c. Normal serum levels of calcium, phosphate, and immunoreactive parathyroid hormone and normal bone biopsy findings after tetracycline double labelling
   d. Low-normal serum level of calcium, low serum level of phosphate, high serum level of immunoreactive parathyroid hormone, and low serum level of 25 (OH)D
   e. Increased serum parathyroid hormone-related protein (PTH-rP)

5. A low radioiodine uptake in a hyperthyroid patient is characteristic of all the following disorders except:
   a. Painless lymphocytic thyroiditis
   b. Surreptitious ingestion of thyroid hormone(s)
   c. Iodide-induced thyrotoxicosis
   d. Graves' disease
   e. Subacute granulomatous thyroiditis

6. Which of the following biochemical abnormalities would *not* occur in a patient with euthyroid sick syndrome?
   a. Low serum level of triiodothyronine (T_3)
   b. Low serum level of thyroxine (T_4)
   c. Low serum value for sTSH
   d. High serum level of T_4
   e. High serum level of T_3

7. Factors that would increase the suspicion of malignancy in a clinically solitary thyroid nodule include:
   a. Young age
   b. Male sex
   c. History of neck irradiation
   d. Family history of thyroid cancer
   e. All the above

8. Low serum value of sTSH may be seen in:
   a. Administration of thyroxine in supraphysiologic doses to a patient with primary hypothyroidism
   b. The acute phase of subacute thyroiditis
   c. Presence of a long-standing multinodular goiter in an elderly patient
   d. Use of such drugs as dopamine, glucocorticoids, and octreotide
   e. All the above

9. All the following statements about diabetic nephropathy are true except:
   a. Important factors in its pathogenesis include duration of diabetes, degree of glycemic control, presence of hypertension, and genetic propensity
   b. Intensive insulin therapy and near normalization of glycemic control decreases the incidence and the rate of progression of microalbuminuria
   c. The use of angiotensin converting enzyme (ACE) inhibitors decreases the risk of progression of nephropathy only in patients with established hypertension
   d. In insulin-dependent diabetes mellitus, microalbuminuria precedes overt proteinuria and can identify patients at risk for progressive nephropathy
   e. Presence of microalbuminuria is an independent risk factor for macrovascular disease

10. All the following statements about the second-generation sulfonylureas glyburide and glipizide are correct except:
    a. They have the same mechanisms of action and effica-

cy as the first-generation sulfonylureas

b. They are nonionically bound to plasma proteins and are not displaced by such ionically charged drugs as warfarin

c. Like the first-generation sulfonylurea tolazamide, they can be associated with the syndrome of inappropriate ADH (SIADH)

d. Transient drug failures may be encountered in the presence of acute medical or surgical illness, failure of adherence to diet and weight gain

e. They are contraindicated in patients with insulin-dependent diabetes mellitus, in pregnant or lactating diabetic women, and in patients with hepatic or renal failure

11. Fasting hypoglycemia may occur in:
    a. Cushing's syndrome
    b. Alcohol intoxication
    c. Primary aldosteronism
    d. Pheochromocytoma
    e. Glucagonoma

12. An 18-year-old man presents with failure of sexual maturation. He is found to be eunuchoidal and to have bilateral gynecomastia and small firm testes. His sense of smell is normal. The serum level of testosterone is low and the serum levels of LH and FSH are increased. The most likely diagnosis is:
    a. Kallmann's syndrome
    b. Prolactin-producing pituitary tumor
    c. Craniopharyngioma
    d. Klinefelter's syndrome
    e. Testicular feminization

13. A 19-year-old woman presents for the evaluation of hirsutism and oligomenorrhea dating since menarche at age 13. A diagnosis of late-onset 21-hydroxylase deficiency is made. Which of the following statements relating to this disorder is correct?
    a. Basal levels of 17-hydroxyprogesterone are usually increased
    b. If basal levels of serum 17-hydroxyprogesterone are normal, they will show an exaggerated response to a cosyntropin stimulation test
    c. The high 17-hydroxyprogesterone production is ACTH-dependent and will suppress with dexamethasone therapy
    d. The disorder is familial and may occur in >5% of patients who have feature of polycystic ovaries
    e. All the above

14. Primary aldosteronism is characterized by all the following except:
    a. Unprovoked hypokalemia due to increased and inappropriate renal potassium loss
    b. Hypokalemic alkalosis
    c. Increased aldosterone levels in the blood and urine that are not suppressed by saline administration
    d. High renin production that is not suppressed by salt loading
    e. Low plasma renin activity that does not respond to stimulation by volume depletion or upright posture

15. Increased urinary free cortisol may be seen in:
    a. Cushing's syndrome
    b. Acute illness
    c. Alcoholism
    d. Depression
    e. All the above

16. Laboratory findings distinctive of primary adrenocortical failure include:
    a. Low plasma level of cortisol that increases in response to the administration of synthetic ACTH (cosyntropin)
    b. Low plasma level of cortisol that increases in response to insulin-induced hypoglycemia
    c. Low plasma level of cortisol that fails to increase in response to administration of cosyntropin or to insulin-induced hypoglycemia
    d. Low plasma level of aldosterone that increases in response to cosyntropin
    e. Hypernatremia, hypokalemia, and suppressed renin

17. Which of the following statements about medullary carcinoma of the thyroid is *not* correct?
    a. It arises from the parafollicular cells of the thyroid and shows distinctive amyloid deposits within the tumor
    b. It may be familial or may occur sporadically
    c. It can present with a thyroid nodule, cervical lymphadenopathy, or hematogenous metastatic disease
    d. Diagnosis can be confirmed by an increased serum level of calcitonin or an exaggerated calcitonin response to calcium or pentagastrin stimulation test
    e. The tumor is TSH-dependent and T_4 suppressive therapy is an integral part of the postoperative management.

True/False (indicate whether each answer is true or false)

18. Thyrotoxicosis due to a thyrotropin-producing pituitary tumor may be associated with:
    a. A "normal" or increased serum level of TSH
    b. High ^{131}I uptake
    c. Diffuse goiter
    d. Infiltrative ophthalmopathy
    e. High α-glycoprotein subunit levels
    f. High serum levels of thyroid-stimulating immunoglobulins

19. Bromocriptine
   a. It suppresses hyperprolactinemia and restores normal gonadal function in 80%-90% of the patients with hyperprolactinemia irrespective of the cause
   b. It may cause regression in tumor size in a significant number of patients who harbor a prolactin-producing pituitary tumor
   c. It is temporizing therapy; discontinuation of its use usually leads to the reemergence of hyperprolactinemia
   d. In the bromocriptine-treated young women who harbor a macroprolactinoma and who desire fertility, use of the drug is stopped at the earliest sign of pregnancy because there is no risk of tumor growth during pregnancy
   e. In patients who have a nonfunctioning pituitary tumor and hyperprolactinemia due to "stalk-effect," bromocriptine can normalize prolactin levels but will not cause regression in tumor size
   f. Because dopamine increases growth hormone secretion in normal persons, bromocriptine is contraindicated in the management of acromegaly

20. Hypoparathyroidism:
   a. May be caused by magnesium intoxication
   b. May be associated with hypocalcemia, hyperphosphatemia, increased serum level of immunoreactive parathyroid hormone, and increased serum level of creatinine
   c. May be associated with other endocrine deficiencies in polyglandular autoimmune disorder (PGA) type I
   d. May be associated with basal ganglia calcification and parkinsonian features
   e. Is characterized by hypocalcemia, hyperphosphatemia, normal serum levels of creatinine, and low or undetectable serum levels of immunoreactive parathyroid hormone
   f. Most commonly occurs as a result of inadvertent damage to the parathyroid glands during thyroid operation

21. T_3 toxicosis:
   a. Occurs in about 20% of all patients with hyperthyroidism
   b. May be the earliest manifestation of hyperthyroidism
   c. May herald relapses and recurrences of hyperthyroidism in patients with Graves' disease
   d. May be associated with normal or low free thyroxine index and suppressed serum sTSH
   e. May be caused by the use of cholestyramine, ferrous sulphate, or sucralfate
   f. Is the most common thyroid function test abnormality in nonthyroidal illness (the euthyroid-sick state)

22. Clinical presentations of primary hypothyroidism may include:
   a. Shortness of stature and failure of sexual maturation in an adolescent
   b. Amenorrhea-galactorrhea and a sellar mass in a young woman
   c. Osteoporosis
   d. Hypercholesterolemia
   e. Pericardial effusion
   f. Normocytic normochromic anemia

23. Insulin-induced hypoglycemia in patients with insulin-dependent diabetes mellitus:
   a. Catecholaminergic symptoms typically appear first, particularly if the rate of decrease in the plasma level of glucose is rapid
   b. Neuroglycopenic symptoms predominate when the rate of decrease in plasma glucose is gradual, when the degree of hypoglycemia is severe, or when the patient has hypoglycemia unawareness
   c. Intensive insulin therapy and near-normal glycemic control are associated with a decreased incidence of hypoglycemia as well as a decreased risk of the development of microvascular complications
   d. Incidence is reduced by heavy exercise and with the use of alcohol
   e. Incidence is increased by the occurrence of renal failure or cortisol deficiency
   f. Is associated with high serum C-peptide (connecting-peptide) levels

24. In Cushing's disease:
   a. Serum levels of ACTH are normal or modestly increased in most patients
   b. In most patients, the hypercortisol state is not suppressed by the administration of a high dose of dexamethasone (8 mg/day for 2 days)
   c. Most patients harbor an ACTH-producing pituitary tumor but imaging of the sella with CT or MRI is negative in >50% of patients
   d. The clinical and biochemical features may be indistinguishable from those of Cushing's syndrome caused by an ectopic ACTH-producing bronchial carcinoid
   e. Petrosal venous sampling with CRH provocative testing shows a central-to-peripheral ACTH gradient >2:1
   f. Hyperpigmentation and hypokalemia are common findings

25. Estrogen therapy in menopause:
   a. Oral and transdermal estrogen are equally effective in the management of hot flashes and genitourinary atrophy
   b. Increases the risk of endometrial cancer; this increased risk is prevented by supplemental progestin
   c. Prevents the rapid phase of bone loss characteristic of

menopause
d. Useful in the management of hypercholesterolemia
e. Useful in the management of hypertriglyceridemia
f. Is contraindicated in patients with active thromboembolic disease and in patients with a previous history of thromboembolic disease that was temporally related to the use of estrogen

26. Secondary causes of diabetes mellitus include:
a. Acromegaly
b. Hemochromatosis
c. Primary aldosteronism
d. Hypopituitarism
e. Pheochromocytoma
f. Cushing's syndrome

27. In pregnancy:
a. Early detection and management of diabetes can significantly decrease perinatal mortality and morbidity
b. Screening for glucose intolerance is advisable in all pregnancies and is usually done at 24-26 weeks of gestation
c. The diagnostic criteria for diabetes in the oral glucose

tolerance test are the same as those for nonpregnant patients
d. The risk of gestational diabetes is increased in patients with obesity, advanced maternal age, and an abnormal obstetric history such as large babies, unexplained stillbirths, and polyhydramnios
e. Gestational diabetes can recur in subsequent pregnancies; ultimately frank diabetes will develop in all patients
f. Gestational diabetes complicates 2%-3% of all pregnancies

28. A 17-year-old female is referred for the evaluation of primary amenorrhea. She is found to be sexually immature. Laboratory studies document low serum levels of estradiol, LH, and FSH. Diagnostic considerations include all the following:
a. Craniopharyngioma
b. Gonadal dysgenesis and 45,XO karyotype
c. Anorexia nervosa
d. Kallmann's syndrome
e. Prolactin-producing pituitary tumor
f. Systemic debilitating disease

ANSWERS

1. Answer e.

In the setting of cortisol deficiency, hyperkalemia is due to associated aldosterone deficiency and points to primary adrenocortisol failure as the cause of the cortisol deficiency. In hypopituitarism, the renin-angiotensin-aldosterone axis is intact (except in rare patients with severe and prolonged ACTH deficiency) and the serum level of potassium is characteristically normal.

2. Answer a.

Normal prolactin secretion by the lactotroph is under dominant hypothalamic inhibition by dopamine. The use of dopaminergic drugs suppresses hyperprolactinemia of diverse causes.

3. Answer c.

MEN I is a familial disorder inherited in an autosomal dominant fashion and characterized by the triad of parathyroid hyperplasia/adenoma and tumors of the endocrine pancreas and anterior pituitary.

4. Answer d.

Diffuse bone pain, weakness, and the presence of pseudofractures point to osteomalacia. A common cause of osteomalacia is vitamin D deficiency. Impaired absorption of calcium by the gut and mobilization of calcium from bone tend to lower serum calcium levels and cause secondary hyperparathyroidism. This compensatory response tends to normalize serum calcium levels; the low serum phosphate level is caused by the phosphaturic effect of parathyroid hormone.

5. Answer e.

Graves' disease, unless associated with iodine exposure and high iodide pool, is characterized by a high radioiodine uptake. In contrast, thyroid inflammation, exposure to exogenous iodides, and TSH suppression by exogenous thyroid hormones are all associated with a suppressed radioiodine uptake.

6. Answer e.

Of the circulating T_3, 80% is derived from the peripheral conversion of T_4 to T_3 in the peripheral tissues by the enzyme deiodinase. In euthyroid sick syndrome, such T_4 to T_3

conversion is suppressed, and the serum triiodothyronine level is characteristically low.

7. Answer e.

All are correct and self-explanatory.

8. Answer e.

All are correct and self-explanatory.

9. Answer c.

The use of ACE inhibitors, even in normotensive diabetics, decreases the risk of development and progression of diabetic nephropathy.

10. Answer c.

Chlorpropamide is the only one among the sulfonylureas whose use has been associated with SIADH. It enhances the secretion and the effect of ADH.

11. Answer b.

The metabolism of alcohol by the liver leads to the suppression of neoglucogenesis and predisposes to hypoglycemia in the fasting alcohol drinker who has exhausted his or her hepatic glycogen stores. All the other disorders are associated with insulin deficiency or resistance and, therefore, with impairment of glucose tolerance and hyperglycemia.

12. Answer d.

Klinefelter's syndrome is characterized by primary gonadal failure and, thus, by hypergonadotropic hypogonadism. In testicular feminization, the phenotype is female and the serum testosterone levels are normal for a male. All the other disorders are characterized by central hypogonadotropic hypogonadism.

13. Answer e.

All are correct and self-explanatory.

14. Answer d.

Primary aldosteronism is characterized by suppressed renin production. Primary excess of aldosterone results in increased renal tubular absorption of sodium, expansion of the extracellular fluid compartment, and suppression of renin production by the juxtaglomerular apparatus.

15. Answer e.

All are correct and self-explanatory. Acute illness, depression, and alcoholism are associated with activation of the CRH-ACTH-adrenal axis and increased production of cortisol. They should enter into the biochemical differential diagnosis of increased urinary free cortisol.

16. Answer c.

In primary adrenocortical failure, the production of cortisol, sex steroids, and aldosterone by the adrenal cortices is decreased. The failed adrenal cortices do not respond to either exogenous ACTH (cosyntropin test) or the increased endogenous ACTH (insulin hypoglycemia test).

17. Answer e.

Medullary carcinoma of the thyroid, unlike the differentiated papillary and follicular cancers of the thyroid follicles, arises from the parafollicular C cells and is not TSH-dependent. After total thyroidectomy, patients with medullary cancer need physiologic replacement and not suppressive doses of thyroid hormone.

18. a, true; b, true; c, true; d, false; e, true; f, false.

Infiltrative ophthalmopathy and high serum levels of thyroid-stimulating immunoglobulins are characteristic of Graves' disease and do not occur with any other cause of the thyrotoxic state.

19. a, true; b, true; c, true; d, false; e, true; f, false.

Bromocriptine is an effective therapy for patients with prolactinomas. It usually suppresses prolactin hypersecretion, and, in a significant number of patients, it causes regression in tumor size. In a female who harbors a prolactinoma, most authorities recommend that use of the drug be stopped at the earliest detection of pregnancy. All such patients with macroprolactinomas who become pregnant during the use of bromocriptine and who stop taking bromocriptine when pregnancy is established should be followed carefully during pregnancy because about 20% may experience clinical effects from regrowth of the pituitary tumor. Bromocriptine, although a dopamine-agonist drug, has a paradoxical suppressive effect on growth hormone secretion in acromegaly. More than 50% of patients with acromegaly experience clinical improvement with use of the drug; only 10% of such patients, however, will have normalization of their growth hormone secretion.

20. a, false; b, false; c, true; d, true; e, true; f, true.

Magnesium is important for PTH production and tissue effect. Magnesium depletion is a common cause of hypoparathyroidism. In hypoparathyroidism, PTH production is decreased and results in the characteristic hypocalcemia and hyperphosphatemia. Immunoreactive parathyroid hormone levels are inappropriately low in the face of hypocalcemia.

21. a, true; b, true; c, true; d, true; e, false; f, false.

Cholestyramine, ferrous sulphate, and sucralfate do not cause T_3 toxicosis. They may interfere with the absorption of orally administered thyroxine. The use of such drugs needs to be kept in mind in the replacement treatment of patients with hypothyroidism. Low serum T_3 levels are the most common thyroid function test abnormality in nonthyroidal illness. This occurs because of decreased conversion of T_4 to T_3 by the peripheral tissues.

22. a, true; b, true; c, false; d, true; e, true; f, true.

Secondary osteoporosis is not characteristic of the untreated hypothyroid state. Careful adjustment of the replacement thyroxine dosage in primary hypothyroidism to achieve a normal sTSH is important; overreplacement exposes the patient to the osteopenic effects of excess thyroid hormones. Normocytic normochromic anemia is a very frequent finding in hypothyroidism and is due to a direct effect of thyroid hormone lack on erythropoiesis; it responds only to thyroid hormone replacement therapy.

23. a, true; b, true; c, false; d, false; e, true; f, false.

Intensive insulin therapy is associated with a twofold or threefold increase in the incidence of significant hypoglycemia. The use of alcohol and heavy exercise predisposes the insulin-treated diabetic patient to hypoglycemia. Exogenous hyperinsulinism, unlike the endogenous type, is associated with very low C-peptide levels. Endogenous insulin is co-secreted with C-peptide, and endogenous hyperinsulinism is associated with high C-peptide levels.

24. a, true; b, false; c, true; d, true; e, true; f, false.

Patients with Cushing's disease harbor an ACTH-producing tumor and have ACTH-dependent hypercortisol state. In two-thirds of these patients, the cortisol production is suppressed by the high-dose dexamethasone suppression test. In the setting of ACTH-dependent Cushing's syndrome, hyper-

pigmentation (due to ACTH excess) and hypokalemia (due to the mineralocorticoid effect of excess cortisol and deoxycorticosterone) reflect very high levels of ACTH overproduction. They usually point away from Cushing's disease and to an ectopic ACTH-producing tumor.

25. a, true; b, true; c, true; d, true; e, false; f, true.

Estrogen therapy increases VLDL production by the liver and may be associated with hypertriglyceridemia. Patients with a known personal or family history of hypertriglyceridemia should be followed closely after the initiation of estrogen therapy. In such patients, estrogen therapy may occasionally induce severe exacerbation of the hypertriglyceridemia and ensuing pancreatitis.

26. a, true; b, true; c, true; d, false; e, true; f, true.

Hypopituitarism, primarily because of lack of the contrainsulin hormone cortisol (and also of GH in children) may be associated with fasting hypoglycemia.

27. a, true; b, true; c, false; d, true; e, false; f, true.

The diagnostic criteria of the oral glucose tolerance test are modified in the pregnant state to fit the criteria established by O'Sullivan and Maher. Two or more of the following plasma glucose values must be met or exceeded: fasting, 105 mg/dL; 1 hour, 190 mg/dL; 2 hours, 165 mg/dL; and 3 hours, 145 mg/dL.

28. a, true; b, false; c, true; d, true; e, true; f, true.

Gonadal dysgenesis in Turner's syndrome is characterized by hypergonadotropic hypogonadism. In all the other disorders, hypogonadism is hypogonadotrophic because of hypothalamic-pituitary disease.

NOTES

CHAPTER 8
GASTROENTEROLOGY

Thomas R. Viggiano, M.D.
John J. Poterucha, M.D.

PART I
Thomas R. Viggiano, M.D.

ESOPHAGUS

Esophageal Function

The upper esophageal sphincter (or cricopharyngeus muscle) and the muscle of the proximal one-third of the esophagus are striated muscle under voluntary control. A transition from skeletal to smooth muscle occurs in the mid-esophagus. In the distal one-third of the organ, the muscle is smooth muscle that is under involuntary control. The lower esophageal sphincter is a zone of circular muscle located in the distal 2-3 cm of the esophagus. To transport food from the mouth through the negative pressured chest into the positive pressured abdomen, the esophagus must transport food against a pressure gradient. To prevent reflux of gastric contents, the lower esophagus has a sphincter for unidirectional flow.

- The esophagus must transport food against a pressure gradient.

Normal Motility

After a person swallows, the upper esophageal sphincter relaxes within 0.5 second. A primary peristaltic wave then passes through the body of the esophagus at a rate of 1-5 cm/sec, generating an intraluminal pressure of 40-100 mm Hg. Within 2 seconds after the swallow, the lower esophageal sphincter relaxes and stays relaxed until the wave of peristalsis passes through it. Then, the lower esophageal sphincter contracts again to maintain its resting tone. Two major symptom complexes result if the esophagus is unable to perform its two major functions: dysphagia (transport dysfunction) and reflux (lower esophageal sphincter dysfunction).

- Dysphagia--transport dysfunction.
- Reflux--lower esophageal sphincter dysfunction.

Dysphagia

Dysphagia is the defective transport of food and is usually described as "sticking." Odynophagia is pain on swallowing. The two causes of dysphagia must be distinguished: mechanical (obstructed lumen) and functional (motility disorder). Answers to three questions frequently suggest the diagnosis: 1) what type of food produces the dysphagia, 2) what is the course of the dysphagia, and 3) is there heartburn (Fig. 8-1)? Dysphagia with an intermittent course is caused by a ring, a web, or a motility disorder.

Mechanical Cause

Mechanical obstruction occurs if the lumen is <12 mm. With mechanical obstruction, the course is progressive; dysphagia for solids is greater than for liquids, and there is associated weight loss.

- Mechanical obstruction: progressive course, weight loss, dysphagia for solids is greater than for liquids.

1. Stricture--Peptic stricture results from prolonged reflux and is usually a short (<2-3 cm long) narrowing in the distal esophagus.

- Peptic stricture results from prolonged reflux, usually in the distal esophagus.

A stricture in the mid-esophagus that may occur with an ulcer is called Barrett's esophagus. This stricture is also due to reflux and, thus, is acquired and not congenital. Normal squamous mucosa is replaced by columnar epithelium, which has 30x increased risk to develop malignancy.

- Barrett's esophagus: a stricture in mid-esophagus.

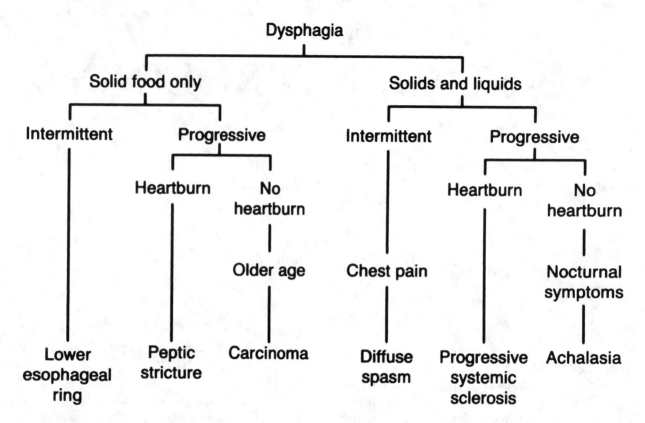

Fig. 8-1. Diagnostic scheme for dysphagia. Obtaining answers to three questions (see text) often yields the most likely diagnosis. (From MKSAP VI: Part 1:44, 1982. American College of Physicians. By permission.)

- It is a complication of chronic reflux.
- It has a 30x increased risk for malignancy

Lye stricture--Alkali is more injurious to the esophagus than acid (in postgastrectomy patients, alkaline reflux can produce severe esophagitis). Do not induce vomiting after lye ingestion. Stricture tends to occur at the three physiologic narrowings where the initial passage of the corrosive may have been delayed. Bougienage after 3-4 weeks may prevent occurrence of stricture. There is increased incidence of cancer.

- Postgastrectomy alkaline reflux can produce severe esophagitis.
- Do not induce vomiting after lye ingestion.
- Lye stricture is associated with increased incidence of cancer.

2. Tumor--Benign. Leiomyoma is the most common benign tumor. It is usually asymptomatic. Recognize the appearance of this tumor on barium swallow fluoroscopy. Perform endoscopy even if classic changes are seen on barium swallow.

Malignant. Recognize the appearance of malignant tumors on barium swallow fluoroscopy. Also, know the conditions that predispose to esophageal (squamous) cancer--achalasia, lye stricture, Plummer-Vinson syndrome, tylosis, smoking, and alcohol. The male:female ratio for esophageal malignancy is 4:1. Of the malignant tumors, 50% are squamous and 50% are adenocarcinoma. Progressive dysphagia with weight loss is usually seen. Diagnosis is established by endoscopy with biopsy and cytology. Prognosis: 5-year survival is only 7%-15%, 28% have lung metastases, and 25% have liver metastases. Treatment: squamous carcinoma is more radiosensitive than adenocarcinoma. Surgery is difficult for proximal lesions. Surgery and preoperative irradiation are used for distal 1/3 lesions. Palliation: laser endoscopy, bougienage, tube placement. Chemotherapy: no agents are known to be beneficial. Squamous carcinoma can produce ectopic parathyroid hormone, thus hypercalcemia does not mean the tumor is unresectable. Barrett's esophagus gives rise to adenocarcinoma.

- Know the radiographic appearance of leiomyoma and esophageal cancer.
- Conditions that predispose to cancer: achalasia, lye stricture, Plummer-Vinson syndrome, tylosis, smoking, and alcohol.
- Esophageal cancers are usually unresectable; palliative treatment.
- 5-Year survival is only 7%-15%.

3. Ring--A mucosal ring is a mucosal membrane that marks the junction of the esophageal and stomach mucosa. Muscular rings are rare. It presents as intermittent dysphagia for solids or as a sudden obstruction from food bolus (steak house syndrome). Know the radiographic appearance. Treatment is dilatation.

- Ring: intermittent dysphagia and food bolus impaction.
- Know its radiographic appearance.
- Treatment is dilatation.

4. Web--A web is a membrane of squamous mucosa that occurs anywhere in the esophagus. It presents as intermittent dysphagia. Plummer-Vinson syndrome: cervical esophageal web, iron deficiency anemia, and 15% chance of oropharyngeal or esophageal cancer.

- Web presents as intermittent dysphagia.
- Plummer-Vinson syndrome: cervical esophageal web, iron deficiency anemia, and 15% chance of oropharyngeal or esophageal cancer.
- Intermittent dysphagia is caused by rings, webs, or motility disorders.

Functional Cause

With functional obstruction (motility disorders), there is dysphagia for solids and liquids, intermittent course, and weight loss may or may not occur. The three important motor abnormalities of the esophagus are achalasia, diffuse esophageal spasm, and scleroderma.

1. Achalasia--Denervated esophagus (degeneration of Auerbach's ganglion cells). Chest radiography shows air fluid level. Barium swallow fluoroscopy shows dilated esophagus with beak-like tapering. Motility pattern: incomplete relaxation of the lower esophageal sphincter (most important); hypertensive lower esophageal sphincter (usually does not have reflux); and aperistalsis in body (a later finding). Always endoscopically examine patients with achalasia. Cancer of the esophagogastric junction may present with the radiographic appearance and motility pattern of achalasia. A clue would be an older patient with dysphagia and heartburn. Treatment is with pneumatic dilatation and not bougienage. Pneumatic dilatation is as effective as Heller myotomy.

In Brazil, the parasite *Trypanosoma cruzi* (Chagas' disease) produces a neurotoxin that destroys the myenteric plexus. Esophageal dilatation identical to achalasia, megacolon, and megaloureter are seen in Chagas' disease.

- Functional obstruction: intermittent dysphagia for solids and liquids.

- Achalasia: chest radiograph shows air fluid level.
- Dilated esophagus with beak-like tapering on barium swallow fluoroscopy.
- Most important motility pattern in achalasia: incomplete relaxation of lower esophageal sphincter.
- Always endoscopically examine patients with achalasia.
- Treat achalasia with pneumatic dilatation and not with bougienage.
- Chagas' disease has esophageal dysfunction identical to that of achalasia.

2. Diffuse esophageal spasm--It usually presents as chest pain but may cause intermittent dysphagia. It is aggravated by stress and hot or cold liquids. Barium swallow fluoroscopy shows corkscrew esophagus, which is normal in the elderly (presbyesophagus). Motility: simultaneous contractions of high amplitude in the body of the esophagus. If the patient is asymptomatic during the test, motility may be normal. The lower esophageal sphincter is hypertensive or has defective relaxation in 1/3 of patients. Medical treatment (nitrates, anticholinergics, nifedipine) has unpredictable results. Surgical treatment is long myotomy.

- Diffuse esophageal spasm usually presents as chest pain.
- It is aggravated by stress and hot or cold liquids.
- Barium swallow fluoroscopy shows corkscrew esophagus.
- Medical treatment has unpredictable results.

3. Scleroderma--Associated with Raynaud's phenomenon or physical findings (skin changes). Barium swallow fluoroscopy shows a common esophagogastric tube. Motility: aperistalsis in the body of the esophagus and incompetence of the lower esophageal sphincter (severe reflux). Scleroderma and mixed connective tissue disease are associated with dysphagia in 75% of patients. Systemic lupus erythematosus and dermatomyositis are associated with dysphagia in only 5% of patients.

- Scleroderma: aperistalsis in the body of the esophagus.
- Scleroderma: incompetence of the lower esophageal sphincter (severe reflux).

Oropharyngeal Dysphagia

Oropharyngeal dysphagia is the result of faulty transfer of a food bolus from the oropharynx to the esophagus caused by disorders of either neural regulation or skeletal muscle (Table 8-1). It presents as high esophageal dysphagia associated with coughing, choking, or nasal regurgitation. Structural causes include cervical osteophytes, goiter, lymphadenopathy, and Zenker's diverticulum. After recognizing that oropharyngeal dysphagia is present, other associated symptoms may lead to diagnosis of the underlying illness (e.g., a young person with

Table 8-1.--Causes of Oropharyngeal Dysphagia

Muscular disorders	Neurologic disorders	Structural causes
Amyloidosis	Amyotrophic lateral sclerosis	Cervical osteophytes
Dermatomyositis	Cerebral vascular accident	Cricopharyngeal dysfunction
Hyperthyroidism	Diphtheria	Goiter
Hypothyroidism	Huntington's disease	Lymphadenopathy
Myasthenia gravis	Multiple sclerosis	Zenker's diverticulum
Myotonia dystrophica	Parkinson's disease	
Oculopharyngeal myopathy	Polio	
Stiff-man syndrome	Tabes dorsalis	
	Tetanus	

oropharyngeal dysphagia, central scotoma, and neurologic symptoms has multiple sclerosis).

- Oropharyngeal dysphagia is the result of faulty transfer of a food bolus from the oropharynx to the esophagus due to neuromuscular disorders.
- It is a high esophageal dysphagia associated with coughing, choking, or nasal regurgitation.

Gastroesophageal Reflux Disease

It is generally accepted that reflux of gastric contents occurs when the lower esophageal sphincter pressure is <10 mm Hg. Internists should know which agents alter lower esophageal sphincter pressure.

Reflux

The lower esophageal sphincter is the major barrier to reflux. This sphincter is a 2- to 4-cm-long specialized segment of circular smooth muscle in the terminal esophagus. The pressure of this sphincter varies markedly during the day, but the normal resting pressure is 15-30 mm Hg. Swallowing causes the pressure to decrease promptly (within 1-2 seconds after the onset of swallowing) and for the sphincter to remain relaxed until the peristaltic wave passes over it. The sphincter then contracts to maintain the increased resting pressure that prevents reflux. Pressure of the lower esophageal sphincter decreases significantly for 2 hours after a meal. Some gastroesophageal reflux occurs in everyone during the day but does not cause symptoms or esophagitis. Patients with clinically symptomatic reflux or inflammation show transient lower esophageal sphincter relaxations of unknown cause and have more frequent and longer lasting episodes of reflux. Various causes of change in lower esophageal sphincter pressure are listed in Table 8-2.

- Reflux of gastric contents occurs when lower esophageal sphincter pressure is <10 mm Hg.

- Lower esophageal sphincter pressure decreases for 2 hours after a meal.
- Patients with clinically symptomatic reflux show transient lower esophageal sphincter relaxations.
- Know which agents decrease lower esophageal sphincter pressure.

The degree of tissue damage is the real concern in gastroesophageal reflux disease. Multiple factors that determine whether reflux esophagitis occurs include 1) lower esophageal sphincter pressure, 2) volume of gastric contents, 3) rate of gastric emptying (if delayed reflux), 4) potency of refluxate (acid, pepsin, bile), 5) efficiency of esophageal clearance (motility, salivary, bicarbonate), and 6) resistance of esophageal tissue to injury and ability to repair.

The evaluation of esophagitis is designed to answer four important questions (Table 8-3): Does the patient have esophagitis and, if so, to what extent? Does the patient have reflux and, if so, how severe? Are the patient's symptoms due to reflux? What is the mechanism of reflux?

Internists should know how to use tests that evaluate reflux in a cost-effective way. In most patients, the medical history is sufficiently typical to warrant a trial of therapy without conducting expensive tests. Additional testing should be performed in patients with an atypical medical history, refractory symptoms, or possible complications of esophagitis.

- In most patients, the medical history is sufficiently typical to warrant a trial of therapy without tests.
- Testing should be performed in patients with an atypical medical history, refractory symptoms, or possible complications of esophagitis.

Esophageal Tests

1. Barium swallow fluoroscopy--Reflux is found in 60% of patients with esophagitis but also in 25% of controls. It is a qualitative test and does not distinguish between "normal"

Table 8-2.--Changes in Lower Esophageal Sphincter Pressure

Increase	Decrease
Endogenous cause	Endogenous cause
Gastrin (pharmacologic doses)	Secretin
Glucagon	Motilin
	Cholecystokinin
	Progesterone (pregnancy)
Exogenous cause	Exogenous cause
Protein meal	Diet
Antacids	Alcohol
Cholinergic drugs	Caffeine
Metoclopramide	Carminatives (spearmint, peppermint)
	Chocolate
	Fatty meal
	Smoking (nicotine)
	Theophylline
	Drugs
	Anticholinergic drugs
	Calcium channel blockers
	Nitrates
	α-Adrenergic antagonists
	β-Adrenergic agonists
	Morphine
	Diazepam
	Benzodiazepine

Table 8-3.--Evaluation of Esophagitis

Question	Tests for reflux (more sensitive one is listed first)
Is reflux present?	pH probe; isotope scan
Is esophagitis present?	Biopsy; endoscopy
Are symptoms due to reflux?	Acid perfusion (Bernstein test)
Mechanism of reflux?	Motility

and abnormal reflux. Upper gastrointestinal radiography is used primarily as a screening test to exclude other diagnoses (e.g., ulcer) and to identify complications of reflux (e.g., strictures, ulcers, Barrett's esophagus). Patients with reflux and dysphagia should have barium esophagography first.

- Reflux is found in 60% of patients with esophagitis but also in 25% of controls.
- Patients with reflux and dysphagia should have barium esophagography first.

2. Esophagoscopy--This is the most definitive test if gross inflammation is present. However, 40% of patients may have symptomatic reflux with no gross inflammation. This is the preferred first test in long-standing cases of reflux to rule out Barrett's esophagus. It is also the first test for patients with reflux without dysphagia.

- Esophagoscopy is the test preferred first in long-standing cases of reflux to rule out Barrett's esophagus.
- It is the first test for patients with reflux without dysphagia.

3. Esophageal biopsy--In patients with reflux but without gross esophagitis, the basal cell layer and papillae are elongated. Esophagoscopy and biopsy are about 100% sensitive for detecting reflux. With Barrett's esophagus, it is important for the biopsy sample to include the mucosa to detect dysplasia (premalignant changes).

- Biopsy may detect esophagitis when gross inflammation is not present.
- With Barrett's esophagus, it is important for the biopsy sample to include the mucosa.

4. 24-Hour pH monitoring--Monitoring the pH in the distal esophagus of patients during a 24-hour period after their normal routine allows a more physiologic evaluation of reflux during daily activities. Reflux is determined by a pH that is <4; findings are positive when the pH is <4 more than 5% of the time. This test is valuable in patients with atypical symptoms, reflux symptoms, a nondiagnostic evaluation, or pulmonary symptoms.

- 24-Hour pH monitoring allows a more physiologic evaluation of reflux during daily activities.
- Positive test: esophageal pH is <4 more than 5% of the time.
- This test is valuable in patients with atypical symptoms.

5. Acid perfusion (Bernstein test)--Saline perfusion for 10 minutes should not cause symptoms; next, switch to 0.1N HCl to see if the pain is reproduced. If heartburn and chest pain occur after acid instillation, treat for reflux.

- If heartburn and chest pain occur after acid instillation, treat for reflux.

6. Esophageal manometry--Manometry is reserved for patients with suspected esophageal motility disorders or with refractory reflux preoperatively.

- Esophageal manometry is reserved for suspected esophageal motility disorders.

Atypical Presentation and Complications of Gastroesophageal Reflux Disease

Atypical presentations include noncardiac chest pain, pulmonary symptoms (asthma and aspiration pneumonia), and hoarseness and cough.

Complications include ulceration, bleeding, stricture, aspiration, Barrett's esophagus, and carcinoma.

Treatment of Reflux

Treatment of gastroesophageal reflux disease is divided into three phases:

Phase 1 therapy--Lifestyle modifications: elevate the head of the bed 6 inches; modify diet so there is less fat and more protein; three meals a day; no eating for several hours before reclining; weight loss if overweight; and avoidance of specific foods (fatty foods, chocolate, alcohol, citrus juices, tomato products, coffee, carminatives). The patient should stop smoking and avoid alcohol. Avoid drugs that decrease lower esophageal sphincter pressure: anticholinergics, sedatives, tranquilizers, theophylline, progesterone or progesterone-containing birth control pills, nitrates, β-adrenergic agonists, and calcium channel blockers. Therapy is with antacids or alginic acid, 30 minutes after meals and at bedtime.

Phase 2 therapy--Therapy includes drugs that decrease gastric acid output: H_2 blockers, all are equally effective. A dose twice daily (bid) is preferable for treating gastroesophageal reflux disease, e.g., cimetidine, 400 mg bid; ranitidine, 150 mg bid; famotidine, 20 mg bid; nizatidine, 150 mg bid. Omeprazole: reserve for cases refractory to H_2 receptor blockers. Drugs that increase the lower esophageal sphincter pressure and esophageal clearance--cisapride, metoclopramide, bethanechol--have a limited role in treating reflux and often cause side effects.

Phase 3 therapy--This therapy includes antireflux surgery, which is reserved for patients who are refractory to medical therapy or who develop complications. Nissen fundoplication is the preferred operation; fundoplication increases lower esophageal sphincter pressure.

- Phase 1 therapy: modify lifestyle, avoid drugs that decrease lower esophageal sphincter pressure, and use antacids as the first line of treatment.
- Phase 2 therapy: H_2 blockers in twice daily doses are effective in most patients; use omeprazole in patients refractory to H_2 blockers.
- Do not use anticholinergics to treat reflux.
- Antireflux surgery is reserved for patients who are refractory to medical therapy or who develop complications.

Noncardiac Chest Pain

Chest pain is a frightening symptom, and patients are often referred to internists and gastroenterologists when cardiac evaluation does not have positive findings. Internists must understand the limitations of the diagnostic studies used to evaluate noncardiac chest pain. First, significant cardiac disease must be ruled out. Esophageal pain may be secondary to a motor disorder or a sensitive mucosa. Gastroesophageal reflux disease is the most common cause of noncardiac chest pain, but the esophagus is only one of several possible causes. Esophageal spasm can closely mimic angina. Esophagogastroduodenoscopy rules out mucosal disease, i.e., inflammation, neoplasms, and chemical injury. Examine esophageal motility to look for motor disorders, e.g., esophageal spasm, "nutcracker esophagus." Therapy for noncardiac chest pain includes avoidance of precipitants. Antacids may be beneficial in patients with inflammation. Sublingual nitroglycerin or calcium channel blockers are sometimes helpful in motor disorders, but their efficacy is unproven. If appropriate, reassure the patient that cardiac disease is not present.

- For noncardiac chest pain, rule out significant cardiac disease.
- Gastroesophageal reflux disease is the commonest cause of noncardiac chest pain.
- Esophageal spasm can closely mimic angina.
- Esophagogastroduodenoscopy rules out mucosal disease.

- Sublingual nitroglycerin or calcium channel blockers sometimes are helpful.

Infections of the Esophagus

Patients with immunodeficiency disorders (AIDS), diabetes mellitus, malignancies (especially lymphoma and leukemia), and esophageal motility disorders are susceptible to opportunistic infections of the esophagus. These infections present as odynophagia. The most important infections to recognize are *Candida*, herpes, and cytomegalovirus. *Candida* infection: barium radiography shows small nodules in the upper 1/3 of the esophagus, and endoscopy shows cottage cheese-like plaques. Diagnosis is made by seeing pseudohyphae on KOH preparations. Treatment is with nystatin or clotrimazole for colonization and ketoconazole or fluconazole for esophagitis. Rarely, amphotericin B is used. Herpes infection: barium radiography and endoscopy show small discrete ulcers without plaques. Diagnosis is based on finding intranuclear inclusions (Cowdry's type A bodies). Treatment is with acyclovir. Cytomegalovirus infection: radiography and endoscopy show severe inflammation with large ulcers. Intranuclear inclusions may be seen but viral cultures are unreliable. Treatment is with ganciclovir.

Other Esophageal Problems

Medication-Induced Esophagitis

Medication-induced esophagitis presents as odynophagia or dysphagia and is more likely to occur if there is abnormal motility, stricture, or compression (left atrial enlargement). It is more common in the elderly and is recognized as inflammation in the mid-esophagus, with sparing of the distal esophagus. Medications commonly associated with esophagitis include tetracycline, doxycycline, quinidine, potassium, ferrous sulfate, and ascorbic acid.

- Mid-esophageal inflammation is associated with abnormal motility, stricture, or compression and is more common in the elderly.
- Medicines responsible for esophagitis: tetracycline, doxycycline, quinidine, ferrous sulfate, and ascorbic acid.

Mallory-Weiss Syndrome

Mallory-Weiss syndrome is mucosal laceration at the esophagogastric junction. It accounts for about 10% of cases of upper gastrointestinal tract bleeding: 75% of patients have a history of retching or vomiting before bleeding, 72% have diaphragmatic hernias, and 90% stop bleeding. Vasopressin, endoscopic injection, or electrocautery may control bleeding. Surgical treatment for persistent bleeding.

- Mallory-Weiss syndrome: mucosal laceration at the esophagogastric junction.

- Accounts for about 10% of cases of upper gastrointestinal tract bleeding.
- 75% of patients have a history of retching and vomiting before bleeding.

Esophageal Perforation

Esophageal perforation commonly occurs after dilatation in an area of stricture. Spontaneous perforation of the esophagus (Boerhaave's syndrome) follows violent retching, often after an alcoholic binge. It also occurs after heavy lifting, defecation, seizures, and forceful labor (childbirth). The most common site of perforation is the left posterior part of the distal esophagus. If pleural fluid is present, it may have an increased concentration of amylase. Zenker's diverticulum, cervical osteophytes (difficult intubations), and endoscopy (intubation) are causes of perforation of the cervical esophagus.

- Esophageal perforation commonly occurs after dilatation.
- Boerhaave's syndrome follows violent retching, often after an alcoholic binge.

STOMACH

Peptic ulcers are defects in the gastric or duodenal mucosa that result from an imbalance between the digestive activity of acid and pepsin in the gastric juice and the host's protective mechanisms to resist mucosal digestion. Recent advances in our understanding of peptic ulcer pathogenesis have caused us to modify our presumption that idiopathic acid hypersecretion is a major etiologic factor. Newer classifications of peptic ulcers categorize ulcers as being associated with three possible etiologic factors: 1) *Helicobacter pylori*, 2) nonsteroidal anti-inflammatory drugs (NSAIDs) or aspirin, or 3) miscellaneous causes. Miscellaneous causes include ulcers due to hypersecretion from gastrinomas (Zollinger-Ellison syndrome), idiopathic hypersecretion, and duodenogastric reflux of gastric mucosal barrier-breaking agents such as bile salts or lysolecithin. Recent reports estimate that <5% of ulcers are due to miscellaneous causes. Thus, at least 95% of peptic ulcers are due to either *Helicobacter pylori* or NSAIDs. The most common cause of duodenal ulcer is *H. pylori*, and the most common cause of gastric ulcer is NSAIDs.

Helicobacter pylori

The Organism

H. pylori is a gram-negative, spiral-shaped, microaerophilic bacillus that contains 4-6 unipolar, sheathed flagella. This fastidious organism resides beneath and within the mucus layer of the gastric mucosa and produces multiple enzymes such as urease and mucolytic proteases that are important for its survival and for its pathogenic effect. After it has been ingested, the organism moves into and through the mucus layer of the stomach. It has been postulated that several virulence factors are needed for successful colonization of the gastric mucosa, including motility, adhesins, proteases, phospholipases, cytokines, cytotoxins, and urease. Urease is thought to protect the organism from the acid environment. After colonization, the organism multiplies in the gastric mucus layer. Defense mechanisms may help control the infection, but unless treated, the organism remains in the gastric mucus layer for life.

H. pylori is a "slow" bacterium that causes persistent gastric infection and chronic inflammation. Ingestion can cause acute symptoms. Within weeks to months after infection, a chronic superficial gastritis develops, and after years to decades, chronic atrophic gastritis or gastric malignancy may develop.

Epidemiology

In the U. S., *H. pylori* has an age-related prevalence, occurring in 10% of the general population younger than age 30 and in 60% of those older than age 60. *H. pylori* is present in 40%-50% of the general population overall; it is more prevalent in Blacks and hispanics, poorer socioeconomic groups, and institutionalized subjects. In developing countries such as India and Saudi Arabia, 50% of the population is infected by age 10, 70% by age 20, and 85%-95% of the population overall is infected. Evidence of person-to-person transmission includes clustering within families, higher than expected prevalence in institutionalized subjects, transmission by endoscopy and biopsy, and a higher prevalence of infection among gastroenterologists. The fecal-oral route of transmission has been postulated, and indeed, *H. pylori* has been isolated from human feces. In the future, detection of the organism in stool may provide a noninvasive approach to the diagnosis of *H. pylori* infection.

Associated Diseases

Active chronic gastritis

In patients with active chronic gastritis that is not associated with immunologic mechanisms (type A gastritis--pernicious anemia) or chemical injury (type C gastritis--alcohol, NSAIDs, aspirin, bile salts), *H. pylori* infection (type B gastritis) is universally found. *H. pylori*-induced active chronic gastritis is the most common type of chronic gastritis, and in some patients, it may progress to chronic atrophic gastritis. An important concept is that *H. pylori*-induced gastritis is the basic disease and the development of duodenal or gastric ulcers or malignancy is a complication of the gastritis.

Duodenal ulcer

H. pylori is found in 90%-95% of patients with duodenal ulcers. The most important link between *H. pylori*-induced gastritis and the development of duodenal ulcers is the presence of gastric metaplasia in the duodenal bulb. Some data suggest that the gastric metaplasia must be infected by *H. pylori* to

permit the development of duodenitis or duodenal ulcer. If *H. pylori*-positive patients with duodenal ulcer do not receive treatment, most have relapse within 1 year. However, if the infection is eradicated, the rate of relapse approaches zero. *H. pylori* infection causes basal and meal-stimulated gastrin release. Asymptomatic carriers of the bacillus may have a protective mechanism that prevents the hypersecretion of gastric acid. Enhanced gastric acid secretion occurs only in ulcer patients.

Gastric ulcer

H. pylori is found in about 80% of patients with gastric ulcer. Eradication of *H. pylori* decreases the relapse rate of gastric ulcers. Adenocarcinoma--Chronic atrophic gastritis is a precursor of gastric cancer. Recently, *H. pylori* has been linked to noncardia gastric adenocarcinoma. Studies from the U. S. and Great Britain have established a strong association between *H. pylori* infection (serum samples) and the emergence of noncardia gastric cancer. It is postulated that *H. pylori* gastritis progresses to atrophic gastritis and, in the presence of other risk factors, gastric adenocarcinoma eventually develops. This appears to be a rare occurrence. The attributable risk of *H. pylori* in gastric cancer has been calculated to be between 35% and 89%, i.e., between 35% and 89% of cancers would not occur if *H. pylori* was not present. A cause-and-effect relationship remains to be established, and further studies are needed to determine the exact role of *H. pylori* in the development of gastric adenocarcinoma. Primary B-cell lymphoma--*H. pylori* has also been associated with primary B-cell lymphoma of the stomach. Of 450 patients with *H. pylori*-positive gastritis, 125 (28%) had mucosal lymphoid follicles and 8 (1.8%) had B lymphocytes infiltrating the epithelium, consistent with the development of early lymphoma.

Nonulcer Dyspepsia

Nonulcer dyspepsia is common, affecting about 20% of the people in the U. S. Of those with functional dyspepsia, approximately 50% are infected with *H. pylori*, similar to the prevalence of *H. pylori* in asymptomatic persons. There is no convincing evidence that treatment of *H. pylori*-positive patients with nonulcer dyspepsia results in significant clinical improvement.

Diagnostic Tests for H. pylori Infection

Various diagnostic tests are available for determining whether *H. pylori* infection is present. The choice of which test to use is determined by the clinical setting of the patient and the cost.

Serology

H. pylori produces not only a local immune response but also a systemic immune response. Current detection methods exist for antibodies of the IgG, IgA, and IgM classes. Serology is the most cost-effective, noninvasive test to diagnose primary *H. pylori* infection, but serology remains positive over time, which limits the usefulness of this test in follow-up evaluation. Its sensitivity is 95% and specificity is 90%-95%; the cost is $40-$100.

Breath test

A radiolabeled dose of urea is given orally to a patient. If *H. pylori* is present, the urease splits the urea and radiolabeled CO_2 is exhaled. The advantage of this test is that it is quick, easy to perform, and does not require endoscopy. As the breath test becomes more widely available, it will be the test of choice for follow-up evaluation. Its sensitivity is 95%-98% and specificity is 95%-98%; the cost is $100-$200.

Biopsy urease tests

A biopsy specimen is impregnated into auger that contains urea and a pH indicator. As the urea is split, the pH of the medium changes the color of the auger from yellow to red. This test depends on the bacterial urease, and the greater the number of organisms, the more rapid the test turns positive. Its sensitivity is 95% and specificity is 98%; the cost is $20.

Histology

An advantage of histology is being able to examine the underlying inflammatory reaction. *H. pylori* can be demonstrated with Gram's stain, hematoxylin and eosin stain, Giemsa stain, and the Warthin-Starry (silver) stain. The sensitivity is 98% and specificity is 98%; the cost is $250 or more.

Culture

Culturing *H. pylori* is tedious and expensive and should be reserved for special circumstances, e.g., when an antibiotic-resistant organism is suspected or if virulence testing is being done. The sensitivity is 90%-95% and specificity 100%; the cost is $150.

Because many symptomatic patients undergo endoscopy, histologic examination and biopsy urease tests are used most commonly in the initial evaluation.

Treatment

The goal of treatment of an *H. pylori*-positive duodenal or gastric ulcer is to heal the ulcer and eradicate (not suppress) the bacteria. Traditionally, eradication of the bacteria has been achieved most effectively with triple antibiotic therapy (the combination of bismuth, metronidazole, and tetracycline achieves 93% eradication). Many other combinations of antibiotics have been recommended but have been less effective. Several studies have reported >80% eradication of *H. pylori* with a combination of omeprazole, 20 mg twice daily, and amoxicillin, 500 mg four times daily for 2 weeks. Several controlled clinical trials are now under way to determine the optimal dose of these two agents, the duration of treatment, and the overall eradication rate. Recently, clarithromycin and omeprazole have been shown to achieve a 78% overall eradication rate in *H. pylori*-positive ulcer patients (85% eradi-

cation rate if no previous treatment and 64% if previous treatment with metronidazole failed). Clarithromycin and omeprazole are recommended as first-line treatment in areas where imidazole-resistant *H. pylori* infections are common; it may also be useful as second-line treatment after failure of conventional triple therapy.

In February 1994, a consensus development panel of the National Institutes of Health recommended that all patients with gastric or duodenal ulcer who are infected with *H. pylori* should receive treatment with antimicrobials. Furthermore, they recommended that *H. pylori*-infected patients with peptic ulcer disease who were in remission on maintenance treatment also receive this treatment. The presence of NSAIDs and aspirin as a contributing factor should not alter treatment with antimicrobials; however, the use of NSAIDs should be discontinued whenever possible. Treatment was not recommended for asymptomatic *H. pylori*-infected patients without ulcers or those with nonulcer dyspepsia.

Nonsteroidal Anti-Inflammatory Drug-Induced Ulcers

NSAIDs inhibit gastroduodenal prostaglandin synthesis, which results in decreased secretion of mucus and bicarbonate and reduced mucosal blood flow. NSAID-induced ulcers occur more commonly in the stomach than in the duodenum, and typically, they are located in the prepyloric area or antrum of the stomach.

The risk of peptic ulcer disease with NSAIDs is dose-dependent. It is important for physicians to understand that the anti-inflammatory properties of NSAIDs predispose to ulceration (prostaglandin inhibition) and that there are different dose-response relationships for analgesia and anti-inflammatory properties of NSAIDs. The maximum analgesic effect plateaus well below the effective anti-inflammatory dose. Low doses of aspirin or NSAIDs give pain relief but have little anti-inflammatory activity. The newer NSAIDs have been marketed with more convenient (less frequent) dosing intervals and in dosages that have marked anti-inflammatory activity. Thus, the use of newer NSAIDs may subject the patient to an increased risk for ulcer without providing increased analgesia. In many instances, the use of NSAIDs can be discontinued and simple analgesic therapy with acetaminophen substituted. For patients who require NSAIDs, an attempt should be made to use the lowest possible dose. It is also important for physicians to know that the risk of peptic ulcer disease with NSAID use is maximal in the first month of treatment and that elderly patients and patients with a previous history of peptic ulcer disease are at highest risk.

H_2-receptor antagonists and sucralfate are ineffective in preventing gastric ulcers and for reducing the frequency of NSAID-induced mucosal erosions. Prostaglandin replacement with the synthetic prostaglandin misoprostol decreases the incidence of NSAID-induced gastric ulcers. However, diarrhea develops in many patients, thus limiting the usefulness of misoprostol.

Gastric Ulcer

In the U.S., duodenal ulcer is 4 times more common than gastric ulcer, which is rare before age 40 and has a peak incidence at age 55-65.

Pathophysiologic abnormalities. NSAID use--Most patients with gastric ulcer have acid secretory rates within the normal range. The exact role of *H. pylori* is unclear.

- Most patients with gastric ulcers have normal acid secretory rates.

Anatomical predisposition--Gastric ulcers usually occur on the lesser curve near the angulus, at the junction of oxyntic and antral mucosa.

- Gastric ulcers usually occur on the lesser curve near the angulus.

Environmental factors--Aspirin, NSAIDs, and bile reflux damage the gastric mucosal barrier. NSAIDs also inhibit prostaglandin synthesis. Smoking--The pathogenesis is unclear. Infectious agents--*H. pylori* and cytomegalovirus. Alcohol causes gastritis, but there is no definite evidence that stress, alcohol, or caffeine causes chronic gastric ulceration.

- NSAIDs, aspirin, bile reflux, and smoking predispose to gastric ulceration.
- No definite evidence that stress, alcohol, corticosteroids, or caffeine causes chronic gastric ulceration.

Natural history--65%-70% of ulcers heal in 12 weeks with placebo, and the rate of recurrence in patients receiving placebo for up to 12 months is 55%-89%. Most ulcers recur in the same area. More than 2-3 recurrences are uncommon. Complications include bleeding, perforation, and obstruction. Clinical manifestations include pain frequently relieved by meals.

Diagnosis--Radiology can detect 90% of gastric ulcers. Criteria suggesting a benign gastric ulcer are Hampton line (a radiolucent line partially or completely traversing the orifice of the ulcer), folds radiating to the edge of an ulcer crater, and an ulcer collar (a translucent band intervening between the ulcer crater and the lumen of the stomach). Criteria suggesting malignancy are negative filling defect in the ulcer crater or at its upper or lower margins and abnormal folds near the base.

- Barium radiography detects 90% of gastric ulcers.
- Negative filling defects in the ulcer crater or at its upper or lower margins suggest malignancy.
- Abnormal folds near the base of the ulcer also suggest malignancy.

Endoscopy is indicated if there is a radiologically diagnosed gastric ulcer (3%-7% of malignant ulcers appear benign), a large ulcer (>2.5 cm), or an appearance not typically benign. It is also indicated after 8 weeks of therapy.

Medical therapy--Healing occurs in 60%-90% of cases treated for 6-8 weeks. Generally, healing rates are similar with H_2 blockers, antacids, sucralfate, and omeprazole. Healing is not increased with combined therapy (e.g., H_2 blockers plus antacids). Medical restrictions include eliminating or decreasing aspirin, NSAIDs, and smoking.

- No increased healing with combination therapy.

Follow-up--If pain is not relieved within 2 weeks, add another medication. Repeat radiography or endoscopy in all patients to document healing. Refer for surgical treatment if ulcer is not healed in 12 weeks (allow 16 weeks if ulcer is large). For recurrent ulcers, the therapy used initially is usually adequate for treating recurrences. Surgical indications are patients with ulcer refractory to therapy, recurrent ulcer on maintenance therapy, complications, or malignancy. Prevention of recurrence: in most patients, recurrence can be treated with separate courses. Chronic maintenance is indicated for patients who would be at high risk if a recurrent ulcer became complicated by perforation or bleeding (e.g., patients with heart disease) and for those with previous complication of a gastric ulcer.

- Repeat radiography or endoscopy in all patients to document healing.
- Surgical treatment is indicated for patients with ulcer refractory to therapy, recurrent ulcer on maintenance therapy, complications, and malignancy.
- Maintenance treatment for patients with previous complication or at high risk for complication with recurrent ulcer.

Duodenal Ulcer

Epidemiology--Lifetime prevalence is about 10% for U.S. males and 4% for females. Risk factors--No convincing data that diet is a factor. Although alcohol is associated with mucosal lesions, it does not cause duodenal ulcer. Aspirin and NSAIDs induce acute injury and cause ulcers, perforation, and bleeding. The effect of corticosteroids is controversial, but the risk seems to be minimal. Cigarette smoking increases risk for duodenal ulcer and impairs ulcer healing. Caffeine causes dyspepsia but not ulcers. *H. pylori* increases risk for duodenal ulcer. There is a higher incidence of these ulcers if there is also chronic lung disease, cirrhosis, or chronic renal failure.

- Prevalence (U.S.): males, 10%; females, 4%.
- Aspirin, NSAIDs, smoking, and *H. pylori* increase risk for duodenal ulcer.
- No evidence that diet, alcohol, corticosteroids, caffeine, or stress increases risk for duodenal ulcer.

- Chronic lung disease, cirrhosis, and chronic renal failure increase the risk for duodenal ulcer.

The pathogenesis and pathophysiology are dependent on acid and peptic activity. The ulcers are rare if acid secretion is <10 mEq/hr, but they can occur in cases of hypersecretion. Mucosal resistance is also a factor. The pathophysiologic abnormalities are complex and likely do not involve a single process. Proposed abnormalities include increased parietal cell and chief cell mass, increased basal secretory drive, increased postprandial secretory drive, rapid gastric emptying, and impaired mucosal defense.

- Duodenal ulcer is rare if acid secretion is <10 mEq/hr.

Diagnosis--80%-90% of ulcer craters can be detected on an optimal radiograph of the upper gastrointestinal tract. With routine radiographic techniques, 50% of duodenal ulcers may be missed. Endoscopy detects 85%-95% of gastroduodenal lesions, with a specificity generally >90%. In patients with simple dyspepsia, a trial of antacids or H_2 blockers for 1-2 weeks is indicated in the appropriate clinical setting. Follow-up endoscopy to document healing in asymptomatic patients is not necessary for duodenal ulcer.

- 80%-90% of ulcer craters can be detected on an optimal radiograph of the upper gastrointestinal tract.
- Specificity is generally >90% with endoscopy.
- Follow-up endoscopy to document healing is not necessary for duodenal ulcer if patient is asymptomatic.

Natural history--Duodenal ulcer is a recurring, chronic disease, and 50%-80% of patients have recurrence within 6-12 months after the initial healing. There is seasonal variation: the ulcers are more common in the fall and spring.

- 50%-80% of patients have recurrence within 6-12 months.

Medical treatment--Eliminate factors impairing healing, including smoking, aspirin, and NSAIDs. All H_2 receptor antagonists are equally effective. Side effects: antiandrogen, gynecomastia, and impotence are usually seen only with high doses of cimetidine. Drug interactions: cimetidine inhibits cytochrome P450 system and increases the therapeutic effects of theophylline, lidocaine, phenytoin, and warfarin. Omeprazole inhibits the H^+/K^+ ATPase pump responsible for acid secretion and irreversibly inactivates the enzyme. In normal subjects, it can produce anacidity. It is the drug of choice in Zollinger-Ellison syndrome and medically refractory reflux esophagitis. Anticholinergics have a limited role in duodenal ulcer. Do not use them in cases of gastroesophageal reflux disease or gastric ulcer. They decrease basal acid secretion by 40%-50% but are limited by their side effects (dry mouth, blurred vision).

The mechanism of antacids may not be entirely secondary to acid neutralization. Other factors may be the binding of bile acids, inactivation of pepsin, or enhanced mucosal resistance to injury. Side effects: Mg^{++}-diarrhea, aluminum hydroxide hypophosphatemia, and constipation. Prostaglandins (e.g., misoprostol) are produced by the gastroduodenal mucosa and have a role in mucosal resistance to injury. Prostaglandins of the E and I groups inhibit acid secretion. They are effective in preventing NSAID-induced ulcers. Side effects: crampy abdominal pain and diarrhea. Sucralfate is a sulfated disaccharide complex with aluminum hydroxide. It does not alter gastric acid or pepsin secretion and is not effective in preventing NSAID-induced ulcers.

- Cimetidine inhibits cytochrome P450; may develop toxicity from theophylline, lidocaine, phenytoin, and warfarin.
- Omeprazole is the drug of choice in Zollinger-Ellison syndrome and refractory gastroesophageal reflux disease.
- Do not use anticholinergics in gastroesophageal reflux disease or gastric ulcer.
- Misoprostol, but not sucralfate, prevents NSAID-induced ulcers.

Refractory Ulcers

Twenty percent of peptic ulcers fail to heal in 4 weeks, but half of these heal with an additional 4 weeks of therapy. They are refractory if healing is not evident after 8-12 weeks, which is the case in 5% of ulcers. Symptoms may persist after healing, so documentation of the ulcer is necessary. Management--Treat for 8 weeks (or longer), check serum level of gastrin and check for *H. pylori*. Prescribe larger doses of H_2 blockers at night or use omeprazole.

- Refractory ulcer: failure to heal after 8-12 weeks of therapy.
- 5% of ulcers are refractory.
- Consider treatment for *H. pylori*.
- Exclude Zollinger-Ellison syndrome.

Recurrent Ulcers

Recurrence does not depend on the length of the initial treatment or on the dose/potency of the agent. Maintenance therapy does reduce recurrences--cimetidine 400 mg at bedtime, 60%-85% without recurrence; placebo, 17%-39% without recurrence. Between 15% and 20% of patients require more antisecretory efficacy than that achieved with cimetidine (400 mg at night) to prevent recurrence. Treatment for *H. pylori* decreases recurrence of duodenal and gastric ulcers.

Complications of Peptic Ulcer Disease and Indications for Surgical Treatment

Intractability is the most common reason for surgical treatment. Confirmation of the presence of ulcer is necessary. Approximately 15% of patients with peptic ulcer disease have severe symptoms requiring surgical treatment.

Table 8-4.--Results of Various Ulcer Operations

Procedure	Mortality, %	% complications	% ulcer recurrence	2nd operation
Gastroenterostomy	...	...	34	70% gastrectomy
Gastrectomy (BI, BII)	3	20% dumping, diarrhea	5	Vagotomy, remove retained antrum
Truncal vagotomy/ pyloroplasty	1	15% dumping, bilious vomiting	15	Re-vagotomize, antrectomy
Truncal vagotomy/ antrectomy*	<1	25% dumping, diarrhea	1	Re-vagotomize
Selective (gastric) vagotomy/pyloroplasty	<1	20% dumping 6% diarrhea	5	Re-vagotomize, antrectomy
Parietal cell vagotomy	<1	5% dumping	5-20 (rising with follow-up)	Re-vagotomize, antrectomy

*Preferred for obstruction and acute hemorrhage.

- Intractability is the common reason for surgical treatment.
- 15% of patients have severe symptoms requiring surgical treatment.

Hemorrhage occurs in 15%-20% of ulcer patients and is most common in those in the 6th decade. Eighty percent of patients relate a history of symptomatic ulcer disease before the onset of bleeding. Hemorrhage is more common with gastric ulcer than with duodenal ulcer, possibly because of an older patient population and the use of NSAIDs. More than 50% of those treated medically hemorrhage again in 10-15 years.

- 15%-20% of ulcer patients hemorrhage.
- Hemorrhage is most common in elderly persons taking NSAIDs.
- >50% of those treated medically hemorrhage again in 10-15 years.

Perforation is a less common complication than hemorrhage and more common than obstruction. Pyloroduodenal perforation is more common than gastric perforation. The preferred procedure for treating perforation is closure of the perforation and proximal selective gastric vagotomy.

- Pyloroduodenal perforation is more common than gastric perforation.

Penetration is the erosion of the ulcer through the wall without leakage of the digestive contents into the peritoneal cavity. The common one is a posterior penetrating ulcer into the pancreas, mimicking pancreatitis. Penetrating ulcers require aggressive treatment and may be refractory.

Gastric outlet obstruction is a complication in 2% of all ulcer patients. In 90% of them, it is caused by duodenal ulcer and in 4%-5%, by gastric ulcer. Only 25%-35% respond to medical management and >90% of responders subsequently require surgical treatment.

- Gastric outlet obstruction is caused by duodenal ulcer in 90% of patients and by gastric ulcer in 4%-5%.

Peptic Ulcer Surgery

The objectives of an operation for peptic ulcer disease are 1) effectiveness (low recurrence rate), 2) safety (low mortality rate), and 3) preservation of the digestive apparatus (low morbidity, few complications). Operations alter the pathophysiology of peptic ulcer disease by: 1) Reducing stimuli for HCl secretion--Vagotomy eliminates the direct cholinergic stimulus. Antrectomy eliminates gastrin-mediated HCl secretion. 2) Reducing parietal cell mass--Antrectomy eliminates gastrin's trophic effect on parietal cells. Subtotal gastrectomy reduces the parietal cell mass by the amount resected. Total gastrectomy is not indicated for peptic disease. It is indicated for cancer and gastric bleeding (previously for Zollinger-Ellison syndrome) (Table 8-4).

- Vagotomy eliminates the direct cholinergic stimulus.
- Antrectomy eliminates gastrin-mediated HCl secretion and eliminates gastrin's trophic effect on parietal cells.
- Parietal gastrectomy reduces parietal cell mass.
- Total gastrectomy is not indicated for peptic disease but is indicated for cancer and gastric bleeding.

Postgastrectomy Syndromes

Early: 1) Duodenal stump leakage--Sudden, severe abdominal pain 3-6 days postoperatively and associated fever, leukocytosis, and abdominal rigidity. The patient is at higher risk if the duodenum is severely inflamed. 2) Bleeding--If within 24 hours: failure to ligate vessel or coagulopathy. If 4-7 days:

anastomotic slough. 3) Gastric retention--Motility disorders may persist for 2 weeks postoperatively. Use gastroscopy to rule out obstruction; treatment is with nasogastric suction.

Late: Recurrent ulcer (anastomotic ulcer) occurs on intestinal side, usually within 2 cm of anastomoses. Differential diagnoses include inadequate vagotomy, inadequate operation, retained antrum, hyperplasia of G cells, and Zollinger-Ellison syndrome.

Work-up includes: 1) Obtain operative and pathology reports--Was stomach resected to the duodenum? Were vagal trunks identified? 2) Perform gastric acid studies--If basal acid output is >2 mEq/hr postoperatively, consider incomplete vagotomy or hypersecretion. 3) Determine gastrin level--Normal is <300 pg/mL; if >1,000 pg/mL, it indicates Zollinger-Ellison syndrome; if 300-1,000 pg/mL, the gastrin stimulation test needs to be performed.

Dumping syndrome--Early: diaphoresis, tachycardia, hypotension, giddiness, abdominal cramps, and diarrhea occur within 15-30 minutes after eating. Vasomotor symptoms are due to release of vasoactive substances (bradykinin, serotonin) into the portal blood and decreased circulating blood volume. Treatment--Frequent small meals low in carbohydrates. Dumping syndrome--Late: faintness, sweating, and coldness occur 1-3 hours after a meal. It resembles insulin reaction because the symptoms are due to a reactive hypoglycemia. Treatment--Frequent small meals low in carbohydrates. Somatostatin relieves the symptoms.

- Dumping syndrome--Early: diaphoresis, tachycardia, hypotension, giddiness, abdominal cramps, and diarrhea.
- Dumping syndrome--Late: faintness, sweating, and coldness due to hypoglycemia.
- Treatment: frequent small meals low in carbohydrates. Trial of somatostatin.

Diarrhea--Postgastrectomy diarrhea may result from many mechanisms. Malabsorption is caused by bacterial overgrowth or unmasking of a latent sprue or lactase deficiency. Postvagotomy diarrhea results from rapid gastric emptying, poor mixing of digestive enzymes, and decreased motility. It may be treated by frequent small meals low in carbohydrate and bulk (cholestyramine may help if rapid transit of bile acids is present). A special cause of diarrhea is gastrocolic fistula.

- Postgastrectomy diarrhea may result from malabsorption and postvagotomy diarrhea.

Gastrocolic fistula or gastrojejunocolic fistula--Abdominal pain that may be relieved by diarrhea, usually malabsorption. The differential diagnosis includes recurrent ulcer, cancer, and Crohn's disease. Colon radiography is the best test (upper gastrointestinal tract radiography detects only 50% of the fistulas).

- Colon radiography is the best test because upper gastrointestinal tract radiography detects only 50% of the fistulas.

Afferent loop syndromes: 1) Early--Postprandial bilious vomiting occurs 15-30 minutes after eating and is associated with nausea and abdominal discomfort. It occurs after Billroth II and results from partial obstruction of the afferent loop. Bile and pancreatic juice accumulate in the afferent loop, which eventually contracts and empties into the stomach. 2) Late (blind loop syndrome)--Bacterial overgrowth occurs in the afferent loop and causes malabsorption, because bile salts are deconjugated, and megaloblastic anemia, because bacteria use vitamin B_{12}. Treatment is to convert Billroth II to Billroth I or Roux-en-Y.

- Afferent loop syndrome (early) occurs after Billroth II and results from partial obstruction of the afferent loop.
- Blind loop syndrome is due to bacterial overgrowth in the afferent loop.

Alkaline reflux gastritis--Abdominal pain, anemia, bilious vomiting. It is caused by the reflux of bile into the stomach. Gastroscopy shows inflammation on the gastric side of anastomoses. It is more frequent with larger resections (i.e., more frequently with Billroth II than with Billroth I than with pyloroplasty). Medical treatment--Aluminum hydroxide gel (Amphojel) and cholestyramine are often unsuccessful. Surgical treatment is conversion to Roux-en-Y (good result in 90%-95% of patients).

- Alkaline reflux gastritis: abdominal pain, anemia, bilious vomiting; caused by reflux of bile.

Anemia--Iron deficiency is the commonest cause of anemia and results from blood loss, bypass of duodenum where iron is absorbed, and decreased acid, which is required to convert the ferric form of iron to the ferrous form, which is better absorbed. Treatment--Ferrous sulfate and vitamin C (also, treat inflammation to prevent blood loss). Vitamin B_{12} deficiency is caused by loss of intrinsic factor with gastric resection, gastritis, or bacterial overgrowth. Folate deficiency is due to poor intake.

- Iron deficiency is the commonest cause of anemia.
- Vitamin B_{12} deficiency: caused by loss of intrinsic factor with gastric resection.
- Folate deficiency: due to poor intake.

Weight loss most commonly is caused by a small gastric reservoir, but always rule out malabsorption and its causes (bacterial overgrowth, sprue, fistula).

Gastric stump cancer occurs 15-20 years postoperatively.

Osteomalacia--Decreased calcium and vitamin D absorption after duodenal bypass.

Susceptibility to infections (especially TB) is due to decreased acid.

Zollinger-Ellison Syndrome

Etiology and Pathogenesis

Zollinger-Ellison syndrome is acid hypersecretion secondary to a gastrinoma usually located in the pancreatic head. The duodenal wall is the most common extrapancreatic site (13%). The gastrinoma is solitary in 50% of cases. Two-thirds of them are malignant but usually indolent. Approximately 25% of patients with gastrinoma have multiple endocrine neoplasia syndrome type I. These patients usually have multiple gastrinomas. Increased gastric parietal cell mass is 2x-3x that of patients with duodenal ulcer.

- Zollinger-Ellison syndrome: acid hypersecretion secondary to gastrinoma.
- The gastrinoma is usually located in the pancreatic head.
- Two-thirds of them are malignant but usually indolent.
- Approximately 25% of the patients have multiple endocrine neoplasia syndrome type I.

Clinical Features

From 90% to 95% of patients with Zollinger-Ellison syndrome develop ulceration, 75% in the duodenal bulb. Diarrhea may precede ulcer symptoms. Diarrhea (present in 1/3 of the patients) is caused by large amounts of HCl secreted into the gastrointestinal tract, increased intestinal secretion, and reduced jejunal absorption. Steatorrhea may occur because of inactivation of pancreatic lipase and precipitation of bile salts. Vitamin B_{12} deficiency occurs secondary to acidic interference with intrinsic factor activity.

- Zollinger-Ellison syndrome: 90%-95% of patients develop ulceration, 75% in the duodenal bulb.
- Diarrhea may precede ulcer symptoms (present in 1/3 of patients).
- Steatorrhea may occur.

Gastrinoma should be considered (check serum level of gastrin) when any of the following are found: multiple ulcers in the upper gastrointestinal tract; ulcers distal to the first portion of the duodenum, intractable ulcers, recurrence postoperatively, unexplained secretory diarrhea, family history of peptic ulcer disease, history of parathyroid or pituitary tumors, gastric acid hypersecretion or hypergastrinemia, ulcer and hypercalcemia, or ulcer and diarrhea.

Diagnosis

Gastric acid secretion--Basal acid output is >15 mEq/hr, and the ratio of basal acid output to maximal acid output is >60%. The increase in acid output is proportionally less than

in normal subjects in response to exogenous stimulation (only 1/3 of patients). In patients who have had a previous ulcer operation, a basal acid output >5 mEq/hr suggests Zollinger-Ellison syndrome. Barium studies show prominent gastric rugal folds. The serum level of gastrin is the most sensitive and specific diagnostic test, but hypergastrinemia is seen in other disorders. Acid hypersecretion should be determined before conducting a provocative test. Secretin test--Normal values in patients with duodenal ulcer. Secretin decreases or has no effect on serum gastrin. In patients with Zollinger-Ellison syndrome, a marked increase in serum gastrin is seen. Levels increase promptly by at least 200 pg/mL. Findings are positive in 95% of those with gastrinoma. Standard meal--In Zollinger-Ellison syndrome, serum levels of gastrin do not increase or increase only slightly, but in gastrin cell hyperplasia, the increase is striking.

- Gastric acid secretion: basal acid output is >15 mEq/hr.
- Barium studies show prominent gastric rugal folds.
- Serum level of gastrin: most sensitive and specific test, but hypergastrinemia is seen in other disorders.
- Secretin test: normal values in patients with duodenal ulcer; in Zollinger-Ellison syndrome, gastrin increases in 95% of patients.

Tumor localization intraoperatively is difficult, and the tumor is not found in 40%-45% of patients. Selective arteriography detects 1/3 of the tumors. Computed tomographic (CT) scanning also detects 1/3 of them. Together, arteriography and CT scanning detect 44% of gastrinomas. Transhepatic portal venous sampling gives results comparable to those of CT.

- Localization of tumor intraoperatively is difficult.
- Selective arteriography detects 1/3 of the tumors.
- CT scanning detects 1/3 of the tumors.

Treatment

Medical treatment--H_2-receptor antagonists induce ulcer healing in 80%-85% of patients, often requiring high doses (5-9 g/day). With long-term treatment, as many as 50% of patients have failure with H_2 blockers. Omeprazole heals 90%-100% of ulcers in 4 weeks. Somatostatin decreases serum levels of gastrin and gastric acid secretion.

- H_2-receptor antagonists produce healing in 80%-85% of patients.
- Omeprazole heals 90%-100% of ulcers in 4 weeks.
- Somatostatin decreases serum levels of gastrin and gastric acid secretion.

Surgical treatment--Approximately 20%-25% of gastrinomas can be completely removed surgically. Surgical exploration, with intent to resect, should be done except in patients with extensive metastatic disease, surgical contraindications, or with multiple endocrine neoplasia type I syndrome. If the gastrinoma cannot be localized or resected, options include total gastrectomy and proximal gastric vagotomy (reduces gastric acid secretion and H_2- blocker requirements).

- 20%-25% of gastrinomas can be completely removed surgically.
- Surgical exploration should be done except in patients with extensive metastatic disease, surgical contraindications, or multiple endocrine neoplasia type I syndrome.

Prognosis

If resection is curative, life expectancy will be normal. If there are sporadic unresectable gastrinomas, the average life expectancy is 2 years.

Stress Ulcers

The underlying conditions for stress ulcers are trauma, sepsis, and serious illness. Most of the hemorrhages occur 3-7 days after the traumatic event. If no prophylactic treatment is given, 10%-20% of patients in Intensive Care Units have hemorrhaging. Burns, especially those involving >35% of the body, cause Curling's ulcer. Central nervous system trauma produces Cushing's ulcer, which is seen in 50%-75% of patients with head injury. Cushing's ulcer tends to be deep and to perforate more often than others.

- Underlying conditions for stress ulcers: trauma, sepsis, serious illness.
- Hemorrhaging occurs 3-7 days after the traumatic event.
- If no prophylactic treatment is given, 10%-20% of patients in Intensive Care Units develop hemorrhaging.
- Burns involving >35% of body have greater tendency to produce Curling's ulcer.
- Stress ulcers are seen in 50%-75% of patients with head injury.

Prophylaxis against bleeding is to keep pH >4.0. Antacids clearly decrease the incidence of bleeding over that of placebo. H_2-receptor antagonists are equally as effective as antacids and sometimes easier to use. Sucralfate is as effective as antacids and H_2 blockers, according to some studies. Also, sucralfate may decrease nosocomial pneumonia in ventilator-dependent patients, because gastric pH is not lowered (decreased bacterial overgrowth). Prostaglandins may have a role in prophylaxis. Enteral feedings can maintain intragastric pH >3.5. If antacids cannot be used, use H_2 blockers or sucralfate; combination treatment may be helpful.

- Prophylaxis: keep pH >4.0.
- Antacids, H_2-receptor antagonists, and sucralfate decrease incidence of bleeding.

- Sucralfate may decrease nosocomial pneumonia in ventilator-dependent patients.

Medical therapy for bleeding, acute gastric mucosal ulcers: correct the underlying predisposing condition. In general, upper gastrointestinal tract bleeding stops about 85% of the time. Some advocate use of iced saline lavage or intragastric levarterenol. Angiographic therapeutic techniques include intra-arterial vasopressin and transcatheter embolization. Endoscopic techniques are electrocautery (bicap heater probe) and laser photocoagulation. Surgical therapy for bleeding acute gastric mucosal ulcers must be considered when blood requirement is >4-6 units per 24-48 hours. The mortality rate for all forms of surgical therapy is 30%-40%.

Nonerosive Nonspecific Chronic Gastritis

Chronic gastritis is divided into two types: type A and type B. Type A, or autoimmune, gastritis involves the body and fundus of the stomach. A subset of patients develops atrophic gastritis (inflammation of the gland zone with variable gland loss). Pernicious anemia with hypochlorhydria or achlorhydria and megaloblastic anemia may result. Antiparietal cell antibodies are found in 90% of patients. Intrinsic factor antibodies are seen less commonly. Other autoimmune diseases such as Addison's disease and Hashimoto's thyroiditis are often present. Gastrin concentrations in the serum are increased. Gastric carcinoid tumors rarely develop. Gastric polyps occur, and intestinal metaplasia may be a precursor to gastric adenocarcinoma.

- Type A gastritis is associated with pernicious anemia and other autoimmune disorders.
- Serum levels of gastrin are increased.
- Type A gastritis is associated with gastric carcinoids, polyps, and adenocarcinoma.

Type B gastritis involves the antrum and is associated with *H. pylori* infection. Serum levels of gastrin are normal. Gastric ulcers and duodenal ulcers occur commonly, and there is increased incidence of gastric adenocarcinoma.

- Type B gastritis is associated with *H. pylori* infection.
- Serum levels of gastrin are normal.
- Type B gastritis is associated with gastric and duodenal ulcers and adenocarcinoma.

Gastric Cancer

In the 1940s, gastric cancer was the most common malignant disease in the U.S. Since then, the decrease in incidence has been dramatic. Japan has the highest mortality rate from gastric cancer. Migration studies show a decrease in incidence in migrants from high-risk areas to low-risk areas and a suggestion of increased risk in persons moving from low-risk to high-risk areas. Environmental factors include diet--increased association with starch, pickled vegetables, salted fish/meat, smoked foods, increased salt consumption, and nitrate and nitrite consumption. Genetic factors include blood group A, which has a 2x-3x greater incidence among relatives. The population at risk are persons older than 50 years. The male:female ratio is as high as 2:1. Also, it is more common in lower socioeconomic groups.

- Dramatic decrease in the incidence of gastric cancer in the U.S. since the 1940s.
- Decreased incidence in migrants from high-risk areas.
- Increased association with starch, pickled vegetables, salted fish/meat, smoked foods, increased salt consumption, and nitrate and nitrite consumption.
- A 2x-3x greater incidence among relatives.

Possible Precancerous Lesions/Situations

1) Chronic atrophic gastritis and intestinal metaplasia are frequently found in patients with gastric cancer (one study showed gastric cancer in 10% of those with atrophic gastritis followed up for 20 years compared with 0.6% in those with normal mucosa or superficial gastritis). However, both conditions are found frequently in older persons without gastric carcinoma. A subtype of intestinal metaplasia, with marked cell differentiation and production of sulfomucin (type IIb), may be the only type associated with gastric cancer. 2) Chronic benign gastric ulcer rarely progresses to cancer. 3) Pernicious anemia--previous autopsy studies showed an incidence of 10%. Recent endoscopic screening study of 123 patients with pernicious anemia showed a prevalence of gastric neoplastic lesions of 8.1%. 4) Postgastrectomy carries increased risk, although surveillance endoscopy is not necessary.

- Chronic atrophic gastritis is found frequently in patients with gastric cancer.
- A subtype of intestinal metaplasia, with production of sulfomucin (type IIb), is associated with gastric cancer.
- Chronic benign gastric ulcer rarely progresses to cancer.
- Pernicious anemia incidence of 10%.
- Postgastrectomy: increased risk.

Clinical Aspects

Gastric cancer is often asymptomatic, but abdominal discomfort and weight loss are the common presenting complaints. Physical examination is often unrevealing, but up to 30% of patients have an epigastric mass. Perform endoscopy, with multiple (7-8) biopsies and CT scanning of abdomen (to identify extragastric extension).

- Abdominal discomfort and weight loss are common presenting complaints.
- 30% of patients have an epigastric mass.
- Perform endoscopy, with multiple (7-8) biopsies.

Treatment and Prognosis

For local disease--Resection, often requires total gastrectomy for tumor-free margins. Omentum and spleen (splenic hilus nodes) are often removed in curative resection. For disseminated disease--Surgical treatment is necessary only for palliation. Response to chemotherapy is generally poor. The only consistent factor is extent of disease. Five-year survival is 90% if the tumor is confined to the mucosa and submucosa, 50% if the tumor is through the serosa, and 10% if the tumor involves lymph nodes.

- Gastric cancer often requires total gastrectomy.
- Surgical treatment is only necessary for palliation.

Gastric Polyps

Gastric polyps are rare; 0.5% incidence in an autopsy series. The two types of polyps are hyperplastic and adenomatous. Hyperplastic polyps are more common and not premalignant. No therapy is needed. Adenomatous polyps are premalignant, especially if >2 cm in size. They occur most often in achlorhydric stomachs, i.e., pernicious anemia, and are usually localized in the antrum. If pedunculated, the polyp can be removed endoscopically.

- Hyperplastic polyps are more common and not premalignant.
- Adenomatous polyps are premalignant, especially if >2 cm in size.

Gastroduodenal Dysmotility Syndromes

Symptoms that suggest abnormal gastric motility (i.e., gastroparesis) include nausea, vomiting, bloating, early satiety, dyspepsia, heartburn, anorexia, weight loss, and food avoidance. The specific cause of abnormal gastric motor function is unknown but is believed to be related to autonomic neuropathy. Diabetes mellitus is probably the most common medical cause of symptomatic gastric motor dysfunction. Conditions causing gastroparesis are listed in Table 8-5.

Table 8-5.--Conditions Causing Gastroparesis

Acute conditions	Chronic conditions
Anticholinergic drugs	Amyloidosis
Hyperglycemia	Diabetes mellitus
Hypokalemia	Gastric dysrhythmias
Morphine	Pseudo-obstruction
Pancreatitis	Scleroderma
Surgery	Vagotomy
Trauma	

- Nausea, vomiting, bloating, early satiety, dyspepsia, heartburn, anorexia, weight loss, and food avoidance suggest abnormal gastric motility.
- It is believed to be related to autonomic neuropathy.
- Diabetes mellitus: most common medical cause of symptomatic gastric motor dysfunction.

Treatment: currently, several prokinetic drugs are available in the U.S. These drugs normalize and/or augment motility, with an accompanying enhancement of aboral movement of luminal contents. Metoclopramide is a dopamine antagonist and a cholinergic agonist that increases the rate and amplitude of antral contractions. It crosses the blood-brain barrier and frequently causes such side effects as drowsiness, athetosis, and prolactin release. Domperidone is a selective dopamine antagonist that works only on peripheral receptors in the gut. It has no cholinergic effects and fewer side effects. Cisapride facilitates the release of acetylcholine from the myenteric plexus (local cholinergic agonist). It does not antagonize dopamine and has few side effects. Bethanechol is a systemic cholinergic agonist with side effects. It may be useful in low dosage in combination with other agents. Erythromycin stimulates both cholinergic and motilin receptors.

- Domperidone is a selective dopamine antagonist.
- Cisapride is a selective cholinergic agonist.
- Erythromycin stimulates both cholinergic and motilin receptors.

Percutaneous endoscopic gastrostomy--Easy to place, allows long-term access for enteral feeding. Complications include aspiration, plugging of the tube, tube migration, and leakage around the tube.

SMALL INTESTINE

Diarrhea

Patients use the term "diarrhea" to refer to any increase in the frequency, fluidity, or volume of the stool or any change in its consistency. Normally, stools are generally solid and brown, but these features may vary with diet. Frequency of stools varies among persons from 1-3 stools daily to 2-3 stools weekly. Blood, pus (leukocytes), and oil are not present in normal stools (Table 8-6).

Physicians define diarrhea as an increase in stool weight or volume. Because a stool is 65%-80% water, stool weight is proportional to stool water. Dietary fiber content influences the water content of the stool and, thus, stool weight can vary according to the diet of a culture. In the U.S., normal daily stool weight is <200 g/day and normal stool volume is <200 mL/day (compared with <400 g/day and 400 mL/day, respectively, in rural Africa).

It is important to understand normal daily intestinal fluid balance. Each day, 9-10 L of isotonic fluid is presented to the proximal small intestine (2 L, diet and 8 L, endogenous secretions). The small bowel absorbs most of the fluid (7-9 L), and the colon absorbs all the 1-2 L presented to it each day except <200 mL and forms a soft solid stool. There is considerable reserve because the maximal absorptive capacity of the small bowel is 12 L/day and 4-6 L/day for the colon.

Mechanisms of Diarrhea

Osmotic diarrhea occurs when water-soluble molecules are poorly absorbed, remain in the intestinal lumen, and retain water in the intestine. Osmotic diarrhea follows ingestion of an osmotically active substance and stops with fasting. Stool volume is <1 L/day, and the stool has an anion gap--stool osmolality is greater than the sum of electrolyte concentrations. Often, stool pH is <7.0. Clinical examples of osmotic diarrhea include lactase deficiency, sorbitol foods, saline cathartics, and antacids.

- In osmotic diarrhea, stool volume is <1 L/day.
- Diarrhea stops with fasting.
- Stool has an anion gap.
- Causes of osmotic diarrhea: lactase deficiency, sorbitol foods, and antacids.

In secretory diarrhea, fluid and electrolyte transport are abnormal, i.e., the intestine secretes rather than absorbs fluid. Stool volume is >1 L/day and its composition is similar to that of extracellular fluid so there is no anion gap. The diarrhea persists despite fasting and often presents with hypokalemia. Clinical examples of secretory diarrhea include bacterial toxins, hormonal tumors, surreptitious laxative ingestion, bile acid diarrhea, and fatty acid diarrhea.

- In secretory diarrhea, stool volume is >1 L/day.
- There is no anion gap.
- Diarrhea persists despite fasting.
- Causes of secretory diarrhea: bacterial toxins, hormonal tumors, surreptitious laxative ingestion, bile acid diarrhea, and fatty acid diarrhea.

Table 8-6.--Normal Stool Composition

		Electrolytes, mEq/L	
Weight	<200 g	Na^+	40
Percent water	65-80	K^+	90
Fat	<7 g	Cl^-	15
Nitrogen	<2.5 g	HCO_3^-	30

In exudative diarrhea, membrane permeability is abnormal, and there is exudation of serum proteins, blood, or mucus into the bowel from sites of inflammation, ulceration, or infiltration. The diarrhea is small volume and may be associated with bloody stools. Examples include invasive bacterial pathogens (*Shigella, Salmonella*, etc.) and inflammatory bowel disease.

- Exudative diarrhea: abnormal membrane permeability.
- Diarrhea is small volume.
- Invasive bacterial pathogens (*Shigella, Salmonella*, etc.) and inflammatory bowel disease.

Motility disorders: both rapid transit (inadequate time for chyme to contact absorbing surface) and delayed transit (bacterial overgrowth) can cause diarrhea. Rapid transit occurs after gastrectomy and intestinal resection and in hyperthyroidism and carcinoid syndrome. Delayed transit occurs with structural defects (strictures, blind loops, small-bowel diverticuli) or underlying illnesses that cause visceral neuropathy (diabetes) or myopathy (scleroderma), i.e., pseudo-obstruction.

- Rapid transit: causes diarrhea because of malabsorption.
- Delayed transit: causes diarrhea because of bacterial overgrowth.

Mixed mechanisms: many disease processes may have more than one mechanism for causing diarrhea, e.g., generalized malabsorption has osmotic and secretory components (fatty acids cause secretion in the colon).

Clinical Approach

It is useful to differentiate small-bowel ("right-sided") diarrhea from colonic ("left-sided") diarrhea (Table 8-7). Right-sided diarrhea is large in volume, with a modest increase in the number of stools. Symptoms attributed to inflammation of the rectosigmoid are absent, and proctoscopic examination findings are normal. Left-sided diarrhea presents as frequent

Table 8-7.--Right-Sided and Left-Sided Diarrhea: Contrasts in Clinical Presentation

Right-sided, or small-bowel, diarrhea	Left-sided, or colonic, diarrhea
Reservoir capacity intact	Reservoir capacity decreased
Large stool volume	Small amounts of stool
Modest increase in number	Frequency
No urgency	Urgency
No tenesmus	Tenesmus
No mucus	Mucus
No blood	Blood

small volume stools with obvious evidence of inflammation, and proctosigmoidoscopic examination usually confirms inflammation. Left-sided diarrhea usually suggests an exudative mechanism, whereas the mechanism for right-sided diarrhea is nonspecific.

Acute Diarrhea

Acute diarrhea is abrupt in onset and usually resolves in several days (3-10 days). It is self-limited, and the cause usually is not found (? viral). No evaluation is necessary unless there are bloody stools and fever or infection is suspected (e.g., travel history, common source outbreak). If these conditions exist, do not treat with antimotility agents. Begin the work-up with stool studies for ova and parasites and proctosigmoidoscopy. Recognize the common situations that predispose to specific infections (see infectious diarrhea below).

- For acute diarrhea, no evaluation is necessary unless there are bloody stools and fever or infection is suspected.
- Do not administer antimotility agents if there are bloody stools and if fever or infection is suspected.

Chronic Diarrhea

Chronic diarrhea is an initial episode lasting longer than 4 weeks or diarrhea that recurs after the initial episode. The most common cause of chronic diarrhea is irritable bowel syndrome, but always rule out lactase deficiency. Be able to differentiate organic diarrhea from functional diarrhea (Table 8-8).

- The most common cause of chronic diarrhea is irritable bowel syndrome.
- Always rule out lactase deficiency in suspected irritable bowel syndrome.
- Differentiate organic diarrhea from functional diarrhea.

Chronic Watery Diarrhea

The evaluation of chronic watery diarrhea usually requires distinguishing secretory diarrhea from osmotic diarrhea (Table 8-9). This can be done by collecting stools and measuring volume, osmolality, and electrolyte content and observing the patient's response to fasting.

- Evaluation of chronic watery diarrhea requires distinguishing secretory diarrhea from osmotic diarrhea.

Anatomy of Nutrient Absorption

The sites of nutrient, vitamin, and mineral absorption are the following: 1) the duodenum absorbs iron, calcium, magnesium, folate, water-soluble vitamins, and monosaccharides; 2) the jejunum absorbs fatty acids, amino acids, monosaccharides, and water-soluble vitamins; and 3) the ileum absorbs monosaccharides, fatty acids, amino acids, fat-soluble vitamins (A, D, E, K), vitamin B_{12}, and conjugated bile salts.

Table 8-8.--Features Differentiating Organic Diarrhea From Functional Diarrhea

	Organic diarrhea	Functional diarrhea
Weight loss	Often present	Not present
Duration of illness	Variable (weeks to years)	Usually long (>6 months)
Quantity of stool	Variable but usually large (>200 g/24 hr)	Usually small (<200 g/24 hr)
Presence of blood in stool	May be present	Never present (unless from hemorrhoids)
Timing when diarrhea occurs	No special pattern	Usually in the morning but rarely wakes patient
Fever, arthritis, skin lesions	May be present	Not present
Emotional stress	No relation to symptoms	Usually precedes or coincides with symptoms
Cramping abdominal pain	Often	May be present

From Matseshe JW, Phillips SF: Chronic diarrhea: a practical approach. Med Clin North Am 62:141-154, Jan 1978. By permission of WB Saunders Company.

Table 8-9.--Typical Findings in Osmotic and Secretory Diarrheas

	Osmotic diarrhea	Secretory diarrhea
Daily stool volume, L	<1	>1
Effect of 48-hr fasting	Diarrhea stops	Diarrhea continues
Fecal fluid analysis		
Osmolality, mOsm	400	290
Na + K x 2,[*] mEq/L	120	280
Solute gap[†]	>100	<50

[*]Multiplied by 2 to account for anions.

[†]Calculated by subtracting ([Na] + [K]) x 2 from osmolality.

From Krejs GJ, Hendler RS, Fordtran JS: Diagnostic and pathophysiologic studies in patients with chronic diarrhea. *In* Secretory Diarrhea. Edited by M Field, JS Fordtran, SG Schultz. Bethesda, MD, American Physiological Society, 1980, pp 141-151. By permission of publisher.

Table 8-10.--Mechanisms of Fat Malabsorption

Alteration	Mechanism	Disease state
Defective digestion	Inadequate lipase	Pancreatic insufficiency
Impaired micelle formation	Duodenal bile salt concentration	Common duct obstruction or cholestasis
Impaired absorption	Small-bowel disease	Sprue and Whipple's disease
Impaired chylomicron formation	Impaired β-globulin synthesis	Abetalipoproteinemia
Impaired lymphatic circulation	Lymphatic obstruction	Intestinal lymphangiectasia and lymphoma

The distal small bowel can adapt to absorb nutrients. The proximal small bowel cannot adapt to absorb vitamin B_{12} or bile salts. Fat absorption is the most complex process. Dietary fat consists mostly of triglycerides that must be digested by pancreatic lipase to fatty acids and glycerol, which are solubilized by micelles for absorption. The fatty acids and monoglycerides are reesterified by intestinal epithelial cells into chylomicrons that are absorbed into the circulation by lymphatic vessels (Table 8-10).

- The distal small bowel can adapt to absorb nutrients.
- The proximal small bowel cannot adapt to absorb vitamin B_{12} or bile salts.

Suspect malabsorption if the medical history suggests steatorrhea, or if there is diarrhea with weight loss (especially if intake is adequate), chronic diarrhea of indeterminate nature, or nutritional deficiency (know the symptoms and signs of malabsorption) (Table 8-11).

Table 8-11.--Causes of Symptoms in Malabsorption

Extra-gastrointestinal symptom	Result of
Muscle wasting, edema	Decreased protein absorption
Paresthesias, tetany	Decreased vitamin D and calcium absorption
Bone pain	Decreased calcium absorption
Muscle cramps	Weakness, excess potassium loss
Easy bruisability, petechiae	Decreased vitamin K absorption
Hyperkeratosis, night blindness	Decreased vitamin A absorption
Pallor	Decreased vitamin B_{12}, folate, or iron absorption
Glossitis, stomatitis, cheilosis	Decreased vitamin B_{12} or iron absorption
Acrodermatitis	Zinc deficiency

Table 8-12.--Associated Symptoms of Systemic Illnesses Causing Diarrhea

Symptom or sign	Diagnosis to be considered
Arthritis	Ulcerative colitis, Crohn's disease, Whipple's disease, *Yersinia* infection
Marked weight loss	Malabsorption, inflammatory bowel disease, cancer, thyrotoxicosis
Eosinophilia	Eosinophilic gastroenteritis, parasitic disease
Lymphadenopathy	Lymphoma, Whipple's disease
Neuropathy	Diabetic diarrhea, amyloidosis
Postural hypotension	Diabetic diarrhea, Addison's disease, idiopathic orthostatic hypotension
Flushing	Malignant carcinoid syndrome
Proteinuria	Amyloidosis
Peptic ulcers	Zollinger-Ellison syndrome
Hyperpigmentation	Whipple's disease, celiac disease, Addison's disease, pancreatic cholera, eosinophilic gastroenteritis

From Fine KD, Krejs GJ, Fordtran JS: Diarrhea. *In* Gastrointestinal Disease: Pathophysiology Diagnosis Management. Fourth edition. Edited by MH Sleisenger, JS Fordtran. Philadelphia, WB Saunders Company, 1989, pp 290-316. By permission of publisher.

- Diarrhea with iron deficiency anemia (evaluation for blood loss is negative) = proximal small bowel, e.g., sprue.
- Diarrhea with metabolic bone disease = decreased calcium and protein, thus, proximal small bowel.
- Hypoproteinemia with normal fat absorption suggests "protein-losing enteropathy." If eosinophilia is present, eosinophilic gastroenteritis; if lymphopenia is present, intestinal lymphangiectasia.
- Oil droplets (neutral fat) or muscle fibers (undigested protein) present in stool = pancreatic insufficiency (maldigestion).
- Serum levels of calcium, magnesium, and iron are usually normal in pancreatic insufficiency. Serum levels of albumin may also be normal.
- Howell-Jolly bodies (if there is no history of splenectomy) or dermatitis herpetiformis suggests celiac sprue (small-bowel biopsy is not diagnostic for sprue, but the response to gluten-free diet is).
- Fever, arthralgias, neurologic symptoms = Whipple's disease.

Helpful hints in the medical history, physical examination, or laboratory results may suggest the possibility of diarrhea or malabsorption (Table 8-12). Other hints in the history might include 1) age--youth suggests lactase deficiency, inflammatory bowel disease, or sprue, 2) travel--parasites, toxigenic agents (exposure to contaminated food or water), 3) drugs--laxatives, antacids, antibiotics, colchicine, lactulose, 4) family history--celiac sprue, inflammatory bowel disease, polyposis coli, lactase deficiency.

Medical history: previous surgery (short-bowel syndrome, dumping syndrome, blind loop syndrome, postvagotomy diarrhea, and ileal resection), radiation, systemic disease.

Diseases Causing Diarrhea

Osmotic Diarrhea

Lactase deficiency: lactose is normally split by lactase into glucose and galactose, which are absorbed in the small bowel. In lactase deficiency, lactose is not absorbed in the small intestine but enters the colon, where it is fermented in the lumen by bacteria to lactic acid. The result is diarrhea of low pH and increased intestinal motility. The most common disaccharidase deficiency is lactase deficiency. "Acquired" lactase deficiency (genetic?) is common in Orientals, blacks, Eskimos, and people from the Middle East. Diarrhea, abdominal cramps, and flatulence occur after ingestion of dairy products. There is improvement with diet. The pH of the stool is <6.0. Lactose tolerance test--Blood sugar increases <20 mg/100 mL after lactose ingestion. Abnormal H_2 breath test. Jejunal biopsy results are normal (disaccharidase levels are decreased). Lactose intolerance can occur in any clinical setting in which the intestinal mucosa is damaged.

- Lactase deficiency: lactose is not absorbed in the small intestine.
- Diarrhea of low pH and increased intestinal motility.
- The most common disaccharidase deficiency is lactase deficiency.
- Diarrhea, abdominal cramps, flatulence occur after ingestion of dairy products.
- Abnormal H_2 breath test.
- Patients on a weight reduction diet who drink diet soda or chew sugarless gum may develop osmotic diarrhea from sorbitol.

Secretory Diarrhea

Watery diarrhea, hypokalemia, achlorhydria--The WHDA or Verner-Morrison syndrome, also called "pancreatic cholera": it is a massive diarrhea (5 L/day) with dehydration and hypokalemia. The patient may have other multiple endocrine tumors (hypercalcemia, hyperglycemia). This diarrhea is associated with a non-beta islet cell tumor of the pancreas. Vasoactive intestinal peptide is the most common mediator, followed by prostaglandin, secretin, and calcitonin. Clinical recognition is by pancreatic scan/angiography and measurement of hormone levels. Treatment is with somatostatin or operation.

- Pancreatic cholera: massive diarrhea, dehydration, hypokalemia.
- Patients may have other multiple endocrine tumors.
- It is associated with a non-beta islet cell tumor of the pancreas.

Carcinoid syndrome: results from tumors of enterochromaffin cells of neural crest origin; 90% of the tumors are in the terminal ileum. There is episodic facial flushing (lasting up to 10 minutes), watery diarrhea, wheezing, right-sided valvular disease (endocardial fibrosis), and hepatomegaly. If the gut is normal, look for bronchial tumors or gonadal tumors. Dietary tryptophan is converted into serotonin (causes diarrhea, abdominal cramps [intestinal hypermotility], nausea, and

vomiting), histamine (responsible for the flushing chemicals (bradykinin, ACTH). Carcinoid syndrom that hepatic metastases are present. The diagnosis of noid syndrome is made by finding increased urinary levels 5-hydroxyindoleacetic acid (5-HIAA) and by liver biopsy. This syndrome is not associated with hypertension. Treatment is with octreotide.

Laxative abuse: of the population over age 60, 15%-30% take laxatives regularly. This is laxative abuse. With surreptitious laxative ingestion, patients complain of diarrhea but do not admit taking laxatives. In referral centers, this is the commonest cause of watery diarrhea. Proctoscopy reveals melanosis coli. Barium enema shows "cathartic colon"--dilated, hypomotile, absent haustra. Laxatives causing melanosis coli include anthracene derivatives (senna, cascara, aloe). Diagnosis--Stool phenophthalein. Address underlying emotional problems.

- Proctoscopy reveals melanosis coli.
- Barium enema shows "cathartic colon," i.e., dilated, hypomotile, absent haustra.
- Address underlying emotional problems.

Bile Acid Malabsorption

Bile acid malabsorption is caused by ileal resection or disease. The diarrhea due to bile acid malabsorption may produce two different clinical syndromes, each requiring a different treatment. 1) Limited resection (<100 cm). Malabsorbed bile acids enter the colon and stimulate secretion. Liver synthesis can compensate, so bile acid concentration in the upper small bowel is greater than the critical micelle concentration. No steatorrhea. Fecal fat is <20 g/24 hr. Treat with cholestyramine, which binds bile acids. 2) Extensive resection (>100 cm)--Bile acids are severely malabsorbed, and enterohepatic circulation is interrupted. This limits synthesis, and the liver cannot compensate. Bile acid concentration is decreased in the upper small bowel, micelles cannot be formed, and fat malabsorption results. The malabsorbed fatty acids themselves stimulate secretion in the colon. Treat with low-fat diet (<50 g/day), medium chain triglycerides. Cholestyramine would further decrease bile acid concentration and increase steatorrhea.

- Limited resection: treat with cholestyramine.
- Extensive resection: treat with low-fat diet, medium chain triglycerides.

Bacterial Overgrowth

The proximal small intestine is usually sterile. The major defense mechanisms in the proximal small bowel are gastric acid, normal peristalsis (the most important defense), and intestinal IgA. When defenses are altered, bacterial overgrowth results. The mechanism of steatorrhea is deconjugation of bile

e not present in the proximal
ile acids changes the ioniza-
ıgated bile acids can be pas-
small bowel. Normally, con-
bsorbed distally in the ileum.
concentration is not reached,
n the intraluminal deficiency
of bile acids.

- Normal peristalsis is the most important defense in the proximal small bowel.
- Deconjugated bile salts can be absorbed passively.
- Mild steatorrhea results from the intraluminal deficiency of bile acids.

Clinical features of bacterial overgrowth are steatorrhea (10-20 g/day), vitamin B_{12} malabsorption (macrocytic anemia), positive jejunal cultures (>10^5 organisms), and abnormal bile acid breath test. Breath test--bile acid breath test--^{14}C-labeled bile acids release $^{14}CO_2$ when deconjugated by bacteria in the gut. This test has low sensitivity (20%-30% false-negative).

Associated conditions--Postoperative (blind loops, enteroenterostomy, gastrojejunocolic fistula), structural (diverticula, strictures, fistulas), motility disorders (scleroderma, pseudo-

obstruction), achlorhydria (atrophic gastritis, gastric resections; achlorhydria corrects with antibiotics), and impaired immunity. Two types of the latter are hypogammaglobulinemic sprue (no plasma cells in lamina propria and flat villi on small-bowel biopsy) and nodular lymphoid hyperplasia associated with IgA deficiency--know radiographic appearance--predisposes to *Giardia lamblia* infection.

- Diarrhea, vitamin B_{12} deficiency, and above conditions suggest bacterial overgrowth.

Infectious Diarrheas

The toxigenic and invasive causes of bacterial diarrhea and the associated features are outlined in Tables 8-13 and 8-14.

Staphylococcus aureus: The diarrhea is of rapid onset; it lasts for 24 hours. There is no fever, vomiting, or cramps. The toxin is ingested in egg products, cream, and mayonnaise. Treatment is supportive.

Clostridium perfringens ("Church picnic"): The toxin is ingested in precooked foods, usually beef and turkey. Heat-stable spores produce toxins. Although the bacteria are killed and the toxin is destroyed, the spores survive. When food is rewarmed, the spores germinate, producing toxin. The diarrhea is worse than the vomiting and is later in onset. It lasts 24 hours. Treatment is supportive.

Table 8-13.--Causes of Bacterial Diarrhea: Toxigenic

Organism	Onset, hr	Mediated by cyclic Amp	Fever	Intestinal secretion
Staphylococcus aureus	1-6	+	-	+
Clostridium perfringens	8-12	-	±	+
Escherichia coli	12	+	+	+
Vibrio cholerae	12	+	Due to dehydration	++++
Bacillus cereus	1-6	+	-	+
	12-24	+	-	++++

Table 8-14.--Causes of Bacterial Diarrhea: Invasive

Organism	Fever	Bloody diarrhea	Bacteremia	Antibiotic effective
Shigella	+	+	+	+
Salmonella	+	-	-	-
Vibrio parahaemolyticus	+	+	-	+(?)
Escherichia coli	+	-	-	-
Staphylococcus aureus (enterocolitis)	+	+	±	+
Yersinia enterocolitica	+	+	+	?
Campylobacter	+	+	±	+
Vibrio vulnificus	+	+	+	+

E. coli ("Traveler's diarrhea"): The toxin is ingested in water and salads. It is a plasmid-mediated enterotoxin. Treatment is supportive. Prophylaxis is with doxycycline and bismuth subsalicylate (Pepto-Bismol). *E. coli* may be important in nursery epidemic diarrhea.

Vibrio cholerae: The toxin is ingested in water. It is the only toxigenic bacterial diarrhea in which antibiotics clearly shorten the duration of the disease. Treatment is with tetracycline.

Bacillus cereus: The source of the toxin is fried rice in oriental restaurants. One type has rapid onset and resembles *S. aureus* infection; the other type has a slower onset and resembles *C. perfringens* infection. The diagnosis is made by isolating the organism from contaminated food and by the medical history. Treatment is supportive.

Other toxigenic bacteria: *C. botulinum* produces a neurotoxin that is ingested in improperly home-processed vegetables, fruits, and meats. It interferes with the release of acetylcholine from peripheral nerve endings. *C. difficile*--See antibiotic/pseudomembranous colitis.

- Toxigenic bacterial diarrhea: watery; no fecal leukocytes.
- *S. aureus*: rapid onset.
- *C. perfringens*: "church picnic diarrhea," precooked foods, later in onset.
- *E. coli*: "traveler's diarrhea."
- *B. cereus*: fried rice in oriental restaurants.

Bacterial Diarrhea (Invasive)

Shigella: It is often acquired outside the U.S. Bloody diarrhea is characteristic, and fever and bacteremia occur. Diagnosis is based on positive stool and blood cultures. Treatment is with ampicillin. Resistant strains are emerging for which chloramphenicol is an alternative. (Plasmids are responsible for antibiotic deactivation resistance.)

Salmonella (non-*typhi*): In U.S., *Salmonella typhimurium* is the most common agent. The toxin is ingested with poultry. Fever is present. The absence of bloody diarrhea is the main characteristic that distinguishes it from *Shigella* infection. Diagnosis is based on positive stool culture. Treatment is supportive. Do not use antibiotics, which prolong the carrier state and do not affect the course of the disease. Use antibiotics only if blood cultures are positive.

Vibrio parahaemolyticus: The toxin is ingested with undercooked shellfish. This infection is increasing in frequency in the U.S. (it is common in Japan). Fever and bloody diarrhea are the chief characteristics. Diagnosis is based on positive stool culture. Antibiotics are of questionable value in treating this infection, but erythromycin may be most effective.

E. coli: Invasive *E. coli* is rare. It presents as fever and bloody diarrhea with profound toxicity.

S. aureus (enterocolitis): Diagnosis is based on positive stool culture or Gram's stain, which shows predominance of gram-positive cocci and a paucity of other organisms.

- Invasive bacterial diarrhea: fever, bloody stools, and fecal leukocytes.
- *Shigella*: bloody diarrhea.
- *S. typhimurium*: no bloody diarrhea; treat with antibiotics only if blood cultures are positive.
- *V. parahaemolyticus*: undercooked shellfish, bloody diarrhea.

"Newer" Enteric Bacterial Pathogens

Yersinia enterocolitica: The spectrum of disease includes acute enteritis and chronic enteritis. Acute enteritis is similar to shigellosis and usually lasts 1-3 weeks. It is characterized by fever, diarrhea, leukocytosis, and fecal leukocytes. Chronic enteritis is found especially in children. There is diarrhea, failure to thrive, hypoalbuminemia, and hypokalemia. Other features are acute abdominal pain (mesenteric adenitis), right lower quadrant pain, tenderness, nausea, and vomiting. It mimics appendicitis or Crohn's disease. This gram-negative rod is hardy and can survive in cold temperatures. It grows on special medium (cold enriched). It is an invasive pathogen. Fecal-oral transmission in water and milk (isolate the patient).

Extraintestinal manifestations are nonsuppurative arthritis and ankylosing spondylitis (in HLA-B27). Skin manifestations are erythema nodosum and multiforme. Thyroid manifestations are Graves' disease and Hashimoto's disease. Multiple liver abscesses and granulomata are present.

Treatment is with aminoglycosides, trimethoprim-sulfamethoxazole (Bactrim). The bacteria are variably sensitive to tetracycline and chloramphenicol. Beta lactamases are frequently produced. Penicillin resistance is common.

- *Y. enterocolitica* infection: acute abdominal pain (differential diagnosis includes appendicitis and Crohn's disease).
- Fecal-oral transmission in water and milk.
- Manifestations include nonsuppurative arthritis and ankylosing spondylitis (in HLA-B27).

Campylobacter jejuni: These are comma-shaped, motile, microaerophilic gram-negative bacilli. Transmission is linked to infected water, unpasteurized milk, poultry, sick dogs, and infected children. The incubation period is 2-4 days before invasion of the small bowel. Infection results in the presence of blood and leukocytes in the stool. It may mimic granulomatous or idiopathic ulcerative colitis. It may also mimic small-bowel secretory diarrhea, with explosive, frequent watery diarrhea due to many species that produce a cholera-type toxin. The diarrhea usually lasts 3-5 days but may relapse. Antibiotic treatment is with erythromycin when severe, but treatment often is not needed. Postdiarrheal illnesses are hemolytic uremic syndrome and postinfectious arthritis.

- *C. jejuni*: transmission linked to infected water, unpasteurized milk, poultry, sick dogs, and infected children.
- May mimic granulomatous or idiopathic ulcerative colitis.

- Diarrhea: usually lasts 3-5 days but may relapse.

Enterohemorrhagic *E. coli*: There is a grossly bloody stool and abdominal pain but no fever. Hemolytic uremic syndrome--large quantities of Shiga-like toxin that is difficult to detect. A useful marker is the inability to ferment sorbitol. Food: hamburger.

- Grossly bloody stool and abdominal pain but no fever.
- May cause hemolytic uremic syndrome.
- Hamburger.

Vibrio vulnificus (noncholera): The organisms are extremely invasive and produce necrotizing vasculitis, gangrene, and shock. They are routinely isolated from seawater, zooplankton, and shellfish along the Gulf of Mexico and both coasts of the U.S., especially in the summer. Two clinical syndromes are 1) wound infection, cellulitis, fasciitis, or myositis after exposure to seawater or cleaning shellfish and 2) septicemia after ingesting raw shellfish (oysters). Patients at high risk for septicemia include those with liver disease, congestive heart failure, diabetes mellitus, renal failure, immunosuppressive states, or hemochromatosis. Treatment is with tetracycline.

- *V. vulnificus* is extremely invasive, producing necrotizing vasculitis, gangrene, and shock.
- Wound infection, cellulitis, fasciitis, or myositis occurs after exposure to seawater or cleaning shellfish.
- Septicemia occurs after ingesting raw shellfish (oysters).

Aeromonas hydrophilia: Previously, the pathogenicity of the bacteria was questioned. Although the infection is often mistaken for that of *E. coli*, *A. hydrophilia* is now recognized as an increasingly frequent cause of diarrhea after swimming in fresh or salt water. The organism produces several toxins. Treatment is with trimethoprim-sulfamethoxazole and tetracycline.

Malabsorption Due to Diseases of the Small Intestine

Celiac Sprue

Celiac sprue is a gluten-sensitive enteropathy. It presents in children as growth retardation, and in adults as an iron deficiency that is unresponsive to iron given orally. Osteomalacia can be present without steatorrhea if the proximal small bowel is involved. Splenic atrophy and abnormal blood smear with Howell-Jolly bodies may be clues to the diagnosis in 10%-15% of patients. Skin manifestation is dermatitis herpetiformis. Small-bowel biopsy is *not* diagnostic, but response to gluten-free diet is diagnostic. If the patient is unresponsive to the diet, review the diet for inadvertent gluten ingestion. If unresponsive after 10-15 years of successful dietary management, rule out lymphoma (especially if there is also abdominal pain).

- Celiac sprue: iron deficiency that is unresponsive to iron given orally; osteomalacia with or without steatorrhea.
- Splenic atrophy and abnormal blood smear with Howell-Jolly bodies may be clues to the diagnosis in 10%-15% of patients.
- Lymphoma is a late complication.

Tropical Sprue

In tropical sprue, diarrhea occurs 2-3 months after travel to the tropics. After 6 months, megaloblastic anemia develops because of folate deficiency and possible coexisting vitamin B_{12} deficiency. The infectious agents are *Klebsiella* and *E. coli*. Small-bowel biopsy shows blunted villi similar to those in celiac sprue. Treatment is with tetracycline (250 mg four times daily) and folate with or without vitamin B_{12}.

- Tropical sprue: diarrhea and megaloblastic anemia after travel to the tropics.
- Cause: coliforms bacteria (*Klebsiella* more than *E. coli*).
- Treatment: tetracycline (250 mg 4 times daily) and folate with or without vitamin B_{12}.

Whipple's Disease

Whipple's disease is a systemic infectious disease involving the CNS, heart, kidneys, and small bowel. It is caused by gram-positive bacilli. Small-bowel biopsy shows PAS-positive granules in the macrophages. Suspect Whipple's disease in patients with recurrent arthritis, pigmentation, adenopathy, or CNS symptoms (dementia, myoclonus, ophthalmoplegia, visual disturbances, coma, seizures). Treatment is with tetracycline or with minocycline if CNS symptoms develop.

- Suspect Whipple's disease in patients with recurrent arthritis, pigmentation, adenopathy, and CNS symptoms.
- Small-bowel biopsy shows PAS-positive granules in the macrophages.
- Treatment: tetracycline or minocycline if CNS symptoms develop.

Eosinophilic Gastroenteritis

Patients with eosinophilic gastroenteritis have a history of allergies (asthma, etc.) and food intolerances and episodic symptoms of nausea, vomiting, abdominal pain, and diarrhea. Laboratory findings include eosinophilia, iron deficiency anemia, and steatorrhea or protein-losing enteropathy. Small-bowel radiographs show coarse folds and filling defects, and biopsy shows infiltration of the eosinophils in the mucosa and, occasionally, absence of villi. Rule out parasitic infection. Treatment with steroids produces a rapid response.

- Mucosal eosinophilic gastroenteritis: allergies, food intolerances, and eosinophilia, and episodic intestinal symptoms.

- Rule out parasitic infection.
- Steroids produce a rapid response.

Systemic Mastocytosis

Systemic mastocytosis is a proliferation of mast cells in the skin (urticaria pigmentosa), bones, lymph nodes, and parenchymal organs. Histamine is released, and 50% of patients have gastrointestinal symptoms, i.e., diarrhea and peptic ulcer. "Bath pruritus" (itching after hot bath) is a clue to the diagnosis.

- Systemic mastocytosis causes urticaria pigmentosa.
- 50% of patients have gastrointestinal symptoms.
- "Bath pruritus" is a clue to the diagnosis.

Intestinal Lymphangiectasia

Intestinal lymphangiectasia is a disorder due to lymphatic obstruction. Hypoplastic lymphatics cause lymph to leak into the intestine. The clinical features are edema (often unilateral leg edema), chylous peritoneal or pleural effusions, and steatorrhea or protein-losing enteropathy. Laboratory findings include lymphocytopenia (average, 600/mm^3) due to enteric loss. All serum proteins are decreased, including immunoglobulins. Small-bowel radiographs show edematous folds, and small-bowel biopsy shows dilated lacteals and lymphatics in the lamina propria that may contain lipid-laden macrophages. The same biopsy findings are seen in obstruction of mesenteric nodes (lymphoma, Whipple's disease, Crohn's disease) and obstruction of venous inflow to the heart (constrictive pericarditis, severe right-sided heart failure). Diagnosis is based on abnormal small-bowel biopsy findings and documented enteric protein loss. Treatment is with low fat diet and medium chain triglycerides (they enter the portal blood rather than lymphatics). Occasionally, surgical excision of the involved segment is useful if the lesion is localized.

- Intestinal lymphangiectasia: unilateral lymphedema of the leg and chylous peritoneal or pleural effusions.
- Lymphocytopenia is universal.
- Decreased serum proteins.
- Small-bowel biopsy shows dilated lacteals and lymphatics.
- Treatment: low fat diet and medium chain triglycerides.

Amyloidosis

Systemic amyloidosis is characterized by a diffuse deposition of an amorphous eosinophilic extracellular protein polysaccharide complex in the tissue. The major sites of amyloid deposition are blood vessel walls and the mucous membranes and muscle layers of the intestine. Any portion of the gut can be involved. Amyloid damages tissues by infiltration (muscle and nerve infiltration causes motility disorders, malabsorption) and ischemia (obliteration of vessels causes ulceration and bleeding). Intestinal dysmotility can produce diarrhea, constipation, pseudo-obstruction, megacolon, and fecal incontinence. Clinical findings in amyloidosis include macroglossia, hepatomegaly, cardiomegaly, proteinuria, and peripheral neuropathy. Pinch (post-traumatic) purpura or periorbital proctoscopic purpura occurs. Diagnosis--Small-bowel radiography shows symmetrical, sharply demarcated thickening of the valvulae conniventes. Fat aspirate confirms the diagnosis in 90%-95% of patients and rectal biopsy in 70%-85%.

Miscellaneous Small-Bowel Disorders

Meckel's diverticulum, the persistence of the vitelline duct, is the most frequent developmental abnormality of the gut. It usually is found within 100 cm from the ileocecal valve on the antimesenteric border of the ileum. It contains all layers of the intestinal wall and so is a true diverticulum. The mucosa is usually ileal but may be gastric (pancreatic, intestinal). Complications include obstruction due to intussusception and volvulus around the band fixing the diverticulum to the bowel wall. Benign (leiomyomas) and malignant (carcinoids, leiomyosarcoma) tumors have been found in diverticula. Diverticulitis is uncommon. Incarceration in an indirect inguinal hernia (Littre's hernia) and perforation that causes peritonitis may occur. Hemorrhage is the common complication and results from ulceration of the ileal mucosa adjacent to the gastric mucosa. This accounts for 50% of the cases of lower gastrointestinal tract bleeding in children and young adults. Radiography usually is not helpful in making the diagnosis. A nuclear scan (parietal cells concentrate technetium) may show the diverticulum, but false-positive and false-negative results can occur.

- Meckel's diverticulum is the most frequent developmental abnormality of the gut.
- It accounts for 50% of the cases of lower gastrointestinal tract bleeding in children and young adults.

Aortoenteric fistula: A history of gastrointestinal tract bleeding in a patient who has had a previous aortic graft demands immediate evaluation to rule out an enteroenteric fistula. If the patient presents with massive bleeding, do not attempt endoscopy or arteriography. Emergency surgery is indicated.

- If a patient presents with massive bleeding, do not attempt endoscopy or arteriography. Emergency surgery is indicated.

Chronic Intestinal Pseudo-Obstruction

Pseudo-obstruction is a syndrome characterized by the clinical findings of mechanical bowel obstruction but without occlusion of the lumen. The two types are primary and secondary. The primary type, also called idiopathic pseudo-obstruction, is a visceral myopathy or neuropathy. The secondary type is due to underlying systemic disease or precipitating causes.

Idiopathic (primary) pseudo-obstruction is associated with recurrent attacks of nausea, vomiting, cramping abdominal pain, distension, and constipation, which are of variable intensity and duration. If it is a familial cause, the patient will have a positive family history and the condition will be present at a young age. Esophageal motility is abnormal (achalasia) in most patients. Occasionally, urinary tract motility is abnormal, and diarrhea or steatorrhea results from bacterial overgrowth. Upper gastrointestinal tract and small-bowel radiographs show dilatation of the bowel and slow transit (not mechanical obstruction).

- Idiopathic pseudo-obstruction is due to a familial cause or to sporadic visceral myopathy or neuropathy.
- Recurrent attacks have variable frequency and duration.
- Abnormal esophageal motility occurs in most patients.
- Steatorrhea is caused by bacterial overgrowth.

Secondary pseudo-obstruction is due to underlying systemic disease or precipitating causes. These causes include the following (significant causes to remember are in italics):

1. Diseases involving the intestinal smooth muscle--*amyloidosis*, scleroderma, systemic lupus erythematosus, myotonic dystrophy, and muscular dystrophy.
2. Neurologic diseases--*Parkinson's disease*, Hirschsprung's disease, Chagas' disease, and familial autonomic dysfunction.
3. Endocrine disorders--*myxedema* and hypoparathyroidism.
4. Drugs--*antiparkinsonian medications* (*L-dopa*), phenothiazines, tricyclic antidepressants, ganglionic blockers, clonidine, and narcotics.

Approach to the Patient With Chronic Intestinal Pseudo-Obstruction

First, a mechanical cause for obstruction must be ruled out. Second, look for an underlying precipitating cause such as metabolic abnormalities, medications, or an underlying associated disease. If a familial idiopathic cause is suspected, assess esophageal motility. Suspect scleroderma if intestinal radiography shows large-mouth diverticula of the small and large intestines. Suspect amyloidosis if the skin shows palpable purpura and proteinuria and neuropathy are present.

- Secondary pseudo-obstruction is due to an underlying systemic disease or precipitating cause.
- Scleroderma presents as large-mouth diverticula of the intestine.
- Amyloidosis presents with palpable purpura, proteinuria, and neuropathy.

Inflammatory Bowel Disease

"Idiopathic inflammatory bowel disease" refers to two disorders of unknown cause: chronic ulcerative colitis and Crohn's disease. Other possible causes of inflammation, especially infection, should be excluded before making the diagnosis of idiopathic inflammatory bowel disease.

Ulcerative colitis is a mucosal inflammation involving only the colon. Crohn's disease is a transmural inflammation that can involve the intestine anywhere from the esophagus through the anus. The rectum is involved in about 95% of patients with ulcerative colitis and in only 50% of those with Crohn's disease. Ulcerative colitis is a continuous inflammatory process extending from the anal verge to more proximal colon (depending on the extent of the inflammation). Crohn's disease is a segmental inflammation in which inflamed areas alternate with virtually normal areas. Ulcerative colitis usually presents as frequent bloody bowel movements with minimal abdominal pain, whereas Crohn's disease presents with fewer bowel movements, less bleeding, and, more commonly, abdominal pain. Crohn's disease is associated with intestinal fistula and fistula to other organs as well as perianal disease. Ulcerative colitis does not form fistulas; perianal disease is uncommon. Strictures of the intestine are common with Crohn's disease but rare in ulcerative colitis (when they are present, they suggest cancer).

- Ulcerative colitis involves only the colon.
- Crohn's disease can involve the intestine anywhere from the esophagus through the anus.
- Ulcerative colitis is a continuous process.
- Crohn's disease is a segmental inflammation.
- Ulcerative colitis has frequent bloody bowel movements.
- Crohn's disease has fewer bowel movements, less bleeding, and more abdominal pain.
- Crohn's disease is associated with intestinal fistula, strictures, and perianal disease.

Extraintestinal Manifestations of Inflammatory Bowel Disease

Arthritis occurs in 10%-20% of patients, usually monoarticular or pauciarticular involvement of large joints. Joint symptoms mirror bowel activity, i.e., joints flare when colitis flares and joints improve as colitis improves. Also, ankylosing spondylitis (relationship with HLA-B27) and sacroiliitis--which are usually progressive and do not improve when colitis improves--can develop.

- The joint symptoms mirror bowel activity.
- Anklyosing spondylitis and sacroiliitis can develop.

Skin lesions occur in 10% of patients. The three types of lesions are erythema nodosum, pyoderma gangrenosum, and aphthous ulcers of the mouth. All these skin conditions usually improve with treatment of colitis. Severe, refractory skin disease is an indication for surgical treatment.

- The skin lesions are erythema nodosum, pyoderma gangrenosum, and aphthous ulcers of the mouth.

Eye lesions occur in 5% of patients. The lesion is usually episcleritis and/or uveitis. These usually improve with treatment of inflammatory bowel disease.

Liver disease also occurs in 5% of patients. Primary sclerosing cholangitis is more common in chronic ulcerative colitis than in Crohn's disease. If the alkaline phosphatase level is increased in a patient with inflammatory bowel disease, the work-up for primary sclerosing cholangitis includes ultrasonography, endoscopic retrograde cholangiopancreatography, and liver biopsy.

- If increased alkaline phosphatase occurs with inflammatory bowel disease, rule out primary sclerosing cholangitis.

Renal stones occur in 5%-15% of patients. In Crohn's disease with malabsorption, calcium oxalate stones occur. In chronic ulcerative colitis, uric acid stones are due to dehydration and loss of bicarbonate in the stool, leading to acidic urine.

Indications for Colonoscopy

Colonoscopy is indicated for evaluating the extent of the disease and for stricture (biopsy) and filling defect (biopsy). It is also indicated for differentiating Crohn's colitis from ulcerative colitis when the two are otherwise indistinguishable. Another indication is for monitoring by random mucosal biopsy the development of dysplasia or cancer.

- Know the indications for colonoscopy in inflammatory bowel disease.

Toxic Megacolon

In patients with active inflammation, avoid the causes of toxic megacolon, including aerophagia, opiates, anticholinergics, hypokalemia, and barium enema.

- In patients with active inflammation, avoid the causes of toxic megacolon.

Treatment of Ulcerative Colitis

Medical: 5-Aminosalicylic acid (ASA) (the active agent) is bound to sulfapyridine (vehicle). Colonic bacteria break the bond, releasing 5-ASA. 5-ASA is not absorbed but stays in contact with the mucosa and exerts its anti-inflammatory action. The efficacy of 5-ASA may be related to its ability to inhibit the lipoxygenase pathway of arachidonic acid metabolism or its ability to function as an oxygen free-radical scavenger (further studies are needed). It is effective in acute disease and in maintaining remission. Side effects (male infertility, malaise, nausea, pancreatitis, rashes, headaches, hemolysis, impaired folate absorption, hepatitis, aplastic anemia, and exacerbation

of colitis) occur in 30% of patients who take sulfasalazine and are related to the sulfapyridine moiety. 5-ASAs are a group of new drugs that deliver 5-ASA to the intestine in various ways. They eliminate sulfa toxicity but are more expensive than sulfasalazine. Two of these drugs are mesalamine and olsalazine. Mesalamine can be given topically (Rowasa suppositories, Rowasa enema) or orally (Asacol, 5-ASA coated with acrylic polymer that releases 5-ASA in the terminal ileum, and Pentasa, ethyl cellulose coating releases 50% of the 5-ASA in the small bowel). Olsalazine consists of two 5-ASA molecules conjugated with each other. Bacteria break the bond, releasing 5-ASA into the colon.

Aminosalicylates are used for mild to moderately active ulcerative colitis and in Crohn's disease. Topical forms are useful in proctitis or left-sided colitis; systemic forms are used for pancolitis. Although 80%-90% of patients do not tolerate sulfasalazine, they do tolerate oral 5-ASA preparations. Side effects include hair loss, pancreatitis (often in patients who developed pancreatitis while taking sulfasalazine), reversible worsening of underlying renal disease, and exacerbation of colitis.

- Sulfasalazine is effective in acute disease and in maintaining remission.
- Sulfasalazine: side effects occur in 30% of patients.
- Aminosalicylates are equally effective but more expensive; they are useful in 80%-90% of patients intolerant to sulfasalazine.

Corticosteroids--Topical preparations should be used twice daily for patients with active mild to moderate disease that is limited to the distal colon. Corticosteroids should be added to the regimen of patients with more proximal disease if sulfasalazine does not control the attacks. Up to 50% of the dose can be absorbed (depending on the preparation used and its vehicle). Oral preparations are indicated in active pancolonic disease of moderate severity in doses of 40-60 mg once daily or 20-40 mg daily in cases of mild disease that are unresponsive to topical steroids and sulfasalazine. Prednisolone, the active metabolite, is the preferred form of drug in patients with cirrhosis (these patients may not be able to convert inactive prednisone to prednisolone). For patients with a prompt response to oral corticosteroids, the dose may be tapered gradually at a rate not to exceed a 5-mg reduction in the total dose every 3-7 days. Intravenous preparations should be used in large doses (prednisolone, 100 mg in divided doses) for up to 10-14 days in severely ill patients. At that time, if there is improvement, it should be possible to convert the medication to oral corticosteroids (60-100 mg/day). If there is no improvement, surgical intervention (colectomy) is required. Corticosteroids are not believed to prevent relapse and therefore should not be used after the patient has complete remission and is symptom-free.

- Prescribe topical preparations twice daily for patients with active mild to moderate disease that is limited to the distal colon.
- Corticosteroids should be added to the regimen of patients with more proximal disease if systemic steroids and sulfasalazine have not controlled the attacks.
- Oral preparations are useful in active pancolonic disease of moderate severity.
- Intravenous preparations are used for severely ill patients.

Total parenteral nutrition does not alter the clinical course of an ongoing attack. Indications for its use include: 1) severe dehydration and cachexia with marked fluid and nutrient deficits, 2) excessive diarrhea that has failed to respond to standard therapy for chronic ulcerative colitis, and 3) debilitated patients undergoing colectomy. Opiates (or their synthetic derivatives) and anticholinergics are contraindicated in chronic ulcerative colitis because they are ineffective and can contribute to the development of toxic megacolon.

- Total parenteral nutrition does not alter the clinical course of the ongoing attack.
- Use of opiates and anticholinergics is contraindicated in chronic ulcerative colitis.

Surgical: Surgical treatment is curative in chronic ulcerative colitis. Indications for colectomy are severe intractable disease, acute life-threatening complications (perforation, hemorrhage, toxic megacolon unresponsive to treatment), symptomatic colonic stricture, and suspected or documented colon cancer. Other indications include intractable moderate to severe colitis, refractory uveitis or pyoderma gangrenosum, growth retardation in pediatric patients, cancer prophylaxis, or inability to taper a regimen to low doses of steroids (i.e., <15 mg/day) over a period of 2-3 months. Procedures include proctocolectomy with ileoanal anastomosis, Koch pouch, or conventional Brooke ileostomy.

- Surgical treatment is curative in chronic ulcerative colitis.

Treatment of Crohn's Disease

Medical: For sulfasalazine, see Treatment of Ulcerative Colitis above. This drug is more effective for colonic disease than for small-bowel disease, although 5-ASA products designed to be released and activated in the small bowel may prove to be effective in the colon. Sulfasalazine does not have an additive effect or a steroid-sparing effect when used with corticosteroids, nor does it maintain remission in Crohn's disease as it does in ulcerative colitis. Nothing is effective in the prophylaxis of Crohn's disease.

- Sulfasalazine is more effective for colonic disease than for small-bowel disease.

- It does not have an additive effect or sparing effect when used with corticosteroids.
- It does not maintain remission in Crohn's disease.

Corticosteroids, see Treatment of Ulcerative Colitis above. The agents that most quickly control an acute exacerbation of Crohn's disease are corticosteroids. They are the most useful drugs for treating small-bowel Crohn's disease.

Azathioprine, in the National Crohn's Disease Cooperative Study, was not significantly different from placebo with regard to therapeutic response. However, this study has been criticized because azathioprine was given for a short period of time and its potential beneficial effect may have been missed--4-6 months are needed to realize any benefit from immunosuppressive drugs like azathioprine or 6-mercaptopurine. Azathioprine is associated with a higher rate of lymphoma than 6-mercaptopurine.

- Azathioprine is not significantly different from placebo with regard to therapeutic response.
- It is associated with a higher rate of lymphoma than 6-mercaptopurine.

6-Mercaptopurine, the active metabolite of azathioprine, has a steroid-sparing effect. Its use should be reserved for patients with active disease who are taking steroids when there is need to reduce the steroid dose (or to maintain a given dose in the face of worsening disease activity).

- 6-Mercaptopurine is the active metabolite of azathioprine.
- It has a steroid-sparing effect.

Metronidazole (at a dose of 20 mg/kg) is quite effective for treating perineal disease. Six weeks may be needed for the therapeutic effect to become manifest; unfortunately, recurrences often occur when the drug dose is tapered or discontinued, leading to chronic therapy. It is as effective as sulfasalazine for disease of the colon. If a patient is unresponsive to sulfasalazine, it is worthwhile switching to metronidazole, but not vice versa. It is less effective for small-bowel disease. Side effects include glossitis, metallic taste, vaginal and urethral burning sensation, neutropenia, dark urine, urticaria, disulfiram (Antabuse) effect, and paresthesias.

- Metronidazole is quite effective for perineal disease.
- Recurrences are frequent when the drug dose is tapered or discontinued.
- It is as effective as sulfasalazine for disease of the colon.

Nutrition--Bowel rest per se does not have any role in achieving remission in Crohn's disease. However, providing adequate nutritional support does help facilitate remission--any form of nutritional support is acceptable as long as it is adequate in amount. Adequate nutrition can be essential in maintaining growth in children with severe Crohn's disease.

Surgical: If Crohn's disease is present during exploration for presumed appendicitis, the acute ileitis should be left alone (many of these patients do not develop chronic Crohn's disease). An appendectomy can be performed if the cecum and appendix are free of disease. Of the Crohn's patients receiving surgical treatment, 70%-90% require reoperation within 15 years (many within the first 5 years after the initial operation). The anastomotic site is the most likely site for recurrence of disease. Indications for surgical treatment include intractable symptoms, acute life-threatening complications, obstruction, unhealed fistulas that cause complications, abscess formation, and malignancy.

- 70%-90% of Crohn's patients operated on require reoperation within 15 years.
- The anastomotic site is the most likely site for disease recurrence.

GASTROINTESTINAL MANIFESTATIONS OF AIDS

Gastrointestinal symptoms occur in 30%-50% of North American and European patients with AIDS and in nearly 90% of the patients in developing countries. The most frequent gastrointestinal tract symptom is diarrhea, which is often chronic and associated with weight loss. Dysphagia, odynophagia, abdominal pain, and jaundice are less frequent. Gastrointestinal tract bleeding is rare. The goal of evaluation is to identify treatable causes of infection or symptoms.

- The majority of AIDS patients with diarrhea have one or more identifiable pathogens.
- Some have no identifiable cause despite extensive evaluation. This may represent idiopathic AIDS enteropathy or, as yet, unidentified pathogens.

The gastrointestinal tract in AIDS is predisposed to a spectrum of viral, bacterial, fungal, and protozoan pathogens.

Viral

Cytomegalovirus

Cytomegalovirus is one of the most common and potentially serious opportunistic pathogens. It most commonly affects the colon and esophagus, although the entire gut, liver, biliary tract, and pancreas are susceptible. There is a patchy or diffuse colitis that may progress to ischemic necrosis and perforation. Symptoms: watery diarrhea and fever; less commonly, hematochezia and abdominal pain. Diagnosis: biopsy specimens show cytomegalic inclusion cells with surrounding inflammation (owl's eye). Treatment: ganci-

clovir, 5 mg per kg twice daily for 14-21 days. If resistant, use foscarnet.

Herpes Simplex Virus

The three gastrointestinal tract manifestations of herpes simplex virus infection in patients with AIDS are perianal lesions (chronic cutaneous ulcers), proctitis, and esophagitis. The organs affected are the colon and esophagus. Symptoms: perianal lesions are painful; proctitis causes tenesmus, constipation, and inguinal lymphadenopathy; and esophagitis causes odynophagia, with or without dysphagia. Diagnosis: cytologic identification of intranuclear (Cowdry's type A) inclusions in multinucleated cells. Diagnosis is confirmed by viral cultures. Treatment: acyclovir given orally or intravenously.

Adenovirus

Adenovirus recently has been reported to cause diarrhea. The organ affected is the colon. Symptoms: watery, nonbloody diarrhea. Diagnosis: culture and biopsy. Treatment: none.

Bacteria

Mycobacterium avium-intracellulare

Infection of the gut occurs in patients with disseminated disease. The small intestine is affected more commonly than the colon. Symptoms: fever, weight loss, diarrhea, abdominal pain, and malabsorption. Diagnosis: acid-fast organisms in the stool and tissue confirmed by culture from stool and biopsy specimens. Treatment: multiple drug therapy with ethambutol, rifampin, ciprofloxacin, and clarithromycin.

Salmonella (typhimurium and enteritidis)

Treatment is with amoxicillin, trimethoprim-sulfamethoxazole, or ciprofloxacin.

Shigella flexneri

Treatment is with trimethoprim-sulfamethoxazole, ampicillin, or ciprofloxacin.

Campylobacter jejuni

Treatment is with erythromycin or ciprofloxacin.

Salmonella, Shigella flexneri, and Campylobacter jejuni have a substantially higher incidence of intestinal infection, bacteremia, and prolonged or recurrent infections in AIDS patients because of antibiotic resistance or compromised immune function or both.

Fungi

Candida albicans

In AIDS patients, Candida causes locally invasive mucosal disease in the mouth and esophagus. Disseminated candidiasis is rare because neutrophil function remains relatively intact. The presence of oral candidiasis in persons at risk for AIDS should alert the physician to possible HIV infection. If oral candidiasis is present, endoscopy is required to confirm esophageal involvement. Symptoms: odynophagia suggests esophageal involvement. Diagnosis: histologic examination shows hyphae, pseudohyphae, or yeast forms. Treatment: nystatin, ketoconazole, fluconazole, or amphotericin.

Histoplasma capsulatum

Histoplasma capsulatum is an important opportunistic infection in AIDS patients who reside in endemic areas. Colonic involvement is more common than small bowel involvement. Symptoms: diarrhea, weight loss, fever, and abdominal pain. The diagnosis is established by culture. Colonoscopy may show inflammation and ulcerations and histologic examination with Giemsa staining shows intracellular yeast-like *Histoplasma capsulatum* within lamina propria macrophages. Treatment: amphotericin or itraconazole.

Protozoa

Cryptosporidium

Cryptosporidium is among the commonest enteric pathogens, occurring in 10%-20% of patients with AIDS and diarrhea in the U.S. and in 50% of those in developing countries. The organs affected are the small and large intestines and the biliary tree. Symptoms: voluminous watery diarrhea, severe abdominal cramps, weight loss, anorexia, malaise, and low-grade fever. Biliary tract obstruction has been reported. Diagnosis: microscopic identification of organisms in stool specimens with modified acid-fast staining or specific *Cryptosporidium* stains. Organisms may also be identified in biopsy specimens or in duodenal fluid aspirates. Treatment: none is known.

Isospora belli

Isospora belli is the more common cause of diarrhea in developing countries. It resembles *Cryptosporidium* oocysts. The small intestine is affected primarily, but the organisms can be identified throughout the gut and in other organs. Symptoms: watery diarrhea, cramping abdominal pain, weight loss, anorexia, malaise, and fever. Diagnosis: oval oocysts in stool seen with modified Kinyoun acid-fast stain. Biopsy specimen from small intestine may show organisms in the lumen or within cytoplasmic vacuoles in enterocytes. *Isospora belli* oocysts contain two sporoblasts and differ from *Cryptosporidium* oocysts, which are small, round, and contain four sporozoites. Treatment: trimethoprim-sulfamethoxazole.

Microsporidia (enterocytozoon bieneuisi)

Microsporidia are emerging as an important pathogen; the organisms have been identified in up to 33% of AIDS patients

with diarrhea. The organ affected is the small intestine. Symptoms: watery diarrhea with gradual weight loss but no fever and no anorexia. Diagnosis: based on electron microscopic identification of round-to-oval meront (proliferative) and sporont (spore-forming) stages of Microsporidia in the villous but not crypt epithelial cells of the duodenum and jejunum. There are reports of positive stool specimens with Giemsa staining. Treatment: none known.

Entamoeba histolytica

Treatment is with metronidazole.

Giardia lamblia

Treatment is with metronidazole.

Blastocystis hominis

Because there is no evidence that *Blastocystis hominis* is pathogenic, it does not need to be treated.

The rates of symptomatic infection with *Entamoeba histolytica, Giardia lamblia,* and *Blastocystis hominis* are not significantly higher than in non-HIV patients. *Entamoeba histolytica* is a nonpathogenic commensal in most patients with AIDS. Giardiasis may require prolonged treatment, as in other immunocompetent persons.

DIAGNOSTIC EVALUATION OF PATIENTS WITH AIDS WHO HAVE DIARRHEA

Initial studies include 1) examination for stool leukocytes; 2) stool cultures for *Salmonella* species, *Shigella flexneri,* and *Campylobacter jejuni* (at least three specimens); 3) stool examination for ova and parasites (using saline, iodine, trichrome, and acid-fast preparations), and 4) stool assay for *Clostridium difficile* toxin. Additional studies include 1) gastroscopy to inspect tissue, aspirate luminal material, and obtain biopsy specimens; 2) examining duodenal aspirate for parasites and culture; 3) duodenal biopsy specimens cultured for cytomegalovirus and mycobacteria; 4) colonoscopy to inspect tissue and obtain biopsy specimens; 5) biopsy specimens cultured for cytomegalovirus, adenovirus, mycobacteria, and herpes simplex virus; 6) biopsy specimens stained with hematoxylin-eosin for protozoa and viral inclusion cells, with methenamine silver or Giemsa stain for fungi, and with Fite for mycobacteria.

If the initial studies and the additional studies listed above do not yield a diagnosis, then there is controversy about further evaluation. Most experts advocate empiric treatment with loperamide (Imodium). Others recommend that biopsy specimens from the duodenum be examined with electron microscopy for Microsporidia or from the colon for adenovirus. I favor empiric treatment with loperamide, because there is no treatment for either Microsporidia or adenovirus.

COLON

Pseudomembranous Enterocolitis

This is a necrotizing inflammatory disease of the intestines characterized by the formation of a membrane-like collection of exudate overlying a degenerating mucosa. Associated conditions are colon obstruction, uremia, ischemia, intestinal surgery, and all antibiotics (except vancomycin).

Antibiotic Colitis

The symptoms of antibiotic colitis are fever, abdominal pain, and diarrhea (mucus and blood), which usually occur 1-6 weeks after antibiotic therapy. Sigmoidoscopy shows pseudomembranes and friability. Biopsy reveals inflammation and microulceration with exudation. The condition usually remits, but it recurs in 15% of cases. Complications include perforation and megacolon. Pathogenesis--The antibiotic alters colonic flora so there is overgrowth of *Clostridium difficile*. The toxin produced by *C. difficile* is cytotoxic, causing necrosis of the epithelium and exudation (pseudomembranes). Diagnosis--Toxin assay is positive in 98% of cases, and cultures are positive in about 75%. Radiography reveals pseudomembranes. Proctoscopic findings may be normal or show classic pseudomembranes. Treatment--Discontinue use of antibiotics and provide general supportive care (fluids, etc.). Avoid use of antimotility agents. If no response, metronidazole, 250 mg three times daily, is 80% effective and inexpensive. Vancomycin, 125 mg four times daily, is also 80% effective but very expensive. If the patient is very ill, cholestyramine binds toxin. For first recurrence, the same antibiotic can be used or the drug can be switched. For multiple recurrences, add cholestyramine and prolong the course of treatment with antibiotics.

- Antibiotic colitis: symptoms include fever, abdominal pain, diarrhea 1-6 weeks after antibiotic therapy.
- Toxin assay is positive in 98% of patients.
- Culture is positive in 75%.
- Metronidazole is the initial treatment.
- 15% have recurrence.

Radiation Colitis

Radiation injury usually affects both the colon and the small bowel. Endothelial cells of small submucosal arterioles are very radiosensitive and respond to large doses of radiation by swelling, proliferating, and undergoing fibrinoid degeneration. The result is an obliterative endarteritis. Disease spectrum--1) Acute disease occurs during or immediately after radiation; the mucosa fails to regenerate, and there is friability, hyperemia, and edema. 2) Subacute disease occurs 2-12 months after radiation. Obliterative endarteritis produces progressive inflammation and ulcer-

ation. 3) Chronic disease consists of fistulas, abscesses, strictures, and bleeding from intestinal mucosal vessels. Predisposing factors include 1) other diseases that produce microvascular insufficiency, e.g., hypertension, diabetes mellitus, atherosclerosis, and heart failure, because they accelerate the development of vascular occlusion; 2) total radiation dose of 40-50 Gy; 3) previous chemotherapy; 4) adhesions; 5) previous surgery and pelvic inflammatory disease; and 6) age, the elderly are more susceptible. Radiography of acute disease shows fine serrations of the bowel, and of chronic disease, stricture of the rectum. Endoscopy shows atrophic mucosa with telangiectatic vessels. Treatment--Endoscopic coagulation is effective.

- Radiation colitis involves both the colon and the small bowel.
- The endothelial cells of the small submucosal arterioles are very radiosensitive.
- The result is obliterative endarteritis.
- Predisposing factors: hypertension, diabetes mellitus, atherosclerosis, chemotherapy, and >40 Gy of radiation.
- The rectum is involved most commonly.

Ischemia

Review of Vascular Anatomy

The celiac trunk supplies the stomach and duodenum. The superior mesenteric artery supplies the jejunum, ileum, and right colon. The inferior mesenteric artery supplies the left colon and rectum.

Acute Ischemia

The symptoms of acute ischemia are sudden severe abdominal pain, vomiting, and diarrhea (with or without blood). Early in the course of ischemia, physical examination findings are normal, but later findings indicate peritonitis. Risk factors include severe atherosclerosis, congestive heart failure, atrial fibrillation (source of emboli), hypotension, and oral contraceptives.

There are several syndromes. 1) Acute mesenteric ischemia is due to obstruction of the superior mesenteric artery in 80% of cases. Most (95%) emboli lodge in this artery because of laminar flow, vessel caliber, and the angle it takes off from the aorta. The clue to search for emboli is atrial fibrillation. This syndrome results in a loss of small bowel and produces short-bowel syndrome. Radiography shows ileus, small-bowel obstruction, and, later, gas in the portal vein. The treatment is embolectomy, which has a 90% mortality rate. 2) Ischemic colitis is due to poor perfusion. It commonly involves areas of the colon between adjacent arteries, i.e., "watershed areas," such as the splenic flexure and rectosigmoid. This syndrome presents with abdominal pain and rectal bleeding. Radiography: thumbprinting of watershed areas is characteristic on radiography. The treatment is supportive and, if the condition deteriorates, surgical resection. 3) Nonocclusive ischemia is due to poor tissue perfusion caused by inadequate cardiac output. It can involve both the small and the large bowel. Its distribution does not conform to an area supplied by a major vessel. It occurs in patients with cardiac failure or anoxia or who are in shock. It is questioned whether digitalis causes mesenteric vasoconstriction.

- Acute superior mesenteric artery syndrome is usually due to emboli.
- Ischemic colitis: diagnosis is based on radiographic finding of thumbprinting of watershed areas.

Chronic Ischemic Colitis

Chronic ischemic colitis is uncommon. Symptoms include postprandial pain and fear of eating (weight loss). At least two of three major splanchnic vessels must be occluded. It is associated with hypertension, diabetes mellitus, and atherosclerosis. Abdominal bruit is a clue to the diagnosis. Angiography is diagnostic in about 50% of cases and shows a stenotic area in two of three major vessels. Treatment is with surgical revascularization.

Occlusion of the superior mesenteric vein accounts for approximately 10% of the cases of bowel ischemia. Risk factors include hypercoagulable states such as polycythemia vera, liver disease, pancreatic cancer, intra-abdominal abscess, and portal hypertension. It presents as abdominal pain that gradually becomes severe. Diagnosis is based on angiographic findings. Treatment is surgical.

- Chronic ischemic colitis is associated with hypertension, diabetes mellitus, and atherosclerosis.
- Mesenteric venous thrombosis occurs with hypercoagulable states.

Amebic Colitis

The colon is the usual site of the disease initially. Symptoms vary from none to explosive bloody diarrhea with fever, tenesmus, and abdominal cramps. Proctoscopy shows discrete ulcers with undermined edges and normal adjacent mucosa. If an exudate is present, swab and make wet mount preparations for trophozoites. Indirect hemagglutination is useful for invasive disease. Radiography shows concentric narrowing of the cecum in 90% of cases. Treat with metronidazole (Flagyl). *Entamoeba histolytica* is the only pathogenic ameba.

- The colon is the initial site of disease.
- Proctoscopy shows discrete ulcers with undermined edges.
- Radiography shows concentric narrowing of the cecum in 90% of cases.
- *Entamoeba histolytica* is the only pathogenic ameba.

Tuberculosis

Tuberculosis presents as diarrhea, a change in bowel habits, and rectal bleeding. The ileocecal area is the most commonly involved site. Radiography shows a contracted cecum and ascending colon and ulceration. Proctoscopy reveals deep and superficial ulcers. The rectum may be spared. A hypertrophic ulcerating mass may be seen. Biopsy samples stained with Ziehl-Neelsen stain are positive for acid-fast bacilli. All cases are associated with pulmonary or miliary tuberculosis.

- Tuberculosis is associated with diarrhea, change in bowel habits, and rectal bleeding.
- The ileocecal area is commonly involved.
- Deep and superficial ulcers are characteristic findings.
- All cases are associated with pulmonary or miliary tuberculosis.

Streptococcus bovis endocarditis is associated with colon disease (diverticulosis or cancer). The colon should be evaluated.

Irritable Bowel Syndrome

Colon motility (and small bowel motility) is the only abnormality. Gas production is not increased. Always rule out lactase deficiency. It is a diagnosis of exclusion (requires negative evaluation).

Nontoxic Megacolon (Pseudo-Obstruction)

Acute pseudo-obstruction of the colon occurs postoperatively (nonabdominal operations) and with spinal cord injury, sepsis, uremia, electrolyte imbalance, and drugs (narcotics, anticholinergics, and psychotropic agents). When the cecum is >13-14 cm in diameter, the risk of perforation increases. Obstruction should be ruled out with Hypaque enema. Treatment includes placement of a nasogastric tube, discontinuation of drug therapy, correction of metabolic abnormalities, and, if needed, colonoscopic decompression or cecostomy.

Chronic pseudo-obstruction of the colon is seen in disorders that cause generalized intestinal pseudo-obstruction.

Congenital Megacolon

Congenital megacolon (Hirschsprung's disease) occurs in 1 of 5,000 births. There is increased incidence with Down syndrome. Congenital megacolon usually becomes manifest in infancy; however, it can present in adulthood. There is a variable length of aganglionic segment from the rectum to the proximal colon (usually confined to rectum or rectosigmoid). The diagnosis is usually made at birth because of meconium ileus or obstipation. If the diagnosis is made in an adult, the patient has a history of chronic constipation. Colon radiographs show a characteristically narrowed distal segment and a dilated proximal colon. Rectal biopsy shows aganglionosis.

Anorectal manometry shows loss of the anorectal reflex. Treatment: sphincter-saving operations.

- Congenital megacolon: increased incidence with Down syndrome.
- In adult, chronic constipation.
- Colon radiographs show characteristically narrowed distal segment and dilated proximal colon.
- Rectal biopsy shows aganglionosis.
- Motility: absent and rectal inhibitory reflex.

Lower Gastrointestinal Tract Bleeding

The evaluation of rectal bleeding should begin with the digital examination, anoscopy, and proctosigmoidoscopy. If a definitive diagnosis cannot be made, next perform a barium enema or arteriography, depending on the nature of the bleeding. The inability to cleanse the colon appropriately during active bleeding makes the barium enema difficult to perform and interpret. Some advocate use of nuclear scanning if the activity of the bleeding is uncertain. With active bleeding, angiography is the diagnostic procedure of choice. It is also indicated for patients with recurrent episodes of rectal bleeding who have had normal results on previous standard tests, i.e., barium enema or colonoscopy. Colonoscopy is not useful if lower gastrointestinal tract bleeding is torrential, but it may be of some benefit if there is a slower rate of bleeding. Colonoscopy is valuable for evaluating patients with unexplained rectal bleeding and persistently positive findings on tests for occult blood in the stool.

- Initial evaluation of rectal bleeding: digital examination, anoscopy, and proctosigmoidoscopy.
- If activity of bleeding is uncertain, try bleeding scan.
- Colonoscopy is not useful if there is torrential lower gastrointestinal tract bleeding.
- Angiography is the procedure of choice for active bleeding.

The important causes of lower gastrointestinal tract bleeding are:

- Angiodysplasia--it usually involves the right colon and small bowel and may respond to endoscopic treatment.
- Diverticular disease--there is usually bleeding without other symptoms.
- Inflammatory bowel disease (colitis)--5% of patients present with this.
- Ischemic colitis--painful and bloody diarrhea.
- Cancer--it rarely causes significant bleeding.
- Meckel's diverticulum--it is the commonest cause of lower gastrointestinal tract bleeding in young patients. It is usually painless.

- Hemorrhoids--they are usually present as rectal outlet bleeding.

Evaluation of lower gastrointestinal tract bleeding: stabilize the patient, perform proctoscopy to rule out rectal outlet bleeding, and obtain nasogastric tube aspirate or use esophagogastroduodenoscopy to rule out upper gastrointestinal tract bleeding. Radionuclide-tagged red blood cell scan may help determine if bleeding is occurring, but it may not precisely localize the bleeding site. If there is active bleeding, perform angiography. If bleeding stops or occurs at a slow rate, perform colonoscopy. If the patient is young, perform Meckel's scan.

Treatment: If angiography localizes the bleeding site, vasopressin, infusion, or embolization may be useful. If the bleeding is found by colonoscopy, epinephrine injection, electrocoagulation, or laser coagulation may be useful. If bleeding is massive or if significant bleeding continues, surgical management is needed.

Diverticular Disease of the Colon

Definitions

Diverticula are acquired herniations of the mucosa and submucosa through the muscular layers of the colonic wall. *Diverticulosis* is the mere presence of uninflamed diverticula of the colon. *Diverticulitis* is the inflammation of one or more diverticula. The diagnosis and management of the complications of diverticular disease are outlined in Table 8-15.

Diverticulitis

Microperforation or macroperforation of the diverticulum with subsequent peridiverticular inflammation is necessary to produce diverticulitis. The severity of the clinical symptoms depends on the extent of the inflammation. Free perforation is infrequent (diverticula are invested by longitudinal muscle and mesentery). Local perforations may dissect along the colon wall and form intramural fistulas. The clinical presentation is left lower quadrant pain, fever, abdominal distension, constipation, and, occasionally, a palpable tender mass. Treatment includes resting the bowel or using a low fiber diet and antibiotics and obtaining an early surgical consultation. Indications for surgical treatment during the acute phase include the development of generalized peritonitis, an enlarging inflammatory mass, fistula formation, colonic obstruction, inability to rule out a carcinoma in an area of stricture, or recurrent episodes of diverticulitis.

- Diverticulitis: the clinical symptoms depend on the extent of inflammation.
- Free perforation is infrequent.
- Clinical presentation: left lower quadrant pain, fever, abdominal distension, constipation, and, occasionally, a palpable tender mass.

- Treatment: rest bowel, give antibiotics, and obtain a surgical consultation.

Angiodysplasia

Angiodysplasia is a common and increasingly recognized cause of lower gastrointestinal tract bleeding in elderly patients. Acquired vascular ectasias are believed to be associated with aging. Angiodysplasia is associated with cardiac disease, especially aortic stenosis. It usually involves the cecum and the ascending colon. There are no associated skin or visceral lesions. The ectasias appear to be due to the chronic, partial, intermittent, and low-grade obstruction of submucosal veins where they penetrate the colon. Obstruction is from muscle contraction and distension of the cecum. Colon radiography is of no diagnostic value. Angiography localizes the extent of involvement. Colonoscopy may show lesions. Apply cautery.

- Acquired vascular ectasias are associated with aging.
- Angiodysplasia is associated with cardiac disease, especially aortic stenosis.
- It usually involves the cecum and ascending colon.
- Colonoscopy may show lesions. Apply cautery.

Colon Polyps

Types of epithelial polyps include: 1) hyperplastic polyps--metaplastic, completely differentiated glandular elements; they are benign. 2) Hamartomatous polyps--mixture of normal tissues; they are benign. 3) Inflammatory polyps--epithelial inflammatory reaction; they are benign. 4) Adenomatous polyps--failure of differentiation of glandular elements. They are the only neoplastic (premalignant) polyp. The three types of adenomatous polyps are tubular adenoma, mixed (tubulovillous) adenoma, and villous adenoma (syndrome of hypokalemia, profuse mucus). The risk of cancer in any adenomatous polyp depends on two features: size >1 cm and presence of villous elements. If a polyp is found on flexible sigmoidoscopy and biopsy shows hyperplastic polyp, no further work-up is needed. If biopsy shows adenomatous polyp, perform colonoscopy to look for additional polyps and to perform polypectomy.

- Adenomatous polyps are the only neoplastic (premalignant) polyp; there are three types.
- The risk of cancer in any adenomatous polyp depends on: size >1 cm and presence of villous elements.
- If biopsy shows adenomatous polyp, perform colonoscopy.

Hereditary Polyposis Syndromes

Only those polyposis syndromes associated with adenomatous polyps have risk of cancer.

Familial polyposis: adenomatous polyps of the colon. More than 95% of the patients develop colorectal carcinoma. There are no extra-abdominal manifestations except for bilateral congenital hyperplasia of the retinal pigment epithelium. Diagnosis

Table 8-15.--Diagnosis and Management of Complications of Diverticular Disease

Complication	Symptoms	Findings	Treatment
Diverticulitis	Pain, fever, and constipation or diarrhea (or both)	Palpable tender colon, leukocytosis	Liquid diet, with or without antibiotics or elective surgery
Pericolic abscess	Pain, fever (with or without tenderness), or pus in stools	Tender mass, guarding leukocytosis, soft tissue mass on abdominal films or ultrasonography	Nothing by mouth, intravenous fluids, antibiotics, early surgical treatment with colostomy
Fistula	Depends on site: dysuria, pneumaturia, fecal discharge on skin or vagina	Depends on site: fistulogram, methylene blue	Antibiotics, clear liquids, colostomy, and, later, resection
Perforation	Sudden severe pain, fever	Septic patient, leukocytosis, free air	Antibiotics, nothing by mouth, intravenous fluids, immediate surgical treatment
Liver abscess	Right upper quadrant pain, fever, weight loss	Tender liver, tender bowel or mass, leukocytosis, alkaline phosphatase, lumbosacral scan (filling defect)	Antibiotics, surgical drainage, operation for bowel disease
Bleeding	Bright red or maroon blood, or clots	Blood on rectal exam, sigmoidoscopy, colonoscopy, angiography	Conservative: blood transfusion if needed, with or without operation

is based on family history and documentation of adenomatous polyps. Screening of all family members is indicated, and colectomy is indicated before malignancy develops.

- More than 95% of patients with familial polyposis develop colorectal carcinoma.
- There are no extra-abdominal manifestations.
- Colectomy is indicated before malignancy develops.

Gardner's syndrome: adenomatous polyps involving the colon, although the terminal ileum and proximal small bowel are rarely involved. More than 95% of the patients develop colorectal cancer. Extraintestinal manifestations include congenital hypertrophy of the retinal pigment epithelium; osteomas of the mandible, skull, and long bones; supernumerary teeth; soft tissue tumors; thyroid and adrenal tumors; and epidermoid and sebaceous cysts. Screening of family members is indicated, and colectomy should be performed before malignancy develops.

- More than 95% of patients with Gardner's syndrome develop colorectal cancer.
- There are extraintestinal manifestations.
- Screening of family members is indicated.

Turcot-Despres syndrome: adenomatous polyps of the colon associated with malignant gliomas and other brain tumors. Autosomal recessive inheritance.

Polyposis Syndromes Not Associated With Risk of Cancer

Peutz-Jeghers syndrome: hamartomas of the small intestine and less commonly of the stomach and colon. Pigmented lesions of the mouth, hands, and feet are associated with ovarian sex cord tumors and tumors of the proximal small bowel.

- Peutz-Jeghers syndrome: hamartomas of the small intestine.
- Pigmented lesions of the mouth, hands, and feet are associated with ovarian sex cord and proximal small bowel tumors.

Juvenile polyposis: hyperplastic polyps involving the colon and, less commonly, the small intestine and stomach. It presents as gastrointestinal tract bleeding or intussusception with obstruction.

- Only adenomatous polyps are premalignant.
- Perform colectomy for diffuse polyposis only if they are adenomatous.
- Screen family of patients with heritable polyposis syndromes only if the polyps are adenomatous.
- All the above syndromes are autosomal dominant except Turcot-Despres syndrome.

Colorectal Cancer

Epidemiology

Epidemiology is important in etiologic theories. Colorectal carcinoma is the second most common cancer in the U.S. There are 100,000 new cases and 60,000 deaths annually. Six percent of Americans eventually develop colon cancer. The mortality rate has not decreased since the 1930s. The incidence varies widely among different populations; it is highest in "westernized" countries. Compared with past rates, rates for cancer of the right colon and sigmoid colon are increased but decreased for the rectum: cecum/ascending colon, 25%; sigmoid, 25%; rectum, 20%; transverse colon, 12%; rectosigmoid, 10%; and descending colon, 6%.

- Colorectal cancer is the second most common cancer in the U.S.
- There are increased rates for cancer of the right colon and sigmoid colon.

Etiology

The role of the environment as a cause of colorectal cancer is supported by regional differences and migrant studies of incidence. Diet--High fat diet increases the risk and may enhance cholesterol/bile acid content of bile which is converted by colonic bacteria to compounds that may promote tumors. High fiber diet is protective. Increased stool bulk may dilute carcinogens/promoters and decrease exposure by decreasing transit time. Fiber components may bind carcinogens or decrease bacterial enzymes that form toxic compounds. Charbroiled meat/fish and fried foods contain possible mutagens. Antioxidants (vitamins A and C), selenium, vitamin E, yellow-green vegetables, and calcium may protect against cancer.

- High fat diet increases the risk of colorectal cancer.
- High fiber diet has a protective effect.
- Charbroiled meat/fish and fried foods contain possible mutagens.

Genetic Factors

Certain oncogenes amplify or alter gene products in colon cancer cells. Aneuploidy is characteristic of more aggressive tumors. The carbohydrate structure of colonic mucus is altered in colon cancer. Cell-cell interaction possibly has a role in cancer development. Also, genetic predisposition has a role in many colon cancer patients. Familial adenomatous polyposis syndromes are autosomal dominant. There is autosomal dominant inheritance of cancer family syndromes (cancer of other sites as well as of the colon) and hereditary site-specific colon cancer. Colorectal cancer appears in the 40-50 age group (20 years earlier than in the general population). Discrete polyps may precede cancer but not diffuse polyposis. Genetic susceptibility in the general population also has a role, e.g., a

3x increased risk of colorectal cancer in first-degree relatives of patients with sporadic colorectal cancer.

- Aneuploidy is characteristic of more aggressive tumors.
- Genetic predisposition to cancer exists in many colon cancer patients.
- Familial adenomatous polyposis is autosomal dominant.
- There is a 3x increased risk of colorectal cancer in first-degree relatives of patients with sporadic colorectal cancer.

Risk Factors for Colorectal Cancer

The risk factors for colorectal cancer include the following: 1) age greater than 40--the risk increases sharply at age 40, doubles each decade until age 60, and peaks at age 80. 2) Personal history of adenoma or colon cancer--the risk increases with the number of adenomas; 2%-6% patients with colon cancer have synchronous colon cancer and 1.1%-4.7% have metachronous cancers. 3) Family history of colon cancer. 4) Inflammatory bowel disease--dysplasia precedes cancer. Cancer rate begins to increase after 7 years of chronic ulcerative colitis and increases 10% per decade of disease. After 25 years the risk is 30%. The risk is greatest for universal colitis. The risk is delayed a decade in left-sided colitis and is negligible in ulcerative proctitis. Cancer risk is *not* related to severity of the first attack, disease activity, or age at onset. Cancer arising in chronic ulcerative colitis has a prognosis similar to that of other colon cancers. The rate of colon cancer is also increased 4x-20x in Crohn's colitis or ileocolitis. 5) Personal history of female genital or breast cancer carries a 2x increased risk of colon cancer.

- Colorectal cancer risk factor: age greater than 40.
- Risk increases with the number of adenomas.
- 2%-6% of patients with colon cancer have synchronous colon cancer and 1.1%-4.7% have metachronous cancers.
- Cancer rate begins to increase after 7 years of chronic ulcerative colitis.
- After 25 years, the risk is 30%.
- The risk is greatest for universal colitis.
- Crohn's colitis: the rate of colon cancer is increased (4x-20x).

Pathology and Prognostic Indicators

Cancer arises in the epithelium and invades transmurally to penetrate the bowel wall and then enters the regional lymphatics to reach distant nodes. Hematogenous spread is via the portal vein to the liver.

Surgical-pathogen stage of primary tumor--The depth of invasion and the extent of regional lymph node involvement are important in determining prognosis.

Modified Dukes' classification (Astler-Coller, 1954): A--mucosa, submucosa (80% 5-year survival); B1--into, not through, the muscularis propria without nodal involvement

(65%); B2--through the bowel wall without regional nodal involvement (43%); C1--B1 with regional nodes involved (53%); C2--B2 with regional nodes involved (15%); and D--distant metastases (5%-10%).

The extent of regional node involvement and prognosis: 1-4 nodes, 35% recur; and >4 nodes, 61% recur.

Other pathologic features and prognosis include: 1) ulcerating/infiltrating tumor is worse than exophytic/polypoid tumor; 2) poorly differentiated is worse than highly differentiated histology; 3) venous/lymphatic invasion has a poor prognosis, as does aneuploidy.

Clinical features and prognosis: a high preoperative level of carcinoembryonic antigen is associated with high recurrence rate and a shorter time before recurrence occurs. Poor prognosis if present with obstruction/perforation. Prognosis is worse in younger than in older patients.

- The depth of invasion and the extent of regional lymph node involvement are important in determining prognosis.
- High preoperative level of carcinoembryonic antigen is associated with high recurrence and a shorter time before recurrence.
- Poor prognosis if present with obstruction/perforation.
- The prognosis is worse in younger than in older patients.

Diagnosis

The clinical presentation is that of a slow growth pattern. Disease may be present for 5 years before symptoms appear. The symptoms depend on the location of the disease. A proximal colon tumor may present with symptoms of anemia, abdominal discomfort, or a mass. The left colon is narrower, and patients may present with obstructive symptoms, change in bowel habits, and rectal bleeding.

If cancer is suspected, perform air-contrast barium enema and flexible sigmoidoscopy or colonoscopy. If cancer is detected with air-contrast barium enema or flexible sigmoidoscopy, colonoscopy is needed to rule out synchronous lesions.

Metastatic survey includes physical examination, evaluation of liver-associated enzymes, and chest radiography. Image the liver if levels of liver-associated enzymes are abnormal. Preoperative level of carcinoembryonic antigen aids in prognosis and follow-up.

- Proximal colon disease: presenting symptoms may be anemia, abdominal discomfort, or mass.
- Left colon disease: obstructive symptoms, change in bowel habits, and rectal bleeding.
- Preoperative level of carcinoembryonic antigen aids in prognosis and follow-up.

Treatment

For most cases, surgical resection is the treatment of choice. This includes wide resection of the involved segment (5-cm margins), with removal of lymphatic drainage. In rectal carcinoma, low anterior resection is performed if an adequate distal margin of at least 2 cm can be achieved; this rectal sphincter-saving operation does not make the prognosis worse in comparison with abdominal perineal resection. The primary tumor is usually resected even if there are distant metastases so as to prevent obstruction/bleeding.

- For most cases, surgical resection is the treatment of choice.

Postoperative Management--No Apparent Metastases

Repeat colonoscopy in 6-12 months and then every 3 years if the findings are negative. Annually test for occult blood in stool.

Adjuvant chemotherapy: 5-fluorouracil and levamisole decrease recurrence by 41% and mortality by 33% in colonic stage C; they may be beneficial for stage B2. Radiotherapy plus 5-fluorouracil decreases the recurrence rate in rectal cancer stages B2 and C, but it is not clear if there is any survival advantage.

- Repeat colonoscopy in 6-12 months and then every 3 years if the findings are negative.
- Annual testing for occult blood in stool.
- 5-Fluorouracil and levamisole decrease recurrence by 41% and mortality by 33% in colonic stage C.

Prevention of Colorectal Carcinoma

Primary prevention--The steps to be taken in primary prevention are not known, although epidemiologic data indicate that a high fiber, low fat diet is reasonable. Secondary prevention--Identify and eradicate premalignant lesions and detect cancer while it is still curable. Screening includes occult blood screening and sigmoidoscopy. With occult blood screening, earlier stage lesions are detected, but this has not decreased mortality. The Hemoccult test has a 20%-30% positive predictive value for adenomas and 5%-10% for carcinomas. With sigmoidoscopy, earlier stage lesions are detected, and the removal of adenomas results in lower than expected incidence of rectosigmoid cancers, but none show decreased mortality. Flexible sigmoidoscopy detects 2x-3x more neoplasms than rigid proctoscopy.

Recommendations for screening--1) For average risk (i.e., anyone not in high-risk group): annual rectal examination after age 40; annual occult blood test after age 50; sigmoidoscopy after age 50 (every 3-5 years after negative findings on two examinations 1 year apart). 2) For prior adenoma or carcinoma: annual occult blood testing; colonoscopy every year until normal x 2, then every 3 years. 3) For familial adenomatous polyposis: annual sigmoidoscopy beginning at puberty until polyposis is diagnosed, then colectomy. 4) For hereditary nonpolyposis cancer syndromes: colonoscopy at age 20;

then annual Hemoccult test and colonoscopy every 3 years. 5) For first-degree relative with colorectal cancer: annual occult blood test and periodic sigmoidoscopy beginning at age 40. 6) For a woman with breast/genital cancer: annual occult blood test and periodic sigmoidoscopy. 7) For ulcerative colitis: annual colonoscopy and multiple biopsies starting after 7 years of universal chronic ulcerative colitis or after 15 years of left-sided chronic ulcerative colitis; dysplasia indicates the need for more frequent endoscopic follow-up and may lead to colectomy.

- Earlier stage lesions can be detected but early detection has not been shown to decrease mortality.
- Flexible sigmoidoscopy detects 2x-3x more neoplasms than rigid proctoscopy.

PANCREAS

Embryology

The pancreas develops in the 4th week of gestation as a ventral and dorsal outpouching or bud from the duodenum. Each bud has its own duct. As the duodenum rotates, the buds appose and join and the ducts anastomose. Pancreas divisum results from the failure of the ducts of the dorsal and ventral pancreas to fuse. This may predispose to acute pancreatitis. In annular pancreas, part of the ventral pancreas encircles the duodenum (usually the second part, proximal to the ampulla) and causes obstruction.

- Pancreas divisum: failure of dorsal and ventral pancreas to fuse. May predispose to acute pancreatitis. Be able to recognize this condition on radiographs.
- Annular pancreas: part of ventral pancreas encircles the duodenum (usually the second part, proximal to the ampulla) and causes obstruction. Be able to recognize this on radiographs.

Classification of Pancreatitis

Acute--reversible inflammation. 1) Interstitial pancreatitis accounts for 80% of cases. Perfusion of the pancreas is intact. It is less severe, with <1% mortality. 2) Necrotizing pancreatitis accounts for 20% of cases. It is more severe, with 10% mortality if sterile and 30% if infected.

Chronic--irreversible (i.e., structural disease, with endocrine or exocrine insufficiency). It is documented by pancreatic calcifications, ductal abnormalities (by endoscopic retrograde cannulization of the pancreas [ERCP]), scarring seen on biopsy, endocrine insufficiency (diabetes), and exocrine insufficiency (malabsorption).

- Acute interstitial pancreatitis: perfusion is intact, mortality is <1%.

- Acute necrotizing pancreatitis: perfusion is compromised, mortality is 10% if sterile and 30% if infected.
- Chronic pancreatitis is documented by pancreatic calcifications, ductal abnormalities, endocrine insufficiency (diabetes), and exocrine insufficiency (malabsorption).

Acute Pancreatitis

In acute pancreatitis, activation of pancreatic enzymes causes autodigestion of the gland. Clinical features are abdominal pain, nausea and vomiting ("too sick to eat"), ileus, peritoneal signs, hypotension, and abdominal mass (pseudocyst).

Etiologic Factors

Alcohol is the most common cause and gallstones the second common cause. The third common cause is idiopathic (approximately 10%). The following drugs cause pancreatitis: azathioprine, 6-mercaptopurine, L-asparaginase, hydrochlorothiazide diuretics, sulfonamides, sulfasalazine, tetracycline, furosemide, estrogens, valproic acid, pentamidine (both parenteral and aerosolized), and the antiretroviral drug dideoxyinosine (ddI). Know these drugs.

The evidence that the following drugs may also cause pancreatitis is less convincing and not definite: corticosteroids, NSAIDs, methyldopa, procainamide, chlorthalidone, ethacrynic acid, phenformin, nitrofurantoin, enalapril, erythromycin, metronidazole, nonsulfa-linked aminosalicylate derivates (such as 5-aminosalicylic acid and interleukin-2).

Other causes: hypertriglyceridemia may cause pancreatitis if the triglycerides are >1,000. Look for types I, IV, and V hyperlipoproteinemia and for associated oral contraceptive use. Hypertriglyceridemia may mask hyperamylasemia. Hypercalcemia may also cause pancreatitis; look for underlying multiple myeloma, hyperparathyroidism, or metastatic carcinoma. In immunocompetent patients, mumps and coxsackievirus cause acute pancreatitis. In AIDS patients, acute pancreatitis has been reported with cytomegalovirus infection. Ductus divisum, or incomplete fusion of the dorsal and ventral pancreatic ducts, may predispose to acute pancreatitis in some people, although this is a controversial matter.

- In nonalcoholic patients with acute pancreatitis, renew all medications, check lipid levels and calcium levels, and rule out gallstones.
- Know which medications definitely cause acute pancreatitis.

Clinical Presentation

Pain may be mild to severe; it is usually sudden in onset and persistent. The pain typically is located in the upper abdomen, with radiation to the back. Relief may be obtained by bending forward or sitting up. Exacerbation of the pain is common with ingestion of food or alcohol. The absence of pain is a poor prognostic feature, because these patients usually present with shock.

Fever, if present, is low grade, rarely exceeding 101°F in the absence of complications.

Volume depletion--Most patients are hypovolemic, because fluid accumulates in the abdomen.

Jaundice--Patients with pancreatitis may have a mild increase in total bilirubin, but they are not usually clinically jaundiced. When jaundice is present, it usually represents obstruction of the common bile duct by stones, compression by pseudocyst, or inflamed pancreatic tissue.

Dyspnea--A wide range of pulmonary manifestations may be seen. In over half of all cases of acute pancreatitis, some degree of hypoxemia is present. This is usually from pulmonary shunting. Patients often have atelectasis and may develop pleural effusions.

- Fever >101°F suggests infection.

Diagnosis of Acute Pancreatitis

Serum amylase--An increase in the serum level of amylase is the most useful test for acute pancreatitis. The level of amylase increases 2-3 hours after an attack and remains elevated for 3-4 days. The magnitude of the elevation does not correlate with the clinical severity of the attack. Serum amylase levels may be normal in some (<10%) patients because of alcohol or hypertriglyceridemia. Persistent elevation suggests a complication, e.g., pseudocyst, abscess, or ascites. Serum amylase is cleared by the kidney. The urine amylase level remains elevated after the serum amylase level returns to normal. Isoenzyme identification may aid in distinguishing between salivary (nonpancreatic) and pancreatic sources. Serum lipase may help distinguish between pancreatic hyperamylasemia and an ectopic source (lung, ovarian, or esophageal carcinoma). Lipase levels are also elevated longer than amylase levels after acute pancreatitis.

Nonpancreatic hyperamylasemia--Parotitis; renal failure; macroamylasemia; intestinal obstruction, infarction, perforation; ruptured ectopic pregnancy; diabetic ketoacidosis; drugs (such as morphine); burns; pregnancy; and neoplasms (lung, ovary, esophagus).

- If presentation for pancreatitis is classic but amylase value is normal, repeat amylase test, check urine amylase and serum lipase levels, and scan the abdomen.
- Persistent hyperamylasemia suggests a complication.
- If amylase is mildly elevated and there is a history of vomiting but no signs of obstruction, perform esophagogastroduodenoscopy to rule out a penetrating ulcer.

Physical findings: 1) Vital signs--tachycardia and orthostasis. 2) Skin--fat necrosis and xanthelasmas. Grey Turner's sign (flank discoloration) or Cullen's sign (periumbilical discoloration) suggests retroperitoneal hemorrhage. 3) Abdomen--often it is less impressive than the amount of pain the patient is having.

- Be able to recognize metastatic fat necrosis.
- Grey Turner's sign and Cullen's sign suggest retroperitoneal hemorrhage.

Laboratory findings: 1) Chest radiography--An isolated left pleural effusion strongly suggests pancreatitis. Infiltrates may represent aspiration pneumonia or adult respiratory distress syndrome. 2) Abdominal flat plate--Look for sentinel loop (dilated loop of bowel over pancreatic area) and colon cutoff sign (abrupt cutoff of gas in the transverse colon). Pancreatic calcifications indicate chronic pancreatitis. 3) Ultrasonography is the procedure of choice in acute pancreatitis, although in the presence of ileus, air in the bowel may obscure visualization of the pancreas. Ultrasonographic examination gives information about the pancreas and is the best method for delineating stones. However, it is not a good method for use in obese patients. 4) CT scan is the next step when visualization of the pancreas is poor with ultrasonography. It gives the same information as ultrasonography, is slightly less sensitive in picking up stones and texture abnormalities, involves radiation, and is more expensive. CT scan is indicated in critically ill patients to rule out necrotizing pancreatitis and is the better imaging choice in obese patients. 5) ERCP has no role in the diagnosis of acute pancreatitis and should be avoided, because it may cause infection. Occasionally, when acute pancreatitis is caused by common bile duct obstruction, endoscopic papillotomy may be performed to relieve the obstruction.

- An isolated left pleural effusion on chest radiography is strongly suggestive of acute pancreatitis.
- On abdominal flat plate, be able to recognize the sentinel loop sign, colon cutoff sign, and pancreatic calcifications.
- Ultrasonographic examination is the procedure of choice in patients with mild acute pancreatitis, in thin patients, and to rule out gallstones.
- CT scan is indicated in seriously ill patients to rule out necrotizing pancreatitis and in obese patients.
- ERCP has no role in the diagnosis of acute pancreatitis.

Treatment

Supportive care is the backbone of treatment, with monitoring for and treatment of complications when they occur. Fluids--Restore and maintain intravascular volume; this usually can be accomplished with crystalloids and peripheral intravenous catheters. Monitor blood pressure, pulse, urine output, daily intake and output, and weight. Eliminate medications that may cause pancreatitis. Use of a nasogastric tube does not shorten the course or severity of pancreatitis. But it should be used in case of ileus or severe nausea and vomiting. Analgesics--Meperidine (Demerol), 75-125 mg given i.m. every 3-4 hours, is preferred, especially over morphine, because it causes less sphincter of Oddi spasm. The efficacy of antisecretory drugs such as H_2 blockers, anticholinergics, somatostatin, or glucagon has not been documented. Total parenteral nutrition is unnecessary in most cases of pancreatitis. Peritoneal dialysis does not change the overall mortality, although it may decrease early mortality in severe pancreatitis.

- Supportive care is the backbone of treatment.
- Eliminate medications that may cause pancreatitis.
- Nasogastric tube does not shorten the course or severity of pancreatitis.
- Meperidine (Demerol) is preferred because it causes less sphincter of Oddi spasm.

Complications

A local complication is phlegmon, a mass of inflamed pancreatic tissue. It may resolve. Pseudocysts, a fluid collection within a nonepithelial-lined cavity, should be expected if there is persistent pain and persistent hyperamylasemia. In 50%-80% of cases, this resolves within 6 weeks without intervention. Pancreatic abscess usually develops 2-4 weeks after the acute episode and presents as fever (>101°F), persistent abdominal pain, and persistent hyperamylasemia. If a pancreatic abscess is not drained surgically, the mortality rate is virtually 100%. Give antibiotics effective for gram-negative and anaerobic organisms. Jaundice is due to common bile duct obstruction. Pancreatic ascites results from disruption of the pancreatic duct or a leaking pseudocyst.

- A local complication of pancreatitis should be suspected if fever, persistent pain, or persistent hyperamylasemia occurs.

A systemic complication is respiratory distress syndrome, a well-recognized complication of acute pancreatitis. Circulating lecithinase probably splits fatty acids off lecithin, producing a faulty surfactant. Pleural effusions occur in approximately 20% of patients with acute pancreatitis. If aspirated, a high amylase content is found. Fat necrosis may be due to elevated levels of serum lipase.

- Adult respiratory distress syndrome is a complication of acute pancreatitis.
- Pleural effusions occur in approximately 20% of patients with acute pancreatitis and have a high amylase content.

Assessment of Severity

Most patients with acute pancreatitis recover without any sequelae. The overall mortality rate of acute pancreatitis is 5%-10%, and death is most often secondary to hypovolemia and shock, respiratory failure, pancreatic abscess, or systemic sepsis. Ranson's criteria are reliable for predicting mortality in acute pancreatitis (Table 8-16). Mortality--less than 3 signs, 1%; 3-4 signs, 15%; 5-6 signs, 40%; and 7 or more signs, 100%.

Table 8-16.--Ranson's Criteria

Admission	48 hours
Age >55 yr	pO$_2$ <60 mm Hg
Leukocyte count >15,000	Hematocrit decrease >10%
Glucose >200	Blood urea nitrogen
Aspartate aminotransferase	increase >5 mg/dL
>250	Calcium <8 mg/dL
Lactate dehydrogenase >350	Estimated fluid
	sequestration >6 L

From Ranson JHC: Acute pancreatitis: surgical management. *In* The Exocrine Pancreas: Biology, Pathobiology, and Diseases. Edited by VLW Go, JD Gardner, FP Brooks, E Lebenthal, EP DiMagno, GA Scheele. New York, Raven Press, 1986, pp 503-511. By permission of publisher.

● Most patients with acute pancreatitis recover without any sequelae.

Chronic Pancreatitis

Chronic use of alcohol (at least 10 years of heavy consumption) is the most common cause of chronic pancreatitis. Gallstones and hyperlipidemia usually do not cause chronic pancreatitis.

Hereditary pancreatitis is autosomal dominant with variable penetrance. Onset is before age 20, although 20% of patients may present later than this. It is marked by recurring abdominal pain, positive family history, and pancreatic calcifications. It may increase the risk for pancreatic cancer.

Trauma with pancreatic ductal disruption causes chronic pancreatitis. Protein calorie malnutrition is the commonest cause of chronic pancreatitis in Third World countries.

● Chronic pancreatitis is commonly caused by alcohol but seldom by gallstones or hyperlipidemia.
● Hereditary pancreatitis is seen in young people with a positive family history and pancreatic calcifications.
● Protein calorie malnutrition is the commonest cause of chronic pancreatitis in Third World countries.

Triad of Chronic Pancreatitis

The triad consists of pancreatic calcifications, steatorrhea, and diabetes mellitus. Pancreatic calcifications--Diffuse calcification is due to heredity, alcohol, or malnutrition. Local calcification is due to trauma, islet cell tumor, or hypercalcemia. By the time steatorrhea occurs, 90% of the gland has been destroyed and lipase output has decreased by 90%.

● Chronic pancreatitis presents as abdominal pain, pancreatic calcification, steatorrhea, and diabetes mellitus.

Laboratory Diagnosis

Amylase and lipase levels may be normal. Stool fat is >10 g per 24 hours on a 48-72-hour stool collection while the patient is on a 100-g fat diet.

Pancreatic function tests: CCK/secretin stimulation--secretin given intravenously and submaximal CCK, with aspiration of duodenal contents and marker.

Bentiromide test--Para-aminobenzoic acid (PABA) conjugated with *N*-benzoyl tyrosine (bentiromide) is given orally. If chymotrypsin activity is adequate, the molecule is cleaved and PABA is absorbed and excreted in the urine. This test requires a normal small intestine (normal D-xylose test) and is useful only in severe steatorrhea.

CT scan shows calcifications, irregular pancreatic contour, dilated duct system, or pseudocysts.

ERCP reveals protein plugs, segmental duct dilatation, and alternating stenosis and dilatation with obliteration of branches of the main duct.

● Amylase and lipase levels may be normal, but evidence for structural disease or endocrine or exocrine insufficiency is present.
● 90% of the gland must be damaged for steatorrhea to occur.

Pain

The mechanism of the pain is not clearly defined; it may be due to ductular obstruction. One-third to one-half of patients have a reduction in pain after 5 years. The possibility of coexistent disease such as peptic ulcer should be considered. Abstinence from alcohol may relieve pain. Analgesics, aspirin or acetaminophen, are used occasionally with the addition of codeine (narcotic addiction is a frequent complicating factor). Celiac plexus blocks relieve pain for 3-6 months, but long-term efficacy is disappointing. A trial of pancreatic enzyme replacement for 1-2 months should be tried. Women with idiopathic chronic pancreatitis are most likely to respond. Surgery should be considered only after conservative measures have failed. Patients with a dilated pancreatic duct may respond favorably to a longitudinal pancreatojejunostomy (Puestow procedure).

● Abstinence from alcohol may relieve pain.
● Narcotic addiction is a frequent complicating factor.
● A 1-2-month trial of pancreatic enzyme replacement is worthwhile. Women are most likely to respond.
● Surgical treatment: only after conservative measures have failed.

Malabsorption

Patients have malabsorption not only of fat but also of essential fatty acids and fat soluble vitamins. The goal of enzyme replacement is to maintain body weight. Diarrhea will not resolve. Enteric-coated or microsphere enzymes are designed to be released at an alkaline pH, thus avoiding degradation by stomach acid. Their advantage is that they contain larger amounts of lipase. The disadvantages are that they are expensive and bioavailability is not always predictable.

Pancreatic Cancer

Pancreatic carcinoma is more common in men than in women. It usually presents between the ages of 60 and 80 years. The 5-year survival rate is <2%. Risk factors include diabetes mellitus, chronic pancreatitis, carcinogens, benzidine, cigarette smoking, and high fat diet. Pancreatic carcinoma usually presents late in the course of the disease. Patients may have a vague prodrome of malaise, anorexia, and weight loss. Symptoms may be overlooked until the development of pain or jaundice.

- Courvoisier's sign: painless jaundice with a palpable gallbladder suggests pancreatic cancer.
- Trousseau's sign: recurrent migratory thrombophlebitis is associated with pancreatic cancer.
- Recent-onset diabetes and nonbacterial (thrombotic) "marantic" endocarditis.

Routine laboratory blood analysis has limited usefulness. Patients may have increased levels of liver enzymes, amylase, and lipase or anemia, although this is variable. Tumor markers are also nonspecific. Ultrasonography is 80% sensitive in localizing pancreatic masses, as is abdominal CT. Either imaging method may be used in conjunction with fine-needle aspiration or biopsy to make a tissue diagnosis. ERCP is used if the ultrasonographic or CT results are inconclusive. It has a sensitivity >90%. ERCP also allows aspiration of pancreatic secretions for cytologic analysis. The "double duct" sign is a classic presentation, with obstruction of both the pancreatic and the bile ducts.

- Ultrasonography and CT are 80% sensitive in localizing pancreatic masses.
- ERCP has a sensitivity >90%.

Surgical treatment is the only hope for cure; unfortunately most lesions are nonresectable. The criteria for resectability are tumor <2 cm, absence of lymph node invasion, and absence of metastasis. Survival is the same for total pancreatectomy and the Whipple procedure: 3-year survival, 33%; 5-year survival, 1%; and operative mortality, 5%.

Radiation therapy may have a role as a radiosensitizer in unresectable cancer. However, survival is unchanged. Chemotherapy has also been disappointing and studies have not consistently shown improved survival.

Cystic Fibrosis

Because patients with cystic fibrosis are living longer, internists should know the common intestinal complications of this disease. Exocrine pancreatic insufficiency (malabsorption) is the common (85%-90%) and most important complication. Endocrine pancreatic insufficiency (diabetes) occurs in 20%-30% of the patients. Rectal prolapse occurs in 20%, and a distal small-bowel obstruction from thick secretions occurs in 15%-20%. Focal biliary cirrhosis develops in 20%.

- Pancreatic insufficiency occurs in 85%-90%.

Pancreatic Endocrine Tumors

Zollinger-Ellison syndrome is a non-beta-cell islet tumor of the pancreas that produces gastrin, causing gastric acid hypersecretion. This results in peptic ulcer disease (see section on Stomach).

Insulinoma is the most common islet cell tumor--a beta-cell islet tumor that produces insulin, which causes hypoglycemia. The diagnosis is based on finding increased fasting plasma levels of insulin and hypoglycemia. CT scanning or arteriography may be useful in localizing the tumor.

Glucagonoma is an alpha-cell islet tumor that produces glucagon. It presents with diabetes, weight loss, and a classic skin rash, migratory necrolytic erythema. The diagnosis is based on finding increased glucagon levels and failure of blood sugar to increase after injection of glucagon.

Pancreatic cholera is a pancreatic tumor that produces VIP, which causes watery diarrhea (see Secretory Diarrhea).

Somatostatinoma is a delta-cell islet tumor that produces somatostatin, which inhibits insulin, gastrin, and pancreatic enzyme secretion. The result is diabetes mellitus and diarrhea. The diagnosis is based on finding increased plasma levels of somatostatin. Octreotide (Sandostatin) is useful in treating these tumors because it prevents the release of hormone and antagonizes target organ effects.

- Zollinger-Ellison syndrome: non-beta-cell islet tumor of the pancreas.
- Insulinoma: commonest islet cell tumor.
- Pancreatic cholera: pancreatic tumor that produces VIP, which causes secretory diarrhea.
- Octreotide prevents hormone release and antagonizes hormone effects.

PART II
John J. Poterucha, M.D.

VIRAL HEPATITIS

Hepatitis A

Hepatitis A virus (HAV) is a small RNA virus that accounts for 20%-25% of cases of acute hepatitis in developed countries. The disease generally is transmitted by the fecal-oral route and has an incubation period of 15-50 days. Spread is more common in overcrowded areas with poor hygiene and poor sanitation. Ingestion of raw shellfish can cause epidemics. Hepatitis caused by HAV is generally mild, especially in children who often have a subclinical or nonicteric illness. Infected adults are more ill and usually develop jaundice. Rarely, HAV may cause fulminant hepatitis. The prognosis is excellent. Chronic liver disease does not develop from HAV. A serum IgM anti-HAV is present during acute illness, generally persists for 2-6 months, and is followed by IgG anti-HAV, which offers immunity from further infection. Because the virus is usually cleared from the feces before onset of jaundice, isolation of patients generally does not halt the spread of infection. Immune serum globulin should be given for household contacts of infected patients. When a common source of food-borne infection is identified, serum globulin should be given to those exposed. A hepatitis A vaccine has been developed and approved for use in the U. S.

- HAV is transmitted by the fecal-oral route.
- Incubation period is 15-50 days.
- Ingestion of raw shellfish can cause epidemics.
- Prognosis is excellent.
- Chronic liver disease does not develop.
- IgM anti-HAV is present during the acute illness.
- Give immune serum globulin for household contacts.
- A vaccine is available.

Hepatitis B

Hepatitis B virus (HBV) is a DNA virus with a surface and core. The core consists of a core antigen and "e" antigen. The disease is transmitted parenterally or by sexual contact. In high prevalence areas, e.g., certain areas of Asia, infants may acquire infection from the mother during childbirth. High-risk groups in the U. S. include intravenous drug users, persons with multiple sexual contacts, and health-care workers. The clinical course of HBV infection varies. Most infections in adults are subclinical, and even when symptomatic, the disease resolves within 6 months. During acute hepatitis, symptoms (when present) are generally more severe than those of HAV. Jaundice rarely lasts >4 weeks. Some patients may have preicteric symptoms of "serum sickness," including arthral-

gias and urticaria. These symptoms may be related to immune complexes, which can also lead to polyarteritis and glomerulonephritis.

- HBV is transmitted parenterally or by sexual contact.
- Infants may acquire infection from mothers.
- High-risk groups: intravenous drug users, persons with multiple sexual contacts, and health-care workers.
- Most infections in adults are subclinical.
- Jaundice rarely lasts >4 weeks.

HBV is not directly cytopathic and hepatocellular necrosis is due to host immune response to viral-infected cells. This inflammatory response accounts for HBV symptoms. Thus, patients with symptomatic HBV are more likely to "clear" the virus than those with subclinical infection. For example, patients with fulminant hepatitis B who recover rarely develop chronic hepatitis B. Viral markers in the blood during self-limited infection with HBV are shown in Figure 8-2.

- Host immune response causes hepatocellular necrosis and accounts for HBV symptoms.
- Patients who recover from fulminant hepatitis B rarely develop chronic hepatitis B.

Time after HBV Infection

Fig. 8-2. Viral markers in blood during self-limited hepatitis B virus infection. (From Robinson WS: Biology of human hepatitis viruses. *In* Hepatology: A Textbook of Liver Disease. Vol 2. Second edition. Edited by D Zakim, TD Boyer. Philadelphia, WB Saunders Company, 1990, pp 890-945. By permission of publisher.)

Note that IgM anti-HBc is nearly always present during acute hepatitis B. Some patients, particularly those with fulminant hepatitis B, may lack hepatitis B surface antigen (HBsAg). HBV-DNA and hepatitis B e antigen (HBeAg) correlate with ongoing viral replication and indicate infectivity. Patients with hepatitis B mutants may have high HBV-DNA levels but lack HBeAg. Commonly encountered serologic patterns of HBV are shown in Table 8-17.

Ten percent of patients acquiring HBV as adults and 90% of those infected as neonates do not clear HBsAg from the serum within 6 months and, thus, become chronically infected. Chronicity is more common in patients with a defect of the immune system. Patients with chronic hepatitis B but normal findings on liver tests and histologic examination of the liver are called carriers and have a good prognosis. Chronic liver inflammation due to HBV may lead to cirrhosis and liver failure. Spontaneous conversion from an HBeAg-positive state to HBeAg-negativity is accompanied by an increase in aminotransferases. Patients with chronic HBV liver disease, particularly if cirrhosis is present, are at high risk for development of hepatocellular carcinoma and should be screened with liver ultrasonography and alpha-fetoprotein determinations every 6 months.

- IgM anti-HBc is nearly always present during acute hepatitis B.
- HBV-DNA and HBeAg correlate with ongoing viral replication and indicate infectivity.
- 10% of patients acquiring HBV as adults and 90% of those infected as neonates do not clear HBsAg.
- Most chronic carriers of HBsAg have essentially a normal liver histologically and a good prognosis.
- Chronic hepatitis due to HBV may lead to cirrhosis.
- Patients with HBV-induced cirrhosis are at high risk for development of hepatocellular carcinoma.

Patients with chronic hepatitis B and active viral replication are candidates for therapy with interferon-α. About 30%-40% will have a response manifested by loss of HBeAg and HBV-DNA. A few patients will also clear HBsAg. Patients more likely to respond to interferon include those with a relatively recent diagnosis of chronic hepatitis B, high serum levels of aminotransferases, active hepatitis without evidence of cirrhosis on biopsy, and low serum levels of HBV-DNA. Those patients with HBV who respond to interferon may have a transient increase in aminotransferases after about 8 weeks of treatment. A brief period of pretreatment with corticosteroids may improve response in those with only mildly elevated levels of aminotransferases. Corticosteroids otherwise have no role in treating hepatitis B.

Table 8-17.--Common Serologic Patterns of Hepatitis B Virus

HBsAg	Anti-HBs	Anti-HBc	HBeAg	Anti-HBe	Interpretation
+	-	IgM	+	-	Acute HBV infection, high infectivity
+	-	IgG	+	-	Chronic HBV infection, high infectivity
+	-	IgG	-	+	Late-acute or chronic HBV infection, low infectivity
+	+	+	±	±	HBsAg of one subtype and heterotypic anti-HBs (common)
					Process of seroconversion from HBsAg to anti-HBs (rare)
-	-	IgM	±	±	Acute HBV infection
					Anti-HBc window
-	-	IgG	-	±	Low-level HBsAg carrier
					Remote past infection
-	+	IgG	-	±	Recovery from HBV infection
-	+	-	-	-	Immunization with HBsAg (after vaccination)
					Remote past infection (?)
					False-positive

From Dienstag JL, Wands JR, Isselbacher KJ: Acute hepatitis. *In* Harrison's Principles of Internal Medicine. Twelfth edition. Edited by JD Wilson, E Braunwald, KJ Isselbacher, RG Petersdorf, JB Martin, AS Fauci, RK Root. New York, McGraw-Hill, 1991, pp 1322-1337. By permission of publisher.

Hepatitis D

The delta agent is a small RNA particle that requires the presence of HBsAg to cause infection. Hepatitis D virus (HDV) infection can occur simultaneously with acute HBV (coinfection) or may infect a chronic HBsAg carrier (superinfection). HDV is strongly associated with intravenous drug abuse in the U.S. Infection with HDV should be considered only in patients with HBsAg and is diagnosed by anti-HDV seroconversion. Acute delta hepatitis is self-limited but may cause fulminant hepatitis. Like HBV, HDV recurs in the transplanted liver.

- Delta agent requires presence of HBsAg to cause infection.
- HDV is strongly associated with intravenous drug abuse.
- HDV infection occurs only in patients with HBsAg.
- Diagnosed by anti-HDV seroconversion.
- HBV and HDV recur in transplanted liver.

Hepatitis C

In the early 1970s, most patients with post-transfusion hepatitis (PTH) lacked serologic markers for either HAV or HBV infection. Thus, PTH was referred to as non-A, non-B hepatitis. In 1989, a single-stranded RNA virus was identified that accounts for most cases of PTH. This is the hepatitis C virus (HCV). In addition to a history of blood transfusions, other risk factors for acquiring HCV infection include parenteral drug abuse and needlestick exposure. However, 30%-40% of HCV patients have no identifiable risk factors and 50%-60% of previously classified "cryptogenic" cirrhosis is due to HCV. The most common presentation of HCV infection is a chronic, asymptomatic increase in aminotransferases. A characteristic feature of chronic HCV is fluctuation in liver enzymes. The correlation between symptoms and degree of hepatic inflammation is poor. The currently used ELISAs have good sensitivity and specificity for HCV infection. The recombinant immunoblot assay (RIBA) is a supplemental test for patients who are anti-HCV positive by ELISA. HCV-RNA can be measured with the polymerase chain reaction and is very sensitive and specific.

- HCV, a single-stranded RNA virus, causes most cases of PTH.
- Risk factors: blood transfusions, parenteral drug abuse, and needlestick exposure.
- 30%-40% of HCV patients have no identifiable risk factors.
- Common presentation: chronic, asymptomatic increase in aminotransferases.
- Characteristic feature: fluctuation in liver enzymes.

Chronic infection develops in 50%-90% of patients with HCV infection, and in at least 20%, it progresses to cirrhosis. Patients with HCV-induced cirrhosis are at increased risk for development of hepatocellular carcinoma. Chronic HCV infection may be associated with cryoglobulinemia and glomerulopathies.

Interferon-α at a dose of 3 million units given subcutaneously three times weekly for 6 months normalizes alanine aminotransferase levels in 40%-50% of patients, but 50% of them have relapse within 6 months after discontinuation of therapy. Patients with cirrhosis are less likely to respond to interferon.

- Chronic infection develops in 50% of infected patients.
- Cirrhosis develops in 20%.
- HCV patients with cirrhosis are at increased risk for hepatocellular carcinoma.
- Chronic HCV infection may be associated with cryoglobulinemia.
- Interferon-α normalizes aminotransferase levels in 40%-50% of patients.
- Patients with cirrhosis are less likely to respond to interferon.

Hepatitis E

Hepatitis E virus (HEV) is an enterically transmitted RNA virus. It can cause acute hepatitis in patients from India, Pakistan, Mexico, Southeast Asia, and travelers returning from these regions. Clinically, hepatitis E resembles hepatitis A. A notable exception is the high risk of fulminant hepatitis E in women who acquire the infection during the third trimester of pregnancy. Chronic hepatitis E does not occur. Hepatitis A, B, and E are compared in Table 8-18.

- HEV is an enterically transmitted RNA virus.
- It resembles hepatitis A.
- High risk of fulminant hepatitis E in women who acquire the infection during the third trimester of pregnancy.

Miscellaneous

Epstein-Barr virus, cytomegalovirus, and herpes viruses can all cause acute viral hepatitis, which is most serious in immune compromised patients.

AUTOIMMUNE HEPATITIS

"Autoimmune hepatitis" (AH) was previously called "autoimmune *chronic* active hepatitis" because it required 3-6 months of abnormal liver enzymes. However, AH can present as acute hepatitis. Classically, AH affects young persons (10-20 years), mainly females. The onset is usually insidious, and initial liver biopsy may show cirrhosis.

By definition, patients with AH should have no history of drug-related hepatitis, HBV, HCV, or Wilson's disease. Immunoserologic markers, including antinuclear antibody (ANA), smooth muscle antibody, soluble liver antigen antibodies, and antibodies to liver/ kidney microsomal (LKM)

Table 8-18.--Comparison of Hepatitis A, B, and E

Feature	Hepatitis A	Hepatitis B[*]	Hepatitis E
Incubation	15-45 days (mean, 30)	30-180 days (mean, 60-90)	14-60 (mean, 40)
Onset	Acute	Often insidious	Acute
Age preference	Children, young adults	Any age	Young adults
Transmission			
Fecal-oral	+++	-	+++
Sexual	±	++	±
Percutaneous	Unusual	+++	-
Severity	Mild	Often severe	Mild
Prognosis	Generally good	Worse with age, debility	Good
Chronicity	None	Occasional (5%-10%)	None
Prophylaxis	Ig	Hepatitis B immune globulin, HBV vaccine	?
Carrier	None	0.1%-30%[†]	None

[*]Concomitant delta hepatitis is similar to hepatitis B, but more severe outcomes are favored.
[†]Varies considerably throughout the world.
From Dienstag JL, Wands JR, Isselbacher KJ: Acute hepatitis. *In* Harrison's Principles of Internal Medicine. Twelfth edition. Edited by JD Wilson, E Braunwald, KJ Isselbacher, RG Petersdorf, JB Martin, AS Fauci, RK Root. New York, McGraw-Hill, 1991, pp 1322-1337. By permission of publisher.

antigens, are usually seen and may help separate patients into certain groups. There is an association with certain HLA types. Associated conditions include Hashimoto's thyroiditis, Coombs' positive hemolytic anemia, diabetes, and glomerulonephritis. Marked increases in serum gamma globulin levels are common, and aminotransferases are generally 4-10 times normal. Corticosteroids (30-40 mg/day) produce improvement in 60%-80% of patients. Changes in results of liver tests and gamma globulin are often dramatic. Azathioprine can be added to allow use of lower doses of prednisone. The prednisone dose should be reduced to control symptoms and maintain serum level of aminotransferases below five times normal. Even after excellent response to corticosteroids, relapse often occurs and control of AH often requires maintenance therapy. Although corticosteroids do not seem to prevent progression to cirrhosis, they improve survival in patients with severe disease.

- Classically, AH affects young persons (10-20 years old), mainly females.
- The onset is usually insidious.
- There should be no history of drug-related hepatitis, HBV, HCV, or Wilson's disease.
- Immunoserologic markers are often seen.
- Marked increases in serum gamma globulin levels are common.
- 60%-80% of patients improve with corticosteroids.
- Changes in results of liver tests and gamma globulin are often dramatic.
- Control of AH often requires maintenance therapy.

ALCOHOLIC LIVER DISEASE

Alcoholic Hepatitis

Alcoholic hepatitis is a histologic diagnosis characterized by fatty change, degeneration, and necrosis of hepatocytes (with or without Mallory bodies) and inflammatory infiltrate of neutrophils. Almost all patients have increased intralobular connective tissue, and they may have cirrhosis. Clinically, patients may be asymptomatic or jaundiced and critically ill. Common symptoms include anorexia, nausea, vomiting, abdominal pain, and weight loss. The most common sign is hepatomegaly, which may be accompanied by ascites, jaundice, fever, splenomegaly, and encephalopathy. AST is increased in 80%-90% of cases but is almost always <400 U/L. Aminotransferases of >400 U/L are not a feature of alcoholic liver disease and a search for other causes (i.e., ingestion of acetaminophen) should be pursued. The AST:ALT ratio is frequently >2. Leukocytosis is seen, particularly in severely ill patients.

- Alcoholic hepatitis is a histologic diagnosis.
- It is characterized by fatty change, degeneration, and necrosis of hepatocytes (± Mallory bodies) and inflammatory infiltrate of neutrophils.
- Common symptoms are anorexia, nausea, vomiting, abdominal pain, and weight loss.
- Common signs are hepatomegaly, ascites, jaundice, fever, splenomegaly, and encephalopathy.
- Increased AST (almost always <400 U/L) in 80%-90% of cases.

- AST:ALT is frequently >2.
- Leukocytosis occurs in severely ill patients.

Poor prognostic markers include encephalopathy, spider angiomata, ascites, renal failure, prolonged prothrombin time, and bilirubin >20 mg/dL. Many patients have progression to cirrhosis, particularly if alcohol intake is not curtailed. Corticosteroids may be beneficial as acute treatment of alcoholic hepatitis, particularly in patients with severe disease characterized by encephalopathy and a markedly prolonged prothrombin time.

- Bad prognostic markers: encephalopathy, spider angiomata, ascites, renal failure, prolonged prothrombin time, and bilirubin >20 mg/dL.
- Corticosteroids may be beneficial in severe disease.

Alcoholic Cirrhosis

Cirrhosis is defined histologically by fibrosis with nodular parenchymal regeneration. Typically, the cirrhosis of alcoholics is micronodular. Only 60% of patients with alcoholic cirrhosis have signs or symptoms of liver disease. Most patients with cirrhosis have no history of alcoholic hepatitis. Women are more predisposed to cirrhosis from alcoholism; this may be related to gastric mucosal levels of alcohol dehydrogenase. Liver enzymes may be relatively normal in cirrhosis without alcoholic hepatitis. Concomitant HCV infection is common in patients with alcoholic liver disease. Prognosis of alcoholic cirrhosis depends on whether patients continue to drink and whether there are symptoms (jaundice, ascites, gastrointestinal bleeding) of chronic liver disease. The 5-year survival for patients without ascites, jaundice, or hematemesis and who abstain is 89%. For those with symptoms and who continue to drink, the 5-year survival is 34%. Liver transplantation is an option for patients with end-stage alcoholic liver disease as long as they have abstained from alcohol for ≥1 year.

- Cirrhosis of alcoholics is micronodular.
- Only 60% of patients with alcoholic cirrhosis have signs or symptoms of liver disease.
- Women are more predisposed to cirrhosis from alcoholism.
- Liver enzymes may be relatively normal.
- 5-Year survival for patients without ascites, jaundice, or hematemesis and who abstain is 89%.
- 5-Year survival for those with symptoms and who continue to drink is 34%.
- Liver transplantation is an option.

NONALCOHOLIC STEATOHEPATITIS

Nonalcoholic steatohepatitis (NASH) is a common cause of abnormal liver tests. About 60% of patients with NASH will have obesity, hyperlipidemia, or diabetes mellitus. The levels of aminotransferases are usually abnormal, whereas the alkaline phosphatase level is increased in about one-third of patients. By definition, all patients have fatty change and inflammation on histologic examination of the liver, and some patients have fibrosis and even cirrhosis. The pathogenesis of NASH is uncertain, and the effect of weight loss and control of hyperlipidemia and hyperglycemia is variable. Of patients with NASH, 20%-30% progress to cirrhosis.

CHRONIC CHOLESTATIC LIVER DISEASES

Primary Biliary Cirrhosis

Primary biliary cirrhosis is a chronic, progressive, cholestatic liver disease primarily affecting middle-aged women. Its cause is unknown but appears to involve an immunologic disturbance resulting in small bile duct destruction. Many patients are identified because of asymptomatic increase of alkaline phosphatase. Common early symptoms are pruritus and fatigue. Patients also may have symptoms due to Hashimoto's thyroiditis or sicca complex. Biochemical features include increased alkaline phosphatase and IgM levels. Later, bilirubin increases, serum albumin decreases, and prothrombin time is prolonged. Steatorrhea may occur because of progressive cholestasis. Fat-soluble vitamin deficiencies and metabolic bone disease are common.

- Primary biliary cirrhosis primarily affects middle-aged women.
- Common early symptoms: pruritus and fatigue.
- Alkaline phosphatase and IgM levels increase.
- Fat-soluble vitamin deficiencies and metabolic bone disease are common.

Circulating antimitochondrial antibodies (AMA) occur in 90%-95% of patients. They are directed against autoantigens, called M2, on inner mitochondrial membranes. The classic histologic lesion is granulomatous infiltration of septal bile ducts. Treatment of primary biliary cirrhosis is generally symptomatic. Cholestyramine may be helpful for itching. Fat-soluble vitamin deficiencies should be addressed. Cyclosporin A, colchicine, and methotrexate are suggested as treatment options to arrest disease progression, but data about them are not conclusive. Ursodeoxycholic acid has recently been shown to delay liver transplantation in patients with primary biliary cirrhosis.

- AMA occur in 90%-95% of patients.
- Classic histologic lesion: granulomatous infiltration of septal bile ducts.
- Treatment: ursodeoxycholic acid.

Primary Sclerosing Cholangitis

Primary sclerosing cholangitis (PSC) is a chronic cholestatic liver disease characterized by obliterative inflammatory fibrosis of extra- and intrahepatic bile ducts. An immune mechanism has been implicated. Patients may have an asymptomatic increase in alkaline phosphatase or progressive fatigue, pruritus, and jaundice. Bacterial cholangitis is uncommon unless biliary tract surgery or instrumentation has been performed previously. Cholangiography establishes the diagnosis of PSC, showing short strictures of bile ducts with intervening segments of normal or slightly dilated ducts, producing a beaded appearance. This cholangiographic appearance can be mimicked by that of AIDS cholangiopathy (due to cytomegalovirus or cryptosporidium) and ischemic cholangiopathy after intra-arterial infusion of fluorodeoxyuridine.

- PSC: obliterative inflammatory fibrosis of extra- and intrahepatic bile ducts.
- Immune mechanism is implicated.
- Asymptomatic increase in alkaline phosphatase.
- Bacterial cholangitis is uncommon.
- Cholangiography establishes diagnosis.
- AIDS cholangiopathy mimics cholangiographic appearance of PSC.

The most commonly associated disease accompanying PSC is chronic ulcerative colitis. Ulcerative colitis occurs in 70% of patients with PSC and may antedate, accompany, or even follow the diagnosis of PSC. Proctocolectomy done for ulcerative colitis has no effect on the development of PSC. Patients with PSC are at higher risk for bile duct cancer; its development may be indicated by rapid clinical deterioration, with jaundice, weight loss, and abdominal pain. Treatment for PSC is generally supportive. Percutaneous or endoscopic balloon dilatation of bile duct strictures may offer palliation, especially in patients with recurrent cholangitis. Many patients have progressive liver disease and require liver transplantation.

- Ulcerative colitis occurs in 70% of patients with PSC.
- Proctocolectomy has no effect on development of PSC.
- PSC patients are at higher risk for bile duct cancer.
- Treatment for PSC is generally supportive.
- Many patients require liver transplantation.

HEREDITARY LIVER DISEASES

Genetic Hemochromatosis

Hemochromatosis is a genetically transmitted disorder of iron metabolism characterized by iron overload. The basic defect may be inappropriately high absorption of iron from the gastrointestinal tract. Because the gene for hemochromatosis is linked closely to HLA loci, HLA typing within a family may help identify susceptible members of a kindred. Genetic hemochromatosis is transmitted in an autosomal recessive manner. In the general population, heterozygote frequency is 10%. Only homozygotes manifest progressive iron accumulation.

- Genetic hemochromatosis is a disorder of iron metabolism.
- High absorption of iron by the gastrointestinal tract.
- Autosomal recessive transmission.
- Only homozygotes have progressive iron accumulation.

Patients usually present with end-stage disease. Peak incidence is between the ages of 40 and 60. Iron overload is manifested more often and earlier in men, because women are somewhat protected by menstrual losses of iron. Clinical features include arthropathy, hepatomegaly, skin pigmentation, diabetes mellitus, cardiac dysfunction, and hypogonadism. Routine liver biochemistry studies generally show little disturbance. Serum level of iron is elevated and transferrin saturation is >60%. Serum levels of ferritin are high, and levels >1,000 suggest hemochromatosis. Increased iron and ferritin levels also occur in other liver diseases, particularly alcoholic cirrhosis. Liver biopsy with quantitation of hepatic iron concentration is the standard method for diagnosing hemochromatosis. Generally, hepatic iron levels in hemochromatosis are >10,000 µg/g dry weight.

- Patients usually present with end-stage disease.
- Iron overload is more common in men.
- Clinical features: arthropathy, hepatomegaly, skin pigmentation, diabetes mellitus, cardiac dysfunction, and hypogonadism.
- Serum levels of ferritin are high.
- Standard for making diagnosis: liver biopsy with quantitation of hepatic iron concentration.

Hemochromatosis is treated with removal of iron by repeated phlebotomies. The standard recommendation is to remove 500 mL per week to the point of mild anemia. A maintenance program of 4-8 phlebotomies per year is required. When initiated in the precirrhotic stage, removal of iron can render the liver normal and may improve cardiac function and diabetes mellitus. Treatment does not reverse arthropathy, hypogonadism, or eliminate increased risk (30%) of hepatocellular carcinoma. All first-degree relatives of patients should be screened for evidence of iron overload.

- Hemochromatosis is treated with repeated phlebotomies.
- Iron removal can render the liver normal.
- Treatment does not reverse arthropathy, hypogonadism, or eliminate increased risk of hepatocellular carcinoma.
- First-degree relatives should be screened.

Wilson's Disease

Wilson's disease is an autosomal recessive disorder characterized by increased amounts of copper in tissues. The basic defect involves an inability to prepare copper for biliary excretion. The liver is chiefly involved in children, but neuropsychiatric manifestations are prominent in older patients. The Kayser-Fleischer ring is a brownish pigmented ring at the periphery of the cornea. It is not invariably present and is more frequent in patients with neurologic manifestations. Hepatic forms of Wilson's disease include fulminant hepatitis (often accompanied by hemolysis and renal failure), chronic hepatitis, and insidiously developed cirrhosis. Development of hepatoma is rare. Neurologic signs include tremor, rigidity, altered speech, and changes in personality. Fanconi's syndrome and premature arthritis may occur.

- Wilson's disease: autosomal recessive disorder characterized by increased copper in tissues.
- Basic defect: inability to prepare copper for biliary excretion.
- Kayser-Fleischer ring: brownish pigmented ring at periphery of cornea.
- Hepatoma is rare.
- Neurologic signs: tremor, rigidity, altered speech, and changes in personality.

Evidence of hemolysis (total bilirubin increased out of proportion to direct bilirubin), low or normal level of alkaline phosphatase, and low serum level of uric acid (due to Fanconi's syndrome) suggest Wilson's disease. The diagnosis is established on the basis of a low serum concentration of copper, a low level of ceruloplasmin, and increased urinary concentration of copper. Ceruloplasmin levels can be misleading--they can be increased by estrogen or biliary obstruction and decreased by liver failure of any cause. High concentrations of copper in the liver are found in Wilson's disease; similarly high values can also occur in cholestatic syndromes. Penicillamine chelates and increases urinary excretion of copper. It is the treatment of choice. Initiate treatment at 1.2 g/day. Failure of treatment should not be considered until 2 years of treatment have been given. All siblings of patients should be screened for copper. Trientine is an alternative to penicillamine. Zinc inhibits gastrointestinal absorption of copper and can be used as adjunctive therapy. Liver transplantation corrects the metabolic defect of Wilson's disease.

- Diagnosis: low serum level of copper, low ceruloplasmin, increased urinary concentration of copper.
- High concentrations of liver copper: Wilson's disease and cholestatic syndromes.
- Penicillamine: treatment of choice; increases urinary excretion of copper.

- Alternative treatment: trientine
- Liver transplantation corrects metabolic defect.

Alpha$_1$-Antitrypsin Deficiency

Alpha$_1$-antitrypsin (AIAT) is synthesized in the liver. The gene is on chromosome 14. M is the common normal allele, and Z and S are frequent abnormal alleles. Intrahepatic accumulation of AIAT in ZZ phenotype causes liver disease; however, disease occurs in only 10%-20% of ZZ patients. During the first 6 months of life, patients often have a history of cholestatic jaundice that resolves. In later childhood or early adulthood, cirrhosis may develop. The prevalence of cirrhosis in patients with MZ phenotype is increased, but the risk is small. Hepatocellular carcinoma can complicate AIAT deficiency, especially in males. Diagnosis of AIAT deficiency is made by determining AIAT phenotype. Serum levels of AIAT may be variable and unreliable. Liver transplantation corrects the metabolic defect and changes the recipient's phenotype to that of the donor.

- Intrahepatic accumulation of AIAT causes liver disease.

Table 8-19.--Common Causes of Fulminant Hepatic Failure

Infective
Hepatitis virus A, B, C(?), D, E
Herpes simplex
Drug reactions and toxins
Halothane
Isoniazid-rifampicin
Antidepressants
Nonsteroidal anti-inflammatory drugs
Valproic acid
Acetaminophen overdose
Mushroom poisoning
Herbal remedies
Ischemic
Ischemic hepatitis
Surgical "shock"
Acute Budd-Chiari syndrome
Metabolic
Wilson's disease
Fatty liver of pregnancy
Reye's syndrome
Miscellaneous (rare)
Massive malignant infiltration
Severe bacterial infection

From Sherlock S, Dooley J: Diseases of the Liver and Biliary System. Ninth edition. Oxford, Blackwell Scientific Publications, 1993, p 102. By permission of publisher.

- During the first 6 months of life, cholestatic jaundice that resolves.
- Hepatocellular carcinoma can complicate AIAT deficiency, especially in males.
- Diagnosis is made by determining AIAT phenotype.
- Liver transplantation corrects the metabolic defect.

FULMINANT HEPATIC FAILURE

Fulminant hepatic failure is defined as hepatic failure with encephalopathy developing <8 weeks after onset of jaundice in patients with no history of liver disease. Its common causes are listed in Table 8-19. Poor prognostic markers include a drug-induced cause (other than acetaminophen), older age, grade 3 or 4 encephalopathy, acidosis, and prothrombin time >50 seconds. Treatment is supportive, and steroids offer no benefit. Patients should be transferred to a medical center where liver transplantation is available.

- Fulminant hepatic failure: hepatic failure with encephalopathy developing <8 weeks after onset of jaundice and no history of liver disease.

- Poor prognostic markers: drug-induced (not acetaminophen), older age, grade 3 or 4 encephalopathy, prothrombin time >50 seconds.
- Steroids offer no benefit.

DRUG-INDUCED LIVER DISEASE

Drugs cause toxic effects in the liver in many ways, often mimicking naturally occurring liver disease. Most drug-induced liver disorders are idiosyncratic and not dose-related; 2% of cases of jaundice in hospitalized patients and 25% of cases of fulminant hepatitis are drug-induced. Consequently, all drugs that have been used by a patient with liver disease must be identified. Histologic classification of drug-induced liver disease and examples are given in Table 8-20.

Acetaminophen toxicity may occur at relatively low doses in alcoholics, because alcohol induces hepatic microsomal P-450 enzymes, which metabolize acetaminophen to its toxic metabolite. Disulfiram can also cause fulminant hepatitis. Amoxicillin-clavulinic acid causes severe cholestatic hepatitis, and valproic acid, tetracycline, and zidovidine can cause severe steatosis. Amiodarone may cause hepatotoxicity, whose

Table 8-20.--Histologic Patterns and Corresponding Examples of Drug-Induced Liver Disease

Pattern	Example
Zonal necrosis	Acetaminophen, carbon tetrachloride
Nonspecific hepatitis	Aspirin, oxacillin
Viral hepatitis-like lesion	Isoniazid, methyldopa
Granulomatous hepatitis	Quinidine, allopurinol
Chronic hepatitis	Methyldopa, nitrofurantoin
Fibrosis	Methotrexate
Cholestasis	
Inflammatory	Chlorpromazine, erythromycin estolate
Bland	Estrogens, anabolic steroids
Fatty liver	
Large globules	Ethanol, corticosteroids
Small droplets	Tetracycline, valproic acid
Vascular lesions	
Hepatic vein thrombosis	Oral contraceptives
Veno-occlusive disease	Certain antitumor agents
Noncirrhotic portal hypertension	Vinyl chloride monomer
Peliosis hepatis	Anabolic steroids
Tumors	
Adenoma	Oral contraceptives, androgens
Focal nodular hyperplasia	Oral contraceptives
Carcinoma	Oral contraceptives, androgens
Angiosarcoma	Vinyl chloride monomer

From Bass NM, Ockner RK: Drug-induced liver disease. In Hepatology: A Textbook of Liver Disease. Vol 2. Second edition. Edited by D Zakim, TD Boyer. Philadelphia, WB Saunders Company, 1990, pp 754-791. By permission of publisher.

histologic features can mimic those of alcoholic liver disease. Methotrexate in a total dose >2 g can cause hepatic fibrosis; some physicians advocate annual liver biopsies in patients receiving long-term methotrexate for psoriasis or rheumatoid arthritis. Intravenous cocaine can cause massive necrosis and death. Adenomas can occur with long-term use of oral contraceptives. Lovastatin commonly causes mild increases in aminotransferases.

- Most drug-induced liver disorders are idiosyncratic, not dose-related.
- 2% of cases of jaundice (hospitalized patients) and 25% of cases of fulminant hepatitis are drug-induced.
- Identify all drugs that have been used by a patient with liver disease.
- In alcoholics, acetaminophen toxicity may occur at relatively low doses.
- Amoxicillin-clavulinic acid causes severe cholestatic hepatitis.
- Amiodarone may cause hepatotoxicity.
- Total dose of methotrexate >2 g can cause hepatic fibrosis.
- Intravenous cocaine can cause massive necrosis.
- Long-term use of oral contraceptives can cause adenomas.

LIVER TUMORS

Hepatocellular Carcinoma

The risk of hepatocellular carcinoma is increased in cirrhosis of nearly any cause but particularly if due to HBV, HCV, hemochromatosis, and alcoholic liver disease. Alpha-fetoprotein is increased in only 50% of patients with hepatocellular carcinoma. Common metastatic sites are lymph nodes, lungs, bone, and brain. Paraneoplastic syndromes include gynecomastia, hypercalcemia, hypoglycemia, polycythemia, and clubbing. Surgical resection is the treatment of choice, presuming that the hepatic reserve is sufficient to permit resection. Liver transplantation is complicated by a high rate of recurrence. Percutaneous alcohol ablation may be useful for small tumors.

- The risk of hepatocellular carcinoma is increased in cirrhosis of nearly any cause.
- Alpha-fetoprotein is increased in 50% of patients with hepatocellular carcinoma.
- Common metastatic sites: lymph nodes, lungs, bone, and brain.
- Paraneoplastic syndromes: gynecomastia, hypercalcemia, hypoglycemia, polycythemia, and clubbing.
- Treatment of choice: surgical resection.
- Liver transplantation is complicated by a high recurrence rate.

Cholangiocarcinoma

The incidence of cholangiocarcinoma is increased in patients with PSC, *Opisthorchis* infection, and a history of choledochal cysts. Cholangiocarcinoma can be difficult to diagnose, especially in patients with PSC.

Adenoma

Adenomas are associated with the use of oral contraceptives. They can present with acute right upper quadrant pain and hemodynamic compromise because of bleeding.

Cavernous Hemangioma

Cavernous hemangioma is the most common benign tumor of the liver. CT scan with contrast agent is often diagnostic.

Metastases

Metastases are more common than primary tumors of the liver. Frequent primary sites are colon, stomach, breast, lung, and pancreas. Surgical resection of isolated colon cancer metastases has limited effect on long-term survival.

COMPLICATIONS OF END-STAGE LIVER DISEASE

Ascites

The pathogenesis of ascites is disputed but probably involves a combination of decreased effective circulatory blood volume (underfill theory) and inappropriate renal sodium retention with expansion of plasma volume (overfill theory). The initial event may be vasodilatation. Patients with ascites generally have a low urinary concentration of sodium. Treatment of ascites involves sodium restriction, diuretics, and (occasionally) fluid restriction. Bed rest is often helpful initially. Generally, spironolactone (100-200 mg/day) is used initially, although a low dose of furosemide (20-40 mg) is often added. The goal is to increase urinary sodium and allow loss of 1 L of ascitic fluid (1 kg weight) per day. Paracentesis is indicated for diagnostic purposes and should be done therapeutically in patients with tense ascites or with respiratory compromise from abdominal distention. Large-volume paracentesis (up to 10 L) combined with 6 g albumin per liter of ascitic fluid removed is safe and well tolerated.

- Pathogenesis of ascites probably involves a combination of decreased effective circulatory blood volume and inappropriate renal sodium retention with expansion of plasma volume.
- Patients generally have a low urinary concentration of sodium.
- Treatment: sodium restriction, diuretics.
- Large-volume paracentesis is safe and well tolerated.

Pleural effusion occurs in 6% of patients with cirrhosis and is right-sided in 67%. Edema usually follows ascites and is related to hypoalbuminemia and possibly increased pressure on the inferior vena cava by intra-abdominal fluid. The sudden onset of ascites in young patients should raise the possibility of hepatic venous outflow obstruction (Budd-Chiari syndrome). Tests most useful for determining the cause of ascites are measurements of total protein and the serum-ascitic fluid albumin gradient [albumin (serum) minus albumin (ascites)]. Albumin gradient >1.1 g/dL almost always indicates portal hypertension. Ascites secondary to portal hypertension induced by congestive heart failure can be distinguished from cirrhotic ascites because congestive heart failure usually has ascitic fluid protein >2.5. Exudative ascites from cancer or tuberculosis generally has ascitic fluid protein >2.5 and albumin gradient of <1.1 (Table 8-21).

Refractory ascites is uncommon. Most physicians advocate therapeutic paracentesis as needed. Peritoneovenous shunts are complicated by disseminated intravascular coagulation and shunt malfunction and, in comparison with diuretics and paracentesis, do not improve survival.

- Pleural effusion occurs in 6% of patients with cirrhosis and is right-sided in 67%.
- Sudden onset of ascites in young patients raises the possibility of hepatic venous outflow obstruction (Budd-Chiari syndrome).

Table 8-21.--Use of Single Measurements to Determine Cause of Ascites

	Serum-ascites albumin gradient, g/dL	Ascites protein, g/dL
Cirrhosis	>1.1	<2.5
Congestive heart failure	>1.1	>2.5
Malignancy	<1.1	>2.5

- Albumin gradient >1.1 g/dL almost always indicates portal hypertension.
- Peritoneovenous shunts do not improve survival.

Spontaneous Bacterial Peritonitis

Spontaneous bacterial peritonitis (SBP) occurs in 10%-20% of cirrhotic patients with ascites. SBP is defined as a bacterial infection of ascitic fluid without any intra-abdominal source of infection. Fever, abdominal pain, and abdominal tenderness are classic symptoms; however, many patients have few or no symptoms. SBP should be suspected in any patient with cirrhotic ascites. For all patients, diagnostic paracentesis is advisable as an initial step. Coagulopathy and thrombocytopenia should not prohibit performing diagnostic paracentesis. Cell count, Gram's stain, and culture of ascitic fluid should be performed on all patients. Bedside inoculation of blood culture bottles with ascites increases the diagnostic yield. SBP is more common in patients with large-volume ascites and those with a low ascitic fluid protein (<1.5 g). Also, blood of all SBP patients should be cultured, because almost 50% will be positive. Variants of SBP are listed in Table 8-22.

SBP and culture-negative neutrocytic ascites should be treated with a third-generation cephalosporin. Response to antibiotics should be assessed by repeat paracentesis 48 hours after the initiation of therapy. The polymorphonuclear count should decrease by 50% and cultures should be sterile. The hospital mortality rate of SBP is 50%-70%, and even if a patient survives hospitalization, the 1-year mortality rate is 60%-80%. A polymicrobial infection of ascitic fluid should prompt a search for an intra-abdominal focus of infection; SBP nearly always involves only one organism. The presence of bacterascites is thought to be due to contamination, and repeat paracentesis is advised.

- SBP occurs in 10%-20% of cirrhotic patients with ascites.
- Classic symptoms: fever, abdominal pain, and abdominal tenderness.
- Many patients have few or no symptoms.
- Bedside inoculation of blood culture bottles with ascites increases the diagnostic yield.

Table 8-22.--Variants of Spontaneous Bacterial Peritonitis

	Ascitic fluid polymorphonuclear cells, mL	Ascitic fluid cultures
Spontaneous bacterial peritonitis	>250	Positive
Culture-negative neutrocytic ascites	>250	Negative
Bacterascites	<250	Positive

- SBP is more common in cases of large-volume ascites and in those with low ascitic fluid protein (<1.5 g).
- SBP nearly always involves only one organism.

Hepatorenal Syndrome

Hepatorenal syndrome, or functional renal failure, consists of renal failure with normal tubular function in patients with cirrhosis. The differential diagnosis is given in Table 8-23. Hepatorenal syndrome is difficult to distinguish from prerenal azotemia; thus, a brief trial of colloid expansion may be needed. Hepatorenal syndrome is often precipitated by vigorous diuretic therapy. Treatment is supportive. After liver transplantation is performed, kidney function returns to normal.

- Hepatorenal syndrome: renal failure with normal tubular function in a cirrhotic patient.
- It is difficult to distinguish from prerenal azotemia.
- It is often precipitated by vigorous diuretic therapy.
- After liver transplantation, kidney function returns to normal.

Portal Systemic Encephalopathy

Portal systemic encephalopathy is a reversible decrease in the level of consciousness in patients with severe liver disease. Disturbed consciousness, personality change, intellectual deterioration, and slowed speech are common manifestations. The electroencephalogram is often abnormal, and patients often have asterixis (flapping tremor). The grading system commonly used for portal systemic encephalopathy is given in Table 8-24.

Table 8-23.--Differential Diagnosis for Hepatorenal Syndrome

	Prerenal azotemia	Hepatorenal syndrome	Acute renal failure
Urinary sodium concentration, mEq/L	<10	<10	>30
Urine to plasma creatinine ratio	>30:1	>30:1	<20:1
Urinary osmolality	At least 100 mOsm > plasma osmolality	At least 100 mOsm > plasma osmolality	Equal to plasma osmolality
Urinary sediment	Normal	Unremarkable	Casts, debris

From Epstein M: Functional renal abnormalities in cirrhosis: pathophysiology and management. *In* Hepatology: A Textbook of Liver Disease. Vol 2. Second edition. Edited by D Zakim, TD Boyer. Philadelphia, WB Saunders Company, 1990, pp 493-512. By permission of publisher.

Table 8-24.--Grading System for Portal Systemic Encephalopathy

Grade of encephalopathy	Level of consciousness	Neurologic abnormalities	EEG abnormalities
0	Normal	None	None
1	Trivial lack of awareness	Slight tremor Uncoordination	Symmetric slowing (5-6 cps)
	Personality change Day-night reversal	Asterixis	Triphasic waves
2	Lethargic	Asterixis	Symmetric slowing
	Inappropriate behavior	Abnormal reflexes	Triphasic waves
3	Asleep but arousable	Asterixis	Symmetric slowing
	Confused when awake	Abnormal reflexes	Triphasic waves
4	Unarousable	Babinski response Decerebrate posture Pupillary responses preserved	Very slow (2-3 cps) delta activity

cps, cycles per second; EEG, electroencephalogram.
From Schafer DF, Jones EA: Hepatic encephalopathy. *In* Hepatology: A Textbook of Liver Disease. Vol 1. Second edition. Edited by D Zakim, TD Boyer. Philadelphia, WB Saunders Company, 1990, pp 447-460. By permission of publisher.

The sudden development of portal systemic encephalopathy in patients with stable cirrhosis should prompt a search for bleeding, infection, or electrolyte disturbances; however, simple precipitating events may include increased dietary protein or constipation. Serum or arterial levels of ammonia are usually increased. Treatment consists of dietary protein restriction and lactulose. Lactulose has a laxative effect to decrease the nitrogenous compounds presented to the liver. It also acidifies the gut contents, thereby "trapping" ammonia as NH^{4+}, but it is unclear whether this is important. Oral neomycin offers no benefit over lactulose.

- Portal systemic encephalopathy: reversible decrease in the level of consciousness in patients with severe liver disease.
- EEG is often abnormal.
- Patients often have asterixis, or flapping tremor.
- Sudden development of portal systemic encephalopathy: look for bleeding, infection, or electrolyte disturbances.
- Treatment: dietary protein restriction and lactulose.

Variceal Hemorrhage

Esophageal varices are collateral vessels that develop because of portal hypertension. Varices can also occur in other parts of the gut. Isolated gastric varices without esophageal varices can occur with sinistral (left-sided) portal hypertension due to splenic vein thrombosis. Most cirrhotic patients with varices do not hemorrhage, but a first hemorrhage has a 30%-50% mortality. Bleeding is generally massive. Early endoscopy is indicated for diagnosis and treatment. Endoscopic therapy consists of sclerotherapy or band ligation. Octreotide alone or vasopressin in combination with nitroglycerin decreases portal venous pressure and may help stop the hemorrhage.

- Esophageal varices are collateral vessels that develop because of portal hypertension.
- Most cirrhotic patients with varices do not hemorrhage.
- First hemorrhage: 30%-50% mortality.
- Bleeding is generally massive.
- Early endoscopy is indicated for diagnosis and treatment.

Recurrent bleeding occurs in 80%-100% of patients. Propranolol given orally can help prevent rebleeding, although most physicians advocate sclerotherapy or banding until varices are obliterated. Patients with refractory bleeding are candidates for shunting. Surgical shunts have a high rate of mortality and morbidity and are complicated by portal systemic encephalopathy. Transjugular intrahepatic portal systemic shunt (TIPS) is a technique performed by vascular radiologists. It involves creating a tract (with expandable stents) between a branch of the hepatic vein and a branch of the portal vein via access from the jugular vein. TIPS is effective in controlling bleeding and has the advantage of avoiding an operation. The incidence of portal systemic encephalopathy after TIPS is 10%-40%, but it usually can be controlled with medical therapy.

- Rebleeding occurs in 80%-100% of patients.
- Patients with refractory bleeding are candidates for shunting.
- Incidence of portal systemic encephalopathy after TIPS is 10%-40%.

CHOLESTASIS AND BILIARY TRACT DISEASE

Cholestasis is broadly defined as a failure of normal bile flow. Alkaline phosphatase levels are usually increased. When alkaline phosphatase is increased without hyperbilirubinemia, the liver origin of the alkaline phosphatase can be confirmed by either alkaline phosphatase isoenzymes or gamma glutamyl transferase elevations. Intrahepatic cholestasis is often due to medications or focal hepatic lesions. Extrahepatic cholestasis can be due to tumors, stones, or benign strictures. Acute biliary obstruction, usually due to a common bile duct stone, may be accompanied by marked transient increases in aminotransferases. Hyperbilirubinemia without other markers of cholestasis may be due to hemolysis, resorption of hematomas, or massive transfusions. The most common cause of isolated indirect hyperbilirubinemia is Gilbert syndrome, which is easily confirmed by showing a decline in bilirubin after the patient has eaten. Usually, the medical history and ultrasonography (to detect dilated biliary system) identify whether cholestasis is intrahepatic or obstructive. Ultrasonography is more likely to show dilated bile ducts in patients with obstruction if bilirubin is ≥10 mg/dL and/or jaundice has been present for ≥10 days.

- Cholestasis is a failure of normal bile flow.
- Alkaline phosphatase levels are usually increased.
- Acute biliary obstruction may be accompanied by marked transient increases in aminotransferases.
- Gilbert syndrome: most common cause of isolated indirect hyperbilirubinemia.
- Medical history and ultrasonography usually identify whether cholestasis is intrahepatic or obstructive.

Gallstones and Cholecystitis

Gallstones can be cholesterol or pigment. Cholesterol gallstones occur when bile is supersaturated with cholesterol relative to bile salts. Excessive cholesterol secretion (females, obesity, exogenous estrogens) or deficient bile acid secretion (terminal ileal disease or resection, bile acid sequestrant therapy) can lead to cholesterol gallstones. Pigment stones can occur with hemolysis or cirrhosis, but usually there is no identifying cause. Ultrasonography is 90%-97% sensitive for detecting gallstones. Cholecystitis may be suggested by gallbladder contraction, marked distention, surrounding fluid, or wall thickening. Ultrasonography also offers the opportunity to detect dilated bile ducts. Radionuclide biliary scanning is helpful in diagnosing cystic duct obstruction with cholecystitis if performed during an episode of pain. Positive test results are marked by nonvisualization of the gallbladder despite biliary excretion of radioisotope.

- Cholesterol gallstones occur when bile is supersaturated with cholesterol.
- Pigment stones can occur with hemolysis or cirrhosis.
- Ultrasonography is 90%-97% sensitive for detecting gallstones.
- Radionuclide biliary scanning helps diagnose cystic duct obstruction with cholecystitis.

Asymptomatic gallstones require no therapy, even in high-risk patients. Patients with episodes of biliary colic or acute cholecystitis should have cholecystectomy. Laparoscopic cholecystectomy is the procedure of choice. High surgical risk patients can undergo percutaneous cholecystostomy as a temporary measure. Nonsurgical therapies for stones include percutaneous extraction, oral dissolution with ursodeoxycholic acid or chenodeoxycholic acid, or direct contact dissolution via gallbladder catheter with methyl-tert butyl ether (MTBE). Ursodeoxycholic acid should be used for only small CT-radiolucent cholesterol stones. It needs to be given for 6-24 months.

- Asymptomatic gallstones require no therapy.
- Procedure of choice: laparoscopic cholecystectomy.
- Use ursodeoxycholic acid for only small CT-radiolucent cholesterol stones.

Bile Duct Stones

Most bile duct stones originate in the gallbladder, although a few patients have primary duct stones. CT and ultrasonography are relatively insensitive for common bile duct stones, and diagnosis usually requires cholangiography accomplished via endoscopic retrograde cholangiopancreatography (ERCP). Patients can have minimal or no symptoms due to common bile duct stone or they can have life-threatening cholangitis with abdominal pain, fever, and jaundice. Patients with common bile duct stones should have them removed. This can be done in 90% of cases via ERCP. Urgency of the procedure depends on the clinical presentation. Patients with minimal symptoms can have elective ERCP, but those with cholangitis and fever unresponsive to antibiotics should have urgent endoscopic treatment. Patients with gallbladder stones who

have papillotomy and clearance of their duct stones have only a 10% chance of having further problems with their gallbladder stones.

- Most bile duct stones originate in the gallbladder.
- Diagnosis of common bile duct stones usually requires cholangiography.
- Common bile duct stones should be removed.
- Urgent endoscopic treatment is needed if cholangitis and fever are unresponsive to antibiotics.

Benign Biliary Tract Strictures

Most benign biliary strictures are iatrogenic. They were especially common in the early days of laparoscopic cholecystectomy. Such strictures are best treated surgically.

Malignant Biliary Obstruction

Malignant biliary obstruction is usually due to carcinoma of the head of the pancreas, bile duct cancer, or metastatic cancer to hilar nodes. If the disease is unresectable, palliative endoscopic or percutaneous stenting is as effective as surgical bypass. One exception is impending duodenal obstruction, at which time operation offers the opportunity for bypass of both biliary and duodenal obstruction. A major complication of stenting is occlusion of the stents, which occurs in 1-6 months.

- Usual causes of malignant biliary obstruction: carcinoma of the head of the pancreas, bile duct cancer, and metastatic cancer to hilar nodes.
- Palliative endoscopic or percutaneous stenting is as effective as surgical bypass.
- Major complication of stenting: occlusion of the stents.

Gallbladder Carcinoma

Gallbladder carcinoma has a strong association with calcified (porcelain) gallbladder. For this reason, cholecystectomy is best for calcified gallbladder.

Sphincter of Oddi Dysfunction

Sphincter of Oddi dysfunction is a poorly defined entity characterized by right upper quadrant pain without any structural cause. Patients with typical biliary-type pain, increased values on liver tests during the pain, a dilated common bile duct, and delayed drainage of contrast after cholangiography often improve after sphincterotomy. Patients without all these criteria generally have a poor or variable response to sphincterotomy.

QUESTIONS

Multiple Choice (choose the one best answer)

1. All the following conditions predispose to the development of esophageal cancer except for:
   a. Lye stricture
   b. Smoking
   c. Alcohol
   d. Diffuse esophageal spasm
   e. Achalasia

2. The symptom complex of oropharyngeal dysphagia is suggested to the clinician by the presence of all the following except for:
   a. High esophageal (cervical) dysphagia
   b. Aspiration
   c. Epigastric pain
   d. Nasal regurgitation with swallowing
   e. Choking with swallowing

3. All the following decrease lower esophageal sphincter pressure except:
   a. Alcohol
   b. Caffeine
   c. Anticholinergic agents
   d. Calcium channel blockers
   e. Protein

4. All the following medications have been implicated in medication-induced esophagitis except for:
   a. Ferrous sulfate
   b. Quinidine
   c. Potassium
   d. Anticholinergic agents
   e. Tetracycline

5. All the following conditions have been associated with an increased frequency of peptic ulcer disease except:
   a. Nonsteroidal anti-inflammatory drugs
   b. Cigarette smoking
   c. Corticosteroids
   d. Cirrhosis
   e. Chronic pulmonary disease

6. All the following clinical entities have an osmotic mechanism for diarrhea except:
   a. Surreptitious laxative ingestion
   b. Saline cathartics
   c. Antacids
   d. Sorbitol foods
   e. Lactase deficiency

7. All the following are seen in malabsorption secondary to pancreatic insufficiency except:
   a. Edema
   b. Bone pain
   c. Alopecia
   d. Easy bruisability
   e. Night blindness

8. Extraintestinal manifestations of inflammatory bowel disease include all of the following except:
   a. Celiac sprue
   b. Arthritis
   c. Primary sclerosing cholangitis
   d. Renal stones
   e. Episcleritis or uveitis

9. All the following are indications for colonoscopy in the evaluation of inflammatory bowel disease except:
   a. To evaluate extent of disease
   b. To perform biopsy of a stricture
   c. To evaluate iron deficiency anemia
   d. To differentiate Crohn's colitis from ulcerative colitis
   e. To monitor for development of dysplasia or cancer.

10. All the following conditions have been associated with the development of pseudomembranous colitis except:
    a. Uremia
    b. Ischemia
    c. Intestinal surgery
    d. Antibiotics
    e. Foreign travel

11. All the following polyps have an increased risk of cancer except for:
    a. A solitary 2-cm tubular adenoma
    b. A solitary 2-cm villous adenoma
    c. Gardner's syndrome
    d. Familial polyposis
    e. Juvenile polyposis

12. All the following have been associated with precipitation of toxic megacolon except:
    a. Proctoscopy
    b. Barium enema
    c. Anticholinergic agents
    d. Opiates
    e. Hypokalemia

13. All the following confirm the diagnosis of chronic pancreatitis except:

a. Pancreatic calcifications
b. Chronic abdominal pain
c. Abnormal pancreatogram
d. Diabetes mellitus
e. Malabsorption

14. All the following drugs have been associated firmly with acute pancreatitis except:
   a. Corticosteroids
   b. 6-Mercaptopurine
   c. Azathioprine
   d. Furosemide
   e. L-Asparaginase

15. All the following are nonpulmonary features of cystic fibrosis except:
   a. Focal biliary cirrhosis
   b. Rectal prolapse
   c. Meconium ileus
   d. Celiac sprue
   e. Pancreatic insufficiency

16. A 42-year-old man presents for an insurance physical examination. He is asymptomatic and is not taking any medication. He had proctocolectomy 4 years ago for ulcerative colitis. Laboratory findings included an alkaline phosphatase level five times the normal value and a twice normal increase in the level of alanine aminotransferase. The most likely diagnosis is
   a. Primary biliary cirrhosis
   b. Primary sclerosing cholangitis.
   c. Acute cholecystitis
   d. Chronic hepatitis C
   e. Autoimmune hepatitis

17. A 38-year-old man presents with fatigue of 2 years' duration. He has no other symptoms and the physical examination findings are normal. The level of alanine aminotransferase is five times the normal value, but the values of alkaline phosphatase, bilirubin, prothrombin time, and albumin are normal. The serologic profile is as follows: HBsAg positive, IgM anti-HBc negative, HBeAg positive, and anti-HCV negative. The most likely diagnosis is:
   a. Acute hepatitis C
   b. Chronic hepatitis C
   c. Acute hepatitis A
   d. Acute hepatitis B
   e. Chronic hepatitis B

18. A 43-year-old alcoholic man presents with jaundice and somnolence. No other history is available. The physical examination findings are notable for a temperature of 38.3°C, somnolence, jaundice, spider angiomata, and ascites. The value for alanine aminotransferase is 53 U/L and for aspartate aminotransferase, 106 U/L. The most likely diagnosis is:
   a. Acute hepatitis A
   b. Acute hepatitis B
   c. Acute hepatitis C
   d. Alcoholic hepatitis
   e. Autoimmune hepatitis

19. A 44-year-old woman comes to the emergency room with abdominal pain. She was well until 5 hours previously, when steady, hard pain in the epigastrium and right upper quadrant developed, accompanied by nausea and an episode of emesis. The pain has started to abate by the time you see her. A similar spell occurred 3 weeks previously. Physical examination findings are notable for only obesity and mild right upper quadrant tenderness. Ultrasonography demonstrates multiple small gallstones. Which one of the following would you advise next?
   a. Endoscopic retrograde cholangiopancreatography
   b. Esophagogastroduodenoscopy
   c. Computed tomography of the abdomen
   d. Oral cholecystography
   e. Laparoscopic cholecystectomy

20. A 55-year-old alcoholic man presents with increasing abdominal distention. He is afebrile and the physical examination findings are consistent with ascites. The serum level of albumin is 2.6 g/dL and the prothrombin time is 18 seconds (INR 1.8). Paracentesis demonstrates 50 neutrophils and a protein value of 1.1 g/dL. Ultrasonography of the abdomen reveals a small liver, splenomegaly, and ascites. Which one of the following would you advise next:
   a. Repeat paracentesis for cytology
   b. Sodium restriction and diuretics
   c. Echocardiography
   d. Hospitalization for intravenous administration of antibiotics
   e. Computed tomography of the abdomen

21. A 43-year-old man presents for an insurance physical examination. Eight years ago he had proctocolectomy for intractable symptoms of ulcerative colitis. The examination findings are normal. Total bilirubin is 2.3 mg/dL and direct bilirubin is 0.1 mg/dL. The values for alkaline phosphatase and hemoglobin are normal. The most likely diagnosis is:
   a. Primary sclerosing cholangitis
   b. Primary biliary cirrhosis

c. Gilbert syndrome

d. Cholangiocarcinoma

e. Choledocholithiasis (common bile duct stones)

22. A 55-year-old man presents with fatigue and pain in the metacarpophalangeal and proximal interphalangeal joints. A grandfather and one brother died of "liver cancer." The physical examination demonstrates hyperpigmentation of the skin, enlargement and deformity of the painful joints, hepatomegaly, and small testes. The value of alanine aminotransferase is 1.5 times normal and glucose is 126, but the results of other tests are normal. Which of the following should you order next:

a. Serum iron and iron-binding capacity

b. Ceruloplasmin

c. Rheumatoid factor

d. Antinuclear antibody

e. Alpha-1-antitrypsin phenotype

True/False (indicate whether each answer is true or false)

23. With regard to *Helicobacter pylori:*

a. Not commonly found in asymptomatic people

b. The most common cause of histologic gastritis

c. A common and important factor in peptic ulcer disease

d. Important for the development of adenocarcinoma of the stomach

e. If eradicated, does not improve healing rate of ulcers

f. If eradicated, prevents recurrence of ulcers

24. Concerning infectious diarrhea:

a. *Bacillus cereus* is associated with fried rice in oriental restaurants

b. *Salmonella* is associated with poultry

c. *Vibrio parahaemolyticus* is associated with ingestion of shellfish

d. Antibiotics shorten the duration of traveler's diarrhea

e. Antibiotics shorten the duration of cholera

f. Antibiotics shorten the duration of *Salmonella* infection

25. With regard to colorectal cancer, indicate whether or not the following are risk factors:

a. Age

b. Hyperplastic polyps

c. Ulcerative colitis

d. Diverticulosis

e. Female genital cancer

f. Breast cancer

26. With regard to treating inflammatory bowel disease:

a. Corticosteroids are useful for maintenance therapy in Crohn's disease and ulcerative colitis

b. Left-sided ulcerative colitis may be treated with topical aminosalicylates or steroids

c. Severe attacks of ulcerative colitis usually require high doses of corticosteroids

d. Immunosuppressive agents may be effective for chronically active steroid-dependent disease

e. Bowel rest is more effective than elemental diet

f. Antibiotic therapy appears to be more effective in ulcerative colitis than in Crohn's disease

27. With regard to malabsorption:

a. The presence of oil droplets in the stool suggests pancreatic insufficiency

b. The presence of undigested meat fibers in the stool suggests intestinal disease

c. Vitamin B_{12} deficiency may be seen in intestinal disease and pancreatic disease

d. Iron deficiency anemia commonly occurs with pancreatic insufficiency

e. Blunted villi on small-bowel biopsy are diagnostic for celiac sprue

f. Small-bowel biopsy that shows PAS-positive organisms in macrophages is seen in Whipple's disease

28. With regard to the hepatitis C virus:

a. It rarely causes chronic infection

b. It leads to an increased incidence of hepatocellular carcinoma

c. Interferon is curative in nearly all patients

d. It accounts for most cases of post-transfusion hepatitis

e. Fluctuating aminotransferase levels are characteristic

f. It has a striking association with inflammatory bowel disease

29. With regard to drug-induced liver disease:

a. Corticosteroids may cause steatosis in the liver

b. Isoniazid hepatotoxicity typically presents with an increased level of alkaline phosphatase

c. The pathogenesis of most drug-induced liver injury is allergic

d. Alcoholic patients are more susceptible to acetaminophen hepatotoxicity than nonalcoholics

e. Rechallenge is recommended in suspected cases of idiosyncratic drug-induced liver disorders

f. Methotrexate hepatotoxicity is always accompanied by abnormal levels of aminotransferases

30. With regard to biliary stone disease:

a. Patients with a previous ileal resection are at increased risk for the development of pigmented gallbladder stones

b. Oral bile acid therapy is useful for large calcified gallbladder stones in high-risk patients

c. Most patients with common bile duct stones also have gallbladder stones

d. Asymptomatic diabetic patients with gallbladder stones should have cholecystectomy

e. Preoperative endoscopic retrograde cholangiopancreatography is indicated in most patients referred for laparoscopic cholecystectomy

f. Patients with ascending cholangitis due to a common bile duct stone should undergo endoscopic retrograde cholangiopancreatography with sphincterotomy and stone extraction

ANSWERS

1. Answer d.

The conditions that predispose to esophageal (squamous) cancer include achalasia, lye stricture, Plummer-Vinson syndrome, tylosis, smoking, and alcohol. Diffuse esophageal spasm is not a premalignant syndrome.

2. Answer c.

Oropharyngeal dysphagia is the result of faulty transfer of the food bolus from the oropharynx to the esophagus. It can be caused by structural causes or by neurologic or muscular disorders. This symptom complex presents as high esophageal dysphagia associated with coughing, choking (aspiration), or nasal regurgitation. It is not associated with epigastric pain.

3. Answer e.

Many dietary substances, including fat, chocolate, caffeine (coffee), theophylline (tea), and carminatives (spearmint, peppermint), decrease lower esophageal sphincter pressure. A protein meal increases lower esophageal sphincter pressure. Of the many drugs that decrease lower esophageal sphincter pressure, anticholinergic agents, calcium channel blockers, and nitrates are the most important.

4. Answer d.

Medications commonly associated with medication-induced esophagitis include tetracycline, doxycycline, quinidine, potassium, ferrous sulfate, and ascorbic acid. Anticholinergic agents have not been implicated in medication-induced esophagitis, but they commonly aggravate gastroesophageal reflux disease.

5. Answer c.

Aspirin and nonsteroidal anti-inflammatory drugs are associated with an increased frequency of peptic ulcer disease. The effect of corticosteroids is controversial, and no clear-cut increased risk has been demonstrated. The incidence of peptic ulcers is higher if there is associated chronic lung disease, cirrhosis, or chronic renal failure.

6. Answer a.

Clinical entities that have an osmotic mechanism for diarrhea include lactase deficiency, food containing sorbitol, saline cathartics, and antacids. Surreptitious laxative ingestion is the commonest cause of unexplained, chronic watery diarrhea of a secretory mechanism.

7. Answer c.

In malabsorption syndrome, edema and muscle wasting are caused by decreased protein absorption. Bone pain is caused by decreased calcium absorption. Easy bruisability and petechiae result from vitamin K malabsorption, and night blindness and hyperkeratosis, from decreased vitamin A absorption. Alopecia is not commonly seen in malabsorption.

8. Answer a.

Extraintestinal manifestations of inflammatory bowel disease include arthritis, skin lesions (erythema nodosum, pyoderma gangrenosum, aphthous ulcer), eye lesions (episcleritis, uveitis), primary sclerosing cholangitis, and renal stones. Celiac sprue is not associated with inflammatory bowel disease.

9. Answer c.

The indications for colonoscopy in inflammatory bowel disease include evaluation of the extent of disease, to evaluate a stricture, to evaluate a filling defect, to differentiate Crohn's disease from ulcerative colitis, and to obtain biopsy specimens to evaluate for dysplasia or precancerous changes. Iron deficiency anemia is not an indication for colonoscopy in active inflammatory bowel disease.

10. Answer e.

Conditions associated with the development of pseudomembranous colitis include intestinal obstruction, uremia, ischemia, intestinal surgery, and all antibiotics except vancomycin. Foreign travel is associated with a number of intestinal infections but not with the overgrowth of *Clostridium difficile*, which produces pseudomembranous colitis.

11. Answer e.

Adenomatous polyps are premalignant polyps, and the risk of cancer increases with increasing size (>1 cm) and increasing villous architecture. Gardner's syndrome and familial polyposis are associated with adenomatous polyps. Juvenile polyposis is associated with hamartomatous polyps, which are not premalignant.

12. Answer a.

Causes of toxic megacolon include aerophagia, opiates, anticholinergic agents, hypokalemia, and barium enema. Proctoscopic examination can be performed safely in a patient with suspected acute colitis to confirm the diagnosis.

13. Answer b.

The diagnosis of chronic pancreatitis is documented by structural abnormalities (pancreatic calcifications, ductal abnormalities by endoscopic retrograde cholangiopancreatography, or scarring on biopsy), endocrine insufficiency (diabetes), or exocrine insufficiency (malabsorption). Abdominal pain is commonly present with chronic pancreatitis, but it does not confirm the diagnosis.

14. Answer a.

Drugs that have been firmly associated with acute pancreatitis include azathioprine, 6-mercaptopurine, L-asparaginase, hydrochlorothiazide diuretics, sulfonamide, sulfasalazine, tetracycline, furosemide, estrogens, valproic acid, pentamidine, and the antiretroviral drug dideoxyinosine (ddI). The evidence that corticosteroids, nonsteroidal anti-inflammatory drugs, methyldopa, procainamide, chlorthalidone, ethacrynic acid, phenformin, nitrofurantoin, enalapril, erythromycin, metronidazole, and aminosalicylates cause pancreatitis is less convincing.

15. Answer d.

Nonpulmonary features of cystic fibrosis include exocrine pancreatic insufficiency (malabsorption), endocrine pancreatic insufficiency (diabetes), rectal prolapse, a distal small-bowel obstruction from thick secretions (meconium ileus equivalent), and focal biliary cirrhosis. Celiac sprue is not associated with cystic fibrosis.

16. Answer b.

This patient has an asymptomatic increase in the alkaline phosphatase level. He also has an increased level of alkaline aminotransferase, an indication that the increased alkaline phosphatase value is almost certainly of liver origin. The more prominent increase of the alkaline phosphatase level indicates a cholestatic process. In a patient with a past history of ulcerative colitis, primary sclerosing cholangitis is the most likely diagnosis. Primary biliary cirrhosis is more common in a woman and is not associated with inflammatory bowel disease.

The patient does not have right upper quadrant pain or fever, which would suggest acute cholecystitis. A patient with chronic hepatitis C and autoimmune hepatitis would present with increased levels of aminotransferases without the prominent increase of the alkaline phosphatase level.

17. Answer e.

This man presents with an increased level of aminotransferase consistent with a hepatitis, and his symptoms of fatigue are consistent with a chronic hepatitis. His serologic profile is most consistent with chronic hepatitis B. Patients with acute hepatitis B generally have more prominent symptoms and also have a positive IgM anti-HBc antibody present. Acute hepatitis C and acute hepatitis A are unlikely because of the clinical presentation. The great majority of patients with chronic hepatitis C are anti-HCV positive.

18. Answer d.

This patient presents with classic physical examination and laboratory findings of alcoholic hepatitis. Note that the aspartate aminotransferase value is twice that of alanine aminotransferase, and both values are only modestly increased. In general, patients with acute viral hepatitis or autoimmune hepatitis present with more prominent increases in the levels of the aminotransferases.

19. Answer e.

This patient presents wtih symptoms of biliary pain. She has risk factors for gallstone disease, including her sex, age, and obesity. Given the symptoms and the cholelithiasis demonstrated on ultrasonography, laparoscopic cholecystectomy is indicated. Endoscopic retrograde cholangiopancreatography to diagnose common bile duct stones may be necessary before or after laparoscopic cholecystectomy. In general, the approach is to proceed with laparoscopic cholecystectomy with cholangiography if clinically indicated. If the cholangiogram demonstrates choledocholithiasis, attempts can be made to remove the stones laparoscopically. If attempts are unsuccessful, postoperative endoscopic retrograde cholangiopancreatography with stone extraction would be performed. Esophagogastroduodenoscopy, computed tomography of the abdomen, and oral cholecystography have no role in the management of this patient.

20. Answer b.

Because the serum level of albumin is 2.6 g/dL and the ascites protein value is 1.1 g/dL, the serum-ascitic fluid albumin gradient is more than 1.5. This is consistent with ascites due to portal hypertension. This patient's history of alcohol abuse and the ultrasonographic findings of a small liver and splenomegaly suggest that he has alcoholic cirrhosis. Treatment for his ascites with sodium restriction and diuretics is in order. Malignant ascites is accompanied by a protein value of more than 2.5 g/dL in the ascitic fluid. In portal hypertension due to congestive failure, the serum-ascitic fluid albumin gradient is more than 1.1, but it is also accompanied by a protein value of more than 2.5 g/dL in the abdominal fluid. Spontaneous bacterial peritonitis is diagnosed on the basis of more than 250 neutrophils/mL in the ascitic fluid, and therefore there is no need for administration of antibiotics. Computed tomography of the abdomen would likely merely confirm what is already known from ultrasonography and the physical examination and is therefore not necessary.

21. Answer c.

This patient has an indirect hyperbilirubinemia. The most common cause of an indirect hyperbilirubinemia in the outpatient setting is Gilbert syndrome. This is a disorder characterized by defective conjugation of bilirubin. The hemoglobin value is normal, and thus no significant hemolysis is indicated. Primary sclerosing cholangitis, primary biliary cirrhosis, cholangiocarcinoma, and choledocholithiasis can also produce an increased level of bilirubin, but all patients with these conditions have an increased level of direct bilirubin, and most have an increased level of alkaline phosphatase. The past history of ulcerative colitis in this patient is of no relevance.

22. Answer a.

This patient has the characteristic history and physical examination and laboratory features of hemochromatosis. The increased level of glucose is consistent with a mild diabetes due to iron excess in the pancreas. The serum iron and iron binding capacity should be measured, and the transferrin saturation will be at least 60% and likely much higher. Measurement of the ceruloplasmin level would be helpful to diagnose Wilson's disease. This patient is old for the diagnosis of Wilson's disease, and Wilson's disease would not explain the small testes and increased level of glucose. An autoimmune hepatitis or α_1-antitrypsin deficiency would not have these characteristic clinical features.

23. a, false; b, true; c, true; d, true; e, false; f, true.

Helicobacter pylori occurs in 10% of the general population younger than age 30 and in 60% of the population older than age 60. Many of these people are asymptomatic without peptic ulcer disease. *H. pylori* is the commonest cause of histologic gastritis and is an important factor in the development of type B antral gastritis, duodenal ulcers, gastric ulcers, and gastric adenocarcinoma. If *H. pylori* is eradicated, the healing of active duodenal ulcers is accelerated and the rate of recurrence of both duodenal ulcers and gastric ulcers decreases.

24. a, true; b, true; c, true; d, false; e, true; f, false.

The organisms that cause infectious diarrhea have been associated with certain foods. *Bacillus cereus* is associated

with fried rice from oriental restaurants; *Salmonella*, with poultry; and *Vibrio parahaemolyticus*, with shellfish ingestion. The only infectious diarrhea for which antibiotics shorten the duration of illness is *Vibrio cholerae*. In *Salmonella* infection, antibiotics may prolong the carrier state and do not affect the course of disease. Antibiotics are indicated in *Salmonella* infection only if the blood cultures are positive. In traveler's diarrhea, treatment is supportive unless there is high fever and toxicity, bloody stools, or positive blood cultures.

25. a, true; b, false; c, true; d, false; e, true; f, true.

Risk factors for colorectal cancer include an age older than 40 years, a medical history of colon adenomatous polyps, a family history of colon cancer, inflammatory bowel disease, and a history of female genital or breast cancer. Hyperplastic polyps are not premalignant and diverticulosis is not associated with colon cancer.

26. a, false; b, true; c, true; d, true; e, false; f, false.

Corticosteroids are useful for suppressing active inflammation, but because of cumulative toxicity, they have little role in maintenance therapy for inflammatory bowel disease. Left-sided ulcerative colitis may be treated with steroid or aminosalicylate enemas. Severe attacks of acute ulcerative colitis usually require high doses of corticosteroids. To minimize the steroid side effects, immunosuppressive agents may be effective for chronically active steroid-dependent patients. Bowel rest has not been shown to be more effective than elemental diet, and antibiotics are more effective in Crohn's disease with perineal involvement than in ulcerative colitis.

27. a, true; b, false; c, true; d, false; e, false; f, true.

The presence of oil droplets and undigested meat fibers in the stool suggests pancreatic insufficiency but not intestinal disease as a cause for malabsorption. Vitamin B_{12} is bound to R protein. In pancreatic disease, this bond may not be cleaved. Thus, vitamin B_{12} cannot bind to intrinsic factor. Therefore, vitamin B_{12} deficiency may be seen in pancreatic insufficiency. Iron is absorbed in the proximal small bowel and is abnormal in small bowel disease but not in pancreatic insufficiency. Blunted small bowel villi are compatible for celiac sprue but may occur in many other conditions and are not diagnostic of celiac sprue. Response to a gluten-free diet is diagnostic of celiac sprue. In Whipple's disease, the characteristic findings on small bowel biopsy are PAS-positive organisms in macrophages.

28. a, false; b, true; c, false; d, true; e, true; f, false.

Hepatitis C results in chronic infection in up to 90% of cases and is associated with an increased incidence of hepatocellular carcinoma. Interferon normalizes aminotransferase values in only about 40%-50% of patients, and most patients will have relapse when use of interferon is discontinued. Hepatitis C is the most common cause of post-transfusion hepatitis, and fluctuating aminotransferase levels are characteristic. Unlike primary sclerosing cholangitis, hepatitis C is not strongly associated with the presence of inflammatory bowel disease.

29. a, true; b, false; c, false; d, true; e, false; f, false.

Corticosteroids, vitamin A, and tetracycline can all cause steatosis. Typically, isoniazid hepatotoxicity presents with increased levels of aminotransferases. Most drug-induced liver injury is idiosyncratic, and rechallenge is not recommended. Alcoholic patients have an increased activity of their cytochrome P-450 system and therefore produce more toxic metabolites of acetaminophen than nonalcoholics. Consequently, in alcoholic patients acetaminophen hepatotoxicity may develop with relatively "nontoxic" doses. Patients with methotrexate hepatotoxicity may have normal values of aminotransferases.

30. a, false; b, false; c, true; d, false; e, false; f, true.

Patients with a prior ileal resection have a relative deficiency of bile salts and therefore are at increased risk for cholesterol gallbladder stones. Oral bile acid therapy is useful for small noncalcified gallbladder stones, and many months of therapy are required. Most patients with common bile duct stones also have gallbladder stones. Prophylactic cholecystectomy is not advised in diabetic patients and in general should be discouraged. Endoscopic retrograde cholangiopancreatography is a useful adjunct in selected patients who have laparoscopic cholecystectomy. The general recommendation is that endoscopic retrograde cholangiopancreatography can follow laparoscopic cholecystectomy if intraoperative cholangiography demonstrates common bile duct stones. Finally, patients with ascending cholangitis are generally ill and can be helped with endoscopic extraction of common bile duct stones.

NOTES

CHAPTER 9

GENERAL INTERNAL MEDICINE

Scott C. Litin, M.D.

INTERPRETATION OF DIAGNOSTIC TESTS

Diagnostic test assessment takes into account two sets of characteristics: those pertaining to the test itself (sensitivity and specificity) and the pretest likelihood that the disease is present in the person being tested (prevalence of disease in a population). When a diagnostic test is applied to a population at risk for the abnormal condition, patients in the studied population can be assigned to one of four groups (Table 9-1):

True-positive = disease present, abnormal test result.

False-positive = disease absent, abnormal test result.

False-negative = disease present, normal test result.

True-negative = disease absent, normal test result.

When data are displayed in a 2-by-2 table, the following test characteristics can be defined (Table 9-1):

1. Sensitivity

   Positive in disease (PID).

   True positivity rate--proportion of patients with the target disorder who have positive test result.

   2-by-2 table definition = $a/(a+c)$.

   "SN out"--a test with 100% sensitivity if negative rules out the disorder.

   Screening tests attempt to maximize sensitivity to avoid missing a person with the disease.

   Characteristic of test--not affected by population characteristics.

2. Specificity

   Negative in health (NIH).

   True negativity rate--proportion of patients without the target disorder who have a negative test result.

   2-by-2 table definition = $d/(b+d)$.

   "SP in"--a test with 100% specificity if positive rules in the disorder.

   Confirmatory tests used in follow-up of screening try to maximize specificity to avoid incorrectly labeling a healthy person as having disease.

   Characteristic of test--not affected by population characteristics.

3. Positive predictive value

   When a patient's illness is evaluated by interpreting a diagnostic test, the 2-by-2 table is read horizontally, not vertically. Therefore, in judging the value of a diagnostic test, it is not essential to know its sensitivity and specificity but whether a patient with positive test results has the disease, i.e., how well the test results predict a disease when compared with the standard for that particular disease. Thus, the horizontal properties of the diagnostic test are of primary interest. Among all patients with a positive diagnostic test result, $(a+b)$, in what proportion, $a/(a+b)$, has the diagnosis been correctly predicted or ruled in? This proportion is the positive predictive value (PPV).

   - PPV is the proportion of patients who test positive who have the disease.
   - This provides information most useful in clinical practice.
   - PPV is affected by the prevalence of the disease in the population.
   - 2-by-2 table definition, PPV = $a/(a+b)$.

4. Negative predictive value

   It is also important to know the percentage of patients with a negative test result, $(c+d)$, who actually do not have the disease. This proportion, $d/(c+d)$, is the negative predictive value (NPV).

   - NPV is the proportion of patients who test negative and have no disease; it is prevalence-dependent.
   - 2-by-2 table definition, NPV = $d/(c+d)$.

5. Prevalence

   The PPV and NPV of a diagnostic test depend on the proportion of persons with the disease among the entire group of persons to whom the test is applied. This proportion, $(a+c)/(a+b+c+d)$, is the prevalence.

Table 9-1.--2-By-2 Table

		Target disorder		
		Present	Absent	
Diagnostic test result	Positive	True + a	False + b	a+b
	Negative	c False -	d True -	c+d
		a+c	b+d	a+b+c+d

Prevalence = (a+c)/(a+b+c+d)
Test characteristics
    Sensitivity = a/(a+c)
    Specificity = d/(b+d)
Frequency-dependent properties
    PPV = a/(a+b)
    NPV = d/(c+d)

How to Construct a 2-By-2 Table

The sensitivity, specificity, and predictive values of normal and abnormal test results can be calculated with even a limited amount of information. For example, suppose a new diagnostic test gives abnormal results in 90% of patients who have the disease and normal results in 95% of patients who are disease-free, and furthermore, the prevalence of the disease in the population to which the test is applied is 10%. This provides the following information:

    sensitivity = 90%
    specificity = 95%
    prevalence = 10%

This test is now ready to be applied to a group of patients by filling in a 2-by-2 table (Table 9-2). The calculation is easier if the test is applied to a large number of patients, e.g., 1,000, and a+b+c+d = 1,000.

Because the prevalence of the disease is 10%, 100 patients have the disease (0.1 x 1,000 = 100, or a+c = 100). Of the patients, 90%, or 900, are disease-free (0.9 x 1,000 = 900, or b+d = 900).

Because the sensitivity of the test is 90%, of the 100 patients with disease, 90% have a positive test result (a = 0.9 x 100 = 90) and 10% have a negative result (c = 0.1 x 100 = 10).

Specificity of 95% means that of the 900 patients who are disease-free, 95% have a negative test result (d = 0.95 x 900 = 855) and 5% have a positive test result (b = 0.05 x 900 = 45).

The 2-by-2 table (Table 9-2) shows that 135 patients (a+b) have an abnormal test result; however, only 90 of these 135 patients actually have the disease. Therefore, the PPV of an abnormal test is a/(a+b) = 90/135 = 66.7%, i.e., only two-thirds of all patients with positive test results will actually have the disease. Similarly, one can determine that 865 patients (c+d)

Table 9-2.--2-By-2 Table for Test With 90% Sensitivity, 95% Specificity, and 10% Prevalence

		Disease present	Disease absent	
Diagnostic test result	Positive	90 a	45 b	135 a+b
	Negative	c 10	d 855	c+d 865
		a+c	b+d	a+b+c+d
Total		100	900	1,000

Prevalence = (a+c)/(a+b+c+d) = 100/1,000 = 10%
Test characteristics
    Sensitivity = a/(a+c) = 90/100 = 90%
    Specificity = d/(b+d) = 855/900 = 95%
Frequency-dependent properties
    PPV = a/(a+b) = 90/135 = 66.7%
    NPV = d/(c+d) = 855/865 = 98.8%

have a negative test result: 855 of these 865 patients are disease-free. Therefore, the NPV of the test is d/(c+d) = 855/865 = 98.8%.

Clinicians should be able to perform these simple calculations. Clinical decision-making by internists is more likely to depend on the PPV and NPV of test results for a given population than on the sensitivity or specificity of the test.

For example, if the prevalence of the disease in the clinician's population is 2% instead of 10%, the PPV and NPV can be recalculated. The PPV of abnormal test results falls to 26.9%, quite different from the 66.7% above, although the sensitivity and specificity of the test (90% and 95%, respectively) have not changed (Table 9-3).

- The most important factor in interpreting an abnormal test result in a patient is the prevalence of the disease in the population being tested.
- High-risk populations (high prevalence of disease) tend to improve the PPV of an abnormal test result.
- Low-risk populations (screening tests) make the NPV of a normal test result look impressive.

PREOPERATIVE MEDICAL EVALUATION

The Art of Medical Consultation

This section is concerned with advice given by an internist to a surgeon in assessing preoperative risk in managing perioperative problems (J Gen Intern Med 2:257-269, 1987). Guidelines for the internist to optimize compliance with the advice are listed below:

Table 9-3.--2-By-2 Table for Test With 90% Sensitivity, 95% Specificity, and 2% Prevalence

		Disease present	Disease absent	
Test result	Positive	18 a	49 b	67 a+b
	Negative	c 2	d 931	c+d 933
		a+c	b+d	a+b+c+d
	Total	20	980	1,000

Prevalence = (a+c)/(a+b+c+d) = 20/1,000 = 2%
Test characteristics
  Sensitivity = a/(a+c) = 18/20 = 90%
  Specificity = d/(b+d) = 931/980 = 95%
Frequency-dependent properties
  PPV = a/(a+b) = 18/67 = 26.9%
  NPV = d/(c+d) = 931/933 = 99.8%

1. Limit the number of recommendations to five or fewer.
2. Focus on crucial recommendations and avoid diluting management plan with trivial suggestions.
3. Be specific, especially regarding drug dosages. Recommend not only which drug to use but specify dose and frequency of administration.
4. Advice about therapy (i.e., initiating or discontinuing drug therapy) is heeded more often than diagnostic suggestions (i.e., ordering tests).
5. Labor-intensive advice that requires the surgeon to do something (look at a blood smear, perform a procedure, etc.) is poorly heeded. If such tasks must be performed, the medical consultant should do them personally.
6. Oral communication with the surgeon usually enhances compliance.
7. Follow-up visits and notes further improve compliance.
Successfully communicating one's assessment and plan is an art. A three-step approach--diagnosis/treatment/prognosis--is often helpful.
1. Diagnosis--the internist creates a problem list that is a table of contents for anyone involved in the care of patient. It is particularly useful to anesthesiologists and surgeons.
2. Treatment--the internist offers recommendations that will diminish the surgical risks associated with the patient's problem. The emphasis is on therapeutics aimed only at diminishing surgical risk.
3. Prognosis--the internist states the surgical and anesthetic risk for each problem (often available in published literature). When this information is lacking, the internist has to substitute personal judgment.
4. The internist should comment on the cumulative risk

for a patient with multiple medical problems, such as cardiac, pulmonary, and liver disease. The risk in such patients may become prohibitive.

- Diagnosis--a problem list.
- Treatment--recommendations only for decreasing surgical risk.
- Prognosis--surgical and anesthetic risk for each problem.
- Internist should comment on cumulative risk for patient with multiple medical problems.

Risks of Anesthesia and the Operation

Operative deaths are uncommon because of the many technical advances made in recent years in surgery and anesthesia. The risk of dying in the perioperative period (i.e., intraoperatively or within 48 hours postoperatively) is about 0.3% when all operations are considered. In major surgical procedures, the mortality risk is still less than 1% in patients younger than 65 years, but it increases to about 5% for those between 65 and 80 years old. Deaths occur in three periods: anesthetic induction (10%), intraoperatively (35%), and in the first 48 hours postoperatively (55%). Postoperative mortality between 48 hours and 6 weeks is usually due to pneumonia, sepsis, cardiac arrest, pulmonary embolus, or renal failure. The American Society of Anesthesiologists (ASA) has published a classification scheme to aid clinicians (Table 9-4). This classification is subjective, and many physicians favor a systematic assessment as opposed to a global impression. However, ASA class IV and V patients have roughly 100 times the mortality of class I patients for a surgical procedure. Also, an emergency procedure roughly doubles the risk in any ASA classification of patients.

- The risk of dying in the perioperative period is 0.3% of all operations.
- Three periods in which deaths (%) occur: anesthetic induction (10%), intraoperatively (35%), and within 48 hours postoperatively (55%).

Many physicians have mistakenly thought that spinal anesthesia is safer than general anesthesia in high-risk patients. From a cardiopulmonary standpoint, this is not true. Spinal anesthesia may be associated with wide fluctuations in blood pressure, anxiety, and less control of the airway and ventilation. Thus, it is inappropriate for the internist to write, "patient too ill for general anesthesia; okay if done under spinal." The final decision about the type of anesthesia is the responsibility of the anesthesiologist.

- From a cardiopulmonary point of view, spinal anesthesia is not safer than general anesthesia.
- Spinal anesthesia may be associated with wide fluctuations in blood pressure.

Table 9-4.--American Society of Anesthesiologists Classification of Anesthetic Mortality Within 48 Hours Postoperatively

Class	Physical status	48-Hour mortality
I	Normal healthy person < 80 years old	0.07%
II	Mild systemic disease	0.24%
III	Severe but not incapacitating systemic disease	1.4%
IV	Incapacitating systemic disease that is a constant threat to life	7.5%
V	Moribund patient not expected to survive 24 hours, regardless of surgery	8.1%
E	Suffix added to any class indicating emergency procedure, e.g., IE, IIE, IIIE	Doubles risk

From MKSAP IX: Part C, Book 4, 1991. American College of Physicians. By permission.

- The final decision about the type of anesthesia is the responsibility of the anesthesiologist.

The type of operation performed is also an important determinant of morbidity and mortality. Procedures associated with low risk include eye surgery, oral surgery, dilatation and curettage, hysterectomy, and herniorrhaphy. Certain other procedures are associated with a higher risk, including craniotomy and cardiovascular operations. Other operations would be considered intermediate risk.

- Low-risk procedures are eye surgery, oral surgery, dilatation and curettage, hysterectomy, and herniorrhaphy.
- Higher risk procedures are craniotomy and cardiovascular operations.
- Other procedures are of intermediate risk.

However, the importance of associated disease in determining surgical risk may outweigh the nature of the procedure or the type of anesthesia used in predicting outcome. The following sections discuss risk assessment and management strategies grouped by organ system.

Pulmonary Risks and Management

Pulmonary complications (hypoventilation, atelectasis, and pneumonia) occur in about one-third of patients postoperatively and account for 50% of overall perioperative mortality. Patients at definite risk for pulmonary complications include smokers, patients with chronic obstructive pulmonary disease, obesity, thoracic surgery, and upper abdominal surgery. Patients with probable increased risk include those >70 years whose duration of anesthesia is >2 hours or who currently have respiratory infection.

- Pulmonary complications account for 50% of overall perioperative mortality.

Preoperative pulmonary function testing should be part of the evaluation of high-risk patients. The interpretation of these tests regarding risk assessment is controversial. However, most authors agree that the simple spirometric measurement of forced expiratory volume in 1 second (FEV_1) is probably as good a predictor as any of surgical risk. If the FEV_1 is >2 L, the patient can safely undergo the surgical procedure. If the FEV_1 is between 1 and 2 L, the risk of postoperative pulmonary complications is increased. An FEV_1 <1 L is indicative of a high risk of postoperative pulmonary complication.

- FEV_1 is a good predictor of surgical risk.
- FEV_1 >2 L, patient can safely undergo procedure.
- FEV_1 <1 L, high risk of postoperative pulmonary complication.

Several measures have been advocated to decrease the pulmonary risks. Preoperative measures to decrease pulmonary risk include instruction in respiratory maneuvers, cessation of cigarette smoking, use of bronchodilators, antibiotic treatment of chronic bronchitis, and chest physiotherapy. Postoperative measures include chest physiotherapy and inspiratory maneuvers, minimization of postoperative narcotic analgesia, and early mobilization of elderly patients.

Cardiac Risks and Management

Each year about 1 out of 10 U.S. citizens undergoes a noncardiac operation. Because of the increasing prevalence of surgical procedures in the elderly, about ⅓ of all noncardiac surgical patients are at risk for cardiac morbidity or mortality after taking into account the prevalence of coronary artery disease or the high risk status in this population. Patients with known or suspected cardiac disease are commonly referred to a general internist or cardiologist for assessment before a noncardiac procedure is performed. Several questions are posed during these consultations:

1. How can the high-risk patient be identified?
2. What selective testing needs to be performed (if any) to further define risk?
3. What intervention or perioperative management is appropriate to decrease cardiac-related morbidity and mortality during noncardiac surgical procedures?

A risk-factor index, the Goldman index, was devised through

a prospective analysis of patients older than 40 years under-going noncardiac general surgery in an attempt to allow clinicians to estimate cardiac risk after clinical assessment (N Engl J Med 297:845-850, 1977). This scale has been validated prospectively and has formed the framework of preoperative cardiac evaluation (Tables 9-5 and 9-6).

Myocardial infarction (MI) is the most feared perioperative complication. Of perioperative MIs, 50% are fatal and 60% are silent. The risk of perioperative MI peaks on the third postoperative day. Patients with recent MIs are at greatest risk for perioperative MIs. The risk of perioperative MI without cardiac disease = 0.2%. Retrospective studies assessed the risk of perioperative MI in patients with recent MI (<3 months) = 27%; if the MI occurred 3-6 months ago, 11%; and if the MI was >6 months ago, 5%. With hemodynamic catheters and aggressive intensive care management, the perioperative MI rate of patients with recent MI could be markedly decreased (MI

<3 months = 5.7%; MI 4 to 6 months = 2.3%). However, the standard recommendation is to delay nonemergent surgery for at least 6 months after MI.

- Of perioperative MIs, 50% are fatal and 60% are silent.
- The risk of perioperative MI peaks on the 3rd postoperative day.
- Patients with recent MI are at greatest risk for perioperative MI, but this rate can be decreased with hemodynamic catheters and aggressive intensive care management.
- Standard recommendation--delay nonemergent surgery for at least 6 months after MI.

Cardiac Evaluation for Patients Undergoing Vascular Surgery

Vascular operations by their nature often place the greatest stress on the heart (cross-clamping abdominal aorta, etc.). The

Table 9-5.--The Goldman Cardiac Risk-Index for Noncardiac Surgery

Clinical variable	Point assessment
History	
Age >70 years	5
Recent myocardial infarction (≤6 mo)	10
Physical examination	
Ventricular gallop or jugular venous pressure ≥12 cm H_2O	11
Significant valvular aortic stenosis	3
Electrocardiogram	
Rhythm other than sinus or atrial ectopy on preoperative tracing	7
More than 5/min ectopic ventricular beats on any tracing preoperatively	7
Poor general medical condition (any of the following)	
Po_2 <60 mm Hg or Pco_2 >50 mm Hg	
Serum potassium <3.0 meq/L or bicarbonate <20 meq/L	
Blood urea nitrogen >50 mg/dL or creatinine >3.0 mg/dL	3
Chronic liver disease	
Noncardiac debilitation	
Surgical procedure	
Intraperitoneal, intrathoracic, aortic	3
Emergency	4
Maximum score	53

From MKSAP IX: Part C, Book 4, 1991. American College of Physicians. By permission. (Modified from Goldman L, Caldera DL, Nussman SR et al: Multifactorial index of cardiac risk in noncardiac surgical procedures. N Engl J Med 297:845-850, 1977.)

Table 9-6.--Cardiac Complications Stratified by the Goldman Risk Index

Risk-index class	Point score	No or minimal complication, %	Severe complications, %	Cardiac death, %
I	0-5	99	0.6	0.2
II	6-12	96	3	1
III	13-25	86	11	3
IV	≥26	49	12	39

From MKSAP IX: Part C, Book 4, 1991. American College of Physicians. By permission. (Modified from Goldman L, Caldera DL, Nussman SR et al: Multifactorial index of cardiac risk in noncardiac surgical procedures. N Engl J Med 297:845-850, 1977.)

prevalence of coronary artery disease (CAD) is much higher in vascular surgical patients (~60%) than in the general surgical population (10%-15%). Thus, the Goldman criteria (Tables 9-5 and 9-6) fail to predict complications accurately in vascular surgical patients. For this group, new predictive rules are needed because of the difference in the prevalence of disease. Adequate exercise levels indicate a low rate of cardiac complications in patients who can exercise on a treadmill to >5 METs or on a bicycle ergometer to >400 kg/m per minute. For those unable to exercise, lack of redistribution on dipyridamole or adenosine thallium scans is predictive of a low rate of complications.

- Vascular operations place the greatest stress on the heart.
- Prevalence of CAD is higher in vascular surgical patients (60%) than in general surgical population (10%-15%).
- Goldman criteria do not accurately predict the complications in vascular surgical patients.
- Adequate exercise levels in these patients indicate a low rate of complication.
- Inability to exercise but lack of redistribution on dipyridamole or adenosine thallium scans indicates a low rate of complications.

To help select patients in need of further study before vascular surgery, five clinical factors have been described: 1) age >70 years, 2) Q-wave on EKG, 3) history of angina pectoris, 4) history of ventricular ectopy requiring treatment, and 5) diabetes mellitus. When these clinical variables were applied to a group of patients, the following complications were noted:
1. No clinical variables--only 3.1% had postoperative ischemic events.
2. Three or more clinical variables--50% had postoperative ischemic events.
3. One or two clinical variables--a further risk subdivision could be made on the basis of the results of a dipyridamole thallium scan.
   a. If scan showed no redistribution--only 3.2% had perioperative ischemic events.
   b. If scan showed redistribution--30% had perioperative ischemic events.

Semiquantitative analysis of dipyridamole scanning improves risk stratification before vascular surgery. This means that for fewer segments or coronary territories involved with thallium redistribution on a scan, perioperative cardiac events are fewer.

On the basis of these factors and the extensive literature on the topic, the algorithm in Figure 9-1 and the following conclusions appear valid:

- Vascular disease is a marker for CAD.
- CAD is a major cause of perioperative and long-term mortality in vascular surgical patients.

- Perioperative cardiac complication rates are low if:
  There are no clinical indicators of CAD.
  The patient can achieve an adequate exercise capacity.
  No redistribution is present on dipyridamole thallium scan.
  Absence of ischemia on preoperative ambulatory ECG monitoring.
- In selected patients, perioperative and long-term mortality is decreased by treatment intervention directed at CAD.

Monitoring for Perioperative Myocardial Ischemia

In high-risk patients undergoing noncardiac operations, early postoperative myocardial ischemia is an important correlate of adverse cardiac outcomes. Patient subgroups who are at high risk for postoperative ischemia and who might benefit most from intensive Holter monitoring in the postoperative period can be identified preoperatively: left ventricular hypertrophy, CAD, diabetes, hypertension, and digoxin use. By identifying high-risk patients and monitoring them postoperatively with real-time monitors with alarms triggered by ST-segment depression, ischemia could be identified instantaneously so rapid intervention could potentially prevent clinical ischemia events. However, this hypothesis is as yet unstudied and unproven, and these interventions, if performed in all at-risk patients, would drive up costs tremendously!

- Early postoperative myocardial ischemia is an important correlate of adverse cardiac outcome in high-risk noncardiac surgical patients.

Valvular Heart Disease

Patients with valvular heart disease present specific risks in noncardiac surgery. Significant aortic stenosis is associated with a "fixed" cardiac output that cannot increase in response to surgical stress. Although such patients have minimal risk with local anesthesia, spinal anesthesia increases the risk because of the frequent induction of vasodilatation, which can cause cardiovascular collapse. Although general anesthesia can be performed with acceptable risks in selected hemodynamically monitored patients with severe aortic stenosis, conventional wisdom is to repair the valve preoperatively (when possible) in patients with critical aortic stenosis.

- Significant aortic stenosis is associated with a "fixed" cardiac output that cannot increase with surgical stress.
- Although selected patients with severe aortic stenosis can tolerate general anesthesia, the valve should be repaired preoperatively when possible in those with critical aortic stenosis.

When mitral regurgitation is present, the status of left ventricular function is of primary importance. Patients with mitral regurgitation tolerate vasodilatation well.

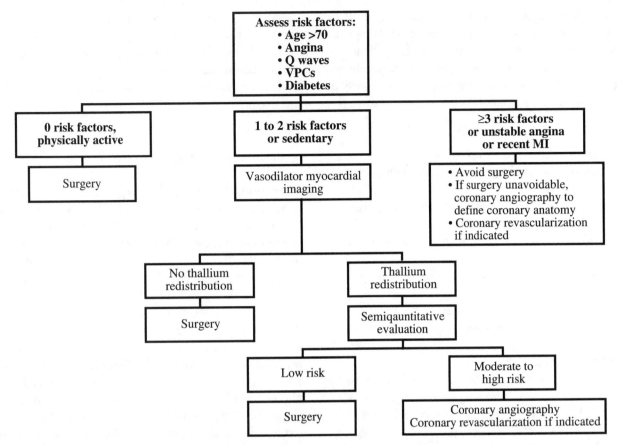

Fig. 9-1. Cardiac evaluation strategy for patients undergoing vascular operations and unable to perform an exercise treadmill test. Carotid endarterectomy is excluded from the evaluation because of low associated morbidity/mortality in absence of accelerating angina or recent myocardial infarction. (From Weitz HH: Cardiac risk stratification prior to vascular surgery. Med Clin North Am 77:377-396, March 1993. By permission of WB Saunders Company.)

- Patients with mitral regurgitation tolerate vasodilatation.
- Patients with valvular heart disease should receive endocarditis prophylaxis in accordance with the standard recommendations of the American Heart Association.

Anticoagulation Issues in Patients With Mechanical Prosthetic Heart Valves Undergoing Noncardiac Operations

No randomized controlled trials have been conducted on anticoagulation in noncardiac surgical patients with mechanical heart valves. However, the following suggestions are offered.

1. Consult with the surgeon to determine whether the intensity of anticoagulation needs to be altered. Procedures such as dental extractions, cataract removal, and other minor operations often can be performed safely with minimal or no decrease in the intensity of anticoagulation.

2. Many factors must be considered when determining a risk-to-benefit assessment of continuous anticoagulation in patients with mechanical prosthetic cardiac valves. Mitral prosthetic values are more thrombogenic than aortic prostheses, regardless of what type of value has been used. In general, the older caged-ball values (Starr-Edwards) are more thrombogenic than bileaflet values

(St. Jude Medical), and *the bioprosthetic valves* are the least thrombogenic. Other factors such as atrial fibrillation, severely impaired left ventricular function, or history of previous thromboembolism also increase the risk of thromboembolism.

3. After a risk-to-benefit assessment has been completed, one of the following strategies can be chosen: a) discontinue warfarin therapy for several days before the procedure to allow the prothrombin time (PT) to normalize (outpatient setting) just before the operation, b) decrease the dose of warfarin (outpatient setting) to maintain the intensity of anticoagulation in a lower or subtherapeutic range during the procedure (discuss this with the surgeon), or c) discontinue warfarin therapy and institute heparin therapy (inpatient setting)--administration of heparin can be discontinued 4 hours before the operation and reinstituted, in conjunction with oral anticoagulant therapy, postoperatively, when it is considered safe.

In most situations, strategy a or b can be undertaken safely at considerable cost advantage (because of the need for fewer hospitalization days) without appreciable increase in risk to the patient. Preoperative heparin therapy during warfarin withdrawal is recommended only for those situations in which the risk of bleeding with anticoagulant therapy and the risk of thromboembolism without anticoagulant therapy are high (for example, major surgical procedure in a patient with mitral valve prosthesis, cardiomyopathy, or previous thromboembolism). Reinstitution of anticoagulation as early as safely possible is appropriate for all three of the strategies mentioned above.

- Teeth extractions, cataract operations, and other minor procedures usually can be performed safely with therapeutic levels of anticoagulation.
- Prosthetic valves in the mitral position are more thrombogenic than aortic prostheses.
- Older ball-cage valves are more thrombogenic than bileaflet valves.
- Bioprosthetic valves are least thrombogenic.
- Anticoagulation in patients with mechanical prosthetic cardiac valves substantially decreases the incidence of thromboemboli but never eliminates it entirely.

Congestive Heart Failure

Patients with congestive heart failure (CHF) have an incidence of perioperative pulmonary edema ranging from 3% (New York Heart Association class I) to 25% (class IV). Patients with a history of CHF but no preoperative evidence of this disorder have a 6% incidence of perioperative pulmonary edema. Although preoperative CHF is the greatest risk factor for development of pulmonary edema, 50% of those who develop this complication have no history of CHF. Most patients who develop CHF perioperatively do so in the first hour after termination of anesthesia. CHF should be aggressively treated preoperatively, and the therapy for chronic compensated CHF should be maintained in the perioperative period.

- Incidence of perioperative pulmonary edema is from 3% to 25% in patients with CHF.
- The greatest preoperative risk for developing pulmonary edema is CHF.
- If CHF develops perioperatively, it usually does so in the 1st hour after anesthesia is terminated.
- Treat CHF aggressively preoperatively, and in the perioperative period, maintain therapy for chronic compensated CHF.

Hypertension

Ideally, patients should have well-controlled hypertension (i.e., $\leq$ 140/90 mm Hg) for several months preoperatively to minimize lability of intraoperative blood pressure as well as postoperative and neurologic complications. However, studies have shown that when hypertension is stable and diastolic blood pressure is $\leq$110 mm Hg, no benefit is derived from postponing elective procedures to achieve better control. If

diastolic blood pressure is >110 mg Hg, it should be stabilized for at least several days preoperatively to diminish risk. Although systolic blood pressure is less well studied, most medical consultants suggest the systolic blood pressure be controlled to <180 mm Hg before the induction of anestheisa for elective procedures.

- If diastolic blood pressure is >110 mm Hg, it should be stabilized for at least several days preoperatively.

Hematologic Risk and Management

Patients with poorly controlled polycythemia vera have a high surgical morbidity and mortality because of an excess of thromboembolic events and decrease in oxygen transport due to high blood viscosity. In polycythemia vera, phlebotomy should be performed to decrease the hematocrit to <45% before elective operations. Platelet counts <50,000/mm^3 or >1,000,000/mm^3 should be evaluated with bleeding times and corrected preoperatively. A platelet count of 50,000/mm^3 usually provides adequate hemostasis for most surgical procedures. If the count is <20,000/mm^3, spontaneous bleeding is common. A bleeding time, activated partial thromboplastin time (APTT), and PT should be determined preoperatively only if the medical history and physical examination results indicate increased bleeding risk, such as previous bleeding with major or minor surgery, easy bruising, or a family history of bleeding disorder.

- Patients with poorly controlled polycythemia vera have high surgical morbidity and mortality because of thromboembolic events and high blood viscosity.
- In polycythemia vera, perform phlebotomy to decrease hematocrit to <45% before elective operation.
- Platelet count of 50,000/mm^3 usually provides adequate hemostasis for most operations.
- Preoperatively determine bleeding time, APTT, and PT only if medical history and physical examination finding indicate increased bleeding risk.

Liver Risks and Management

Patients with chronic liver disease, particularly those with progressive hepatic failure, possess a high operative risk. Preoperatively, the internist should concentrate on correcting electrolyte abnormalities and abnormal clotting variables, reducing ascites, treating encephalopathy, and improving the patient's nutritional status.

Endocrinologic Risks and Management

Thyrotoxic patients are at high risk for surgical complications, such as arrhythmias, high output CHF, and death. Thyroid storm occurs in 20%-30% of these patients. Thus, elective surgery should be postponed and treatment (antithyroid drugs or radioiodine) should be given for at least 3 months until the patient is euthyroid. If an operation is emergent, a thyrotoxic patient should be pretreated with propranolol, propylthiouracil, potassium iodide, and hydrocortisone. The hypothyroid patient can undergo surgical procedures at very low risk. Severely myxedematous patients should receive thyroxine replacement therapy, careful monitoring, and supportive therapy, including free water restriction and diuretics.

- Thyrotoxic patients are at high risk for surgical complications.
- This condition should be treated for 3 months or until patient is euthyroid before any elective operation is performed.
- In case of an emergency operation, pretreat with propranolol, propylthiouracil, potassium iodide, and hydrocortisone.

Patients with diabetes mellitus have a greater risk of surgical complications due to underlying cardiovascular and cerebrovascular disease. It is preferable to have the patient in moderate diabetic control preoperatively to diminish the risk of infection. Remember that the patient may not be able to recognize the signs and symptoms of hypoglycemia in the perioperative period. Thus, oral hypoglycemic agents are withheld, the insulin dose is cut in half on the day of the operation, and the serum glucose level should be maintained in the 150-250 mg/dL range in the perioperative period.

- In cases of diabetes mellitus, there is greater risk of surgical complications because of underlying cardiovascular and cerebrovascular disease.
- Withhold oral hypoglycemic agents, cut insulin dose in half on the day of the operation, and maintain the serum glucose level at 150-200 mg/dL in the perioperative period.

To be on the safe side, adequate preoperative and perioperative corticosteroid replacement prep should be given to any patient who has received suppressive doses of corticosteroids for 2 weeks or more during the past year.

Nutrition

Perioperatively, malnourished patients have increased complications related to wound infection, pneumonia, respiratory insufficiency, and adversely affected cellular and humoral immune function. In nutritional assessment, clinical judgment of malnutrition is as accurate as objective measurements. Thus, detailed laboratory measurements of albumin and other substances are not usually necessary. There is some rationale in giving preoperative nutritional supplementation to malnourished patients, and continuing support through the perioperative period.

Thromboembolism Prophylaxis

Although all surgical patients are at some risk for venous thromboembolic disease, certain patients form a high-risk subset, including elderly patients, patients undergoing prolonged anesthesia or operation, patients with previous venous thromboembolic disease, prolonged immobilization or paralysis, malignancy, obesity, varicosities, or estrogen use. Reasonable guidelines for thromboembolism prophylaxis in surgical patients to decrease the overall risk of deep venous thrombosis or pulmonary embolism are given in Table 9-7.

Perioperative Antibiotic Prophylaxis

Antibiotics are given perioperatively to prevent infection of normal sterile tissues by direct contamination during the surgical procedure. The risk of wound infection depends largely on the type of operation. "Clean" operations are ones in which the gastrointestinal, genitourinary, and respiratory tracts are not entered and there is no surrounding inflammation. Previously, antibiotic prophylaxis was not required for this type of procedure because the risk of infection was about only 5%, as opposed to a much higher risk in other procedures, which required prophylactic treatment with antibiotics to prevent wound infection (clean-contaminated, contaminated, and dirty operations). However, antibiotic prophylaxis is now recommended for simple clean procedures such as inguinal hernia repair and breast surgery. A short course of prophylactic therapy (one dose of antibiotic preoperatively and no more than one dose postoperatively) is as effective as longer regimens and is less likely to be associated with toxicity or development of resistant organisms in clear or clean-contaminated operations. Technically, the antibiotics used in dirty or contaminated procedures are for treatment of established infection rather than for prophylaxis and are often continued for 5 to 10 days postoperatively.

Preoperative Laboratory Tests

Few laboratory tests should be ordered solely because an operation is planned. In the absence of symptoms, signs, or risk factors for a disease, results of routinely ordered tests are usually normal, and when abnormal, they are usually ignored. Authors looking at specific preoperative tests have suggested that chest radiography, ECG, PT, APTT, and bleeding time are not justified as "routine" preoperative tests in young healthy persons. In the cost-effective climate of modern medical practice, tests should be performed for specific clinical indications and not because a patient is being seen in the outpatient clinic, hospital, or operating room (Table 9-8).

Because ECG abnormalities increase with age and certain abnormalities are related to major perioperative morbidity, most medical consultants suggest a routine ECG in all patients >50 years old before elective operations. Although the relationship between chest radiographic findings and perioperative morbidity is not well-defined, elderly patients frequently need postoperative chest radiographs performed because of pulmonary complications, and a baseline preoperative radiograph is to be helpful in patients >60 years.

Table 9-7.--Prophylaxis for Deep Venous Thrombosis

Clinical setting	Recommended prophylaxis
General surgery patients	
<40 years old, no risk factors	Early ambulation
>40 years old, no additional risk factors	Elastic stockings or low-dose heparin (every 12 hours) or intermittent pneumatic compression
>40 years old, with additional risk factors	Low-dose heparin (every 8 hours) or low-molecular-weight heparin
>40 years old with additional risk factors and with high potential for wound hematomas or infection	Dextran or intermittent pneumatic compression
>40 years old with multiple risk factors	Intermittent pneumatic compression *plus* low-dose heparin or low-molecular-weight heparin or dextran
Orthopedic surgery	
Hip replacement	Warfarin or low-molecular-weight heparin or low-dose heparin (dose adjusted to APTT at upper limit of control range)
Hip fracture	Warfarin or low-molecular-weight heparin
Knee surgery	Intermittent pneumatic compression or low-molecular-weight heparin
Neurosurgery	Intermittent pneumatic compression
Medical conditions	
Myocardial infarction	Low-dose heparin if full-dose heparin is not already being administered
Congestive heart failure and/or pulmonary infections	Low-dose heparin
Ischemic stroke with lower extremity paralysis	Low-dose heparin or low-molecular-weight heparin
Nonambulatory patients or patients with venous stasis	Low-dose heparin
Long-term indwelling central venous catheters	Warfarin, 1 mg daily

APTT, activated partial thromboplastin time.
From MKSAP X: Part A, Book 3, 1994. American College of Physicians. By permission.

Table 9-8.--Indications for Standard Preoperative Tests in Nonemergency Situations

Test	Indications
Hematocrit	All women; men >60 years old; anticipated blood loss
Electrolytes	Patients >60 years or with renal disease or diabetes, or who take diuretics, steroids, bowel preparations
Prothrombin and partial thromboplastin times, platelet count	Patients with liver disease, bleeding, or malignancy, or who take anticoagulants
Electrocardiography	Patients >50 years or with cardiovascular disease, lung disease, peripheral vascular disease, or diabetes
Chest radiography	Patients >60 years or with pulmonary or cardiovascular disease or acute pulmonary symptoms

Modified from MKSAP X: Part A, Book 3, 1994. American College of Physicians. By permission.

- Chest radiography, ECG, PT, APTT, and bleeding time are not "routine" preoperative tests in young healthy persons.
- Tests should be performed for specific clinical indications.

Geriatric Surgical Patients

The number of surgical procedures performed on elderly patients has steadily increased. Elderly patients comprise 15% of the population but account for one-third of all surgical procedures, half of all emergency surgical procedures, and three-quarters of overall surgical mortality. Age is an independent risk factor for perioperative cardiovascular morbidity. The Goldman index scale (Tables 9-5 and 9-6) also underestimates the cardiac risk in geriatric patients, who, like vascular surgical patients, have a much higher prevalence of CAD. Also, as with patients undergoing vascular operations, geriatric patients scheduled for a high-risk procedure should have a thoughtful cardiac evaluation. In certain instances, this might include exercise assessment to provide guidance. Most elderly patients have at least one associated chronic medical illness. This fact and the pathophysiologic effects of aging on the cardiovascular and pulmonary systems probably explain why geriatric patients have a higher perioperative mortality rate than younger patients. Intervention aimed at meticulously looking for and treating perioperative complications (anemia, infection, pneumonia) leads to improved outcomes (less post-operative delirium, fewer hospital days, etc.) in geriatric patients.

- Elderly patients account for one-third of all surgical procedures.
- Age is an independent risk factor for perioperative cardio-vascular morbidity.
- Geriatric patients have a much higher prevalence of CAD.
- Geriatric patients have a higher perioperative mortality rate.

Perioperative Medication Management

The internist tailors perioperative drug therapy to individual circumstances with particular attention to three factors:
1. Have the indications and doses for the specific drug been clearly defined?
2. What are the likely anesthetic and surgical interactions and complications?
3. Is a clinically important withdrawal syndrome likely, and how can it be managed safely?

Most drugs used in managing chronic medical conditions can and should be continued through the perioperative period. Often, patients can receive medications with sips of water on the morning of the operation and resume oral medications or parenteral substitution later in the day. Should particular questions occur about the continuation of a specific drug, communicate with the anesthesiologist.

- Most drugs for chronic medical conditions should continue to be used through the perioperative period.

CURRENT CONCEPTS IN ANTICOAGULATION THERAPY

International Normalized Ratio

What Is Its Significance?

The international normalized ratio (INR) was developed to standardize reporting of the PT assay test results. Standardization was necessary because of the variability in the responsiveness of the different thromboplastins used as reagents throughout the world. The international sensitivity index (ISI) is the value representative of the responsiveness of a given thromboplastin to the reduction of vitamin K-dependent coagulation factors. The variations in ISI between different thromboplastins are due to differences in their manufacture and source and in the method of preparation. A more responsive thromboplastin produces less rapid stimulation of coagulation factors,

producing a greater prolongation of the PT for a given reduction in clotting factors. A less responsive thromboplastin activates residual clotting factors more rapidly and results in a less prolonged PT, despite a comparable decrease in clotting factors. Therefore, with use of a more responsive thromboplastin, a lower dose of warfarin is required to maintain the PT at a desired ratio than the dose required with a less responsive thromboplastin--i.e., an acceptable PT ratio using a very responsive thromboplastin might give a false sense of security in a patient who is actually at risk for clotting. If a less responsive thromboplastin were used, that same ratio might give a false sense of security in a patient who is actually at risk for major bleeding. The INR is simply an exponential mathematical transformation of PT (usually reported in seconds) into a "corrected" ratio value.

- INR standardizes reporting of PT assay test results.

How Can the INR be Calculated?

The INR is calculated from the patient's PT ratio, which is a simple calculation, and the ISI, which is more complicated. The ISI is calculated by the manufacturer of the thromboplastin or by the laboratory performing the test. The formula is

$$INR = \left(\frac{Patient\ PT}{Mean\ control\ PT}\right)^{ISI}$$

How Does the INR Help in Clinical Practice?

The ISI of most thromboplastins used in the U.S. varies from 1.8 to 2.8. Because there is no "typical" North American thromboplastin, the earlier habit of using PT ratios has inadvertently left many patients at risk due to over or under anticoagulation. The use of the INR offers several advantages listed below:

- Smooth regulation of anticoagulant therapy.
- Benefit to patients who travel, because there is consistency among laboratories using different types of thromboplastin.
- Standardization of anticoagulant therapy in clinical trials and scientific publications.
- Potentially decreased risk of bleeding or thrombotic complications associated with oral anticoagulant therapy.

What Are Recommended INR Therapeutic Ranges for Oral Anticoagulant Therapy?

The INR therapeutic ranges recommended by the American College of Chest Physicians (October 1992) are summarized in Table 9-9. In short, an INR of 2.0-3.0 is used for all indications except for mechanical prosthetic heart valves, which require a slightly higher INR of 2.5-3.5.

Table 9-9.--Recommended INR Therapeutic Ranges for Oral
Anticoagulant Therapy

Indication	INR
Prophylaxis of venous thrombosis	
(high-risk surgical procedure)	2.0-3.0
Treatment of venous thrombosis	2.0-3.0
Treatment of pulmonary embolism	2.0-3.0
Prevention of systemic embolism	2.0-3.0
Tissue heart valves	2.0-3.0
Acute myocardial infarction (to	
prevent systemic embolism)	2.0-3.0
Valvular heart disease	2.0-3.0
Atrial fibrillation	2.0-3.0
Recurrent systemic embolism	2.0-3.0
Mechanical prosthetic heart valves	
(high risk)	2.5-3.5

From Litin SC, Gastineau DA: Current concepts in anticoagulant therapy.
Mayo Clin Proc 70:266-272, 1995.

Antithrombotic Therapy for Venous Thromboembolic Disease

Guidelines for anticoagulation in patients with venous thromboembolic disease are summarized in Table 9-10.

Anticoagulation in Prosthetic Heart Valves

What Are the Recommendations for Anticoagulation in Patients With Mechanical Prosthetic Heart Valves?

It is strongly recommended that all patients with mechanical prosthetic heart valves receive warfarin. Levels of warfarin that prolong INR to 2.5-3.5 are recommended. Levels of warfarin producing an INR <1.8 have a high risk of thromboembolic events, and levels that increase INR to >4.5 have a high risk of excessive bleeding. Dipyridamole (375-400 mg/day) in addition to warfarin may have an additive effect without any increase in bleeding. Aspirin (100 mg/day) in addition to warfarin may have an additive effect without increasing the risk of major bleeding, although minor bleeding may be increased.

- All patients with mechanical prosthetic heart valves should receive warfarin.
- Use warfarin levels that prolong INR to 2.5-3.5.
- Warfarin levels that 1) decrease INR <1.8 have high risk of thromboembolic events or 2) increase INR >4.5 have high risk of excessive bleeding.
- Dipyridamole plus warfarin may have additive benefit without increased bleeding.
- A low dose of aspirin plus warfarin may have additive benefit without causing major bleeding (may increase minor bleeding).

What Is Recommended if a Patient With a Prosthetic Heart Valve Has a Systemic Embolism Despite Adequate Therapy With Warfarin (INR 2.5-3.5)?

Such patients might benefit from the addition of aspirin (100-160 mg/day) to the warfarin. Dipyridamole (400 mg/day) in addition to warfarin is an alternative option. Finally, some patients may respond to a slight increase in the warfarin dose, thus increasing the INR to 3.0-4.5.

- No regimen ever eliminates the risk of systemic embolization or the risk of bleeding!

Table 9-10.--Guidelines for Anticoagulation in Adult Patients With Venous Thromboembolic Disease

Deep venous thrombosis or pulmonary embolus	Guidelines for anticoagulation
Suspected	Administer bolus of heparin (5,000 U i.v.) and perform imaging study
Confirmed	Rebolus with heparin (5,000-10,000 U i.v.) and start maintenance infusion at 1,300 U/hour (heparin 20,000 U in 500 mL 5% dextrose in H_2O, infused at 33 mL/hour), or use a weight-based heparin nomogram
	Check activated partial thromboplastin time at 6 hours and adjust to maintain its value between 1.5 and 2.5 times control value
	Check platelet count daily
	Begin warfarin therapy on day 1 at 10 mg daily for first 2 days, then administer warfarin daily at estimated daily maintenance dose (consider beginning with low doses in elderly patients and those with malnourished states, liver disease, etc.)
	Stop heparin therapy after 5 to 7 days of joint therapy when INR is 2.0-3.0 off heparin
	Anticoagulate with warfarin for 3 months, maintain INR of 2.0-3.0

From Litin SC, Gastineau DA: Current concepts in anticoagulant therapy. Mayo Clin Proc 70:266-272, 1995.

What Are the Recommendations for Anticoagulation in Patients With Bioprosthetic Heart Valves?

It is recommended that all patients with bioprosthetic valves in the mitral position receive warfarin therapy (INR, 2.0-3.0) for the first 3 months. Anticoagulant therapy of patients with bioprosthetic valves in the aortic position who are in sinus rhythm is optional during the first 3 months. Certain patients with bioprosthetic valves have underlying conditions (i.e., atrial fibrillation, left atrial thrombus) that require long-term warfarin therapy to prevent systemic emboli. Among patients with bioprosthetic heart valves who are in sinus rhythm, long-term therapy with aspirin (325 mg daily) may offer protection against thromboembolism and appears reasonable for patients without contraindication.

- Patients with bioprosthetic valves in the mitral position receive warfarin therapy (INR, 2.0-3.0) for 1st 3 months.
- Patients with bioprosthetic valves who have atrial fibrillation or left atrial thrombus require long-term warfarin therapy to prevent systemic emboli.
- Long-term therapy with aspirin may protect patients with bioprosthetic heart valves who are in sinus rhythm against thromboembolism.

Hemorrhagic Complications of Anticoagulation

When the Anticoagulant Effect of Warfarin Needs to Be Reversed, What Is the Best Way to Do This?

The anticoagulant effect of warfarin can be reversed by stopping treatment, administering vitamin K, or replacing vitamin K-dependent coagulation factors with fresh frozen plasma. When warfarin therapy is discontinued, no significant effect is seen on the INR for 2 or more days because of the half-life of warfarin (36 to 42 hours) and the delay before newly synthesized functional coagulation factors replace dysfunctional coagulation factors.

Administering vitamin K lowers the INR more rapidly, depending on the dosage of vitamin K and severity of the anticoagulant effect. When high doses of vitamin K are used, reversal is rapid and seen by about 6 hours. The disadvantage is that patients often remain resistant to warfarin for up to a week, making continued warfarin treatment difficult. This problem can be overcome by using much lower dosages of vitamin K given subcutaneously (0.5-1.0 mg) or by slow intravenous infusion.

- Anticoagulant effect of warfarin can be reversed by stopping treatment, giving vitamin K, or replacing vitamin K-dependent coagulation factors with fresh frozen plasma.
- Replacement of vitamin K-dependent coagulation factors with fresh frozen plasma produces an immediate effect and is the treatment of choice in cases of life-threatening bleeding or serious warfarin overdosages.

Are There Certain Patient Characteristics That Increase the Risk of Hemorrhagic Complications of Anticoagulant Treatment?

A strong relationship between intensity of anticoagulant therapy and risk of bleeding has been reported in patients receiving treatment for deep venous thrombosis and prosthetic heart valves. The concurrent use of drugs that interfere with hemostasis and produce gastric erosions (aspirin, nonsteroidal anti-inflammatory drugs) increases the risk of serious upper gastrointestinal tract bleeding. Other drugs such as trimethoprim-sulfamethoxazole and disulfiram inhibit the clearance of warfarin, thus potentiating its effect. Still other agents such as broad-spectrum antibiotics have the potential of augmenting the anticoagulant effect of warfarin by eliminating bacterial flora, thereby producing vitamin K deficiency. Several comorbid disease states associated with increased bleeding during warfarin therapy are treated hypertension, renal insufficiency, hepatic insufficiency, and cerebrovascular disease.

- The relationship between the intensity of anticoagulant therapy and the risk of bleeding is strong.
- Concurrent use of drugs that interfere with hemostasis and produce gastric erosions increases the risk of serious upper gastrointestinal tract bleeding.
- Trimethoprim-sulfamethoxazole and disulfiram inhibit the clearance of warfarin, potentiating its effect.
- Broad-spectrum antibiotics eliminate bacterial flora, thus augmenting warfarin's anticoagulant effect.

Cerebrovascular Disorders

What Are the Recommendations for Patients With Symptomatic Carotid Stenosis?

Carotid endarterectomy performed by experienced surgeons is superior to medical therapy for preventing stroke after an anterior circulation transient ischemic attack (TIA) or minor stroke in appropriately selected patients. In several trials, patients with >70% carotid stenosis without major operative risk factors had a significant reduction in their risk of stroke over the subsequent 2 years compared with that of medical controls.

What Is the Recommended Mode of Therapy for TIAs and Minor Strokes?

Aspirin is effective in doses from 75 mg to 1,300 mg/day in preventing recurrent symptoms or stroke. For patients who are not candidates for carotid endarterectomy (posterior circulation symptoms, major medical problems, unfavorable anatomy), aspirin treatment is strongly recommended. Ticlopidine is slightly more effective than aspirin but is significantly more expensive and more toxic. At this time, ticlopidine is recommended only for patients who are aspirin-sensitive or for those having recurrent ischemic events during aspirin therapy.

What Is Appropriate Therapy During a Progressing Ischemic Stroke?

No therapy is known to have a positive effect during these situations. Many physicians believe it might be reasonable to anticoagulate with heparin for 3-5 days in this setting, especially if the ischemic stroke involves the vertebrobasilar circulation. Others simply recommend aspirin.

What Therapy Is Suggested After a Completed Thrombotic Stroke?

Use of anticoagulants in patients with completed thrombotic strokes has not been shown to be effective. Some studies support aspirin therapy after minor thrombotic stroke. One study reported ticlopidine, 500 mg/day, was superior to placebo in patients with moderate to severe strokes. However, because of the cost and toxicity of ticlopidine, aspirin is recommended initially. Ticlopidine should be considered only for aspirin-intolerant patients or patients with ischemic symptoms during aspirin therapy.

What Is Recommended Therapy After Acute Cardioembolic Stroke?

In nonhypertensive patients with small to moderate-sized embolic strokes, a computed tomographic scan should be done 48 hours or more after the onset of stroke to document the absence of spontaneous hemorrhagic transformation. If no hemorrhage is seen, institute heparin therapy followed by warfarin, at a dose that prolongs the PT to an INR of 2.0-3.0. If the patient had a large embolic stroke but is deemed a potential anticoagulation candidate, anticoagulant therapy should be postponed 7-14 days because of the predisposition in these patients to hemorrhagic transformation.

COMMON CLINICAL PROBLEMS IN GENERAL INTERNAL MEDICINE

Treatment of Hyperlipidemia

Case

A 55-year-old man with stable class II angina is referred for consideration of drug treatment for hyperlipidemia. He is otherwise healthy. He quit smoking cigarettes 2 years previously and has no other known risk factors for CAD. He has closely followed the advice of a dietitian for the past 6 months, but his cholesterol levels have shown no significant decrease. His most recent values are: total cholesterol, 240 mg/dL; HDL-C, 35 mg/dL; and triglycerides, 75 mg/dL.

Discussion

The evidence is that lowering the cholesterol level also lowers the risk of CAD and is associated with decreased progression of coronary artery lesions as well as increased regression of these lesions.

The second report of the National Cholesterol Education Program defined high-risk status as definite CAD and/or atherosclerotic disease or two of the following risk factors: Positive risk factors--

- Male ≥45 years old.
- Female ≥55 years old or premature menopause without estrogen replacement.
- Family history of CAD (definite MI or sudden death before 55 years of age in father or other first-degree male relative or before 65 years of age in mother or other first-degree female relative).
- Current cigarette smoker.
- Hypertension (blood pressure ≥140/90 mm Hg or taking antihypertension medications).
- Low HDL cholesterol (<35 mg/dL).
- Diabetes mellitus.

Negative risk factor--

- High HDL cholesterol ≥60 mg/dL (if HDL cholesterol level is ≥60 mg/dL, subtract one risk factor).

LDL-cholesterol is used to monitor patients with hypercholesterolemia and is calculated from the following formula:

$$LDL\text{-}C = (\text{total cholesterol}) - (\text{HDL cholesterol}) - (\text{triglycerides}/5)$$

In this patient, LDL-C = (240) - (35) - (75/5) = 190 mg/dL.

Secondary causes of hyperlipidemia should be ruled out in all patients. Secondary causes of hyperlipidemia may be caused by diseases (hypothyroidism, diabetes, uremia, obstructive liver disease), drugs (corticosteroids, progestins, thiazides, beta-blockers), or diet (alcohol abuse, increased saturated fats).

- Rule out secondary causes of hyperlipidemia in all patients.

After secondary causes are ruled out, the next line of treatment involves weight reduction in overweight patients, increased physical activity, and dietary therapy (Table 9-11). Both weight reduction and exercise not only promote lowering of cholesterol levels but have other benefits, such as decreasing triglycerides, increasing HDL cholesterol, decreasing blood pressure, and decreasing the risk of diabetes mellitus.

Dietary therapy to decrease elevated serum levels of cholesterol is initiated in patients without CAD or risk factors if LDL-C is ≥160 mg/dL, for patients without CAD but at least two risk factors if LDL-C is ≥130 mg/dL, and for patients with CAD if LDL-C is >100 mg/dL. Generally, a minimum of 6 months of intensive dietary therapy and counseling should be carried out in primary prevention before initiating drug therapy; shorter periods can be considered in patients with severe increases of LDL cholesterol (220 mg/dL) or known CAD. If drug therapy is initiated, it should be added to dietary therapy and not substituted for it. Drug treatment should be considered in patients without CAD and with fewer than two risk factors if LDL-C ≥190 mg/dL, without CAD but with two or more risk factors if LDL-C ≥160 mg/dL, or with CAD if LDL-C is ≥130 mg/dL (Table 9-11).

- If at least 6 months of dietary therapy fail to lower cholesterol to goal level, consider drug therapy.

If hypolipidemic drugs are used, the choice of drug depends on the mechanism of action, side-effect profile, efficacy, and cost. The following discussion considers the most common classes of drugs used in the treatment of hyperlipidemia.

Bile acid sequestrants (e.g., cholestyramine and colestipol)-- Clinical trials have documented their benefit and safety. Their mechanism of action involves removing plasma LDL by depleting the bile acid pool, which causes an increase in hepatic LDL receptors. These drugs are often used alone (in patients with mild increases in LDL cholesterol levels) or in combination with other drugs (in patients with greater increases in LDL cholesterol levels). Side effects include gastrointestinal symptoms, binding of other concurrently administered drugs, constipation, and increased triglyceride levels, especially in patients who begin with increased levels.

Nicotonic acid (niacin)--This agent is effective in decreasing total cholesterol and triglyceride levels as well as increasing HDL cholesterol levels. In a large secondary prevention trial, it was shown to reduce total mortality. Side effects are common and, thus, limit the use of this drug in many patients. Side effects can include flushing, nausea, abdominal discomfort, and skin itching. Increased levels of plasma glucose, uric

acid, and hepatic enzymes may also occur. Slow-release preparations reduce the side effect of flushing, but the incidence of liver dysfunction increases significantly, especially with higher doses. Small doses of aspirin taken before the niacin can also block flushing.

3-Hydroxy-3-methylglutaryl-coenzme A (HMG-CoA) reductase inhibitors, or "statins" (e.g., lovastatin, pravastatin, simvastatin, and fluvastatin)--These drugs are highly effective in decreasing LDL cholesterol by blocking hepatic cholesterol synthesis, which causes an increase in LDL liver receptors. They have few side effects, although myalgias, myopathy, and increase in hepatic enzymes may occur. Myopathy can increase with concurrent use of cyclosporine, niacin, erythromycin, and fibrates (fibric acid derivatives). Long-term safety remains to be demonstrated; therefore, these drugs should be used with particular caution in young men and premenopausal women. At least one secondary prevention study has shown decreased mortality risk with the use of statins. They are attractive for treatment of severe forms of hypercholesterolemia.

Fibrates (e.g., gemfibrozil)--These are the drugs of choice for decreasing increased levels of triglycerides. In some patients, these drugs slightly lower LDL cholesterol and raise HDL cholesterol levels. However, they do not usually produce substantial decreases in LDL cholesterol levels. Side effects are rare and mostly related to the gastrointestinal tract. These drugs may also increase the risk of gallstones. Therapeutically, they are most useful for disorders of hypertriglyceridemia, especially in patients with diabetes mellitus.

All the above-mentioned drugs have the potential to interact with warfarin (bile acid sequestrants can bind the drug, thus decreasing the PT, and the other hypolipidemic drugs may potentiate warfarin, thus increasing the PT). Therefore, when they are used in anticoagulated patients, close monitoring is indicated.

In general, the following drugs alone or sometimes in combination are recommended.

Table 9-11.--Treatment Decisions Based on LDL Cholesterol Level

Patient category	Initiation level	LDL goal
Dietary therapy		
Without CAD and with fewer than two risk factors	≥ 160 mg/dL	< 160 mg/dL
Without CAD and with two or more risk factors	≥ 130 mg/dL	< 130 mg/dL
With CAD	> 100 mg/dL	≤ 100 mg/dL
Drug treatment		
Without CAD and with fewer than two risk factors	≥ 190 mg/dL	< 160 mg/dL
Without CAD and with two or more risk factors	≥ 160 mg/dL	< 130 mg/dL
With CAD	≥ 130 mg/dL	≤ 100 mg/dL

CAD, coronary artery disease.
From Expert Panel on Detection, Evaluation, and Treatment of High Blood Cholesterol in Adults: Summary of the second report of the National Cholesterol Education Program (NCEP) Expert Panel on Detection, Evaluation, and Treatment of High Blood Cholesterol in Adults (Adult Treatment Panel II). JAMA 269:3015-3023, 1993.

1. For patients with increased levels of LDL cholesterol: bile acid sequestrants, HMG CoA reductase inhibitors, and nicotinic acid.
2. For patients with increased levels of LDL cholesterol and triglycerides: nicotinic acid, fibrates, and HMG CoA reductase inhibitors.
3. For patients with isolated hypertriglyceridemia if treatment is indicated: fibrates and nicotinic acid.
4. Estrogen replacement in postmenopausal women is potential alternative or adjunct to drug therapy in those with increased levels of LDL cholesterol.

Drug therapy for hyperlipidemia must be individualized. In general, a positive effect is gained and fewer side effects experienced by starting therapy with low doses of medication and increasing the dose slowly, if necessary. No studies have supported or condemned the use of drug therapy in the elderly.

Tobacco Abuse

Case

A 60-year-old woman comes to your office for her annual mammogram, breast examination, and pelvic examination. You note from the preexamination questionnaire that she is a current smoker and has smoked one pack per day for 30 years. Examination of the lungs reveals scattered rhonchi and wheezes with a prolonged expiratory phase. You broach the subject of smoking cessation with the patient, but she quickly and defensively counters with a number of statements. She states that after 30 years of smoking "the damage is done" and there is no sense in quitting. She also fears gaining weight after quitting and says that when she did try to quit several years ago, she quickly became so nervous and edgy that she could not sleep and was unpleasant to be around. How might you devise a plan to deal effectively with this patient's tobacco abuse problem?

Discussion

Tobacco use is the leading cause of preventable premature death in the U.S. In addition to being the causative factor for nearly 90% of all cases of lung cancer, smoking is associated with cancer of the oral cavity, larynx, esophagus, stomach, pancreas, uterine cervix, and genitourinary tract. However, among ex-smokers abstinent for 15 years or longer, the incidence of lung cancer is reduced to the rates seen in nonsmokers.

Smokers are 2 to 6 times as likely to have an MI as are nonsmokers, and 20% of all deaths due to cardiovascular disease are attributable to smoking. After several years of abstinence, the cardiovascular risk of ex-smokers is not significantly different from that of those who have never smoked.

Compared with smokers, ex-smokers have less phlegm production and wheezing, greater FEV_1 and vital capacity, better immune function, and lower mortality from pulmonary infections, bronchitis, and emphysema. Although some lung damage is irreversible, ex-smokers have significant improve-

ment in their pulmonary function during the first year of cessation. After that, the decline in lung function stabilizes at a nonsmoker's rate. Smokers continue to show a decline in lung function at twice the rate of ex-smokers.

Often, one of the most compelling arguments for a patient to stop smoking is that it harms others. It is estimated that >50,000 people die annually in the U.S. from medical complications of passive smoking. Most of these deaths are from accelerated heart disease, although the number of lung cancer deaths is also significant. Studies have estimated that nonsmoking spouses of smokers have an all-cancer risk about 1.5 times that of nonsmoking spouses of nonsmokers.

The National Cancer Institute advises physicians to use an easy-to-remember four-step approach in counseling their patients in smoking cessation.

1. **Ask** about smoking at every opportunity.
   The physician should question patients about smoking at any new encounter, inquiring not only if they smoke, but how much they smoke. It is also helpful to ask whether they have ever tried to stop smoking and if so, what happened.
2. **Advise** all smokers to stop.
   Less than two-thirds of physicians report advising their patients to stop smoking and only two-thirds of patients report receiving smoking cessation advice from their physician. This counsel can often be an influential message to patients. The physician should state the advice clearly; for example, "As your physician, I must advise you to stop smoking now." It helps to personalize the "quit smoking" message by referring to other illnesses the patient has, family history, passive smoking issues, etc.
3. **Assist** the patient in stopping to smoke.
   Set a quit date with the patient. Try to do it within 4 weeks, acknowledging with the patient that the time never is ideal. Provide self-help materials. Consider prescribing nicotine gum or nicotine patches, especially for highly addicted patients (those who smoke more than one pack per day or have their first cigarette within 30 minutes of awakening). Consider signing a stop-smoking contract with the patient. Finally, if the patient is not willing to quit at this time, provide motivating literature and bring the topic up again at the next visit.
4. **Arrange** follow-up visits.
   Set up a follow-up visit within 1-2 weeks after the quit date. Counseling programs and behavioral therapy programs can be effective in smoking cessation. A transdermal nicotine patch together with behavioral therapy results in significantly higher cessation rates than transdermal nicotine alone. If during follow-up visits, you discover the patient has relapsed, advise them that this is not uncommon. Encourage the patient to try again immediately.

Several other important concerns that patients have can be addressed and answered. For those worrying about weight gain with smoking cessation, it is useful to let them know that although the majority of patients do gain weight, the average weight gain is only 5 lb, and this can be anticipated and dealt with effectively. For patients who have noted difficulties with nervousness and poor sleep after smoking cessation, advise them that these symptoms are related to nicotine withdrawal and usually resolve after 2 or 3 weeks. Nicotine gum or patches can often help control these symptoms. Some patients notice an increase in coughing after they stop smoking. This can be explained as a temporary response caused by an increase in the lung's ability to remove phlegm and, thus, represents recovery of the lungs' own defense mechanisms. After cessation has been achieved, the patient should be advised to refrain from having even an occasional cigarette, because nicotine addiction seems to be triggered quickly in most ex-smokers.

Acute Low Back Pain

Case

A 55-year-old man comes to your office with a 3-day history of severe low back pain in the lumbosacral area. He recalls no specific trauma, and the review of systems is negative for fever, weight loss, or other constitutional symptoms. He complains of no numbness, tingling, or weakness in his legs and has no bladder or bowel symptoms. He works in a factory, and his job requires some minor lifting and bending. Make a diagnostic assessment, therapeutic plan, and suggestions about levels of activity.

Discussion

In December 1994, the Agency for Health Care Policy and Research published clinical practice guidelines relating to adult patients with acute low back problems. The following discussion focuses on suggestions from these Guidelines.

Acute low back problems are one of the most common reasons for patients to visit a physician's office. Acute low back problems are defined as activity intolerance due to lower back or back-related leg symptoms of less than 3 months' duration. It is important to know that 90% of patients with acute low back problems have a spontaneous recovery and return to previous levels of activity within 1 month. On the initial assessment of such a patient, a focused medical history and physical examination should be performed so that a potentially dangerous underlying condition is not overlooked. Based on this evaluation, low back symptoms can be classified into one of three working categories:

1. *Potentially serious spinal conditions*--This category includes tumor, infection, fracture, or major neurologic disorder. One would look for "red flags" in the history or examination that would point to these conditions, i.e., a history of trauma (fracture) or cancer (spinal epidural metastases), risk factors for spinal infection and/or fever/chills (infection), saddle anesthesia or bladder and

bowel dysfunction (cauda equina syndrome), etc.
2. *Sciatica*--This category includes back-related lower limb symptoms suggestive of lumbosacral nerve root compromise. Sciatica would be further suggested by a positive straight leg raise, as defined by pain below the knee at <70° of leg elevation, aggravated by dorsiflexion of the ankle. Crossover pain (i.e., eliciting pain in the leg with sciatica by straight raising of the unaffected leg) is an even stronger indication of nerve root compression. Correlative findings on sensory examination, specific muscle strength loss, and reflex changes can be used to further diagnose sciatica and to localize the nerve root suspected to be involved.
3. *Nonspecific back symptoms*--This category includes low back pain without signs or symptoms of a serious underlying condition or nerve root compression.

The patient in the case example appears to have nonspecific back discomfort. After this diagnosis is made, the physician could educate the patient about this problem, reassuring him that the evaluation results do not suggest a dangerous problem and that a rapid recovery can be expected. Should the patient not recover within a month, a more extensive evaluation may be needed, including radiography and special studies.

In the interim, the physician must address the need for symptom control measures. This can include oral medications. The safest effective medication for acute low back problems appears to be acetaminophen, which has a low side-effect profile. Nonsteroidal anti-inflammatory drugs can be used, but the disadvantages are cost and side-effect profile (gastrointestinal tract irritation/ulceration, etc.). Muscle relaxants seem to be no more effective than nonsteroidal anti-inflammatory drugs in treating low back symptoms and even a combination of relaxants and NSAIDs has not demonstrated benefit. They also can produce significant drowsiness. Opioids appear no more effective than safer analgesics and should be avoided if possible. If opioids are chosen, they should be used for only a short time and the patient must be warned of the potential side effects of drowsiness, cloudy mentation, and constipation and the potential for dependency.

Physical methods are often used in the treatment of acute back problems; however, most of these methods, including traction, massage, ultrasound, and trigger point injections, have not been proven effective in symptomatic treatment. Some have suggested that spinal manipulation is safe and might be effective for appropriate patients who have acute low back symptoms but no radiculopathy.

Activity alteration is a balance between avoiding undue back irritation and preventing debility due to inactivity. Most patients do not require bed rest. In fact, it has been suggested that patients with acute low back pain who continue ordinary activities within the limits permitted by the pain recover more rapidly than those treated with bed rest or back-mobilizing exercises. If bed rest is used, it should be used for only 2 or 3 days, because prolonged bed rest has a potential debilitating effect and its efficacy in treatment is unproven. Bed rest generally is reserved for patients with severe limitations due to sciatica. Certain postures and activities can increase stress on the back and aggravate the symptoms. Patients must be taught to minimize the stress of lifting by keeping the object being lifted close to the body at the level of the naval. Lifting with the legs as opposed to the back must be emphasized. Prolonged sitting can sometimes aggravate problems, and patients should be encouraged to change their position frequently. Until the

patient returns to normal activity, aerobic conditioning may be recommended to help avoid debilitation from inactivity. When requested, it may be appropriate for the physician to offer specific instructions about activity at work for patients with acute limitations due to low back symptoms. The physician should make it clear to both the patient and the employer that even moderately heavy unassisted lifting may aggravate back symptoms and that any restrictions are intended to allow for spontaneous recovery or for time to build activity tolerance through exercise.

QUESTIONS

Multiple Choice (choose the one best answer)

1. A test for fecal occult blood has a sensitivity of 33% and a specificity of 95% in the diagnosis of colon cancer. Of every 100 patients without colon cancer tested for fecal occult blood, how many will have positive findings?
    a. 5
    b. 33
    c. 67
    d. 95
    e. 100

2. Assume fecal occult blood testing has a sensitivity of 33%, a specificity of 95%, and there is a 1% prevalence of colon cancer in your geriatric population. If a patient had positive findings on a test for fecal occult blood, what is the positive predictive value of that test in judging whether the patient truly has colon cancer?
    a. 1%
    b. 6%
    c. 9%
    d. 33%
    e. 87%

3. Which of the following statements about the positive predictive value of a test is correct?
    a. It represents the proportion of patients with a target disorder who have a positive test result
    b. 2-by-2 table definition = a/(a+c)
    c. It provides little use in clinical practice
    d. It is affected by the prevalence of disease in the population
    e. 2-by-2 table definition = d/(c+d)

4. A 40-year-old man about to have hernia repair presents for a preoperative evaluation. His medical history and physical examination results are unremarkable. Which of the following studies are indicated before he has general anesthesia?
    a. Chest radiography and electrocardiography
    b. Complete blood cell count
    c. PT and APTT
    d. Blood glucose level
    e. No studies are indicated

5. Which of the following statements about perioperative management is *not* correct?
    a. It is reasonable to proceed with the operation if diastolic blood pressure is ≤110 mm Hg

b. Thyrotoxic patients are at high risk for perioperative complications

c. If polycythemia vera is not controlled, surgical morbidity and mortality are increased

d. Most cardiac and antihypertensive medications should be withheld on the morning of the operation

e. A platelet count of 50,000/mm^3 usually provides adequate hemostasis for most procedures

6. A 70-year-old man who takes warfarin for chronic atrial fibrillation presents with a significant acute hemorrhage of the lower gastrointestinal tract. His INR is 8.0. Which of the following is the best management option?

a. Withhold warfarin therapy until the INR normalizes, then perform diagnostic work-up for gastrointestinal tract bleeding

b. Give fresh frozen plasma to normalize the INR, then perform diagnostic work-up for gastrointestinal tract bleeding

c. Give a low dose of vitamin K to lower INR, then perform diagnostic work-up for gastrointestinal tract bleeding

d. Give a high dose of vitamin K to normalize INR. No diagnostic work-up for gastrointestinal tract bleeding is indicated, because it would not be cost-effective when associated with an elevated INR

e. Give fresh frozen plasma to normalize the INR. No diagnostic work-up for gastrointestinal tract bleeding is indicated, because it would not be cost-effective when associated with an elevated INR

7. A 59-year-old man with known coronary artery disease has total cholesterol of 250 mg/dL, HDL cholesterol of 30 mg/dL, and triglycerides of 150 mg/dL. Which statement pertaining to his hyperlipidemia is *not* correct?

a. His calculated LDL cholesterol is 190 mg/dL

b. He should be examined for secondary causes of hyperlipidemia

c. He should be treated with intensive diet therapy, and if an inadequate response is achieved, drug therapy should be instituted with a goal LDL cholesterol ≤100 mg/dL

d. He should immediately start receiving drug therapy with a goal LDL cholesterol of ≤130 mg/dL

e. Because he has coronary artery disease, no computation of other risk factors needs to be performed to classify him into high-risk status

True/False (indicate whether each answer is true or false)

8. The following statements relate to drug therapy for hyperlipidemia.

a. Bile acid sequestrants, fibrates, and HMG CoA reductase inhibitors can all potentiate the action of warfarin, thus increasing prothrombin time

b. Bile acid sequestrants are a poor drug choice in patients with increased triglycerides

c. Niacin is the drug of choice for diabetic patients with hyperlipidemia

d. Niacin is effective in decreasing LDL cholesterol and triglycerides while increasing HDL cholesterol

e. HMG CoA reductase inhibitors have few side effects, but myopathy can be seen, especially with concurrent use of cyclosporine, erythromycin, or fibrates

f. Fibrates are the drug of choice for treating increased triglycerides

9. The following statements pertain to tobacco abuse.

a. Smoking is the causative factor for nearly half of all lung cancers

b. Smoking has been implicated as a causative factor in pancreatic and esophageal cancer

c. Passive smoking has not been implicated in causing medical complications or deaths

d. Ex-smokers experience improvement in pulmonary function, but little improvement is seen in the first year after cessation

e. The N.C.I. has a four-step approach to counsel patients in smoking cessation, including the "buzz words" *Ask, Advise, Assist,* and *Arrange*

f. The average weight gain experienced by patients after smoking cessation is 20 pounds

10. The following statements pertain to the evaluation and treatment of acute low back pain.

a. Of patients with acute low back problems, 90% return to previous levels of activity within 30 days

b. A lumbar spine radiograph should be performed routinely at the first visit to rule out potentially serious spinal conditions

c. Crossover pain, elicted by raising the normal leg and producing pain in the leg with sciatica, is a strong indication of nerve root compression

d. Bed rest for 5-7 days has proven efficacy in treating acute low back pain

e. Nonsteroidal anti-inflammatory drugs are the safest, most economical medication for treating acute low back problems

f. Traction and massage are two treatment modalities with proven effect in acute low back problems

ANSWERS

1. Answer a.

The question relates to how many false-positive results will be seen in a test whose specificity is 95%. Therefore, in testing patients without disease, 95 will have negative tests (true negatives) and 5 will have positive tests (false positives).

2. Answer b.

		Disease present	Disease absent	
Diagnostic test result	Positive	33 a	495 b	528 a+b
	Negative	c 67	d 9,405	c+d 9,472
		a+c	b+d	a+b+c+d
	Total	100	9,900	10,000

The above diagram correctly fills in the numbers for this question. Question 2 asks you to determine the positive predictive value of the fecal occult blood test, or a/(a+b), i.e., 33/528 = 6%.

3. Answer d.

Sensitivity represents the proportion of patients with a target disorder who have a positive test result; a/(a+c) also refers to sensitivity. Positive predictive value is a useful determinant in clinical practice. Positive predictive value *is* affected by the prevalence of disease in the population. Negative predictive value: d/(c+d).

4. Answer e.

In an otherwise healthy patient in this age group, no laboratory studies would be indicated.

5. Answer d.

It is most appropriate to administer cardiac and blood pressure medications with small sips of water by mouth before the operation, and it may be dangerous to withhold them. All the other statements in this question are true.

6. Answer b.

When a patient receiving anticoagulation therapy has a sig-nificant acute hemorrhage, it is most appropriate to administer fresh frozen plasma to quickly reverse the anticoagulation. Even when gastrointestinal tract bleeding is associated with a markedly increased INR, it is appropriate to evaluate the patient for the source of bleeding, because a significantly accountable lesion will be found in approximately 1/3 of the patients.

7. Answer d.

LDL cholesterol = (total cholesterol - HDL cholesterol - triglycerides/5), or 190 mg/dL. All patients should be examined for secondary causes of hyperlipidemia before treatment. Patients with coronary artery disease should be treated by diet and later by drug therapy if diet alone proves inadequate to achieve goal LDL cholesterol ≤100 mg/dL. Patients with known coronary artery disease need not have other risk factors added up for classification, because they are already in the highest risk group.

8. a, false; b, true; c, false; d, true; e, true; f, true.

Fibrates and HMG CoA reductase inhibitors can potentiate the action of warfarin; bile acid sequestrants can bind warfarin and, thus, decrease prothrombin time. Because bile acid sequestrants can increase triglycerides, they are a poor choice for patients with elevated triglycerides. Niacin can aggravate hyperglycemia and generally is not used in patients with diabetes mellitus.

9. a, false; b, true; c, false; d, false; e, true; f, false.

Smoking is the causative factor for nearly 90% of all lung cancers. Passive smoking has been implicated as a cause of medical complications and deaths. Ex-smokers show marked improvement in pulmonary function during the first year after cessation. The average weight gain experienced by patients after smoking cessation is about 5 pounds.

10. a, true; b, false; c, true; d, false; e, false; f, false.

There is no indication to routinely perform lumbar spine radiography in acute low back problems without signs in the medical history or physical examination that point to potentially serious spinal conditions. Prolonged bed rest (5-7 days) has not been proven effective in treating acute low back problems and may lead to deconditioning, etc. Acetaminophen is the safest and most economical medication for treating acute low back problems. Traction and massage have not been proven to be effective in treating acute low back problems.

CHAPTER 10
GENETICS

Virginia V. Michels, M.D.

Genetic factors play a role in the development of many types of human disease. Genetic determinants may be single gene defects, mitochondrial mutations, chromosome abnormalities, or multifactorial.

CHROMOSOME ABNORMALITIES

Approximately a sixth of all birth defects and cases of congenitally determined mental retardation are due to chromosome abnormalities. Chromosome abnormalities occur in about 1 in 180 live births. One-third of these abnormalities involve an abnormal number (aneuploidy) of non-sex chromosomes (autosomes). Factors known to result in a higher-than-average risk for having a child with autosomal aneuploidy are maternal age ≥35 years and having previously had an affected child. Prenatal diagnosis by karyotyping of fetal cells obtained by amniocentesis or chorionic villus sampling can be offered to pregnant women who are at increased risk.

- Chromosome abnormalities occur in 1 in 180 live births.
- Risk factors for autosomal aneuploidy: maternal age ≥35 years and having had an affected child.

Down Syndrome

The most common autosomal aneuploidy syndrome in term infants is Down syndrome (incidence, 1 in 880). The most serious consequence of Down syndrome is mild-to-moderate mental retardation (average IQ, about 50). Forty percent of patients with Down syndrome have a congenital heart defect, most frequently ventricular septal defect or atrioventricular canal defect, although other congenital heart defects may occur. Thyroid disease is frequent, and Alzheimer's disease develops at a relatively early age in many. A few patients have hypoplasia of the odontoid, which is important to diagnose before participation in certain sports. Males with Down syndrome are usually sterile, but affected females are fertile

and have a very high risk of having an affected child. Most persons with Down syndrome have trisomy 21 as a result of a new mutation nondisjunctional event; in these cases, the risk to the parents of having another affected child is 1%-2% or higher, depending on maternal age. In 3% of persons with Down syndrome, a translocation chromosome abnormality is present, in which the extra chromosome 21 is attached to another chromosome, most commonly 14 (Fig. 10-1). These translocation chromosomes may be inherited in an *unbalanced* form from a parent carrying a *balanced* form of the translocation; these parents have a 5%-15% risk of having another affected child. For identification of these high-risk families, chromosome analysis should be done on all patients with Down syndrome. Even if the parents have completed their childbearing, the karyotype of the affected individual should be determined so that other relatives (e.g., adult siblings) can be counseled. The same principles are presumed to be true for other autosomal aneuploidy syndromes.

- Most common autosomal aneuploidy syndrome in term infants is Down syndrome.
- Most serious consequence of Down syndrome is mild-to-moderate mental retardation.
- Most frequent heart defect in Down syndrome is ventricular septal defect or atrioventricular canal defect.
- Males with Down syndrome are usually sterile, but females are fertile.
- Most persons with Down syndrome have trisomy 21.

Sex Chromosome Aneuploidy Syndromes

Approximately 35% of chromosome abnormalities in liveborn infants involve sex chromosome aneuploidy. These infants may have an additional X or Y chromosome or be lacking one. Patients with 47,XXX or 47,XYY karyotypes usually have no major birth defects or mental retardation, although the mean IQ may be 90 rather than 100. Patients with 47,XYY usually are detected incidentally. Patients with a 47,XXY karyotype

Fig. 10-1. Karyotype 46,XY,-14,+t(14;21)(p11;q11) from patient with Down syndrome. Extra chromosome 21 material is translocated to a chromosome 14. Result is robertsonian translocation. (Karyotype courtesy of G. Dewald, Ph.D.)

(Klinefelter syndrome) have small testes, infertility, and a tall eunuchoid body habitus. Patients with a 45,X karyotype (Turner syndrome) or its variants--one structurally abnormal X, such as 46,X,r(X) (Fig. 10-2)--or mosaicism for an X or Y chromosome--such as 45,X/46,XX--usually are mentally normal but have a risk of approximately 30% for a congenital heart defect. Bicuspid aortic valve with or without coarctation of the aorta is particularly common. Short stature, webbed neck, increased number of pigmented nevi, failure to develop secondary sexual characteristics, short 4th or 5th metacarpals or metatarsals, renal malformations, and increased risk for thyroid disease are also variably present. Ordinarily, parents of patients with sex chromosome aneuploidy are not at increased risk for having another affected child, and these parents do not routinely need chromosome analyses.

- 47,XXY karyotype (Klinefelter syndrome): small testes, infertility, tall eunuchoid body habitus.
- 45,X karyotype (Turner syndrome): short stature, lack of secondary sex characteristics, usually mentally normal, 30% risk of congenital heart defect, and commonly bicuspid aortic valve.
- Other possible features of 45,X karyotype: webbed neck, increased number of pigmented nevi, short 4th or 5th metatarsals or metacarpals.

Other Chromosome Abnormalities

Thirty-four percent of chromosome abnormalities involve structural changes such as deletions, duplications, inversions, or translocations. The translocations may be balanced (no net

loss or gain of genetic material) or unbalanced. People with balanced translocations are usually phenotypically normal and healthy but may be at increased risk for miscarriages or their children may have birth defects. Patients with net loss or gain of genetic material by any of the mechanisms listed above have phenotypic abnormalities that usually include mental retardation and frequently other major or minor birth defects. Parents of all patients with a structural chromosome abnormality should have chromosome analyses to determine whether they are carriers of a balanced translocation.

- Parents of all patients with a structural chromosome abnormality should have chromosome analyses.

Fragile X-Linked Mental Retardation

The fragile X-linked mental retardation syndrome occurs in about 1 in 1,000 males. This unusual chromosome abnormality is characterized by a visible fragile site on the long arm of an X chromosome at band q27 when the lymphocytes are cultured in media deficient in folic acid (Fig. 10-3). The fragile site is never observed in all cells, and the frequency may be as low as 4%. Affected males may be physically normal or have a long, thin face with prominent jaw, large simplified ears, and enlarged testes. The degree of mental retardation ranges from mild to profound. An occasional male is clinically normal and is referred to as a "transmitting" male. Carrier females may be phenotypically normal or mildly retarded and dysmorphic; occasionally they are moderately or severely retarded. Some carrier females do not express the fragile site cytogenetically. Initially puzzling aspects of this syndrome

Fig. 10-2. Karyotype 46,X,r(X) from patient with Turner syndrome. (Karyotype courtesy of G. Dewald, Ph.D.)

included the observations that transmitting males had daughters who, although obligate carriers, rarely showed signs of the disease. However, these daughters could have typically affected sons. This now can be explained by the discovery of a DNA trinucleotide repeat (CGG) that is more likely to expand and thereby become more abnormal during transmission through a female. Direct DNA analysis of the size of the trinucleotide repeat is a more accurate method than standard cytogenetic analysis for detection of carrier females.

- Fragile X: fragile site on long arm of X chromosome at band q27.
- Males with fragile X: may be physically normal or have long, thin face, prominent jaw, large ears, enlarged testes, mild to profound mental retardation.
- Carrier females: phenotypically normal or mildly retarded and dysmorphic.
- To detect carrier females: direct DNA analysis of trinucleotide repeat is most accurate.

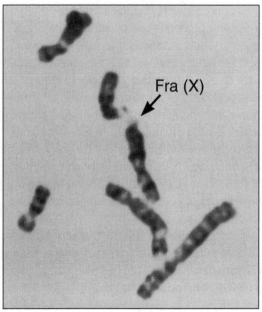

Fig. 10-3. Chromosome analysis from patient with fragile X syndrome. Fragile site is visible on long arm of X chromosome at band q27 when lymphocytes are cultured in media deficient in folic acid. (Photograph courtesy of G. Dewald, Ph.D.)

PATTERNS OF INHERITANCE

Autosomal Dominant

In autosomal dominant inheritance, the responsible gene is located on one of the autosomes and the gene overrides its homologue in terms of clinical effect. Therefore, one copy of the gene is sufficient for the trait to be expressed or for the disease to be present, and heterozygotes have the disease. There is a 50% chance that any child born to an affected person will inherit the abnormal gene.

- Autosomal dominant inheritance: responsible gene is located on autosome and overrides its homologue.
- 50% chance that child of affected person will inherit abnormal gene.

The severity of the disease caused by the abnormal gene may be uniform for some conditions, such as achondroplasia, but the severity may be variable for other conditions, such as neurofibromatosis and Marfan syndrome. This difference of severity is referred to as "variable expression." In contrast, the term "incomplete penetrance" means that some persons who have inherited the gene show no signs of it. Obviously, the clinical decision regarding whether a person has signs of the gene defect depends on the thoroughness of the examination and the sensitivity of the investigative techniques. For example, many families with hypertrophic cardiomyopathy were thought to include members with incomplete penetrance until asymptomatic patients were examined with echocardiography. Although transmission of a disease through members of either sex through multiple generations of a family strongly suggests autosomal dominant inheritance, it is important to remember that autosomal dominant diseases can occur without a positive family history. This can occur because of incomplete penetrance, incorrect assignment of paternity, new mutation, or somatic mosaicism. New mutation events represent changes in the genetic material of the individual egg or sperm that gives rise to the fetus. Although the risk for siblings of a person whose disease arose by new mutation is not increased over that of the general population, the risk for the offspring still is 50%. Somatic mosaicism refers to the possibility that one of the parents has the gene defect in only some cells, including the reproductive cells (germinal mosaicism), such that the person has no or few signs of the disease but potentially can transmit the disease to one or more children.

- In autosomal dominant inheritance, disease severity may be uniform or variable.
- Incomplete penetrance: no signs of abnormal gene in a person who has inherited it.
- Somatic mosaicism: person has gene defect in only some cells.

Some of the diseases with autosomal dominant inheritance are listed in Table 10-1 and summarized on the following pages.

Ehlers-Danlos Syndromes

Type I

There may be up to 15 forms of Ehlers-Danlos syndrome. Type I, or gravis type, was the first described and serves as a prototype for discussion of this group of genetically heterogeneous disorders. The syndrome is inherited as an autosomal dominant condition, and the basic defect in type I disease has not been defined. The disorder is characterized by velvety textured, hyperextensible, fragile skin that splits easily and heals poorly, resulting in wide, thin scars. Many tissues are friable, which is an important consideration when surgical procedures are considered. Even fetal membranes are affected and frequently rupture before term, resulting in premature birth. "Molluscoid pseudotumors" are areas of sagging, wrinkled, redundant skin that may develop over the knee and elbow joints. Small fat- or mucin-containing spherules may be present in the subcutaneous tissue and may be calcified. The joints are hyperextensible and prone to dislocations. Pes planus, scoliosis, degenerative arthritis, visceral diverticulosis, and spontaneous pneumothorax may occur.

- Ehlers-Danlos type I is an autosomal dominant condition.
- Features: velvety textured, hyperextensible, fragile skin.
- Joints are hyperextensible and prone to dislocation.
- Associated conditions: pes planus, scoliosis, degenerative arthritis, visceral diverticulosis, spontaneous pneumothorax.

Involvement of small blood vessels results in easy bruisability. Mitral valve prolapse may occur in 50% of patients. Dilatation of the aortic root or pulmonary artery and prolapse of the tricuspid valve may occur. Vascular rupture is relatively rare.

- Ehlers-Danlos type I: mitral valve prolapse in 50%.
- Vascular rupture is uncommon.

Type II

Ehlers-Danlos syndrome type II, or mitis type, is similar to type I but milder; it also is inherited as an autosomal dominant disorder. A significant number of patients have mitral valve prolapse. It is uncertain whether this disorder results from a mutation at the same locus as for type I.

- Ehlers-Danlos type II is milder than type I.

Type III

The joint hypermobility of Ehlers-Danlos syndrome type III, or benign familial hypermobility syndrome, is similar to that in type I and may result in joint dislocations. However, skin

Table 10-1.--Diseases With Autosomal Dominant Inheritance

Achondroplasia

Amyloidosis (many types)

Ehlers-Danlos syndrome, types I, II, III, VIII, some type IV, VI, and VII

Huntington disease

Hypertrophic cardiomyopathy

LEOPARD syndrome

Low-density lipoprotein (LDL) receptor deficiency (hypercholesterolemia)

Marfan syndrome

Multiple endocrine neoplasia, types I, IIa, and IIb

Myotonic dystrophy

Neurofibromatosis, types 1 and 2

Noonan syndrome[*]

Osler-Weber-Rendu disease (hereditary hemorrhagic telangiectasia)

Osteogenesis imperfecta, types I and IV, most type II

Polycystic kidney disease (some forms are autosomal recessive)

Porphyria (several types)

Pseudoxanthoma elasticum (some forms are autosomal recessive)

Spherocytosis

Tuberous sclerosis

Von Hippel-Lindau disease

Von Willebrand disease

---

[*]Most cases are sporadic, but there is good evidence that they have new mutation autosomal dominant disease.

hyperextensibility and scarring are minimal or absent. There is a wide range of expression both within and between families. Families with the mildest manifestations merge with the general population in terms of normal variation in joint mobility. It is an autosomal dominant disorder.

- In Ehlers-Danlos type III, joint hypermobility is similar to that in type I.
- Skin hyperextensibility and scarring are minimal or absent.

Type IV

Ehlers-Danlos syndrome type IV, or vascular type, may be genetically heterogeneous with both autosomal dominant and, perhaps less commonly, autosomal recessive forms. It is usually due to deficiency of type III collagen synthesis or secretion in skin, aorta, uterus, and intestine. This is the most severe form of Ehlers-Danlos syndrome and is characterized by rupture of large arteries, the colon, or the gravid uterus. Angiography and other invasive procedures may precipitate vascular or organ rupture and should be done only after careful consideration of the risk:benefit ratio. Mitral valve prolapse frequently is present. In some patients the skin is extremely

thin, allowing visualization of the underlying venous network (Fig. 10-4). Despite this, there is a tendency to form keloid scars and contractures. In contrast to other forms of Ehlers-Danlos syndrome, the skin and connective tissues may not be hyperextensible. Occasional complications include spontaneous pneumothorax and severe periodontal disease. This defect is expressed in cultured skin fibroblasts, so prenatal diagnosis theoretically is possible. Although it has been suggested that type III collagen also is deficient in some patients with congenital cerebral aneurysms or acquired abdominal aortic aneurysms who do not have classic Ehlers-Danlos syndrome, demonstrable defects occur in only a very small proportion of patients.

Fig. 10-4. Thin, prematurely aged-appearing skin in young man with Ehlers-Danlos syndrome type IV.

- Ehlers-Danlos type IV has autosomal dominant and possibly autosomal recessive forms.
- It is due to deficiency of type III collagen synthesis.
- Angiography and other invasive procedures may precipitate vascular or organ rupture.
- Mitral valve prolapse is frequently present.
- Occasional complications: spontaneous pneumothorax and severe periodontal disease.

Type V

Ehlers-Danlos syndrome type V is an X-linked recessive disease that may be associated with lysyl oxidase deficiency, although this has not been a universal finding. Skin hyperextensibility is severe, but joint hypermobility is mild to moderate. Mitral and tricuspid valve prolapse or insufficiency may be present.

- Ehlers-Danlos type V is X-linked recessive disease.

Type VI

Ehlers-Danlos syndrome type VI is called the ocular type because blindness from retinal detachment or ocular rupture is a serious complication. In some cases the disease is due to an autosomal recessively inherited deficiency of procollagen lysyl hydroxylase. Severe scoliosis, recurrent joint dislocations, aortic rupture, and gastrointestinal hemorrhage also can occur. Prenatal diagnosis is possible only in families with a documented biochemical defect.

- Ehlers-Danlos type VI is called ocular type.
- Blindness from retinal detachment is a complication.
- Some cases are autosomal recessive.
- Scoliosis, joint dislocations, aortic rupture, and gastrointestinal hemorrhage occur.

Type VII

Ehlers-Danlos syndrome type VII, or arthrochalasis multiplex congenita, is characterized by extreme joint laxity and dislocations. Some patients might have defective conversion of procollagen to collagen, which is an autosomal recessive defect. However, more commonly, others have structural abnormalities of half their α-2 chains of type I collagen which interfere with the enzymatic conversion of procollagen to collagen. This is an autosomal dominant condition that sometimes arises as a new mutation.

- Ehlers-Danlos type VII usually is autosomal dominant.

Type VIII

Ehlers-Danlos syndrome type VIII is similar to types I and II but includes particularly severe periodontal disease. It is an autosomal dominant disorder, and the basic defect is unknown.

- Ehlers-Danlos type VIII is autosomal dominant.

There is marked genetic heterogeneity in all the Ehlers-Danlos syndromes that have been chemically defined. An equal degree of heterogeneity probably will be found in the more common types I, II, and III.

Hypertrophic Cardiomyopathy

Isolated hypertrophic cardiomyopathy frequently is inherited as an autosomal dominant disorder. Penetrance ranges from more than 75% to 100% in different families when relatives are studied with electrocardiography and echocardiography. Investigation of first-degree relatives is necessary. Even if parents are normal by echocardiography, the possibility of new mutation cannot be excluded, and children born to an affected parent must be considered to be at risk and should be evaluated. The possibility of an autosomal dominant disorder can never be excluded on the basis of a negative family history.

- Isolated hypertrophic cardiomyopathy is autosomal dominant.
- Investigation of first-degree relatives is necessary.
- Children of affected parents are at risk.

As with any autosomal dominant disorder, the risk of passing the abnormal gene to each child is 50%. The course of the disease may be variable, even within a family; therefore, the age at onset cannot be predicted precisely. It is not rare to study a child who presents with symptoms and to discover, after family investigations, that an asymptomatic parent is affected.

- In hypertrophic cardiomyopathy, the risk of passing the gene to each child is 50%.
- Course of disease is variable.
- Age at onset cannot be predicted.

Hypertrophic cardiomyopathy with or without outflow obstruction has been observed within single families. This is compelling evidence that they are different manifestations of the same disease.

Approximately 50% of families with hypertrophic cardiomyopathy have a defect in the β cardiac myosin heavy-chain gene on chromosome 14q. However, other families have not shown linkage to this locus, a finding demonstrating genetic heterogeneity. Other gene defects that may cause hypertrophic cardiomyopathy include cardiac troponin T, tropomyosin, and others that remain unidentified.

- About 50% of families with hypertrophic cardiomyopathy have defect in β cardiac myosin heavy-chain gene.

Marfan Syndrome

The Marfan syndrome is relatively common; its incidence is 1 in 20,000. It is an autosomal dominant disorder with extremely variable expression, and approximately 20% of cases arise by new mutation. There are no well-documented instances of nonpenetrance.

- Marfan syndrome is relatively common--1 in 20,000.
- It is an autosomal dominant disorder.
- About 20% of cases arise by new mutation.

The disease involves the musculoskeletal, cardiovascular, and ocular systems. Skeletal abnormalities include tall stature, a low upper:lower segment ratio because limbs are relatively long compared with the trunk, scoliosis or kyphosis, and pectus deformities. These features result from overgrowth of the tubular bones. Increased joint laxity and hyperextensibility are common, but occasionally patients have limited extension of fingers and elbows. The face may be long and the palate highly arched. This "marfanoid habitus" may be present in patients with other disorders such as other connective tissue dysplasias, mucosal neuroma syndrome (multiple endocrine neoplasia type IIb), Stickler syndrome, and homocystinuria. The characteristic body habitus is never sufficient evidence for making the diagnosis of Marfan syndrome in the absence of other characteristic features or a well-documented family history of Marfan syndrome.

- Marfan syndrome involves the musculoskeletal, cardiovascular, and ocular systems.
- Skeletal abnormalities: tall stature, low upper:lower segment ratio, scoliosis or kyphosis, pectus deformities.
- Increased joint laxity and hyperextensibility are common.

The ocular abnormalities associated with Marfan syndrome include subluxation of the lenses, myopia, and retinal detachment. As the most specific ocular feature, dislocation of the lenses is very helpful in making the diagnosis of Marfan syndrome, although ectopia lentis also can occur in other disorders such as homocystinuria and Weill-Marchesani syndrome. Dislocations occur in 50%-80% of patients; the lens frequently is displaced upward, but this is not always the case. Gross dislocations may be evident without the aid of special equipment, but lesser degrees of dislocation may be evident only by slit-lamp examination. Therefore, all patients suspected of having Marfan syndrome must have a complete ophthalmologic evaluation, including slit-lamp examination. Patients with Marfan syndrome should have frequent ophthalmologic examinations to permit early detection of complications such as retinal detachment or glaucoma.

- Ocular abnormalities of Marfan syndrome: subluxation of lenses, myopia, retinal detachment.

- Dislocation of lenses is helpful for diagnosis; ectopia lentis can occur in homocystinuria and Weill-Marchesani syndrome.
- Dislocations occur in 50%-80% of cases.
- All patients must have ophthalmologic evaluation.

The life expectancy of patients with Marfan syndrome is shortened because of cardiovascular disease. The most common manifestation is mitral valve prolapse with or without mitral regurgitation. Dilatation of the ascending aorta is the next most common cardiovascular disorder; it may lead to aortic regurgitation, aortic rupture, or dissecting aneurysm. Although <70% of patients have evidence of cardiovascular disease on physical examination, >80% have abnormalities detected by echocardiography.

- Life expectancy in Marfan syndrome is shortened by cardiovascular disease.
- Most common cardiovascular manifestations are mitral valve prolapse and dilatation of ascending aorta.
- More than 80% of patients have abnormalities found on echocardiography.

Mitral valve prolapse in patients with Marfan syndrome initially may involve only the posterior leaflet; it may be late systolic or pansystolic and often is progressive. Prophylactic antibiotic therapy for bacterial endocarditis is warranted. The prevalence of mitral valve prolapse is similar in males and females. In one retrospective series of 166 patients who had had echocardiography before age 22 years, 8 patients died as a result of mitral valve regurgitation and the complication developed in an additional 15 patients. Mitral insufficiency may be present in infants with Marfan syndrome. Acute onset of severe mitral regurgitation due to rupture of chordae tendineae may occur even in childhood. Mitral valve prolapse in a patient with a "marfanoid" body habitus is not a sufficient basis for the diagnosis of Marfan syndrome in the absence of a positive family history of Marfan syndrome or other characteristic findings. Patients with some forms of Ehlers-Danlos syndrome and nonspecific connective tissue dysplasias can have a similar body habitus, joint laxity, and mitral valve prolapse.

- Mitral valve prolapse in Marfan syndrome is progressive.
- Prophylactic antibiotic for bacterial endocarditis is warranted.

In two series, aortic abnormalities were found in 60%-90% of patients with Marfan syndrome. In children and adults, the diameter of the aortic root usually is abnormal in proportion to body surface area. Aortic dilatation is progressive, with symmetric involvement in the region of the sinus of Valsalva and sinotubular ridge. The maximal aortic root diameter is several centimeters superior to the level of aortic leaflet insertion. A greater degree of aortic root dilatation is positively correlated with aortic regurgitation and dissection. Progression of aortic root dilatation may be due to the strain of left ventricular ejection, and β-adrenergic blockers may protect against progressive dilatation. In a controlled study, patients with aortic root dilatation who were given propranolol to decrease left ventricular inotropy by 30% had a significantly lesser degree of dilatation and less morbidity.

- Aortic abnormalities occur in 60%-90% of cases of Marfan syndrome.
- Aortic dilatation is progressive.

Although surgical risks are increased in patients with Marfan syndrome because of tissue friability, surgical treatment frequently is successful for mitral and aortic regurgitation and for aortic dissection. In one series of 41 patients who had a total of 79 operations for aneurysms or valvular insufficiencies, the early mortality rate was 3%; 62% survived at least 15 years. This study spanned 16 years, and 7 of the 11 late deaths may have been prevented by surgical techniques that now are available.

- Surgical risks are increased in Marfan syndrome.
- Surgical treatment is often successful for mitral and aortic regurgitation and aortic dissection.

Patients with Marfan syndrome are prone to traumatic aortic rupture, so contact sports and strenuous exercise should be avoided. The risk of cardiovascular complications during pregnancy poses a special problem for women with Marfan syndrome. Acute aortic dissection may occur before, during, or after labor. A retrospective review of one series of patients suggested that the risk of maternal death was "low in patients with minimal preexisting vascular disease" but the risk may be "significant" in those with moderate degrees of aortic root dilatation. Therefore, aortic root diameter must be considered when counseling women who are considering childbearing. Some physicians advise women with aortic root dilatation not to become pregnant. Those who decide to become pregnant should receive care appropriate for high-risk obstetric patients.

- Patients with Marfan syndrome should avoid contact sports and strenuous exercise (risk of aortic rupture).
- In pregnant women with Marfan syndrome, aortic dissection may occur before, during, or after labor.
- Some physicians advise women with aortic root dilatation not to become pregnant.

Additional features sometimes associated with Marfan syndrome include decreased amounts of subcutaneous tissue, skin striae, inguinal hernias, pneumothorax, and degenerative joint disease.

In addition to physical examination, the diagnostic evaluation of patients suspected of having Marfan syndrome should include chest radiography, ophthalmologic examination (including slit-lamp evaluation of the lenses), and echocardiography. A thorough family history should be obtained. For patients with a well-documented family history of Marfan syndrome, characteristic involvement of the skeletal, cardiovascular, or ocular organ systems may be sufficient for the diagnosis to be made. However, in patients without a positive family history, the patient must have the characteristic body habitus and either aortic root dilatation or ectopia lentis. In those with ectopia lentis, homocystinuria must be excluded. In patients with the characteristic body habitus and mitral valve prolapse but without aortic root dilatation, the diagnosis cannot be made definitely. If skin hyperextensibility, poor skin and wound healing, or atrophic skin scarring is present, the patient probably has a form of Ehlers-Danlos syndrome. If no other abnormality is present, it may be impossible to exclude the diagnosis of Marfan syndrome, and subsequent evaluations are warranted.

- Diagnostic evaluation for Marfan syndrome includes chest radiography, ophthalmologic evaluation, and echocardiography.

First-degree relatives should be evaluated even if they have no obvious stigmata of Marfan syndrome. Families have been observed in which a child presented with obvious phenotypic features of Marfan syndrome and a parent was found to be affected only after echocardiography revealed aortic dilatation or slit-lamp examination revealed ectopia lentis.

The basic cause of Marfan syndrome is a defect in fibrillin; the gene encoding fibrillin is on chromosome 15q15-21. This discovery potentially makes presymptomatic and prenatal diagnosis possible in families known to have the disease, and in the near future it also may allow for diagnostic testing in patients with equivocal signs of the disease.

- Cause of Marfan syndrome is a defect in fibrillin.

Myotonic Dystrophy

Myotonic dystrophy, the most common form of muscular dystrophy in adults, has an incidence of approximately 1 per 8,000-20,000. The inheritance pattern is autosomal dominant with extremely variable expression. Although average age at onset is in the second to third decade of life, the disease may be evident at birth or first be noticed in the seventh decade. The disease is characterized by myotonia, muscle atrophy and weakness, ptosis of the eyelids, and expressionless facies resulting from particularly severe involvement of facial and temporal muscles. Rate of progression of the disease is variable, but disability is usually severe within 15-20 years after onset. Associated abnormalities may include premature frontal baldness, testicular atrophy or menstrual irregularities, gastrointestinal symptoms related to smooth muscle involvement, and cardiac disease. Distinctive refractile posterior subcapsular cataracts often are evident by slit-lamp examination. Although glucose intolerance is common, overt diabetes mellitus occurs in only about 6% of patients.

- Myotonic dystrophy is most common form of muscular dystrophy in adults.
- Incidence is 1 in 8,000-20,000.
- Autosomal dominant inheritance with extremely variable expression.
- Age at onset is usually second to third decade of life.
- Characteristics: myotonia, muscle atrophy and weakness, ptosis of eyelids, expressionless facies.
- Disability is severe within 15-20 years after onset.
- Associated abnormalities: premature frontal baldness, testicular atrophy or menstrual irregularities, gastrointestinal symptoms, cardiac disease.
- Diabetes mellitus occurs in 6% of patients.

The diagnosis is based on clinical findings and a typical electromyographic pattern characterized by prolonged rhythmic discharges. The gene for myotonic dystrophy is located on chromosome 19 at band q13, and genetic counseling is warranted for the patient and family. First-degree relatives should be investigated. The risk for children born to an affected parent is 50%. The molecular basis of most cases of myotonic dystrophy is expansion of a CTG trinucleotide repeat sequence in a gene encoding a protein kinase. Thus, direct DNA-based diagnosis of the disease is possible in most cases. The size of the DNA repeat expansion tends to increase during transmission from one generation to the next. This increasing size correlates with worsening disease severity in subsequent generations, a phenomenon known as "anticipation." Affected females also need to be aware of the additional risk of having an affected infant with severe, sometimes fatal, hypotonia and mental deficiency. This infantile form of the disease does not occur when the father is the affected parent.

- Diagnosis of myotonic dystrophy is based on clinical and electromyographic findings or DNA analysis.
- Genetic counseling is warranted for patients and family members with myotonic dystrophy.
- First-degree relatives should be investigated.

Cardiac disease is present in approximately two-thirds of patients with myotonic dystrophy, and sudden death may occur. There is prolongation of the P-R or QRS interval, and there are changes in the T wave and ST segment. Intra-atrial and His-Purkinje conduction may be prolonged, and heart block may require implantation of a pacemaker. There seems to be degeneration of the conducting tissue before other cardiac muscle is involved. If general anesthesia is required, caution must be taken. Many affected patients have central and alveolar hypoventilation resulting in a serious risk of postanesthetic respiratory depression,

which can occur several hours after the patient seems to be alert and stable.

- Cardiac disease occurs in 2 of 3 patients with myotonic dystrophy, and sudden death may occur.
- Many patients have central and alveolar hypoventilation.

Neurofibromatosis

Type 1

Neurofibromatosis type 1 is an autosomal dominant disorder with an incidence of approximately 1 in 3,000-4,000. Approximately 50% of patients have the disease because of a new mutation. The disorder has markedly variable expression but very high penetrance. The diagnosis is based on two or more of the following clinical criteria: six or more café-au-lait macules of ≥1.5 cm in diameter (in a child, five or more that are 0.5 cm), axillary or inguinal freckling, two or more Lisch nodules of the iris, two or more neurofibromas or one plexiform neurofibroma, a definitely positive family history, or one of these and one of the uncommon characteristic manifestations such as orbital or sphenoid wing dysplasia, optic or other central nervous system glioma, renal artery dysplasia with or without abdominal aorta coarctation, or tibial pseudofracture. Additional, less specific signs of the disease may include pheochromocytoma and scoliosis. Fewer than 10% of patients develop malignancy, often neurofibrosarcoma. The gene has been identified and is a GTPase-activating protein involved in the *ras* signaling process. The gene is very large, and multiple different mutations have been identified; there is no evidence for non-allelic heterogeneity. Because of the multitude of different mutations, there is no clinically practical DNA-based test for direct diagnosis. However, linkage analysis can be used for presymptomatic or prenatal diagnosis in informative families (see Linkage Analysis, page 371).

- Neurofibromatosis type 1 is autosomal dominant.
- Incidence is 1 in 3,000-4,000.
- Disorder has markedly variable expression but very high penetrance.
- Fewer than 10% of patients develop malignancy (often neurofibrosarcoma).
- Multiple different mutations have been identified.

Type 2

Neurofibromatosis type 2 is an autosomal dominant disorder that is genetically distinct from neurofibromatosis type 1. The gene has been identified and is localized to the long arm of chromosome 22. It has been referred to as either "merlin" or "schwannomin." In addition to occuring in the germline of neurofibromatosis type 2 patients, acquired mutations in this gene occur in some sporadic meningiomas and schwannomas. DNA-based diagnosis is available by linkage analysis in some familial cases or by direct mutation analysis in some patients. The disorder is characterized by acoustic neuromas, usually bilateral, with or without other central nervous system gliomas, subcapsular posterior cataracts, and café-au-lait macules.

- Neurofibromatosis type 2 is autosomal dominant.
- Characteristics: acoustic neuromas, sometimes nervous system gliomas, subcapsular cataracts, café-au-lait macules.

Osteogenesis Imperfecta

Historically, osteogenesis imperfecta has been divided into four types. Type I is the most common form of osteogenesis imperfecta tarda, and type IV tends to be more severe. Osteogenesis imperfecta congenita includes types II and III. Type II is lethal in the perinatal period, whereas type III may be compatible with prolonged survival with extreme crippling and short stature. The disease is characterized by multiple bone fractures, and some patients have opalescent teeth, blue sclerae, and child- or adult-onset hearing loss. Some patients have increased bruisability. The clinical expression is extremely variable between and within families. Multiple defects in the genes encoding the α-1 and α-2 chains of type I collagen have been reported, and thus the disease is extremely heterogeneous at the DNA level.

Types I and IV, most type II, and some type III osteogenesis imperfecta cases are autosomal dominant. Mitral valve prolapse is increased in frequency but infrequently progresses to significant regurgitation. The mean aortic root diameter is slightly but significantly increased, and aortic regurgitation occurs in 1%-2% of patients.

Tuberous Sclerosis

Tuberous sclerosis is an autosomal dominant disorder with variable expression and high penetrance. Approximately 50% of cases arise by new mutation. It is characterized by cortical or retinal tubers, seizures, mental retardation in <50%, depigmented "ash leaf" macules, facial angiofibromas, dental pits, subungual or periungual fibromas, shagreen patches, and renal cysts or angiomyolipomas. Cardiac rhabdomyomas are more frequent in the fetus and infant and often resolve with age. Pulmonary fibrosis resulting in a "honeycomb" appearance by radiography is more frequent in young women and tends to progress rapidly. Central nervous system astrocytomas may occur. There is non-allelic heterogeneity, with one gene defect that causes tuberous sclerosis on chromosome 9 and another on chromosome 16. Although the gene on chromosome 9 has not yet been identified, that on chromosome 16 (tuberin) is a tumor suppressor gene.

- Tuberous sclerosis is autosomal dominant and has high penetrance.
- About 50% of cases arise by new mutation.
- Characteristics: cortical or retinal tubers, seizures, mental

retardation in <50%, "ash leaf" macules, angiofibromas, subungual or periungual fibromas, shagreen patches, renal cysts or angiomyolipomas.

Von Hippel-Lindau Disease

Von Hippel-Lindau disease is characterized by retinal, spinal cord, and cerebellar hemangioblastomas, cysts of the kidneys, pancreas, and epididymis, and renal cysts and cancers. Other manifestations include hemangioblastomas of the medulla oblongata, cysts and hemangiomas of other visceral organs, pancreatic cancer, and pheochromocytomas.

- Characteristics of von Hippel-Lindau disease: retinal, spinal cord, and cerebellar hemangioblastomas; cysts of kidneys, pancreas, and epididymis.

Retinal hemangioblastomas often are the earliest manifestation of von Hippel-Lindau disease. The mean age at diagnosis is 21-28 years, but they can occur as early as 4 years. Initially, the lesion appears as a small red dot that may enlarge at a variable rate to appear as a gray disk or globular, red tumor. The lesions leak, and localized retinal detachment is frequent. Large lesions may be obscured by exudate or gliosis, or they may calcify. Multiple or bilateral lesions occur in 20%-58% of patients, and 16%-36% of those with retinal lesions have diminished vision.

- Retinal hemangioblastomas may be earliest manifestation of von Hippel-Lindau disease.

Hemangioblastomas of the central nervous system in von Hippel-Lindau disease are benign, and associated morbidity is due to space-occupying effects. They occur most frequently in the cerebellum and spinal cord but also can be in the medulla oblongata and rarely in the cerebrum. The average age at onset of symptoms is 30 years.

- Hemangioblastomas of central nervous system in von Hippel-Lindau disease are benign tumors with morbid effects.

Renal cysts, hemangiomas, and benign adenomas are usually asymptomatic. Rarely, cysts are so extensive as to mimic polycystic kidney disease and cause renal failure. The cysts vary in size from a few millimeters to >2 cm; they are bilateral in 60% and frequently multiple. Renal clear cell cancers are bilateral or multiple in 40%-87% of cases. They are the leading cause of death, which occurs at a mean age of 44 years.

- Renal cysts, hemangiomas, and benign adenomas are usually asymptomatic in von Hippel-Lindau disease.
- Renal cancer is a major cause of death.

Most pancreatic cysts are asymptomatic. They rarely lead

to diabetes mellitus or steatorrhea. Pancreatic disease, including cystadenocarcinoma or islet cell tumors, tends to cluster in certain families.

Adrenal cysts, adenomas, and cortical hyperplasia are asymptomatic. Pheochromocytomas are bilateral in 17%-34% of patients, and the average age at diagnosis is 25-34 years. Pheochromocytomas tend to cluster within certain families, but linkage studies have shown that families with and without pheochromocytomas have defects of the same gene.

- Pheochromocytomas of von Hippel-Lindau disease cluster within certain families.

Many male patients with von Hippel-Lindau disease have benign, asymptomatic epididymal lesions, although occasionally fertility is impaired. An epididymal cyst in a relative at risk is not sufficient by itself to diagnose von Hippel-Lindau disease.

Inheritance is autosomal dominant, and the risk for any child born to an affected person is 50%. Expression is variable, but penetrance is complete in thoroughly evaluated families. Males and females are affected equally.

- Von Hippel-Lindau disease is autosomal dominant.

Patients with a hemangioblastoma should have a review of the family history, computed tomography or magnetic resonance imaging of the head and upper spine, ophthalmologic examination, and computed tomography or ultrasonography of the abdomen. Patients with bilateral epididymal cysts or polycystic pancreas should also be screened, and it should be considered in patients with pheochromocytomas, polycystic kidneys, or renal cancer. Patients with von Hippel-Lindau disease need annual physical and ophthalmologic examinations, peripheral blood cell count, urinalysis, computed tomography or magnetic resonance imaging of the head, and computed tomography or ultrasonography of the abdomen. Evaluation of urinary catecholamines is reasonable, particularly if the patient is hypertensive or has a family history of pheochromocytoma. Patients should have genetic counseling, and first-degree relatives should have physical and ophthalmologic examinations beginning at age 4 years, imaging of the head and spine at 11 years, and imaging of the abdomen at 18 years. It is unknown at what age one can safely discontinue screening for at-risk members. Presymptomatic and prenatal diagnosis by use of linked DNA markers is available in some families. The gene that causes von Hippel-Lindau disease was recently identified and is localized to chromosome 3p25-26. The normal gene acts as a tumor suppressor, and more than 18 different mutations have been detected in this gene in patients with von Hippel-Lindau disease. The large number of mutations makes DNA diagnosis by direct mutation analyses impossible on a routine basis for all patients. Acquired mutations in this gene also have been found in sporadic renal cell carcinomas.

Autosomal Recessive

Autosomal recessive disease occurs because of abnormal genes that are located on the autosomes. However, one copy of the abnormal gene is not sufficient to cause disease, and heterozygotes (carriers) are not clinically different from the general population. When two persons who are heterozygotes for a given gene defect mate, the children are at 25% risk of inheriting the abnormal gene from both parents and, thus, of having the disease.

- Autosomal recessive inheritance: abnormal genes are located on autosomes, but one copy of gene is not sufficient to cause disease.
- Heterozygotes (carriers) are not clinically different from the general population.

Because the heterozygous state may be transmitted silently through many generations before the chance mating of two heterozygotes occurs, it is not surprising that there rarely is a family history of the disease in previous generations. The occurrence of multiple affected siblings within a family suggests autosomal recessive inheritance; however, because of the small average family size in this country, many autosomal recessive diseases seem to occur as isolated cases.

The risk for the children of a person who has an autosomal recessive disease depends on the frequency of the abnormal gene in the population. Except for common diseases such as cystic fibrosis or sickle cell anemia, the risk is usually small, provided that this person does not marry a relative or a person who has a family history of the same disease.

Many diseases that are caused by an identified metabolic defect, such as homocystinuria, are autosomal recessive diseases due to an enzyme deficiency. When the enzymatic defect is established, carrier testing and prenatal diagnosis sometimes are possible.

Some of the diseases with autosomal recessive inheritance are listed in Table 10-2 and summarized on the following pages.

Friedreich Ataxia

This is an autosomal recessive disorder. The first sign of the disease is ataxic gait. The mean age at onset is approximately 12 years. Dysarthria, hypotonic muscle weakness, loss of vibration and position senses, and loss of deep tendon reflexes develop subsequently. In some patients, diabetes mellitus, nystagmus, optic atrophy, dementia, respiratory dysfunction due to kyphoscoliosis, and decreased sensory nerve conduction velocities also develop.

Table 10-2.--Diseases With Autosomal Recessive Inheritance

Alkaptonuria
α_1-Antitrypsin deficiency
Cystic fibrosis
Familial Mediterranean fever
Friedreich ataxia
Gaucher disease
Glycogen storage disease, types I, II, III, IV, V, VII
Hemochromatosis
Homocystinuria
Oculocutaneous albinism
Phenylketonuria
Pseudoxanthoma elasticum (some forms are autosomal
　　dominant)
Refsum disease
Sickle-cell disease
Tay-Sachs disease
α- and β-Thalassemia
Wilson disease

- Friedreich ataxia is autosomal recessive.
- First sign of disease is ataxic gait.
- Mean age at onset is 12 years.
- Dysarthria, hypotonic muscle weakness, loss of vibration and position senses, and loss of deep tendon reflexes develop subsequently.

In one series, 60 of 82 patients with Friedreich ataxia had clinical evidence of cardiac dysfunction 4 months to 4 years before death, and 56% died of heart failure. The mean age at death was 36.6 years. Cardiac arrhythmias, particularly atrial fibrillation, were common and occurred in 50% of fatal cases. At autopsy, most cases had marked thickening of the left ventricle with extensive interstitial fibrosis and focal degeneration of muscle fibers. Muscle fibers were hypertrophied and many had large nuclei. The cardiomyopathy may be of the hypertrophic type with subaortic stenosis.

- Cardiac arrhythmias occur in 50% of fatal cases of Friedreich ataxia.

The risk for a sibling being affected is 25%. The basic biochemical defect remains unknown. However, the gene has been localized to chromosome 9q12-21.1 by genetic linkage studies of affected families. This evaluation potentially allows for prenatal or presymptomatic diagnosis of cases in which one affected child already has been diagnosed.

- Risk of Friedreich ataxia in sibling of affected person is 25%.

Gaucher Disease

Gaucher disease is an autosomal recessive disorder due to deficiency of the enzyme glucocerebrosidase, which results in lipid storage in the spleen, liver, bone marrow, and other organs. Type 1 (non-neuronopathic) disease is most frequent in Ashkenazi Jews (carrier frequency, 1 in 10). The disease may be asymptomatic at any age or present in childhood or adulthood with splenomegaly, hepatosplenomegaly, thrombocytopenia, anemia, degenerative bone disease, or pulmonary disease. Type 2 (infantile, neuronopathic) has no ethnic predisposition, and type 3 (juvenile form) has intermediate clinical signs. The first sign of neurologic involvement in types 2 and 3 is supranuclear ophthalmoplegia.

- Gaucher disease is autosomal recessive.
- Disease is due to deficiency of the enzyme glucocerebrosidase.
- Type 1 is most frequent in Ashkenazi Jews.
- Type 2 has no ethnic predisposition.
- First sign of neurologic involvement in types 2 and 3 is supranuclear ophthalmoplegia.

Enzyme replacement is effective treatment for non-neuronopathic forms of the disease, but it is not yet known whether it is effective for patients with neurologic involvement.

- Enzyme replacement therapy is effective for non-neuronopathic Gaucher disease.

Glycogen Storage Diseases

Glycogen storage disease type I is due to deficiency of the enzyme glucose-6-phosphatase. It is characterized by hypoglycemia, hypercholesterolemia, hyperuricemia, lactic acidosis, short stature, hepatomegaly, and delayed onset of puberty. Adults with this disease may develop malignant hepatomas, premature coronary disease, pancreatitis, gout, and renal disease.

- Glycogen storage disease type I is due to deficiency of the enzyme glucose-6-phosphatase.
- Characteristics: hypoglycemia, hypercholesterolemia, hyperuricemia, lactic acidosis, short stature, hepatomegaly, delayed puberty.

Glycogen storage disease type II (Pompe disease) is an autosomal recessive disorder due to deficiency of the lysosomal enzyme α-1,4-glucosidase (acid maltase). The infantile form is characterized by hypotonia, macroglossia, and progressive cardiomyopathy resulting in death within the first year of life. The electrocardiogram is characterized by high-voltage QRS complexes in all leads and a short P-R interval. Cardiac catheterization frequently reveals biventricular hypertrophy with left outflow tract obstruction. The myocardium is different histologically from the myocardium in isolated hypertrophic cardiomyopathy. There is evidence of glycogen storage with vacuolation of heart muscle. Histologic examination of tissues such as liver and kidney may reveal engorged lysosomes, but in muscle the lysosomes may have ruptured and cytoplasmic glycogen is seen. The diagnosis can be confirmed by determination of α-1,4-glucosidase activity in skeletal muscle or cultured fibroblasts. Prenatal diagnosis through enzyme analysis of amniotic fluid cells is possible.

- Glycogen storage disease type II is autosomal recessive.
- Disease is due to deficiency of the enzyme α-1,4-glucosidase.
- Characteristics of infantile form: hypotonia, macroglossia, progressive cardiomyopathy.

Juvenile and adult forms of glycogen storage disease type II also exist. The presenting characteristic is skeletal muscle weakness, and cardiac involvement usually is absent or minimal. At least one patient had a cardiac arrhythmia that required implantation of a ventricular pacemaker, but her echocardiogram showed no cardiomegaly.

- Characteristics of juvenile and adult forms of glycogen storage disease: skeletal muscle weakness, minimal or absent cardiac involvement.

Glycogen storage disease type III is due to an autosomal recessively inherited deficiency of amylo-1,6-glucosidase (debrancher) activity. The enzyme is deficient in liver, and in some patients also in skeletal muscle, cultured skin fibroblasts, and leukocytes. Clinically, the disorder is characterized by hepatomegaly and growth retardation that resolves at puberty. There may be hypoglycemia and hyperlipidemia. Skeletal muscle weakness may develop in adult life. Cardiomyopathy, when present, may be life-threatening and mimic hypertrophic cardiomyopathy. Histologic evaluation of cardiac tissue reveals increased intracellular glycogen with no disarray of myofibers or myofibrils. Deficiency of the enzyme has been documented in cardiac muscle from one patient.

- Glycogen storage disease type III is autosomal recessive.
- Disease is due to deficiency of amylo-1,6-glucosidase activity.
- Characteristics: hepatomegaly, growth retardation that resolves at puberty.

Hemochromatosis

Clinical features of the disease may be gray-brown skin pigmentation, cardiomyopathy, hepatomegaly with fibrosis or cirrhosis, diabetes mellitus, hypogonadism, and bone demineralization. The disease is due to tissue damage by iron overload, although the extent of iron overload in an organ does not always correspond to the severity of tissue damage. Biochemical abnormalities include increased serum iron and ferritin levels, increased transferrin saturation, and increased urinary iron excretion, especially in response to deferoxamine administration. The hemochromatosis gene is linked to the HLA complex on chromosome 6, and this linkage association was instrumental in proving the autosomal recessive inheritance pattern.

- Features of hemochromatosis: gray-brown skin pigmentation, cardiomyopathy, hepatomegaly, diabetes mellitus, hypogonadism, bone demineralization.
- Disease is due to tissue damage by iron overload.
- Disease is autosomal recessive.

The risk for siblings of an affected patient is 25%, and therefore all should be screened for biochemical evidence of the disease. Patients with iron overload should have phlebotomy until the excess iron is removed, regardless of whether clinical signs of the disease are present. The risk for children of affected individuals is relatively low (approximately 1 in 36) but is not negligible because of the relatively high gene frequency in the general population. Therefore, children should be screened to determine whether they are at risk for the disease. Some advocate population screening.

- Siblings of patients with hemochromatosis have risk of 25% for the disease.
- Children of patients with hemochromatosis need to be screened.

Heart disease occurs in 15%-20% of patients with clinically evident hemochromatosis, and the earliest signs may be electrocardiographic changes characterized by decreased QRS amplitude and T-wave flattening or inversion. Later, congestive heart failure and arrhythmias may occur. The heart condition sometimes resolves after phlebotomy.

- Heart disease occurs in 15%-20% of patients with hemochromatosis.

Homocystinuria

The classic form of homocystinuria is due to autosomal recessively inherited deficiency of cystathionine β-synthase. The gene is expressed in skin fibroblasts and amniocytes, so prenatal diagnosis by determination of enzyme activity in amniocytes is feasible.

- Homocystinuria is autosomal recessive disease.
- Disease is due to deficiency of cystathionine β-synthase.

The incidence of the disease is approximately 1 per 200,000. Clinically, it is characterized by tall stature with a low upper segment:lower segment ratio, pectus deformities, scoliosis, genu valgum, pes planus, and a highly arched palate. Lens dislocation is progressive, and the direction of displacement is usually, but not always, downward. Myopia, retinal detachment, secondary glaucoma, fair hair and skin, cutaneous flushing, and hernias may be present. Approximately 50% of patients are mentally retarded, but this is variable even within a sibship. The electroencephalogram may be abnormal, and some patients have seizures, focal neurologic signs, and hemiatrophy of the brain. Acute episodes of "nervousness" or schizophrenic behavior may occur. Osteoporosis with a tendency to fractures and "codfish"-shaped, collapsed vertebrae may be evident radiographically. None of the features are present consistently in all patients, and some affected individuals appear normal.

- Incidence of homocystinuria is about 1 per 200,000.
- Clinical features: tall stature, pectus deformities, scoliosis, genu valgum, pes planus, highly arched palate.
- Lens dislocation is progressive.
- About 50% of patients are mentally retarded.
- "Nervousness" or schizophrenic behavior may occur.
- Osteoporosis and "codfish"-shaped, collapsed vertebrae may be seen on radiographs.

Cardiovascular abnormalities include arterial or venous thrombosis, angina pectoris, coronary occlusions at a young age, renal artery narrowing resulting in hypertension and renal atrophy, cerebrovascular accidents, thrombophlebitis, and pulmonary emboli. Dilatation of the pulmonary artery and left atrial endocardial fibroelastosis have been reported. Thrombi are particularly likely to occur after operation, venipuncture, or catheterization.

- Cardiovascular abnormalities of homocystinuria: arterial or venous thrombosis, angina pectoris, coronary occlusions at young age.
- Thrombi are likely after operation, venipuncture, catheterization.

Histologic examination of the arteries reveals marked fibrous thickening of the intima. Aortic intimal fibrosis may be severe enough to mimic coarctation. Medial changes consist of thrombosis and dilatation with widely spaced, frayed muscle fibers. The elastic fibers of the large arteries may be fragmented, and dilatation of the ascending aorta has been observed. No consistent platelet defect has been noted.

The disease sometimes may be diagnosed by positive results of urinary nitroprusside test and confirmed by the more sensitive method of elevated urinary homocystine excretion by amino acid chromatography. Levels of plasma homocystine

and its precursor, methionine, are increased. The goal of treatment is to lower the plasma homocystine level, which seems to result in slower progression and fewer symptoms of the disease; 50% of patients respond to pyridoxine therapy (25-1,000 mg/day). Supplemental folate also should be given because patients who are potentially capable of responding to pyridoxine may not do so in the presence of folate deficiency. A low-protein, low-methionine diet can be useful, but adults find it difficult to comply with this. For infants, a low-methionine formula is available. Betaine and penicillamine also have been reported to be of benefit in decreasing plasma homocystine levels.

- In homocystinuria, levels of plasma homocystine and its precursor, methionine, are increased.
- Goal of treatment: lower plasma homocystine level.

A rare form of homocystinuria is due to deficiency of *N*-methyltetrahydrofolate-homocysteine methyltransferase. Affected patients have additional neurologic symptoms, and the plasma methionine levels may be normal. Patients with homocystinuria due to abnormal cobalamin metabolism also have normal plasma methionine levels and may have methylmalonic acidemia and megaloblastic anemia.

Pseudoxanthoma Elasticum

There are two hereditary forms of pseudoxanthoma elasticum: autosomal dominant and autosomal recessive. Both forms are characterized by yellowish skin papules, especially on the neck and flexural areas, angioid streaks and choroiditis of the retina, and vascular complications, including angina pectoris, claudication, calcification of peripheral arteries, and renal vascular hypertension. In one series of patients, 19% had angina pectoris, 14% had calcification of peripheral arteries, and 18% had intermittent claudication. The age at onset of complications is variable, and they may occur in early adolescence. Endocardial thickening may result in deformity of the valves, and the conduction system also may be involved, resulting in arrhythmias. Histologically, the arteries show fragmented elastic fibers with granular deposits in place of amorphous elastin. The basic defect is not known.

- Two hereditary forms of pseudoxanthoma elasticum: autosomal dominant and autosomal recessive.
- Characteristics: yellowish skin papules, angioid streaks and choroiditis of retina, vascular complications.

Refsum Disease

Refsum disease is an autosomal recessive neurodegenerative disease characterized by cerebellar ataxia, hypertrophic polyneuropathy, and retinitis pigmentosa. Deafness, ichthyosis, and cardiac conduction defects are frequently present. Onset of the disorder may be in infancy or middle age, and the course is progressive. Cerebrospinal fluid protein concentration is increased, and phytanic acid accumulates in serum and organs. Hypertrophic interstitial neuritis and degenerative changes of nuclei and fiber tracts are observed histologically in the brain stem. The electrocardiogram is characterized by a prolonged P-Q interval and ST-segment and T-wave changes. Impaired atrioventricular conduction, bundle branch block, and sudden death from cardiac arrhythmia may occur. Myocardial fibrosis has been reported.

- Refsum disease is autosomal recessive.
- Characteristics: cerebellar ataxia, hypertrophic polyneuropathy, retinitis pigmentosa.
- Frequently present: deafness, ichthyosis, cardiac conduction defects.

Phytanic acid is a fatty acid present in dairy products and fat from grazing animals. Patients with Refsum disease are deficient in the catabolic enzyme phytanic acid α-hydroxylase, which results in accumulation of ingested phytanic acid in fatty deposits in the involved organ systems. The enzyme deficiency is expressed in cultured skin fibroblasts, and prenatal diagnosis is possible.

- Patients with Refsum disease are deficient in phytanic acid α-hydroxylase.

Dietary restriction of phytanic acid results in clinical improvement and stabilization of the disease. Electrocardiographic changes sometimes resolve after treatment. Plasmapheresis removes phytanic acid from the body and may allow liberalization of the diet; it can be extremely valuable in the management of acutely ill patients.

Tay-Sachs Disease

Tay-Sachs disease is an autosomal recessive disease due to deficiency of hexosaminidase A. The classic infantile form of the disease is rapidly fatal and is due to storage of ganglioside GM_2 in neural tissue. It is particularly common in people of Ashkenazi Jewish ancestry; the carrier frequency is 1 in 30. Therefore, screening for carriers by determination of enzyme activity in serum (or leukocytes, particularly in pregnant women, in whom the serum level is unreliable) is recommended in this population. Prenatal diagnosis is available when both the mother and the father are carriers.

- Tay-Sachs disease is autosomal recessive.
- Disease is due to deficiency of hexosaminidase A.

Rare juvenile and adult forms of the disease exist and may present with ataxia, upper motor neuron disease, or other neurologic disorders. These late-onset variants have less of an ethnic predisposition.

X-Linked Recessive

X-linked recessive diseases are caused by abnormal genes located on the X chromosome. Female heterozygotes, who have one abnormal gene on one X chromosome and one normal gene on the other X chromosome, usually are clinically normal. Exceptions may occur because of the phenomenon of lyonization, in which one X chromosome is inactivated at random early in fetal life; if the normal gene is inactivated in a critical number of cells, the woman may have symptoms or clinical signs of the disease. However, the disease usually is less severe than in males. The likelihood of clinical signs of the disease developing in a female varies by disease. For example, it is rare for female carriers of hemophilia VIII to have severe bleeding problems, but it is relatively common for carriers of ornithine carbamoyltransferase (ornithine transcarbamoylase) deficiency to have intermittent symptoms.

- X-linked recessive diseases are caused by abnormal genes on X chromosome.
- Development of clinical signs of disease in female varies by disease.

Males who inherit the abnormal gene have no corresponding genetic loci on the Y chromosome and therefore are referred to as "hemizygotes." Any male child born to a heterozygous female is at 50% risk for having the disease; female children are at 50% risk for inheriting the gene and being carriers. All the daughters of affected males are carriers, and all the sons are unaffected (i.e., male-to-male transmission cannot occur).

- Males with abnormal gene are called "hemizygotes."
- Male child of heterozygous female has 50% risk of disease.
- Female child is at 50% risk of inheriting the gene.

X-linked recessive diseases also may arise by new mutation affecting either the mother or the afflicted son. Genetic counseling is difficult in these situations because if the mother represents the new mutation the risk for her future male children is 50%. However, if the child represents the new mutation, there is no significant risk for siblings of that child. New advances in DNA-based diagnosis have resulted in opportunities for carrier detection for some diseases, which circumvent problems created by lyonization.

Some of the conditions with X-linked recessive inheritance are listed in Table 10-3 and summarized on the following pages.

Duchenne and Becker Muscular Dystrophies

Duchenne muscular dystrophy is one of the most common types of muscular dystrophy; its incidence is approximately 1 in 3,500 newborn males. It is an X-linked recessive disease, and approximately a third of the cases arise by new mutation. Progressive skeletal weakness beginning at 2 to 5 years of age,

Table 10-3.--X-Linked Recessive Conditions

Adrenoleukodystrophy ("X-linked" form)

Chronic granulomatous disease (many cases; autosomal recessive forms are less common)

Color blindness

Duchenne and Becker muscular dystrophies

Fabry disease

Glucose-6-phosphate dehydrogenase deficiency

Hemophilia A and B

Ocular albinism

Rickets, hypophosphatemic

Testicular feminization

---

with death in the late teens or 20s, is characteristic. The diagnosis is made on the basis of clinical findings and markedly increased creatine kinase levels. The muscle biopsy findings are relatively nonspecific. Becker muscular dystrophy has later onset.

- Incidence of Duchenne muscular dystrophy is 1 in 3,500 newborn males.
- Duchenne muscular dystrophy is X-linked recessive.
- Skeletal weakness at 2 to 5 years of age is characteristic.

The genetic defect that results in both Duchenne and Becker muscular dystrophies involves the dystrophin gene located on chromosome X at band p2l. Approximately two-thirds of patients have a submicroscopic partial gene deletion, and the rest have undetected deletions, duplications, or other abnormalities. The dystrophin gene is very large, consisting of at least 60 exons and 1,800 kilobases. The entire gene has been cloned. The protein product of this gene, dystrophin, is a rod-shaped cytoskeletal protein that is predominantly localized to the surface membrane of striated muscle cells. Identification of the molecular defect has resulted in improved ability to determine carrier status in female relatives by DNA analysis. This is a significant improvement over carrier testing by measurement of creatine kinase levels, because levels are increased in only 70% of obligate carriers. DNA analysis also can be used for prenatal diagnosis. All mothers, sisters, and children of patients with Duchenne or Becker muscular dystrophy should have genetic counseling.

- Mothers, sisters, and children of patients with Duchenne or Becker muscular dystrophy need genetic counseling.

The heart disease in patients with Duchenne muscular dystrophy is characterized by significant changes in systolic time intervals suggestive of compromised left ventricular function. There are histologic changes characterized by multifocal dystrophic areas with fibrosis and loss of myofilaments. These changes are most marked in the posterobasal segment and contiguous lateral and inferior walls of the left ventricle.

- Heart disease in Duchenne muscular dystrophy involves changes in systolic time intervals.

Fabry Disease

Fabry disease is a lysosomal storage disease due to deficiency of α-galactosidase A. The inheritance pattern is X-linked recessive, although females may have less severe signs of the disease than males. Glycosphingolipids accumulate in the endothelium, perithelium, and smooth muscle of blood vessels. There is less accumulation in ganglion cells, myocardial cells, reticuloendothelial cells, and connective tissue cells.

- Fabry disease is due to deficiency of α-galactosidase A.
- Disease is X-linked recessive.
- Females may have less severe signs than males.

The first signs of the disease may be telangiectatic angiokeratomas of the skin and mucous membranes. Acroparesthesias and episodes of severe burning pain in the palms and soles with proximal radiation also may occur in childhood and adolescence. Whorl-shaped corneal opacities and cataracts develop. In adulthood, cardiovascular and renal diseases are the major causes of morbidity and mortality. Cardiac problems, including ischemia, infarction, congestive heart failure, mitral insufficiency, and aortic stenosis, may result from progressive glycosphingolipid infiltration. Systemic hypertension due to infiltration of renal parenchymal vessels may aggravate the cardiac disease. Electrocardiography may show signs of left ventricular hypertrophy, ST-segment changes, and T-wave inversion. Occasionally, patients have arrhythmias and a short P-R interval.

- First signs of Fabry disease may be telangiectatic angiokeratomas of skin and mucous membranes.
- Acroparesthesias may occur in childhood and adolescence.
- Whorl-shaped corneal opacities and cataracts develop.
- In adults, cardiovascular and renal diseases develop.

The interventricular septum and posterior left ventricular wall may be thickened. Cardiomegaly, especially involving the left atrium and ventricle, is observed. The right atrium and ventricle may be dilated. Myocardial cells show extensive glycosphingolipid deposited around the nucleus and between myofibrils. Endothelial cells and smooth muscle cells are hypertrophied. The mitral valve frequently is thickened and has normal or thick papillary muscles; the tricuspid valve may be involved, but the aortic and pulmonary valves usually are normal. Lipid-filled cells are seen within the fibrous tissue of involved valves.

Neurologic signs result from small-vessel involvement in the brain. The most frequent cause of death is renal failure.

Dilantin and carbamazepine are useful for treating the pain. Renal transplantation can prolong life. The gene has been cloned, and prenatal diagnosis is possible.

MITOCHONDRIAL MUTATIONS

Mitochondria each contain several circular copies of their own genetic material, mitochondrial DNA. This mitochondrial DNA is approximately 16,000 base pairs in length and encodes for transfer-RNAs and several proteins involved in the mitochondrial respiratory chain. Many mitochondrial enzymes, including some others of the respiratory chain complex, are encoded by nuclear DNA and transported into the mitochondria. Mitochondrial DNA mutations cause Leber's optic atrophy and the multisystem syndromes of multiple episodes of lactic acidosis and stroke (MELAS) and myoclonic epilepsy with ragged red fibers (MERRF). Many cases of Kearns-Sayre syndrome (cardiomyopathy and ophthalmoplegia) are due to mitochondrial mutations. Mitochondrial disorders can arise as new mutations or be maternally inherited; only the egg contributes mitochondria to the zygote, the sperm does not. Mitochondrial mutations may be homoplasmic (present in all mitochondrial DNA) or heteroplasmic (present in only some of the mitochondrial DNA). Accumulation of acquired mutations may contribute to the aging process, and mitochondrial mutations may play a role in the pathogenesis of ischemic heart disease.

- Mitochondrial DNA mutations cause Leber's optic atrophy and multisystem syndromes.
- Many cases of Kearns-Sayre syndrome are due to mitochondrial mutations.
- Only the egg contributes mitochondria to the zygote; sperm does not.

MULTIFACTORIAL CAUSATION

Multifactorial means that the disease or trait is determined by the interaction of environmental influences and a polygenic (many gene) predisposition. Human conditions that may have multifactorial causation include many common birth defects--such as congenital heart defects, cleft lip and palate, and neural tube defects--and many common diseases--such as diabetes mellitus, asthma, hypertension, and coronary artery atherosclerosis.

- Multifactorial causation: disease or trait is due to environmental influences and polygenic predisposition.
- Birth defects that may have multifactorial causation: congenital heart defects, cleft lip and palate, neural tube defects.

- Diseases that may have multifactorial causation: diabetes mellitus, asthma, hypertension, coronary artery atherosclerosis.

The multifactorial model predicts that there will be a tendency for familial aggregation of the condition but without a strict mendelian pattern of inheritance. Familial aggregation also can be due to common environmental factors, so familial aggregation by itself is not sufficient to prove multifactorial causation.

Because familial aggregation exists for multifactorial disorders, it is implicit that the occurrence risk will be increased for members of an affected family over that of the general population. As expected, the risk is highest for first-degree relatives (parents, siblings, children), who have half of their genes in common. The risk is less for second-degree relatives (grandparents, aunts, uncles, grandchildren, nephews, nieces), who share one-quarter of their genes. The risk decreases exponentially thereafter; third-degree relatives (great-grandparents, cousins, great-grandchildren) share only one-eighth of their genes. Empiric (observed) risk figures for some well-studied multifactorial disorders fit well with the predicted risks.

The genetic liability in multifactorial causation is due to the cumulative effect of many genes, each having a small effect, rather than to the effect of one major gene. These genes create a liability that presumably is continuously distributed within the population. If the genetic liability is strong enough, under an unfortunate set of environmental circumstances the disorder will occur.

- Genetic liability in multifactorial causation is due to cumulative effect of many genes.

For many multifactorial conditions, there is a difference in predilection between males and females which could result directly from genetic differences or from different internal (e.g., hormonal) or external environmental factors. Furthermore, if a member of the less commonly affected sex has the condition, his or her genetic liability was probably greater and therefore the risk for his or her relatives is greater. Similarly, if a person has a more severe form of the disease, the risk for relatives is higher. For disorders in which disease frequency increases with age, earlier onset sometimes implies a greater risk for relatives. Finally, the greater the number of affected individuals within the family, the higher the risk for other relatives. There also are racial differences in the frequency of many disorders of multifactorial causation.

When the inheritance pattern of any disease is being determined, the possibility of genetic heterogeneity always must be considered. For example, there are both autosomal dominant and multifactorial causes of atrial septal defect which may be indistinguishable clinically. Failure to recognize that different genetic diseases can cause the same or similar clinical entities can result in confusion when determining risks.

Table 10-4 lists some conditions of multifactorial causation.

PRESYMPTOMATIC AND PRENATAL DIAGNOSIS OF GENETIC DISEASE BY DNA ANALYSIS

Presymptomatic and prenatal diagnosis of genetic diseases utilizing peripheral blood specimens or specimens obtained by amniocentesis or chorionic villus sampling has become a routine part of clinical practice because of the identification of the basic genetic defect underlying numerous mendelian conditions and the capability for direct DNA diagnosis. In addition, even when the causative genetic defect has not yet been identified, knowledge of its chromosome localization may allow for diagnosis by linkage analysis. Because individual genes are too small to be seen microscopically, standard chromosome analysis generally is not helpful even when the gene has been localized to a specific chromosome region.

The DNA-based laboratory procedures used for diagnosis, the limitations of the tests, and the importance of an accurate clinical diagnosis and family history are described below. A discussion of the prenatal diagnosis of Duchenne muscular dystrophy (DMD) provides an excellent example of these issues. Although the following examples describe prenatal diagnosis, the same principles apply to presymptomatic diagnosis.

Importance of an Accurate Clinical Diagnosis and Family History

The importance of a correct diagnosis in the index patient when diagnosis by DNA analysis is being contemplated cannot be overemphasized. This criterion is in contrast to many instances of genetic diagnosis by chromosome analysis in which the cytogeneticist usually can be relied on to note most abnormalities (fragile X and subtle deletions are examples of

Table 10-4.--Conditions of Multifactorial Causation

Atherosclerosis

Atopic disease or allergy

Cancer

Cardiac defects (congenital)

Cleft lip or palate

Diabetes mellitus

Hypertension

Neural tube defects

Schizophrenia

---

exceptions) regardless of the exact indication for the study. This approach is possible because the procedure of chromosome analysis involves examination of all 46 chromosomes in a given cell to look for gross structural changes. In contrast, it is impossible to systematically examine each of a person's 100,000 genes to detect all abnormalities.

● It is impossible to systematically examine each of a person's 100,000 genes.

The laboratory's process of detection of even one abnormal gene must be directed by the precise clinical diagnosis. The DNA-based assays are specific for the disease being studied, and abnormalities elsewhere in the genome will not be detected. Thus, if the incorrect assay is chosen because of an incorrect clinical diagnosis, the disease-causing mutation will not be detected. For example, if a pregnant woman's brother and uncle are believed to have DMD but the correct diagnosis is X-linked Emery-Dreifuss muscular dystrophy, the wrong DNA analysis will be performed and may result in an erroneous prediction as to whether the fetus is affected. It is the responsibility of the physician to obtain medical records or to arrange for one of the affected relatives to be examined to confirm the reported diagnosis, and the physician may want the assistance of a medical geneticist or other specialist in this process.

In addition to confirmation of the diagnosis, an accurate family pedigree is necessary. It is important to know whether the index patient represents a sporadic case or whether other family members also are affected. This information must be considered in the determination of whether DNA diagnosis is possible and in the interpretation of the results of DNA analysis. In sporadic cases, diagnosis by linkage analysis (see below), which is based on tracking the mutation through the family, may be impossible.

● Accurate family pedigree is necessary for diagnosis.

In these sporadic cases, diagnosis often can be established only for diseases for which direct DNA diagnosis is possible. In contrast, in families with multiple affected members, direct DNA diagnosis is the first diagnostic choice when possible, followed by linkage analysis if the mutation cannot be directly identified. For other diseases, linkage studies are the only option. For example, in DMD, approximately 60% of patients have a deletion identifiable by techniques in routine use for clinical testing. If a deletion is detected in a sporadic patient with DMD, it usually is possible to determine whether the mother is a carrier and, if so, direct DNA diagnosis can be applied for her male fetuses. If a deletion cannot be detected in a sporadic patient with DMD, then specific prenatal diagnosis is not possible for the mother's future children, although exclusion of a disease may still be possible by use of linked markers. The mother of a sporadic patient with DMD has a prior risk for being a carrier of approximately 2 in 3, and the options include fetal sex determination followed by termination of all male fetuses, although at least 2 of 3 would be expected to be unaffected, or termination of fetuses that inherited the same markers as the index patient, in which at least 1 of 3 would be unaffected.

● In families with multiple affected members, direct DNA diagnosis is first diagnostic choice.

Alternatively, if there are multiple affected family members with DMD, the issue of new mutation is not a concern. If a deletion is detected in these multiplex families, this is the simplest approach for testing male fetuses of women at risk within the family. However, if a deletion is not detected, then blood specimens can be collected from multiple family members for linkage analysis (Fig. 10-5).

Linkage Analysis

Linkage analysis for prenatal diagnosis is based on the biologic fact that individual units of genetic material (genes) are situated in linear order on one of the 24 types of chromosomes (22 autosomes plus the X and Y chromosomes). The word "alleles" refers to the different forms of genetic material at the same gene locus, for example, the A and B alleles at the ABO blood group locus. Genes located on different chromosomes segregate independently, so there is a 50% chance that an individual egg or sperm will contain the same or different alleles encoded within these two chromosomal loci (Fig. 10-6).

● "Alleles" are different forms of genetic material at the same gene locus.

Genes located on the same chromosome are *syntenic*. During the pairing of homologous chromosomes during meiosis, crossovers can occur between genes even if they are located on the same chromosome. The average number of crossovers per chromosome per meiosis is two. Genes located far apart on the same chromosome are more likely to be separated by crossovers than are genes located close together. If the genes are so far apart that they are separated by crossovers at least 50% of the time, then these genes are not linked even though they are syntenic, and they exhibit random segregation (Fig. 10-7).

● Genes located on same chromosome are *syntenic*.

Of course, linkage is not an all-or-none phenomenon. There is the potential for crossover to occur between any two gene loci, and this could happen in 20% of meioses, 2% of meioses, or 0.2% of meioses, for example, depending on the "distance" between them. Although physical distance is correlated with the likelihood of crossover, other factors such as location of the genes adjacent to the chromosome centromere and sex of

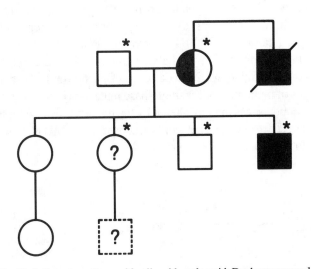

Fig. 10-5. Sample pedigree of family with males with Duchenne muscular dystrophy (shaded symbols). Carrier females are shown with half-shaded symbols. Members for whom blood was requested for DNA linkage analysis are marked with an asterisk. Squares, males; circles, females; line through square indicates that person is deceased; dashed-line square indicates male fetus. Note that blood for DNA from pregnant woman's father and unaffected brother is helpful for DNA linkage studies. Most laboratories offering these tests assist the referring physician in determining which family members need testing.

Fig. 10-6. Random segregation of gene locus on chromosome 1 in relation to gene locus on chromosome 18. There is a 50% chance that allele A will segregate with allele B or allele b. These loci are not syntenic and do not demonstrate linkage.

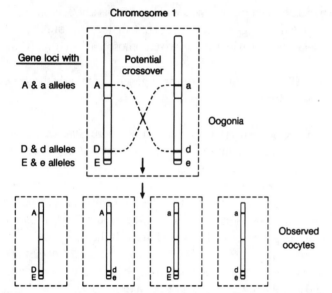

Fig. 10-7. Three gene loci on chromosome 1. Locus with allele A and allele a is located at sufficient distance from loci with alleles D/d and E/e that random segregation occurs. However, loci with alleles D/d and E/e always show D and E together or d and e together (not drawn to scale). Loci for D/d and E/e do not show random segregation and thus are linked.

the individual also influence the likelihood of crossover. Therefore, a measure of the functional likelihood of crossover, a centimorgan (cM), is used to describe the observed recombination rate. Thus, if crossovers occur in 10% of meioses, the loci are said to be 10 cM apart. On average, 1 cM corresponds to approximately 1,000 kilobases of DNA. The degree of linkage of specific genes must be generated from clinical observations in numerous families.

For tests used in clinical practice, it is important to know the frequency of crossovers occurring between the disease gene and the marker gene, because this is one factor that limits the accuracy of the test. If the disease gene and the marker gene are 2 cM apart, it is important for the patient to know that the accuracy will be less than 98%. The use of flanking markers, i.e., markers on both sides of the gene, if available, can help circumvent the problem of undetected

crossovers. Although known genes sometimes are used for markers, more commonly DNA segments of unknown function are used for markers. These "anonymous" DNA segments, like genes themselves, can be highly variable in their nucleotide sequence. These normal variations are located extensively throughout the genome and can be recognized by one of many different kinds of bacterial enzymes that cut DNA at specified sites. DNA polymorphisms located within the gene of interest are less likely to show recombination with the mutation site than those located adjacent to the gene (Fig. 10-8).

- The accuracy of linkage-based diagnosis is variable from one disease to another, depending on how tightly the disease gene and marker DNA are linked.

The size of the DNA fragments generated by these cutting enzymes varies among individuals because of normal variations in our DNA sequences. These different-sized fragments are referred to as restriction fragment length polymorphisms. These can be separated by size by electrophoresis on a gel. Once separated by size, the DNA fragments can be transferred to a nylon membrane as part of the procedure known as Southern blot analysis.

Southern Blot Procedure

After a patient's DNA has been extracted from peripheral blood lymphocytes, subjected to enzyme cutting, and electrophoresed to separate different sizes of DNA fragments, a radioactive probe for the disease gene or for the marker DNA segments is applied and hybridizes to the complementary DNA sequences of interest. The fragments then can be visualized on x-ray film. An example of linkage analysis by Southern blotting in a family with DMD is shown in Figure 10-9.

In addition to linkage analysis, Southern blotting can be used in some cases for direct detection of deletion or duplication types of mutations, or for single-base mutations if the enzyme restriction site is directly altered by the mutation. An example of direct detection of a deletion in a patient with DMD is shown in Figure 10-10.

Fig. 10-8. Bacterial restriction enzyme *HAE* III. There are hundreds of types of bacterial enzymes that recognize and cleave specific DNA sequences. Appropriate enzyme that provides most information for DNA markers near disease gene of interest will be selected by the laboratory performing the test. Resulting fragments of differing sizes in different persons are restriction fragment-length polymorphisms.

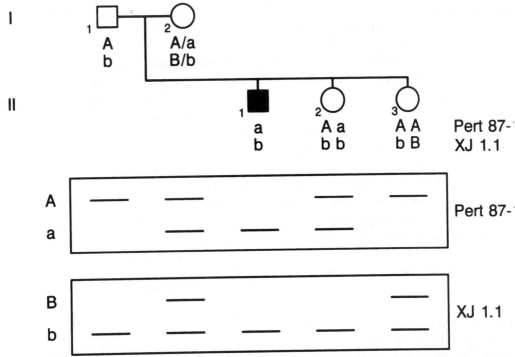

Fig. 10-9. Representation of a family segregating for Duchenne muscular dystrophy and data for two probes that detect restriction fragment-length polymorphism, Pert 87-1 and XJ 1.1. Bottom half of figure represents Southern blot analysis of these two probes with arbitrary designation of alleles A/a for Pert 87-1 and B/b for XJ 1.1. Square, normal male; circle, female; shaded symbol, affected individual. Sister II.3 of affected male II.1 inherited Ab haplotype from her father and AB haplotype from her mother. Because her brother has ab haplotype, it can be predicted that she is not a carrier and her fetus is not at increased risk. Although sister II.2 did inherit the ab haplotype, it cannot be determined with certainty that she is a carrier because it is not known whether the mutation arose in brother or whether mother is a carrier. Sister II.2 could elect prenatal diagnosis, with the realization that males who inherit the ab haplotype might be affected or unaffected, whereas those who inherit the Ab haplotype would most likely be unaffected.

Fig. 10-10. Mother (I.1) of this patient (II.1) with sporadic Duchenne muscular dystrophy wanted to know whether she was a carrier or whether a new mutation had occurred in her son, because of her concern for the risk for future children. Southern blot analysis detected a deletion in her son (II.1) (lane 2 as compared to control in lane 1). By densitometry, the mother seemed to have less than the expected amount of DNA (not shown) corresponding to her son's deletion. Thus, she was diagnosed as being a carrier for the dystrophy and can be offered specific prenatal diagnosis. If no deletion had been detectable (by various methods), then her carrier status could not have been determined.

Polymerase Chain Reaction

Another method of DNA diagnosis that has had great impact on clinical practice is the polymerase chain reaction (PCR). The PCR involves replication of a specific, relatively small segment of DNA in an exponential fashion, so that up to a billion copies are produced. One uses known DNA sequences from within the area of interest, and these known DNA sequences allow creation of synthetic oligonucleotides that serve as primers to hybridize with the patient's DNA sequence to initiate the amplification process (Fig. 10-11).

The multiple copies of the DNA segment that are produced by the PCR then can be identified by various techniques, including direct visualization after gel electrophoresis. This allows detection of mutations in the patient's DNA. For example, the PCR can be used for detection of mutations in specific regions of the dystrophin gene for the diagnosis of DMD and other diseases.

Diseases Amenable to DNA Diagnosis

The number of diseases diagnosable by DNA analysis is increasing as additional disease genes are localized or identified and cloned. Humans are believed to have approximately 100,000 genes; currently, approximately 2,000 genes have been mapped. Some diseases for which DNA diagnosis is available are listed in Tables 10-5 through 10-7, but these lists will change rapidly and are not meant to be all-inclusive.

Furthermore, when diagnosis is based on linkage, some families may not have the necessary number of family members available to allow for informative DNA analysis.

Table 10-5.--Some Autosomal Dominant Diseases Diagnosable by DNA Analysis

Amyloidosis, some forms
Familial adenomatous polyposis coli
Familial hypercholesterolemia (low-density lipoprotein receptor defects)
Huntington disease
Marfan syndrome
Multiple endocrine neoplasia, types I, II, and IIb
Myotonic dystrophy
Neurofibromatosis, types 1 and 2
Osteogenesis imperfecta, some forms
Polycystic kidney disease
Spinocerebellar ataxia, type I
Retinoblastoma
Von Hippel-Lindau disease
Von Willebrand disease

Other families may have a sufficient number of family members who are willing to participate but the DNA markers in common usage to study their specific gene defect may not be informative in a particular family. An example of this problem is shown in Figure 10-12.

Thus, the physician who encounters a clinical situation for the first time which may be amenable to DNA-based diagnosis should discuss the testing procedure and its limitations with the laboratory personnel or a geneticist familiar with the details

Fig. 10-11. PCR is used to make multiple copies of short segment of DNA of interest. DNA from patient is denatured to single-stranded DNA in the presence of oligonucleotide primers. DNA sequences of these primers are made to specification to anneal with DNA sequences on both sides of DNA segment of interest. DNA between these primers is then synthesized, and entire process can be repeated automatically.

Table 10-6.--Some Autosomal Recessive Diseases Diagnosable
by DNA Analysis

α_1-Antitrypsin deficiency
Congenital adrenal hyperplasia (21-hydroxylase deficiency)
Cystic fibrosis
Gaucher disease
Hemochromatosis
Phenylketonuria
Sickle-cell disease
Spinal muscular atrophy, infantile form
Tay-Sachs disease
α- and β-Thalassemia

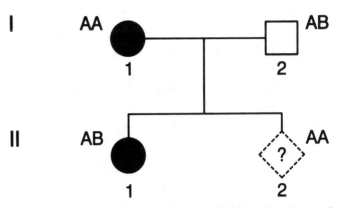

Fig. 10-12. Mother (I.1) and first child (II.1) are affected by autosomal dominant disease. Marker alleles linked to this disease are shown next to each person's symbol. Because mother's genotype is AA, it cannot be determined whether the fetus inherited the chromosome with the A marker and the disease gene or the other A marker without the disease gene. This family is said to be noninformative.

Table 10-7.--Some X-Linked Diseases Diagnosable by DNA
Analysis

Alport syndrome (X-linked form)
Duchenne and Becker muscular dystrophies
Fragile X-linked mental retardation
Hemophilia A and B
Kennedy spinobulbar atrophy
Lesch-Nyhan syndrome
Ornithine transcarbamoylase deficiency
Wiskott-Aldrich syndrome
X-linked ichthyosis
X-linked lymphoproliferative disease

of the specific disease testing before a detailed discussion of the prenatal diagnosis with the patient. Ideally, these discussions should take place before a woman becomes pregnant. For example, if a woman provides a family history of a brother with DMD and she is deciding whether to have a child, it would be prudent to confirm the diagnosis and get a detailed family history to determine whether prenatal diagnosis seems feasible rather than simply stating that prenatal diagnosis is possible. This woman would be in a difficult situation if she became pregnant while assuming that prenatal diagnosis was possible only to find out later that prenatal diagnosis was not possible because her brother was a sporadic case or is deceased and she has no detectable deletion. Parenthetically, deletions can be much more difficult to detect in a woman heterozygous for an X-linked disease than in a hemizygous affected male.

● DNA-based diagnoses cannot be used for all families, even when DNA tests for a specific disease are available.

An example of an X-linked disease has been used throughout this discussion, but the same general principles apply to autosomal dominant and recessive diseases. Prenatal diagnoses of cystic fibrosis, sickle-cell disease, and the thalassemias are particularly important because of their high frequency. Virtually all cases of sickle-cell disease and most cases of thalassemia can be diagnosed by direct DNA analysis with the PCR without the need for linkage analysis. Direct DNA analysis with the PCR of the phenylalanine 508 mutation, which accounts for approximately 70% of cystic fibrosis mutations, is possible; however, the remaining 30% of mutations are so diverse that more extensive gene testing or linkage analysis is necessary.

Occasionally, linkage analysis can be applied even if the affected family member is deceased or represents a sporadic case. If multiple alleles are analyzed that flank the site of the gene defect, it may be possible to deduce the marker genotype of the deceased person by studying other family members.

Another potential pitfall in prenatal diagnosis by DNA analysis is genetic heterogeneity. For example, most patients with autosomal dominant polycystic kidney disease have a gene defect linked to markers on chromosome 19. However, up to 10% of families have a phenotypically similar disease due to a different, nonallelic genetic mutation that does not show linkage to these markers. Thus, in the minority of families linkage cannot be performed for presymptomatic or prenatal diagnosis; if the family is not recognized to be one of the "unlinked" families, an erroneous diagnosis may be made. There are numerous other examples of this type of genetic heterogeneity, including retinitis pigmentosa, spinocerebellar ataxias, and Charcot-Marie-Tooth disease.

It is anticipated that the rapid advances made in molecular genetics in the past several years will accelerate as the genetic bases of additional diseases are identified and newer techniques for molecular diagnosis become available.

● Genetic heterogeneity can confound DNA linkage studies.

GLOSSARY

Autosome: Chromosome other than sex chromosome.

Chromosome: Long strands of double-stranded DNA that encode genes and that are associated with a protein framework. Normal human has 46 chromosomes per cell.

Deletion: Structural abnormality in which part of a chromosome is missing.

Duplication: Structural abnormality in which an extra copy of part of a chromosome is present.

Gene: A portion of DNA molecule that codes for a specific RNA or protein product.

Hemizygote: A person who has a gene form on one chromosome but no homologous chromosome with a corresponding gene site. The term usually refers to males because they have only one X chromosome.

Heterozygote: A person who has different gene forms at a given site on two homologous chromosomes.

Homozygote: A person who has the same gene forms at a given site on two homologous chromosomes.

Inversion: Structural abnormality characterized by reversal of a segment within the chromosome.

Karyotype: The chromosome complement of an individual person.

Linkage (genetic linkage): Physical proximity of two gene loci on the same chromosome such that segregation is nonrandom.

Phenotype: The observable biochemical or physical characteristics of an individual as determined by genetic material and environment.

Proband: The index patient.

Recurrence: Occurrence of another case of a specific condition in the same family.

Translocation: Structural abnormality characterized by transfer of a piece of one chromosome to another chromosome.

QUESTIONS

Multiple Choice (choose the one best answer)
1. Patients with fragile X-linked mental retardation
   a. Are always male
   b. Are always female
   c. May be male or female
   d. Have a 46,XX genotype with male phenotype
   e. Have a 46,XY genotype with female phenotype

2. Familial hypertrophic cardiomyopathy
   a. Is always due to myosin gene mutations
   b. Is due to myosin gene mutations in approximately 50% of cases
   c. Is always due to hypertrophin gene mutation
   d. Is due to hypertrophin gene mutations in approximately 50% of cases
   e. Has no known gene defect associations

3. Neurofibromatosis type 1 is characterized by variable combinations of
   a. Cerebellar hemangioblastomas and renal cysts
   b. Subependymal tubers and renal angiomyolipomas
   c. Café-au-lait macules and bilateral acoustic neuromas
   d. Café-au-lait macules and cataracts
   e. Café-au-lait macules and iris Lisch nodules

4. Osteogenesis imperfecta type I
   a. Usually is associated with mild-to-moderate disease and a variable number of fractures
   b. Is lethal in the newborn period
   c. Is a genetic lethal (i.e., is lethal before reproductive age)
   d. Is autosomal recessive
   e. Is often associated with aortic aneurysm and rupture

5. Genetic hemochromatosis is
   a. A benign genetic trait

b. More common in persons of Mediterranean ancestry
c. Autosomal dominant
d. Amenable to presymptomatic diagnosis
e. Characterized by renal cysts

6. Gaucher disease type 1
   a. Should be treated with splenectomy as soon as diagnosed.
   b. Often presents with mild splenomegaly and thrombocytopenia
   c. Occurs only in adults
   d. Is autosomal dominant
   e. Has no ethnic predisposition

7. Becker muscular dystrophy
   a. Is lethal in early childhood
   b. Is due to an unknown X-linked gene defect
   c. Is due to dystrophin gene defects
   d. Is characterized only by skeletal muscle involvement
   e. Cannot be diagnosed by DNA analysis

True/False (indicate whether each answer is true or false)
8. Mitochondrial mutations
   a. Can cause Leber's optic atrophy
   b. Can cause cardiomyopathy
   c. Can cause muscle weakness
   d. Can cause lactic acidosis
   e. Can cause retinal pigment degeneration
   f. Can cause ophthalmoplegia

9. For genetic diseases in which the causative gene has been identified
   a. DNA diagnosis is always possible
   b. DNA diagnosis is always possible if affected family members are available
   c. DNA analysis is a powerful diagnostic tool that can be used to simultaneously screen a person for most genetic diseases
   d. DNA-based linkage analysis can be used for diagnosis of sporadic genetic disease
   e. DNA-based linkage analysis can be used for diagnosis of some genetic diseases when affected family members are available
   f. DNA direct mutation analysis can be used for diagnosis of some genetic disorders regardless of whether family members are available

10. Down syndrome
   a. Is due to trisomy 21 in most cases
   b. Is usually familial
   c. Is the most common autosomal aneuploidy syndrome
   d. Is associated with Alzheimer's disease at a relatively early age
   e. Is potentially heritable when the karyotype is 46,XX,t(14;21)
   f. Is associated with an increased risk for thyroid disease

ANSWERS

1. Answer c.
Although X-linked, some carrier women with the fragile X mutation are mentally retarded. The standard karyotype reveals the appropriate 46,XX or 46,XY chromosomes as appropriate for sex.

2. Answer b.
Hypertrophic cardiomyopathy is due to myosin gene mutations in approximately 50% of cases. Currently, there is not a gene called hypertrophin. There are at least two other mutations that can cause hypertrophic cardiomyopathy, tropomyosin and troponin T.

3. Answer e.
Cerebellar hemangioblastomas and renal cysts are characteristic of von Hippel-Lindau disease. Subependymal tubers and renal angiomyolipomas are characteristics of tuberous sclerosis. Café-au-lait macules and bilateral acoustic neuromas are characteristic of neurofibromatosis type 2. Café-au-lait macules and cataracts are also characteristic of neurofibromatosis type 2.

4. Answer a.
Osteogenesis imperfecta type I is a mild-to-moderate disease. The lethal form is referred to as type II. It is inherited as an autosomal dominant disease. Although there may be mild aortic dilatation, aneurysm and rupture would be very rare.

5. Answer d.

Genetic hemochromatosis can result in cardiomyopathy, diabetes mellitus, and hepatic cirrhosis. It may be more common in persons of Western European ancestry, and it is an autosomal recessive disorder. It is not characterized by renal cysts. It is important to rememer that presymptomatic diagnosis and treatment to alleviate iron overload may prevent complications of the disease.

6. Answer b.

Gaucher disease type 1 should not be treated with splenectomy because there is evidence that splenectomy may worsen the bone disease. It may present with mild splenomegaly and thrombocytopenia, or the splenomegaly may be severe. The presentation can be in childhood or adulthood. It is an autosomal recessive disorder and has an ethnic predisposition in Ashkenazi Jews. It is amenable to treatment by intravenous enzyme replacement.

7. Answer c.

Becker muscular dystrophy is usually compatible with survival to adulthood and is due to the X-linked dystrophin gene defect. Although predominant symptoms generally relate to the skeletal muscle, there may be significant cardiomyopathy, and occasionally this is the presenting sign of the illness. It often can be diagnosed by DNA analysis.

8. a, true; b, true; c, true; d, true; e, true; f, true.

Mitochondrial mutations can result in all of the listed complications. Mitochondrial mutations result in extremely variable disease that is not always predictable by the exact mutation and may be related to other nuclear or mitochondrial mutations and to whether the mutation is homoplasmic or heteroplasmic.

9. a, false; b, false; c, false; d, false; e, true; f, true.

When a gene defect has been identified to cause a specific disease, this does not necessarily mean that DNA diagnosis is possible. This may result from the fact that the gene is very large; mutations may be spread throughout the gene and may not be readily detectable. For example, in neurofibromatosis, only about 15% of patients have mutations that are detectable with current techniques. DNA diagnosis is not always possible even if affected family members are available; it also requires either direct mutation analysis or appropriate markers that can be used for linkage. It is not a general screening tool that can be used to screen persons for multiple different genetic diseases; rather, one must target the specific genetic disease(s) of interest for testing.

10. a, true; b, false; c, true; d, true; e, true; f, true.

Down syndrome is usually due to trisomy 21 and this is generally sporadic. It is the most common autosomal aneuploidy syndrome, and Alzheimer's disease may develop in early adulthood in up to 30%-40% of patients. Heritable forms may be due to chromosome rearrangements that can be present in the carrier parent in a balanced state. Persons with Down syndrome have an increased risk for hypothyroidism.

CHAPTER 11
GERIATRICS

Darryl S. Chutka, M.D.

DEMOGRAPHICS

The age at which a person becomes elderly is not fixed. People age at different rates and at times, and the chronologic age does not match the physiologic age. The process of aging begins when one is born, and from that time on, a combination of changes takes place--both anatomically and physiologically--that results in the changes of aging. In addition to these changes, various disease states occur and result in further changes in the person. Most organs have the reserve capability to handle the changes due to normal aging and to many disease states.

The demographics of aging suggest that with time those older than 65 years will represent a larger proportion of our population. Currently, the elderly (>65 yr) represent about 12% of the U.S. population. If current trends continue, this number is expected to double during the next 40 years. Based on current projections, the most rapid increase in the elderly population is expected between the years 2010 and 2030, the years that those born between 1945 and 1965 ("baby boomers") reach age 65. The "old-old" population, those over age 85, is growing faster than other segments of the population. The significance of this relates to the greater likelihood of health problems for this segment of the population and the greater expense generated for the care of the old-old.

- The elderly (>65 years) represent about 12% of the U.S. population.
- The population of those older than 85 is growing faster than other segments of the population.

Two important terms to understand are "life expectancy" and "life span." Life expectancy has increased as our culture has progressed through time. Currently, life expectancy is about 84 years for women and 80 years for men. Primarily, this increase is due to improved nutrition, sanitation, and immunization. Much of the increase in life expectancy is due to the decrease in premature mortality in children and young adults

and not to a decrease in the mortality of the elderly. Although life expectancy has shown an increase with time, life span has remained fixed at approximately 100-110 years. More people are living closer to the end of their life span and fewer are dying prematurely. This is known as the "rectangularization of the survival curve." The elderly can be divided into three groups: the "young-old" (65-75 years), "middle-old" (75-85 years), and "old-old" (>85 years). The poorest segments of the population include the old-old, elderly widows, and the elderly with little formal education. Social security is the primary source of income for approximately one third of the elderly in the U.S.

The sex ratio (M:F) decreases with advancing age. Of the group of persons >65 years, there are about 75 men for every 100 women. Among those >85 years, there are only 50 men for every 100 women. Only 5% of those >65 years reside in a nursing home, although with advancing age, this percentage increases (20% of those >85 years). More than two thirds of the elderly live in a family setting with their spouse or children. It is more common for women (40%) than for men (16%) to live alone in the community.

- Life expectancy has increased primarily because of improved nutrition, sanitation, and immunizations.
- Life expectancy has increased with time; life span has not.
- Only 5% of those >65 years live in a nursing home.

HEALTH CARE FINANCING

The cost of health care for the elderly is substantial. It is estimated that the elderly account for 36% of U.S. health care costs. Those >65 years have four times the number of physician visits and four to five times the length of hospital stays as those <65 years. Most of the health care cost for the elderly is for hospital care (40%). The costs for physician visits (20%) and long-term care (20%) are also significant. Financing long-term care can be particularly difficult for the elderly. Many assume Medicare will provide coverage, but in fact it covers little (2%). Half of all long-term care financing is provided by individual patients or their families and 40% is provided by Medicaid, medical assistance for those demonstrating financial need. Long-term care insurance provides only 5% of the cost.

- The elderly account for 36% of U.S. health care costs.
- The elderly have 4x the number of physician visits and 4x-5x the length of hospital stays.
- Most of the financing for long-term care is by private pay. Medicare provides coverage for only 2%.

REHABILITATION/ASSISTIVE DEVICES

Rehabilitation is important to many elderly and may be either restorative (to improve a loss in function) or maintenance (to prevent loss of function currently present). The importance of improving or maintaining one's functional status cannot be overstated, because functional status often determines whether a person can safely live independently in the community or requires nursing home placement. A significant number of nursing home admissions are for rehabilitation, with the expectation the person will eventually leave the facility and return home after some recently lost function is regained. The need for rehabilitative services can be determined by reviewing one's ability to perform activities of daily living, such as dressing, eating, bathing, toileting, transferring, and ambulation.

- Rehabilitation is important to many of the elderly.
- A significant number of nursing home admissions are for rehabilitation.

Often, assistive devices are prescribed to assist a person in gaining functional status in one or more activities of daily living. Assistive devices are important for many of the elderly, allowing them to maintain their mobility. These devices often allow many to live independently and to delay or prevent institutionalization. Before recommending an assistive device, several factors need to be taken into account. Patients must accept the fact that they have an impairment and that the assistive device will help. Also, the device must be affordable, properly fitted, and easy to use.

- Assistive devices are important for many of the elderly.

Walkers and canes are useful for elderly patients with sensory impairments, problems maintaining balance, or weakness/pain of the lower extremities. Canes can support up to 25% of the body weight and are most useful for those with difficulties with balance or unilateral leg weakness or pain.

The cane should be fitted to the proper length so that the elbow is flexed at a 20°-30° angle. Walkers are useful for persons who have a more significant balance problem or greater weakness than can be managed effectively with a cane. Walkers are useful for persons with bilateral lower extremity weakness and can support up to 50% of the body weight, depending on the type of device used. Parkinsonian patients often have a tendency to fall backward and usually do best with walkers that have wheels on the front. Persons with significant upper extremity weakness often do best with four-wheeled walkers, because they may be unable to lift the walker as they ambulate. Wheelchairs are commonly prescribed for the elderly, both for short-term and long-term use. It is extremely important for the wheelchair to be properly fitted to the individual patient by a trained therapist. Both the height and width of the chair need to be assessed carefully. An improperly sized wheelchair can contribute to pressure sores, deep venous thrombosis, falls, and serious injury.

- Canes benefit persons with unilateral disabilities of the lower extremities or sensory impairments and can support up to 25% of the body weight.
- Walkers benefit those with bilateral lower extremity weakness or pain and can support up to 50% of the body weight.

VISION CHANGES

A combination of anatomical and physiologic changes related to aging and various disease states that are common in the elderly frequently cause decreased vision. Vision loss increases with advancing age, and more than one quarter of those >85 years report significant visual impairment. Over 90% of the elderly wear glasses. It is estimated that at least 25% of nursing home residents are legally blind. The most common eye problem in the elderly population is presbyopia, causing difficulty with close focus. It is a result of decreased lens flexibility from continued addition of cells to the lens throughout life. Cataracts also become more common with advancing age; in fact, they begin forming fairly early in life, but the progression varies from person to person. There is evidence of a relationship between exposure to ultraviolet light throughout one's lifetime and the development of cortical cataracts. Cataract operation with intraocular lens implantation is effective in restoring visual acuity; however, it is less effective in those of advanced age or who have other preexisting eye disease.

- One quarter of those >85 years report significant visual impairment.
- At least 25% of nursing home residents are legally blind.
- There is a relationship between exposure to ultraviolet light and development of cortical cataracts.

Chronic open-angle glaucoma produces a slow progressive loss of peripheral vision that often is not noticed by the person until a significant amount of vision is lost. Vision loss occurs as a result of increased intraocular pressure damaging the optic nerve. In addition to visual field defects, examination reveals atrophy and cupping of the optic disc. Open-angle glaucoma rarely produces symptoms until peripheral vision is lost. If this disease is watched for, it can be diagnosed and effectively treated before significant vision loss occurs. The decision to treat glaucoma is not based solely on the degree of ocular tension. Treatment is started when there is evidence of vision loss or physical evidence of ocular damage, such as cupping of the optic disks. The options for the treatment of glaucoma are several. Pilocarpine causes pupillary constriction and opens the trabecular meshwork, increasing the flow of aqueous humor. β-Blockers such as timolol decrease the production of aqueous humor. Epinephrine decreases the production of aqueous humor and increases its flow. Carbonic anhydrase inhibitors act by decreasing the production of aqueous humor. Trabeculoplasty by laser is often performed when glaucoma cannot be adequately controlled medically. It results in the increased outflow of aqueous humor. Acute angle-closure glaucoma is much less common than chronic open-angle glaucoma and accounts for about only 5% of glaucoma cases. Patients present to physicians much sooner with acute angle-closure glaucoma because of the associated symptoms. Obstruction to aqueous humor outflow results in a rapid increase in intraocular pressure, producing symptoms of eye pain, blurred vision with halos around lights, headache, and nausea. The pupil dilates and is unresponsive to light. Urgent treatment is needed to prevent vision loss.

- Open-angle glaucoma rarely produces symptoms until peripheral vision is lost.
- Treatment is started when there is evidence of vision loss or physical evidence of ocular damage, such as cupping of the optic disks.

Macular degeneration is associated with the gradual and progressive loss of central vision but the sparing of peripheral vision. It is associated with aging, tobacco use, and, possibly, hypertension. A relationship with chronic exposure to sunlight has not been proven. More often, the disease is unilateral in younger persons and bilateral in older ones. Laser treatment in some types of macular degeneration is somewhat beneficial; however, most cases are managed with devices used to assist vision, such as increased lighting and magnifying lenses.

- Macular degeneration: gradual, progressive loss of central vision and sparing of peripheral vision.
- Macular degeneration: associated with aging, tobacco use, and possibly hypertension.

HEARING CHANGES

Hearing loss in the elderly is commonly caused by a central auditory processing disorder, a problem resulting in difficulty with speech perception due to a disorder in the central nervous system. The ability to discriminate speech is worse than predicted for the amount of pure tone lost. The prevalence of hearing loss, especially of high frequencies (presbycusis), increases significantly among persons >65 years, approaching 50% of those >80 years. Noise-induced hearing loss produces a similar high-frequency hearing loss. Elderly patients with a high-frequency hearing loss usually have the most difficulty in appreciating consonant sounds. Causes of conductive hearing loss include cerumen impaction, perforation of the tympanic membrane, cholesteatoma, Paget's disease, and otosclerosis. Hearing aids may benefit many elderly with hearing loss, and many improvements have been made in those devices. The goal of hearing amplification is to provide a high signal-to-noise ratio. Some models are able to select the range of frequency amplification to the specific environment, others can be programmed to amplify the specific frequencies for which the patient has the greatest hearing loss. A less expensive version amplifies the higher frequencies, the frequencies most commonly lost with aging. Hearing aids are most beneficial when used in an environment with minimal background noise, such as a one-on-one conversation. They will be least helpful when used in crowded rooms, with many others speaking.

- Hearing loss secondary to a central auditory processing disorder results in difficulty with speech perception worse than predicted for the amount of pure tone lost.
- Chronic exposure to loud noise can result in a high-frequency hearing loss.
- The prevalence of hearing loss increases significantly among persons >65 years, approaching 50% of those >80 years.
- Causes of conductive hearing loss: cholesteatoma, Paget's disease, and otosclerosis.

RHEUMATOLOGIC PROBLEMS

Rheumatologic problems are among the commonest complaints of the elderly. These diseases tend to be chronic, and they often accumulate with time. Although most of these diseases are not life-threatening, they commonly cause an alteration in lifestyle and lead to significant disability. Osteoarthritis is extremely common among the elderly and is present in >80%. It produces joint symptoms that vary with time and degree of activity. Osteoarthritis usually can be differentiated from rheumatoid arthritis by the medical history and findings on physical examination. Osteoarthritis does not tend to produce systemic symptoms, which are common in rheumatoid arthritis. Joint inflammation, although seen in osteoarthritis, is much more pronounced in rheumatoid arthritis. Osteoarthritis and rheumatoid arthritis both are chronic diseases. Although patients have variability in their disease activity, acute worsening of a specific joint should make a physician suspicious of a superimposed crystalline arthritis (gout or pseudogout) or septic arthritis, which are seen occasionally in those with underlying chronic joint disease.

- Osteoarthritis is extremely common among the elderly and is present in >80%.
- Acute joint symptoms in patients with osteoarthritis or rheumatoid arthritis may represent crystalline or septic arthritis.

Osteoarthritis

Osteoarthritis results in asymmetrical loss of articular cartilage, causing asymmetrical narrowing of the joint space. It has a predilection for the hands (distal and proximal interphalangeal joints, first carpometacarpal joint of the thumb), hips, knees, and feet (first tarsometatarsal joint), with relative sparing of the elbow, wrist, metacarpophalangeal joints of the hand, and ankle. Osteoarthritis has a typical radiographic appearance that includes asymmetrical narrowing of the joint space, presence of osteophytes, subchondral sclerosis, and cystic changes in the bone. Systemic symptoms do not occur. Joint pain is common with joint use and weight-bearing activity. Rest usually provides relief from this pain. The treatment of osteoarthritis includes adequate rest, local heat, and exercise to strengthen periarticular muscles, occasionally injections of steroids into inflamed joints, and analgesics. Because significant joint inflammation is rare in osteoarthritis, an analgesic such as acetaminophen should be tried initially for pain relief. Nonsteroidal anti-inflammatory drugs (NSAIDs) can be used quite effectively; however, they carry a risk of more significant adverse effects, especially when used chronically.

- Osteoarthritis produces asymmetrical narrowing of the joint space.
- Osteoarthritis has a predilection for the hands, hips, knees, and feet.

Rheumatoid Arthritis

Rheumatoid arthritis is often found in elderly patients, most commonly as a chronic disease that was acquired earlier in life. It can also develop later in life and falls into one of two groups. As in younger individuals, it may present with symmetrical inflammation of distal joints, positive rheumatoid factor, and a propensity to progress with time. Another presentation is rather common in the elderly, acute onset of proximal joint pain and stiffness, very similar to polymyalgia rheumatica. Rheumatoid factor is often negative, and rheumatoid nodules are often absent. In contrast to osteoarthritis,

patients with rheumatoid arthritis have systemic symptoms. Extra-articular manifestations are occasionally present in rheumatoid arthritis and may include the skin (rheumatoid nodules), lung (fibrosis, rheumatoid nodules, pleural effusions), blood vessels (vasculitis), nervous system (mononeuritis multiplex), and hematologic system (Felty's syndrome). Sjögren's syndrome (splenomegaly, leukopenia) also occasionally accompanies rheumatoid arthritis. Radiographs of joints involved with rheumatoid arthritis characteristically show symmetrical narrowing of the joint space. Diagnosis is usually made by physical examination revealing an inflammatory, symmetrical arthritis. Laboratory test results can often be misleading. The rheumatoid factor is often negative in many elderly patients with rheumatoid arthritis. False-positive results for rheumatoid factor can also be found in many elderly who do not have the disease, although usually in a low titer. Elderly patients with rheumatoid arthritis receive the same therapeutic agents as younger patients: NSAIDs, chloroquine, methotrexate, gold, and low doses (5 to 7.5 mg/day) of steroids.

- About 10% of cases of rheumatoid arthritis develop in persons >65 years.
- Radiographs of rheumatoid arthritis show symmetrical narrowing of the joint space.
- Elderly persons with rheumatoid arthritis often are negative for rheumatoid factor, whereas other elderly persons without rheumatoid arthritis may have false-positive results for rheumatoid factor.

Crystalline Arthropathy

Crystalline arthropathy is common in the elderly population. Whereas gout tends to be more common in men and to involve more distal joints, especially the great toe, pseudogout is more common in women and tends to involve more proximal joints, especially the knee.

Gout is a monoarticular arthritis caused by intra-articular deposition of uric acid crystals. It is associated with the hyperuricemia produced by thiazide diuretics. Gouty attacks may be precipitated by stressful events such as a surgical procedure, severe illness, or trauma. Although the diagnosis of gout is usually made on the basis of the medical history and physical examination findings, it is confirmed by microscopic evaluation of the synovial fluid from an affected joint. Urate crystals have a long needle-like shape and are negatively birefringent with polarizing light. Treatment for an acute attack of gout is NSAIDs. Colchicine given orally or intravenously may be used in patients who should not receive NSAIDs. Long-term suppressive therapy usually is not initiated until after several acute episodes of gout have occurred. Suppressive therapy may include daily allopurinol, probenecid, or low doses of oral colchicine. Treatment of asymptomatic hyperuricemia is rarely necessary, although it is initiated in patients with uric acid renal stones or occasionally when starting chemotherapy for various hematologic malignancies.

- Gout: a monoarticular arthritis, more common in men.
- Gout: associated with the use of thiazides.
- Urate crystals are long and needle-like and negatively birefringent with polarizing light.
- Initial treatment of an acute attack of gout is with NSAIDs.

Pseudogout (calcium pyrophosphate deposition disease) is also a monoarticular arthritis; it most frequently involves the knee and wrist. As with gout, an acute attack can occur with a stressful event such as a surgical procedure, trauma, or illness. Radiographs of joints with pseudogout often show linear articular calcification, although about 25% of the elderly have articular calcification with no clinical evidence of the disease. The calcium pyrophosphate crystals are rectangular and exhibit positive birefringence with polarizing light. Treatment of an acute attack is with NSAIDs or steroids given intra-articularly in the affected joints. Daily therapy with low doses of colchicine may decrease the frequency of the attacks.

- Pseudogout is a monoarticular arthritis and commonly involves the knee.
- Calcium pyrophosphate crystals are rectangular and positively birefringent with polarizing light.
- Treatment of an acute attack of pseudogout is with NSAIDs or steroids injected intra-articularly.

Polymyalgia Rheumatica and Temporal Arteritis

Polymyalgia rheumatica and temporal arteritis occur more commonly in women than in men and are seen in persons >50 years. Patients with polymyalgia rheumatica describe stiffness, aching, and weakness of proximal muscles (shoulders, hips), especially in the morning. This is thought to be due to synovitis of the shoulder and hip joints. Patients may also complain of nonspecific malaise, fatigue, low-grade fever, and anorexia with weight loss. Although the patients commonly describe weakness, muscle strength is normal when tested. The diagnosis is usually suspected on the basis of the classic history obtained from the patient; no specific laboratory test is diagnostic for the disease. Patients usually have an increased erythrocyte sedimentation rate and, occasionally, mild anemia. The levels of muscle enzymes (creatinine kinase, aspartate aminotransferase) are not increased. The response to treatment is characteristic and often can be used to support the diagnosis. Treatment with low doses of steroids (prednisone, 15-20 mg/day) results in dramatic symptomatic improvement, often within 24 hours. After treatment has been initiated, the steroid dose can be tapered gradually, using the patient's clinical response and erythrocyte sedimentation rate as indicators of disease activity.

- Polymyalgia rheumatica is more common in women.
- Although patients complain of weakness, muscle strength is normal.
- Laboratory findings include an increased erythrocyte sedimentation rate and, occasionally, mild anemia.
- Patients respond dramatically to treatment with steroids.

Temporal arteritis develops in about 15% of the patients with polymyalgia rheumatica. Pathologically, there is inflammation of the medium-sized arteries that arise from the aortic arch. Systemic symptoms include low-grade fever and fatigue; anorexia with weight loss is also common. More than 50% of the patients have unilateral or bilateral headache. Many patients also have scalp and bitemporal tenderness and jaw claudication due to involvement of the facial artery. Vision loss, including unilateral or bilateral visual blurring, visual field loss, diplopia, and blindness due to ischemic optic neuritis, may occur and is the most worrisome symptom. As with polymyalgia rheumatica, temporal arteritis is usually suspected on the basis of the patient's description of the symptoms. Few findings are documented on physical examination. Some patients have tender, swollen, or pulseless temporal arteries. Rarely, bruits may be heard over medium-sized arteries involved with disease. Although no diagnostic laboratory test is specific for temporal arteritis, almost all patients have a significantly increased erythrocyte sedimentation rate, often >100 mm/hour. Mild anemia may also be present. After temporal arteritis is suspected, the diagnosis should be confirmed with temporal artery biopsy. A generous piece (4-5 cm) of the temporal artery should be obtained, initially on the side of the patient's symptoms. If the findings are negative, a similar biopsy should be performed on the contralateral side. The inflammatory changes in the artery may be spotty or confined to a small portion of the artery, occasionally causing difficulty in confirming the diagnosis pathologically. Treatment consists of high doses of steroids (prednisone, 60 mg/day), and it may be started before the biopsy sample is obtained, assuming it is to be done in the next 24-48 hours. Prednisone should be tapered by assessing the patient's clinical response to treatment and the erythrocyte sedimentation rate.

- Temporal arteritis develops in about 15% of patients with polymyalgia rheumatica.
- Temporal artery biopsy should not be performed in patients with polymyalgia rheumatica unless they have symptoms of temporal arteritis.
- Temporal arteritis commonly presents with a unilateral or bilateral headache.
- Vision loss is the most worrisome symptom.
- The erythrocyte sedimentation rate is usually increased.
- Treatment with high doses of steroids should be initiated when the disease is suspected and can be started before the temporal artery biopsy is performed.

THYROID DISEASE

Thyroid disease becomes more common with advancing age. Most elderly patients with hyperthyroidism present with the typical findings; however, a significant minority have somewhat atypical symptoms. Some of the elderly have anorexia with weight loss, altered stool frequency (either diarrhea or constipation), or cardiovascular abnormalities, including hypertension, increased angina, myocardial ischemia, congestive heart failure, and atrial fibrillation. Other symptoms that may develop include apathy, depression, tremor, and myopathy. Bone density loss is also accelerated with hyperthyroidism. Ophthalmopathy, lid lag, tachycardia, and increased perspiration are relatively uncommon in the elderly. The development of a goiter with hyperthyroidism is noted in only about 60% of the elderly. The commonest cause of hyperthyroidism in the elderly is Graves' disease. Radioiodine therapy is the safest and most economical treatment for hyperthyroidism in elderly patients.

- Hyperthyroidism associated with goiter is uncommon in the elderly.
- Graves' disease is the commonest form of hyperthyroidism in the elderly.
- Radioiodine therapy is the safest treatment for hyperthyroidism in the elderly.

The diagnosis of hypothyroidism in elderly patients is often made by finding low levels of total serum thyroxine (T_4) or an increased sTSH on laboratory testing of asymptomatic patients. The common symptoms of hypothyroidism are vague (constipation, cold intolerance, dry skin) and often attributed to the many "symptoms of aging." Almost all the patients have hypothyroidism due to primary thyroid failure rather than to pituitary or hypothalamic insufficiency. The commonest cause of hypothyroidism in the elderly is Hashimoto's thyroiditis. Treatment should begin with a low dose of thyroid supplement (25-50 µg/day), increasing the dose by 25 µg every 3-4 weeks. Patients with coronary artery disease should receive an even lower starting dose and more gradual dose increments. It takes approximately 6-8 weeks for a given dose of thyroid supplement to equilibrate. The sTSH should be checked after about 8 weeks to assess whether the supplement dose is correct. Thyroid hormone requirements decrease with advancing age, most elderly persons require 75-100 µg/day; however, some require as little as 50 µg/day. Subclinical hypothyroidism can be found in about 15% of the elderly. These patients are clinically euthyroid and have a low-normal total (serum) T_4 level and a slightly increased sTSH level. Whether to treat these patients is a matter of controversy. Most physicians do not treat unless symptoms of hypothyroidism develop or the sTSH level continues to increase.

- Hypothyroidism is often difficult to detect in the elderly.
- Most cases of hypothyroidism are due to primary thyroid failure rather than to pituitary or hypothalamic disease.
- Hashimoto's thyroiditis is the commonest cause of hypothyroidism in the elderly.
- Very low starting doses and very gradual dose increments should be prescribed in hypothyroid patients with coronary artery disease.

Euthyroid sick syndrome is common in elderly hospitalized patients. The patients are clinically euthyroid, but with low serum levels of T_3 and T_4 and a low-normal level of sTSH. Laboratory values tend to return to normal after the patient has recovered from the illness. The syndrome may be caused by a decreased amount of thyroid-binding protein and a substance that inhibits T_4 binding.

- Euthyroid sick syndrome is common in elderly hospitalized patients.

The prevalence of thyroid nodules increases with age. The best way to determine whether the nodule is malignant is to perform fine needle aspiration. Thyroid cancer in older patients carries a poorer prognosis than in younger ones.

DEMENTIA

Dementia represents an acquired cognitive impairment that affects all spheres of the intellect. It is a gradually progressive disorder and becomes more common with advancing age. About 10%-20% of the population >65 years have some degree of dementia. The number of dementia patients increases with time, and the percentage of the population with dementia has been reported to be as high as 50% in those >90 years. The commonest form of irreversible dementia is Alzheimer's disease (50%-70%), followed by multi-infarct dementia (15%-25%). Up to 30% of elderly patients referred for memory impairment have a treatable condition, most often depression (pseudodementia). Other potentially reversible dementias include drugs, toxic agents (heavy metals, alcohol, various solvents), hypothyroidism, vitamin B_{12} deficiency, normal-pressure hydrocephalus, subdural hematoma, and neurosyphilis. Dementia involves considerably more than loss of memory. Other cognitive functions that are affected include judgment, abstract thinking, attention, ability to learn new material, and, eventually, recognition and production of speech. Personality changes frequently accompany dementia, and patients may have paranoia and delusional thoughts and show agitation and aggressiveness.

- 10%-20% of persons >65 years have some form of dementia (50% of those >90 years).
- 30% of the elderly referred for memory impairment have a

treatable, potentially reversible condition, often depression.
- The commonest cause of irreversible dementia is Alzheimer's disease.

The diagnosis of Alzheimer's disease cannot be confirmed until postmortem examination; no laboratory test, including computed tomographic (CT) scan of the head, is specific for the disease. The diagnosis of Alzheimer's is made primarily by history, usually from family members, and a determination of the cognitive status of the patient. Physicians have been shown to have an accuracy of up to 95% in diagnosing Alzheimer's disease. Alzheimer's disease represents a gradually progressive cognitive impairment. Eventually, behavior problems are common, including the tendency to wander, develop paranoia, agitation, delusions, or hallucinations (or a combination). Typically patients with Alzheimer's disease have little insight into the disease process and are often brought to the physician by a family member. Pathologically, central nervous system findings in Alzheimer's disease include neuronal plaques, which represent extracellular deposits of protein containing amyloid, and neurofibrillary tangles, which are intracellular protein bound to microtubules. Neuronal plaques and neurofibrillary tangles are also found in nondemented persons but in much smaller numbers. The amount of acetylcholine, a neurotransmitter, is decreased, as is choline acetyltransferase activity.

- No laboratory test is specific for Alzheimer's disease.
- Alzheimer's disease: a gradually progressive cognitive impairment.

The evaluation of a demented patient involves establishing the existence and degree of cognitive impairment, ruling out reversible dementias, and performing baseline tests to follow future deterioration. This is accomplished by taking a medical history and performing a physical examination (including neurologic examination) and general laboratory tests. Accepted laboratory tests include complete blood cell count, electrolytes, liver function, serum level of creatinine, blood glucose, vitamin B_{12} level, thyroid function, syphilis serology, chest radiography, electrocardiography, and CT of the head. CT scanning of the head is done to rule out various types of central nervous system lesions, such as mass lesions, and not to check for cerebral atrophy. Psychometric evaluation is also useful, especially when following the progress of the patient. Electroencephalography (EEG), magnetic resonance imaging (MRI) of the head, and lumbar puncture are performed only in unusual circumstances and are rarely necessary.

- Evaluation of a demented person involves ruling out reversible dementias.

- CT scanning of the head is done to rule out various types of central nervous system lesions.
- EEG, MRI, and lumbar puncture are rarely necessary.

Up to the present time, the treatment of Alzheimer's disease has been limited to controlling the abnormal behavior of those with the disease. None of the neurotropic medications commonly used in the management of demented patients markedly improves cognitive function. Medications such as sedative-hypnotics or major tranquilizers frequently improve some of the abnormal behaviors (agitation, delusions, hallucinations, etc.), but they often worsen memory and orientation. Major tranquilizers may also cause movement disorders (tardive dyskinesia), thus contributing to falls. The recent availability of tacrine, a cholinesterase inhibitor, has given physicians their first true option for treatment. When tacrine is given in doses of 80-120 mg/day, cognitive improvement may occur in some patients. Patients often do not have significant improvement in their functional status; however, many do not receive or are unable to tolerate the doses of medication required. Tacrine commonly causes gastrointestinal disturbance and liver function test abnormalities.

- Evaluation is important for ruling out reversible dementias.
- Medications commonly used in the management of dementia (major tranquilizers, sedative/hypnotics) do not improve memory or orientation.
- Tacrine may produce cognitive improvement in some patients with Alzheimer's disease.

In addition to Alzheimer's disease, several other types of dementia exist. Multi-infarct dementia is common and, at times, can be difficult to differentiate from Alzheimer's disease. The patient usually demonstrates a stepwise progression consistent with the multiple ischemic infarcts, often with focal neurologic deficits also produced by the ischemic CNS events. Several types of vascular dementias are possible, including cortical multi-infarct, subcortical multi-infarct, and small-vessel ischemia with demyelination (Binswanger's disease). Dementia associated with Parkinson's disease is another type of dementia. Dementia develops in up to 40% of parkinsonian patients, many indistinguishable from patients with Alzheimer's disease. These patients have the features typical of Parkinson's disease: resting tremor, rigidity, and bradykinesia in addition to the intellectual impairments of the dementia. In some, the cognitive deficit is thought to be secondary to a deficiency of dopamine, and in these patients, effective treatment of Parkinson's disease can improve cognition. In others with a more severe dementia, treatment of the parkinsonian symptoms does not affect the cognitive status. Pick's disease is an uncommon cause of dementia, with an early age of onset, usually in the fifth or sixth decade. Pick's disease is characterized by prominent changes in personality and behavior, with less prominent disturbance of memory. Pathologically, the frontal and temporal lobes of the brain are involved. Swollen neurons called "balloon cells" and argentophilic inclusion bodies are seen microscopically. Creutzfeldt-Jakob disease is another uncommon cause of dementia which has an earlier onset than Alzheimer's disease, usually in the sixth decade. The patient's condition rapidly deteriorates, eventually to a vegetative state with myoclonic jerks and seizures. The cause is thought to be infectious and due to an unidentified slow virus. Huntington's disease is autosomal dominant and has early onset of symptoms (usually in the fourth or fifth decade). Choreiform movements eventually develop in these patients. AIDS dementia affects up to 50% of people with AIDS and is uncommon in the elderly.

- Multi-infarct dementia is characterized by a stepwise progression; several forms exist.
- Dementia associated with Parkinson's disease may improve with the treatment of Parkinson's disease.
- Pick's disease is associated with personality changes.
- Creutzfeldt-Jakob disease is associated with early onset of dementia, with rapid progression and development of myoclonic jerks.
- Dementia associated with AIDS is uncommon among the elderly.

Delirium is an acute confusional disorder that is frequently mistaken for dementia. It is associated with a decreased level of consciousness, hallucinations, and delusions. Its several causes include 1) many common medical illnesses (urinary tract infection, sepsis, pneumonia, etc.) in patients with limited organ reserve function or organ failure; 2) drugs, including sedative-hypnotics, anticholinergic agents, NSAIDs, β-blockers, and antipsychotic agents; 3) metabolic disturbances, such as hyper- or hypoglycemia and hypercalcemia; 4) hypoxia; and 5) hypotension. Patients with delirium frequently have a preexisting mild (often unrecognized) dementia.

- Delirium is frequently mistaken for dementia.

PULMONARY CHANGES

Pulmonary function declines with advancing age, likely because of a combination of the normal anatomical and physiologic changes of aging, injury from various environmental exposures (tobacco, air pollution), and disease states that affect the lung. Changes in the shape of the lungs contribute to the changes in pulmonary physiology. The apical-to-base length of the lungs decreases as the anterior-to-posterior length increases with age. The bronchioles and alveolar ducts increase in diameter, decreasing alveolar surface area. The aged lungs also have reduced compliance because of decreased lung elas-

ticity. These anatomical and physiologic changes result in a decrease in efficiency of air exchange, reduced air flow rates, and alterations in lung volumes. The changes that occur include decreases in mucociliary clearance, vital capacity, 1-second forced expiratory volume, maximal breathing capacity, and diffusing capacity. The lung residual volume and alveolar-arterial oxygen gradient increase with age. The total lung capacity remains unchanged.

Because of the potential for frequent adverse effects and toxicity from several of the drugs used in treating chronic obstructive pulmonary disease (COPD), the recommendations for treatment have gradually changed. Theophylline can produce cardiac arrhythmias, seizures, and gastrointestinal symptoms, and drug levels need to be measured periodically to minimize drug toxicity. Several commonly used medications (e.g., erythromycin) can cause altered theophylline metabolism, potentially leading to adverse effects from drug toxicity. For these reasons, the use of theophylline in patients with COPD has decreased. Also, β-agonist inhalers can have systemic effects, and they do not alter the course of bronchial reactivity or decrease bronchial inflammation. The recent trend for treatment of COPD has been toward the chronic use of inhaled corticosteroids, with supplemental use of β-agonist inhalers as needed. Recent evidence shows that inhaled corticosteroids produce some systemic steroid effects on bone density.

- Pulmonary function declines with age because of a combination of changes due to aging, environmental exposure, and disease.
- Changes in lung shape contribute to changes in pulmonary physiology.
- Changes in pulmonary physiology include a reduction in VC, FEV_1, MVV, and DLCO, and an increase in RV and $(A-a)O_2$ gradient.

RESPIRATORY DISEASE

Pneumonia is one of the top 10 causes of death among the elderly and is the cause of death in 15% of nursing home residents. The bacterial organisms that cause pneumonia change with advancing age. Elderly patients have increased numbers of gram-negative bacteria as part of their normal oral flora. They also have an increased likelihood of aspirating their oral secretions, which probably contribute to the increased incidence of pneumonia caused by gram-negative and anaerobic bacteria. The likely cause of pneumonia depends on the setting in which the patient acquired the infection. Overall, *Streptococcus pneumoniae* is the commonest etiologic organism, but *Haemophilus influenzae*, other gram-negative bacteria, and anaerobes are more common among those in nursing homes and hospitals. Organisms such as *Legionella*, *Chlamydia*, and *Moraxella catarrhalis* are also seen in the elderly. Treatment must reflect the most likely etiologic agent.

In recent times, a significant percentage of *S. pneumoniae* organisms have become penicillin-resistant. Appropriate treatment for pneumonia acquired in an outpatient setting or nursing home is a second-generation cephalosporin. For pneumonia acquired in a hospital, additional coverage is needed for gram-negative and atypical bacteria. Acceptable treatment includes a third-generation cephalosporin, with erythromycin given intravenously. Because of the high mortality of pneumonia, many believe that elderly nursing home patients should be hospitalized to initiate treatment. If the patient's condition is not toxic and appears stable, pneumonia can be treated in the nursing home (providing that the patient is observed closely).

- Pneumonia is among the top 10 causes of death among the elderly.
- Elderly patients have a greater number of gram-negative bacteria as part of their normal oral flora.
- *Streptococcus pneumoniae* is the commonest etiologic organism.
- Aspiration is more likely to occur in elderly persons.
- Treatment must reflect the likely causal organisms.

Tuberculosis, after declining in frequency for many years, is increasing in frequency. The number of reported cases has increased 20% in the last 10 years. Tuberculosis is more common with advancing age, with the elderly having two to four times the case rate of those <65 years. Those residing in nursing homes have from two to six times the case rate of the general population. Most cases of tuberculosis in the elderly are due to reactivation of a previous infection rather than being newly acquired disease. It is thought that active tuberculosis eventually develops in about 4% of patients with a positive tuberculin skin test (PPD). Tuberculosis is suspected on the basis of clinical findings, which may be subtle and include fatigue, anorexia with weight loss, and cough. Chest radiography may also help in suspecting the disease. Confirmation of the disease requires evaluation of sputum and gastric washings for the presence of acid-fast organisms. Cultures may take up to 6 weeks to become positive. Increasing numbers of multidrug-resistant *Mycobacterium tuberculosis* are being found, but this is not true in most cases involving the elderly, because most of their cases are due to reactivation of the disease acquired many years earlier.

- Tuberculosis is increasing in frequency.
- Tuberculosis is more common with advancing age.
- Persons residing in nursing homes have from two to six times the case rate of the general population.
- In the elderly, most cases of tuberculosis are due to reactivation of a previous infection.

Without symptoms, the PPD is the only test available to determine the possibility of tuberculosis. Intermediate strength tuberculin (5 TU) is administered intradermally, and the degree of induration (not erythema) is read. The Centers for Disease Control and the American Thoracic Society have developed recommendations for the interpretation and determination of a positive PPD. Three groups representing positive tests have been defined:

- **>5 mm**--Close contacts of those with active disease, those clinically suspected of having tuberculosis, and those with HIV or at risk for HIV.
- **≥10 mm**--Foreign persons with a high prevalence of tuberculosis in their home country, intravenous drug users, medically underserved persons, those who live or work in institutions (nursing homes, group homes, correctional facilities), and those with medical problems associated with an increased risk of developing tuberculosis.
- **≥15 mm**--The rest of the population.

The PPD may be falsely negative in several instances, including malnutrition, immunosuppression, lymphatic disease, acute infections, recent infection with *M. tuberculosis*, recently administered live viral vaccination, or an improperly administered skin test.

On admission to a nursing home, the patient should be administered a 2-stage PPD. The first skin test should be read 7 days after it is administered. The second test is administered on the 7th day if the patient shows <10 mm of induration. The second test is interpreted 2 days after it is applied. Up to 15% of additional positive reactors are identified with this method. In those with a positive PPD, chest radiography should be performed. If the findings are negative and the patient is asymptomatic, no treatment should be initiated unless it can be shown that the patient has converted to a positive PPD within the last 2 years. If the chest radiographic findings are abnormal, sputum and gastric washings should be obtained and cultured.

- Patients admitted to a nursing home should have a 2-stage PPD test.

Chemoprophylaxis for persons >35 years consists of isoniazid for 6-12 months. It is indicated if the PPD is positive and the patient 1) has been converted to a positive PPD within the last 2 years, 2) is an intravenous drug user, 3) has a coexisting medical problem (silicosis, various malignancies such as leukemia or lymphoma, chronic renal failure, diabetes mellitus) or is HIV-positive, 4) has had a recent, rapid weight loss, 5) is immunocompromised (including patients taking steroids), 6) has been in a household with or has had close contact with a tuberculosis patient, or 7) has an abnormal chest radiographic finding.

Elderly patients with proven tuberculosis who reside in an area of high antituberculin drug resistance should be started on treatment with three or possibly four antituberculin drugs until the sensitivity results are known. If the tuberculosis organism is not a resistant strain, the patient may receive treatment with two drugs, usually isoniazid and rifampin. Isoniazid-induced hepatotoxicity is common with advancing age and develops in up to 5% of those >65 years. A baseline level and periodic checks of aspartate aminotransferase levels should be done in elderly patients taking isoniazid. Elderly patients treated with isoniazid should also receive vitamin B_{12} (pyridoxine) supplements of 10 to 25 mg/day to prevent peripheral neuropathy.

- Isoniazid can produce liver toxicity in the elderly, and liver function should be monitored.
- Elderly patients taking isoniazid should receive pyridoxine to prevent peripheral neuropathy.

IMMUNIZATIONS

Pneumococcal pneumonia vaccine is effective against 23 of the strains of *S. pneumoniae*, which account for 80% of the strains that commonly cause pneumonia. Because of decreasing effectiveness with time, revaccination is now being advised by some after 6 years. The influenza vaccine is changed on a yearly basis, depending on the prevalent strain. It should be given annually to high-risk persons, those >65 years, and those in frequent close contact with the elderly. It takes about 2-3 weeks to develop immunity to influenza after receiving the vaccine. Any of the elderly who are unvaccinated during an influenza epidemic should be given amantadine or rimantadine.

- Consideration should be given to revaccinating with pneumococcal vaccine to high-risk groups after 6 years.
- The influenza vaccine should be administered to the elderly annually in the autumn.

OSTEOPOROSIS

Osteoporosis and its complications are extremely common in the elderly. Osteoporosis results in a loss of bone density, with a normal bone-to-mineral ratio. Hip, wrist, and vertebral compression fractures are common causes of morbidity and mortality. Peak bone density is achieved at about age 30, with men having a higher bone density than women at all ages. After age 30, bone density gradually declines throughout the rest of one's lifetime. Loss of estrogen, either because of an operation (oophorectomy) or menopause, causes a more rapid decline in bone density. The diagnosis of osteoporosis is usually made clinically, and it is often difficult to know when bone density loss is more than acceptable for one's age. The following help to establish the diagnosis: 1) presence of multiple risk factors (advanced age; female; caucasian; low calcium intake through much of one's lifetime; thin build; a history of steroid, tobacco, or alcohol use; northern European ancestry; prolonged inac-

tivity; and family history positive for osteoporosis); 2) ruling out secondary causes (glucocorticoid excess, hypogonadism, hyperthyroidism, hyperparathyroidism, osteomalacia, myeloma); 3) physical examination findings (loss of height, increased thoracic kyphosis); and 4) radiographic findings of osteopenia or vertebral compression fractures. Bone density can be measured by several techniques (single- or dual-photon absorptiometry, quantitative CT scan). Bone density can be used to assess the risk of fractures, to check progression of disease, and to assess response to treatment. No simple laboratory tests are available that can confirm the diagnosis of osteoporosis.

- Osteoporosis: extremely common in the elderly.
- Bone density can be used to assess the risk of fractures, to check progression of disease, and to assess response to treatment.

The treatment of osteoporosis is disappointing and, currently, is best aimed at prevention. Premenopausal women require 1,000 mg/day of elemental calcium, and postmenopausal women require 1,500 mg/day. Currently, the most effective treatment is adequate calcium intake, weight-bearing exercise, adequate vitamin D (600-800 IU/day), and estrogen replacement therapy, especially when initiated shortly after menopause. Progestin should be used with estrogen to decrease the risk of endometrial cancer. Progestin is not necessary in those who have had a hysterectomy. In addition to showing a decrease in bone loss after menopause, starting hormonal treatment in those with osteoporosis reduces the rate of fractures. Calcitonin and etidronate slow the progressive decrease in bone density by inhibiting bone resorption; however, long-term studies are needed to determine if this results in a reduction in the fracture rate. Fluoride can increase bone density; however, there is a question of increased bone fragility.

- Hip and vertebral compression fractures are common causes of morbidity and mortality.
- No simple laboratory tests are available to confirm the diagnosis of osteoporosis.

OSTEOMALACIA

Osteomalacia results from defective bone mineralization and is caused most commonly by a deficiency of vitamin D. It may be due to inadequate intake of vitamin D, lack of exposure to the sun, malabsorption, chronic liver disease, or chronic renal disease (resulting in inadequate conversion of 25-hydroxyvitamin D to 1,25-dihydroxyvitamin D). Radiographically, the bone appears osteopenic and can look like osteoporosis. Laboratory findings include decreased serum levels of calcium, phosphorus, and 1,25-dihydroxyvitamin D and increased levels of alkaline phosphatase. Defective bone mineralization may also be caused by very low levels of phosphate, which can be due to excessive use of aluminum-containing antacids, tumor effect, or renal tubule disorders.

- Osteomalacia: the commonest cause is inadequate vitamin D_2, which results from various mechanisms.
- Osteomalacia can appear like osteoporosis.
- Unlike osteoporosis, osteomalacia has abnormal laboratory findings, including low serum levels of calcium and phosphorus and increased alkaline phosphatase.

URINARY INCONTINENCE

Urinary incontinence is common among the elderly, affecting at least 15% of those living independently and about 50% of those in institutions. It causes multiple medical, social, and economic complications and is a common reason for nursing home placement. Incontinence may lead to urinary tract infection, skin breakdown, social isolation, and depression. Understanding urinary incontinence requires a knowledge of the anatomy of the urinary tract and the physiology of micturition. Failure to appreciate this information can result in inaccurate diagnosis and ineffective treatment.

- Urinary incontinence affects at least 15% of the elderly who live independently and about 50% of those in institutions.

Anatomy

The detrusor muscle consists of three muscular layers. Its functions include urine storage (relaxed detrusor) and urine emptying (detrusor contraction). Both sympathetic and parasympathetic nerves innervate the detrusor muscle. Stimulation of the sympathetic nerves causes relaxation of the detrusor muscle, whereas stimulation of the parasympathetic nerves produces contraction of the detrusor muscle. The internal sphincter is a smooth muscle under involuntary (sympathetic nerves) control. Sympathetic stimulation produces increased internal sphincter tone. The external sphincter is striated muscle under voluntary (pudendal nerve) control. It contracts in response to transient increases in intra-abdominal pressure (cough, sneeze, etc.). The external sphincter rapidly fatigues and has little importance in maintaining continence.

Stretch receptors located in the detrusor wall send information to the central nervous system. The spinal cord transmits sensory (ascending) signals to the brain and motor (descending) signals to the bladder. The brain causes stimulation of the sympathetic nerves when urine storage is desired (relaxation of the detrusor and contraction of the internal sphincter) and stimulation of the parasympathetic nerves when bladder emptying is desired (contraction of the detrusor). The internal sphincter relaxes with inhibition of the sympathetic nerves.

- The urinary bladder receives both sympathetic and parasym-

pathetic innervation, relaxing and filling with sympathetic stimulation and contracting and emptying with parasympathetic stimulation.
- The internal urinary sphincter contracts with sympathetic stimulation, promoting bladder filling, and relaxes with bladder emptying, because of inhibition of the sympathetic nerves.

Effects of Age

The changes in the urinary system that occur with aging do not cause urinary incontinence: incontinence is not a normal result of aging. However, the changes that occur can contribute to the problem of incontinence. These changes include smaller bladder capacity, early contractions of the detrusor muscle, decreased ability to suppress contractions of the detrusor muscle and postpone urination, and increased nocturnal production of urine.

Medications Affecting Urination and Continence

Medications that can affect urination and continence include 1) potent diuretics, which cause brisk filling of the bladder; 2) anticholinergic agents that can impair detrusor muscle contraction; 3) sedative-hypnotics that may cause confusion; 4) narcotics that impair detrusor muscle contraction; 5) α-adrenergic agonists that increase internal sphincter tone; 6) α-adrenergic antagonists that decrease internal sphincter tone; and 7) calcium channel blockers that decrease detrusor muscle tone.

- Medications that affect urination: diuretics, anticholinergic agents, sedative-hypnotics, narcotics, α-adrenergic agonists, α-adrenergic antagonists, and calcium channel blockers.

Established Incontinence

Patients are more likely to have reversible incontinence if it is of recent onset. Although established incontinence is more difficult to treat, it can be managed with significant benefit to the patient. In the elderly, overactivity of the detrusor muscle (urge incontinence) is a common cause of established incontinence, accounting for 40%-70% of cases. It causes early contractions of the detrusor muscle at low bladder volumes. Symptoms include urinary frequency and urgency, with losses of small-to-moderate urine volumes. Nocturia often occurs. Detrusor overactivity is seen with central nervous system disease (mass lesion, Parkinson's disease, stroke) or bladder irritation (infection, benign prostatic hyperplasia, fecal impaction, atrophic urethritis).

Overflow incontinence is uncommon. It is seen with urinary outflow obstruction (benign prostatic hyperplasia, tumor) or detrusor underactivity/hypotonic bladder (autonomic neuropathy). Symptoms are low urine flow and frequent urinary dribbling.

Outlet incompetence (stress incontinence) is common in women and rare in men (unless sphincter damage has occurred).

It is caused by laxity of pelvic floor muscle and lack of bladder support, resulting in small losses of urine with transient increases in intra-abdominal pressure (cough, sneeze, etc.).

- Detrusor overactivity is common in the elderly, accounting for 40%-70% of cases of urinary incontinence.
- Detrusor overactivity may occur with central nervous system disease or disorders that cause bladder irritation.
- Overflow incontinence is uncommon. It is seen with urinary outflow obstruction or a hypotonic detrusor muscle.
- Outlet incompetence is common in women and rare in men.

Functional incontinence is the inability of persons who are normally continent to reach toilet facilities in time. Often, it is due to various medications (e.g., potent diuretics) and some limitation of mobility (restraints, hemiparesis).

Evaluation of Incontinence

Evaluation of incontinence includes taking a medical history and performing a physical examination and several simple laboratory tests. The medical history should include the amount of urine lost, precipitating factors, whether symptoms of obstruction exist, and the patient's functional status. Also, document symptoms of neurologic disease, associated disease states, menstrual status and parity, and medications used.

Physical examination of the abdomen should evaluate bladder distention and possible abdominal masses. In examining the pelvis, check for uterine, bladder, or rectal prolapse; atrophic vaginitis; and pelvic masses. The rectal examination should document any masses, fecal impaction, sphincter tone, and prostate enlargement or nodules. A neurologic examination should be performed to search for disease of the central nervous system or of the spinal, autonomic, or peripheral nerves.

Laboratory tests that should be conducted include 1) urinalysis and urine culture to check for infection, pyuria, and hematuria; 2) blood urea nitrogen and creatinine determination to assess renal function; 3) calcium and glucose measurements to assess polyuric states; 4) occasionally, intravenous pyelography and/or renal ultrasonography may be performed to check for hydronephrosis, which may occur with chronic bladder outlet obstruction; and 5) postvoid residual bladder volume to estimate the degree of bladder emptying. Urodynamics usually are not necessary to establish the diagnosis of incontinence. Often, the urodynamic test results do not fit the clinical picture. Many elderly persons with no incontinence have abnormal urodynamics, and occasionally, those with incontinence have normal urodynamics. These studies are often indicated when patients have medically confusing histories or more than one type of incontinence. Cystometry measures bladder volume and pressure and can be used to detect uninhibited contractions of the detrusor muscle, lack of bladder

contractions, and bladder sensation. Voiding cystourethrography measures the urethrovesical angle and residual urine volume. Uroflow measures urinary flow rate, and electromyography evaluates the external sphincter and detects detrusor-sphincter dyssynergia.

- In most cases, urinary incontinence can be diagnosed on the basis of the medical history and physical examination findings.
- Common laboratory tests that may help in the diagnosis include urinalysis, urine culture, blood urea nitrogen, creatinine, serum calcium, and blood glucose.
- A postvoid residual bladder volume may be helpful in determining the degree of bladder emptying.
- Urodynamic studies are not usually necessary to establish the diagnosis of urinary incontinence.

Treatment of Incontinence

The treatment of detrusor overactivity is aimed at suppressing the early contractions of the detrusor muscle. Behavioral training is often successful. Also, medications that inhibit parasympathetic stimulation of the bladder muscle are effective. The anticholinergic drugs that are used include oxybutynin, flavoxate, and imipramine. Calcium channel blockers, used as smooth muscle relaxants, may also be tried.

- Behavior training is often successful in treating incontinence.
- Anticholinergic drugs that are used: oxybutynin, flavoxate, and imipramine.

The treatment of overflow incontinence is aimed at providing complete drainage from a bladder that either is not adequately contracting or has significant outflow obstruction. When treating a hypotonic bladder, medications that increase the tone of the detrusor muscle can be tried. These include cholinergic agonists (bethanechol). Treatment of obstruction includes operation (transurethral resection of the prostate) and use of α-adrenergic antagonists (prazosin, terazosin, or doxazocin), which decrease the tone of the internal sphincter. An external urinary catheter is of little benefit, because it does not drain the bladder. An indwelling catheter or intermittent catheterization is occasionally necessary.

The treatment of outlet incompetence is aimed at surgically restoring the normal posterior urethrovesical angle of 90°-100°. Increasing the tone of the internal sphincter with α-adrenergic agonists (pseudoephedrine, phenylpropanolamine, and imipramine) may also be of benefit. Hormonal therapy (topical estrogen) helps restore the mucosa of the urethra, increasing its resistance. Pelvic floor (Kegel) exercises are also useful.

- The tone of the internal sphincter can be increased by administering α-adrenergic agonists.

Urologic Consultation

In most elderly patients, the diagnosis of urinary incontinence can be established without the need for evaluation by a urologist. The following conditions indicate the need for urologic evaluation: high postvoid residual urine volume, outflow obstruction, significant uterine or bladder prolapse, abnormal findings on prostate examination, recurrent urinary tract infections, hematuria, unknown diagnosis, or failure to improve with treatment.

Use of Urinary Catheters

External (condom) catheters have a slight risk of infection and problems with long-term use. They have minimal benefit in overflow incontinence. Intermittent catheterization has a small risk (from 1%-20% depending on patient setting) of infection with each insertion. It is useful with temporary incontinence. Postvoid residual volumes should be used as a guide in determining the frequency of catheterization. Intermittent catheterization has limited use in the management of chronic incontinence of nursing home patients because of expense, and self-catheterization will be limited in those living independently if they have poor manual dexterity or poor vision. Eventually, significant bacteriuria develops in essentially all patients with indwelling catheters. The chronic use of suppressive antibiotics is not recommended because it does not prevent long-term suppression of bacteriuria and results in infections caused by resistant organisms. Antibiotic treatment should be reserved for symptomatic infections only.

- Intermittent catheterization has a 1%-20% risk of infection with each insertion.
- Postvoid residual volumes should be used as a guide in determining the frequency of catheterization.
- The chronic use of suppressive antibiotics is not recommended.

URINARY TRACT INFECTIONS

Urinary tract infections become more common with advancing age and cause a wide spectrum of disease. They are the most common infection in nursing home residents and the most common cause of sepsis in the elderly; yet, they may also produce the syndrome of asymptomatic bacteriuria. Incomplete emptying of the bladder, which is commonly found in the elderly (cystocele, benign prostatic hyperplasia), urinary instrumentation, and chronic catheterization all predispose the elderly to urinary tract infection. The elderly have various bacterial organisms that produce urinary tract infections. *E. coli*, the most common organism to cause these infections in the younger population, causes only about half of the infections in the elderly. Other gram-negative organisms such as *Enterococcus, Proteus, Klebsiella*, and *Pseudomonas* are more

common in the elderly. Because of the wide variety of organisms, urine cultures should be obtained when evaluating elderly patients who have urinary tract infection. Treatment may be started with typical antibiotics (e.g., trimethoprim-sulfamethoxazole, amoxicillin, cephalosporins) pending urine culture results. Those who have potential for resistant organisms or who have had an indwelling urinary catheter should receive an antibiotic with a wider spectrum of coverage, such as a quinolone.

- Urinary tract infection: most common infection in nursing home residents.
- Urinary tract infection; most common cause of sepsis in the elderly.
- *Enterococcus, Proteus, Klebsiella*, and *Pseudomonas* are more common in the elderly.
- The elderly have a wider variety of bacteria causing urinary tract infections than younger persons; therefore, urine cultures should be obtained in elderly patients with urinary tract infection.

Asymptomatic bacteriuria is more common with age and has been associated with increased mortality; however, the mortality appears to be unrelated to the bacteriuria and is likely a marker for increased severity of illness and debility. Asymptomatic bacteriuria should not be treated unless there is a history of chronic urinary obstruction.

- Asymptomatic bacteriuria does not lead to increased morbidity and mortality as a result of infection and should not be routinely treated.

Patients with chronic indwelling catheters eventually have bacteriuria. The bacterial organisms change with time. Routine surveillance cultures should not be done in these patients, and the bacteriuria should not be treated unless the patient is symptomatic. In those who have had urinary catheters removed, bacteriuria should be treated if the urine remains bacteriuric for more than 48 hours. In some patients, removal of the urinary catheter alone will result in resolution of the bacteriuria.

- Patients with chronic indwelling catheters eventually have bacteriuria. Surveillance cultures should not be obtained, and the bacteriuria should not be treated unless the patient becomes symptomatic.

USE OF MEDICATIONS IN THE ELDERLY

More than 30% of all prescriptions are written for persons >65 years old. Medications are a common cause of iatrogenic disease in the elderly, and they are handled differently in the elderly because of various changes in pharmacokinetics and pharmacodynamics. The overall result is a longer duration of activity of many drugs, lower doses needed to achieve desired therapeutic effects, more frequent adverse drug effects of drug-drug interactions, and greater likelihood of drug toxicity. Thus, it is important to know the changes in pharmacokinetics and pharmacodynamics, how to dose elderly patients, and a selection of drugs that are better tolerated by the elderly.

- More than 30% of all prescriptions are written for persons >65 years old.
- Changes occur in the pharmacokinetics and pharmacodynamics in the elderly.

Pharmacokinetics includes drug absorption, distribution, metabolism, and elimination. There are age-related changes that have an effect on each of these factors, affecting several more than others. Age-related changes that could have an effect on drug absorption include decreased blood supply to the small bowel, villous atrophy resulting in a decreased surface area for the absorption of drugs, and decreased gastric acidity. There is little evidence that drug absorption is significantly decreased with advancing age. Drug distribution does play a major role in altered pharmacokinetics and changes significantly with age, because of alterations in the various volumes of distribution in the elderly. These changes include an increase in adipose tissue, a decrease in total body water and lean body mass, and for many, a change in levels of plasma protein. The result of increased adipose tissue is an increase in the volume of distribution for lipid-soluble drugs; this can result in an increase in drug half-life, especially of lipid-soluble drugs. The decrease in body water results in a smaller volume of distribution for water-soluble drugs, potentially leading to a higher than expected drug concentration. A decrease in plasma protein (e.g., albumin) results in less protein-bound (inactive) acidic drugs and a greater amount of free (active) drug. α1-Acid glycoproteins are acute phase reactants and increase in persons with significant inflammation. This can produce an increase in basic drug (lidocaine, propranolol) protein-binding and less free drug.

- Pharmacokinetics includes drug absorption, distribution, metabolism, and elimination.
- There is little evidence that drug absorption is significantly decreased with advancing age.

Drug metabolism is performed primarily by the liver. With advanced age, the ability of the liver to metabolize drugs is decreased because of various factors, including a decrease in the number of functioning hepatocytes, decreased hepatic blood flow, and decreased hepatic enzymatic activity. Phase I metabolism involves the oxidation or reduction of a drug, using the cytochrome P450 system. This type of metabolism produces active metabolites and slows with age. Phase II

metabolism involves acetylation and produces inactive metabolites. It shows no change with advancing age. It is extremely difficult to predict a patient's ability to metabolize a specific drug because there is no simple test to perform.

- With advanced age, the ability of the liver to metabolize drugs is decreased.

Drug elimination refers to the ability of the renal system to excrete drugs from the circulation. In general, there is a reduction in renal function with age, with a decrease in both renal plasma flow and glomerular filtration rate (up to 30%), although the variability among persons is great. The serum level of creatinine is not a good measure of renal function in the elderly, because creatinine is a product of muscle breakdown. The elderly have decreased lean body mass with advancing age; therefore, less creatinine is produced. Thus, it is possible to have a normal serum level of creatinine in an elderly patient who has as much as a 30% reduction in renal function. A reasonably accurate estimate of renal function is the following:

-
$$\text{Creatine clearance (mL/min)} = \frac{(140 - \text{age}) \times \text{weight (kg)}}{72 \times \text{serum creatinine (mg/dL)}} \quad [\times 0.85 \text{ for women}]$$

Pharmacodynamic changes also occur with aging and have an effect on the action of medications. Pharmacodynamics refers to drug sensitivity, which can change with age. These changes may reflect an alteration of receptor number, receptor sensitivity to drug, or an altered receptor response to a drug. Less is known about altered pharmacodynamics than about pharmacokinetics; however, the pharmacodynamic changes for several drugs have been identified. There is a decreased responsiveness of β-adrenergic drugs (e.g., less tachycardia with isoproterenol, less bradycardia with β blockers), increased sedation with benzodiazepines, and greater analgesia with opiates.

Adverse drug effects are common in the elderly and frequently cause serious complications. Elderly patients often have limited organ reserve function and are unable to respond, as younger persons can, to the adverse effect.

As a result of altered pharmacokinetics and pharmacodynamics with aging, one needs to use medications carefully in the elderly, avoiding polypharmacy whenever possible and watching for evidence of adverse drug effects and drug-drug interactions, both of which increase in frequency with age.

- Alteration in drug absorption is the least important in alterations in pharmacokinetics.
- Drug distribution includes an increase in adipose tissue, decrease in body water, and in many persons, a change in plasma protein.
- Drug metabolism and clearance tend to decrease with age but are difficult to predict.

SLEEP DISORDERS IN THE ELDERLY

Changes occur in sleep with aging. Some of these changes are due to the normal physiology of aging, others to associated disease states, and some to specific sleep disorders that are more common among the elderly.

Sleep Physiology

Sleep stages I and II are the light stages of sleep. The percentage of sleep spent in these stages increases with age. As a result, the elderly are aroused more easily by noise, light, or various disease symptoms (e.g., pain) and have an increased number of nighttime awakenings. Sleep stages III and IV are considered the deep stages of sleep. Deep-stage sleep decreases with age. Rapid eye movement (REM) sleep also decreases with age, with fewer and shorter REM periods. As a result of these changes, the elderly have a less restful sleep. Sleep latency (the time required to fall asleep) increases with age, making it increasingly difficult for elderly persons to fall asleep.

- Sleep stages I and II are the light stages of sleep and tend to increase with age, whereas stages III and IV, the deeper stages of sleep, tend to decrease with age.
- REM sleep tends to decrease with age.

Sleep Disorders

Some sleep disorders increase in frequency with age. Nocturnal myoclonus is the unilateral or bilateral twitching of the legs that occurs after a person is asleep. Although a person usually is not aware of these twitchings, the bed partner is. Nocturnal myoclonus results in multiple nocturnal awakenings, often interrupting and shortening deep-stage sleep.

Restless leg syndrome is an uncomfortable sensation in the legs that occurs before a person falls asleep. This sensation is relieved by moving the legs or by walking. It results in increased sleep latency. Restless leg syndrome is often associated with nocturnal myoclonus.

Sleep apnea has three forms: obstructive, central, and mixed. The obstructive form is relatively common in the elderly. Sleep apnea causes multiple nighttime awakenings (it can be hundreds of episodes). It is more common in males (30:1) and obese persons. In addition to interfering with sleep, it may produce pulmonary and systemic hypertension. Currently, the most effective treatment is nasal continuous positive airway pressure.

- The elderly tend to have specific sleep disorders more commonly than younger persons, including nocturnal myoclonus, restless leg syndrome, and sleep apnea.

Medications for Insomnia

Medications for insomnia, although commonly prescribed for the elderly with insomnia, are useful for short-term use only. They are not beneficial for chronic insomnia. Most result in tolerance with nightly use, can produce habituation, produce rebound insomnia when discontinued, and may increase apneic spells in those with sleep apnea. If a sedative-hypnotic medication is to be used in an elderly patient, short-acting or intermediate-acting drugs are advised (Table 11-1). Drugs with longer half-lives tend to be more lipid-soluble, and they often have active metabolites. They may accumulate when used on a nightly basis and produce daytime somnolence. Drugs with shorter half-lives tend to be less lipid-soluble and to have minimally active or inactive metabolites. Any of the sedative-hypnotic medications may worsen confusion and/or memory, especially in patients with some underlying cognitive impairment.

Table 11-1.--Sedative-Hypnotic Drugs for Elderly Patients

Long-acting	Intermediate-acting	Short-acting
Diazepam	Temazepam	Oxazepam
Flurazepam	Lorazepam	Triazolam
Clonazepam	Estazolam	
Chlordiazepoxide		

QUESTIONS

Multiple Choice (choose the one best answer)

1. Which of the following is true of life expectancy?
   a. It is the same as life span
   b. It has remained stable and fixed at approximately 100 to 110 years
   c. The increase in life expectancy is due to a decrease in the mortality of the elderly
   d. The increase in life expectancy is due to increased use of high-technology equipment and resuscitation techniques
   e. The increase in life expectancy is due to a decreased infant mortality

2. Which of the following is true of closed-angle glaucoma?
   a. It is associated with chronic ultraviolet light exposure
   b. It can be precipitated by medications with anticholinergic effects
   c. Peripheral vision is slowly lost, often without the patient being aware of vision loss
   d. It is slightly more common than open-angle glaucoma
   e. It is chronic and slowly progressive

3. An 86-year-old woman residing in a nursing home has a cough productive of yellow sputum, dyspnea, and a temperature of 38.6°C. She is hospitalized with presumed pneumonia. Assuming the patient has no drug allergies, the best choice of intravenous antibiotic(s), pending results of sputum and blood cultures, would be:
   a. Pencillin G
   b. Pencillin G, gentamicin, and erythromycin
   c. Erythromycin
   d. Cefuroxime and erythromycin
   e. Ciprofloxacin

4. A 74-year-old woman complained of aching and weakness of her shoulders, neck, and hips. She noted stiffness in the mornings, anorexia and weight loss. Laboratory tests revealed a hemoglobin level of 10.2 g/dL and an erythrocyte sedimentation rate of 82 mm/hr. Which of the following is true about this disease state?
   a. A temporal artery biopsy should be performed immediately because of the likelihood of temporal arteritis
   b. A high dose (60 mg/day) of corticosteroids should be started for treatment
   c. If the aspartate aminotransferase (AST) level is checked, it will likely be increased
   d. Colchicine will produce marked relief from symptoms
   e. Rheumatoid arthritis is a possible cause of the patient's symptoms

5. A 67-year-old man presented with right knee pain and swelling of 8 hours' duration. He recalled a similar episode 8 years earlier. Which of the following diseases is least likely to cause these symptoms?
   a. Gout
   b. Rheumatoid arthritis
   c. Septic joint
   d. Pseudogout
   e. Joint trauma

6. Which of the following is true about Alzheimer's disease?
   a. Head CT scan showing cerebral atrophy confirms the diagnosis
   b. Neuronal plaques and neurofibrillary tangles are specific to Alzheimer's disease
   c. Patients have decreased choline acetyltransferase activity
   d. The disease is due to inadequate cerebral perfusion from atherosclerotic disease
   e. Tacrine arrests the progression of the disease

True/False (indicate whether each answer is true or false)

7. A 68-year-old man complained of urinary incontinence. Which of the following is/are true regarding this patient?
   a. Urodynamic studies will likely be necessary to establish a specific diagnosis
   b. Statistically the most likely cause in an elderly man is detrusor overactivity
   c. Before any studies are performed, the patient should be given an empiric trial of oxybutinin
   d. If the patient has overflow incontinence, an external catheter may be helpful
   e. Even though the patient has no irritative symptoms, if bacteriuria is found, antibiotic treatment will likely relieve the urinary incontinence

8. If a patient with urinary urgency and obstructive urinary symptoms is given a medication with anticholinergic effects, which of the following is/are true?
   a. The patient will likely have improved urinary flow
   b. It may precipitate urinary retention, with inability to void
   c. The symptoms of urgency may improve
   d. The postvoid urinary residual volume may increase
   e. The obstructive symptoms are likely to improve, but not the symptoms of urgency

9. Which of the following is true regarding medication use in the elderly?
   a. Decreased drug absorption plays a major role in altered pharmacokinetics in older patients

b. Phase I metabolism involves the cytochrome P450 system and often slows with age

c. A normal serum level of creatinine implies normal renal function

d. Pharmacodynamic changes may result in a decreased effect of medications in older patients

e. A smaller volume of distribution should result in a smaller loading dose of a medication

ANSWERS

1. Answer e.

Life expectancy and life span are different. Life expectancy has increased with time; life span is fixed at the approximate age of 100 to 110 and represents the ultimate age that we can achieve. The increase in life expectancy is not due to our increase in technology or to keeping our elderly alive longer, but rather improvement in nutrition, sanitation, and immunizations, and decreased infant mortality.

2. Answer b.

Closed-angle glaucoma is much less common than open-angle glaucoma. It is not associated with ultraviolet light exposure; however, it can be precipitated by anticholinergic drugs in persons with narrow angles. Closed-angle glaucoma is an acute process and can result in permanent vision loss if not treated promptly.

3. Answer d.

The treatment of pneumonia in the elderly must take into account the setting in which it is acquired and the likely bacterial organism involved. This patient needs treatment with antibiotics that cover *S. pneumoniae* and *H. influenzae*, with increased suspicion of other common gram-negative and atypical organisms. Neither penicillin G nor erythromycin covers a broad enough spectrum of bacteria to be used as the initial antibiotic for this patient. Penicillin G, erythromycin, and gentamicin would cover an appropriate spectrum of bacteria; however, gentamicin is potentially quite toxic to the elderly. Ciprofloxacin would not be the best choice because its coverage of *S. pneumoniae* is suboptimal. The best choice among the options listed is cefuroxime plus erythromycin. It covers both gram-positive, common gram-negative, and atypical organisms and is relatively safe and well tolerated by elderly patients.

4. Answer e.

The patient is likely to have polymyalgia rheumatica (PMR). Although there is a relationship between PMR and temporal arteritis, only 15% of those with PMR have temporal arteritis and temporal artery biopsy should be performed only if there are symptoms of temporal arteritis. The disease responds dramatically to steroids; however, high doses are not necessary. Colchicine is not used to treat PMR. Despite patient complaints that sound as though there is muscle involvement, muscle enzyme levels are normal. At times, PMR can look like rheumatoid arthritis in the elderly.

5. Answer b.

Monoarticular arthritis is likely to represent a crystalline arthritis (gout or pseudogout) or septic joint or to be the result of trauma.

6. Answer c.

Head CT should be done in the evaluation of Alzheimer's disease, but not to look for cerebral atrophy. The test is done to look for potentially reversible diseases such as mass lesions, evidence of normal pressure hydrocephalus, or a previous stroke. Although neuronal plaques and neurofibrillary tangles are seen in patients with Alzheimer's disease, they are also seen in others without dementia, although in smaller numbers. Patients with Alzheimer's disease have a decrease in the neurotransmitter acetylcholine and a decrease in choline acetyltransferase activity. Although tacrine can result in cognitive improvement in some patients with Alzheimer's disease, it does not arrest the progression of the disease.

7. a, false; b, true; c, false; d, true; e, false.

In most cases of urinary incontinence, the diagnosis can be established with a thorough medical history and physical examination; only occasionally will urodynamic studies be necessary. Oxybutynin is a useful medication for detrusor overactivity; however, if the patient has significant obstruction from benign prostatic hyperplasia, increased urinary retention may result. An external catheter is not useful with overflow incontinence because there is a problem with bladder emptying and an external catheter will not drain the bladder in these patients. Treating bacteriuria in patients with symptomatic urinary symptoms will often result in resolution of incontinence. However, treating asymptomatic bacteriuria rarely cures urinary incontinence.

8. a, false; b, true; c, true; d, true; e, false.

The detrusor is innervated by parasympathetic nerves, with acetylcholine as the neurotransmitter. Anticholinergic medications help suppress early detrusor contractions and reduce symptoms of urgency by inhibiting acetylcholine. In patients with some obstruction to urinary outflow, an anticholinergic drug can result in a bladder that does not contract sufficiently to overcome the urinary outflow obstruction, and urinary retention and/or decreased urinary flow may result.

9. a, false; b, true; c, false; d, true; e, true.

Absorption is the least important of the pharmacokinetic changes associated with aging. There is no critical evidence to suggest that drug absorption decreases with age. Phase I metabolism involves the oxidation or reduction of a drug that uses the cytochrome P450 system. For many elderly persons, this mechanism slows with age. Because creatinine is a product of muscle breakdown and because there is decreased muscle mass associated with aging, the serum level of creatinine often underestimates renal function. An elderly patient can still have a significant decrease in renal function (up to 30%) with a normal serum level of creatinine. Creatinine clearance is a better measure of renal function in the elderly. Not all pharmacodynamic changes reflect a decrease in drug effect. Benzodiazepines have increased sedating ability and opiates have greater analgesic activity in the elderly, because of pharmacodynamic factors. The volume of distribution helps determine the loading dose of a drug, whereas the rate of elimination of a drug helps determine its maintenance dose.

CHAPTER 12

HEMATOLOGY

Thomas M. Habermann, M.D.

ANEMIAS

Evaluation of Anemias

The causes of anemia are complex. The World Health Organization has stated that the lower limit of normal for venous hemoglobin concentration in males older than 14 years living at sea level is 13 g/dL and in nonpregnant females is 12 g/dL. A defined, organized approach to the anemias is essential. Because the initial evaluation of anemia after the history and physical examination begins with the complete blood count, one way to classify anemia is by the mean corpuscular volume (MCV): microcytic, macrocytic, and normocytic anemia.

The complete blood cell count (CBC) is the most commonly ordered blood test. The measured values of the CBC include the total counts for red blood cells (RBCs), platelets, and white blood cells (WBCs) and the volumes of RBCs, platelets, WBCs, and hemoglobin. The calculated values include the hematocrit, MCV, mean corpuscular hemoglobin, mean corpuscular hemoglobin concentration, and red cell distribution width. These values help to differentiate thalassemia from iron deficiency anemia (Tables 12-1 and 12-2).

The differential diagnosis of hypochromic microcytic anemias includes iron deficiency, thalassemic syndromes, anemia of chronic disease, sideroblastic anemias, hemoglobin E, unstable hemoglobins, and lead poisoning. The causes of iron deficiency include blood loss, increased requirements (as in pregnancy), and decreased absorption (partial gastrectomy and malabsorption syndromes). Disorders associated with blood loss include gastrointestinal (ulcers, malignancy, telangiectasia, hiatal hernia, and long-distance runner's anemia), respiratory (malignancy, pulmonary hemosiderosis), menstruation, phlebotomy (blood donor, diagnostic phlebotomy, polycythemia rubra vera, and self-inflicted), trauma, and surgery.

In a nonreferral practice, iron deficiency anemia is the cause of up to 90% of all hypochromic-microcytic anemias (color plate 12-1). Of the remaining 10%, the thalassemic syndromes are more common than the other rare forms of the hypochromic-microcytic anemias. However, the anemia of chronic disease is variable, depending on whether the setting is inpatient or outpatient and whether a community-based or a referral center. The CBC and other laboratory values provide further information for differentiating these entities (Table 12-2). These studies often provide the major clues to the type of anemia. One must always be concerned about blood loss. The evaluation of stool for blood loss is essential in the initial work-up and may also provide clues to a combined anemia. A laboratory approach to microcytic anemias is outlined in Figures 12-1

Table 12-1.--Differentiation of Microcytic Anemias on Basis of Blood Values

	Type of anemia	
	Thalassemia	Iron-deficiency
RBC count	>5.0 x 10^{12}/L	<5.0 x 10^{12}/L
Red cell distribution width	<16	>16
MCV-RBC-(5 x Hb)-3.4	Negative	Positive

Hb, hemoglobin; MCV, mean corpuscular volume; RBC, red blood cell.

Table 12-2. Comparison of Hypochromic-Microcytic Anemias

Disease state	MCV	Red blood cells	% transferrin saturation	Ferritin, µg/L	Marrow iron
Iron deficiency anemia	Decreased	Decreased	<15	Low	Absent
Anemia of chronic disease	Normal or decreased	Decreased	<15 or normal	Normal or increased	Normal or increased
Thalassemia minor	Decreased	Usually increased	Normal	Normal or increased	Normal

MCV, mean corpuscular volume.
Modified from Savage RA: Cost-effective laboratory diagnosis of microcytic anemias of complex origin. ASCP check sample H84-10(H-153). By permission of American Society of Clinical Pathologists.

and 12-2. The serum ferritin test is the most useful initial test in documenting iron deficiency, but the values obtained may be increased in the presence of iron deficiency and coexistent inflammatory states, liver disease, hepatocellular carcinoma, and malignancy.

Confusing problems in iron deficiency include patient compliance, wrong dosage schedules, wrong treatment (enteric-coated iron preparations), diminished absorption (previous surgery and mucosal disease of the small bowel), competitive interference with antacids, blood loss in excess of treatment, other causes of anemia, and physician impatience with response. Oral replacement treatment is the treatment of choice in iron deficiency. Ferrous sulfate three times a day at a dose of 325 mg orally 1 hour before or 2 hours after meals is the initial treatment. The CBC should be rechecked 4 weeks after starting iron therapy. Correction of the anemia would be anticipated in 6 weeks. Another 6 months of treatment is necessary to replenish bone marrow reserves.

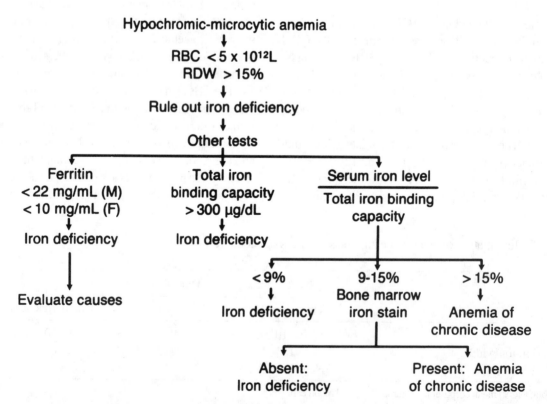

Fig. 12-1. Algorithm for approach to diagnosis of hypochromic-microcytic anemias with normal or decreased red blood cell (RBC) counts. RDW, red cell distribution width. (Modified from Savage RA: Cost-effective laboratory diagnosis of microcytic anemias of complex origin. ASCP check sample H84-10(H-153). By permission of American Society of Clinical Pathologists.)

Hypochromic-microcytic anemia

↓

RBC >5 x 10^{12}/L
RDW normal

↓

Differential diagnosis:
β-thalassemia,
α-thalassemia,
abnormal hemoglobin

↓

Hb A$_2$

>4.0%
β-Thalassemia trait

<4.0%
↓
Hemoglobin electrophoresis
Southern blot

Fig. 12-2. Algorithm for approach to diagnosis of hypochromic-microcytic anemias with an increased total red blood cell (RBC) count. Hb, hemoglobin. (Modified from Savage RA: Cost-effective laboratory diagnosis of microcytic anemias of complex origin. ASCP check sample H84-10(H-153). By permission of American Society of Clinical Pathologists.)

Thalassemia is the most common single gene disorder in the world. β-Thalassemia results when β-globulin chains are absent, resulting in an excess of α-globulin chains in the RBCs. β-Thalassemia can be identified by simple screening methods (Tables 12-1 and 12-2 and Fig. 12-2). Genetic counseling is indicated when a diagnosis of α- or β-thalassemia is established.

The differential diagnosis of the macrocytic anemias includes vitamin B$_{12}$ deficiency, folate deficiency, chemotherapy agents, myelodysplasia, liver disease, alcohol abuse, hypothyroidism, cold agglutinin disease, smoking, and hemolysis. A laboratory approach to macrocytic anemias is outlined in Figure 12-3. The pathophysiology of drug-induced macrocytosis includes marrow toxicity with interference with folate metabolism (alcohol), marrow toxicity with chemotherapy drugs (cyclophosphamide, methotrexate, hydroxyurea, etc.), marrow toxicity with other drugs (zidovudine), altered folate metabolism with anticonvulsants (phenytoin, primidone, and phenobarbital), and altered folate metabolism from other drugs (oral contraceptives, triamterene, sulfasalazine, and sulfamethoxazole). Patients with achlorhydria of any cause do not absorb vitamin B$_{12}$, because hydrochloric acid is required to free vitamin B$_{12}$ from food. A normal functioning pancreas is required. The causes of vitamin B$_{12}$ deficiency are many and

include pernicious anemia, total or partial gastrectomy, ileal resection, bacterial overgrowth syndromes, achlorhydria, and chronic pancreatitis.

The symptoms and signs of vitamin B$_{12}$ deficiency include paresthesias, gait disturbance, mental status changes, vibratory/position sense impairment, and the absence of ankle reflexes and extensor plantar responses. A low serum level of vitamin B$_{12}$ confirms the diagnosis of a deficiency state. A low intrinsic factor antibody confirms the diagnosis of pernicious anemia. The serum level of vitamin B$_{12}$ may rarely be normal in pernicious anemia. Serum gastrin levels are high in pernicious anemia. The serum level of methylmalonic acid is increased in vitamin B$_{12}$ deficiency states. The Schilling test may be required after these tests. True-negative results in part I of the Schilling test include dietary deficiency and cobalamin-binding-protein abnormalities, and false-negative results occur in food-bound malabsorption due to achlorhydria. In part II of the Schilling test, false-positive results occur in cases attributable to mucosal megloblastosis. Antibiotics are given in part III of the Schilling test, and the differential diagnosis of a positive result includes ileal malabsorption and defective intrinsic factor in the test. A negative test result in this stage of the test occurs in the blind loop syndrome. The treatment of pernicious anemia is vitamin B$_{12}$, 1,000 µg intramuscularly for 5 days, followed by 500-1,000 µg intramuscularly every month. Alternatively, vitamin B$_{12}$ may be given orally at a dose of 500-1,000 µg/day.

The normochromic-normocytic group of disorders present the greatest challenge in differential diagnosis. The differential diagnosis of the normochromic-normocytic anemias includes stem cell dysfunction (aplastic anemia and red cell aplasia), marrow replacement (tumor and fibrosis), renal disease, hemolysis, acute hemorrhage, mixed nutritional deficiency, myelodysplasia, chemotherapy, anemia of acute disease, anemia of chronic disease (acute infections, chronic infections, neoplasia, rheumatoid arthritis, polymyalgia rheumatica, etc.), and erythropoietin deficiency. The anemia of renal failure and liver disease is important in this differential diagnosis. The anemia of renal disease may be related to decreased erythropoietin or shortened RBC survival. It is important to obtain a reticulocyte count to exclude hemolysis early on in the evaluation in patients with normochromic-normocytic anemias. It is essential to exclude blood loss from the gastrointestinal tract that may be acute and not manifested by a microcytic blood picture.

Erythropoietin

Erythropoietin is a glycoprotein that acts through specific receptors on RBC precursors. It is produced primarily in the kidneys, although a small amount is produced in the liver. There are no preformed stores. The gene is located on chromosome 7. Recombinant human erythropoietin is

Fig. 12-3. Laboratory approach to macrocytic anemias. MCV, mean corpuscular volume. (Modified from Colon-Otero G, Menke D, Hook CC: A practical approach to the differential diagnosis and evaluation of the adult patient with macrocytic anemia. Med Clin North Am 76:581-597, May 1992. By permission of WB Saunders Company.)

identical to native erythropoietin, and antibodies have not been reported. There is an inverse relationship between the circulating concentration of erythropoietin and the hemoglobin or hematocrit value. Regulation is linked to an oxygen sensor, not to peripheral catabolism. Erythropoietin production increases with hypoxia. The serum levels of erythropoietin are not influenced by age or sex. The higher hemoglobin value in men seems to be due to androgenic steroids. The serum levels of erythropoietin are low, never absent, in chronic renal failure, polycythemia rubra vera, rheumatoid arthritis, and human immunodeficiency virus (HIV) infection. Zidovudine can increase the serum erythropoietin value. High erythropoietin levels are present in marrow hypofunction (pure red cell aplasia), deficiency states (iron deficiency), tumor, autonomous production (hepatocellular carcinoma), and high altitude.

Anemias of malignancy and the use of neoplastic agents may respond to erythropoietin, particularly multiple myeloma, lymphoma, and solid tumors. It is also useful after bone marrow transplantation. Erythropoietin has been used with efficacious results in the autologous blood donor setting, especially in women and in persons who donate >4 units Approved indications are end-stage renal disease, the anemia of HIV infections, the anemia of malignancy, and the anemias caused by neoplastic agents.

- Erythropoietin: a glycoprotein produced in kidney; production increases with hypoxia.
- Its level is low in renal failure, polycythemia rubra vera, rheumatoid arthritis, and HIV infection.
- Its level is high in pure red cell aplasia, iron deficiency, tumors, and high altitude.
- Indications include end-stage renal disease, the anemia of HIV, and the anemias of malignancy and neoplastic agents.

In evaluating patients with erythrocytosis, a normal or low erythropoietin value associated with an increased RBC mass does not prove autonomous erythropoiesis.

Patients must have adequate iron stores to respond to erythropoietin. If erythropoietin is given to healthy individuals, the hematocrit can increase dramatically. As the hematocrit increases above 60%, the viscosity of the blood rapidly increases. Myocardial infarction or strokes may occur with the misuse of erythropoietin.

Hemolytic Anemia

First, it is essential to determine the presence of hemolytic anemia as manifested by laboratory evidence of an increased rate of erythropoiesis and laboratory evidence of increased RBC destruction. Second, specific causes should be sought. Hemolytic anemias may be Coombs-negative or Coombs-positive.

The initial evaluation includes a history and physical examination, CBC, morphology, and reticulocyte count. Conditions found during the work-up that can be mistaken for hemolysis include hemorrhage, recovery from deficiency states, metastatic carcinoma, and myoglobinuria. Studies of a family's hematologic history are important. The differential diagnosis of hemolytic anemia is outlined in Figure 12-4.

Inheritance Patterns

Membrane defects and unstable hemoglobin diseases are autosomal dominant. Most enzymopathies are autosomal recessive. The most common enzymopathy, glucose-6-phosphate dehydrogenase deficiency, is sex-linked, as is phosphoglycerate kinase deficiency.

- Membrane defects and unstable hemoglobin diseases are autosomal dominant.
- Most enzymopathies are autosomal recessive.
- Glucose-6-phosphate dehydrogenase deficiency is sex-linked.

Laboratory Findings

The CBC abnormalities in autoimmune hemolytic anemia include anemia, thrombocytosis, or thrombocytopenia. The presence of autoimmune hemolytic anemia and autoimmune thrombocytopenia is called Evans's syndrome. The reticulocyte value is usually persistently increased, reflecting an enhanced bone marrow response. The bilirubin value is usually 1 to 5 µg/dL and almost exclusively unconjugated or indirect. The direct bilirubin should be less than 15% of total if the bilirubin value is >4 µg/dL. The haptoglobin concentration is usually low, with no compensatory increased rate of synthesis, and the lactate dehydrogenase level is increased.

Peripheral Smear (Differential Diagnosis)

Spherocytes (color plate 12-2) are associated with hereditary spherocytosis, burns, *Clostridium* infections, autoimmune hemolytic anemia, and hypophosphatemia. Basophilic stippling occurs in lead poisoning, β-thalassemia, and arsenic poisoning. Hypochromia occurs in thalassemia and lead poisoning. Target cells are present in thalassemia, hemoglobin C and E, obstructive jaundice or hepatitis, lecithin-cholesterol-acyltransferase deficiency, and the splenectomy state (color plate 12-3). Agglutination is present in cold agglutinin disease (color plate 12-4). Stomatocytes are associated with acute alcoholism and are also found as an artifact. Acanthocytes (color plate 12-5) are present in chronic liver disease, abetalipoproteinemia, malabsorption, and anorexia nervosa. Heinz bodies are present in glucose-6-phosphate dehydrogenase deficiency.

Schistocytes: Microangiopathic Hemolytic Anemia

In microangiopathic hemolytic anemia, the RBCs are fragmented and deformed in the peripheral blood (color plate 12-6). The fragmentation is caused by fibrin deposits in small blood vessels leading to mechanical hemolysis. The results of the Coombs' test are negative. Patients with microangiopathic hemolytic anemia are often thrombocytopenic.

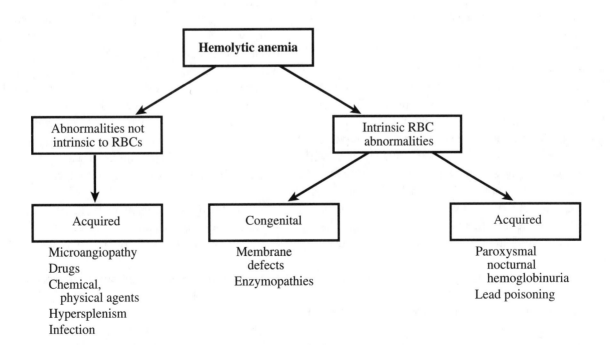

Fig. 12-4. Differential diagnosis of hemolytic anemia.

Microangiopathic hemolytic anemia is associated with thrombotic thrombocytopenic purpura, hemolytic uremic syndrome, malignant hypertension, pulmonary hypertension, acute glomerulonephritis, acute renal failure, renal allograft rejection, preeclampsia, eclampsia, disseminated intravascular coagulopathy, collagen vascular diseases, scleroderma, systemic lupus erythematosus, Wegener's syndrome, periarteritis nodosa, carcinomatosis, small gastric carcinomas, hemangiomas, Kasabach-Merritt syndrome, viral infections (HIV), and bacterial infections and as a toxic effect of mitomycin C.

Differential Diagnosis of Intravascular Hemolysis

The differential diagnosis includes transfusion reactions from ABO antibodies, microangiopathic hemolytic anemia, paroxysmal nocturnal hemoglobinuria, paroxysmal cold hemoglobinuria, autoimmune hemolytic anemia (uncommon), cold agglutinin syndrome, immune complex drug-induced hemolytic anemia, infections (including falciparum malaria and clostridial sepsis), and glucose-6-phosphate dehydrogenase deficiency.

- Most hemolysis is extravascular.

In intravascular hemolysis, hemoglobin is released into the plasma. It combines rapidly with haptoglobin, which transports it to the liver. When haptoglobin is depleted, hemoglobinemia results, and plasma turns pink-red in color at concentrations of 50-100 mg/dL.

Hemoglobinuria occurs when the plasma hemoglobin is >25 mg/100 mL. The urine may become pink, red, brown, or black. Other causes of red urine include beets, phenazopyridine (Pyridium), porphyrinuria, and myoglobinuria. Hemosiderinuria is the result of desquamation of renal tubular cells.

Coombs-Positive Hemolytic Anemia

Positive results with Coombs' test indicate the presence of C3 and/or IgG on RBCs. Twenty percent to 80% of warm antibody autoimmune hemolytic anemias are secondary. Malignancies that may be associated with Coombs-positive hemolytic anemia are many and include chronic lymphocytic leukemia, non-Hodgkin's lymphoma, and ovarian carcinoma. The Coombs' test gives positive results in 8%-15% of all hospitalized patients, and studies reveal no cause in 95% of these patients. Hemolytic transfusion reactions and drug-related causes are important causes of a positive Coombs' reaction.

- Coombs' test: detects the presence of C3 and/or IgG on RBCs.
- The cause of positive findings on Coombs' test is unknown in 95% of hospitalized patients.
- Transfusion-related and drug-related causes are important causes of a positive Coombs' reaction.

Drug-Induced Hemolytic Anemia (Mechanisms)

Autoantibody mechanism (methyldopa)--This is dose-related, and about 0.3%-0.8% of patients develop hemolysis. Hemolysis occurs in 18 weeks to 4 years after ingestion of the drug. The direct Coombs' test becomes positive in 3-6 months and is IgG in high titer. There is no anamnestic response to rechallenge. Discontinuation of use of the drug usually leads to a rapid reversal in hemolysis. The mechanism of action is related to an altered cellular immune system, with a block in the activation of suppressor T cells. Other drugs with a similar mechanism known to cause autoimmune hemolytic anemia include procainamide, ibuprofen, and cimetidine.

Drug-adsorption (hapten) immunohemolytic anemia (penicillin)--This complication requires high doses of drug for >7 days. The onset is subacute at 7-10 days. A high titer of penicillin antibody is always present in the serum. A positive Coombs' test develops in 3% of patients and is related to dose in that at 2 million units per day 30% of patients are positive and at 10 million units per day, 100% of patients are positive. A penicillin allergy is not necessarily present. Drug-absorption hemolytic anemia may be fatal if not detected early. Other drugs, including cephalosporins, tetracycline, quinidine, and cisplatin, may cause autoimmune hemolytic anemia by the same mechanism.

Immune-complex mechanism (innocent bystander) (stibophen)--An antidrug antibody forms first and reacts with the drug to form an immune complex. The antidrug antibody complex is then absorbed on the RBCs. The cell-bound complex may activate complement, causing intravascular hemolysis. The Coombs' test is positive because of the presence of complement on the RBC surface. Clinically, a small quantity of drug is sufficient to cause autoimmune hemolytic anemia if there is previous exposure. Acute intravascular hemolysis with hemoglobinemia and hemoglobinuria is the usual clinical course. Drugs implicated in this type of autoimmune hemolytic anemia include quinidine, quinine, phenacetin, acetaminophen, aminosalicylate (PAS), isoniazid (INH), streptomycin, rifampin, methadone, probenecid, insulin, sulfonylureas, hydralazine, hydrochlorothiazide, sulfa drugs, triamterene, and melphalan. Immune hemolytic anemia and renal failure are seen in patients taking captopril, hydrochlorothiazide, rifampin, dipyrone, and mitomycin C.

- Autoantibody mechanism: methyldopa.
- Drug-adsorption mechanism: penicillin.
- Immune-complex mechanism: stibophen, quinine, and quinidine.
- Some drugs produce autoimmune hemolytic anemia by more than one mechanism.

The treatment of warm autoimmune hemolytic anemia includes the following. The first general principle is to treat the underlying disease and discontinue the use of drugs that have been implicated in hemolysis. If the patient is clinically stable, do not transfuse blood. Avoid transfusion in patients with autoimmune hemolytic anemia. If the patient is symptomatic and studies show improvement in symptoms if the hemoglobin is >8 g/dL, transfuse with packed RBCs only if angina, cardiac decompensation, or neurologic symptoms (e.g., lethargy, weakness, confusion, or obtundation) are present. If transfusion is required, then transfuse with the most compatible RBCs by crossmatch with type-specific ABO and Rh blood. The major risk of transfusion is the formation of autoantibodies to foreign RBC antigens by previous transfusions and pregnancies.

If steroids are given, the dose of prednisone should be 60-80 mg/day. Most patients respond in 7 days. If the patient has a relapse during tapering of the drug, return to the previous dose. About 50% of patients with idiopathic autoimmune hemolytic anemia require other therapy. Splenectomy is required in about 60% of cases. Immunosuppressive drugs such as cyclophosphamide (60 mg/m^2 per day) or azathioprine (80 mg/m^2 per day) are the next line of therapy.

Cold Agglutinin Syndrome (Primary Cold Agglutinin Disease)

Cold agglutinin syndrome is characterized by the presence of agglutination, hemolytic anemia, a positive Coombs' test response, chronic anemia, and a "monotonous" prognosis. Autoantibodies are maximally reactive at low temperatures. The degree of hemolysis depends on the thermal amplitude: the higher the titer, the more likely to bind complement. The clinical signs and symptoms are related to small vessel occlusion and include acrocyanosis of the ears, tip of the nose, toes, and fingers. Hepatosplenomegaly is uncommon. Skin color is dusky blue and then turns normal or blanches. All digits may be affected equally. This should be differentiated from Raynaud's phenomenon, in which one or two fingers turn white to blue to red.

The peripheral blood smear shows agglutination of RBCs that disappears if prepared at 37°C (color plate 12-4). Agglutinated RBCs clump together. In rouleaux, the cells stack up on one another (color plate 12-7). The anemia is mild to moderate, and the Coombs' test is positive. The cold agglutinin titer is >1:1,000. Therapy includes avoidance of the cold. Steroids are less effective in cold than in warm autoimmune hemolytic anemia. Splenectomy is generally ineffective. Some patients may respond to immunosuppressive drugs such as cyclophosphamide or chlorambucil. Plasma exchange is not very effective but should be considered if the patient is acutely ill, because IgM is intravascular.

- Cold agglutinin syndrome: agglutination and hemolytic anemia.
- Acrocyanosis of the ears, tip of the nose, toes, fingers; differentiate from Raynaud's phenomenon.

- Positive Coombs' test response and cold agglutinin titer >1:1,000.

Immunology of Cold Agglutinins

An IgM antibody exhibits a reversible thermal-dependent equilibrium reaction with RBCs and is favored at lower temperatures. A monoclonal kappa protein is seen in cold agglutinin syndrome, chronic lymphocytic leukemia, multiple myeloma, lymphoma, and Waldenström's macroglobulinemia. In secondary diseases, there is a polyclonal light chain reaction with a high thermal cold agglutinin of anti-I specificity (*Mycoplasma pneumoniae*) or anti-I specificity (infectious mononucleosis, cytomegalovirus, and lymphoma).

Mycoplasma pneumoniae (anti-I)--In patients with *Mycoplasma pneumoniae*, 50% have cold agglutinins >1:64, most have splenomegaly, and acrocyanosis is unusual. The course of this complication generally resolves in 2-3 weeks, but fatalities have been reported. Treatment includes keeping the patient warm and treating the infection with tetracycline or erythromycin.

Infectious mononucleosis (anti-I)--Of patients with infectious mononucleosis, 40%-50% have cold agglutinins and 3% have autoimmune hemolytic anemia. The onset occurs by 13 days in 67% of patients. The duration of hemolysis is <1 month in 75% of patients and 1-2 months in 25%. Hepatosplenomegaly is present in 71% of patients. Steroids are of distinct value in treating this disorder, as may be splenectomy.

Paroxysmal Cold Hemoglobinuria (Complement-Mediated Lysis)

Paroxysmal cold hemoglobinuria is the least common cause of autoimmune hemolytic anemia. Results of the Donath-Landsteiner test are positive. This condition can be idiopathic or secondary. The secondary causes include syphilis (congenital and late), mononucleosis, mycoplasma, chickenpox, mumps, and measles. Measles is the most common secondary cause. Clinical manifestations include shaking chills, fever, malaise, abdominal pain, back pain, and leg pain. There is rapid and severe anemia. The prognosis is good. This condition resolves after the infection clears. Treatment includes protection from the cold, treatment of the underlying disease, and possibly a short course of steroids.

Coombs-Negative Hemolytic Anemias

The differential diagnosis includes the enzymopathies, glucose-6-phosphate dehydrogenase deficiency, pyruvate kinase deficiency, paroxysmal nocturnal hemoglobinuria, hereditary spherocytosis, and thrombotic thrombocytopenic purpura.

Glucose-6-Phosphate Dehydrogenase Deficiency

This is the most common RBC enzyme deficiency. It is inherited on the X chromosome and is sex-linked. All enzymopathies are autosomal recessive except glucose-6-phosphate dehydrogenase and phosphoglycerate kinase, which are sex-linked. In males, it is present in 12% of U.S. blacks, 20%-32% of Greeks, and 0.4% of Italians. In females, one X chromosome is inactivated, and the gene is present on both, so the activity ranges from 0%-100% with a mosaic population. Female heterozygotes with falciparum malaria have a selective advantage. This selective advantage has been attributed to the inhibition of parasite growth and replication through the mechanism of increased oxidant stress. The oxidation of hemoglobin leads to the formation of methemoglobin, and sulfhemoglobin may be a product, with precipitation, condensation, and attachment of the denatured portion to the inside of the membrane-forming Heinz bodies. The normal enzyme has a half-life of 62 days, but reticulocytes have a half-life of 124 days and aged cells have a half-life of 31 days. Therefore, in an acute hemolytic state, the glucose-6-phosphate level may be within normal limits. There is individual variability to oxidant stress. It is not possible to stimulate the enzyme with methylene blue or ascorbic acid to counteract the formation of methemoglobin; these drugs may actually exacerbate the anemia.

- Glucose-6-phosphate dehydrogenase deficiency: the most common RBC enzyme deficiency; inherited on the X chromosome.
- Falciparum malaria provides some protection.
- Half-life: normal, 62 days; reticulocytes, 124 days; and aged cells, 31 days.

In the steady state, there is no anemia or RBC defect. There is an increased risk of hemolysis in patients with concurrent renal or hepatic disease, viral and bacterial infections, diabetic acidosis, and low levels of blood glucose. Even a mild infection can produce hemolytic anemia, and this is more common than drug provocation. The organisms commonly associated with this complication are *Salmonella*, *Escherichia coli*, pneumococcus, *Rickettsia*, and viral hepatitis. Favism is seen only in Caucasians and not in blacks.

- No anemia or RBC defect occurs in the steady state.

Drugs commonly causing hemolytic anemia in glucose-6-phosphate dehydrogenase deficiency include antimalarial agents (primaquin and chloroquine), dapsone, sulfonamides (sulfanilamide, sulfamethoxazole, sulfapyridine, and sulfasalazine), nitrofurantoin, diazoxide, and nitrites (which are derived from nitrates from nitroglycerin, fertilizer-contaminating home wells, and amyl nitrite).

- Important to look for cause, particularly drugs.
- Infection is more common than drug provocation.

Abnormal laboratory findings include intravascular hemolysis, methemoglobinemia, and methemalbuminenia (highly specific for intravascular hemolysis). The presence of Heinz bodies on supravital staining is a good screening test, but the absence of these bodies does not rule out the diagnosis. Reticulocytosis rarely masks the deficiency in Caucasians but it may in blacks and heterozygous females. The glucose-6-phosphate dehydrogenase assay is the definitive test. Treatment includes treating the underlying infection and withdrawing use of the offending drug.

- Heinz bodies seen on supravital staining of the peripheral blood is a good screening test.
- Treat underlying infections and withdraw the use of offending drugs.

Other Enzymopathies

About 35 distinct enzymopathies have been identified, and most of them are accepted as an etiologic basis for RBC dysfunction. Two deficiency states comprise the largest number: glucose-6-phosphate dehydrogenase and pyruvate kinase. With the exception of glucose-6-phosphate dehydrogenase deficiency, potentially symptomatic enzymopathies are uncommon. Treatment is supportive and empirical. Other enzymopathies include unstable hemoglobins, glucose phosphate isomerase, pyrimidine 5'-nucleotidase, and triose phosphate isomerase deficiencies. In a study conducted on a referral population, only 35% of patients who were referred for an enzyme deficiency work-up had an identifiable enzyme deficiency.

Paroxysmal Nocturnal Hemoglobinuria

Paroxysmal nocturnal hemoglobinuria is a chronic disease caused by an unidentifiable RBC defect. Patients with this condition have a median survival of 10 years. It is a clonal disorder in which blood cells are unusually sensitive to activated complement and are lysed. Lysis is complement-mediated. Hemolysis occurs at night because this is when people become more acidotic. The disorder is characterized by abnormal pluripotent stem cells, reticulocytopenia, leukopenia, or thrombocytopenia due to lysis by complement. Normal and abnormal cells occur simultaneously in most patients. A distinct class of membrane proteins is selectively deleted from the plasma membranes of maturing cells. Defects that affect cells in paroxysmal nocturnal hemoglobinuria are related to the omission of membrane lipid phosphotidylinositol membrane proteins. This involves deficiencies in the surface molecules that normally regulate activation of C3B and C5-9 in the complement cascade. There is a decrease in a membrane protein (decay-accelerating factor) that regulates the alternate complement pathway on normal blood cells. Also, the activity of RBC acetylcholinesterase is decreased.

Clinically, paroxysmal nocturnal hemoglobinuria is characterized by a chronic hemolytic anemia with hemoglobinuria and hemoglobinemia (intravascular hemolysis). Venous thrombosis of the portal system, brain, and extremities is associated with 50% of the deaths in paroxysmal nocturnal hemoglobinuria. Episodes of severe pain may occur in the abdomen and back in conjunction with painful or difficult swallowing.

Complications include acute nonlymphocytic leukemia in 5%-10% of patients (paroxysmal nocturnal hemoglobinuria clone disappears), aplastic anemia (association of aplastic anemia, splenomegaly, and relative reticulocytosis suggests diagnosis), and venous thrombosis (Budd-Chiari syndrome is the major cause of death). Budd-Chiari syndrome is manifested by abdominal pain, tender hepatomegaly, nausea, vomiting, fever, and increased levels of lactate dehydrogenase, serum glutamic-oxaloacetic transaminase, gamma-glutamyl-transferase, and conjugated bilirubin. Hepatic ultrasonography and venography are important in making the diagnosis. Treatment includes emergent heparinization, a long-term course of anticoagulation, and fibrinolytic therapy.

Diagnosis--The sucrose hemolysis test can give false-positive results but is a good inexpensive screening test. The Ham test (acid hemolysis test) is the best confirmatory test.

Treatment--Iron therapy: a burst of erythropoiesis can be seen if the patient is iron deficient; however, in most patients, iron may be given safely. Androgen therapy stimulates bone marrow and is of most benefit if the bone marrow is hypoplastic. Prednisone (alternate-day therapy, 15-40 mg) may inhibit activation of complement by the alternate pathway. Prednisone is of no benefit if the bone marrow is hypoplastic or there is mild hemolysis. Discontinue treatment with steroids if no effect occurs in 6 weeks. Transfusions: initially, transfuse with packed RBCs. If complicated by hemolysis, washed or frozen RBCs should be given. A hemolytic crisis may be initiated by infections. Treatment may include steroids, transfusion, and hydration to prevent renal failure. For venous thrombosis, the treatment of choice is heparin, which may activate alternate pathway of complement. Painful episodes are managed with narcotics and rehydration. Bone marrow transplantation is indicated in severe aplastic anemia. Antithymocyte globulin is effective in the management of paroxysmal nocturnal hemoglobinuria.

- Paroxysmal nocturnal hemoglobinuria: a chronic disease caused by an unidentifiable RBC defect.
- Venous thrombosis is associated with 50% of deaths.
- Intravascular hemolysis with hemoglobinuria and hemoglobinemia.
- Leukemia occurs in 5%-10%; aplastic anemia.
- Diagnosis: Ham test and sucrose hemolysis test.

Hereditary Spherocytosis

Hereditary spherocytosis is an autosomal dominant disorder in which splenomegaly is invariably present. It is caused by an underlying defect in the RBC membrane cytoskeleton caused by a partial deficiency in one or more of the components called spectrin and band 4.1. Osmotic fragility of RBCs is increased. The clinical features include jaundice, splenomegaly, negative results with Coombs' test, spherocytes, and increased osmotic fragility. Gallstones are present in 43%-85% of patients. Treatment is splenectomy, which invariably causes cessation of hemolysis. It should be performed after the first decade of life.

- Hereditary spherocytosis: autosomal dominant as well as sporadic.
- Splenomegaly occurs in most patients; cholelithiasis in 43%-85%.
- Other features: negative results with Coombs' test and increased osmotic fragility.
- Treatment: splenectomy after the first decade of life.

Thrombotic Thrombocytopenic Purpura

Thrombotic thrombocytopenic purpura is a syndrome rather than a disease. Classically, it is characterized by the pentad of anemia, thrombocytopenia, neurologic signs, fever, and renal abnormalities. The anemia is normochromic-normocytic, with microangiopathic hemolytic features (color plate 12-6). The Coombs' test gives negative results. The results of coagulation studies are normal or only mildly abnormal, in contrast to disseminated intravascular coagulopathy. The cause of this syndrome is unknown in more than 90% of patients. It is related to pregnancy and the use of oral contraceptives.

Clinically, thrombocytopenia is associated with bleeding in 96% of cases--petechiae and purpura, retinal bleeding, hematuria, gingival bleeding, melena, menorrhagia, hematemesis, and hemoptysis. Neurologic signs consist of remittent and frequent changes, including headache, coma, mental changes, paresis, seizure/coma, aphasia, syncope, visual symptoms, dysarthria, vertigo, agitation, confusion, and delirium. Renal abnormalities include a creatinine level of >1.5 in less than 20% of cases. Azotemia is an unfavorable prognostic sign. An abnormal urinary sediment with proteinuria, hematuria, pyuria, or casts was present in 82% of patients in one series.

The pathologic findings are characterized by widespread intraluminal hyaline vascular occlusions with platelet aggregates and fibrin, with no inflammatory changes in terminal arterioles or capillaries in virtually any organ. The preferred biopsy site is the bone marrow. Other sites to consider for biopsy are the gingiva, skin, petechial spot, muscle, and lymph nodes.

Without treatment, >90% of patients die of multiorgan failure. With treatment, 70%-80% of patients survive the disease with little or no sequelae. The treatment of choice is plasmapheresis with the replacement of fresh frozen plasma (plasma exchange). Other ancillary treatments include dipyridamole (400-600 mg/day), aspirin (with a dose from 300 mg twice a week to 600-1,200 mg/day), and prednisone (dose of 60 mg/kg per day). The overall response rate to therapy is 80%-90%.

- Thrombotic thrombocytopenic purpura: the pentad of anemia, fever, thrombocytopenia, neurologic signs, and renal abnormalities.
- Its cause is unknown; exclude oral contraceptives and pregnancy as etiologic factors.
- Features: Coombs' test gives negative results, microangiopathy, normal prothrombin time, normal activated partial thromboplastin time, and normal fibrinogen.

Adult Hemolytic Uremic Syndrome

Adult hemolytic uremic syndrome is characterized by microangiopathic hemolytic anemia (anemia and thrombocytopenia) with a creatinine level >3 mg/dL. There is no fever or neurologic sign. The pathologic findings are similar to those in thrombotic thrombocytopenic purpura but are limited to only the kidneys. It is often preceded by an acute infective process. There is a much higher morbidity and mortality rate in adults, and adult hemolytic uremic syndrome is best managed as thrombotic thrombocytopenic purpura is in adults. This may be associated with *E. coli* O 157:H7 diarrhea. The management of the hemolytic-uremic syndrome is supportive in this situation. Dialysis may be necessary. The efficacy of plasmapheresis and plasma exchange has not been proved.

Sickle Cell Anemia

Sickle cell anemia is the most common heritable hematologic disease affecting humans. The gene must be inherited from both parents. It occurs in black Africans and rarely in Caucasians. About 8% of blacks carry the sickle cell gene, with the disease occurring in 1/625 of them. There is a selective advantage from *Plasmodium falciparum* malaria, with preferential sickling of only the parasitized cells. Hemoglobin S is different from hemoglobin A in the substitution of valine for glutamic acid at the sixth position, resulting in abnormalities in polymerization (or gelation), with deoxygenation that leads to sickling. The end result of the polymerization is a permanently altered membrane protein. Two-thirds of the RBCs are removed by extravascular mechanisms.

Sickling is promoted by low oxygen tension, low pH, increased 2,3-diphosphoglycerate, high cellular concentration of hemoglobins, loss of cell water, hemoglobin D, and HbO-ARAB. Sickling is retarded by hemoglobin F.

Symptoms are not present until the patient is older than 6 months. Vaso-occlusive disease develops between the ages of 12 months and 6 years. Acute crises are due to recurrent obstruction of the microcirculation by intravascular sickling. Laboratory testing is not helpful. Atypical symptoms should suggest pneumonia, pulmonary infarct, acute pyelonephritis, or cholecystitis.

Bone and joint crises: bone and joint symptoms include gnawing pain and swelling of the elbows and knees. Radiographs may show bone infarcts and periostitis, but these do not appear until symptoms subside. Infarcts and periostitis may be documented with bone scans. Abdominal crises: small infarcts of mesentery and abdominal viscera with symptoms of 4-5 days' duration. This is a nonsurgical problem if bowel sounds are present.

Central nervous system crises: children and young adults are more susceptible. Children have infarcts, and adults characteristically have hemorrhages. Do not perform angiographic procedures unless the patient has been prepared with RBCs. The therapy for these crises is immediate exchange transfusion. Chronic transfusion therapy is indicated in this complication to maintain hemoglobin S <30%, because the risk of recurrent episodes is >50%.

Pulmonary crises: acute chest syndrome accounts for 20% of deaths. Clinical aspects include fever, chest pain, tachypnea, increased WBC count, and pulmonary infarcts. Age makes a difference in cause. In children, infected segments enhance local sickling, so sickling is a secondary phenomenon. The causative organisms include pneumococcus, *Mycoplasma*, *Haemophilus*, *Salmonella*, and *E. coli*. In adults, sickling tends to be a primary event, with no signs of infection.

Aplastic crises: usually follow a febrile illness, with disappearance of reticulocytes and normoblasts. They last 5-10 days. Hemolytic crises: may occur in patients with concomitant glucose-6-phosphate dehydrogenase deficiency, hereditary spherocytosis, and mycoplasmal pneumonia.

Infectious crises are the most frequent cause of death of patients younger than 5 years. The organisms include *Streptococcus pneumoniae* of the blood and spinal fluid (70% of patients). Normally, 80% of the cases of meningitis are caused by *Haemophilus influenzae* in this age group. At ages older than 5 years, gram-negative bacteria predominate, with osteomyelitis caused by *Staphylococcus*, pneumococcus, and *Salmonella*. The causes of infections/infectious crises include decreased IgM, defective alternate pathway, deficiency phagocytosis-promoting peptide tuftsin, and impaired splenic function. The challenge with *Streptococcus pneumoniae* is not followed by appropriate opsonin production.

Chronic manifestations--There is a progressive lag in growth and development after the first decade of life and a chronic destruction of bone and joints, with ischemia and infarction of the spongiosa. The vertebrae become fish-mouthed. Avascular necrosis is common in multiple joints. Ocular manifestations include stasis and occlusion of small vessels that is nonproliferative or proliferative. They may require laser photocoagulation. Cardiovascular manifestations include cardiomegaly, flow murmurs, and a pansystolic murmur with click that mimics mitral regurgitation. Restrictive lung disease may develop. Hepatobiliary manifestations include hepatomegaly with the pathologic features of distended sinusoids, periportal fibrosis, and hemosiderin pigment. Marked hyperbilirubinemia may be due to hepatitis, intrahepatic sickling, choledocholithiasis, or coexistent glucose-6-phosphate dehydrogenase deficiency. There is an increased incidence of pigmented gallstones in 30%-60% of adults, with symptoms in 10%-15%. Renal manifestations include papillary necrosis, hyposthenuria by age 6-12 months (disruption of countercurrent multiplier system, nocturia, enuresis), hematuria (ulcer in renal pelvis, urate stones), nephrotic syndrome secondary to focal segmental glomerulonephropathy, tubular damage secondary to small infarcts, and priapism. Leg ulcers may occur.

In pregnancy, there is no increase in disease manifestations, but there is an increase in maternal mortality of 20% and fetal mortality of 20%. Early complications of pregnancy include thrombophlebitis, pyelonephritis, and hematuria. Late complications include major infarcts of the lung, kidney, and brain; toxemia; congestive heart failure; and postpartum endometritis.

Laboratory findings include anemia (range, 5.5-9.5 g/dL), sickled cells, cigar cells, ovalocytes, targets, basophilic stippling, polychromatophilia, reticulocytes (8%-12%), and hyposplenia with Howell-Jolly bodies. A persistent increase in the WBC count of 12,000-15,000 is characteristic. On hemoglobin electrophoresis, hemoglobin S moves more slowly than hemoglobin A.

Treatment--The primary treatment is prevention. Infection, fever, dehydration, acidosis, hypoxemia, cold, and high altitude should be avoided. Acetaminophen is indicated for fever because aspirin contributes to an acid load. A temperature >105°F means infection, and infection is uncommon if the temperature is <102°F. Prophylactic use of penicillin is beneficial. Vaccines, including pneumococcal, influenza A, and *Haemophilus*, are indicated, as is folate supplementation, especially in pregnancy. Iron chelation is recommended if the transfusion requirement is high. Splenectomy is recommended for those children who survive the initial splenic sequestration crisis. This is the only indication for splenectomy. Blood transfusion and exchange transfusion are the most effective means of treatment available. The hemoglobin S cells should be decreased to <30%. These modalities are especially indicated for the following: history of cerebral vascular accidents, progressive retinopathy, renal or cardiac decompensation preoperatively, and pregnancy (at 30-34 weeks, maintain hemoglobin >10 g/dL). Short-term transfusion therapy is indicated in acute chest syndrome. Other indications for transfusion are priapism, protracted hematuria, and chronic skin ulcers. In vaso-occlusive crises, the cornerstone of treatment includes fluids and correction of urinary sodium losses. Other important considerations are treatment of infections: penicillin in children and coverage for *Staphylococcus* in adults. Analgesics are essential. Blood transfusions do not modify the course. Prenatal diagnosis may be made by analysis of amniotic fluid or chorionic villi biopsy, which is preferred to fetal blood sampling. In the Multicenter Study of Hydroxyurea in Sickle Cell Anemia, which was a double-blinded, placebo-controlled trial, hydroxyurea decreased the frequency of painful

vaso-occlusive crises by about 50%. In patients with severe recurrent episodes, the frequency of the acute chest syndrome was decreased and patients required fewer transfusions. Hydroxyurea increases fetal hemoglobin and may prevent the cells from becoming rigid, preventing vaso-occlusion.

The Cooperative Study of Sickle Cell Disease reported in a prospective analysis that 50% of patients with sickle cell anemia survived beyond the fifth decade. Few patients survive into their 60s. Symptomatic patients had the highest early mortality. A high level of fetal hemoglobin predicted improved survival in young patients. Acute chest syndrome, renal failure, seizures, a baseline WBC count >15 x 10^9/L, and a low level of fetal hemoglobin were associated with the risk of early death in patients 20 years of age or older. In adults, 78% of patients died during an acute sickle cell crisis. Acute pain and chest syndrome was the most common cause of death, and stroke was the next most common cause. This was followed by infection (*E. coli*, *Staphylococcus aureus*, HIV, tuberculosis, malaria, pneumococcus, and hepatitis). In children younger than 5 years, the cause of infection is almost universally pneumococcal sepsis.

Sickle cell trait occurs in 8% of American blacks. There is no anemia, RBC abnormalities, increased risk of infections, or increased mortality; 35%-45% of hemoglobin is hemoglobin S. Associations with sickle cell trait include hematuria, splenic infarction at high altitude (over 10,000 feet), hyposthenuria, bacteriuria, pyelonephritis in pregnancy, and reduced mortality from *Plasmodium falciparum* infection.

In hemoglobin SC disease, patients have only hemoglobin S and C, with an absence of hemoglobin A and normal or increased levels of hemoglobin F. Patients with sickle cell hemoglobin C survive longer than those with sickle cell anemia. The sickle cell hemoglobin C disorder is less severe than sickle cell disease with three exceptions: proliferative retinopathy, aseptic necrosis of femoral heads, and acute chest syndrome secondary to fat emboli in the final months of pregnancy. There is mild anemia; in 10% of patients, the hemoglobin is <10 g/dL. Sickle cells are rare on the peripheral blood smear, and 50% of the cells in the peripheral blood are target cells. The spleen remains functional.

Hemoglobin S/β-thalassemia is less severe than sickle cell disease. The spleen remains functional, but retinopathy is more common.

- Hydroxyurea decreases the frequency of painful vaso-occlusive crises by 50%.
- Acute chest syndrome, renal failure, seizures, a baseline WBC count >15,000/mL, and a low level of fetal hemoglobin are associated with a risk of early death in adults.
- Death is associated with acute pain and chest syndrome, stroke, and infection.
- Patients with sickle cell hemoglobin C survive longer than those with sickle cell anemia.

MALIGNANCIES

Chronic Lymphocytic Leukemia

Chronic lymphocytic leukemia is a lymphoproliferative disorder of mature lymphocytes (color plate 12-8). It is the commonest form of leukemia in patients 60 years and older in the Western world; 90% of patients are older than 50. Chronic lymphocytic leukemia is more of an accumulative than a proliferative disorder of long-lived immunologically incompetent cells. It is rare in the Orient. The two staging classifications are outlined in Tables 12-3 and 12-4.

Predictors of survival include stage, response to initial treatment, WBC count >50,000/mL, abnormal chromosomes, and lymphocyte doubling time (unfavorable if <12 months).

Complications include recurrent infection; 50% of patients have hypogammaglobulinemia. Fever in chronic lymphocytic leukemia is secondary to infection and not to chronic lymphocytic leukemia. The exception is Richter's syndrome. Immunologic complications include autoimmune hemolytic anemia (in 10% of patients); immune-mediated thrombocytopenia (in <5%), which is IgG-mediated and is treated with steroids; and pure RBC aplasia.

- In chronic lymphocytic leukemia, fever = infection (except for Richter's syndrome).
- Hypogammaglobulinemia in 50% of patients with recurrent infection.
- Autoimmune hemolytic anemia in 10%.
- Thrombocytopenia in <5%.

- Prophylactic gamma globulins are indicated for gamma globulin levels <0.3 g/dL with or without previous infection.

Chronic lymphocytic leukemia is associated with increased incidence of solid tumors of the lung and skin (basal cell, squamous cell). Other hematologic malignancies associated with chronic lymphocytic leukemia include Richter's syndrome, which is chronic lymphocytic leukemia that has transformed into large cell lymphoma and is characterized by fevers, massive asymmetrical adenopathy, splenomegaly, and a poor outcome. Also, patients may develop secondary drug-induced acute nonlymphocytic leukemia. Infectious complications include *Staphylococcus aureus*, pneumococci, *Pseudomonas*, *Klebsiella*, *Pneumocystis*, cytomegalovirus, *Candida*, herpes simplex, and herpes zoster.

Laboratory findings: lymphocytes are usually monotonous, small, and may be clefted; 97% express common B-cell antigens CD19 and CD20, surface immunoglobulins IgM or IgM and IgD, and coexpress T-cell-specific antigen CD5. Chromosomal abnormalities are found in 55% of patients. Of these, trisomy 12 is the common one. Structural abnormalities of chromosomes 13 and 14 are also seen. Patients with chromosome abnormalities are likely to have a worse prognosis. To date, there is no evidence of pure clonal remissions or cure with treatment. The median survival time is 5 years from the onset of treatment.

- Trisomy 12 is the most common chromosomal abnormality.

Table 12-3.--Staging: Rai Classification

Stage	Characteristics	No. patients	Median survival time, mo	No. patients[*]	Median survival time, mo
0	Peripheral (>15 x 10^9/L) lymphocytosis, bone marrow lymphocytosis (>40%)	22	>150	79	129
I	Lymphocytosis, lymphadenopathy	29	101	154	74.4
II	Lymphocytosis, splenomegaly	39	71	203	58.2
III	Lymphocytosis, anemia with hemoglobin <11, excluding AIHA	21	19	127	28.1
IV	Lymphocytosis, thrombocytopenia	14	19	105	19.3

[*]Six combined series.

Data from Rai KR, Sawitsky A, Cronkite EP, Chanana AD, Levy RN, Pasternack BS: Clinical staging of chronic lymphocytic leukemia. Blood 46:219-234, 1975.

Table 12-4.--Classification of International Workshop on Chronic Lymphocytic Leukemia

Clinical stage	Features
A	No anemia or thrombocytopenia and fewer areas of lymphoid enlargement. (Spleen, liver, and lymph nodes in cervical, axillary, and inguinal regions.) A(0), A(I), or A(II).
B	No anemia or thrombocytopenia with three or more involved areas. B(I) or B(II).
C	Anemia (<10 g/dL) and/or thrombocytopenia regardless of the number of areas of lymphoid enlargement. C(III) or C(IV).

From International Workshop on CLL: Chronic lymphocytic leukaemia: proposals for a revised prognostic staging system. Br J Haematol 48:365-367, 1981. By permission of Blackwell Scientific Publications.

Specific treatment--A French study compared treatment versus no treatment in early stage disease, and there was no difference in survival. In contrast, survival in patients with advanced stage disease is better if the chronic lymphocytic leukemia responds to treatment, with a median response duration of 4 years versus 1 year in nonresponders. Chlorambucil and/or prednisone is the initial treatment of choice. The overall response is 60%-70%. Prednisone alone is indicated in immune-related anemia and thrombocytopenia. Fludarabine is the treatment of choice for chronic lymphocytic leukemia in relapse. Fludarabine induces an overall response rate of 50%-60% in previously treated patients and 80% in previously untreated ones. The dose-limiting toxicity of fludarabine is myelosuppression, which predisposes to opportunistic infections secondary to a quantitative suppression in T-helper (CD4) lymphocytes. Splenectomy is recommended for refractory immune complications, massive splenomegaly, and hypersplenism. Other options include systemic chemotherapy with cyclophosphamide, vincristine, doxorubicin (Adriamycin), and prednisone.

Treatment guidelines--Rai classification:
Stage 0--No treatment.
Stage I and stage II--Treat only if symptomatic from bulky lymphadenopathy or hepatosplenomegaly or WBC count is >50 x 10^9/L. If the disease is stable and there is no impairment of job status, no treatment is necessary. There is no documentation of an increase in survival with early treatment. In fact, one study has shown an increased risk of secondary malignancies with no increase in survival.

Stage III and stage IV--Short median life expectancy, invariably symptomatic. Treat all patients to alleviate symptoms and to improve life expectancy.

Treatment guidelines--International Workshop classification:
Stage A--Observe.
Stage B--Some patients will need treatment, as outlined in stages I and II indications above.
Stage C--Treat all patients.

- Observe stage 0 or stage A patients.
- Treat patients with Rai stages III and IV disease and International Workshop stages B and C.
- Overall response rate to chlorambucil and/or prednisone is 60%-70%.
- Fludarabine is the treatment of choice for patients who have relapse.

Hairy Cell Leukemia

Hairy cell leukemia is characterized by an insidious onset of cytopenias without constitutional symptoms. At some time during the course of the disease, 90% of patients have splenomegaly. The hairy cell cytoplasmic projections are "hairy" with multiple, thin, or blunt projections (color plate 12-9). The cells contain tartrate-resistant acid phosphatase (positive TRAP stain). Most are B-cell in nature and clonal, as demonstrated by light- and heavy-chain immunoglobulin gene rearrangements. Hairy cell leukemia accounts for <2% of all cases of leukemias. The cause is not known.

- Hairy cell leukemia: cytopenias.
- Splenomegaly is common.
- Hairy cells have cytoplasmic projections.
- B-cell in nature and clonal.
- Constitutes <2% of all cases of leukemias.

Clinical characteristics--The symptoms are related to cytopenias, infections, and splenomegaly.

- Middle-aged patients.
- Splenomegaly in 90% of patients.
- Infections are related to cytopenias.

Laboratory findings reveal anemia, thrombocytopenia, neutropenia, and pancytopenia. More than 75% of patients have anemia, thrombocytopenia, and neutropenia. The bone marrow yields a dry tap on bone marrow aspiration; biopsy specimens are hypercellular with diffuse infiltration. Hairy cells may or may not be seen in the peripheral blood.

- Cytopenias in 75% of patients with hairy cell leukemia.
- Bone marrow: dry tap.

- Hairy cells may not be seen in peripheral blood smear.
- Infection is related to granulocytopenia and impaired cell-mediated immunity.

Complications--Infection is the major cause of death. Infection should be considered when a previously stable patient develops new symptoms. Fever is not a manifestation of the disease but indicates an underlying infection. Localized pyogenic infections are more common, e.g., bacterial pneumonia, urinary tract infections, and infections of the skin. The incidence of atypical mycobacterial infections is increased. There is a higher incidence of viral infections, fungal infections, parasitic diseases, toxoplasmosis, histoplasmosis, coccidiosis, and pneumocystis. Bleeding and vasculitis (skin, joint, erythema nodosum) are other complications.

- Hairy cell leukemia: Infection is the major cause of death.
- Fever denotes infection.
- Atypical mycobacterial infections.

Treatment--Observation may be indicated for patients who are asymptomatic with very mild cytopenias. Indications for intervention include significant cytopenia, serious or recurrent infections associated with neutropenia, bleeding secondary to thrombocytopenia, splenic infarction, vasculitis, and increasing number of hairy cells. 2-Chlorodeoxyadenosine produces complete remission in 85%-88% of patients after a single 7-day continuous, intravenous infusion. Other treatments include interferon alfa-2a or 2b recombinant, which produces a 13% complete remission after 18 months of subcutaneous treatments and a partial remission rate of 66%. 2'-Deoxycoformycin produces complete remission rates in 75% of patients, with a relapse rate of 10%. Splenectomy only improves peripheral blood cell counts and has no effect on the bone marrow. The only indications for splenectomy are a very large spleen and patchy bone marrow involvement in a young patient, splenic infarct, and profound life-threatening bleeding secondary to thrombocytopenia.

- 2-Chlorodeoxyadenosine is the treatment of choice in hairy cell leukemia.
- Other treatments include 2'-deoxycoformycin, interferon alfa-2a or 2b recombinant, and splenectomy.

Lymphadenopathy

The differential diagnosis of lymphadenopathy is very broad. The differential diagnosis of lymphadenopathy and fever with or without splenomegaly includes the following:

1. Infectious mononucleosis, Epstein-Barr virus, cytomegalovirus, and toxoplasmosis.
2. Syphilis, subacute bacterial endocarditis, sarcoidosis, *Salmonella*, tuberculosis, and acquired immune deficiency (AIDS).
3. Hodgkin's disease, non-Hodgkin's lymphoma, angioimmunoblastic lymphadenopathy, mixed essential cryoglobulinemia, systemic mastocytosis, chronic lymphocytic leukemia, myelofibrosis, Waldenström's macroglobulinemia, and multiple myeloma.
4. Systemic lupus erythematosus and rheumatoid arthritis.
5. Kawasaki disease, Whipple's disease, serum sickness, and Kaposi's sarcoma.

Hodgkin's Disease

The diagnosis of Hodgkin's disease is based upon the presence of Reed-Sternberg cells, which typically have two or more nuclei with prominent nucleoli, giving the cells the appearance of owl's eyes (color plate 12-10).

The Rye classification divides Hodgkin's disease into four subtypes: nodular sclerosing Hodgkin's disease (40%-70%), mixed cellularity Hodgkin's disease (20%-40%), lymphocyte-depleted Hodgkin's disease (rare), and lymphocyte-predominant Hodgkin's disease (5%). Lymphocyte-predominant Hodgkin's disease has distinctive histologic and immunologic features. Polymerase chain reaction detects Epstein-Barr virus in 60%-80% of cases. The staging classification is outlined in Table 12-5, and the staging procedures in Table 12-6.

Disease stage is the principal factor in selecting treatment for patients with Hodgkin's disease. Lymphangiography complements computed tomography. Special procedures include formal staging laparotomy, magnetic resonance imaging, gallium scan, bone scan, and liver/spleen scan. Prognostic factors in limited stage Hodgkin's disease include age <40, more than three sites of disease involvement, mixed cellularity, lymphocyte-depleted Hodgkin's disease, and B symptoms.

Staging laparotomy may be performed if radiation therapy is the treatment of choice, if detection of intra-abdominal disease would alter the choice of therapy, and if there are not adverse factors for relapse, such as a large mediastinal mass. Staging laparotomy is not indicated in clinical stage IIIB to IVB patients. The risk of abdominal involvement in patients younger than 35 years with nodular sclerosing Hodgkin's disease and high cervical neck nodes is low, and staging laparotomy may not be indicated in this setting.

Currently, the treatment for patients who are not part of a clinical trial and who have pathologic stage IA or IIA disease above the diaphragm without a bulky mediastinal mass and less than five nodules in the spleen is mantle field radiation, with radiation fields extended to include all nodes above the diaphragm and the para-aortic regions at a dose of 35-44 Gy. The freedom from progression and survival rates at 14 years were 93% and 83%, respectively, in one series. Most relapses after radiation therapy occur within 2 years after treatment. Approximately 66% of patients who have relapse after radiation therapy are long-term survivors after chemotherapy treatment.

The treatment of choice in patients with stages IIB, III2A, IIIB, or IV disease is chemotherapy. The most important factor

Table 12-5.--The Cotswolds Staging Classification of Hodgkin's Disease

Classification	Description
Stage I	Involvement of a single lymph node region or lymphoid structure
Stage II	Involvement of two or more lymph node regions on the same side of the diaphragm (the mediastinum is considered a single site, whereas hilar lymph nodes are considered bilaterally)
Stage III	Involvement of lymph node regions or structures on both sides of the diaphragm
Stage III-1	With or without involvement of splenic, hilar, celiac, or portal nodes
Stage III-2	With involvement of para-aortic, iliac, and mesenteric nodes
Stage IV	Involvement of one or more extranodal sites in addition to a site for which the designation "E" has been used
	Designations applicable to any disease stage
A	No symptoms
B	Fever (temperature >38°C), drenching night sweats, unexplained loss of >10% of body weight within the preceding 6 months
X	Bulky disease (a widening of the mediastinum by more than 1/3 or the presence of a nodal mass with a maximal dimension >10 cm)
E	Involvement of a single extranodal site that is contiguous or proximal to the known nodal site
CS	Clinical stage
PS	Pathologic stage (as determined by laparotomy)

From Lister TA, Crowther D: Staging for Hodgkin's disease. Semin Oncol 17:696-703, 1990. By permission of WB Saunders Company.

Table 12-6.--Staging Procedures for Hodgkin's Disease

History and examination: identification of B symptoms

Imaging procedures: plain chest radiography, computed tomography of the thorax, computed tomographic scan of the abdomen and pelvis, and bipedal lymphangiography

Hematologic procedures: full blood cell count with differential, determination of erythrocyte sedimentation rate, and bilateral bone marrow aspiration and biopsy

Biochemical procedures: tests of liver function and measurement of serum albumin, lactate dehydrogenase, and calcium

Special procedures: laparotomy, ultrasonographic scanning, magnetic resonance imaging, gallium scanning, technetium bone scanning, and liver-spleen scanning

Staging laparotomies: performed only if radiation therapy is the desired treatment, so is not indicated in clinical stage IIIB to IVB patients; the detection of intra-abdominal disease would alter the choice of therapy. Patients should not have adverse features for relapse, such as a large mediastinal mass. The risk of abdominal involvement in females younger than 35 years with nodular sclerosing Hodgkin's disease and high cervical neck nodes is low

Modified from Lister TA, Crowther D: Staging for Hodgkin's disease. Semin Oncol 17:696-703, 1990. By permission of WB Saunders Company.

influencing the outcome after chemotherapy is the intensity of the dose. Multiple regimens have been evaluated and are effective. In a three-arm trial, the Cancer and Leukemia Group B (CALGB) compared MOPP (nitrogen mustard, vincristine [Oncovin], procarbazine, and prednisone) with ABVD (doxorubicin [Adriamycin], bleomycin, vinblastine, dacarbazine) and MOPP/ABVD. MOPP/ABVD was administered for 12 months. ABVD and MOPP/ABVD were superior to MOPP. The complete remission rates in stages IIIA2, IIIB, and IV were 83%, with 65% of patients alive and disease-free at 5 years (Table 12-7).

Salvage therapy for patients who have relapse consists of conventional-dose chemotherapy or autologous bone marrow transplantation. The National Cancer Institute reported that a second complete remission was seen in 93% of patients who had initial remissions of at least 12 months compared with 29% of those whose initial remissions were of shorter duration. The first randomized trial comparing high-dose chemotherapy followed by autologous bone marrow transplantation with conventional-dose salvage chemotherapy in patients with relapse and refractory Hodgkin's disease revealed that the 3-year event-free survival was 53% for the transplanted group versus 10% for the conventional chemotherapy group. These results were significantly different statistically, and the trial was closed early. These and other data suggest that autologous bone marrow or peripheral blood stem-cell

Table 12-7--Initial Treatment of Hodgkin's Disease

Stage	Type	Response
IA	Radiation therapy (mantle and para-aortic)	93% freedom from progression
IIA	Radiation, extended field (mantle and para-aortic)	82% freedom from progression
IIIA1	Radiation	
IIIA2, IIIB, IV	Chemotherapy	65% of patients receiving ABVD or MOPP/ABVD were alive and disease-free at 5 years

ABVD, doxorubicin, bleomycin, vinblastine, and dacarbazine; MOPP, nitrogen mustard, vincristine, procarbazine, and prednisone.

transplantation is indicated after first relapse from any front-line Hodgkin's disease chemotherapy regimen irrespective of the duration of remission.

Late complications of Hodgkin's disease are significant. The risks include infertility, amenorrhea, pneumococcal sepsis in 7% of patients following splenectomy, hypothyroidism, thyroid carcinoma, avascular necrosis, cardiomyopathy secondary to doxorubicin or radiation therapy, radiation pneumonitis, pulmonary fibrosis, and secondary cancers. The secondary cancers include acute nonlymphocytic leukemia, myelodysplastic syndromes, non-Hodgkin's lymphoma, and solid tumors. ABVD is less leukemogenic than MOPP. Patients at highest risk are those who have received multiple courses of chemotherapy. The risk of non-Hodgkin's lymphoma is 4% at 10 years. Radiation therapy increases the risk of solid tumors. After 15 years, the risk of secondary solid tumors is 13%; these tumors include cancers of the stomach, breast, lung, thyroid, skin, and head and neck.

- Polymerase chain reaction detects Epstein-Barr virus in 60%-80% of cases of Hodgkin's disease.
- Disease stage is the principal factor in selecting treatment for patients with Hodgkin's disease.
- The treatment of choice for patients who are not part of a clinical trial and who have pathologic stage IA or IIA disease above the diaphragm without a bulky mediastinal mass and <5 nodules in the spleen: mantle field radiation, with radiation fields extending to include the para-aortic regions.
- The treatment of choice for patients with pathologic stage IIB, III2A, IIIB, or IV disease: chemotherapy.
- Autologous bone marrow or peripheral blood stem-cell transplantation is indicated after first relapse from any front-line chemotherapy for Hodgkin's disease.
- Complications of survival include acute nonlymphocytic leukemia, solid tumors, and cardiomyopathy.

Non-Hodgkin's Lymphoma

Non-Hodgkin's lymphomas are clinically, pathologically, cytogenetically, and immunologically a diverse group of lymphoproliferative disorders. The prognosis depends on the histologic subtype, stage, and other clinical and laboratory features. At least eight different classification schemes are used world-wide; not all of them are derived from information on cytochemistry, chromosomes, or oncogenes. Not all subcategories can be translated from one classification scheme to another. The Working Formulation for Clinical Usage, which groups non-Hodgkin's lymphomas by natural history and response to therapy, has been the most widely used scheme in the U.S. (Table 12-8). This and other existing schemas are based on morphologic patterns only. These morphologic patterns have characteristically associated cytogenetic abnormalities and oncogene associations. The Revised European-American Lymphoma Classification is the most recently proposed classification (Table 12-9).

The low-grade non-Hodgkin's lymphomas are a group of lymphoproliferative disorders that 1) are not curable (unless pathologic stage I disease), 2) present with advanced stage III and IV disease, 3) are very treatable with simple programs, 4) occur in older patients, and 5) have a long survival. Often patients die of causes other than lymphoma. The paradox of the non-Hodgkin's lymphomas is that the low-grade non-Hodgkin's lymphomas are not curable, but patients live for a long time. In contrast, the intermediate and high-grade lymphomas are potentially curable, but the length of survival is short if the patient does not go into remission. Patients may progress to a more aggressive lymphoma, with a risk that ranges from 10% to 70% in reported series, depending on frequency of new biopsies at the time of progression, follow-up duration, and post-mortem data. The median age is 50-60 years. The median survival rates exceed 10-15 years.

Because the low-grade non-Hodgkin's lymphomas are not curable, the most reliable end points are progression-free survival and overall survival. Achievement of a complete remission is not a viable end point in low-grade lymphomas, because marrow infiltration is difficult to evaluate. Immunoglobulin kappa/lambda light chain restriction studies in peripheral blood and flow cytometry demonstrate circulating cells in peripheral blood after treatment in patients who

Table 12-8.--Non-Hodgkin's Lymphomas

Classification	
Low grade	Malignant lymphoma: small lymphocytic
	Malignant lymphoma: follicular, predominantly small cleaved cell
	Malignant lymphoma: follicular, mixed small cleaved and large cell
Intermediate grade	Malignant lymphoma: follicular, predominantly large cell
	Malignant lymphoma: diffuse, small cleaved cell
	Malignant lymphoma: diffuse, mixed small and large cell
	Malignant lymphoma: diffuse large cell
High grade	Malignant lymphoma: large cell immunoblastic
	Malignant lymphoma: lymphoblastic
	Malignant lymphoma: small noncleaved cell
Miscellaneous	Composite malignant lymphoma
	Mycosis fungoides
	Extramedullary plasmacytoma
	Unclassified
	Other

Modified from The Non-Hodgkin's Lymphoma Pathologic Classification Project: National Cancer Institute sponsored study of classification of non-Hodgkin's lymphoma: summary and description of a working formulation for clinical usage. Cancer 49:2112-2135, 1982. By permission of American Cancer Society.

have been deemed to be in remission, and polymerase chain reaction studies have demonstrated abnormal cell populations in patients believed to be in complete remission.

Most patients with low-grade non-Hodgkin's lymphoma have stage II or IV disease, which is not curable with standard treatment regimens. Observation is the initial treatment of choice in asymptomatic patients. The Stanford group reported on 83 patients with advanced disease who were not treated initially and had an actuarially predicted survival of 82% at 5 years and 73% at 10 years. At median follow-up of 50 months, 51 of the 83 patients (61%) required therapy at a median interval of 3 years from the time of diagnosis. Spontaneous regression was observed in 19 patients, partial remission in 13, and complete remission in 6. In a randomized trial in selected asymptomatic patients who were randomized to ProMACE-MOPP plus total lymphoid irradiation or to observation, there was no survival difference between the two groups.

For those patients with symptoms, bulky disease, or progressive disease, options with the goal of achieving complete remission include oral chlorambucil taken daily, intravenous CVP (cyclophosphamide, vincristine, and prednisone), CVP with total lymphoid irradiation, or CHOP (cyclophosphamide, doxorubicin, vincristine, and prednisone).

In patients with the histologic features of intermediate-grade non-Hodgkin's lymphoma, anthracycline chemotherapy regimens are the hallmark of therapy, with complete remission rates of 60%-80% of patients with stage II to IV disease, with the long-term disease-free survival as predicted by the International Index. The intergroup trial in the U.S. compared CHOP (cyclophosphamide, doxorubicin, vincristine, and prednisone), m-BACOD (methotrexate, bleomycin, doxorubicin, cyclophosphamide, vincristine, and dexamethasone), ProMACE-CytaBOM (cyclophosphamide, doxorubicin, etoposide, prednisone, cytarabine, bleomycin, vincristine, methotrexate, and leucovorin), and MACOP-B (methotrexate, doxorubicin, cyclophosphamide, vincristine, bleomycin, and prednisone) and found no statistically significant difference in the 3-year disease-free survival. The mortality rates were higher in m-BACOD and MACOP-B. Trials are now under way comparing standard treatment with the incorporation of autologous bone marrow transplantation as primary treatment. Currently, CHOP is the reference standard of treatment for intermediate-grade non-Hodgkin's lymphoma.

In nonrandomized studies of patients with relapse who received very high doses of therapy and autologous bone marrow transplant, the overall cure rates have been reported to be 20%. In patients who had relapse after complete remission and who are sensitive to retreatment with standard chemotherapy regimens, the reported cure rates are 35%-40%.

In a trial comparing autologous bone marrow transplantation with sequential chemotherapy for intermediate-grade and high-grade non-Hodgkin's lymphoma in first complete remission in a study of 464 patients, the LNH-84 regimen was compared with high-dose cyclophosphamide, carmustine, and etoposide (CBV) followed by autologous bone marrow transplantation. There was no improvement in disease-free or overall survival in this study. A more productive approach may be to select those patients with adverse prognostic factors who are in complete remission to proceed with autologous bone marrow transplantation therapy. In this study, only 44% of patients were considered high-intermediate or high risk by the age-adjusted index. This and other studies show the difficulties of demonstrating a role for autologous bone marrow transplantation as part of the initial management of non-Hodgkin's lymphoma.

Preliminary information on patients who have not entered complete remission with initial chemotherapy is more interesting. In an Italian study, patients who achieved partial remission were randomized to either chemotherapy with DHAP (dexamethasone, high-dose cytarabine, and cisplatin) or

Table 12-9.--Lymphoid Neoplasms Recognized by the International Lymphoma Study Group

B-cell neoplasms

I. Precursor B-cell neoplasm: precursor B-lymphoblastic leukemia/lymphoma

II. Peripheral B-cell neoplasms
1. B-cell chronic lymphocytic leukemia/prolymphocytic leukemia/small lymphocytic lymphoma
2. Lymphoplasmacytoid lymphoma/immunocytoma
3. Mantle cell lymphoma
4. Follicle center lymphoma, follicular
   Provisional cytologic grades: I (small cell), II (mixed small and large cell), III (large cell)
   Provisional subtype: diffuse, predominantly small cell type
5. Marginal zone B-cell lymphoma
   Extranodal (MALT-type with or without monocytoid B cells)
6. Provisional entity: Splenic marginal zone lymphoma (with or without villous lymphocytes)
7. Hairy-cell leukemia
8. Plasmacytoma/plasma cell myeloma
9. Diffuse large B-cell lymphoma*
10. Burkitt's lymphoma
11. Provisional entity: high-grade B-cell lymphoma, Burkitt-like*

T-cell and putative natural killer-cell neoplasms

I. Precursor T-cell neoplasm: precursor T-lymphoblastic lymphoma/leukemia

II. Peripheral T-cell and natural killer-cell neoplasms
1. T-cell chronic lymphocytic leukemia/prolymphocytic leukemia
2. Large granular lymphocytic leukemia (LGL)
   T-cell type
   NK-cell type
3. Mycosis fungoides/Sézary syndrome
4. Peripheral T-cell lymphomas, unspecified*
   Provisional cytologic categories: medium-sized cell, mixed medium and large cell, large cell, lymphoepithelioid cell
   Provisional subtype: hepatosplenic γδ T-cell lymphoma
   Provisional subtype: subcutaneous panniculitic T-cell lymphoma
5. Angioimmunoblastic T-cell lymphoma (AILD)
6. Angiocentric lymphoma
7. Intestinal T-cell lymphoma (with or without enteropathy associated)
8. Adult T-cell lymphoma/leukemia (ATL/L)
9. Anaplastic large-cell lymphoma (ALCL), CD30+, T and null-cell types
10. Provisional entity: anaplastic large-cell lymphoma, Hodgkin's-like

Hodgkin's disease

I. Lymphocyte predominance

II. Nodular sclerosis

III. Mixed cellularity

IV. Lymphocyte depletion

V. Provisional entity: lymphocyte-rich classic Hodgkin's disease

*These categories are thought likely to include more than one disease entity.

From Harris NL, Jaffe ES, Stein H, Banks PM, Chan JKC, Cleary ML, Delsol G, De Wolf-Peeters C, Falini B, Gatter KC, Grogan TM, Isaacson PG, Knowles DM, Mason DY, Muller-Hermelink HK, Pileri SA, Piris MA, Ralfkiaer E, Warnké RA: A revised European-American classification of lymphoid neoplasms: a proposal from the International Lymphoma Study Group. Blood 84:1361-1392, 1994. By permission of American Society of Hematology.

autologous transplantation. After 48 months, the survival was statistically significantly better in the transplanted group. Prognostic factors are important in lymphoma.

The International Index is based on clinical pretreatment characteristics and the relative risk of death. Clinical features that were associated with survival included age (≤60 versus >60 years), LDH (normal or greater), performance status (0,1 versus 2-4), stage (I/II versus III/IV), and extranodal involvement (≤1 site versus >1 site). Patients were divided into different risk groups based on the number of risk factors, with predicted 5-year survivals in the low-risk group (with zero or one factor) of 73%; in the low-intermediate group (with two factors), 51%; in the high-intermediate group (with three factors), 43%; and in the high group (with four or five factors), 26%.

- Non-Hodgkin's lymphomas are diverse.
- The Working Formulation for Clinical Usage has been the most commonly used classification scheme.
- The Ann Arbor Staging System has traditionally been used in lymphoma.
- The most predictive pretreatment characteristics for the risk of death are age, LDH, performance status, stage, and extranodal involvement.
- Exceptions to the standard management programs in non-Hodgkin's lymphoma include primary bone, isolated gastric, central nervous system, testicular, bowel, orbital, pulmonary, and cutaneous lymphomas.
- Most patients with low-grade lymphoma are not curable but have a long survival time.
- Of patients with the histologic features of advanced intermediate-grade non-Hodgkin's lymphoma, 30%-40% are cured of their disease with anthracycline regimens.
- Patients with HIV-related lymphoproliferative disorders with a CD4 count <200/mL receive different treatment.
- Low-grade lymphomas may transform into intermediate-grade and high-grade lymphomas.

Monoclonal Gammopathies

The differential diagnosis of monoclonal gammopathies includes monoclonal gammopathies of undetermined significance and malignant monoclonal gammopathies. The malignant gammopathies include multiple myeloma (IgG, IgA, IgD, IgE, and free light chains): overt multiple myeloma, smoldering multiple myeloma, plasma cell leukemia, nonsecretory myeloma, osteosclerotic myeloma, plasmacytoma (solitary plasmacytoma of bone, extramedullary plasmacytoma), malignant lymphoproliferative diseases (Waldenström's [primary] macroglobulinemia, malignant lymphoma), heavy chain diseases, and amyloidosis (primary, with myeloma).

Monoclonal Gammopathies of Undetermined Significance

In this condition, the M-protein level is <3 g/dL in the serum, and there are <10% plasma cells in the bone marrow. The serum level of creatinine is normal, and either a small amount of M protein or no M protein occurs in the urine. There is no anemia or osteolytic bone lesions. Twenty-three percent of the patients may have progression to a malignant monoclonal gammopathy. Population-based studies have demonstrated that 1% of adults older than 50 and 3% of those older than 70 have a monoclonal protein in the serum. Of monoclonal gammopathies, 60% are IgG, 20% are IgM, 10% are IgA, and 7% are free light chains. In most patients, serum protein electrophoresis should be followed at 6- to 12-month intervals indefinitely.

Multiple Myeloma

In multiple myeloma, 10% or more plasma cells are found in the bone marrow (color plate 12-11). At least one of the following must be present: M protein in the serum >3 g/dL, M protein in the urine, osteolytic bone lesions. Anemia, hypercalcemia, or increased creatinine level are present in variable numbers of patients.

Clinical features include bone pain (66% of patients), renal insufficiency (50%), hypercalcemia (30%), and weakness, fatigue, and spinal cord compression (5%). The incidence of pneumococcal pneumonia, gram-negative infections, and herpes zoster is increased. The CBC resembles that of normochromic-normocytic anemia. Radiographs show punched-out lytic lesions, osteoporosis, and fractures. A beta$_2$-microglobulin >2.7 μg/mL or a plasma cell labelling index ≥0.8% are adverse prognostic factors.

Treatment--Because multiple myeloma is not curable, treatment should be delayed until evidence of progression develops, the patient becomes symptomatic, or treatment is necessary to prevent imminent complications. Controversy exists as to whether melphalan and prednisone taken orally or a combination of intravenously and orally administered alkylating agents should be used (M2 protocol melphalan, cyclophosphamide, carmustine, vincristine, and prednisone). With melphalan and prednisone, 50%-60% have an objective response and all have relapse, with a median survival of 2-3 years. The standard treatment for most patients remains melphalan and prednisone given for 4-7 days every 4-6 weeks. Current comparative trials are evaluating the roles of high-dose cyclophosphamide, autologous bone marrow or stem cell transplantation, and interferon alfa-2a or 2b recombinant. Fifty percent of patients respond to erythropoietin. Studies have demonstrated that interferon alfa-2a or 2b recombinant is capable of prolonging the duration of remission in comparison with patients who have received no maintenance, but survival differences have not been consistently demonstrated. There may be survival benefit with autologous marrow or peripheral stem cells.

- Plasma cells: <10% in monoclonal gammopathies of undetermined significance; >10% in myeloma.
- M protein: <3 g/dL in monoclonal gammopathies of undetermined significance; ≥3 g/dL in myeloma.
- Myeloma: bone pain (66% of patients), renal dysfunction (50%), hypercalcemia (30%), spinal cord compression (5%).
- Myeloma: punched-out bone lesions, pneumococcal infection.

Waldenström's Macroglobulinemia

Waldenström's macroglobulinemia is characterized by an increase in the IgM paraprotein >3.0 g/dL, lymphadenopathy, or splenomegaly. In 20%-40% of patients, bone marrow involvement with well-differentiated plasmacytoid lymphocytes occurs. Another characteristic is anemia, and Bence Jones proteinuria may be present in 55% of patients. Hyperviscosity syndrome occurs in 15% of patients. Other problems include cryoglobulinemia, sensorimotor peripheral neuropathy, cold agglutinin hemolytic anemia, and renal disease (nephrotic syndrome).

Many patients have only an IgM monoclonal gammopathy of undetermined significance, with no signs or symptoms, and should be monitored without initial treatment.

Hyperviscosity syndrome is characterized by fatigue, dizziness, blurred vision, bleeding from mucous membranes, sausage-shaped retinal veins, and papilledema. The plasma volume is expanded with an increase in serum viscosity. Because 80% of IgM is intravascular, plasmapheresis with albumin and saline replacement is the initial treatment of choice followed by chemotherapy. The disorder most commonly has been treated with chlorambucil (8 mg/m^2) and prednisone (40 mg/m^2 for 10 days at 6-week intervals); 60% of patients respond, with a median survival of 5 years. 2-Chlorodeoxyadenosine administered as a 7-day continuous infusion is the treatment of choice for patients who have not responded to chlorambucil and prednisone; it is also being evaluated in newly diagnosed patients.

Amyloidosis

Patients with amyloidosis present with fatigue, weight loss, hepatomegaly, macroglossia, renal insufficiency, proteinuria, nephrotic syndrome, congestive heart failure, orthostatic hypotension, carpal tunnel syndrome, and peripheral neuropathy. Amyloidosis is classified as primary (90% of patients in U.S.), secondary (chronic infections, autoimmune disease), familial, associated with aging, localized (skin, bladder, etc.), amyloidosis of endocrine glands with medullary carcinoma, and amyloidosis with multiple endocrine neoplasia type II. The most common system involved in patients with primary amyloidosis is the kidney, followed by congestive heart failure secondary to an infiltrative cardiomyopathy (25%), carpal tunnel (20%), peripheral neuropathy, and orthostatic hypotension.

The diagnosis is first established by finding a monoclonal protein in the serum or urine that is confirmed by immunofixation. Initial biopsies should include fat aspiration of the abdominal wall (80% positive), rectum (75%), or bone marrow (56%). Nearly 90% of patients with primary systemic amyloidosis have a detectable monoclonal protein in the serum or urine on immunoelectrophoresis and immunofixation of the serum and urine. This is the most important screening test when the diagnosis is expected. Four of 10 patients present with nephrotic syndrome, 1 in 6 with congestive or restrictive cardiomyopathy, and about 1 in 7 with a sensorimotor peripheral neuropathy. Unexplained hypercholesterolemia may be a manifestation of the nephrotic syndrome. The echocardiogram is abnormal in 60% of patients. The neuropathy is progressive, painful, symmetrical, and demyelinating. Peripheral neuropathy is often associated with autonomic failure, as manifested by diarrhea, pseudo-obstruction, or orthostatic syncope. About 50% of patients with amyloid neuropathy have carpal tunnel syndrome.

The median survival of all patients is 24 months: for those with overt congestive heart failure, <6 months; with nephrotic syndrome, 27 months; and with peripheral neuropathy, 42 months.

Treatment with melphalan and prednisone has a response rate of 18%. Pathologic characteristics--Primary amyloidosis consists of the variable region of immunoglobulin light chains; secondary amyloidosis consists of protein A.

Acute Leukemias

The cause of acute leukemia is unknown in most cases, but there are many associations, including idiopathic aplastic anemia, paroxysmal nocturnal hemoglobinuria, myeloproliferative disorders, preleukemic syndromes, radiation, benzene, cytotoxic chemotherapy, Down syndrome, Fanconi's syndrome, and ataxia-telangiectasia. The classic syndrome of patients who have been exposed to alkylating agents (melphalan, cyclophosphamide, chlorambucil) is pancytopenia in 10-36 months, with the chromosome abnormalities of monosomy 5 and 7. It is refractory to standard treatment regimens.

- Alkylating agents should be used in benign diseases, with consideration of the risk of development of acute myelogenous leukemia, non-Hodgkin's lymphoma, bladder cancer, and other solid tumors.
- Recently described secondary leukemias are those related to topoisomerase II inhibitor agents (etoposide).
- High incidence of neoplasms in Down syndrome, Fanconi's syndrome, and ataxia-telangiectasia.

Acute Nonlymphocytic Leukemia (Acute Myelogenous Leukemia)

The median age of patients with acute nonlymphocytic leukemia (color plate 12-12) is 65 years. Fifty percent of patients have symptoms for >3 months. Good prognostic signs include age <40 years old; chromosome abnormalities of t(8,21), t(15,17), inversion 16, or normal chromosomes; and obtaining complete remission with one cycle of induction chemotherapy. Poor prognostic signs include age >40; preleukemic phase; the chromosome abnormalities of monosomy 5, monosomy 7, t(9,22), trisomy 8, 11q-, and complex cytogenetic patterns; and poor general physical condition or underlying health problems.

For patients who present with extreme leukocytosis (WBC >100 x 10^9/L) with acute leukemia, the initial complication of most concern is cerebral hemorrhage. Emergency treatment includes hydration, alkalinization of urine, allopurinol (600 mg), hydroxyurea (6-8 g orally), cranial irradiation (4-6 Gy), and leukopheresis followed by the treatment of the specific type of leukemia.

- Acute nonlymphocytic leukemia: median age of patients is 65 years; 50% have symptoms >3 months.
- Good prognosis in patients <40 years old, chromosomal abnormalities t(8,21), t(15,17), inv16, or normal chromosomes, and obtaining complete remission with one cycle of induction chemotherapy.

Therapy--Platelet transfusions are required throughout the course of the treatment. Early empiric broad-spectrum antibiotic coverage for fevers is essential.

Induction chemotherapy:
1. Cytarabine (cytosine arabinoside) with an anthracycline agent (daunorubicin or idarubicin)--The complete remission rate is 70%-75% in patients ≤60 years and 35%-50% for those >60 years, with the potential for cure in 20% of patients. Despite substantial recent advances, most patients with acute myelogenous leukemia eventually have relapse and most do so within 1 year. Of patients who have relapse after induction and consolidation therapy, 30%-50% achieve a second remission.
2. *Trans*-retinoic acid (Atra)--M3 acute myelogenous leukemia (promyelocytic acute nonlymphocytic leukemia) (color plate 12-13) with a t(5,17) translocation: *trans*-retinoic acid results in a 90% complete remission rate. These patients then need to be treated with cytarabine or a daunorubicin-type program. After remission is achieved, disease-free survival is excellent, with 76% of patients surviving 6 years as compared with 12% in other acute nonlymphocytic leukemia studies. This is the first malignancy in which a chromosomal alteration has served as the target for induction chemotherapy.

There are three types of postremission therapy. Maintenance therapy uses low doses of chemotherapy, which avoids severe bone marrow suppression. Consolidation therapy uses regimens similar to those used for induction therapy. Intensification therapy uses more intensive therapy than that used during remission induction. Postremission therapy includes chemotherapy and transplantation. Low-dose combination Ara-C and 6-thioguanine are superior to no further treatment in prolonging disease-free survival after achievement of complete remission. High-dose cytarabine improves remission duration in patients younger than 60 years as compared with conventional-dose cytarabine with or without 6-thioguanine.

The following generalizations may be made about allogeneic bone marrow transplantation in acute nonlymphocytic leukemia. Generally, after 2 years of complete remission, the risk of relapse is lower. Transplantation in cases of relapse is age-dependent: patients <30 years old have a better prognosis than those >30. Allogeneic bone marrow transplantation in early relapse or in second remission is almost as efficacious as transplantation in first complete remission. Recommendations--If the patient is <55 years old, consider bone marrow transplant in first remission of HLA match with poor prognostic factors. In those patients without poor risk factors and not on study, perform transplantation in early relapse or second remission. Results--Currently, the disease-free survival at 5 years for patients undergoing allogeneic transplantation in first remission is 50%; in first relapse, 30%; and in second remission, 28%. Early results of autologous transplantation are encouraging.

Acute Lymphoblastic Leukemia

Acute lymphoblastic leukemia (color plate 12-14) is most common in children with complete remission rates >90% and with long-term disease-free survivals of 60%-70%. In adults, this leukemia is less common, with remission rates of up to 75%; however, most patients will have relapse. Of adult acute lymphocytic leukemia, 80% of cases are B cell in origin, 20% have T-cell markers, and 1%-2% express surface immunoglobulin. Most B-cell leukemias express CD10, the common ALL antigen (cALLa). Early pre-B-acute lymphocytic leukemia patients are cALLa negative. Early pre-B acute lymphocytic leukemia is also known as "null acute lymphocytic leukemia." Clinical presentation--One-third of patients present with bleeding, and 25% have symptoms for >3 months. Bone pain, lymphadenopathy, splenomegaly, and hepatomegaly are more common in acute lymphoblastic leukemia than in acute nonlymphocytic leukemia. Splenomegaly, lymphadenopathy, and hepatomegaly occur in 3/4 of the patients (compared with 1/2 of patients with acute myelogenous leukemia).

Prognostic factors--The best prognosis is in children 3-10 years old. After the age of 20, survival time continues to decrease with increasing age and shorter complete remission durations. Poor prognostic factors include age, WBC count

>30 x 10^9/L, null cell phenotype, specific chromosome abnormalities, and achievement of remission after >4 weeks of intensive chemotherapy. Chromosomal abnormalities--80%-90% of adults have chromosome abnormalities. Normal chromosomes have the best prognosis. The poorest prognosis is associated with t(9,22); t(4,11); t(8,14); and t(1,19). These patients have lower complete remission rates, shorter remission duration, and very poor survival. Also, t(9,22) has <15% survival at 5 years and is present in 25% of adults but only 2%-3% of children. Chromosome abnormalities are independent of age, WBC count, immunotype.

Treatment:

1. Induction--The three agents commonly used include vincristine, prednisone, and anthracyclines along with one or more of the following: L-asparaginase, cytarabine, methotrexate, or cyclophosphamide. The complete remission rate is 70%-90%. The addition of L-asparaginase, cytarabine, or cyclophosphamide may improve remission duration.
2. Intensification/postinduction therapy is commonly used. Long-term relapse-free survival of 10%-42% in adults. The use of allogeneic bone marrow transplant in first complete remission results in a 21%-71% disease-free survival at 2-10 years, with relapse rates of 10%-40%. Trials are under way for evaluating autologous bone marrow transplant.
3. Relapse--Allogeneic or autologous bone marrow transplants are of benefit in patients who achieve a second complete remission. After a second complete remission and then allogeneic transplant, the disease-free survival ranges from 26% to 54% at various time periods. At second complete remission and then autologous transplant, the disease-free survival ranges from 23% to 31% at various periods of time.
4. Recent results of unrelated allogeneic donor transplants reveal a 45% leukemia-free survival for patients in first remission, but there are significant logistical and age restrictions. Trials are under way evaluating autologous transplantation. Indications for bone marrow transplantation include high-risk cytogenetic abnormalities

in first remission and patients in second or subsequent remission.

Myelodysplastic Syndromes

Myelodysplastic syndromes, as classified by the French-American-British Group (with median survival time), are refractory anemia (26 months), refractory anemia with ringed sideroblasts (34 months), refractory anemia with excess blasts (9 months), refractory anemia with excess blasts in transformation (5 months), and chronic myelomonocytic leukemia (12 months). These disorders present with anemia and other cytopenias. The most life-threatening complication is transformation to acute leukemia. This occurs in 12% of patients with refractory anemia, 8% with refractory anemia with ringed sideroblasts, 44% with refractory anemia with excess blasts, 14% with chronic myelomonocytic leukemia, and 60% with refractory anemia with excess blasts in transition. A significant proportion of patients die of cytopenic complications, most commonly leukopenia. The standard of care in most patients with this disorder is supportive. Patients younger than age 55 should be considered for allogeneic bone marrow transplantation.

Myeloproliferative Disorders

The myeloproliferative disorders are polycythemia rubra vera, agnogenic myeloid metaplasia, essential thrombocythemia, and chronic granulocytic leukemia. Their characteristic features are given in Table 12-10. The myeloproliferative disorders are interrelated: polycythemia rubra vera converts to agnogenic myeloid metaplasia in 10% of cases. Essential thrombocythemia converts to agnogenic myeloid metaplasia in 5% of cases. Acute myelogenous leukemia is a complication of polycythemia rubra vera (10% of cases), essential thrombocythemia (15%), agnogenic myeloid metaplasia (20%), and chronic myelogenous leukemia (70%).

- The myeloproliferative disorders are polycythemia rubra vera, agnogenic myeloid metaplasia, essential thrombocythemia, and chronic granulocytic leukemia.
- Myeloproliferative disorders are interrelated.

Table 12-10.--Characteristic Features of Chronic Myeloproliferative Disorders

Characteristic	Polycythemia rubra vera	Agnogenic myeloid metaplasia	Primary thrombocythemia	Chronic granulocytic leukemia
Increased red cell mass	Yes	No	No	No
Myelofibrosis	Later	Yes	Rare	Later
Thrombocytosis	Variable	Variable	Yes	Variable
bcr-abl Oncogene	No	No	No	Yes

From Petitt RM, Silverstein MN: Current clinical management of primary thrombocythemia. Contemp Intern Med Jan 1991, pp 46-52. By permission of Aegean Communications.

Chronic Myelogenous Leukemia (Chronic Granulocytic Leukemia)

Chronic myelogenous leukemia constitutes 20%-30% of all leukemias and is characterized by an acquired defect of clonal origin at the pluripotential cell level. There is a pool of granulocyte precursors with the capacity for normal maturation (color plate 12-15). The Philadelphia chromosome, t(9,22), is the hallmark of this disease. The translocation results in the formation of a chimeric *bcr-abl* oncogene. The disease terminates in a maturation block or blast crisis. New chromosomal abnormalities appear and reappear. Different cell types can be seen, including myeloblasts (50%-60% of patients), megakaryoblasts (15%), B lymphoblasts, erythroblasts (10%), monoblasts, myelomonocytic blasts, and basophilic blasts.

Clinical features--Before the advent of allogeneic bone marrow transplantation and interferon alfa-2a or 2b recombinant, the median survival was 3.5 years after diagnosis. Prognostic factors are different in multiple series. In one study, a good prognosis (61-month median survival versus 34 months) was associated with a spleen size of 0-6 cm and 0%-10% circulating blasts. A poor prognosis was associated with an age >45 years, platelet count >700 x 10^9/L, splenomegaly, and circulating blasts. The chronic phase is characterized by <10% blasts in blood and bone marrow and is of 2-3 years' duration. Symptoms include malaise, dyspnea, anorexia, fever, night sweats, weight loss, abdominal fullness, easy bruising, bleeding, gout, priapism, and hypermetabolism. Splenomegaly is present in 85% of patients.

Laboratory findings--Leukocytosis with <10% blasts in the chronic phase of disease and WBC count of 100,000 are common. Granulocytes in all stages of maturation are present on peripheral blood smear, with basophilia and eosinophilia. The number of platelets is increased, with large bizarre forms present on peripheral blood smears. The hemoglobin concentration ranges from 9 to 12 g/dL. The leukocyte alkaline phosphatase score is low or absent. The differential diagnosis of a low or absent leukocyte alkaline phosphatase score includes paroxysmal nocturnal hemoglobinuria, infectious mononucleosis, and aplastic anemia. The vitamin B_{12} level is increased because of increased transcobalamin I. Other findings include pseudohyperkalemia, pseudohypoglycemia, and false-positive increase in acid phosphatase in the serum. The bone marrow is hyperplastic, with myelofibrosis in 10%-40% of patients.

- Chronic myelogenous leukemia: acquired defect of clonal origin.
- Philadelphia chromosome, t(9,22), is the hallmark of the disease.
- WBC count is usually >100,000; granulocytes in all stages of maturation.
- Bone marrow shows hyperplasia; myelofibrosis in 10%-40% of patients.

- The leukocyte alkaline phosphatase score is low or absent in chronic myelogenous leukemia, paroxysmal nocturnal hemoglobinuria, infectious mononucleosis, and aplastic anemia.
- Increased vitamin B_{12}; increased acid phosphatase.

Treatment--Conventional chemotherapy has not appreciably prolonged survival. There is little evidence that any patient has been cured with conventional therapy, including hydroxyurea and multiagent regimens. The three agents used in the initial treatment of chronic myelogenous leukemia are hydroxyurea, busulfan, and interferon alfa-2a or 2b recombinant. Hydroxyurea is used more commonly, with response rates of 85%-90%. A recent study demonstrated that both overall and post-transplant survival are inferior for patients treated with busulfan as compared with hydroxyurea. Hydroxyurea is the treatment of choice for high blast counts and leukostasis lesions, and it is safe in thrombocytopenia. Moreover, it has fewer side effects than busulfan. Recovery after an overshoot is more rapid than with busulfan. Continued maintenance therapy is necessary. Megaloblastic RBCs appear in the peripheral blood. Hydroxyurea should be used in all patients who are considered candidates for bone marrow transplantation, because of the risk of interstitial pneumonitis and veno-occlusive disease with busulfan. The dose of busulfan must be reduced by 50% at a WBC count of 20,000, and its use must be stopped when the WBC count reaches 10,000-12,000. Other side effects of busulfan include thrombocytopenia, leukopenia, prolonged bone marrow myelosuppression, increased skin pigmentation, pulmonary toxicity, amenorrhea, germinal cell atrophy, fetal malformations, veno-occlusive disease of liver, and a wasting syndrome.

Interferon alfa-2a or 2b recombinant suppresses the Philadelphia chromosome. Hematologic responses are 40%-80%, with cytogenetic remissions in the range of 10%-40%. The median survival is >60 months. One randomized trial has demonstrated an improvement in survival and remission duration in patients treated with interferon alfa-2a or 2b recombinant in comparison with hydroxyurea.

The treatment of "blast crisis" includes allopurinol, fluids, hydroxyurea, cranial radiation, and leukocyte apheresis.

- Accelerated phase at 30-36 months; the chronic phase converts to an accelerated or blast phase (75%), which is characterized by blast counts >20%; increase in anemia, thrombocytopenia, basophilia, and leukocyte alkaline phosphatase score; splenomegaly; lymphadenopathy; bone pain; cerebral hemorrhage; fever; headache; and myelofibrosis. Cytogenetic abnormalities precede condition by 6 months.
- If treated with busulfan or hydroxyurea, 10%-15% of patients die in the first year and about 26% per year thereafter.

- Toxicity of busulfan: prolonged myelosuppression, pulmonary toxicity, veno-occlusive disease of the liver.
- Interferon alfa-2a or 2b recombinant suppresses the Philadelphia chromosome.
- Intensive treatment in patients with chronic granulocytic leukemia does not postpone or prevent blast crisis or appreciably improve survival.

Allogeneic bone marrow transplantation should be performed in the chronic phase, within the first 12 months in young patients who have an HLA-identical match or an identical twin. The only curative regimen to date is high-dose chemotherapy with total body irradiation followed by transplantation of allogeneic bone marrow from HLA-compatible siblings. Hematologic relapses occur in 10%-20% of patients receiving a transplant in the chronic phase. The long-term disease-free survival rates are 40%-60%.

- Currently, the only curative regimen is HLA-compatible allogeneic bone marrow transplantation.

Agnogenic Myeloid Metaplasia

Clinical features--Splenomegaly occurs in 100% of the patients and is the hallmark of agnogenic myeloid metaplasia. Other features are leukoerythroblastic peripheral blood smear (96% of patients), teardrop cells, and hypocellular marrow (85%). The basic event is the fibroblastic proliferation in bone marrow (color plate 12-16). Anemia may be caused by expanded plasma volume, ineffective erythropoiesis, blood loss, or hemolysis.

Pathologic features--The bone marrow reveals panhyperplasia with modest fibrosis to osteosclerosis. The spleen is pathologically characterized by extramedullary hematopoiesis in the sinusoids of red pulp. Hepatomegaly may occur in 70% of patients because of engorgement by blood, extramedullary hematopoiesis, or hemosiderosis.

- Agnogenic myeloid metaplasia: splenomegaly is its hallmark.
- Leukoerythroblastic peripheral blood smear in 96% of patients.
- Teardrop cells.
- Basic event: fibroblastic proliferation of bone marrow.

Treatment--Observe the 20% of asymptomatic patients (80% will remain asymptomatic at 5 years). Medical therapy for anemia with symptoms includes the following:

1. Transfusion with packed RBCs if RBC mass is low (check RBC mass and plasma volume).
2. Androgens for ineffective erythropoiesis: testosterone enanthate (400-600 mg/week) or fluoxymesterone (10 mg three times daily). Response occurs in 40% of males and 32% of females. Poor response in long-existing

disease and massive splenomegaly. Side effects are hirsutism and fluid retention.
3. Corticosteroids for hemolysis.
4. Check stool for occult blood loss due to esophageal varices and microinfarcts of the gut.
5. Treat vitamin B_{12} and folate deficiency if indicated.

Pressure symptoms occur in 23% of patients and may be managed with hydroxyurea or splenic irradiation.

1. 63% of patients respond to splenic irradiation but the response duration is short (3.5 months). Indications for splenic irradiation include splenic infarct, perisplenitis, and ascites from peritoneal implants.
2. Bleeding with or without thrombocytopenia may be managed with platelet transfusions.
3. Treat disseminated intravascular coagulopathy appropriately if present (may be present in up to 40% of patients).
4. Splenectomy is indicated in major hemolysis, pressure symptoms, life-threatening thrombocytopenia, portal hypertension, and life-threatening bleeding.

Prognosis--Overall survival is 60% at 5 years. The prognosis is good if the patient is asymptomatic, hemoglobin concentration is >10, platelet count is >100,000, and the liver is <5 cm below the costal margin.

Essential Thrombocythemia (Primary Thrombocythemia)

Essential thrombocythemia is a clonal hematologic disorder in which patients present with asymptomatic thrombocytosis, thrombotic disorders, or hemorrhage. The median survival is >10 years, with 80% of patients alive at 5 years. The overall risk of bleeding is 3% and of thrombosis, 20%. The risk factors include age, previous thrombosis, and short remission. The risk of acute leukemic transformation is <2%.

Diagnosis--Platelet count is >600 x 10^9/L; megakaryocytic hyperplasia in the bone marrow; splenomegaly; absence of the Philadelphia chromosome, which is a translocation between chromosome 9 and 22 or M*bcr* rearrangement (100% of patients); normal RBC mass (100%); no collagen fibrosis and stainable iron in the bone marrow. Also, there is no other secondary cause of thrombocytosis, including acute or chronic inflammatory disease; acute or chronic bleeding; iron deficiency; chronic bone marrow stimulation (e.g., hemolysis); rebound after thrombocytopenia; disseminated malignancy; splenectomy, congenital asplenia, or functional hyposplenism; postoperative state; and intense exercise, parturition, trauma, and epinephrine. An increased C-reactive protein level in patients with thrombocytosis suggests a reactive process.

Treatment--Platelet apheresis should be used in the emergent management of acute bleeding or thrombosis. Patients <30 years old may be observed if there are no hemorrhagic or thrombotic problems, no significant trauma, and no emergency or elective surgery. Platelet apheresis is indicated in cases of elective surgery for patients of any age and in pregnant women during the course of delivery. Treatment is recommended for patients with thrombotic symptoms, a previous history of thrombotic events, cardiovascular risk factors, and those older than 60 who have a platelet count >600 x 10^9/L. Currently, hydroxyurea is the treatment of choice for most patients. Patients who are asymptomatic and have a platelet count <600 x 10^9/L and asymptomatic and of childbearing age may be observed. Chronic treatments available for the management of essential thrombocythemia include hydroxyurea; anagrelide; antiaggregating agents for mild thrombotic symptoms, including aspirin and dipyridamole; radioactive phosphorus at a dose of 2.7 mCi/m^2; and interferon alfa-2a or 2b recombinant.

Erythrocytosis

Polycythemia--The history, physical examination, CBC, arterial blood gases, leukocyte alkaline phosphatase score, and the marrow can determine the diagnosis in a high percentage of patients, as shown in Table 12-11. Every patient with unexplained erythrocytosis should have an intravenous pyelogram or CT scan of the abdomen.

The differential diagnosis of erythrocytosis with a normal oxygen saturation value includes the following: hypernephroma, renal adenoma, hydronephrosis, renal cyst, transplantation, Bartter's syndrome, cerebellar hemangioblastoma, adrenal cortical adenoma or hyperplasia, ovarian carcinoma, hepatoma, pheochromocytoma, uterine fibroids, and hemoglobinopathies. Administration of erythropoietin to healthy persons may cause erythrocytosis.

● Polycythemia rubra vera: very low erythropoietin.

Table 12-11.--Differential Diagnosis of Erythrocytosis

	Polycythemia rubra vera	Apparent or stress erythrocytosis	Anoxic polycythemia	Tumor
History	Multiple symptoms	Nervous Hypertension Obesity	High-altitude COPD Fibrosis Congenital heart disease Sleep apnea Hemoglobinopathy	
Gout	Occasionally	Occasionally		
Other history	Postbathing pruritus[*]			
Examination	Plethora skin, mucous membrane	±Plethora	Cyanosis	No cyanosis, clubbing, or COPD
	Distention of retinal vein		Clubbing[*]	Mass in left upper quadrant
	Hepatomegaly (50%) Splenomegaly (75%);[*] not others			
Laboratory				
Oxygen saturation	Normal	Normal	<88% (±88%-92%)[*]	Normal
LAP score	+++ (almost invariably)[*]	Normal	Normal	Normal
Red blood cell mass	++	Normal	+ to ++	+ to ++
Plasma volume	Normal or slightly increased	Reduced	Normal	Normal
Excretory urogram	Normal	Normal	Normal	Tumor
Erythrocyte sedimentation rate	0-1[*]	Normal	Normal, low	
Bone marrow	Pancytosis	Erythrocytosis	Erythrocytosis	Erythrocytosis
Platelets	+ to ++ (50%)	Normal	Normal	± Normal

COPD, chronic obstructive pulmonary disease; LAP, leukocyte alkaline phosphatase.
[*]Most important differentiating factors.
Modified from Dameshek W: Comments on the diagnosis of polycythemia vera. Semin Hematol 3:214-215, 1966. By permission of WB Saunders

- Cerebral blood flow decreases at a hematocrit of >46.
- Smoking 1.5 packs of cigarettes per day can raise hematocrit to 60% (check carboxyhemoglobin).
- RBC mass returns to normal when smoking is stopped.

Polycythemia Rubra Vera

Clinical features include weakness, postbathing pruritus, headache, dizziness, weight loss, joint symptoms, dyspnea, and epigastric distress. Classification: category A, increased RBC mass, splenomegaly, normal arterial oxygen saturation; category B, platelet count >400 x 10^9/L, WBC >12 x 10^9/L (no fever or infection), leukocyte alkaline phosphatase score >100, serum level of vitamin B_{12} >900 ng/L. The presence of all three criteria in category A establishes the diagnosis. If the patient has increased RBC mass (category A) with either of the other two category A criteria, then two of the four category B criteria are necessary to establish the diagnosis. Unfavorable prognostic signs are previous thrombotic disease, age >60 years, diabetes mellitus, vascular diseases, and hypertension.

Laboratory findings--The bone marrow is normal in up to 10% of patients; 90%-95% have absent iron stores in the bone marrow even if not phlebotomized. Cytogenetic abnormalities are present in 11%. The erythropoietin level is low. The Philadelphia chromosome in the bone marrow is negative. Morphologically, the bone marrow may resemble chronic myelogenous leukemia in 10%-40% of patients. The leukocyte alkaline phosphatase score is increased.

- The leukocyte alkaline phosphatase score may be increased in polycythemia rubra vera, leukemoid reactions, agnogenic myeloid metaplasia, idiopathic thrombocytopenic purpura, pregnancy, pyogenic infections, and stress erythrocytosis.
- Think of polycythemia rubra vera with microcytosis, absent iron stores, and splenomegaly.

Treatment in patients who are asymptomatic is phlebotomy to maintain the hematocrit <42-45. Phlebotomize every 2-4 months, because there is 250 mg of iron in 1 pint of blood. If the normal daily absorption is 4 mg, then phlebotomizing every 2 months will maintain the hematocrit in an appropriate range. Start at 500 mL every other day for 3-6 phlebotomies and maintain the hematocrit at 42-45 every 2-4 months. In the elderly, start at 250 mL phlebotomies. There is a risk of thrombosis in older patients with vascular lesions, with the rate and volume of phlebotomy, and in patients with a history of thrombosis. In patients with asymptomatic thrombocytosis, anagrelide decreases the platelet count in 96% of those treated. Other agents available include hydroxyurea and interferon alfa-2a or 2b recombinant.

In patients who are symptomatic or who are at risk for thrombosis, hydroxyurea, anagrelide, and ^{32}P are the treatment approaches. Hydroxyurea is the treatment of choice. All patients 60 years and younger with cardiovascular risk factors or a previous history of thrombosis should be considered for treatment. With ^{32}P, the number of platelets decreases in 2 weeks and the number of RBCs decreases in 1 month. This treatment is indicated for patients older than 60, because of the 2.3-fold risk of acute nonlymphocytic leukemia in younger patients treated with ^{32}P. Chlorambucil is not indicated because of a 5.3-fold risk of developing acute nonlymphocytic leukemia when compared with phlebotomy.

- Sequence of ordering tests in erythrocytosis. CBC: if the hematocrit is >58% in males or >52% in females, then proceed with erythrocytosis evaluation. Arterial oxygen saturation: if oxygen saturation >92%, then check carboxyhemoglobin (smoker's polycythemia). If the arterial blood gases are normal, measure the erythropoietin level. If the hematocrit is 54%-58% in males and 45%-52% in females and there is microcytosis and/or splenomegaly, measure the erythropoietin level. Determining the RBC mass and plasma volume may aid in diagnosis, especially in the more difficult cases.

Oncogenes

Oncogenes are gene loci that have the potential to affect neoplastic transformation of cells. They were originally defined in viral systems. Most oncogenes identified to date have been detected in tumors induced by acute transforming viruses. Alkylating agents and radiation involve activation of many of the same cellular oncogenes that are homologous to the oncogenes carried by retroviruses. Many oncogenes have been shown to be associated with specific chromosomal breakpoints or translocations (Table 12-12). Therefore, a silent oncogene can come to be involved at an active chromosomal site, resulting in unregulated expression (cell division) or expression of an inappropriate cell type (cell differentiation). Also, there are proteins that convert an extracellular signal into an intracellular biochemical event, leading to a neoplastic event such as epidermal growth factor. Oncogenesis is likely a multistep process.

Oncogenes in virus-induced transformation--Retroviruses: viral gene sequences encode a product thought to activate transcription of many different cellular genes. Examples include HTLV-I, causative agent in adult T-cell leukemia; HTLV-II, associated with one T-cell hairy-cell leukemia line; and Epstein-Barr virus infection in Burkitt's lymphoma, nasopharyngeal carcinoma, Hodgkin's disease, and post-transplantation lymphoproliferative disorders. Oncogene activation may occur with rearrangements of an oncogene, mutation of an oncogene, or through altered expression of an oncogene.

- Oncogenes are gene loci with the potential to affect neoplastic transformation of cells.
- Most known oncogenes have been detected in tumors

Table 12-12.--Chromosome Rearrangement and Increase of Specific Oncogenes

Disease	Rearrangement	Oncogene
Burkitt's lymphoma	t(8,14)	c-*myc*
	t(8,22)	Translocation into transcriptionally active immunoglobulin heavy or light chain loci
Acute lymphocytic leukemia	t(8,14)	c-*myc*
Chronic granulocytic leukemia	t(9,22)	c-*abl*
Follicular small cleaved cell lymphoma	t(14,18)	*bcl*-2
Diffuse large cell non-Hodgkin's lymphoma	---	*bcl*-6

induced by viruses.
- Many oncogenes are associated with chromosomal breakpoints or translocations.

COAGULATION

Prolonged Bleeding Time

The coagulation mechanism does not participate in the bleeding time. An abnormal bleeding time is a reflection of vascular defects, quantitative disorders of platelets (including thrombocytopenia and thrombocytosis), or functional disorders of platelets. Qualitative platelet defects result in an abnormal bleeding time but normal partial thromboplastin time, prothrombin time, thrombin time, and platelet count (except von Willebrand's disease and disseminated intravascular coagulopathy).

- Prolonged bleeding time differential diagnosis includes Glanzmann's thrombasthenia, von Willebrand's disease, Bernard-Soulier syndrome, disseminated intravascular coagulopathy, thrombocytopenia, storage pool disease, drugs (aspirin, etc.), and uremia.

von Willebrand's disease

von Willebrand's disease is the most common inherited bleeding disorder; at least 20 subtypes have been described. In most subtypes of von Willebrand's disease, the inheritance pattern is autosomal dominant with incomplete penetrance (parent of either sex). The bleeding is usually mild, but hemorrhage postoperatively can be severe. Mucocutaneous bleeding, epistaxis, easy bruising, and menorrhagia are characteristic, with occasional gastrointestinal tract bleeding, hematuria, and, rarely, hemarthroses.

To understand von Willebrand's disease, it is helpful to review platelet activity. The initial step of adhesion is followed by aggregation. Collagen and factor VIII-related antigen are involved in adhesion. Factor VIII-related antigen is found in plasma, platelets, and endothelial regions and is detected functionally by its ability to cause aggregation of washed platelets when ristocetin is administered. Aggregation requires ADP and thromboxane A_2. The activation of the clotting mechanism and generation of thrombin seem to result from the activation of the platelet membrane during adhesion and aggregation. Platelets make available platelet factor III and catalyze the activation of other coagulation factors. von Willebrand factor (vWF) is contained in endothelial cells, platelets, and plasma. The factor VIII complex is composed of the following: 1) VIII:C, the coagulant activity which is missing in hemophiliac plasma; this is decreased in hemophilia and von Willebrand's disease and circulates in the plasma with von Willebrand factor VIII (VIII vWF). 2) VIII C:Ag, antigenic determinants of VIII:C; this is decreased in von Willebrand's disease and is normal in hemophilia. 3) VIII vWF antigen (vWF:Ag): Willebrand factor (vWF); this serves as a carrier for VIII:C and is the mediator of the initial platelet adhesion to the blood vessel wall. It is produced by megakaryocytes and vascular endothelial cells. The adhesive function is contained largely within large multimers. 4) VIII vWF activity: ristocetin cofactor, the activity necessary for ristocetin-induced platelet aggregation that is not present in von Willebrand's disease. 5) VIII R:Ag, antigenic determinant of VIII R:vWF and/or VIII R:RCo; factor VIII-related antigen is important in adherence, and it is likely that the activities of VIII R:vWF and VIII R:RCo are properties of this protein. All platelet-related activities of the VIII molecule are referred to as "vWF." vWF plays an essential role in the adhesion of platelets to the subendothelium. Factor VIII coagulant activity and vWF activity reside in two separate molecules that are noncovalently bound in the plasma. Therefore, von Willebrand's disease represents a defect in hemostasis involving the interaction of the platelet membrane glycoprotein, subendothelial tissues, and vWF. There is either decreased synthesis, decreased release, or abdominal production of vWF.

The many distinct variants can be divided into different subtypes. Type I is characterized by a quantitative abnormality in vWF. It is the most common type and is autosomal dominant in inheritance pattern. The total amount of circulating vWF multimers are ≤50%. The distribution and function of vWF are normal. Type II is characterized by a qualitative dysfunctional abnormality in vWF. Type IIA and IIB are characterized by an absence of more functionally potent, large high molecular weight vWF multimers from plasma. There is a decrease in the total vWF and VIII:C levels. A number of variants exist. Type IIC is characterized by quite abnormal multimers. Heterozygous vWD disease is characterized clinically by mild to moderate bleeding. It is autosomal dominant in inheritance pattern. The laboratory diagnosis of von Willebrand's disease includes prolonged bleeding time, reduced VIII:C, VIII:vWF antigen (vWF:Ag), vWF activity (ristocetin-cofactor activity), normal platelet aggregation except in the presence of ristocetin, and a mildly prolonged partial thromboplastin time.

- The tests essential for the diagnosis and exclusion of von Willebrand's disease are: plasma vWF antigen, plasma vWF activity, and plasma factor coagulant activity.
- Supplementary tests that may be needed for the type of von Willebrand's disease: activated partial thromboplastin time, bleeding time, platelet count, vWF multimer analysis, and ristocetin-induced platelet aggregation response.

Treatment--Mild and moderate cases of von Willebrand's disease require treatment only at the time of an operation or bleeding. For menorrhagia, birth control pills are effective. For dental extractions, local hemostasis and local fibrinolytic agents are effective. In pregnancy, there is no need to transfuse in mild to moderate cases of the disease, because the levels of vWF increase with the duration of pregnancy. The mainstays of treatment are 1-desamino-8-D-arginine vasopressin (DDAVP), factor VIII concentrates rich in vWF, and cryoprecipitate. DDAVP causes the release of preformed vWF multimers from the subendothelium and is useful in type I von Willebrand's disease. Repeated injections of this agent may cause hyponatremia. Rapid tachyphylaxis may develop. A trial should be conducted before it is used as primary therapy. The levels increase for 4-8 hours. This usually is effective only in type I von Willebrand's disease. For patients with type IIB and III von Willebrand's disease or for those with type I disease who have become transiently unresponsive to DDAVP, viral-inactivated factor VIII preparations rich in vWF are recommended. Cryoprecipitate from carefully selected and repeatedly tested donors is more desirable than cryoprecipitate from random donors.

Glanzmann's Thrombasthenia

Glanzmann's thrombasthenia results from a defect in the first phase of platelet aggregation, secondary to marked reduction or absent platelet glycoproteins IIb and IIIa. It is autosomal recessive in inheritance pattern. Early hemorrhagic complications occur in the neonatal period, and epistaxis, purpura, petechiae, and ecchymoses persist throughout life. The laboratory findings include no clumping of platelets on the peripheral blood smear, normal platelet number and morphology, and no aggregation with ADP, epinephrine, thrombin, or collagen. There is aggregation with ristocetin/factor VIII R:vWF. Treatment consists of nasal packing, local measures, and cryoprecipitate, with or without platelets, when local measures are not successful.

Bernard-Soulier Syndrome

Bernard-Soulier syndrome is the result of the absence of glycoprotein Ib complexes on the surface of human platelets that mediate ristocetin-induced vWF-dependent platelet aggregation. Glycoprotein Ib is the platelet receptor for vWF. It is more common in whites and blacks and is autosomal recessive in inheritance pattern. This disorder is characterized by moderate to severe bleeding with surgery and menstruation. Bleeding typically is from mucous membranes, the gums, and the gastrointestinal tract. The bleeding time is markedly prolonged. Characteristically, there is thrombocytopenia with giant platelets. The aggregation pattern is the opposite of that of Glanzmann's thrombasthenia with normal platelet aggregation with ADP, collagen, epinephrine, and thrombin but no aggregation with ristocetin.

Storage Pool Disease

Normally, ATP, ADP, serotonin, and calcium are stored by platelets and released from them. In storage pool disease, there is a marked decrease in platelet ADP and a lesser decrease in ATP. Because of the profound decrease in ADP, the amount released from the platelets is insufficient to bring uninvolved platelets into larger aggregates.

Disseminated Intravascular Coagulopathy

Disseminated intravascular coagulopathy is characterized by a dynamic process caused by many diseases with microvascular clotting secondary to thrombin deposition. The laboratory findings are variable. No single laboratory test can confirm or exclude the diagnosis, which depends on the clinical setting and laboratory findings. The manifestations vary from patient to patient and from time to time in the same patient. These may be of little clinical significance or cause life-threatening bleeding or clotting. The mortality rates of severe disseminated coagulopathy range from 50% to 85%.

The pathophysiology of disseminated intravascular coagulopathy is complex. Thrombin is formed in the vascular system and alters platelets. The platelets aggregate, agglutinate, and secrete many products, resulting in thrombocytopenia and platelets that do not function well. Plasmin circulates systematically degrading fibrin and fibrinogen, creating the D-dimer and X, Y, D, and E fragments known as fibrinogen degradation products. Thrombin cleaves fibrinopeptides A and B from fibrinogen to form fibrin monomers. These monomers may complex with fibrinogen (polymerization) to form insoluble fibrin, which is deposited in capillaries and small blood vessels, resulting in microangiopathy. Activated factor XIII cross-links fibrin to make it more resistant to fibrinolysis. Thrombin increases the activity of factors V and VIII. Therefore, thrombin accounts for the decreased fibrinogen, platelets, and factors II, V, VIII, and XIII. Secondary fibrinolysis may occur. Bleeding occurs because the coagulation factors are depleted or fibrinolysis with vessel damage results in decreased control proteins, such as antithrombin III and protein C. Activated factor XII leads to kallikrein production, resulting in the conversion of plasminogen to plasmin, which is capable of digesting fibrinogen, clotting factors, and complement. The clinical picture depends on a balance: if thrombin activity is greater than plasmin activity, there is thrombosis; or, if plasmin activity is greater than thrombin activity, there is hemorrhage.

The following occur in acute disseminated intravascular coagulopathy: bleeding from wounds and perivenipuncture sites, ecchymoses, petechiae, hematomas, hematuria, intracranial hemorrhage, intrapleural hemorrhage, intraperitoneal hemorrhage, hemoptysis, vaginal melena, and hematemesis. Thromboembolic complications, as manifested by necrotic skin lesions, pulmonary emboli, acute arterial occlusions, ischemia, stroke, and myocardial infarction, may occur in 8% of patients. Thrombosis is more common than bleeding in chronic disseminated intravascular coagulopathy.

Causes--Malignancies are the most common cause: prostate, breast, lung, leukemia (acute progranulocytic [M3]), pancreas, and lymphoma. Infections are the second most common cause (gram-negative and gram-positive organisms, e.g., *Staphylococcus*, *Streptococcus*, pneumococcus, typhoid, *Rickettsia*, viral, fungal, histoplasmosis, *Aspergillus*). Surgery/trauma is the third leading cause. Other causes are liver disease, pregnancy, acute renal failure associated with cardiogenic shock, gun shots, endothelial injury (giant hemangiomas, aortic aneurysms, angiography), hemolytic transfusion reactions, burns, crush injuries, acidosis, and alkalosis.

Tests--The best screening study results are thrombocytopenia in 90% of patients, increased prothrombin time in 90% of patients, and hypofibrinogenemia in 70% of patients. The best available confirmatory test is the fibrin D-dimer assay, which detects fibrinogen fragments that are formed by the lysis of cross-linked fibrin. More sensitive techniques include detection of products of fibrinolysis or fibrin degradation products (D-dimer products) and coagulation activation (soluble fibrin monomers). The values obtained with these two tests may be increased in the postoperative state and in patients with recent thrombi, because of fibrinolysis that may not be a reflection of a pathologic state.

● Screening tests for disseminated intravascular coagulopathy: thrombocytopenia (90%), increased prothrombin time (90%), and hypofibrinogenemia (70%)

Treatment--The first goal in treatment is to treat the underlying disease. Next, the approach depends on the clinical situation. If the patient has a low level of fibrinogen, low platelet count, and/or low levels of clotting factor and is not bleeding or undergoing a surgical procedure, no treatment is necessary. If the patient is bleeding or undergoing a surgical procedure, treat with cryoprecipitate, fresh frozen plasma, and platelets. Monitoring the effect of replacement therapy with platelet and fibrinogen levels 30 minutes-1 hour after transfusion and every 4-6 hours thereafter provides a guide to further replacement therapy. If the patient continues to bleed and the above measures do not cause an increase in coagulation factors, it may be necessary to continue factor and platelet replacement therapy and to start a continuous infusion of heparin. If there is evidence of fibrin deposition or thrombosis (such as dermal necrosis in purpura fulminans, acral ischemia, livedo reticularis, or venous thromboembolism), heparin therapy is indicated. Both full-dose therapy (a loading dose of 5,000 units followed by 1,000 units per hour) and subcutaneous heparin have been advocated. Monitoring is a problem. The initial approach is to follow the prothrombin time, fibrinogen level, and platelet count. A heparin assay to achieve a level of 0.2-0.4 M/mL is an alternative approach that is not advocated as a routine practice. The thrombotic events of disseminated intravascular coagulopathy in solid tumor malignancy can be treated effectively with heparin, but warfarin anticoagulation may not be as effective. Other instances in which heparin is indicated are retained dead fetus with hypofibrinogenemia before induction of labor, excessive bleeding associated with giant hemangioma, promyelocytic leukemia, and mucinous adenocarcinoma. Heparin is not indicated in >95% of patients.

Coagulation and Liver Disease

The most important factor is the condition of the blood vessels. There is no tendency to bleed unless and until blood vessels are damaged, such as by needle, surgical procedure, or gastric acid. The three main coagulation patterns are: 1) portal hypertension, which is characterized by thrombocytopenia and normal coagulation factor synthesis; 2) cholestasis, which results in impaired absorption of fat-soluble vitamins and an increase in prothrombin time and activated partial thromboplastin time; and 3) acute and chronic hepatocellular disease, which is characterized by a normal fibrinogen level (until late in the course of the disease), thrombocytopenia, and an increase

Table 12-13.--Differences in Laboratory Findings Between Liver Disease and Disseminated Intravascular Coagulopathy

Tests	Liver disease	Disseminated intravascular coagulopathy
Thrombocytopenia	Mild, decreased in 50% of patients, <50,000 uncommon	90% of patients
Increased prothrombin time	Common	90% of patients
Decreased fibrinogen	Late in disease	70% of patients
Factor V	Decreased	Regularly decreased
Factor VIII	Normal	Regularly decreased
Factors VII, X	Decreased	Normal

in prothrombin time and activated partial thromboplastin time because of multiple factor deficiencies. Table 12-13 contrasts liver disease with disseminated intravascular coagulopathy.

Factor-Deficiency States

Factor XI Deficiency (Hemophilia C)

This disorder is autosomal dominant in inheritance pattern and more common among persons of Jewish descent. Bleeding occurs after injury or operation. Laboratory findings include prolonged partial thromboplastin time and activated partial thromboplastin time but a normal prothrombin time. The treatment of choice is fresh frozen plasma.

Factor IX Deficiency (Christmas Disease, Hemophilia B)

This X-linked disorder accounts for 15% of all cases of hemophilia. It is clinically indistinguishable from factor VIII deficiency. The laboratory abnormalities include an abnormal partial thromboplastin time. The treatment for mild cases is fresh frozen plasma. Patients undergoing a surgical procedure or who have major bleeding should receive purified factor IX complex. There may be an increased risk of thrombosis, because of the presence of activated factors VII and X. Three other available products are KONȳNE, Proplex, and Profilnine, which are factor IX-complex products developed from a monoclonal antibody purifying process. They are safe from contamination with the AIDS virus, and the risk of hepatitis is significantly reduced.

Factor VIII Deficiency (Hemophilia A)

This disease results from a defect in factor VIII:C, is X-linked recessive in inheritance pattern, and accounts for 85% of cases of hemophilia. If a hemophiliac male has children from a normal female, all daughters are obligatory carriers and all sons are normal. If a normal male marries a carrier, each daughter has a 50% chance of being a carrier and each son has a 50% chance of having hemophilia. At birth, there are no bleeding manifestations; however, 50% of males bleed at the time of circumcision. Bleeding occurs in 75% of severely affected infants by age 18 months. The severity of hemophilia runs true in families. Severe hemophiliacs have less than 1% factor VIII and clinically have hemarthroses, atrophied muscles, subcutaneous hematomas in the tongue and neck, and hematomas in the genitourinary and gastrointestinal tracts. Mild hemophiliacs have factor VIII levels of 5%-25% (55%-145%) and may bleed heavily, even fatally, postoperatively or after dental extractions unless the factor is adequately replaced.

Laboratory studies reveal an abnormal partial thromboplastin time, abnormal factor VIII:C, normal prothrombin time, normal bleeding time, and normal thrombin time. Treatment consists of factor VIII concentrate, which has a half-life of 8-12 hours. Current factor VIII:C concentrates are regarded as safe from HIV transmission. However, three highly purified products, all produced by monoclonal antibodies, are available and no cases of AIDS or hepatitis B or C have been reported with the use of these products. There have been no seroconversions to HIV with any of the products in the U.S., including products that have been heated in aqueous solution, solvent-detergent treated, and/or immunoaffinity purified. Heat and solvent-detergent treated concentrates appear to be free from transmission of hepatitis B, hepatitis C, and HIV. Hepatitis A and parvovirus are not inactivated by these techniques. Recombinant factor VIII products are also available and appear to be free from human virus transmission. Always check Bethesda unit assay before any general surgery in patients with hemophilia. From 5% to 20% of hemophiliacs develop inhibitors (IgG antibodies) that inactivate factor VIII:C (Bethesda units). If the inhibitor is <3 Bethesda units/mL, then treat with higher doses or replacement therapy. If the value is higher (>10 Bethesda units), one can attempt to use prothrombin complex concentrates (II, VII, IX, X) to "bypass." Table 12-14 contrasts hemophilia A with von Willebrand's disease.

- Management of hemophilia A: a desmopressin trial should be undertaken in cases of mild-to-moderate hemophilia A.
- For other patients, factor VIII products that are heat treated, solvent-detergent treated, immunoaffinity purified, or produced by recombinant techniques.
- Recombinant techniques appear to be free from human virus transmission.

Table 12-14.--Differences Between Hemophilia A and von
Willebrand's Disease

	Hemophilia A	von Wille-brand's disease
Inheritance	Sex-linked	Autosomal
Bleeding time	Normal	Prolonged
Factor VIII:C	Decreased	Decreased
Factor VIII rag	Normal	Decreased
Ristocetin cofactor	Normal	Decreased

Acquired factor VIII deficiency states may occur and are secondary to the following causes: idiopathic, postpartum, collagen vascular diseases (rheumatoid arthritis, systemic lupus erythematosus, temporal arteritis), drug hypersensitivity (penicillin, sulfonamides), malignancies (lymphoproliferative, solid tumors), and old age. Clinically, bleeding is intramuscular, retropharyngeal, retroperitoneal, and cerebral. Also, hematuria occurs. The treatment is very difficult and requires the combination of steroids, cyclophosphamide, plasmapheresis, prothrombin-complex concentrate, activated prothrombin-complex concentrate, and porcine factor VIII. The combination of cyclophosphamide and prednisone may be effective in the outpatient setting in patients with an acquired factor VIII inhibitor.

Factor XII deficiency is an autosomal recessive disorder in which thromboembolic complications are more important than bleeding complications. The activated partial thromboplastin time is abnormal, and the prothrombin time is normal.

Factor VII deficiency is characterized clinically by epistaxis, gingival bleeding, bleeding after trauma, menorrhagia, and hemarthroses. The activated partial thromboplastin time is normal, and the prothrombin time is abnormal.

Factor X deficiency is characterized by bleeding that is the same as that in factor VII deficiency. An acquired factor X deficiency state may occur in amyloidosis. The activated partial thromboplastin time and prothrombin time are abnormal.

Factor V deficiency may be acquired in myeloproliferative disorders. Bruising occurs with severe bleeding postoperatively and at the onset of menstruation. Treatment consists of administering platelets and fresh frozen plasma.

In factor XIII deficiency, there is a history of umbilical cord bleeding, ecchymoses, and prolonged hemorrhage from cuts. It is autosomal recessive in inheritance. All routine clotting tests, including bleeding time, may give normal results. Treatment is with fresh frozen plasma. Table 12-15 summarizes the hemorrhagic disorders.

Treatment of Factor Deficiency States

Circulatory overload problems must be taken into consideration when transfusing into patients materials used to treat deficiency states. The composition of these materials is given in Table 12-16. To control major bleeding or to prepare patients for a surgical procedure, it is advised that the plasma level of factor VIII be increased to 60% in patients with factor VIII deficiency. The number of factor VIII units is calculated by multiplying the patient's weight in pounds by 12 (example, 160 pounds x 12 = 1,920 units of factor VIII).

Fresh frozen plasma is a good source of all factors. It is used in treating congenital deficiencies in factors II, V, VII, IX, X, XI, and XIII and multiple coagulation deficiencies, including oral anticoagulant overdose, liver disease, massive transfusion, disseminated intravascular coagulopathy, plasmapheresis, and vitamin K deficiency. One should suspect multiple coagulation factor deficiencies in patients with prolonged prothrombin times and partial thromboplastin times >1.5 times normal if not due to known coagulation factor deficiency or

Table 12-15.--Summary of Test Results in Hemorrhagic Disorders and Anticoagulant Therapy

	Prothrombin time	Activated partial thromboplastin time	Thrombin time	Fibrinogen	Bleeding time
Classic hemophilia A	Normal	Abnormal	Normal	Normal	Normal
von Willebrand's disease	Normal	Normal or abnormal	Normal	Normal	Abnormal
Afibrinogenemia	Abnormal	Abnormal	Abnormal	Absent	Normal
Hypofibrinogenemia	Normal	Normal	Normal	Low	Normal
Dysfibrinogenemia	Normal or abnormal	Normal or abnormal	Abnormal	Normal	Normal
Factor XIII deficiency	Normal	Normal	Normal	Normal	Normal
Heparin	Slightly abnormal	Abnormal	Abnormal	Normal	Normal or abnormal
Warfarin (Coumadin)	Abnormal	Normal or abnormal	Normal	Normal	Normal

Table 12-16.--Composition of Materials Used to Treat Factor Deficiency States

Type	Volume, mL	Factor VIII units per container	Amount of protein per 100 factor VIII units, mg
Fresh frozen plasma	180-250	160-225	3,300
Cryoprecipitate	10-30	75-120	900
Antihemophilic factor	10-25	250-500	500

Modified from Huestis DW, Bove JR, Busch S: Practical Blood Transfusion. Third edition. Boston, Little, Brown and Company, 1981, p 295. By permission of authors.

circulating lupus-like anticoagulant. In dosing fresh frozen plasma, 1-2 units is usually not sufficient to replace coagulation factors, as in liver disease, which requires 3-9 units. The maximal effect declines 2-4 hours after transfusion. Purified antihemophilic concentrates are derived from fresh frozen plasma of paid donors and are lyophilized or freeze-dried in form. Complications include hepatitis and factor VIII inhibitors. Cryoprecipitate is a good source of factors V, VIII, and fibrinogen. The activity per gram of protein is 12-60 times that of fresh frozen plasma. One bag will increase the factor VIII level 2.5% or one bag per 6 kg of body weight twice a day in factor VIII deficiency. Factor IX complex contains factors II, VII, IX, and X. Activated factor IX-complex products include KONỹNE and anti-inhibitor coagulant complex, heat treated (Autoplex T). This is indicated in severe factor IX deficiency and in the management of factor VIII inhibitors. Complications include hepatitis, disseminated intravascular coagulopathy, and thrombosis.

Hypercoagulable States

Risk factors for thrombosis are noncongenital, congenital, and acquired. Noncongenital risk factors include age, trauma, obesity, immobilization, pregnancy, diabetes mellitus, and oral contraceptive pills. Congenital causes include the deficiency states of protein S, protein C, and antithrombin III. Acquired conditions include lupus anticoagulant, disseminated intravascular coagulopathy, paroxysmal nocturnal hemoglobinuria, pregnancy, malignancy, inflammatory bowel disease, myeloproliferative disorders, cryoglobulinemia, and aberrant blood flow. Protein S deficiency is more common than deficiency of protein C or antithrombin III. Routine coagulation assays fail to detect these patients. A 50% decrease in either protein S or C increases thrombotic tendencies. Family studies are requisite. Assays are available for all three. Protein S is a vitamin K-dependent factor that is required for expression of activated protein C anticoagulant activity. There is an increased incidence of thrombosis, with venous complications greater than arterial. Activated protein C destroys activated factors V and VIII and, thus, is a potent plasma anticoagulant. Activated protein C requires a second vitamin K-dependent factor, or cofactor, protein S. Antithrombin III deficiency is an uncommon

cause of venous thromboembolism. The management of protein S deficiency, protein C deficiency, and antithrombin III deficiency requires heparin and oral anticoagulant agents. There is an increased incidence of warfarin (Coumadin) necrosis that is a rare complication in nonhospitalized patients and occurs 2-10 days after initiating treatment with warfarin.

The antiphospholipid antibodies include anticardiolipin antibodies, lupus anticoagulants, protein-phospholipid reactivity, and anti-reagin antibodies. The lupus anticoagulant is an immunoglobulin (IgG, IgA, or IgM) that interferes with in vitro phospholipid steps of coagulation, causing a prolonged clotting time in the activated partial thromboplastin time, Dilute Russell Viper Venom Time, or plasma clot time. Patients with the lupus anticoagulant are at a higher risk for thrombosis. This is an interfering inhibitor of the activated partial thromboplastin time that does not correct with equal volumes of normal plasma. These react with anionic phospholipids, prothrombin, and β_2 glycoprotein 1. The screening test is the prolonged activated partial thromboplastin time. Clinically, venous thrombosis of the lower extremities is more common than arterial thrombosis.

The clinical syndromes of the antiphospholipid antibody syndromes include major (venous and arterial thromboses, spontaneous abortions, and thrombocytopenia) and minor (livedo reticularis, multistroke dementia, and chorea) components. The thrombotic manifestations are venous (deep venous thrombosis, cutaneous thrombosis, renal vein thrombosis, and Budd-Chiari syndrome) or arterial (central nervous system, coronary thrombosis, and renal artery or vein thrombosis). Hematologic associations include thrombocytopenia, hemolysis, and hypocomplementemia. Obstetrical associations are maternal (deep venous thrombosis, chorea, eclampsia, and pulmonary embolus) and fetal (spontaneous abortion, fetal death, and second and third trimester premature birth).

There is no indication for the treatment of asymptomatic patients without a history of associated conditions. Initial treatment with heparin followed by anticoagulation with warfarin with an International Normalized Ratio (INR) >3.0 is the treatment for thrombosis. Low doses of aspirin and heparin are recommended for the management of pregnant patients.

Who should be tested? Patients who should be considered for further testing include persons <40 years old with thrombotic events and those with a strong family history of thrombosis, recurrent thromboses at different sites, skin necrosis, recurrent fetal loss, and thrombosis at unusual sites (sagittal sinus thrombosis, mesenteric thrombosis, etc.).

Warfarin

Warfarin limits the gamma-carboxylation of the vitamin K-dependent coagulation proteins II, VII, IX, and X and anticoagulant proteins C and S, impairing their biologic function in blood coagulation. This drug is contraindicated in pregnancy and in patients with a hemorrhagic tendency such as thrombocytopenia or coagulation factor abnormalities, diastolic blood pressure >110 mm Hg, gastrointestinal tract lesions liable to bleed, severe liver disease, severe renal disease, malabsorption, subacute bacterial endocarditis, diverticulosis, or colitis. It is also contraindicated if the patient recently had a surgical procedure performed on the central nervous system or eye. The appropriate dose of warfarin for preventing systemic embolism, valvular heart disease, and myocardial infarction, for prophylaxis for venous thrombosis, and for treating venous thrombosis and pulmonary embolism is that which maintains the prothrombin time at an INR of 2-3, which corresponds to a prothrombin time ratio of 1.3 to 1.5. An INR of 3.0-4.5 is recommended for patients with recurrent pulmonary emboli or patients with mechanical prosthetic heart valves. The main complication is bleeding, which occurs in 2%-4% of patients. In patients with a prolonged prothrombin time with or without bleeding, use of the drug should be stopped for 24-72 hours. In patients who have taken a suicidal dose or have a suspected cerebral hemorrhage and who need no further anticoagulation, vitamin K given intravenously at a dose of 20-30 mg may be administered with fresh frozen plasma. Fresh frozen plasma may be administered to patients taking warfarin who require continued anticoagulation but who have life-threatening bleeding. Drugs that potentiate warfarin include those that prolong the prothrombin time, such as phenylbutazone, metronidazole, sulfinpyrazone, trimethoprim/sulfamethoxazole, and disulfiram. Drugs that inhibit platelet function, such as aspirin, may also potentiate the toxic effects of warfarin. Some drugs antagonize warfarin; e.g., cholestyramine decreases the absorption of warfarin. Other drugs, such as barbiturates, carbamazepine, and rifampin, increase the clearance of warfarin.

Heparin

Heparin inhibits thrombin by forming a heparin-antithrombin III complex. The heparin is then reused. In the initial treatment of deep venous thrombosis or pulmonary embolus, the goal is to prolong the activated partial thromboplastin time at a level of 1.5-2.5 times normal within the first 24 hours of treatment. If this is not accomplished, the risk of recurrent thromboembolism is 15-fold, and the risk persists for weeks. Heparin and warfarin may be given simultaneously and be overlapped for 5 days, after which treatment should be warfarin alone.

Warfarin treatment should be maintained for 3 months if there are no risk factors. Prolonged treatment may be indicated when risk factors such as prolonged immobilization, hypercoagulable state, and recurrent deep venous thrombosis exist.

Heparin is indicated for the treatment of venous thrombosis and pulmonary emboli. It is also used to prevent venous thrombosis and pulmonary emboli (prophylactic doses of 5,000 U subcutaneously every 8-12 hours in cases of abdominal surgery or for medical patients with a history of thrombosis, prolonged bed rest, congestive heart failure, or cancer). A dose of 12,000 U is administered subcutaneously twice a day for the prevention of mural thrombosis after myocardial infarction. Heparin is indicated in the prevention of coronary artery rethrombosis after thrombolysis, and it is the treatment of choice in venous thrombosis and pulmonary emboli in pregnancy (15,000 U subcutaneously twice a day). Impedance plethysmography, ultrasonography, or venography may document this complication of pregnancy. (Warfarin is contraindicated in pregnancy because of the risks of embryopathy, including nasal hypoplasia and central nervous system abnormalities.) Heparin is indicated after treatment with thrombolytic therapy. The normal dose is a 5,000-U bolus followed by 30,000 to 35,000 U/24 hours by continuous infusion. Side effects include hemorrhage (which occurs in 6.8% of patients treated by continuous infusion), osteoporosis, and skin necrosis. A hypersensitivity reaction may convert antithrombin III from a slow inhibitor to a very rapid inhibitor.

Thrombolytic Therapy

The thrombolytic agents are streptokinase, urokinase, recombinant tissue plasminogen activator and urokinase-like activator, and anisolyated streptokinase-plasminogen activator complex. Fibrin is the major target of thrombolytic therapy. Anticoagulation does *not* dissolve or prevent the growth of thrombi (even at recommended doses), eliminate the source of subsequent emboli in the deep veins during an acute attack, alleviate hemodynamic problems, prevent valvular damage, prevent persistent venous hypertension, or prevent persistent pulmonary hypertension. The primary role of anticoagulation is prophylaxis against further propagation of the clot.

Thrombolytic therapy lyses thrombi and emboli and restores the circulation to normal, normalizes hemodynamic disturbances, reduces morbidity, decreases systemic and mean pulmonary artery pressures at 72 hours, prevents venous vascular damage and subsequent venous hypertension in the lower extremities, and prevents permanent damage to the pulmonary vascular bed, reducing the likelihood of persistent pulmonary hypertension. Residual emboli usually persist with heparin therapy alone. Tissue plasminogen activator has a relative fibrin specificity; yet, significant fibrinolysis and bleeding may occur. There is an initial fibrinolysis of the plug followed by proteolysis of fibrinogen and factors V and VIII. In general, venous thrombi are rich in fibrin and are potentially more suitable than platelet thrombi to fibrinolytic therapy. The age of the thrombus is also important in that it is essential to start these agents within 48 hours in cases of pulmonary emboli and in <7 days in cases of deep venous thrombosis. In cases of pulmonary emboli, this treatment improves hemodynamics and pulmonary perfusion; it may be indicated with more lobar pulmonary arteries or an equivalent amount of emboli in other vessels with or without shock or submassive emboli accompanied by shock or impending shock or persistent hypotension. In deep venous thrombosis, these agents may minimize valvular dysfunction and decrease the risk of recurrent and postphlebitic syndrome. At this time, these agents are not recommended for routine use in pulmonary emboli and deep venous thrombosis.

If the timing is appropriate, these agents may be administered in thrombosis of the hepatic, renal, mesenteric, cerebrovenous, sinus, and central retinal veins. Of arterial disorders, acute myocardial infarction has been the most excessively studied. The SCAT 1 trial demonstrated that mortality was significantly lower in patients randomized to heparin after thrombolytic therapy in acute myocardial infarction. The GUSTO trial revealed that a rapid infusion of tissue plasminogen activator with intravenously given heparin was most favorable.

Thrombolytic therapy is monitored with fibrinogen levels. The absolute contraindications to this therapy include active internal bleeding and a cerebral vascular accident within the preceding 2 weeks. Relatively major contraindications include the following if they have occurred within <10 days: major surgical procedure, obstetrical delivery, pregnancy, the first 10 days post partum, organ biopsy, burns, skin grafts, previous puncture of noncompressible vessels, thoracentesis, paracentesis, gastrointestinal tract bleeding, ulcerative colitis, diverticulosis, serious trauma, systolic blood pressure >200 mm Hg, diastolic pressure >110 mm Hg, intracranial neoplasms, or thrombocytopenia. Relatively minor contraindications include a high likelihood of left-sided heart thrombus such as mitral stenosis with atrial fibrillation, subacute bacterial endocarditis, severe hepatic or renal disease, age >75 years, diabetic hemorrhagic retinopathy, active and progressive cavitating lung lesions, ulcerative cutaneous and mucous membrane lesions, recent intra-arterial diagnostic procedure except arterial blood gases. Bleeding may be superficial or internal; it occurs because of the indiscriminate lysis of fibrin. Thrombolytic agents are not substitutes for heparin and warfarin and, therefore, the morbidity is additive. Approaches to hemorrhage control include volume replacement, manual techniques, and RBC transfusions. If bleeding is massive, replace with cryoprecipitate and fresh frozen plasma and discontinue use of heparin. With central nervous system bleeding, discontinue fibrinolytic therapy, administer cryoprecipitate and fresh frozen plasma, and avoid anticoagulants and antiplatelet agents.

Aplastic Anemia

Aplastic anemia may develop as a consequence of a defect in the stem cell population, defective marrow environment, or immune suppression. This group of disorders with failure of hematopoiesis is characterized by peripheral pancytopenia, bone marrow hypocellularity, and absence of malignant or myeloproliferative diseases. No primary disease of hematopoietic tissue is evident.

Natural history--Before the use of allogeneic bone marrow transplantation and antithymocyte globulin, 80% of patients with severe aplastic anemia were not alive at 1-2 years, and 20% had partial recovery.

- Aplastic anemia: pancytopenia, hypocellular bone marrow, and absence of primary disease of hematopoietic tissue.
- Full recovery is uncommon without allogeneic bone marrow transplantation or antithymocyte globulin.

Clinical features include weakness, fatigue, easy bruising or bleeding, fever, and infections. Lymphadenopathy and splenomegaly are uncommon. In 40%-70% of patients, the cause of aplastic anemia is idiopathic. This is more frequent in adults. Drugs are the second most common cause of aplastic anemia. These include chloramphenicol, phenylbutazone, methylphenylethylhydantoin, trimethadione, sulfonamides, gold, and benzene. Paroxysmal nocturnal hemoglobinuria and infections are the third and fourth most common causes, respectively. Infectious hepatitis is the most common infection to cause aplastic anemia. Non-A, non-B, non-C hepatitis followed by hepatitis A are the most common types of hepatitis to cause aplastic anemia. Hepatitis B is the least common hepatitis that causes aplastic anemia. These patients have a poor prognosis. Other infectious agents causing aplastic anemia include Epstein-Barr viral infections, influenza, and mycobacterial infections. Ionizing irradiation may also be a cause.

If transfusion is needed, select nonrelated donors and use leukocyte-poor RBC transfusions and single-donor platelet transfusions. Transfusions should be given with considerable care and concern. Family members should not be donors, because they are more likely to sensitize the patient to minor histocompatibility antigens present in the donor but absent in the patient. The survival rate is better for those not receiving transfusion.

Immunosuppressive treatments include antithymocyte globulin and steroids with or without cyclosporine. These are not curative. In a trial of moderate to severe aplastic anemia patients, 11 of the 21 treated with antithymocyte globulin alone had sustained improvement, whereas none of the 21 in the control population improved.

The German Aplastic Anemia Study Group reported that treatment with antithymocyte, methylprednisolone, and cyclosporine was more effective than treatment with antithymocyte globulin and methylprednisolone and may represent the treatment of choice in patients not eligible for bone marrow transplantation. The allogeneic bone marrow transplantation success rate is 66% in young patients. This is the therapy of choice in all patients with a homozygous twin and should be considered immediately for all patients younger than age 20, and this treatment should be considered in high-risk patients between the ages of 20 and 45 with an HLA-match. A trial of immunosuppressive therapy is indicated in other patients, including those with moderate disease and those 45-55 years old. Cyclosporine or corticosteroids, at a dose of 0.2-1.0 mg/kg daily, and androgens are other therapeutic modalities. Androgens are not effective in severe aplastic anemia. The toxic effects include virilization and hepatic toxicity. The 17-alpha derivative is responsible for hepatic adenomas and hepatocellular carcinoma.

- With severe aplastic anemia, avoid transfusions.
- If the patient is younger and has an HLA-matched donor or identical twin, consider bone marrow transplantation with cyclophosphamide alone or cyclophosphamide plus irradiation in previously transfused patients as preconditioning. If the patient is older or has no HLA match, treat with a combination of antithymocyte globulin and methylprednisolone with or without cyclosporine.
- Long-term survival in patients with severe disease has increased from <25% in patients treated with androgens to 75% in those treated with intensive immunosuppressive therapy and to 66% in those treated with bone marrow transplantation.

Neutropenia

The causes of neutropenia are multiple. Drug-induced neutropenia is associated with sulfonamides, semisynthetic penicillins (nafcillin, ampicillin), phenothiazines, nonsteroidal anti-inflammatory agents (indomethacin), and antithyroid medications (propylthiouracil, methimazole). Cyclic neutropenia is characterized by oscillations in the neutrophil counts every 19-23 days. It is a disorder of neutrophil production at a regulation phase. The typical clinical syndrome is manifested as furuncles, cellulitis, chronic gingivitis, and abscesses. Patients can predict the timing of successive episodes. Treatment involves timely antibiotics, avoidance of dental and surgical work at nadirs, oral hygiene, and dental care. Granulocyte colony-stimulating factor (filgrastim) may be effective in increasing the neutrophil count.

Neutropenia in the black population is common, and if patients are asymptomatic, this need not be evaluated further. Other causes of neutropenia include autoimmune neutropenia (which is secondary to an antibody), antigens, rheumatoid arthritis, and chronic active hepatitis.

Thrombocytopenia

The causes of thrombocytopenia in adults are multiple and broadly include autoimmune idiopathic thrombocytopenic purpura, drug-induced thrombocytopenia, pseudothrombocytopenia, refractoriness to platelet transfusion therapy, post-transfusion purpura, and secondary causes. Secondary causes include systemic lupus erythematosus (in which 14%-26% of patients develop thrombocytopenia), infections (HIV, rubella, infectious mononucleosis), chronic lymphocytic leukemia, non-Hodgkin's lymphoma, sarcoidosis, ovarian carcinoma, and purpura of septicemia.

The diagnosis of pseudothrombocytopenia should be excluded with examination of a peripheral blood smear. Causes of pseudothrombocytopenia include EDTA-induced platelet clumping, platelet satellitosis, May-Hegglin anomaly, Bernard-Soulier syndrome, and large platelets in myeloproliferative disorders. A spuriously low platelet count may be reported in EDTA-induced platelet agglutination. This is an antibody-mediated phenomenon caused by antibodies that bind to the patient's platelets after withdrawal of calcium.

Post-transfusion purpura occurs 7-10 days after blood transfusion and is a complication of the transfusion of blood products from donors positive for the platelet antigen P1A[1] into P1A[1]-negative recipients previously sensitized to this antigen by pregnancy or transfusions. Treatment includes plasmapheresis or exchange transfusion; prednisone may be added to the regimen.

Idiopathic thrombocytopenic purpura is an autoimmune disease characterized by thrombocytopenia with a normal WBC count and hemoglobin (Table 12-17). The clinical

Table 12-17.--Idiopathic Thrombocytopenic Purpura

Characteristics	Acute	Chronic
Presentation	Abrupt onset of petechiae, purpura, mucosal bleeding	Insidious petechiae, menorrhagia
Usual age	Children (2-6 years old)	Adults (20-40 years old)
Sex	Male = female	Female:male = 3:1
Antecedent infection	Common 85%	Uncommon
	Typically an upper respiratory tract infection	
Platelet count, x10^9/L	<20 x 10^9/L	30-80 x 10^9/L
Duration	2-6 weeks	Months to years
Spontaneous remission	80% within 6 months	Uncommon, fluctuates

From Lee GR, Bithell TC, Foerster J, Athens JW, Lukens JN: Wintrobe's Clinical Hematology. Vol 2. Ninth edition. Philadelphia, Lea & Febiger, 1993, p 1331. By permission of publisher.

manifestations include purpura, mucous membrane hemorrhage, and cerebromeningeal bleeding. From 7% to 28% of children and up to 40%-60% of adults progress to a chronic state of idiopathic thrombocytopenic purpura. In most patients, the platelet count is <50,000/μL, and 30% are <10,000/μL. The mean platelet volume is increased. Splenomegaly is present in only 10% of patients. If it is present, one should think of other causes. Bone marrow examination reveals a normal to increased number of megakaryocytes. Antibodies to specific platelet-membrane glycoproteins, usually the IIb-IIIa complex, and platelet IgG (erroneously called antiplatelet-antibody tests) measurements are detected in most patients but are not essential in the diagnosis or treatment. Up to 10% of patients with chronic ITP may have accessory spleens. The absence of Howell-Jolly bodies on a peripheral blood smear of patients who have previously undergone splenectomy suggests the diagnosis, which is confirmed by radionuclide imaging or CT scan. Surgical removal may be beneficial.

Corticosteroids are the mainstay of initial treatment; 70% of patients initially respond, with about a 40% chance of long-term remission at an initial dose of prednisone of 1 mg/kg daily for up to 1 month. Steroids decrease antibody production in the reticuloendothelial system and decrease reticuloendothelial clearance. Splenectomy removes the predominant site of antibody production and platelet destruction and is followed by a 75% chance of long-term remission. Dexamethasone (40 mg/day for 4 sequential days every 28 days for 12 months) is indicated for the treatment of resistant or relapsed idiopathic thrombocytopenic purpura. Danazol decreases the number of phagocytic cell IgG Fc receptors. A slow infusion of vincristine or vinblastine may be given to patients who do not respond to the above measures. A high dose of gamma globulin, which blocks the Fc receptors of phagocytic cells, followed by platelet transfusion is used in emergency bleeding in acute idiopathic thrombocytopenic purpura, e.g., central nervous system bleeding. Other agents used in refractory cases include azathioprine (Imuran), cyclophosphamide, colchicine, cyclosporine, and immunoadsorption apheresis on staphylococcal protein A columns.

In drug-induced thrombocytopenia, the pathophysiology is secondary to haptens bound to a carrier protein. Clinically, there is acute bleeding with a hemorrhage syndrome characterized by bleeding from mucous membranes, petechiae, and oozing after brushing the teeth. These problems subside after use of the drug is discontinued. Drug-induced thrombocytopenia subsides in 4-14 days except for gold, which may take much longer. In contrast, viral-induced thrombocytopenia resolves in 2 weeks to 3 months. Drugs implicated include heparin, quinidine, quinine, gold salts, sulphonamides, procainamide, and rifampin. Heparin-induced thrombocytopenia has a variable incidence of 1%-30%. Heparin may enhance platelet aggregation; this mechanism has been implicated in thrombocytopenia and thrombosis. Venous thrombosis is more common than arterial thrombosis. The mechanism of action is immunologic, with heparin-specific IgG antibody and antibodies against a platelet-heparin complex. This complication is usually mild, and the patients are asymptomatic. It develops 3-15 days after therapy, with a median time of 10 days. It is not dose-related and can occur at very low doses. There are no reliable risk factors. Patients are at higher risk if there is a history of this problem. It is essential to pay attention to any substantial decrease in platelet number while patients are taking heparin.

- 6%-8% of pregnant women at term and 25% of women with preeclampsia have mild thrombocytopenia with platelets >80,000/μL.
- Drug-induced thrombocytopenia subsides in 4-14 days except with gold.
- Viral-induced thrombocytopenia resolves in 2 weeks to 3 months.
- Heparin-induced thrombocytopenia is not dose-related.

Postsplenectomy State

Postsplenectomy complications include sepsis secondary to pneumococcus, meningococcus, *Haemophilus influenzae*, *Escherichia coli*, and *Staphylococcus aureus*. Hematologic features include such RBC abnormalities as Howell-Jolly bodies present on the peripheral blood smear. Leukocytes show a postsplenectomic surge and then return to normal numbers. Platelets also show a postsplenectomic surge; the value usually returns to normal in 1 month. If there is a history of splenectomy but no Howell-Jolly bodies on a peripheral blood smear, suspect an accessory spleen and confirm it with a liver-spleen scan.

Spontaneous Splenic Ruptures

Spontaneous splenic ruptures have been reported to occur in infectious mononucleosis (color plate 12-17), cytomegalovirus infections, acute and chronic myelogenous leukemia, acute and chronic lymphocytic leukemia, myeloproliferative diseases, and non-Hodgkin's lymphoma.

Transfusion Reactions

The major transfusion reactions include acute hemolytic transfusion reactions, transfusions associated with anti-IgA antibodies, transfusion-associated adult respiratory distress syndrome, delayed hemolytic transfusion reactions, febrile transfusion reactions, urticarial transfusion reactions, and circulatory overload. Acute hemolytic transfusion reactions are the most life-threatening. The most common cause is human error (51%), especially when blood is released on an emergency basis, and these are secondary to ABO mismatches. Other causes include antibodies not detected before transfusion, such as Kell, Duffy, and Kidd. ABO mismatches are less frequent when compared with Kell, Duffy, and Kidd and have virtually disappeared from transfusion reaction complications, but clerical error may play a role in these reactions. Intravascular hemolysis is caused by problems related to ABO, Kell, Duffy, and Kidd. Females are at greater risk than males, because sensitization through pregnancy leads to a higher frequency of preformed antibodies. Obstetrical complications with massive bleeding also predispose females. Age is a factor because older people receive more transfusions. Transfusion of large amounts of blood products given urgently also increases the risk. Clinically, there is pain at the intravenous site, apprehension, back pain, abdominal pain, fever, chills, chest pain, hypotension, nausea, flushing, and dyspnea. The Coombs' test gives positive results in all but anti-A. Complications include oliguria in 33.3% of patients, acute postischemic renal failure, and disseminated intravascular coagulopathy in 4%. In one series, the mortality rate was 17%. Treatment includes immediate termination of the transfusion, intravenous access, vigorous administration of fluids, and furosemide to increase renal cortical blood flow. It is difficult to distinguish between an acute hemolytic transfusion reaction and a febrile non-hemolytic transfusion reaction at the time fever occurs. Therefore, fevers occurring during transfusion should be worked up for hemolysis.

Transfusion reactions associated with anti-IgA antibodies and anaphylactic reactions are secondary to IgA deficiency, the development of a class-specific anti-IgA antibody, normal IgA levels with anti-IgA antibodies acquired through pregnancy or previous transfusions, and ataxia telangiectasia, in which 44% of patients have class-specific anti-IgA antibodies. The pathogenesis is secondary to anti-IgA antibodies of IgG type that are capable of binding complement. Clinically, patients develop apprehension, hives, hypotension, chest pain, abdominal pain, lumbar pain, flushing of the face and neck, dyspnea, and cyanosis. Wheezing, diarrhea, vomiting, unconsciousness, and chills may occur. Fevers are uncommon. The treatment includes stopping the transfusion and giving antihistamines and conventional anti-anaphylactic drugs. Transfusion policy for patients with this problem includes washed RBCs, frozen RBCs, and IgA-deficient plasma.

Transfusion-associated adult respiratory distress syndrome or transfusion-related acute lung injury is a complication of transfusion, with respiratory distress in 6 hours, hypotension, bilateral pulmonary infiltrates, normal pulmonary capillary wedge pressure, and fever. Recovery is rapid, occurring in 24-48 hours. Most blood donors implicated in this complication have had multiple pregnancies. Possible mechanisms include leukoagglutinating and lymphocytotoxic antibodies passively transfused from the donor to the recipient, resulting in polymorphonuclear-leukocyte-complement-triggered pulmonary edema. The treatment is supportive. Many patients require a ventilator with positive end-expiratory pressure, furosemide, and dopamine. This disorder may be misdiagnosed as circulatory overload.

Delayed hemolytic transfusion reactions occur because of the inability to detect clinically significant recipient antibodies before transfusion. This is less dramatic and less dangerous than acute hemolytic reactions and is more common in females. The recipient's plasma already contains antibody before transfusion because of previous transfusion, or previous pregnancy. It usually involves the Rh or Kidd systems, which become rapidly undetectable and increase quickly in titer on rapid stimulation. Results of the Coombs' test are positive. There is evidence of hemolysis. One-third of patients are asymptomatic, and the others present with anemia, chills, jaundice, and fever. Management consists of monitoring hemoglobin and renal output. Urticarial reactions are a complication of 1%-3% of all transfusions. Glottal edema and asthma are rarely associated. The cause is an antibody in the recipient against foreign-donor serum proteins. Treatment consists of stopping the transfusion, which is not absolutely necessary, and giving antihistamines (premedication with antihistamines if patient had previous reaction).

Febrile reactions are characterized by chills and fever an hour after the transfusion starts, with accompanying flushing, headache, tachycardia, and discomfort lasting 8-10 hours. This occurs in 1% of all transfusions. The causes include previous transfusions or pregnancy with acquired antibodies against donor leukocyte antigens, antiplatelet antibodies, and antiserum protein antibodies. Treatment consists of stopping the transfusion to evaluate the problem further, because one cannot initially distinguish a febrile reaction from a hemolytic transfusion reaction because both conditions may present with fever.

Circulatory overload may cause tightness in the chest, dry cough, and acute edema in patients with an already increased intravascular volume or decreased cardiac reserve. Management includes slowing the transfusion to 100 mL/hour, placing the patient in the sitting position, and giving diuretics.

Gaucher's Disease

Adults have type I Gaucher's disease, with no neurologic symptoms, splenomegaly, and no symptoms; 50% have anemia or thrombocytopenia. Bone lesions are present in 75%, with the femur being most common with an Erlenmeyer flask deformity. Avascular necrosis and pathologic fractures may occur. The pathogenesis is related to an accumulation of glucosylceramide due to deficient β-glucuronidase. The Gaucher cell is large and has an eccentric nucleus and fibrillar cytoplasm that is wrinkled like tissue paper (color plate 12-18). Treatment options include alglucerase (Ceredase) (an enzyme replacement therapy that is extraordinarily expensive), hemisplenectomy, and allogeneic bone marrow transplantation.

- Differential diagnosis of asymptomatic massive spleno-megaly includes Gaucher's disease, agnogenic myeloid metaplasia, portal hypertension, splenic cyst, non-Hodgkin's lymphoma, and hairy-cell leukemia.

Porphyria

The porphyrias are enzyme disorders, which are autosomal dominant with low disease penetrance, except for congenital erythropoietic porphyria, which is autosomal recessive. Disease manifestation depends on the type of the excess porphyrinogen intermediate and related porphyrin. When there is an excess of the earlier precursor molecules (δ-aminolevulinic acid and porphobilinogen), the clinical manifestations are neuropsychiatric. These symptoms include autonomic dysfunction (abdominal pain, vomiting, constipation, tachycardia, and hypertension), psychiatric symptoms, fever, leukocytosis, syndrome of inappropriate antidiuretic hormone, and neurologic symptoms (proximal paresis and paresthesias). If the excess is in the distal intermediates (uroporphyrins, coproporphyrins, and protoporphyrins), then the manifestations are cutaneous (photosensitivity, blister formation, facial hypertrichosis, and hyperpigmentation). If the excess is early and late, then there are neuropsychiatric and cutaneous manifestations. Porphobilinogen production and excretion are invariably increased during significant symptoms caused by the three neuropathic porphyrias, which include acute intermittent porphyria, hereditary coproporphyria, and porphyria variegata. In hereditary coproporphyria and porphyria variegata, there is an accumulation of coproporphyrinogen/coproporphyrin or protoporphyrinogen/protoporphyrin and a concomitant increase in δ-aminolevulinic acid and porphobilinogen. In the acute porphyrias, porphobilinogen is increased during the attacks. Acute intermittent porphyria lacks skin lesions. It is important to check fecal porphyrins in protoporphyria, variegate porphyria, and coproporphyria. The porphyrias are compared in Table 12-18. Secondary coproporphyrinuria has multiple causes, including impaired hepatobiliary transport of coprophyrin (steroids) or increased hepatic or erythroid synthesis (alcohol, liver disease, or hemolytic anemia).

Table 12-18.--Comparison of Porphyrias

Porphyria cutanea tarda	Acute intermittent porphyria	Porphyria variegata
Features		
Most common Iron overload Skin lesions on light-exposed areas Hypertrichosis Increased uroporphyrins in urine No neuropathic features	Increased urinary δ-aminolevulinic acid (ALA) and porphobilinogen (PBG) Triad: abdominal pain of 3-5 days' duration, neurologic problems of polyneuropathy and motor paresis, psychiatric problems with hallucinations, confusion, psychosis, seizures Decreased uroporphyrinogen I synthase	Clinically: skin, sun-exposed, mechanical fragility; abdominal pain; neurologic problems (e.g., acute intermittent porphyria) Increased protoporphyrin and coproporphyrin in stool
Associations		
Alcoholic liver disease Estrogens: females, males treated for prostatic carcinoma Hexachlorobenzene	Drugs: sulfonamides, barbiturates, alcohol Menstrual cycle Infection Decreased food intake	Common in South Africa, Holland
Treatment		
Phlebotomy, to remove iron	Large amounts of glucose (400 g/day) Luteinizing hormone Avoid prolonged fasting and crash diets	Glucose Avoid prolonged fasting and crash diets

- Determine the 24-hour urinary porphobilinogen during the acute episode.

Cardiac Toxicity of Chemotherapeutic Agents

Doxorubicin (Adriamycin) has the greatest potential for cardiac toxicity. It is dose-limited at a dose of 450 mg/m^2 to 500 mg/m^2. The course is characterized by cardiomyopathy to congestive heart failure to death. The pathologic features are characterized by a diffuse patchy myocardial cell degeneration that antedates any alteration in left ventricular function. Risk factors include age >70 years, coronary artery disease, hypertension, and the use of other cardiotoxic agents. Weekly and prolonged continuous infusion schedules may decrease the risk of toxicity. Acutely, there may be transient and reversible nonspecific ST-segment changes, decrease in ejection fraction, or arrhythmias. The dilated cardiomyopathy is dose-dependent: a 3.5% risk at a total dose of 400 mg/m^2 and 7% at a dose of 550 mg/m^2. The clinical features of the cardiomyopathy vary widely. Follow-up examination requires evaluating left ventricular ejection fraction by radionuclide ventriculography or echocardiography. The former is more sensitive.

- Doxorubicin has the greatest potential for cardiac toxicity.
- Incidence of cardiomyopathy is dose-dependent.
- Age >70 years, coronary artery disease, and previous radiation may potentiate toxicity.

Superior Vena Cava Syndrome

Most cases (78%) of superior vena cava syndrome are caused by malignancy. Extrinsic compression of the thin superior vena cava, which has a low intravascular pressure, in a rigid compartment contributes to the pathophysiology of this syndrome. The causes include bronchogenic carcinoma (75% of cases, with small cell and squamous cell carcinoma most common), lymphoma (15%), testicular carcinoma (consider this if biopsy shows anaplastic or undifferentiated carcinoma; check β-subunit of human chorionic gonadotropin and alpha-fetoprotein), carcinoma, and adenocarcinoma of undetermined primary. The symptoms include suffusion of face and conjunctiva, dyspnea, facial swelling, other swelling, cough, dysphagia, syncope, orthopnea, stridor, and lethargy. Physical examination reveals thoracic vein distention, neck vein distention, facial edema, cyanosis, edema of upper extremities, paralyzed vocal cord, Horner's syndrome, and heart murmurs. The diagnosis is established by the history and physical examination. Superior vena cava venography is not useful. A tissue diagnosis is essential to establish a diagnosis precisely. Mediastinotomy is the safest way to obtain histologic diagnosis. If the syndrome is rapid in onset, then treatment must be rapid. In patients with lymphoma, testicular carcinoma, or small cell carcinoma of the lung, treat the underlying disease initially with chemotherapy. If life-threatening problems are present, such as tracheal obstruction or increased intracranial pressure, emergency radiation therapy may be necessary in any disorder presenting with superior vena cava syndrome. Steroids may be helpful. Initial treatment with radiation therapy is indicated in solid tumors, with a total dose of 30-50 Gy or a single dose of 7-12 Gy. Anticoagulation is indicated only if a blood clot has been implicated in the pathophysiology. Diuretics and surgical decompression are not indicated.

- For superior vena cava syndrome, establish a tissue diagnosis.
- Features: edema of the face and neck and venous engorgement of the upper torso.
- Medical emergency in certain situations; may require immediate radiation.

Hypercalcemia in Malignant Disease

Virtually any malignancy may lead to hypercalcemia. Specific causes include carcinomas of the breast and lung (squamous and large cell carcinoma are common and adenocarcinoma and small cell carcinoma are uncommon causes), hypernephroma, other tumors (head and neck, cervix, prostate, neuroblastoma, hepatoma, and melanoma), lymphoma, Burkitt's lymphoma, multiple myeloma, Hodgkin's disease, and Waldenström's macroglobulinemia.

- Hypercalcemia in malignancy does not always denote advanced stage cancer.
- Lung malignancies of squamous cell and large cell cancer and myeloma are common causes.

Nonmalignant causes include primary hyperparathyroidism, thyroid disease (Graves' disease, myxedema), renal disease, acute renal failure, chronic renal failure, rhabdomyolysis, drugs (thiazides, lithium, calcium carbonate, tamoxifen, hypervitaminosis A and D), bed rest (fracture), trauma, watery diarrhea, miliary tuberculosis, hypophosphatasia, histiocytosis X, diuretic phase of acute tubular necrosis, granulomatous disorders (tuberculosis, sarcoid, cocci, berylliosis), adrenal insufficiency, acromegaly, pheochromocytoma, immobilization, hyperalimentation, familial, idiopathic mild alkali syndrome, and addisonian crisis.

The signs and symptoms include lassitude, somnolence, weakness, anorexia, nausea, vomiting, constipation, abdominal pain, peptic ulcer, pancreatitis, polyuria, polydipsia, poor intake, renal failure, hyporeflexia, Babinski's sign, myopathy, stupor, coma, occasional localizing signs, visual abnormalities, psychotic behavior, bradycardia, tachycardia, shortened QT interval, digitalis sensitivity, arrhythmias, hypertension, fractures, pain, skeletal deformities, loss of height, poor skin turgor, calcinosis, and band keratopathy. It is misdiagnosed as terminal disease, brain metastases, drug toxicity, renal failure, diabetes insipidus, acute abdomen, and intractable peptic ulcer disease. The diagnosis can be confirmed by measuring serum levels of parathyroid hormone (PTH). In cancer, these levels are low, and in primary hyperparathyroidism, the level is increased.

- Misdiagnoses include terminal disease, brain metastases, drug toxicity, renal failure, diabetes insipidus, acute abdomen, and intractable peptic ulcer disease.

The mechanisms of action of hypercalcemia are multiple. Osteolytic metastases may produce accelerated skeletal resorption. The tumor may secrete a polypeptide with PTH-like activity without osseous metastases. Local osteolytic factors can cause direct pressure. Prostaglandin PGE_2 is associated with the hypercalcemia of renal carcinoma, tumors of the parotid gland, lung cancer, adenocarcinoma of the pancreas, and metastatic carcinoma of unknown primary tumor. In these cases, there are no bone metastases, and the PTH levels are undetectable. Treatment includes indomethacin at a dose of 15-50 mg/day or aspirin at a dose of 1-4.8 g/day. Osteoclast activating factors are associated with multiple myeloma, lymphoma, and Burkitt's non-Hodgkin's lymphoma. There are non-PTH extracts from tumor in vitro that cause active bone resorption and regress with specific anti-tumor activity. Other factors include dehydration, mobilization, adrenal insufficiency secondary to tumor metastases, estrogens, androgens, progestins, and tamoxifen.

Most hypercalcemia is related to increased bone resorption. Intestinal absorption is low or low-normal in most cases. There usually is no increase in renal tubular reabsorption, but the kidney may be involved in hyperparathyroidism, breast cancer, metabolic alkalosis, and salt depletion. The course is short and rapidly progressive. There may be moderate to severe weight loss and no renal calculi; pancreatitis is rare. The serum level of calcium is >14 mg/dL in 75% of patients. The serum level of alkaline phosphatase may be increased, normal, or decreased. Anemia and metabolic alkalosis may be present. The alkaline phosphatase level is increased in 50% of patients but can be increased in primary hyperparathyroidism. Hypophosphatemia can occur whether or not there is a PTH-secreting tumor. Hypoalbuminemia must be considered, and for every gram of albumin below 4, add 1 to the ionized calcium.

Treatment is multifaceted. The use of such precipitating factors as vitamins A and D, lithium, thiazides, absorbable antacids, and estrogens should be discontinued. The patient should be mobilized. Also, the patient should be hydrated with a minimum of 2.5-4 L of fluid in the first 24 hours. To each liter of normal saline, add 20-40 mEq of KCl and 10-20 mEq of magnesium. Experimentally, if the sodium is increased from 25 mEq to 250 mEq, calcium excretion is increased three-fold and is not related to the glomerulofiltration rate. Treat the

underlying disease. Glucocorticoids are especially efficacious in multiple myeloma, breast cancer, and non-Hodgkin's lymphomas. The typical dose is 80 mg of prednisone in divided doses daily. The mechanisms of action include antitumor effects, an antivitamin D effect, inhibition of prostaglandin synthesis or release, inhibition of osteoclast activating factor production, anti-PTH activity, and an inhibitory effect on osteoprogenitor cells. Furosemide should be administered after 2 L of fluid. The dosages are variable, ranging from 20 mg to 40 mg up to every 4 hours. Furosemide blocks the tubular reabsorption of calcium, depletes sodium, depletes potassium, and depletes magnesium. The biphosphonates have an inhibitory effect on osteoclast function and viability. Etidronate at a dose of 7.5 mg/kg over 4 hours is given intravenously up to 7 days. This decreases calcium within 2 days. Pamidronate is given by intravenous infusion at a dose of 15-45 mg/day for up to 6 days. Alternatively, 90 mg may be given over 24 hours or it may be administered orally at a dose of 1,200 mg for up to 5 days. In general, the biphosphonates are more potent than calcitonin and less toxic than plicamycin. Plicamycin inhibits RNA synthesis in osteoclasts. There may be subjective improvement within 12 hours and improvement in the serum levels of calcium in 36 hours. The dose is 25 µg/kg over 4 hours and may be repeated once if necessary. Side effects include thrombocytopenia, hemorrhage, renal complications, increased liver enzymes, sudden arterial occlusion, and toxic epidermal necrolysis. Contraindications include thrombocytopenia and coagulopathy. Calcitonin may be administered subcutaneously or intramuscularly in the form of salmon calcitonin at a dose of 4 U/kg every 12 hours. The onset is rapid, but the response is moderate and unsustained. Gallium nitrate decreases the solubility of hydroxyapatite crystals to inhibit bone resorption. The dose is 200 mg/m^2 in 1 L of fluid intravenously over 5 days. This may be nephrotoxic. The use of phosphate should be restricted to extreme life-threatening hypercalcemia. Calcium phosphate complexes are deposited in vessels, lungs, and kidneys.

HEMOCHROMATOSIS

Hemochromatosis is the end result of a pathologic process that evolves over years and is secondary to the excessive absorption of dietary iron.

- Endocrine dysfunction: 50% with diabetes mellitus at presentation and a minority have vascular sequelae; hypogonadism (decreased libido, impotence, and amenorrhea); hypopituitarism.
- Cardiac: congestive heart failure and arrhythmias.
- Skin: bronze, "slate gray."
- Arthropathy: chondrocalcinosis, bone cysts, and irregularity.
- Hepatomegaly, cirrhosis, and hepatocellular carcinoma.

- Lethargy, weight loss.
- Transferrin saturation >55% on at least two occasions should raise clinical suspicion.
- After an index case is identified, family members must be screened.

The gene responsible for hereditary hemochromatosis is coinherited with the HLA A3 antigen. It is inherited as an autosomal recessive trait and involves 1/20,000 hospital admissions; 2-8/1,000 are affected in the general population. Males present in the fourth to fifth decade. The transferrin saturation is >55% even early in life and before tissue iron loading occurs. The causes of hemochromatosis include hereditary hemochromatosis (idiopathic), secondary anemia and ineffective erythropoiesis (thalassemia major, thalassemia minor), hereditary spherocytosis, idiopathic refractory sideroblastic anemia and myelodysplasia, oral intake of iron (medicinal), liver disease (alcoholic cirrhosis, portal caval anastomosis), drugs (isoniazid, chloramphenicol), and copper deficiency. Screening appears to be effective and should be considered at about age 30 in men.

The best screening test is a transferrin saturation >55%; it is reliable in identifying homozygotes. Urine iron is increased in the range of 5-20 mg/24 hours (normal, <2 mg/24 hours). The reference standard for diagnosis is liver biopsy, and hepatic iron by dry weight is markedly increased at 200-1,800 µg/100 ng dry weight (normal, 30-140). The goal of treatment is to improve prognosis and the clinical course in patients with established liver damage. The mainstays of treatment are phlebotomy and chelation; 224 mg of iron are removed per phlebotomy unit. Patients initially have venesection once to twice weekly. Maintenance phlebotomies are required. Deferoxamine (10 mg/day by continuous infusion) is the chelation agent used most often. Timely diagnosis and therapy can prevent irreversible organ failure. Features not altered by chelation include arthropathy, hypogonadism, development of hepatocellular carcinoma, and hepatic cirrhosis.

HEMATOLOGY OF ACQUIRED IMMUNE DEFICIENCY

In acquired immune deficiency (AIDS), lymphocytopenias are the hallmark of the disease. There is an absolute reduction of T4 lymphocytes, with a relative reduction of the T4 to T8 ratio. Also, there is functional impairment of T4 lymphocytes. Whereas T8 lymphocytes may increase early in the disease in infections, they decrease in number late in the disease. Neutropenia occurs in 50%-75% of the patients. Natural killer cells are normal in number but altered in function. Neutropenia may be due to autoimmune destruction with antigranulocyte antibodies in two-thirds of patients, decreased production, zidovudine (AZT), ganciclovir, trimethoprim-sulfamethoxazole, pentamidine, coexisting infections, non-Hodgkin's lymphoma, or antineoplastic chemotherapy. Neutrophil dysfunction is also manifested by decreased chemotaxis, granulation, and phagocytosis.

Anemia is a significant problem in HIV-infected patients. Most commonly, the anemia is normochromic normocytic. The degree of anemia is a prognostic factor in the patients. Anemia occurs in 10% of asymptomatic HIV-positive patients, 50% of patients with AIDS-related complex, and >75% of patients with overt AIDS. HIV-associated RBC problems include decreased RBC production; 70% of AIDS patients have decreased erythropoietin levels. Approximately 25% of patients have positive results on the Coombs' test, but significant hemolysis is not common. Of patients treated with zidovudine, 30% develop significant anemia, which is characteristically macrocytic. Decreased RBC production is a principal cause. Erythropoietin has been used successfully in those with an erythropoietin level <500 IU/mL. Anemia is also associated with infections from *Mycobacterium avium* complex, parvovirus, B19, *Mycobacterium tuberculosis*, and histoplasmosis. Anemia may be malignancy-related. Decreased vitamin B_{12} levels are present in 20% of HIV-infected patients and are due to altered serum transport of vitamin B_{12} and not to a deficiency in body stores unless there has been prolonged malabsorption.

Thrombocytopenia occurs in 5%-15% of HIV-infected patients and is often detected early in the disease. The serum and cell-bound antibodies are frequently positive. Circulating complexes are either the cause of or are associated with immune cytopenias. Idiopathic thrombocytopenic purpura is usually accompanied by platelet-associated antibodies and responds to zidovudine (80% of patients), prednisone (90%), danazol, dapsone (60%), immunoglobulin given intravenously, and splenectomy (80%). Other HIV associations include thrombotic thrombocytopenic purpura, decreased platelet production, and peripheral platelet sequestration. Other non-HIV associations include therapy, infection, and malignancy. Coagulation disorders may complicate HIV disorders. The lupus-like anticoagulant is present in 20% of HIV patients, usually in association with opportunistic infections, and is rarely associated with thrombosis or bleeding. Vitamin K deficiencies due to nutritional abnormalities, drugs, or hepatic dysfunction may occur. Other problems include increased vWF:Ag levels (with a poor prognosis if >200%), elevated level of tissue plasminogen activator (with a poor prognosis if >20 ng/mL), and an elevated fibrinogen level.

Non-Hodgkin's lymphoma is the second most common HIV-associated malignancy, occurring in 0.5%-1.0% of patients. Extranodal disease occurs in 66.6% of patients. Up to one-third of patients with lymphoma may have bone involvement. There is also an increased risk of Hodgkin's disease among HIV patients.

PARVOVIRUS INFECTION

Parvovirus infection (B19), or fifth disease, is a highly contagious disease in children. Adults with this infection may develop a polyarthralgia syndrome or cytopenia. Abnormalities in the erythroid line include severe anemia, reticulocytopenia, and RBC hypoplasia in the marrow. Pancytopenia may occur. Immunoglobulin therapy administered intravenously may be of benefit.

REVIEW OF CHEMOTHERAPEUTIC AGENTS

Chemotherapeutic agents--alkylating agents, antibiotics, and hormones--and their effects are reviewed in Table 12-19.

Table 12-19.--Chemotherapeutic Agents

Drug	Toxic effects	Other
	Alkylating agents	
Carmustine	Delayed marrow suppression, nausea, vomiting, pulmonary, hepatic toxicity, secondary leukemia	Cumulative marrow suppression, crosses blood-brain barrier
Busulfan	Pulmonary fibrosis	Hepatic metabolism, renal excretion
Carboplatin	Marrow suppression, nausea and vomiting, less nephrotoxicity and neurotoxicity than cisplatin	Renal excretion
Chlorambucil	Pulmonary, secondary leukemia	Hepatic metabolism
Cisplatin	Nephrotoxicity, peripheral neuropathy, ototoxicity, magnesium depletion	Renal excretion
Cyclophosphamide	Acute nonlymphocytic leukemia and dysmyelopoietic syndromes (monosomy 5 and 7), bladder cancer, leukopenia, cystitis, pulmonary fibrosis, syndrome of inappropriate ADH secretion, alopecia, nausea, vomiting	Hepatic metabolism to active compound, renal excretion, lower dose with renal failure, late transitional cell carcinoma of bladder
Dacarbazine	Marrow suppression, flu-like syndrome, severe nausea and vomiting, fever	
Melphalan	Marrow suppression, secondary leukemia	Renal excretion, erratic oral absorption
Nitrogen mustard	Marrow suppression, nausea and vomiting, sterility, secondary leukemia	
Streptozocin	Diabetes, marrow suppression, severe nausea and vomiting, renal	Leads to pancreatic and endocrine insufficiency

Table 12-19 (continued)

Drug	Toxic effects	Other
Antibiotics		
Bleomycin	Pulmonary fibrosis (threshold 400 µg/lifetime) but may recur at lower doses, fever and chills, myalgias, skin pigmentation, alopecia, adult respiratory distress syndrome with oxygen	Lower dose with renal insufficiency
Dactinomycin	Marrow suppression, radiation recall, nausea and vomiting, mucositis, alopecia	
Daunorubicin	Marrow suppression, radiation recall, cardiomyopathy, mucositis, nausea and vomiting, alopecia, acute nonlymphocytic leukemia	Decrease dose by 50% if bilirubin >1.5 mg/dL or by 75% if bilirubin >3.0 mg/dL
Doxorubicin	Dose-related cardiomyopathy, marrow suppression, alopecia, nausea and vomiting, stomatitis, radiation recall, acute nonlymphocytic leukemia	Hepatic metabolism, biliary excretion, decrease dose by 50% if bilirubin >1.5 mg/dL or by 75% if bilirubin >3.0 mg/dL
Mitomycin C	Delayed marrow suppression, nausea and vomiting, alopecia, hepatic toxicity, microangiopathic hemolytic anemia	Vesicant, alkylator, forms free radicals
Mitoxantrone	Marrow suppression, cardiac toxicity, nausea and vomiting, mucositis, alopecia, blue sclera and urine	
Hormones		
Corticosteroids	Diabetes, hepatic toxicity, aseptic necrosis, adrenal insufficiency, myopathy, infection, osteoporosis, peptic ulcer disease, hypokalemia, psychosis, cataract	
Diethylstilbestrol (estrogen)	Feminization, hypertension, irregular menses, hepatic toxicity, thrombotic complications, fluid retention, morning sickness	
Flutamide	Gynecomastia, hepatic toxicity	
Fluoxymesterone	Masculinization, fluid retention, hepatic toxicity, irregular menses, erythrocytosis	
Leuprolide	Tumor flare, hot flashes, impotence, amenorrhea	LHRH agonist
Megestrol acetate	Thrombosis, menstrual irregularities, male impotence	
Podophyllotoxin		
Etoposide (VP-16)	Acute nonlymphocytic leukemia t(11q23)	
Adenosine deaminase inhibitors		
2'-Deoxycoformycin, Fludarabine, 2-Chlorodeoxyadenosine	Myelosuppression, Opportunistic infections	

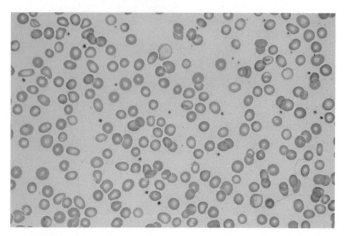

Color plate 12-1. Hypochromic-microcytic anemia. Small cells, <6 µm in diameter, with increased central pallor and assorted aberrations in size (aniso-cytosis) and in shape (poikilocytosis). (Courtesy of Curtis A. Hanson, M.D., Mayo Clinic.)

Color plate 12-2. Spherocytes. Smooth, small, and spheroidal darkly stained cells with minimal or no central pallor. (Courtesy of Curtis A. Hanson, M.D., Mayo Clinic.)

Color plate 12-3. Target cells. Red blood cells with a broad diameter and a dark center. (Courtesy of Curtis A. Hanson, M.D., Mayo Clinic.)

Color plate 12-4. Agglutination. Clumping of red blood cells.

Color plate 12-5. Acanthocytes. Note the thin, thorny, or finger-like pro-jections. (Courtesy of Curtis A. Hanson, M.D., Mayo Clinic.)

Color plate 12-6. Schistocytes. Fragmented red blood cells shaped like hel-mets, triangles, or kites. (Courtesy of Curtis A. Hanson, M.D., Mayo Clinic.)

Color plate 12-7. Rouleaux. Stacking of red blood cells. (Courtesy of Curtis A. Hanson, M.D., Mayo Clinic.)

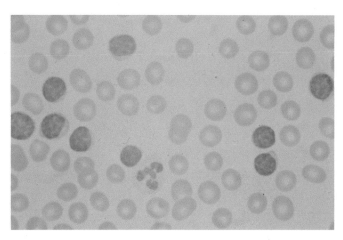

Color plate 12-8. Chronic lymphocytic leukemia. Large number of small and agranular mature lymphocytes whose nuclei are approximately the same size as red blood cells.

Color plate 12-9. Hairy-cell leukemia. Mature lymphocytes with eccentrically placed nuclei and pale cytoplasm that have characteristic projections.

Color plate 12-10. Hodgkin's disease. A Reed-Sternberg cell, a binucleate large cell. (Courtesy of Curtis A. Hanson, M.D., Mayo Clinic.)

Color plate 12-11. Plasma cell. Note the eccentrically placed round nucleus; the copious, dark blue cytoplasm has a characteristic pale-staining area adjacent to the nucleus.

Color plate 12-12. Acute nonlymphocytic leukemia. Large pleomorphic cells with large nuclei and a barely visible nuclear membrane.

Color plate 12-13. Acute promyelocytic leukemia. Note the large nuclei; more than half of the leukemic cells have large atypical granulations. (Courtesy of Curtis A. Hanson, M.D., Mayo Clinic.)

Color plate 12-14. Acute lymphocytic leukemia. Large, rounded, and indented nuclei with diverse shapes and scant, darker blue cytoplasm.

Color plate 12-15. Chronic myelogenous leukemia. Normal-appearing myeloid cells representing all stages of maturation, with a decreased number of erythropoietic cells and one basophil precursor in the center. (Courtesy of Curtis A. Hanson, M.D., Mayo Clinic.)

Color plate 12-16. Fibrosis. Bone marrow biopsy showing core diffusely replaced by fibrosis, with minimal normal hematopoietic elements present.

Color plate 12-17. Infectious mononucleosis. Large atypical lymphocyte has a large amount of pale cytoplasm, which may be vacuolated, and a large oblong nucleus.

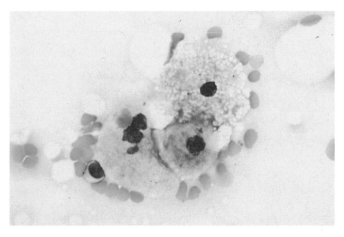

Color plate 12-18. Gaucher's cells. Large cell with characteristic pale, foamy, and fibrillar cytoplasm. (Courtesy of Curtis A. Hanson, M.D., Mayo Clinic.)

QUESTIONS

Multiple Choice (choose the one best answer)

1. High serum levels of erythropoietin occur in all of the following except:
   a. Iron deficiency
   b. High altitude
   c. Hepatocellular carcinoma
   d. Pure red cell aplasia
   e. Untreated polycythemia rubra vera

2. Which disorder is sex-linked in inheritance pattern?
   a. Unstable hemoglobin disease
   b. Hereditary spherocytosis
   c. Sickle cell anemia
   d. Glucose-6-phosphate dehydrogenase deficiency
   e. Pyruvate kinase deficiency

3. Target cells are least likely to be seen in which of the following?
   a. Thalassemia syndromes
   b. Hemoglobin C
   c. Postsplenectomy
   d. Iron deficiency
   e. Obstructive jaundice

4. In glucose-6-phosphate dehydrogenase deficiency:
   a. Drugs are the most common precipitating factor
   b. Diabetic acidosis and hypoglycemia do not precipitate hemolysis
   c. A normal glucose-6-phosphate dehydrogenase level during the acute episode of hemolysis excludes the diagnosis
   d. In the steady state, there may be no anemia
   e. Heinz bodies are present on a Wright-stained peripheral blood smear

5. In thrombotic thrombocytopenic purpura:
   a. Coombs' test is usually positive
   b. The treatment of choice is plasmapheresis and plasma exchange
   c. The fibrinogen level is decreased and prothrombin time is increased
   d. The natural history of the disorder is not affected by therapeutic intervention
   e. Females should continue to take the oral contraceptives that they were taking before diagnosis and management

6. In sickle cell anemia:
   a. Hydroxyurea decreases the frequency of painful vaso-occlusive crisis by approximately 50%
   b. In adults with a pulmonary crisis, sickling is a secondary event and frequently is caused by infection
   c. Abnormalities on bone radiographs demonstrate infarcts, and periostitis appears during the acute symptomatic period
   d. Older adults are most susceptible to central nervous system crises
   e. Acute chest syndrome is not a common cause of death

7. Predictors of survival in chronic lymphocytic leukemia include all the following except:
   a. Stage
   b. Lymphocyte doubling time
   c. Age
   d. Abnormal chromosomes
   e. Response to initial therapy

8. A 65-year-old woman has a white blood cell count of 30,000, 95% mature lymphocytes on the peripheral blood smear, platelet count of 214 x 10^9/L (150-450), and hemoglobin of 13.4 g/dL (normal, 12.0 to 15.5). Physical examination revealed no evidence of lymphadenopathy or hepatosplenomegaly. The treatment of choice is:
   a. Fludarabine
   b. Observation
   c. CHOP
   d. CVP
   e. Chlorambucil/prednisone

9. A 24-year-old woman has asymptomatic bilateral cervical lymphadenopathy. Lymph node biopsy specimen revealed nodular sclerosing Hodgkin's disease. CT revealed small mediastinal nodes. A staging laparotomy was negative. The treatment of choice is:
   a. Observation, because the patient is asymptomatic
   b. MOPP
   c. ABVD
   d. Radiation therapy in mantle and para-aortic fields
   e. Radiation therapy with a mantle and inverted Y

10. A 69-year-old woman has lymphadenopathy. Lymph node biopsy specimen revealed follicular small cleaved cell non-Hodgkin's lymphoma. The bone marrow demonstrated involvement with small cleaved cells. CT of the abdomen revealed minimal retroperitoneal lymphadenopathy. The treatment of choice is:
    a. CHOP
    b. Chlorambucil orally
    c. Interferon alfa-2a or 2b recombinant subcutaneously
    d. CVP
    e. Observation

11. A 62-year-old woman was found to have an IgG kappa M spike of 1.6 g/dL on serum protein electrophoresis. She was asymptomatic. The complete blood cell count and serum levels of creatinine and calcium were normal. The treatment of choice is:
    a. VBMCP
    b. VBMCV followed by autologous bone marrow transplantation
    c. Observation
    d. Melphalan/prednisone
    e. VAD (vincristine, doxorubicin [Adriamycin], dexamethasone)

12. A 20-year-old woman has a white blood cell count of 74 x 10^9/L (normal, 4 to 10.4), hemoglobin of 7.4 g/dL (11.6 to 14.9), and platelet count of 2,000 x 10^9/L (184-370). The spleen was 10 cm below the costal margin. Bone marrow examination revealed panhyperplasia with a t(9;22) chromosome abnormality. The treatment of choice is:
    a. Autologous bone marrow transplantation
    b. Hydroxyurea, long-term
    c. Interferon alfa recombinant, long-term
    d. ^{32}P
    e. Hydroxyurea or interferon alfa-2a or 2b recombinant followed by allogeneic bone marrow transplantation in the first 6 to 12 months, because she has an HLA-identical sibling

13. Prolonged bleeding time is not found in which of the following disorders?
    a. Bernard-Soulier syndrome
    b. Uremia
    c. Platelet counts <50 x 10^9/L
    d. Factor IX deficiency
    e. Glanzmann's thrombasthenia

14. In von Willebrand's disease:
    a. The inheritance pattern is autosomal recessive
    b. The treatment of choice is fresh frozen plasma
    c. Platelet transfusions are indicated when there is active bleeding
    d. Type I von Willebrand's disease is characterized by a quantitative abnormality in von Willebrand factor
    e. Pregnant patients with mild-to-moderate type I von Willebrand's disease require DDAVP treatment during pregnancy

15. In the treatment of hemophilia A, which therapeutic option is not appropriate?
    a. Cryoprecipitate
    b. DDAVP in patients with mild-to-moderate disease who were tested previously
    c. Highly purified factor VIII concentrates produced by monoclonal antibodies
    d. Heat-treated factor VIII concentrates
    e. Solvent-treated factor VIII concentrates

16. All the following statements regarding warfarin therapy are true except for:
    a. Warfarin limits the gamma-carboxylation of the vitamin-K-dependent coagulation proteins II, VII, IX, and X
    b. Warfarin limits the gamma-carboxylation of anticoagulant proteins C and S
    c. Metronidazole and trimethoprim/sulfamethoxazole may antagonize warfarin
    d. Warfarin is contraindicated in pregnancy
    e. Cholestyramine reduces the clearance of warfarin

17. Which of the following is not associated with the antiphospholipid syndrome in pregnancy?
    a. Positive findings on a laboratory test alone are sufficient for the diagnosis
    b. Ongoing pregnancies are associated with thrombosis, including peripheral vein thrombosis and Budd-Chiari syndrome
    c. Thrombocytopenia
    d. Fetal distress and death
    e. Preeclampsia

18. The recommended INR is 2.0 to 3.0 in all the following except:
    a. Treatment of deep venous thrombosis
    b. Treatment of pulmonary embolus
    c. Prevention of systemic embolism in myocardial infarction
    d. Prevention of systemic embolism in mechanical prosthetic heart valves
    e. Prevention of systemic embolism in tissue heart valves

19. A 79-year-old woman presented with recurrent ventricular tachycardia. A platelet count of 20 x 10^9/L (normal, 196 to 451) was reported. The next best test to perform is:
    a. Bone marrow aspiration and biopsy
    b. Serum antiplatelet antibody assay
    c. Antinuclear antibody assay
    d. Platelet aggregation studies
    e. Review of the peripheral blood smear to evaluate for platelet clumping or repeating the complete blood cell count in EDTA.

20. A 58-year-old man had severe pancytopenia. Bone marrow examination revealed a cellularity-to-fat ratio of 5:95. The treatment of choice is:
    a. Allogeneic bone marrow transplantation

b. Cyclophosphamide
c. Antithymocyte globulin
d. Steroids
e. Lithium

21. A 35-year-old female presented with purpura. She was not taking any medication. The complete blood count revealed: hemoglobin, 13.5 g/dL (normal, 12 to 15.5); white blood cell count, 5.2×10^9/L (normal, 3.5 to 10.5); and platelet count, 5×10^9/L (normal, 150 to 450). The treatment of choice is:
    a. Intravenous immunoglobulin
    b. Oral prednisone
    c. Danazol
    d. Cyclophosphamide
    e. Splenectomy

22. All the following statements are true about transfusion reactions except for:
    a. The most common cause of acute hemolytic transfusion reaction is human error
    b. In acute hemolytic transfusion reactions, ABO mismatches are less frequent when compared with reactions to Kell, Duffy, and Kidd
    c. Transfusion-related adult respiratory distress syndrome (ARDS) may be misdiagnosed as circulatory overload
    d. Fever occurs only in acute hemolytic transfusion reactions
    e. Delayed hemolytic transfusion reactions usually involve Rh and Kidd systems

23. Which of the following is not found in adults with type I Gaucher's disease?
    a. Splenomegaly
    b. Neurologic symptoms
    c. Bone lesions in 75% of patients
    d. Thrombocytopenia
    e. Pathologic bone fractures

24. Which drug is most commonly associated with secondary leukemias?
    a. Daunorubicin
    b. Methotrexate
    c. Cyclophosphamide
    d. Cisplatin
    e. Busulfan

True/False (indicate whether each answer is true or false)
25. The following are consistent with a diagnosis of β-thalassemia:
    a. Red blood cell count $>5 \times 10^{12}$/L
    b. Mean corpuscular volume of 105 fL in a 50-year-old man

c. Ferritin of 3 mg/mL
d. Hemoglobin A_2 levels <4%
e. Transferrin saturation level of 2%
f. Mean corpuscular volume of 65 fL

26. The following statements are consistent with a diagnosis of thrombotic thrombocytopenic purpura:
    a. Schistocytes on the peripheral blood smear
    b. Decreased fibrinogen
    c. Prolonged prothrombin time
    d. Increased serum level of creatinine
    e. Thrombocytopenia
    f. Spherocytes seen on the peripheral blood smear

27. In paroxysmal nocturnal hemoglobinuria:
    a. The sugar water test has few false-positive results
    b. Venous thrombosis of the portal system or brain is associated with 50% of the deaths
    c. The disorder is characterized by a chronic hemolytic anemia with hemoglobinuria
    d. Budd-Chiari syndrome is the major cause of death
    e. Complications of the disorder include acute nonlymphocytic leukemia and aplastic anemia
    f. Iron stain performed on bone marrow biopsy specimen reveals the presence of iron

28. The major criteria for polycythemia rubra vera include:
    a. Erythrocyte sedimentation rate of 0.1 mm/hour (normal, 0 to 29)
    b. Increased red blood cell mass
    c. Splenomegaly
    d. Increased vitamin B_{12}
    e. Low leukocyte alkaline phosphatase score
    f. A decreased erythropoietin level

29. A 35-year-old man with a 14-year history of recurrent transitional cell carcinoma of the bladder presented with a white blood cell count of 126×10^9/L (normal, 4.1 to 10.9). The white blood cell differential count was normal. CT revealed a large mass in the wall of the bladder. A preoperative consultation was obtained.
    a. The patient must undergo leukopheresis
    b. The patient should be treated with hydroxyurea
    c. The patient must have a bone marrow examination
    d. Cytogenetic studies of peripheral blood should be performed preoperatively
    e. The next best step is to measure the leukocyte alkaline phosphatase score
    f. The patient should receive treatment with busulfan

30. With regard to the following:
    a. HTLV-I is the causative agent in adult T-cell leukemia

b. The Epstein-Barr virus is associated with post-transplantation lymphoproliferative disorders

c. The t(9;22) translocation is associated with chronic lymphocytic leukemia

d. The *bcl-2* oncogene is associated with follicular small cleaved cell lymphoma

e. Trisomy 12 is the most common chromosome abnormality in chronic lymphocytic leukemia

f. The t(9;22) translocation is associated with chronic myelogenous leukemia

31. The results of the following laboratory tests are abnormal in von Willebrand's disease:
   a. Bleeding time
   b. Activated partial thromboplastin time
   c. Fibrinogen
   d. VIII:C
   e. Prothrombin time
   f. Thrombin time

32. The results of the following laboratory tests typically are normal in patients taking warfarin:
   a. Bleeding time
   b. Fibrinogen
   c. The activated partial thromboplastin time may be normal or abnormal
   d. Thrombin time
   e. Prothrombin time
   f. Assays for factors II, VII, IX, and X

33. With regard to various factor deficiencies:
   a. In factor XII deficiency, thromboembolic complications are more common than bleeding complications
   b. In factor VII deficiency, prothrombin time is abnormal
   c. In factor X deficiency, the activated partial thromboplastin time and prothrombin time are abnormal
   d. In factor XIII deficiency, all routine clotting tests are normal

e. Factor V deficiency may be acquired in myeloproliferative disorders

f. In patients with mild factor VIII deficiency, bleeding may occur only at the time of a surgical procedure or major trauma

34. With regard to thrombocytopenia:
   a. Post-transfusion purpura occurs 7 to 10 days after blood transfusions
   b. Severe hemorrhage is normal in idiopathic thrombocytopenic purpura
   c. Drug-induced thrombocytopenia subsides in 4 to 14 days except when due to gold
   d. Viral-induced thrombocytopenia resolves in 4 to 14 days
   e. The treatment of choice in post-transfusion purpura includes plasmapheresis or a high dose of gamma globulin
   f. The incidence of heparin-induced thrombocytopenia is 1% to 30%

35. In tumor lysis syndrome:
   a. Hyperkalemia (>6 mEq/L) may cause arrhythmias
   b. Hyperphosphatemia (>10 mg/dL) can lead to secondary hypocalcemia
   c. Calcium phosphate may be deposited at extraskeletal sites
   d. Hyperuricemia (>10 mg/dL) can occur
   e. Hemodialysis may be required
   f. Patients may be hypocalcemic

36. With regard to parvovirus (B19) infections:
   a. Adults may present with a polyarthralgia syndrome
   b. Severe anemia and reticulocytopenia may occur
   c. Aplastic crises may occur in hereditary spherocytosis, sickle cell disease, and thalassemia major
   d. Pancytopenia may be present
   e. Immunoglobulin given intravenously may be of benefit
   f. Are highly contagious in children

ANSWERS

1. Answer e.

High serum levels of erythropoietin are present in marrow hypoproliferative states (such as pure red cell aplasia), deficiency states (such as iron deficiency), autonomous production (such as hepatocellular carcinoma), and high altitude. In untreated polycythemia rubra vera, the serum levels are low.

2. Answer d.

Glucose-6-phosphate dehydrogenase deficiency is sex-linked. Hereditary spherocytosis is an autosomal dominant disorder. The membrane defects and unstable hemoglobin diseases are autosomal dominant. Most enzymopathies are autosomal recessive, with the exception of glucose-6-phosphate dehydrogenase deficiency and phosphoglycerate kinase deficiency.

3. Answer d.

Significant numbers of target cells are seen in hemoglobin C disorders. Target cells are also common in thalassemia syndromes, postsplenectomy, and obstructive jaundice. Target cells are least likely to be present in iron deficiency.

4. Answer d.

In the study state, the patient may not be anemic. Heinz bodies are present in supravital stained peripheral blood specimens. Glucose-6-phosphate dehydrogenase levels may be normal during the acute attack because of the half-life of glucose-6-phosphate dehydrogenase. Infection is the most common precipitating factor. Hyperglycemia and hypoglycemia may precipitate hemolysis. Normally, the half-life of glucose-6-phosphate dehydrogenase is 62 days, but in reticulocytes it is 124 days and in aged cells 31 days.

5. Answer b.

Thrombotic thrombocytopenic purpura is a Coombs'-negative hemolytic anemia of undetermined cause in a large number of patients. Pregnancy and the use of oral contraceptives have been associated with the disease. Before the advent of plasmapheresis and plasma exchange, the survival rate was very low. These therapeutic interventions have resulted in favorable clinical responses in 80%-90% of patients.

6. Answer a.

In a recent randomized trial, hydroxyurea decreased the frequency of painful vaso-occlusive crises by 50%. In adults with a pulmonary crisis, sickling is a primary event. Plain bone radiographs do not demonstrate abnormalities during the acute symptomatic period. Acute chest syndrome is a common cause of death.

7. Answer c.

Age is not a predictor of survival in chronic lymphocytic leukemia.

8. Answer b.

This patient has Rai stage 0 disease with lymphocytosis only. These patients should be observed until they are symptomatic, have bulky disease, a platelet count <100 x 10^9/L or hemoglobin <11.0 g/dL.

9. Answer d.

Hodgkin's disease is a curable disease. This patient has pathologic stage II disease. The treatment of choice is radiation therapy in a mantel field, with radiation to include the upper abdominal field, which is the para-aortic area.

10. Answer e.

This patient has low-grade non-Hodgkin's lymphoma, which is pathologic stage IVA because of bone marrow involvement.

Because the patient is asymptomatic and does not have bulky disease, observation is recommended. There is no evidence that early treatment improves survival. Currently, this disease is not curable in this patient.

11. Answer c.

This patient has a monoclonal gammopathy of undetermined significance. The patient should be observed at this time. Twenty-three percent of patients may have progression to a malignant monoclonal gammopathy, which would include multiple myeloma, Waldenström's macroglobulinemia, amyloidosis, and non-Hodgkin's lymphoma.

12. Answer e.

This young woman has chronic myelogenous leukemia. In patients who have an HLA-identical sibling, treatment for 6-12 months with hydroxyurea or interferon alfa-2a or 2b recominant followed by allogeneic bone marrow transplantation offers the potential for cure.

13. Answer d.

In hemophilia, bleeding time is normal. Bernard-Soulier syndrome and Glanzmann's thrombasthenia have associated inherited defects of platelet receptors. After the platelet count is <75 x 10^9/L, bleeding time may be prolonged.

14. Answer d.

The inheritance pattern in von Willebrand's disease is autosomal dominant. Fresh frozen plasma is not indicated as a treatment of choice in von Willebrand's disease or the hemophilias because of the risk of volume overload and infectious complications. Active bleeding should be treated with replacement therapy and not with platelets. In pregnancy, there is a progressive increase in factor VIII in patients with type I von Willebrand disease, and patients with type I von Willebrand's disease do not require replacement therapy.

15. Answer a.

In the management of hemophilia A, the most specific treatment is indicated. In addition, treatments that are least likely to transmit viruses are the treatments of choice.

16. Answer c.

Drugs that potentiate warfarin include those that prolong prothrombin time, such as phenylbutazone, metronidazole, sulfinpyrazone, trimethoprim/sulfamethoxazole, and disulfiram.

17. Answer a.

In the antiphospholipid syndrome in pregnancy, clinical findings must accompany positive findings on a laboratory test.

18. Answer d.

Recommended INR for recurrent systemic pulmonary

emboli and mechanical prosthetic values is 3.0 to 4.5.

19. Answer e.

The initial test in the evaluation of thrombocytopenia should include a peripheral blood smear to rule out EDTA-induced platelet clumping. This is the most common cause of pseudothrombocytopenia. No treatment is required.

20. Answer c.

This patient has aplastic anemia. Because of his age, the treatment of choice is antithymocyte globulin with or without cyclosporine.

21. Answer b.

This patient has idiopathic autoimmune thrombocytopenic purpura. The initial treatment of choice is oral prednisone at a dose of 1 mg/kg daily.

22. Answer d.

Fever occurs in acute febrile transfusion reactions and acute hemolytic transfusion reactions. Because fever occurs in acute hemolytic transfusion reactions, transfusions are stopped when patients become febrile. Patients are evaluated for this problem.

23. Answer b.

Neurologic symptoms are not found in type I Gaucher's disease.

24. Answer c.

Of the drugs listed, cyclophosphamide is the most common drug associated with secondary leukemias.

25. a, true; b, false; c, false; d, false; e, false; f, true.

β-Thalassemia typically has a microcytic anemia, normal ferritin level, red blood cell count $>5 \times 10^{12}/L$, hemoglobin A_2 level $>4\%$, and a normal transferrin saturation.

26. a, true; b, false; c, false; d, true; e, true; f, false.

Thrombotic thrombocytopenic purpura is a nonspherocytic Coombs'-negative hemolytic anemia accompanied by thrombocytopenia. In contrast to disseminated intravascular coagulopathy, the fibrinogen and prothrombin time are typically normal.

27. a, false; b, true; c, true; d, true; e, true; f, true.

Because the sugar water test has a significant number of false-positive results, the acid hemolysis test classically has been used to confirm the diagnosis.

28. a, false; b, true; c, true; d, false; e, false; f, false.

The major criteria for polycythemia rubra vera include a red blood cell mass, splenomegaly, and normal oxygen saturation.

29. a, false; b, false; c, false; d, false; e, true; f, false.

This patient has a leukamoid reaction. The most expeditious way to distinguish this from chronic myelogenous leukemia is with a leukocyte alkaline phosphatase score. This score is increased in leukamoid reactions and low in chronic myelogenous leukemia.

30. a, true; b, true; c, false; d, true; e, true; f, true.

The t(9;22) translocation is associated with chronic myelogenous leukemia and not with chronic lymphocytic leukemia.

31. a, true; b, true; c, false; d, true; e, false; f, false.

Von Willebrand's disease is characterized by an increased activated partial thromboplastin time, which is secondary to a decreased VIII:C and prolonged bleeding time

32. a, true; b, true; c, true; d, true; e, false; f, false.

Prothrombin time is abnormal in patients taking warfarin. Because warfarin affects the vitamin K-dependent factors, factor II, VII, VIII, and X are abnormal. The activated partial thromboplastin time may be normal or abnormal.

33. a, true; b, true; c, true; d, true; e, true; f, true.

In factor XIII deficiency, all routine clotting tests are normal. Thromboembolic complications may be associated with factor XII deficiency.

34. a, true; b, false; c, true; d, false; e, true; f, true.

Severe hemorrhage is not common in idiopathic thrombocytopenic purpura. Viral-induced thrombocytopenia resolves in 2 weeks to 3 months. Drug-induced thrombocytopenia subsides in 4 to 14 days except when due to gold.

35. a, true; b, true; c, true; d, true; e, true; f, true.

Tumor lysis syndrome is a potentially life-threatening complication characterized by hyperkalemia, hyperphosphatemia, and hypocalcemia. Hemodialysis may be required.

36. a, true; b, true; c, true; d, true; e, true; f, true.

The manifestations of parvovirus infections in adults are different from those in children and include polyarthralgia syndrome and cytopenias. Immunoglobulin therapy may be of benefit.

CHAPTER 13

HYPERTENSION

Gary L. Schwartz, M.D.

HYPERTENSION

Definition

Systolic blood pressures between 130 and 139 mm Hg and diastolic blood pressures between 85 and 89 mm Hg are considered high-normal. Hypertension is defined as average blood pressure ≥140/90 mm Hg. It is stratified further on the basis of pressure level (Table 13-1).

- Hypertension is average blood pressure ≥140/90 mm Hg.

Isolated systolic hypertension, mainly a problem of the elderly, is defined as systolic blood pressure ≥140 mm Hg with diastolic blood pressure <90 mm Hg. Secondary causes of isolated systolic hypertension include disorders associated with either increased cardiac output (anemia, thyrotoxicosis, arteriovenous fistula, Paget's disease of bone, beriberi) or increased cardiac stroke volume (aortic insufficiency, complete heart block).

- Isolated systolic hypertension affects mainly the elderly.
- Secondary cause: increased cardiac output (anemia, thyrotoxicosis, arteriovenous fistula, Paget's disease of bone, beriberi).
- Secondary cause: increased cardiac stroke volume (aortic insufficiency, complete heart block).

Epidemiology

Blood pressure increases with age. Systolic blood pressure increases throughout the seventh decade but diastolic blood pressure plateaus in the fifth decade. Hypertension is a major risk factor for cardiovascular morbidity and mortality (myocardial infarction, congestive heart failure, stroke, and renal disease). Risk is continuous and proportionate over both systolic and diastolic blood pressure levels. Systolic blood pressure is as good or better a predictor of risk than diastolic blood pressure. In young adulthood and early middle age, high blood pressure is more common in men than in women. In older persons, the reverse is true. It is more common in blacks than in whites at all ages, and in both races, it is more common in less-educated persons than in more educated ones. For any given level, men have greater morbidity and mortality than women and blacks greater than whites. It is estimated that 50 million Americans have hypertension or are taking medication to lower blood pressure.

- Hypertension is a major risk factor for cardiovascular morbidity and mortality.
- Risk is continuous and proportionate over both systolic and diastolic blood pressure levels.
- Men and blacks have greater morbidity and mortality.

In hypertensive persons, the most common causes of death are due to complications of coronary artery disease. Factors that add to this risk are tobacco use, hyperlipidemia, diabetes mellitus, obesity, sedentary lifestyle, and family history of premature cardiovascular disease. Target organ damage (stroke, left ventricular hypertrophy, ischemic heart disease, congestive

Table 13-1.--Stages of Hypertension

Stage[*]	Degree	Blood pressure, mm Hg	
		Systolic	Diastolic
1	Mild	140-159	90-99
2	Moderate	160-179	100-109
3	Severe	180-209	110-119
4	Very severe	≥210	≥120

[*]Stage is defined by systolic *or* diastolic blood pressure.

Modified from Joint National Committee on Detection, Evaluation, and Treatment of High Blood Pressure: The Fifth Report of the Joint National Committee on Detection, Evaluation, and Treatment of High Blood Pressure (JNC V). Arch Intern Med 153:154-183, 1993.

heart failure, and renal disease) increases the risk of cardio-vascular events even if blood pressure is controlled. This fact argues for early treatment of mild hypertension. Therefore, in addition to the level of blood pressure, risk in the individual patient is determined by the presence of additional cardio-vascular risk factors and target organ damage.

- The most common causes of death in hypertensive persons are related to complications of coronary artery disease.
- Other risk factors for coronary artery disease: tobacco use, hyperlipidemia, diabetes mellitus, obesity, sedentary lifestyle, and family history of premature cardiovascular disease.
- Target organ damage increases the risk of cardiovascular events even if blood pressure is controlled.

Left ventricular hypertrophy is a powerful predictor of sudden death and myocardial infarction in hypertensive persons. Other factors associated with increased left ventricular muscle mass include increasing age, obesity, and increased physical activity. Echocardiography is more sensitive than electro-cardiography in detecting left ventricular hypertrophy.

- Left ventricular hypertrophy is a powerful predictor of sudden death and myocardial infarction in hypertensive persons.
- Echocardiography is more sensitive than electrocardiography in detecting left ventricular hypertrophy.

Diagnosis

Because blood pressure varies, the diagnosis of hypertension requires several measurements made on different occasions. The person should be at rest in the sitting position for at least 5 minutes before the measurement. Recent physical activity, use of tobacco or caffeine, or a full urinary bladder can transiently increase blood pressure. Some persons have increased blood pressure when it is measured in a physician's office but have normal blood pressure at all other times. This is called "office hypertension" or "white coat hypertension." Whether these people suffer the adverse consequences of hypertension is uncertain; therefore, they usually require no treatment initially but need to be followed and periodically assessed for target organ damage. Older persons may have pseudohypertension, a falsely increased systolic and diastolic blood pressure when measured by the cuff method; it is the result of a stiff vascular tree caused by atherosclerosis. Pseudohypertension may exist if the radial artery remains palpable after brachial artery occlusion by inflating the blood pressure cuff above systolic blood pressure level (Osler maneuver).

- The diagnosis of hypertension requires several measurements made on different occasions.
- Recent physical exercise, use of tobacco or caffeine, or a full urinary bladder can increase blood pressure.

- Office (white coat) hypertension: increased blood pressure only when measured in a physician's office.
- Older patients may have pseudohypertension, the result of a stiff vascular tree.

Evaluation

After the diagnosis of hypertension is established, 1) determine, if possible, the duration and severity of hypertension and any previous therapies and reasons for discontinuation, 2) assess for target organ damage, 3) identify associated cardiovascular risk factors, and 4) consider the possibility of secondary hypertension. Secondary hypertension accounts for <5% of all cases of increased blood pressure.

- Secondary hypertension explains <5% of all cases of increased blood pressure.

Clues to secondary hypertension are features that are not consistent with essential hypertension. Essential hypertension usually occurs in the fourth or fifth decade. There is often a family history of hypertension. Usually, blood pressure is mildly increased initially and easily controlled with one or two medications. Target organ damage is rare and routine laboratory findings are normal. Blood pressure does not progress to higher levels over a short period of time. Factors inconsistent with essential hypertension are listed in Table 13-2.

- Recognition of secondary hypertension is important.

Table 13-2.--Factors Inconsistent With Essential Hypertension

---

Age at onset--before 30 or after 50 years
Blood pressure >180/110 mm Hg at time of diagnosis
Significant target organ damage at time of diagnosis
Hemorrhages and exudates on funduscopic examination
Renal insufficiency
Cardiomegaly
Features suggesting secondary hypertension
    Primary aldosteronism (unprovoked hypokalemia, Chvostek's sign, Trousseau's sign)
    Pheochromocytoma (labile blood pressure with sweating, tremor, tachycardia, pallor, neurofibromatosis, orofacial neuromas [MEN II])
    Renovascular disease (abdominal bruits)
    Cushing's disease (truncal obesity, pigmented stria)
    Coarctation of aorta (delayed/absent femoral pulses)
    Polycystic kidney disease (abdominal or flank masses, family history of renal disease)
Poor response to appropriate three-drug therapy

Drugs

Certain drugs can cause or aggravate hypertension or interfere with the action of antihypertensive medications. These drugs and their mechanism of action are listed in Table 13-3.

- Certain drugs can cause or aggravate hypertension or interfere with the action of antihypertensive medications.
- Oral contraceptives induce sodium retention, increase renin substrate, and facilitate the action of catecholamines.
- Nonsteroidal anti-inflammatory drugs induce sodium retention by blocking the formation of vasodilating, natriuretic prostaglandins.

- Tricyclic antidepressants block the uptake of guanethidine and inhibit the action of centrally acting agents (methyldopa, clonidine).

Laboratory Studies

Routine laboratory tests should include: complete blood cell count, potassium, glucose, creatinine or BUN, uric acid, calcium, cholesterol (total and HDL), triglycerides, urinalysis, and electrocardiography (ECG). Additional studies should not be performed unless abnormalities are identified on initial screening tests or the history or examination suggests a secondary form of hypertension.

Table 13-3.--Drugs That Can Increase Blood Pressure or Interfere With Antihypertensive Therapy

Drug	Mechanism
Oral contraceptives	Induce sodium retention Increase renin substrate Facilitate action of catecholamines
Alcohol (>2 oz daily)	Activation of sympathetic nervous system Increase cortisol secretion Increase intracellular calcium levels
Sympathomimetics and amphetamine-like substances (cold formulas, allergy medications, diet pills)	Increase peripheral vascular resistance Interfere with action of guanethidine and guanadrel
Nonsteroidal anti-inflammatory drugs	Induce sodium retention by blocking formation of vasodilating, natriuretic prostaglandins, thus interfering with action of diuretics, β-blockers, and angiotensin converting enzyme inhibitors
Corticosteroids	Iatrogenic Cushing's disease
Tricyclic antidepressants	Block uptake of guanethidine Inhibit action of centrally acting drugs such as methyldopa and clonidine
Ephedrine	Competitive antagonist of guanethidine
Monoamine oxidase inhibitors (in combination with tyramine--found in aged cheeses and some red wines)	Prevent degradation and metabolism of norepinephrine released by tyramine-containing foods Increase blood pressure when combined with reserpine/guanethidine
Cocaine	Vasoconstriction Interferes with action of adrenergic inhibitors
Marijuana	Increases systolic blood pressure

Treatment

The goal of therapy is to eliminate the cardiovascular morbidity and mortality attributable to hypertension by decreasing blood pressure to <140/90 mm Hg.

Lifestyle Modifications

Lifestyle modifications may be sufficient for patients with stage 1 hypertension. It is adjunctive therapy for those with more severe hypertension. Restriction of daily sodium intake to 100 mEq (2 g sodium, 4 g salt) decreases blood pressure in some but not all hypertensive persons. Although salt sensitivity is more common among persons who are black, obese, elderly or who have low renin hypertension or higher blood pressure levels, the antihypertensive effect of many medications is enhanced by sodium restriction. Also, sodium restriction minimizes diuretic-induced potassium losses. The prevalence of hypertension is increased in the obese. An increase in blood pressure often parallels weight gain. Weight loss may decrease blood pressure. Weight reduction to within 15% of ideal body weight is the goal, although losses of as little as 10 lb may produce a decrease in blood pressure. Restriction of daily alcohol intake to <2 oz is often associated with a decrease in blood pressure. Alcohol is a source of calories, and its use is often associated with poor compliance. Excessive alcohol intake may cause labile hypertension that is difficult to control in association with other symptoms (flushing, tachycardia) that suggest pheochromocytoma. Regular aerobic exercise may decrease blood pressure directly and by facilitating weight loss. Because coronary artery disease is the most common cause of mortality in hypertensive persons, all cardiovascular risks need to be addressed. The benefits of blood pressure reduction are diminished in smokers. Dyslipidemia (increased LDL cholesterol, decreased HDL cholesterol, increased triglycerides) and glucose intolerance coexist more often in hypertensive than in normotensive persons.

- Restriction of daily sodium intake to 100 mEq decreases blood pressure in some, not all, hypertensive persons.
- Weight reduction to within 15% of ideal body weight is the goal.
- Restriction of alcohol intake to <2 oz daily is often associated with a decrease in blood pressure.
- Regular aerobic exercise may decrease blood pressure directly.
- Address all cardiovascular risk factors.

Short-term trials have shown that biofeedback and relaxation training decrease blood pressure in a subset of hypertensive persons. Long-term effects of these modalities on blood pressure reduction have not been assessed. Short-term studies have shown that dietary supplementation with potassium, calcium, and magnesium decreases blood pressure; however, potential dangers of long-term supplementation are unknown.

Thus, the role of these cations in the treatment of hypertension is unclear.

A 3-6-month trial of lifestyle modifications is appropriate for stage 1 hypertension. If lifestyle modifications fail to decrease blood pressure to <140/90 mm Hg, drug treatment should be considered, especially in patients at increased risk because of additional cardiovascular risk factors or target organ changes. Also, significant changes in lifestyle (weight reduction, exercise, limitation of alcohol intake, and sodium restriction) may allow tapering of an established drug program.

- A 3-6-month trial of lifestyle modifications is appropriate for stage 1 hypertension.
- If this fails to decrease blood pressure to <140/90 mm Hg, consider drug treatment.

Pharmacologic Therapy

More than 50% of cases of stage 1 hypertension can be controlled with one drug. Important factors in selecting a drug for initial therapy are its 1) effectiveness as monotherapy, 2) side-effects, and 3) cost. Proper drug selection is important in maintaining long-term compliance.

Drugs appropriate for monotherapy are diuretics, β-blockers, calcium channel antagonists, angiotensin converting enzyme (ACE) inhibitors, α-blockers, and α-β-blockers. Centrally acting α-agonists (clonidine, methyldopa, guanfacine, guanabenz) and traditional vasodilators (hydralazine, minoxidil) may be associated with pseudotolerance--i.e., reflex stimulation of the renin-angiotensin-aldosterone system and/or the sympathetic nervous system that causes fluid retention, increased vascular resistance, or increased cardiac output and loss of efficacy with prolonged use--and so ordinarily are not used as monotherapy. Centrally acting α-agonists are appropriate when used in combination with diuretics, whereas traditional vasodilators are best as a third drug in combination with diuretics and adrenergic inhibitors. Additional important factors influencing drug selection include the recognition that certain drugs work better according to a person's age and race (diuretics and calcium antagonists are more effective in blacks and the elderly; β-blockers and ACE inhibitors are more effective in whites and younger patients), the presence of concomitant diseases, and drug-drug interactions. If the first drug chosen fails to control blood pressure, discontinue its use and substitute a drug of a different class or add a second drug to the first. With combination therapy, make certain that the chosen drugs work in combination and that two drugs of the same class are not used simultaneously. Fatigue and impotence are potential side effects of all antihypertensive drugs.

- Drugs for monotherapy: diuretics, β-blockers, calcium channel antagonists, ACE inhibitors, α-blockers, α-β-blockers.
- Centrally acting α-agonists ordinarily are not used as monotherapy but are appropriate in combination with diuretics.

- Traditional vasodilators are best as a third drug in combination with diuretics and adrenergic inhibitors.

Thiazide Diuretics

Thiazide diuretics have been the mainstay of treatment of mild-to-moderate hypertension. Concomitant diseases for which these drugs should be considered are edema states and congestive heart failure due to systolic dysfunction. Metabolic disturbances associated with their use are hypokalemia, hyperuricemia, hypercalcemia, hypomagnesemia, hyponatremia, glucose intolerance, hypochloremic metabolic alkalosis, and increase of LDL cholesterol and triglycerides. Because of these potential adverse effects, relative contraindications to the use of thiazide diuretics include the coexistence of diet-controlled type II diabetes, gout, hyperlipidemia, cardiac arrhythmias, and ischemic heart disease. Drug interactions include potentiation of lithium toxicity (thiazides decrease renal clearance of lithium), lessening of the anticoagulant effect of warfarin, enhancement of digitalis toxicity, and enhancement of the effects of skeletal muscle relaxants. Nonsteroidal anti-inflammatory drugs decrease the antihypertensive effect of thiazide diuretics. Use of these diuretics is associated with volume depletion pancreatitis, vasculitis, mesenteric infarction hepatitis, intrahepatic cholestasis, interstitial nephritis, and photosensitivity. Rarely, they cause blood dyscrasias. Thiazide diuretics are usually ineffective when serum creatinine is >2.0 mg/dL. An exception is indapamide, a thiazide-like diuretic that is effective in states of decreased renal function and that is less likely to increase blood lipids. When serum creatinine is >2.0 mg/dL, a more potent loop diuretic or metolazone is more effective. Volume expansion is often important etiologically in hypertension associated with renal insufficiency.

- Metabolic disturbances associated with diuretics: hypokalemia, hyperuricemia, hypercalcemia, hypomagnesemia, hyponatremia, glucose intolerance, hypochloremic metabolic alkalosis, and increased LDL cholesterol and triglycerides.
- Drug interactions: potentiation of lithium toxicity, lessening of anticoagulant effect of warfarin, enhancement of digitalis toxicity, and enhancement of effects of skeletal muscle relaxants.
- Use of diuretics is associated with pancreatitis, vasculitis, mesenteric infarction, hepatitis, and photosensitivity.

Furosemide

The major indication for furosemide is hypertension associated with renal insufficiency. Similar to thiazide diuretics, furosemide can cause volume depletion, hypokalemia, hyperuricemia, increased fasting blood glucose, hypochloremic alkalosis, and can decrease lithium clearance. Unlike thiazide diuretics, furosemide causes calciuresis. Potential adverse effects include reversible deafness, postural hypotension (especially in older patients), photosensitivity, pancreatitis, blood dyscrasias, nephrocalcinosis, and interstitial nephritis. Furosemide decreases salicylate and lithium clearance and enhances the effects of skeletal muscle relaxants. It is synergistic when used with metolazone. Avoid using with aminoglycosides or other ototoxic drugs. Nonsteroidal anti-inflammatory drugs reduce the antihypertensive response.

- Major indication for furosemide: hypertension associated with renal insufficiency.
- Furosemide can cause: hypokalemia, hyperuricemia, increased fasting blood glucose, decreased lithium clearance, enhanced salicylate clearance, and enhanced effect of skeletal muscle relaxants.
- Adverse effects: reversible deafness and postural hypotension.

Bumetanide

The actions (including adverse effects, electrolyte alterations, and drug interactions) of bumetanide are identical to those of furosemide; however, bumetanide is a more potent diuretic on a milligram-per-milligram basis (1 mg is equivalent to 40 mg furosemide).

Ethacrynic Acid

The actions of ethacrynic acid are similar to those of furosemide. Although permanent hearing loss is a risk, ethacrynic acid is an alternative diuretic for patients with sulfa sensitivity.

Potassium-Sparing Diuretics

1. Spironolactone. Spironolactone is an aldosterone antagonist used specifically in persons with primary aldosteronism or with severe secondary aldosteronism. Its diuretic effect is antagonized by the concomitant use of salicylates. Adverse effects include hyponatremia, hyperkalemia, hyperchloremic acidosis, gynecomastia (but not breast cancer), and skin rash. Spironolactone is usually combined with thiazides to limit hypokalemia.

- The diuretic effect of spironolactone is antagonized by the concomitant use of salicylates.
- Adverse effects: hyperkalemia, gynecomastia, and skin rash.

2. Triamterene. Triamterene inhibits renal potassium-wasting independent of aldosterone. Side effects include hyperkalemia and skin rash.

- Triamterene inhibits renal potassium-wasting independent of aldosterone.

3. Amiloride. The actions of amiloride are similar to those of triamterene. Side effects are hyperkalemia, gastrointestinal distress, and skin rash.

Of the potassium-sparing diuretics, only spironolactone causes gynecomastia. In general, these drugs should be avoided in cases of renal failure and when ACE inhibitors are used.

- Avoid potassium-sparing diuretics in renal failure and when ACE inhibitors are used.

Adrenergic Inhibitors

When a diuretic alone fails to control blood pressure, an adrenergic inhibitor can be added. Adrenergic inhibitors are divided into centrally acting and peripherally acting drugs.

1. Peripherally acting inhibitors.
   a. Reserpine. Reserpine blocks the transport of norepinephrine into storage granules in peripheral neurons, causing decreased sympathetic nervous system tone. Side effects include depression, nasal congestion, and stimulation of gastric acid secretion, which can precipitate or aggravate peptic ulcer disease. A history of depression or peptic ulcer disease should contraindicate its use.

- Major side effects of reserpine: depression, nasal congestion, and stimulation of gastric acid secretion.

   b. Guanethidine. Guanethidine generally is used only as part of a combination drug program to treat resistant hypertension. It decreases blood pressure by causing degranulation of catecholamine storage granules in nerve endings. It does not enter the central nervous system. It has a long half-life. The maximal hypotensive effect of a given dose may not be manifested for 2-3 weeks. It should be given only once daily, and titration requires several weeks. Major side effects are postural hypotension, fluid retention, diarrhea, and retrograde ejaculation. Tricyclic antidepressants, antihistamines, and ephedrine interfere with its action. Guanadrel, a short-acting form of guanethidine, is easier to titrate to an effective dose because it has a shorter half-life.

- Major side effects of guanethidine: postural hypotension, fluid retention, diarrhea, and retrograde ejaculation.
- Tricyclic antidepressants, antihistamines, and ephedrine interfere with its action.

   c. Prazosin. Prazosin blocks α_1-adrenergic receptors on vascular smooth muscle cells to blunt catecholamine-induced vasoconstriction. The first dose can precipitate hypotension and syncope; therefore, it should be given before bedtime. Longer acting peripheral α_1-blockers (doxazocin, terazosin) that allow single daily dosing are available. These drugs may lessen voiding symptoms associated with benign pro-

static hypertrophy. Although the use of α_1-blockers in the elderly is frequently associated with orthostatic hypotension, they do not have adverse metabolic side effects. Other side effects include gastrointestinal distress and, rarely, sedation and dry mouth.

- Because the first dose of prazosin can cause hypotension and syncope, it should be given before bedtime.
- Use in the elderly is often associated with orthostatic hypotension but no adverse metabolic side effects.

   d. β-Blockers. Many β-blockers are available, differing in cardioselectivity (affinity for cardiac β_1 receptors greater than for noncardiac β_2 receptors), lipid solubility, and whether they have partial intrinsic (agonist) sympathomimetic activity (ISA). Non-ISA β-blockers decrease blood pressure by reducing cardiac output, inhibiting sympathetically mediated renin release from the kidneys, and inhibiting central sympathetic outflow. β-Blockers with ISA activity do not decrease cardiac output and cause mild peripheral vasodilatation. As lipid solubility increases, more drug is metabolized by the liver, more of it enters the brain, and its duration of action is shorter. As lipid solubility decreases, the drug is mainly eliminated by renal excretion, less of it enters the brain, and its duration of action is longer. Very lipid-soluble drugs are propranolol, metoprolol, and timolol. Intermediate lipid-soluble drugs are pindolol and acebutolol. The least lipid-soluble drugs are atenolol and nadolol.

- As lipid solubility increases, more drug is metabolized by the liver, more of it enters the brain, and its duration of action is shorter.
- As lipid solubility decreases, the drug is eliminated mainly by renal excretion, less enters the brain, and its duration of action is longer.
- Very lipid-soluble drugs: propranolol, metoprolol, and timolol.
- Least lipid-soluble drugs: atenolol and nadolol.

Cardioselective β-blockers include acebutolol, atenolol, and metoprolol. Cardioselectivity is relative; at high doses, all β-blockers are nonselective (block both cardiac β_1 and noncardiac β_2 receptors). β-Blockers with ISA activity are pindolol and acebutolol. Three β-blockers--propranolol, timolol, and metoprolol--prevent sudden death and myocardial infarctions in patients with a history of myocardial infarction. β-Blockers should be considered for use in hypertensive patients with concomitant angina, supraventricular arrhythmia, glaucoma, migraine headaches, or hypertrophic cardiomyopathy. Contraindications to the use of β-blockers are asthma, congestive heart failure with decreased systolic function, disease of the conduction system of the heart, angina due to coronary vasospasm, Raynaud's phenomenon, severe occlusive peripheral vascular disease, pheochromocytoma (in absence of alpha blockade), and depression. Because β-blockers may mask the symptoms of hypoglycemia and delay recovery from it, caution is required when used in diabetics taking hypoglycemic drugs or insulin. Side effects include cold extremities (non-ISA β-blockers), fatigue, insomnia, nasal congestion, and, possibly, depression.

- Cardioselectivity is relative; all β-blockers are nonselective at high doses.
- Propranolol, timolol, and metoprolol prevent sudden death and myocardial infarction in persons with a history of myocardial infarction.
- Contraindications: asthma, congestive heart failure with decreased systolic function, disease of the conduction system of the heart, angina due to coronary vasospasm, Raynaud's phenomenon, severe occlusive peripheral vascular disease, pheochromocytoma, and depression.
- β-Blockers may mask hypoglycemia and delay recovery from it, so use them carefully in diabetics taking insulin or oral hypoglycemic drugs.
- Side effects: cold extremities, fatigue, insomnia, nasal congestion, and, possibly, depression.

   e. Labetalol. Labetalol is a combination of a nonselective β-blocker and a postsynaptic α_1-blocker. The ratio of α-to-β blocking action is between 1:3 and 1:7. It induces decreased cardiac output and peripheral vascular resistance. Labetalol can be used intravenously to treat hypertensive crisis. All the precautions applying to β-blockers apply to this drug. Orthostatic hypotension and scalp itching are its most common side effects. It may interfere with metanephrine and catecholamine assays.

- Labetalol can be used intravenously.
- All precautions applying to β-blockers apply to labetalol.
- Common side effects: orthostatic hypotension and scalp itching.
- It may interfere with metanephrine and catecholamine assays.

   2. Centrally acting inhibitors.
      a. Methyldopa. Methyldopa inhibits central sympathetic outflow. Its side effects include sedation, dry mouth, hepatitis, fever, positive Coombs' test, hemolytic anemia, leukopenia, thrombocytopenia, and antinuclear antibody positivity. Doses should not exceed 3 g/day. Hemoglobin and liver enzymes should be checked periodically. Methyldopa potentiates lithium and haloperidol toxicity, increases

prolactin levels with consequent breast stimulation, interferes with metanephrine assays, and can induce orthostatic hypotension (especially in the elderly).

- Methyldopa side effects: sedation, dry mouth, hepatitis, fever, positive Coombs' test, hemolytic anemia, leukopenia, thrombocytopenia, and antinuclear antibody positivity.
- It potentiates lithium and haloperidol toxicity and increases prolactin levels.
- It can induce orthostatic hypotension, especially in the elderly.

      b. Clonidine. Clonidine also inhibits central sympathetic outflow and has the side effects of dry mouth and sedation, but it is not associated with liver toxicity or positive Coombs' test. Because sudden discontinuation of clonidine may induce rebound hypertension, accompanied by symptoms of tachycardia, flushing, and diaphoresis, it should be slowly tapered. (Rebound hypertension can occur with all centrally acting agents and with β-blockers.) Taper and discontinue use of clonidine preoperatively for anticipated surgical procedures in which the patient will not be able to take the medication. Alternatively, patients can be converted preoperatively to the transdermal form of clonidine. Treatment of rebound hypertension usually involves reinstituting clonidine therapy (or whatever agent was discontinued suddenly).

- Sudden discontinuation of clonidine may induce rebound hypertension.
- It should be tapered slowly.
- Taper and discontinue it preoperatively.

      c. Guanabenz. Guanabenz, a newer centrally acting α_2 agonist, is similar in action to clonidine and methyldopa. It may also have weak peripheral neuronal blocking properties. Its side effects are similar to those of clonidine and methyldopa, but, unlike methyldopa, it is not associated with liver toxicity or positive Coombs' test.

- Side effects of guanabenz are similar to those of clonidine and methyldopa.

      d. Guanfacine. Guanfacine, another new clonidine-like drug, can be given once daily and may have fewer central nervous system side effects.

Vasodilators
   Vasodilators are usually used as step 3 agents in combination with a diuretic and an adrenergic inhibitor.

1. Hydralazine. Hydralazine decreases blood pressure by directly dilating arterioles. Doses should not exceed 200 mg daily. Its side effects include headache, palpitations, tachycardia, fluid retention, lupus-like syndrome, and peripheral neuropathy. Hydralazine should not be used in patients with a recent cerebral hemorrhage or a dissecting aortic aneurysm because of its tendency to increase cardiac output and cerebral blood flow.

- Hydralazine: direct dilatation of arterioles.
- Dose should not be >200 mg daily.
- Side effects: headache, palpitations, tachycardia, fluid retention, lupus-like syndrome, and peripheral neuropathy.
- Do not give to patients with recent cerebral hemorrhage or dissecting aortic aneurysm.

2. Minoxidil. Minoxidil is a very potent, direct vasodilator used to treat severe hypertension with or without renal insufficiency. Its side effects include significant volume expansion with edema, hirsutism, and pericardial effusion. It may cause atrial fibrosis and pulmonary hypertension, but this has not been proved.

- Side effects: volume expansion with edema, hirsutism, and pericardial effusion.

ACE Inhibitors

ACE inhibitors decrease blood pressure by inhibiting the enzyme that converts angiotensin I to angiotensin II, a potent vasoconstrictor. These drugs are appropriate initial therapy for hypertension and work well in combination with other antihypertensive agents, particularly diuretics. Captopril is the only sulfhydryl-containing ACE inhibitor. Because it is eliminated by renal excretion, dose reduction is necessary in cases of renal insufficiency (this is true for most available ACE inhibitors). Side effects presumed to be due to the sulfhydryl group in captopril are skin rash, loss of taste, proteinuria with membranous glomerulonephropathy, and leukopenia. Leukopenia is more likely to occur in patients with collagen vascular disease and renal insufficiency. Side effects shared by all ACE inhibitors are orthostatic hypotension, hyperkalemia, cough, angioedema, and loss of renal function. In patients with bilateral renal artery stenosis, ACE inhibitors can precipitate acute renal failure because of disruption of autoregulation of glomerular filtration in the setting of severe renal ischemia.

- ACE inhibitors inhibit the enzyme that converts angiotensin I to angiotensin II.
- ACE inhibitors are appropriate initial therapy for hypertension.
- Dose reduction is necessary in renal insufficiency.
- Side effects of captopril: skin rash, loss of taste, proteinuria with membranous glomerulonephropathy, and leukopenia.

- Side effects of all ACE inhibitors: orthostatic hypotension, hyperkalemia, cough, angioedema, and loss of renal function.

Calcium Channel Antagonists

Calcium channel antagonists are direct vasodilators. They are divided into dihydropyridines (nifedipine, nicardipine, isradipine, felodipine, and amlodipine) and nondihydropyridines (verapamil, diltiazem). These drugs can be used as initial therapy for hypertension in patients with concomitant ischemic heart disease and angina, variant angina due to coronary vasospasm, supraventricular arrhythmias (verapamil), Raynaud's phenomenon (nifedipine), and migraine headaches (verapamil). Verapamil (and to a lesser extent, diltiazem) has a negative effect on the proximal cardiac conduction system and is a negative inotrope. Verapamil should not be used in patients with conduction system disease (sick sinus syndrome, second degree or greater heart block) and should be avoided in patients with congestive heart failure (ejection fraction <40%). Verapamil in combination with β-blockers can produce profound cardiodepression. Because it decreases the renal and nonrenal elimination of digoxin, verapamil increases the risk of digoxin toxicity. Quinidine and verapamil in combination can cause serious hypotension in patients with idiopathic hypertrophic subaortic stenosis.

- Calcium channel antagonists are direct vasodilators.
- Verapamil should not be used in sick sinus syndrome or second degree or greater heart block.
- Avoid using verapamil with congestive heart failure (ejection fraction <40%).
- Verapamil increases the risk of digoxin toxicity.

Verapamil and other calcium channel antagonists can cause an increase in liver enzymes associated with hepatic necrosis. The most common side effect of verapamil is constipation. Most of the side effects associated with nifedipine and other dihydropyridine calcium channel antagonists are related to their potent peripheral vasodilator properties. These side effects include headache, tachycardia, flushing, and edema. Cimetidine and other drugs decreasing blood flow to the liver may increase the biologic effects of calcium channel antagonists. All calcium channel antagonists are metabolized by the liver, and dose adjustments may be necessary in the presence of liver disease. They can safely be used in renal insufficiency.

- Calcium channel antagonists can cause an increase in liver enzymes associated with hepatic necrosis.
- The most common side effect of verapamil: constipation.
- Other side effects: headache, tachycardia, flushing, and edema.
- Calcium channel antagonists are metabolized by the liver, so dose adjustments are necessary in liver disease.

CAUSES OF SECONDARY HYPERTENSION

Renovascular Hypertension

Renovascular hypertension is the most common form of potentially curable secondary hypertension. It occurs in 1%-2% of the hypertensive population. Stenosis of a renal artery increases renin production from the ischemic kidney. Renin acts on circulating renin substrate to produce angiotensin I, which is converted to angiotensin II, a potent vasoconstrictor, by ACE found in lung and other tissues. In addition to vasoconstriction, angiotensin II stimulates aldosterone production, which causes renal sodium retention and volume expansion. Angiotensin II also stimulates thirst and release of vasopressin.

- Renovascular disease: the most common form of potentially curable secondary hypertension.
- Renal artery stenosis increases renin production.
- Renin increases angiotensin II.
- Angiotensin II is a potent vasoconstrictor and stimulates aldosterone production, causing renal sodium retention and volume expansion.

Correcting renal ischemia eliminates the stimulus for excess renin release and often cures or lessens hypertension. In unilateral renal artery stenosis, prolonged hypertension eventually causes nephrosclerosis in the nonischemic kidney. If this occurs, relieving renal arterial stenosis may not cure hypertension. The longer the duration of hypertension before diagnosis, the less likely that correction of renal ischemia will be beneficial for blood pressure control.

- Correcting renal ischemia eliminates excess renin release.
- The longer the duration of hypertension, the less likely that correction of renal ischemia will be beneficial.

Fibromuscular dysplasia is the most common cause of renovascular hypertension in younger persons, especially women. Lesions usually affect the middle and distal portions of the main renal vessels, often extending into branches. Medial fibroplasia, the most common subtype in adults, has a classic string-of-beads appearance on angiography. Except for rare subtypes, fibromuscular dysplasia progresses slowly over time; however, dissection and thrombosis can occur.

- Fibromuscular dysplasia: the common cause of renovascular hypertension in younger persons.
- It progresses slowly over time.

Atheromatous disease is the most common cause of renovascular hypertension in older persons. Lesions usually are in the proximal third of the renal artery, often near the orifice. Although atheromatous renal artery disease may occur in 50%-75% of older persons with hypertension, it causes or aggra- vates hypertension less frequently. The disease is frequently bilateral and, in 50% of cases, progresses over time, even if blood pressure is controlled. Bilateral disease can progress and lead to end-stage renal disease.

- Atheromatous disease: the common cause of renovascular hypertension in older persons.
- The disease is frequently bilateral and, in 50% of cases, progresses over time.

Clinical clues suggesting renovascular hypertension include: onset of hypertension before age 30 (consider fibromuscular dysplasia, especially in women); onset of hypertension after age 50 (consider atherosclerotic renal vascular disease); presentation of accelerated or malignant hypertension; sudden worsening of hypertension (renovascular hypertension superimposed on essential hypertension). The most important physical finding is an abdominal bruit, especially a high-pitched systolic/diastolic bruit in the upper abdomen or flank. However, 50% of patients with renovascular hypertension do not have this finding. Other physical clues include severe retinopathy of accelerated malignant hypertension (hemorrhages, exudates) or evidence of occlusive disease in other vascular beds. Laboratory abnormalities consistent with renovascular hypertension include hypokalemia (due to secondary aldosteronism) and, rarely, ischemia-induced polycythemia or nephrotic range proteinuria.

- For hypertension before age 30, consider fibromuscular dysplasia, especially in women.
- The most important physical finding: abdominal bruit.
- Laboratory abnormalities: hypokalemia, ischemia-induced polycythemia, and nephrotic range proteinuria.
- For hypertension after age 50, consider atherosclerotic renovascular disease.

Decline of renal function with the use of an ACE inhibitor or after a sudden decrease in blood pressure may indicate bilateral renal artery disease or small vessel disease of the kidneys (nephrosclerosis). Atheroembolic renal disease may present with a sudden onset or worsening of hypertension and a subacute decline in renal function. Historical clues (e.g., occurrence after angiography or aortic surgery), physical findings (livedo reticularis, peripheral emboli), and laboratory abnormalities (increased erythrocyte sedimentation rate, anemia, hematuria, eosinophilia, eosinophiluria) help identify these patients.

- Sudden decline in renal function with the use of an ACE inhibitor may indicate bilateral renal artery disease.
- Sudden onset or worsening of hypertension and subacute decline in renal function may be due to atheroembolic renal disease.

In young persons with hypertension (even if not severe) of short duration who have suggestive clinical features, evaluation for renovascular hypertension is indicated, because identification and correction of renal artery stenosis can be performed with low risk of morbidity and mortality, and correction is associated with a high probability of cure. Evaluation for renovascular hypertension in older patients must be done on a selective basis. Selection should be restricted to those patients with suggestive clinical features whose blood pressure cannot be controlled medically or who have an unexplained, observed decline in renal function and who are considered reasonable risks for (and are willing to undergo) interventional therapy.

- In young patients with hypertension of short duration, evaluate for renovascular hypertension.
- Evaluation for renovascular hypertension in older patients must be done on a selective basis.

Screening Tests

Intravenous Pyelography

Intravenous pyelography has been replaced by captopril renography as the initial screening test of choice. Characteristic abnormalities are: 1) unilateral reduction in renal mass, with the pole-to-pole diameter of the smaller kidney decreased by ≥1.5 cm; 2) delayed appearance of contrast agent in the collecting system of the ischemic kidney; 3) hyperconcentration of contrast agent in the ischemic kidney on delayed films; 4) ureteral scalloping by collateral vessels; and 5) cortical thinning or irregularity. Sensitivity is 70%-75%; thus, normal findings on intravenous pyelography do not exclude the diagnosis. Specificity is 85%. It is a reasonable choice if renal obstruction, infarction, calculus disease, or parenchymal disease is of concern.

- Abnormalities on intravenous pyelography: unilateral reduction in renal mass (≥1.5-cm decrease in pole-to-pole diameter of the smaller kidney), delayed appearance of contrast agent in the collecting system of the ischemic kidney (hyperconcentration of this agent in the ischemic kidney), ureteral scalloping by collateral vessels, and cortical thinning or irregularity.

Captopril Radionuclide Renal Scan

Many consider the captopril radionuclide renal scan the screening method of choice. Sensitivity of captopril renography is 90%; specificity is 90%-95%. Pretest treatment of patients with captopril increases the sensitivity of the scan compared with that of standard renography. The rationale is that glomerular filtration in an ischemic kidney depends on the vasoconstricting effect of angiotensin II on the efferent arteriole of the nephron. Acute treatment with an ACE inhibitor causes efferent arteriolar dilatation, with loss of filtration pressure in the nephron. This causes a decline of glomerular filtration in the ischemic kidney, with less of an effect on renal blood flow. These changes are identified with the scanning technique. Radionuclides most commonly used are ^{131}I orthoiodohippuric acid (OIH), which is a marker for renal blood flow, and ^{99m}Tc diethylenetriamine pentaacetic acid (DPTA), which is a marker for glomerular filtration rate. The criteria for a positive test with DPTA are time to peak activity in the kidney ≥11 minutes and a ratio of the glomerular filtration rate between the kidneys ≥1.5. The criterion for a positive test with OIH is residual cortical activity at 20 minutes ≥30% of peak activity. The renal scan is safe for patients with renal insufficiency or a history of contrast allergy. Its interpretive value is reduced by azotemia and bilateral or branch renal artery disease. Urinary outflow obstruction may mimic renal artery stenosis.

- Many consider captopril radionuclide scan the screening method of choice.
- Sensitivity of 90% and specificity of 90%-95%.
- It is safe for patients with renal insufficiency or a history of contrast allergy.
- Urinary outflow obstruction may mimic renal artery stenosis.

Digital Venous Subtraction Angiography

Digital venous subtraction angiography uses contrast media, but access to the circulation is through a peripheral vein. Thus, it can be performed safely as an outpatient procedure. It allows visualization of the proximal main renal arteries (usual location of atherosclerotic disease) in 90% of patients but is not good for assessing distal or branch renal arteries (usual location of fibromuscular dysplasia). This technique is expensive, and in 20%-30% of cases, renal arteries are not identified because of superimposition of abdominal vessels or patient motion. Sensitivity is 85%-90% and specificity is 85%-90%.

- Digital venous subtraction angiography: the proximal main renal arteries are visible in 90% of patients.
- It is not good for assessing distal or branch renal arteries.
- It is expensive.
- Renal arteries not identified in 20%-30% of cases.
- Sensitivity of 85%-90% (same for specificity).

Duplex Ultrasonography

Duplex ultrasonography is noninvasive and does not use contrast media. It should be considered for patients with renal insufficiency or a history of contrast allergy. This method measures flow-velocity changes in renal vessels that occur with renal artery stenosis. Criteria for a positive test are 1) a ratio of peak flow velocity in the renal artery to peak flow velocity in the aorta >3.5 and 2) renal artery peak systolic flow ≥180 cm/sec. In up to 50% of cases, one or both renal arteries cannot be visualized because of technical problems. Sensitivity is 80%-90% and specificity is 90%.

- Consider duplex ultrasonography for patients with renal insufficiency or a history of contrast allergy.
- In up to 50% of cases, one or both renal arteries cannot be visualized.
- Sensitivity of 80%-90% and specificity of 90%.

Captoptil Test

Acute blockade of angiotensin II formation by ACE inhibitors produces a reactive increase in plasma renin activity. The magnitude of this increase is greater in patients with renovascular hypertension than in those with essential hypertension. This is the basis for the captopril test. Use of antihypertensive agents that influence the renin-angiotensin-aldosterone axis must be discontinued several days before the test. Plasma renin activity is measured at baseline and at 60 minutes after administering captopril orally. Criteria for a positive test include: 1) post captopril plasma renin activity >12 ng/mL per hour, 2) absolute increase in plasma renin activity over baseline of ≥10 ng/mL per hour, and 3) ≥150% increase in plasma renin activity if baseline plasma renin activity is >3 ng/mL per hour or ≥400% if baseline renin activity is <3 ng/mL per hour. Results are compromised in the presence of renal insufficiency. Sensitivity is 39%-100% and specificity is 72%-100%.

- Plasma renin activity is measured at baseline and at 60 minutes after administering captopril orally.
- With renal insufficiency, the results are compromised.
- Sensitivity of 39%-100% and specificity of 72%-100%.

Renal Vein Renins

Lateralization of renal vein renins is the best predictor of a good interventional outcome in unilateral renal artery stenosis; however, because many factors can influence renin secretion and are difficult to control for, this is not a good screening test. It is invasive and expensive. Lateralization is present if the ratio of renin activity on the affected side compared with that on the normal side is 1.5:1.0 or greater. Sensitivity is 63%-77% and specificity is 60%-95%.

- Lateralization of renal vein renins: the best predictor of good interventional outcome in unilateral renal artery stenosis.
- It is invasive and expensive.
- Lateralization is present if the ratio of renin activity of the affected side to the normal side is 1.5:1.0 or greater.

Renal Arteriography

Renal arteriography is the standard method for identifying renal arterial lesions. Renal artery stenosis must be demon-strated in combination with clinical features and, in some cases, renal vein renins. If there are good clinical reasons to suspect disease, proceeding directly to arteriography is appropriate.

- Renal arteriography: the standard method for identifying renal arterial lesions.

Therapy for Renovascular Hypertension

Options for management of renovascular hypertension include medical and interventional therapies. Percutaneous balloon angioplasty and surgical procedures to relieve renal ischemia are the nonmedical treatments. Goals of interventional therapy are to cure or improve hypertension and to preserve renal function. Interventional therapy should be reserved for good surgical candidates. Medical therapy is reserved for patients not considered candidates for interventional therapy (because of the extent or location of the vascular lesions, medical/surgical risk, uncertainty about causative significance of the lesion).

Percutaneous transluminal angioplasty is the treatment of choice for amenable lesions due to fibromuscular dysplasia. Its role in the management of atherosclerotic renovascular lesions is less well defined. Complications of angioplasty include groin hematoma, dye-induced azotemia, dissection of the renal artery, renal infarction, and, rarely, rupture of the renal artery, with loss of the kidney and the need for immediate surgery. Cholesterol embolization is a risk in older patients with diffuse atherosclerosis.

- Angioplasty is the treatment of choice for amenable lesions due to fibromuscular dysplasia.
- Its complications: groin hematoma, dye-induced azotemia, dissection of the renal artery, renal infarction, and, rarely, rupture of the renal artery.

Surgical treatment is best for cases of atheromatous renal artery disease. Kidneys ≤8 cm in pole-to-pole length should be removed, not revascularized, if intervention is indicated and removal will not jeopardize overall renal function.

- Surgical treatment is best for most cases of atheromatous renal artery disease.

Medical treatment of renovascular hypertension differs little from that of essential hypertension. Volume retention and vasoconstriction (due to activation of the sympathetic nervous system and angiotensin II) both contribute to the hypertension. ACE inhibitors can precipitate acute renal failure if unrecognized bilateral renal artery stenosis is present. Medical treatment does not correct the underlying ischemia of the affected kidney, and decreasing systemic blood pressure without correcting renal vascular stenosis may aggravate further loss of renal function.

guanadrel, α-blockers, or calcium channel antagonists may be used. After a high salt diet for 3 days (and with concomitant vigorous potassium supplementation), patients should submit a 24-hour urine collection for measurement of sodium, potassium, creatinine, and aldosterone. Creatinine can be used as an approximation of the adequacy of the collection. A 24-hour urine aldosterone >12 ng (when urine sodium is >200 mEq/24 hours) confirms the diagnosis of primary aldosteronism.

- In a hypokalemic, hypertensive patient, a PAC-to-PRA ratio >20 suggests primary aldosteronism.
- The diagnosis of primary aldosteronism: hypokalemia, renin suppression, and increased aldosterone secretion in a sodium replete state in a hypertensive patient.
- Before diagnostic evaluation: discontinue interfering drugs and assess plasma volume status.
- After a 3-day high salt diet, measure sodium, potassium, creatinine, and aldosterone in a 24-hour urine collection.
- 24-Hour urine aldosterone >12 ng (if urine sodium is >200 mEq/24 hr) confirms the diagnosis of primary aldosteronism.

Adenoma and bilateral hyperplasia must be distinguished. Removing an aldosterone-producing adenoma normalizes blood pressure and hypokalemia in 70% of cases. Unilateral or bilateral adrenalectomy seldom corrects hypertension when bilateral adrenal hyperplasia is present. Adrenal CT scan is the initial study for distinguishing between subtypes. CT is effective in localizing adenomas >1 cm in diameter when the adrenal glands are imaged at 0.3-cm intervals. Generally, if a single adenoma >1 cm in diameter is clearly identified, surgical treatment is the choice. If no mass is identified, assume the diagnosis of bilateral hyperplasia and prescribe spironolactone or other potassium-retaining diuretics. Often, additional medications are needed for blood pressure control.

- Removing aldosterone-producing adenoma normalizes hypertension and hypokalemia in 70% of cases.
- Unilateral or bilateral adrenalectomy seldom corrects hypertension in cases of bilateral adrenal hyperplasia.
- Adrenal CT scan is the initial study for distinguishing between subtypes.
- If a single adenoma is >1 cm in diameter, treatment is surgical.
- If no mass is seen, prescribe spironolactone or other potassium-retaining diuretics.

If the results are equivocal or the gland opposite that containing the presumed adenoma is abnormal or if CT findings are normal in a young patient with severe hypertension and hypokalemia, sampling blood from the adrenal veins may distinguish between subtypes. In these settings, subspecialty consultation should be sought.

- If the results are equivocal, sampling blood from the adrenal veins may distinguish between subtypes.

Pheochromocytoma

Pheochromocytomas are tumors of chromaffin cell origin that produce paroxysmal or sustained hypertension. A "rule of 10" is often quoted for this tumor: 10% are extra-adrenal (90% are located in one or both adrenal glands), 10% occur in children (90% in adults between the third and fifth decades of life; equal occurrence in males and females), 10% are multiple or bilateral, 10% recur after the initial resection, 10% are malignant, and 10% are familial. Extra-adrenal pheochromocytomas may occur anywhere along the sympathetic chain and occasionally in aberrant sites (superior para-aortic region [46%], inferior para-aortic region [29%], bladder [10%], and thorax [10%]). Chromaffin cells synthesize catecholamines from tyrosine. Norepinephrine is the end product in all sites except in the adrenal medulla, where 75% of norepinephrine is metabolized further to epinephrine. Extra-adrenal tumors produce only norepinephrine, whereas adrenal pheochromocytomas may produce an excess of one or both chemicals. Patients with tumors that secrete predominantly epinephrine tend to have mainly systolic hypertension, tachycardia, sweating, flushing, and tremulousness and may present with hypotension. Patients with tumors that secrete mainly norepinephrine tend to have both diastolic and systolic hypertension, less tachycardia, and fewer paroxysms of anxiety and palpitations.

- Remember the "rule of 10."
- 80%-90% of pheochromocytomas are in the adrenal glands.
- They may occur anywhere along the sympathetic chain.
- They are malignant in up to 10% of cases.
- Extra-adrenal tumors produce only norepinephrine.
- Adrenal pheochromocytomas produce an excess of epinephrine or norepinephrine or both.

Familial pheochromocytomas tend to be bilateral. Familial syndromes include: a simple form inherited as an autosomal dominant trait unassociated with other glandular abnormalities; multiple endocrine neoplasia type IIA (medullary carcinoma of the thyroid [increased plasma level of calcitonin], pheochromocytoma, hyperparathyroidism) and type IIB (pheochromocytoma, medullary carcinoma of the thyroid, mucosal neuromas, thickened corneal nerves, intestinal ganglioneuromatosis, marfanoid body habitus); neurofibromatosis (café au lait spots); and von Hippel-Lindau disease (pheochromocytoma, retinal hemangiomatosis, cerebellar hemangioblastomas, renal cell carcinoma).

- Familial tumors: tend to be bilateral.
- Multiple endocrine neoplasia type II: medullary carcinoma of the thyroid, pheochromocytoma, and hyperparathyroidism.

- Pheochromocytoma associated with neurofibromatosis and von Hippel-Lindau disease (retinal angiomas, cerebellar hemangioblastomas, and renal cell carcinoma).

Symptoms

Headache, sweating, or palpitations are common, and all may occur in paroxysms. Paroxysms of hypertension occur in <50% of persons; most persons have sustained hypertension. Exercise, bending, urination, defecation, induction of anesthesia, smoking, or infusion of intravenous contrast media can induce a paroxysm. Some patients have a history of weight loss and hypermetabolism. Others have both hypertension and orthostatic hypotension, and some have retinopathy of accelerated hypertension.

- Common symptoms of pheochromocytoma: headache, sweating, and palpitations.
- Exercise, bending, urination, defecation, induction of anesthesia, smoking, or infusion of contrast media can induce a paroxysm.
- Some patients have a history of weight loss and hypermetabolism; others have both hypertension and orthostatic hypotension.

Screening

Patients who should be screened for pheochromocytoma are those with a history of paroxysmal hypertension, progressive or treatment-resistant hypertension, hypertension with diabetes mellitus, hypermetabolism and weight loss, marked hypertension in response to anesthesia induction, neurocutaneous lesions and hypertension, family history of pheochromocytoma, medullary carcinoma of the thyroid or hyperparathyroidism, and orthostatic hypotension. Patients with a history of paroxysmal symptoms and hypertension should also be screened for pheochromocytoma, as should children with hypertension. The best screening test is 24-hour urine metanephrine concentration. Because pheochromocytomas may secrete intermittently, multiple samples may be required. Urine should be collected immediately after a paroxysm. In addition to urine metanephrine concentration, urine VMA and catecholamine concentrations should be measured in selected patients. Medications that can interfere with these assays are listed in Table 13-4.

- Screening for pheochromocytoma: history of paroxysmal hypertension, progressive or treatment-resistant hypertension, hypertension with diabetes mellitus, hypermetabolism and weight loss, and marked hypertension in response to anesthesia induction.
- Screen children with hypertension.
- Best screening test is 24-hour urine metanephrine concentration.

- Medications interfering with assays: sympathomimetics, methyldopa, phenothiazines, tricyclic antidepressants, labetalol, levodopa.

Diagnosis and Treatment

Computerized abdominal imaging (CT or MRI) is the initial test used to locate a tumor. The treatment is surgical. Preoperatively, administer α-blockers followed by β-blockers if needed for blood pressure and cardiac rhythm control. Patients with hypertensive crisis can be given α-blockers intravenously. β-Blockers can be used if tachycardia is excessive.

- Use computerized abdominal imaging to locate tumor.
- Treatment is surgical.
- Preoperatively, administer α-blockers followed by β-blockers.

Coarctation of the Aorta

Coarctation of the aorta is commonly just beyond the take off of the left subclavian artery. It is detected most often in childhood but may escape detection until adulthood. The classic feature of coarctation is increased blood pressure in the upper extremities, with low or unobtainable blood pressure in the lower extremities. The mechanism of hypertension involves volume expansion and inappropriate renin secretion. Symptoms of coarctation include headache, cold feet, and exercise-induced leg pain (claudication). Clinical signs include hypertension, murmurs in the front or back of the chest, visible pulsations in the neck or chest wall, and weak femoral pulses or delay

Table 13-4.--Medications That Interfere With Results of Catecholamine and Metabolite Measurements

Associated with increased values
Amphetamines
Phenothiazines
Labetolol
Drugs containing catecholamines (decongestants)
Levodopa
Methyldopa
Withdrawal from clonidine or related drugs
Ethanol
Tricyclic antidepressants
Benzodiazepines
Sotalol
Associated with decreased values
Central α$_2$ agonists (clonidine and related drugs)
Metyrosine
Reserpine
Guanethidine
Methylglucamine (iodinated contrast medium)

when simultaneously palpating the radial and femoral pulse. Chest radiography can be diagnostic. A characteristic "3 sign" due to dilatation above and below the constriction plus notching of the ribs by enlarged collateral vessels may be identified. The diagnosis is proved by aortography, and the treatment is surgical. Postoperative hypertension is usually transient and may be associated with mesenteric vasculitis and bowel infarction. Plasma renin activity levels are usually high. β-Blockers or ACE inhibitors are recommended treatments.

- Coarctation of the aorta is usually just beyond the take off of the left subclavian artery.
- Usually, it is detected in childhood but may not be detected until adulthood.
- Classic feature: increased blood pressure in the upper extremities and low/unobtainable blood pressure in the lower extremities.
- Mechanism: volume expansion and inappropriate renin secretion.
- Symptoms: headache, cold feet, and exercise-induced leg pain.
- Signs: hypertension, murmurs in front or back of the chest, visible pulsations in the neck or chest wall, and weak femoral pulses.
- Chest radiography can be diagnostic.

Hypertension in Pregnancy

Normally, blood pressure decreases early in pregnancy and then gradually increases to pre-pregnant levels toward term. During pregnancy, renin substrate, renin activity, and aldosterone levels increase. Vessels during normal pregnancy are hyporesponsive to angiotensin, perhaps because of prostaglandins produced by the uteroplacental unit. Although aldosterone levels increase, renal sodium retention is not marked, probably because progesterone and prostaglandins are natriuretic. Progesterone is also a vasodilator. During normal pregnancy, plasma volume and cardiac output increase 50%-60% of baseline. The renal blood flow and glomerular filtration rate increase by 35%. Blood pressure decreases in normal pregnancy because of reduced peripheral vascular resistance. Other substances that increase during normal pregnancy are estrogen, deoxycorticosterone, and vasodilating prostaglandins produced by the uteroplacental unit.

- Blood pressure decreases early in pregnancy, gradually increasing to pre-pregnant levels toward term.
- Renin substrate, renin activity, and aldosterone increase.
- During pregnancy, vessels are hyporesponsive to angiotensin.
- Renal sodium retention is not marked, probably because progesterone and prostaglandins are natriuretic.
- In normal pregnancies, blood pressure decreases because of reduced peripheral vascular resistance.

Definition

Hypertension during pregnancy is when systolic blood pressure increases ≥30 mm Hg and diastolic blood pressure increases ≥15 mm Hg, as compared with values before 20 weeks' gestation. When previous blood pressure levels are unknown, a pressure of ≥140/90 mm Hg is abnormal. Four major hypertensive syndromes in pregnancy are 1) chronic hypertension--high blood pressure known to be present before pregnancy or diagnosed before the 20th week of gestation, 2) preeclampsia-eclampsia (described below), 3) chronic hypertension with superimposed preeclampsia, and 4) transient hypertension (or gestational hypertension)--increase in blood pressure without significant edema or proteinuria, with return of blood pressure to normal within 10 days after delivery. This is a predictor for the future development of essential hypertension.

- Hypertension: systolic blood pressure increases ≥30 mm Hg and diastolic blood pressure increases ≥15 mm Hg, as compared with values before 20 weeks' gestation.
- Transient hypertension is a predictor for future development of essential hypertension.

Preeclampsia is characterized by the triad of hypertension, edema, and proteinuria developing after the 20th week of gestation. Eclampsia consists of these symptoms plus convulsions. Warning symptoms of eclampsia include headache, blurring of vision, epigastric pain, hyperreflexia, or cerebral symptoms. The risk of developing eclampsia is markedly increased in women with severe proteinuria (>5 g), oliguria, or absolute blood pressures >160/110 mm Hg. Preeclampsia occurs more commonly in women who are relatively young or old to be pregnant, first pregnancy, twin pregnancy, obesity, diabetes mellitus, family history of eclampsia or preeclampsia in mother, renal disease, or pregnancy in the setting of chronic hypertension. Preeclampsia developing before the 20th week of gestation suggests the possibility of molar pregnancy, fetal hydrops, α-thalassemia, or renal disease.

- Preeclampsia: characteristic triad of hypertension, edema, and proteinuria after the 20th week of gestation.
- Eclampsia: same symptoms as preeclampsia plus convulsions.
- Preeclampsia is more common in women relatively young or old for pregnancy, first or twin pregnancy, obesity, diabetes mellitus, family history of eclampsia or preeclampsia in mother, renal disease, pregnancy in setting of chronic hypertension.

The cause of preeclampsia is not well known. The best hypothesis involves underperfusion of the uteroplacental unit. Unlike normal pregnant women, those with preeclampsia are sensitive to the pressor effects of angiotensin. There is a marked increase in peripheral resistance. Renal blood flow and glomerular filtration rate are decreased. Vascular volume is decreased. There is often hemoconcentration. Placental prostaglandin levels decrease. Uric acid is most often increased and distinguishes patients with preeclampsia from those with chronic hypertension in pregnancy.

- Unlike normal pregnant women, those with preeclampsia are sensitive to the pressor effects of angiotensin.
- Peripheral resistance markedly increases.
- Uric acid is most often increased: this distinguishes women with preeclampsia from those with chronic hypertension in pregnancy.

Treatment of Hypertension in Pregnancy

For previously untreated women, consider drug therapy if diastolic blood pressure is ≥100 mm Hg. Methyldopa (most completely studied) is recommended as initial therapy. If this drug is ineffective or not tolerated, consider other drugs. Except for ACE inhibitors, none of the currently available drugs are known to increase perinatal morbidity or mortality. Most of the concern about these drugs is theoretical. There is evidence that β-adrenergic blocking drugs and α-β-blocking drugs are safe and effective for treating chronic hypertension in pregnancy. There is some concern that the use of β-adrenergic blockers early in pregnancy can retard fetal growth and in late pregnancy could slow fetal heart rate.

- For previously untreated women, use drug therapy if diastolic blood pressure is ≥100 mm Hg.
- Recommended initial therapy: methyldopa.
- ACE inhibitors are contraindicated during pregnancy.

Treatment of Preeclampsia-Eclampsia

Prevention strategies for preeclampsia have limited value. It is important to identify the high-risk woman and to monitor her closely to identify preeclampsia early. Low doses of aspirin have received much attention as a possible agent for preventing preeclampsia, but currently its use is investigational. Early recognition of preeclampsia is based primarily on diagnostic blood pressure increases in the late second or early third trimester of pregnancy. Proteinuria is an important sign of progression, usually warranting hospitalization. The woman should be kept at rest in bed. Monitor blood pressure, urine output, and fluid retention (estimated by daily weights) daily. Periodically determine the platelet count, creatinine level, uric acid level, and urine protein excretion. Evidence of central nervous system involvement (headache, disorientation, visual symptoms) or hepatic distention (abdominal pain, hepatic tenderness) are important findings that suggest progression of preeclampsia. Hepatic rupture is associated with a 65% mortality and can be prevented only by delivery of the fetus. Evidence of progressive preeclampsia after the 30th week of gestation is an indication for delivery. When gestational age is critical (25-30 weeks), delivery is indicated by worsening maternal symptoms, laboratory evidence of end-organ dysfunction, or deterioration of fetal condition. If a fetus is immature and preeclampsia is nonprogressive, a period of observation is warranted. Hypertension should be treated with drugs if diastolic blood pressure is >100 mm Hg. The treatment of choice is methyldopa. Calcium channel antagonists, β-adrenergic blockers, or hydralazine are reasonable alternatives.

- Proteinuria is an important sign of progression, usually warranting hospitalization.
- Keep the woman at bed rest.
- Central nervous system progression or hepatic distention suggests progression of preeclampsia.
- Progressive preeclampsia after the 30th week of gestation is an indication for delivery.
- Delivery is indicated by worsening maternal symptoms, laboratory evidence of end-organ dysfunction, or deterioration of the fetal condition.
- If diastolic blood pressure is >100 mm Hg, treat with drugs.
- Treatment of choice: methyldopa.

Magnesium sulfate is the treatment of choice for impending eclampsia. It can be administered intravenously as 20 mL of 20% solution over 4 minutes. Intermittent doses of a 50% solution given intramuscularly every 4 hours can also be used. Monitor the patient's patellar reflex, urine output, and respirations while giving magnesium. Calcium gluconate is the treatment of choice for magnesium toxicity.

- Magnesium sulfate: treatment of choice for impending eclampsia.
- Calcium gluconate: treatment of choice for magnesium toxicity.

Treatment of Hypertensive Crisis

The drug of choice for the treatment of a hypertensive crisis during pregnancy is hydralazine administered intravenously. Initially administer a 5-mg bolus. This can be followed by 5-10 mg every 20-30 minutes. Side effects include tachycardia and headache. For hypertension refractory to hydralazine, diazoxide is recommended. Miniboluses (30 mg) should be used. Side effects include arrest of labor and neonatal hyperglycemia. Labetalol may replace diazoxide as the second-line drug. Calcium antagonists can be used, but the concomitant use of magnesium sulfate may cause severe hypotension. Diuretics and sodium nitroprusside (cyanide poisoning in the fetus) should be avoided. However, maternal well-being may override these concerns.

- The drug of choice for treating hypertensive crisis: hydralazine given intravenously.

- For hypertension refractory to hydralazine, use diazoxide.
- Avoid diuretics and sodium nitroprusside.

Hypertensive Urgencies and Emergencies

Acute, severe increases in blood pressure are a medical emergency; prompt therapy may be lifesaving.

Definitions

Malignant hypertension is a sudden severe increase in blood pressure associated with acute injury to target organs (brain, heart, kidneys, retina). Parenteral antihypertensive therapy to decrease blood pressure immediately is required. Retinal examination reveals hemorrhages, exudates, and papilledema. Hypertensive encephalopathy may be present; it is cerebral edema due to breakthrough hyperperfusion of the brain caused by severely increased blood pressure. Manifestations include papilledema, headache, confusion, gastrointestinal distress, and seizures. The term "hypertensive emergency" implies malignant hypertension or impending malignant hypertension.

- Malignant hypertension: sudden severe increase in blood pressure associated with acute injury to target organs.
- Parenteral therapy to decrease blood pressure immediately is required.
- Retinal hemorrhages, exudates, and papilledema occur.
- Hypertensive encephalopathy: papilledema, headache, confusion, gastrointestinal distress, and seizures.

Accelerated Hypertension

Accelerated hypertension is a sudden increase in blood pressure to less severe levels. It is not associated with acute target organ damage. Retinal examination reveals hemorrhages and exudates but not papilledema. If left untreated, it may progress to malignant hypertension. Blood pressure usually can be decreased to safer levels with oral or parenteral medications over several hours. The term "hypertensive urgency" implies accelerated hypertension or severe increases in blood pressure without evidence of acute target organ damage occurring in a setting in which it is important to decrease blood pressure over several hours.

- Accelerated hypertension: sudden increase in blood pressure to less severe levels.
- It is not associated with acute target organ damage.
- Retinal hemorrhages and exudates occur but not papilledema.
- Blood pressure can be decreased with oral or parenteral medications.

Causes

Causes of hypertensive urgencies and emergencies include the development of accelerated malignant hypertension on the background of neglected essential hypertension, sudden discontinuation of antihypertensive therapy (especially cloni-

dine and β-blockers), renovascular disease, collagen diseases (especially scleroderma), monoamine oxidase inhibitors and tyramine-containing foods, intracerebral or subarachnoid hemorrhage, acute aortic dissection, pheochromocytoma crisis, acute head injury, and acute stroke.

- Causes of hypertensive urgencies and emergencies: neglected essential hypertension, discontinuation of antihypertensive therapy, renovascular disease, collagen diseases, pheochromocytoma crisis, and stroke.

Pathophysiology

Malignant hypertension is a rapidly progressive vasospastic disorder associated with marked increase in peripheral vascular resistance and increased levels of renin and angiotensin. Locally generated vasoconstricting factors such as endothelin may be important. If not reversed, necrosis of blood vessel walls occurs (fibrinoid necrosis), with severe damage to organs, particularly the brain and kidneys. With progressive increases in blood pressure, autoregulation of cerebral blood flow breaks down. Normally, as blood pressure increases, cerebral blood vessels constrict to maintain constant blood flow. When blood pressure increases to a critical level, cerebral blood vessels suddenly dilate, causing marked hyperperfusion of the brain and leakage of fluid. This leads to cerebral edema and the clinical presentation of hypertensive encephalopathy.

- Malignant hypertension: a rapidly progressive vasospastic disorder.
- Renin and angiotensin levels are increased.
- If not reversed, necrosis of blood vessel walls occurs.

Evaluation and Management

Patients with hypertensive emergencies and evidence of acute organ injury should be hospitalized in an intensive care unit. An arterial catheter should be established to monitor blood pressure closely. Initial studies should include chest radiography, ECG, creatinine or BUN, urinalysis, glucose, sodium, potassium, and hemoglobin. Studies to determine the underlying cause should be deferred; however, a spot urine for catecholamines is reasonable. The challenge of treating hypertensive emergencies is to decrease blood pressure promptly without compromising the function of vital organs. Blood pressure should be decreased quickly to a diastolic level of approximately 110 mm Hg, after which the patient should be monitored for evidence of worsening cerebral, renal, or cardiac status. Blood pressure is then gradually decreased to a diastolic level of 90-100 mm Hg. Ischemic pancreatitis and intestinal infarction are complications in some patients.

Generally, sodium nitroprusside is the drug of choice. It must be given in an intensive care setting, with an arterial catheter in place. This balanced arterial and venous dilator decreases both preload and afterload. The initial dose is 0.5-

10.0 µg/kg per minute. It is titrated to a maximal dose of 500 µg/kg per hour. The infusion must be protected from light. Toxicity is related to the development of cyanide in erythrocytes, and thiocyanate levels should be monitored every 48 hours. Therapy should be discontinued if the blood level is >12 mg/dL. Sodium nitrate or hydroxycobalamin can be infused in case of toxicity. Side effects of sodium nitroprusside include nausea, vomiting, agitation, muscular twitching, coarse tremor, and flushing. Frequently, patients with malignant hypertension are volume constricted because of pressure natriuresis. However, as blood pressure decreases, fluid retention occurs and the addition of a loop diuretic is often required.

- Sodium nitroprusside: the drug of choice.
- Toxicity is related to the development of cyanide in erythrocytes.
- Monitor thiocyanate levels every 48 hours.
- In case of toxicity, infuse sodium nitrate or hydroxycobalamin.
- Sodium nitroprusside side effects: nausea, vomiting, agitation, muscular twitching, coarse tremor, and flushing.

Diazoxide is an alternative therapy and should be given by minibolus techniques (50-100-150 mg every 5-10 minutes). This method avoids excessive hypotension with the initial dose. Blood sugar should be monitored in diabetics. Side effects include nausea, hypotension, flushing, tachycardia, and chest pain.

- Diazoxide is an alternative therapy.
- Side effects: nausea, hypotension, flushing, tachycardia, and chest pain.

Hydralazine can be used (usually in preeclampsia). It is slower acting than the other agents. Its side effects include tachycardia, flushing, headache, vomiting, and aggravation of angina.

Adrenergic inhibitors include phentolamine and trimethaphan. Phentolamine is administered intravenously in doses of 5-15 mg. Its side effects include tachycardia and flushing. Trimethaphan is administered as an infusion at rate of 0.5-5 mg/minute. Its side effects include paresis of bowel and bladder, orthostatic hypotension, blurred vision, and dry mouth.

- Adrenergic inhibitors: phentolamine and trimethaphan.
- Side effects (trimethaphan): bowel and bladder paresis, orthostatic hypotension, blurred vision, and dry mouth.

Labetalol is administered by repetitive intravenous minibolus injections. It has the advantage of being available orally for the ease of conversion. The precautions applying to β-blockers also apply to this drug.

Conditions Requiring Avoidance of Specific Drugs
- Acute myocardial infarction or angina--hydralazine (increases cardiac work), diazoxide (increases cardiac work).
- Dissecting aortic aneurysm--hydralazine (increases cardiac output), diazoxide (increases cardiac output).
- Stroke, head injury, hypertensive encephalopathy--methyldopa (sedation, increases cerebral blood flow), diazoxide (decreases cerebral blood flow).

As soon as possible, initiate regular oral treatment and taper intravenous treatment. After blood pressure is controlled, search for secondary causes of hypertension.

QUESTIONS

Multiple Choice (choose the one best answer)
1. The oral drug of choice for treating hypertension during pregnancy is:
   a. Hydrochlorothiazide
   b. Captopril
   c. Methyldopa
   d. Hydralazine
   e. Propranolol

2. Which blood study best distinguishes primary aldosteronism from secondary aldosteronism due to diuretic use?
   a. Potassium concentration
   b. Sodium concentration
   c. Bicarbonate concentration
   d. Glucose concentration
   e. Blood pH

3. A 24-year-old woman presents with new onset headaches. Her blood pressure is 220/130 mm Hg. Hemorrhages without papilledema are noted on examination of the fundi. Auscultation of the abdomen reveals the presence of a loud systolic-diastolic bruit audible in the right upper quadrant of the abdomen. The *most* appropriate test to further evaluate the cause of her hypertension is:
   a. Intravenous pyelography
   b. Captopril radionuclide scan
   c. Duplex ultrasonography of the renal arteries
   d. Renal angiography
   e. Digital venous angiography

4. All the following statements about drugs used for the treatment of hypertension are true except:

   a. Angiotensin converting enzyme inhibitors are contraindicated in pregnancy

   b. Verapamil may cause an increase in blood levels of digoxin

   c. Diuretics may interfere with the elimination of lithium

   d. Hydrochlorothiazide increases urinary calcium

   e. Methyldopa can cause a hemolytic anemia

5. A 42-year-old business executive was found to have a blood pressure of 140/100 mm Hg during a community screening, and this value was confirmed at several subsequent office visits. His father and an older sibling have hypertension. Findings on physical examination were normal. Appropriate laboratory tests to perform would include all the following except:

   a. Plasma cholesterol and triglyceride concentrations

   b. Electrocardiography

   c. Intravenous pyelography

   d. Urinalysis

   e. Fasting plasma glucose concentration

6. Compared with nonpregnancy, the physiologic characteristics of normal pregnancy include all but one of the following:

   a. Increased plasma renin activity

   b. Increased plasma aldosterone concentration

   c. Increased peripheral vascular resistance

   d. Increased plasma volume

   e. Increased cardiac output

7. A 54-year-old man reported to the emergency room with a severe headache. His wife reported that he had been mildly confused at times. He has a history of chronic hypertension but has not taken his medications for the last week. On examination, his blood pressure was 230/150 mm Hg. Retinal examination was inadequate. No focal neurologic findings were noted. Initial laboratory findings: EKG showed LVH with atypical T-waves, serum creatinine was 2.0 mg/dL, and urinalysis showed erythrocytes and protein. The most appropriate next step is:

   a. Administer nifedipine (10 mg sublingually), and if blood pressure responds, arrange for follow-up evaluation by personal physician

   b. Restart previous oral therapy, and if blood pressure responds, arrange for follow-up evaluation by personal physician

   c. Admit the patient to the intensive care unit and begin parenteral antihypertensive therapy

   d. Arrange for emergency renal ultrasonographic examination to exclude urinary tract obstruction

   e. Measure cardiac enzymes and arrange for coronary angiography

True/False (indicate whether each answer is true or false)

8. A 56-year-old woman complains of a nonproductive, nocturnal cough for the past three months. She denies having fever. She is a nonsmoker, and there is no previous history of lung disease. She has hypertension that is controlled with captopril and hydrochlorothiazide/triamterene. She has a history of type II diabetes mellitus associated with hypertriglyceridemia and mild renal insufficiency. She takes indomethacin for osteoarthritis.

   a. She is at risk for developing hyperkalemia

   b. Hydrochlorothiazide may aggravate glucose intolerance

   c. Indomethacin may increase her risk for hyperkalemia and interfere with the antihypertensive effect of both hydrochlorothiazide and captopril

   d. Her cough may be a side effect of captopril therapy

   e. Hydrochlorothiazide may increase the plasma levels of triglycerides and cholesterol

   f. A loop diuretic may be a more effective antihypertensive drug if her creatinine level is >2 mg/dL or creatinine clearance is <30 mL/min

9. Regarding the drug treatment of hypertension:

   a. Amitriptyline may interfere with the blood pressure-lowering action of clonidine

   b. The dose of lithium may need to be increased if hydrochlorothiazide is used because this drug enhances the renal elimination of lithium

   c. Hydralazine could be the cause of a lupus syndrome

   d. Verapamil would be a good choice for a patient who has had a recent myocardial infarction and persistent angina

   e. A history of depression or peptic ulcer disease would be a relative contraindication for the use of reserpine

   f. Methyldopa can cause hepatitis

10. Regarding secondary hypertension:

    a. A patient with a cerebellar hemangioblastoma should be screened for pheochromocytoma

    b. Renovascular hypertension should be considered in a patient who presents with accelerated or malignant hypertension

    c. Appropriate initial drug treatment for a patient with a pheochromocytoma would be a β-blocker followed by an α-blocker if needed

    d. A potential side effect of triamterene therapy for primary aldosteronism in men is painful gynecomastia

    e. An acute decline in renal function after treatment with an angiotensin converting enzyme inhibitor suggests the possibility of bilateral renal artery stenosis

    f. Hypertension due to the use of oral contraceptives will usually resolve within 1 month after discontinuing use of the drug

ANSWERS

1. Answer c.

Methyldopa is the oral drug of choice for the treatment of hypertension in pregnancy. The only drugs absolutely contraindicated in pregnancy are the angiotensin converting enzyme inhibitors. Generally, diuretics are avoided in the treatment of preeclampsia.

2. Answer b.

Patients with primary aldosteronism often have mild hypernatremia because of both decreased vasopressin production (because of volume expansion) and decreased vasopressin action on the kidney (i.e., mild nephrogenic DI). Patients with secondary aldosteronism as occurs with diuretics often have mild hyponatremia as a consequence of increased vasopressin production due to volume depletion. Both primary aldosteronism and secondary aldosteronism are characterized by hypokalemia, metabolic alkalosis and, occasionally, glucose intolerance.

3. Answer d.

This clinical presentation strongly suggests secondary hypertension, likely due to renal vascular stenosis. In a young female, the renal artery stenosis is likely due to fibromuscular dysplasia. Identification of this disorder is important because interventional treatment, if technically possible, may cure the hypertension. Because all the screening methods are associated with false-negative results and because the pre-test clinical suspicion is high in this case, it would be most appropriate to proceed directly to renal angiography.

4. Answer d.

Hydrochlorothiazide is associated with hypercalcemia and decreased urinary calcium. This provides a rationale for its use in the treatment of calcium nephrolithiasis.

5. Answer c.

This presentation is entirely consistent with essential hypertension. Therefore, no screening tests for secondary hypertension are indicated.

6. Answer c.

Pregnancy is characterized physiologically by vasodilatation and decreased peripheral vascular resistance. Blood pressure often declines with the onset of pregnancy and returns to pre-pregnant levels only near term. This is observed despite the recognition that plasma volume and cardiac output both increase. Blood vessels are resistant to the constrictor actions of angiotensin II, which is often increased in pregnancy. Although aldosterone levels are increased, sodium retention is not as great as would occur with similar levels in a non-pregnant person.

7. Answer c.

This patient presents with hypertensive crisis. He has a severe increase in blood pressure and possible hypertensive encephalopathy. In addition, he may have acute renal and cardiac injury. This patient needs to be admitted to an intensive care setting and have his blood pressure decreased carefully and immediately, and he needs to be observed for the effects of decreased blood pressure on target organ function.

8. a, true; b, true; c, true; d, true; e, true; f, true.

This patient has several risk factors for hyperkalemia, including renal disease, use of a potassium-sparing diuretic, use of an angiotensin converting enzyme inhibitor, use of a nonsteroidal anti-inflammatory drug, and diabetes mellitus, with an impairment of the insulin mechanism to control blood levels of potassium. Hydrochlorothiazide can impair glucose tolerance and increase plasma cholesterol and triglyceride levels. Indomethacin interferes with the production of renal prostaglandins and can interfere with the antihypertensive action of diuretics and angiotensin converting enzyme inhibitors. A nonproductive cough is a potential side effect of angiotensin converting enzyme inhibitors. A loop diuretic is preferred in patients with significant renal insufficiency.

9. a, true; b, false; c, true; d, false; e, true; f, true.

Hydrochlorothiazide impairs the renal elimination of lithium and the plasma level of lithium may increase with concomitant diuretic therapy. A better choice for drug therapy in a patient with hypertension, recent myocardial infarction, and angina would be a β-blocker. This class of drugs provides secondary protection against recurrent myocardial infarction.

10. a, true; b, true; c, false; d, false; e, true; f, false.

Cerebellar hemangioblastoma suggests the possibility of von Hippel-Lindau disease, which is associated with pheochromocytoma. One possible cause for hypertensive crisis is renovascular hypertension and should be considered along with several other potential causes. The drug treatment for pheochromocytoma is α-blockers. β-Blockers are used after α-blockade to treat tachycardia if necessary. The only potassium-sparing diuretic associated with the potential for gynecomastia is spironolactone. Because angiotensin converting enzyme inhibitors can disrupt autoregulation of glomerular filtration in the setting of renal ischemia from renal artery stenosis, a sudden decline in renal function with their use suggests the possibility of bilateral renal artery stenosis. It may take 3-6 months for hypertension due to oral contraceptives to resolve.

CHAPTER 14

INFECTIOUS DISEASES

Zelalem Temesgen, M.D.
Douglas R. Osmon, M.D.
William F. Marshall, M.D.

This chapter is not inclusive. Topics that should be common knowledge have been omitted. The emphasis is uncommon manifestations of common infectious diseases and important points covered in the infectious disease literature during the past several years.

EMERGING PATHOGENS

Hantavirus Infection, *Hantavirus* Pulmonary Syndrome

In May 1993, an outbreak of an acute illness consisting of fever, rapid development of respiratory failure, and death was reported in the four-state area of New Mexico, Arizona, Colorado, and Utah. Most of the initial cases occurred in young Navajo Indians.

The causative agent was a virus belonging to the genus *Hantavirus* (family Bunyaviridae). This virus is tentatively named Muerto Canyon or Sin Nombre virus. Infection is thought to be through inhalation of aerosolized secretions from the common deer mouse (*Peromyscus maniculatus*).

Since the early reports, cases have also been identified in many other states and Canada. The clinical manifestation begins with a prodrome of fever and generalized myalgia, followed in 4-5 days by respiratory symptoms of cough, dyspnea, and tachypnea. Respiratory symptoms progress very rapidly to a picture resembling that of adult respiratory distress syndrome. Diagnosis is possible with serologic studies (i.e., enzyme-linked immunosorbent assay for antivirus IgM and IgG antibodies). Treatment is mainly supportive. Ribavirin, a guanosine analog, has been used effectively for treating hemorrhagic fever with renal syndrome caused by other related Hantaviruses, but its efficacy in *Hantavirus* pulmonary syndrome is not yet established.

Ehrlichia Infections

Ehrlichia species are gram-negative intracellular bacteria that resemble *Rickettsia* species and preferentially infect lymphocytes, monocytes, and neutrophils. The species that cause human ehrlichiosis are *E. chaffeensis* and another as yet unnamed *Ehrlichia* species with affinity to granulocytes (hence, the disease is called human granulocytic ehrlichiosis). Human ehrlichiosis is a tick-borne disease. Tick exposure is reported by as many as 83% of patients.

The disease is seasonal and the peak incidence is from May through July. The vector is uncertain but includes the common dog tick, *Dermacentor variabilis*, and the lone star tick, *Amblyomma americanum*. The incubation period is approximately 7 days, followed by fever, chills, malaise, headache, and myalgia. Less than 50% of patients have a rash. Important laboratory features include leukopenia, thrombocytopenia, and increased levels of hepatic transaminases.

The severity of the disease is variable, but severe complications including death can occur. Diagnosis is serologic (indirect immunofluorescent assay); a polymerase chain reaction (PCR) method is being developed. Treatment is with tetracycline, 25 mg/kg per day in four equally divided doses, or doxycycline, 100 mg twice a day. Chloramphenicol is not effective.

Cat-Scratch Disease

Bartonella henselae (formerly *Rochalimaea henselae*) has been identified as the primary causative agent of cat-scratch disease (Table 14-1). The disease is characterized by a papule or pustule at the site of inoculation followed by tender enlargement of the regional lymph nodes draining an extremity. Low-grade fever and malaise may also be present. Exposure to domestic cats (especially kittens) is the main risk factor. About 10% of patients may have extranodal manifestations. Disseminated infection has been described in patients with acquired immunodeficiency syndrome (AIDS).

Diagnosis is based on the clinical picture and serologic evidence of antibodies to *B. henselae*. Biopsy finding of organisms positive for Warthin-Starry stain or culture can also be helpful. Treatment is indicated in patients with symptoms and bothersome adenopathy. The antibiotic of choice is ciprofloxacin, 500 mg twice daily for 10-14 days. Trimethoprim-sulfamethoxazole, rifampin, and gentamicin are alternative agents.

Invasive Group A Streptococcal Infection

Since the mid 1980s, there have been increasing reports of severe group A streptococcal infection, including necrotizing fasciitis, myonecrosis, toxic shock-like syndrome, and severe joint, lung, heart, and brain infections. Overall mortality has been 30% despite previous good health and appropriate treatment. Many patients have had amputation of extremities or major tissue loss.

The explanation for this resurgence is unclear, but some investigators have postulated that the presence of virulent strains (especially M1 and M3), virulence factors such as streptococcal pyrogenic exotoxin, and protease production, in association with a lack of immunity to these strains in the affected patients, may play a role. Treatment should consist of early intervention in the form of admission to an intensive care unit, management of shock, prompt initiation of antibiotics, and early and aggressive operation when indicated. The antibiotic of choice remains high-dose penicillin given intravenously.

SPECIFIC MICROORGANISMS

STREPTOCOCCI

These organisms may be divided into groups (Lancefield) by carbohydrates in cell wall: group A, B, C, etc. Group A may be further divided into types by differences in M proteins--types 1-49+, etc. The M protein is a virulence factor. All streptococci are susceptible to penicillin, except enterococci and penicillin-resistant strains of pneumococci.

- All streptococci are susceptible to penicillin, except enterococci and penicillin-resistant strains of pneumococci.

Group A β-Hemolytic: *Streptococcus pyogenes*

Infections

Impetigo is caused by group A β-hemolytic streptococci (color plate 14-1). If *Staphylococcus aureus* is present, it probably plays no role in the pathology or pathogenesis. Antibiotic therapy shortens the duration of infection and prevents suppurative complications but probably does not prevent acute glomerulonephritis.

- Antibiotic probably does not prevent acute glomerulonephritis.

Pharyngitis is a self-limited infection. Antibiotic therapy prevents acute rheumatic fever and shortens the duration of infec-

Table 14-1.--Features of Cat-Scratch Disease and Bacillary Angiomatosis

Variable	Cat-scratch disease	Bacillary angiomatosis
Predominant host	Immunocompetent	Immunosuppressed (AIDS)
Vector	Cats and dogs	Cats
Demonstrated cause	*Bartonella henselae* (majority)	*B. henselae*
	Afipia felis	*R. quintana*
Pathology	Lymphoid hyperplasia, granulomas, abscess formation	Ectatic capillaries surrounded by neutrophilic infiltrate
Clinical presentation	Papule or pustule at inoculation site, regional lymphadenopathy, fever, and malaise in 30%	Cutaneous nodules (do not confuse with Kaposi's sarcoma), visceral peliosis
Natural history	Self-limited (2-4 months)	Progressive
Diagnosis	Histopathology (Warthin-Starry stain), skin test, lymph node culture, serology, analysis of 16S rDNA	Histopathology, blood culture (lysis centrifugation, prolonged incubation), tissue culture, serology
Treatment	Efficacy unclear; rifampin, ciprofloxacin, gentamicin	Doxycycline, erythromycin

From Tompkins DC, Steigbigel RT: *Rochalimaea's* role in cat scratch disease and bacillary angiomatosis. Ann Intern Med 118:388-390, 1993. By permission of American College of Physicians.

tion if it is given within the first 24 hours of infection. Rapid diagnostic tests for streptococcal pharyngitis are specific but not sensitive (50%-70%). Common complications are otitis media and sinusitis.

● Common complications are otitis media and sinusitis.

Erysipelas is an acute inflammation of the skin with involvement of cutaneous lymphatic vessels; it usually occurs on the face. It has a sharp border; is raised, violaceous, and painful; and most often occurs in the elderly. It has recently been associated with toxic strep syndrome.

Cellulitis is an acute inflammation of the skin and subcutaneous tissue and occurs in tissue damaged by trauma, in operative wounds, and in tissue with poor venous and lymphatic drainage (postmastectomy cellulitis of the arm and cellulitis of the leg after saphenous vein harvest for coronary artery bypass grafting may recur). Tinea pedis may also serve as a portal of entry.

Group A streptococcal pneumonia is rare but can be extremely severe. It is frequently associated with preceding viral infections, including influenza, measles, and chronic lung disease. There has been a recent increase in group A streptococcal bacteremia in children and adults. Changes in virulence mechanism may be responsible.

Penicillin is the drug of choice for treatment of group A streptococcal infection. Cephalosporins (first-generation), erythromycin, and vancomycin are alternatives. There are no reports of penicillin resistance to date. There have been reports of an increased prevalence of erythromycin-resistant strains.

● There are no reports of penicillin resistance to date.

Toxins

Group A streptococci produce many toxins. Scarlet fever may develop in patients with no previous immunity to erythrogenic toxin. Production of hyaluronidase causes the rapidly advancing margins characteristic of cellulitis due to β-hemolytic streptococci. Exotoxin A is similar to the toxin that causes toxic shock syndrome in patients with *S. aureus* infection (toxic strep syndrome).

Nonsuppurative Complications

The nonsuppurative complications of group A streptococcal infection are acute rheumatic fever and acute glomerulonephritis. There has been a resurgence of acute rheumatic fever among children (urban and rural) and in military recruits. It occurs only after pharyngitis, never after skin infections. Recently, the diagnostic criteria for rheumatic fever were revised (Table 14-2). Treatment is with aspirin and steroids depending on clinical circumstances and the severity of symptoms and organ involvement.

● Resurgence of acute rheumatic fever among children (urban and rural) and in military recruits.

The approach to prophylaxis is controversial. One approach, if a murmur is present, is indefinite prophylaxis with penicillin G, preferably benzathine penicillin 1.2 million units monthly (alternative, oral penicillin V potassium 250 mg twice a day). If the patient is allergic to penicillin, alternatives are sulfonamides and erythromycin. If there is no murmur, prophylactic antibiotics are given until age 25. If there is no murmur, no attack within previous 5 years, and no carditis with previous attack, prophylaxis may be discontinued. Prophylactic antibiotics are used to prevent recurrent acute rheumatic fever, not for prevention of subacute bacterial endocarditis (SBE). SBE prophylaxis differs.

Acute glomerulonephritis may occur after both skin infections and pharyngitis, but it is more common after skin infections (Table 14-3).

● Prophylactic antibiotics are used to prevent recurrent acute rheumatic fever, not for prevention of subacute bacterial

Table 14-2.--Jones Criteria for Diagnosis of Initial Attack of Rheumatic Fever* (1992 Update)

Major manifestations
  Carditis
  Polyarthritis
  Chorea
  Erythema marginatum
  Subcutaneous nodules
Minor manifestations
  Clinical findings
    Arthralgia
    Fever
  Laboratory findings
    Elevated acute-phase reactants (erythrocyte sedimentation rate, C-reactive protein)
    Prolonged P-R interval
Supporting evidence of antecedent group A streptococcal infection
  Positive throat culture or rapid diagnostic test
  Elevated or rising streptococcal antibody titer

*If supported by evidence of recent group A streptococcal infection, two major, or one major and two minor, criteria are enough for diagnosis. Three exceptions in which Jones criteria do not need to be fulfilled: 1) recurrent rheumatic fever (single major or several minor criteria in patient with a reliable history of previous rheumatic fever if supporting evidence of recent group A streptococcal infection), 2) isolated chorea, and 3) indolent carditis.
From Special Writing Group of the Committee on Rheumatic Fever, Endocarditis, and Kawasaki Disease of the Council on Cardiovascular Disease in the Young of the American Heart Association: Guidelines for the diagnosis of rheumatic fever: Jones Criteria, 1992 update. JAMA 268:2069-2073, 1992. By permission of American Medical Association.

Table 14-3.--Differences Between Acute Glomerulonephritis and Acute Rheumatic Fever Caused by Group A Streptococcal Infection

| | After infection | | Recurrence of disease | Antibiotics prevent disease |
	Skin	Pharynx		
AGN	Yes	Yes (<skin)	Rare, if ever	?
ARF	No	Yes	Often	Yes

AGN, acute glomerulonephritis; ARF, acute rheumatic fever.

endocarditis.
- Acute glomerulonephritis may occur after both skin infections and pharyngitis.

Group B: *Streptococcus agalactiae*

This organism is an important cause of maternal and neonatal bacteremia and neonatal meningitis. It is part of normal flora of the female genital tract and gastrointestinal tract. It is more resistant to penicillin than group A streptococci, although penicillin is still the treatment of choice. Treatment of meningitis is with penicillin or ampicillin plus gentamicin.

Group C

Group C streptococci may be β-hemolytic and may cause pharyngitis; but unlike group A streptococci, they do not cause nonsuppurative complications. Bacteremia may be associated with the presence of malignancy and altered immune systems.

Group D Streptococci and Enterococci

Enterococci are no longer considered group D streptococci. The taxonomy differences are also reflected in the differences in susceptibility to penicillin between enterococci and group D streptococci (Table 14-4). Both can cause endocarditis. *Streptococcus bovis* endocarditis and bacteremia may be associated with carcinoma of the colon or other colonic disease. Consider SBE in anyone with a blood culture positive for group D streptococci or enterococci. SBE often occurs in elderly men (prostatism). The source is the genitourinary tract.

- *S. bovis* endocarditis and bacteremia may be associated with

Table 14-4.--Classification of Group D Streptococci and Enterococci

Group D streptococci	*Enterococcus* (note name change)
S. bovis	*E. faecalis* (80%-90%)
S. equinis (rare)	*E. faecium* (5%-10%)
Penicillin MIC	Penicillin MIC
≤0.1 µg/mL	≥1 µg/mL

MIC, minimal inhibitory concentration.

carcinoma of the colon or other colonic disease.

An increasing number of nosocomial bacteremias and urinary tract infections are due to enterococci. Sources are the genitourinary tract, intra-abdominal infection, and intravenous lines. Endocarditis rarely complicates nosocomial enterococcal bacteremia. Nosocomial-acquired strains are more likely to have unusual resistance patterns.

Treatment of *S. bovis* and *S. equinis* is with penicillin alone or penicillin plus streptomycin or gentamicin. If the patient is allergic to penicillin, a cephalosporin or vancomycin is used.

- Treatment of *S. bovis* and *S. equinis* is with penicillin alone or penicillin plus streptomycin or gentamicin.

In regard to the in vitro susceptibility of enterococci, they are only inhibited, not killed, by penicillin alone. They are resistant to all cephalosporins. Increasing numbers of enterococci are resistant to aminoglycosides (aminoglycoside-modifying enzymes), produce β-lactamase, or are resistant to glycopeptides (i.e., vancomycin, particularly among *Enterococcus faecium*) (plasmid-mediated alteration in enzyme that produces peptidoglycan). Nosocomial transmission of these resistant strains has occurred. It is imperative that in vitro susceptibility testing for these drugs be performed on enterococcal isolates causing serious infections.

- Enterococci are resistant to all cephalosporins.

For treatment of SBE, a combination of penicillin (or ampicillin) plus streptomycin or gentamicin must be used for isolates that do not produce β-lactamase and that do not have high-level aminoglycoside resistance. Short-course (2-week) therapy cannot be used for enterococcal endocarditis. If the patient is allergic to penicillin, use vancomycin plus streptomycin or gentamicin. Tobramycin and amikacin are not synergistic with either penicillin or vancomycin. High-level gentamicin resistance (>500 µg/mL) implies a lack of synergism. Susceptibilities to streptomycin should then be checked. Optimal regimens for isolates resistant to both gentamicin and streptomycin are unknown.

- For SBE, a combination of penicillin (or ampicillin) plus streptomycin or gentamicin must be used for isolates that do not produce β-lactamase.

Urinary tract infections and bacteremia without evidence of endocarditis can usually be treated with penicillin, ampicillin, or vancomycin alone as long as the strains are susceptible in vitro. Options for treatment of uncomplicated urinary tract infection in penicillin-allergic patients are ciprofloxacin, nitrofurantoin, or vancomycin, depending on clinical circumstances.

E. faecium may be more resistant to penicillin. In one study, 35% of *E. faecium* organisms were reported to be resistant. The most effective therapy is vancomycin plus gentamicin. *E. faecium* organisms are resistant to all aminoglycosides except streptomycin and gentamicin. Optimal regimens for vancomycin-resistant strains are unknown.

Group F and Group G

These organisms occasionally cause pharyngitis and bacteremia. They may be β-hemolytic and do not cause nonsuppurative complications. Group G bacteremias have been associated with the presence of malignancy and altered immune systems.

Streptococcus pneumoniae

Complications of pneumococcal pneumonia include empyema and pericarditis from direct extension of infection. Empyema occurs in <1% of patients and should be suspected when there is persistent fever despite appropriate antibiotic therapy. Pericarditis often causes precordial pain and a friction rub.

S. pneumoniae is the most common cause of bacterial meningitis in adults (color plate 14-2). Furthermore, suspect it in any patient with recurrent meningitis. If there is recurrent meningitis, always consider the patient to have a cerebrospinal fluid leak. These patients frequently give a history of previous head trauma. Therapy for pneumococcal meningitis is with high-dose cefotaxime or ceftriaxone *with or without* vancomycin until susceptibility test results are available. If the patient is allergic, vancomycin or chloramphenicol may be used.

- *S. pneumoniae* is the most common cause of bacterial meningitis in adults.
- Always consider patient to have cerebrospinal fluid leak if recurrent *S. pneumoniae* meningitis is present. These patients frequently give a history of previous head trauma.

S. pneumoniae is one of the most common causes of otitis media, especially in children. Spontaneous peritonitis is frequently caused by *S. pneumoniae*, especially in patients with nephrotic syndrome and in the pediatric age group. Endocarditis

is rare. Acute bacterial arthritis can also occur.

- Spontaneous peritonitis is frequently caused by *S. pneumoniae*, especially in patients with nephrotic syndrome and in the pediatric age group.

Certain patients are at high risk for infection with *S. pneumoniae*. After splenectomy, fulminant, usually fatal, pneumococcal bacteremia with disseminated intravascular coagulation and severe bleeding may develop. *S. pneumoniae* infections are more frequent and unusually severe in patients with sickle cell anemia. Patients with multiple myeloma, alcoholism, and hypogammaglobulinemia are also at increased risk.

S. pneumoniae is the leading cause of invasive bacterial respiratory disease in patients with human immunodeficiency virus (HIV) infection. They have a high incidence of pneumonia and bacteremic pneumococcal pneumonia. Diagnosis of pneumococcal bacteremia precedes diagnosis of HIV infection in 50%-80% of cases. Recurrent invasive disease occurs in 8%-25% of cases. Serotypes causing the invasive disease are similar to those causing invasive disease in normal hosts. Clinical presentation and treatment are similar to those in normal hosts. Secondary prophylaxis for recurrent episodes (penicillin) may be necessary. Prophylaxis for *Pneumocystis carinii* pneumonia with trimethoprim-sulfamethoxazole may provide effective primary or secondary prophylaxis.

- After splenectomy, fulminant, usually fatal, pneumococcal bacteremia with disseminated intravascular coagulation and severe bleeding may develop.
- *S. pneumoniae* infections are more frequent and unusually severe in patients with sickle cell anemia.
- Patients with multiple myeloma, alcoholism, and hypogammaglobulinemia are also at increased risk of infection.
- *S. pneumoniae* is the leading cause of invasive bacterial respiratory disease in patients with HIV.

Treatment is with penicillin G; if patients are allergic to penicillin, a cephalosporin, vancomycin, or erythromycin may be used. Do not use ciprofloxacin or other fluoroquinolones. From 0.2% to >2% of strains in the United States are highly resistant to penicillin (minimal inhibitory concentration >2 μg/mL). Vancomycin, cefotaxime, or ceftriaxone may be effective. The mechanism of resistance is thought to be alterations in the penicillin-binding proteins. Risk factors for development of penicillin-resistant pneumococci are previous β-lactam antibiotic use, nosocomial acquisition, and multiple previous hospitalizations.

- Do not use ciprofloxacin or other fluoroquinolones to treat pneumococcal disease.

The pneumococcal vaccine is polyvalent, containing capsular polysaccharide from the 23 serotypes that most commonly cause pneumococcal infection. It is used in adults with chronic lung or heart disease and immunosuppressed patients, especially after splenectomy and in patients with sickle cell disease and hereditary spherocytosis. It can be given simultaneously with influenza virus vaccine. Antibody levels may not be detectable for 5-6 years after vaccination in older adults, and therefore vaccination may have to be repeated.

STAPHYLOCOCCI

Staphylococcus aureus

Toxins

Preformed enterotoxins produced by S. aureus are a common cause of food poisoning in the United States. The toxin is heat stable; therefore, the toxin is not destroyed by cooking food. An exotoxin, exfoliatin is produced by S. aureus belonging to phage group II and produces "scalded skin syndrome," an erythematous rash that progresses to bullous lesions. It should be differentiated from toxic epidermal necrolysis (skin biopsy). It occurs most frequently in pediatric patients and is rare in adults. Therapy is with local skin care and antistaphylococcal antibiotics. Toxic shock syndrome is due to an exotoxin (TSST-1) usually produced by S. aureus.

- Preformed enterotoxins produced by S. aureus are not destroyed by cooking food.
- Toxic shock syndrome is due to an exotoxin (TSST-1) usually produced by S. aureus.

Clinical Syndromes

Superficial infections include folliculitis (infection of hair follicles without involvement of skin or subcutaneous tissues), furuncle (more extensive follicular infection, often involves subcutaneous tissues and occurs in areas of friction and poor personal hygiene), carbuncle (infection in thick inelastic tissues of the scalp or upper back), and impetigo (much less common than group A β-hemolytic streptococci). Treatment is moist heat to promote drainage. Personal hygiene also needs to be improved. Drainage occasionally is required, as are antistaphylococcal agents for severe infection.

S. aureus is the most common cause of acute hematogenous osteomyelitis in pediatric patients and is a common cause of chronic osteomyelitis in adults. It is the second most common cause of prosthetic joint infection, after coagulase-negative staphylococci.

- S. aureus is a common cause of chronic osteomyelitis in adults.
- It is the second most common cause of prosthetic joint

infection.

All cases of community-acquired S. aureus bacteremias must be treated for 4-6 weeks with parenteral antibiotics because of the potential for 1) metastatic abscesses and 2) infective endocarditis. If nosocomial S. aureus bacteremias have a removable focus (i.e., intravenous catheter), it should be removed and treatment given for 10-14 days. Staphylococcal pneumonia is an infrequent cause of community-acquired disease. It is more frequent after influenza. It is a common cause of nosocomial disease in intubated patients, along with hospital-acquired aerobic gram-negative rods. If S. aureus is isolated in cases of urinary tract infection, consider S. aureus bacteremia with seeding of the kidneys.

- All cases of community-acquired S. aureus bacteremias must be treated for 4-6 weeks with parenteral antibiotics.
- Staphylococcal pneumonia is an infrequent cause of community-acquired disease. It is more frequent after influenza.

Mechanisms of Resistance

Mechanisms of resistance for S. aureus include β-lactamase production for methicillin-susceptible, penicillin-resistant isolates and intrinsic chromosomal resistance that is not plasmid-mediated for methicillin-resistant isolates. This intrinsic resistance is related to a decrease in the affinity of β-lactam antibiotics for penicillin-binding proteins. Methicillin resistance is often associated with resistance to multiple agents including quinolones.

Treatment

If S. aureus is penicillin-susceptible (rare), penicillin G is preferred. Alternatives are cefazolin and vancomycin. If the isolate is methicillin-susceptible, nafcillin, oxacillin, cephalosporins (first-generation), vancomycin, and imipenem are effective.

MRSA Infections

Nosocomial infections caused by methicillin-resistant S. aureus (MRSA) are increasing in frequency and are associated with previous use of multiple antibiotics, intravenous drug abuse, burns, and other hospital-acquired infections. The drug of choice for treatment is vancomycin alone or in combination with gentamicin or rifampin. MRSA may also be susceptible to cotrimoxazole and ciprofloxacin or minocycline with or without rifampin. Emergence of resistance to fluoroquinolone agents is common.

- Nosocomial infections caused by MRSA are increasing in frequency and are associated with previous use of multiple antibiotics, intravenous drug abuse, burns, and other hospital-acquired infections.

MRSA Carrier State

This is a difficult problem in hospitals and long-term-care

facilities. The use of mupirocin ointment or other therapies (cotrimoxazole with or without rifampin) is successful for temporarily eradicating the nasal carrier state, but relapse is common.

Coagulase-Negative Staphylococci (*Staphylococcus epidermidis*)

Clinical Syndromes

S. epidermidis is a common cause of prosthetic valve endocarditis, osteomyelitis (usually after joint arthroplasty or other prosthetic implantations), and meningitis after neurosurgical procedures and is associated with wound infection. Treatment often requires removal of the foreign body and administration of appropriate antibiotics. Peritonitis can occur in patients on chronic ambulatory peritoneal dialysis. Bacteremia occurs in patients with infected intravascular devices.

Treatment

For treatment of serious coagulase-negative staphylococcal infection, in vitro susceptibility testing is mandatory. If methicillin resistance is present, the treatment of choice is vancomycin. For treatment of prosthetic valve endocarditis, the regimen should be vancomycin plus rifampin for 6 weeks and gentamicin for at least the first 2 weeks. Ciprofloxacin is also active against some strains, but when used alone emergence of resistance occurs rapidly. The combination of ciprofloxacin and rifampin seems promising.

- If methicillin resistance is present, the treatment of choice is vancomycin.

GRAM-NEGATIVE BACILLI

Escherichia coli Infections

E. coli is part of the normal flora of the gastrointestinal tract. Focal infection is due to ascending infection (urinary tract) or a break in a mucosal barrier (intra-abdominal infection). Bacteremia is often secondary to focal infection elsewhere.

Clinical syndromes associated with *E. coli* include urinary tract infection; it is the most common cause of uncomplicated urinary tract infections in women. Intra-abdominal infections are also associated with *E. coli* and are often a result of perforated appendix, diverticulitis, and cholangitis. These infections are often polymicrobial. *E. coli* is the most common cause of spontaneous bacterial peritonitis. Bacteremia is often a result of pyelonephritis, cholangitis, and intra-abdominal abscess. It can also occur spontaneously in patients with cirrhosis without a portal of entry. *E. coli* gastroenteritis and hemorrhagic colitis also occur.

- Bacteremia is most commonly a result of pyelonephritis, cholangitis, and intra-abdominal abscess.

Treatment is surgical drainage when appropriate and antibiotics chosen on the basis of in vitro sensitivity testing. *E. coli* is often susceptible to ampicillin, cephalosporins (including first-generation agents), trimethoprim-sulfamethoxazole, and aminoglycosides.

Proteus, Morganella, Providencia Infections

P. mirabilis is indole-negative and causes 75%-90% of *Proteus* infections. *P. vulgaris* is indole-positive and is a less common cause of infection. *M. morganii* and *P. rettgeri* also cause infection. They are all part of the normal fecal flora and can also be found in soil and water. Urinary tract infections with or without secondary bacteremia are the most common clinical manifestations. Urinary tract infections are often associated with an alkaline urine, which enhances production of ammonium-magnesium phosphate stones. Wound infections, sinusitis, corneal ulceration, and peritonitis are much less common clinical infections produced by these organisms.

P. mirabilis is sensitive to ampicillin. The others are not sensitive to ampicillin but are usually susceptible to gentamicin, ticarcillin, mezlocillin, third-generation cephalosporins, imipenem, and ciprofloxacin.

Klebsiella, Enterobacter, Serratia Infections

K. pneumoniae causes both community-acquired and nosocomial pneumonia. It is often associated with alcoholism, diabetes mellitus, and chronic obstructive pulmonary disease. Red currant jelly sputum is characteristic. Lung abscess and empyema are more frequent than with other community-acquired pneumonias. *Enterobacter* and *Serratia* are associated with nosocomial infection, including pneumonia and bacteremia.

- Lung abscess and empyema are more frequent than with other community-acquired pneumonias.

Klebsiella is often sensitive to cephalosporins (including first-generation agents), aminoglycosides, trimethoprim-sulfamethoxazole, imipenem, and ciprofloxacin. *Enterobacter* and *Serratia* are usually resistant to first-generation cephalosporins (sensitive to gentamicin and extended-spectrum penicillins, third-generation cephalosporins, imipenem, and ciprofloxacin). The drug of choice depends on results of in vitro sensitivity testing. Recent reports have suggested an increase in resistance to third-generation cephalosporins in certain strains of *Enterobacter*. Third-generation cephalosporins, despite in vitro data suggesting sensitivity, may not be the drug of choice for *Enterobacter* infections because of high rates of emergence of resistance. Quinolones or imipenem may be effective therapy in this setting.

- *Klebsiella* is often sensitive to cephalosporins.
- *Enterobacter* and *Serratia* are usually resistant to first-generation cephalosporins.

Pseudomonas Infections

P. aeruginosa

This organism predominantly causes nosocomial infection. Hospital water supplies are often a source of infection. *Pseudomonas*, together with *Staphylococcus aureus*, is the most frequent cause of infections complicating massive burns. It is a cause of folliculitis associated with hot tubs, osteomyelitis (particularly in injection drug users or in osteomyelitis complicating a nail puncture wound), and malignant otitis externa in patients with diabetes mellitus. Complicated urinary tract infections are often due to this organism. *P. aeruginosa* is a common cause of nosocomial pneumonia. Patients with cystic fibrosis have an especially high frequency of pulmonary infections with *Pseudomonas*. Meningitis caused by *Pseudomonas* can develop after neurosurgical procedures. Patients with neutropenia are also at particularly high risk of infection, especially bacteremia. In neutropenic patients with bacteremia due to *P. aeruginosa,* ecthyma gangrenosum may occur.

- *Pseudomonas*, together with *S. aureus*, is most frequent cause of infections complicating massive burns.
- It is a cause of malignant otitis externa in patients with diabetes mellitus.
- In neutropenic patients with bacteremia due to *P. aeruginosa,* ecthyma gangrenosum may occur.

Pseudomonas organisms are often resistant to many antibiotics. Extended-spectrum penicillins plus an aminoglycoside are synergistic against most *P. aeruginosa*. Ceftazidime plus an aminoglycoside may be the most effective combination for life-threatening infections. Aztreonam, imipenem, and ciprofloxacin are also active against most strains.

Stenotrophomonas (Xanthomonas) maltophilia

This organism causes nosocomial infections, pneumonia, and wound infections, most often in patients in intensive care units. It is associated with person-to-person transmission, especially from failure of adequate hand washing. Multiple drug resistance is common. It may be susceptible to trimethoprim-sulfamethoxazole, ticarcillin/clavulanate, and moxalactam. It is often resistant to aminoglycosides, imipenem, ceftazidime, and ciprofloxacin.

- *S. maltophilia* is associated with person-to-person transmission, especially from failure of adequate hand washing.

Salmonella typhi

S. typhi causes various clinical syndromes, including gastroenteritis, bacteremia with and without suppurative complications, a chronic asymptomatic carrier state, and typhoid fever.

In patients with typhoid fever, findings on physical examination include fever with relative bradycardia and rose spots (50%). The leukocyte count may be decreased. Blood cultures are usually positive within approximately 10 days of symptom onset, whereas stool cultures are positive after 10 days of symptoms. Bone marrow biopsy and culture may also reveal the diagnosis.

- In typhoid fever, findings on physical examination include fever with relative bradycardia and rose spots (50%).

The traditional therapy for typhoid fever has been chloramphenicol or ampicillin. Alternatives are cotrimoxazole, third-generation cephalosporins, and ciprofloxacin. There is increasing resistance to chloramphenicol and ampicillin. Once susceptibility results are obtained, appropriate directed therapy can be used.

- The traditional therapy for typhoid fever has been chloramphenicol or ampicillin.

Other Salmonella Infections

S. choleraesuis causes chronic bacteremia and mycotic aneurysms. *S. typhimurium* and *S. enteritidis* produce gastroenteritis and occasionally bacteremia. *Salmonella* urinary tract infections occur in patients from the Middle East who are infected with *Schistosoma haematobium*.

Haemophilus influenzae

The incidence of disease caused by *H. influenzae* has decreased significantly in children because of the institution of the *H. influenzae* vaccine. Adult cases represent approximately 25% of invasive *H. influenzae* disease. Approximately 50% are serotype B. Nontypable strains may be more common in pneumonia, tracheobronchitis, and upper respiratory tract infection. Bacteremic pneumonia makes up 70% of invasive disease in adults. Other infections include meningitis, obstetrical infections, epiglottitis, and primary bacteremia. Chronic lung disease, pregnancy, human immunodeficiency virus (HIV) infection, splenectomy, and malignancy are risk factors for invasive disease. β-Lactamase production is found in up to 40% of isolates recovered from adults with invasive disease. Overall mortality rate is 28%.

- Adult cases represent approximately 25% of invasive *H. influenzae* disease.
- Chronic lung disease, pregnancy, HIV infection, splenectomy, and malignancy are risk factors for invasive disease.
- β-Lactamase production is found in up to 40% of isolates recovered from adults with invasive disease.

Otitis media, sinusitis, conjunctivitis, and epiglottitis are common in pediatric patients. *H. influenzae* is a common cause of sinusitis in adults. Ampicillin resistance is related to production of β-lactamase. If a strain is β-lactamase negative, ampicillin can be used. *Haemophilus* infections that are β-lactamase positive or negative can be treated with cotrimoxazole, cefuroxime, third-generation cephalosporins, imipenem, ciprofloxacin, aztreonam, or a β-lactam-β-lactamase inhibitor combination.

- *H. influenzae* is a common cause of sinusitis in adults.
- Ampicillin resistance is related to production of β-lactamase.

If *H. influenzae* meningitis occurs in adults, consider hypogammaglobulinemia, asplenia, or cerebrospinal fluid leak. Treatment is based on results of susceptibility testing. Resistance to ampicillin is increasing. A third-generation cephalosporin is the drug of choice. Cefuroxime is not as effective. Alternative treatment is chloramphenicol plus ampicillin until susceptibility results are known. Prophylactic treatment with rifampin is recommended for all household contacts and children in day care centers.

For epiglottitis, do not use ampicillin as empiric therapy. Therapy is third-generation cephalosporin or ampicillin/sulbactam.

Endocarditis is caused by *H. parainfluenzae* and *H. aphrophilus*. It is often associated with large systemic emboli. Treatment is with ampicillin alone if the organism is susceptible or with third-generation cephalosporin for 3 weeks.

Most cases of pneumonia and tracheobronchitis are caused by nontypable β-lactamase negative strains of *Haemophilus*. Most are susceptible to ampicillin.

The vaccine is useful for prevention and should be given to all children. It may be useful in patients at increased risk of invasive disease, including patients with HIV.

Bordetella pertussis

This organism is the cause of whooping cough in children. It may cause severe lymphocytosis (>100,000 lymphocytes/mm^3). The number of reported cases is increasing. There were 27,826 cases in the United States from 1980-1989; 12% were in patients >15 years old. *B. pertussis* is the cause of prolonged bronchitis in older children and adults. Atypical symptoms are common. As many as 50 million adults are now susceptible to infection as a result of waning immunity.

- *B. pertussis* may cause severe lymphocytosis (>100,000 lymphocytes/mm^3).
- It is the cause of prolonged bronchitis in older children and adults.

Diagnosis is made from nasopharyngeal culture. Direct fluorescence antibody testing is relatively insensitive. Treatment is with erythromycin and supportive care. Isolates resistant to erythromycin are becoming increasingly common.

Brucellosis

Brucellosis occurs most frequently in persons exposed to livestock or persons who drink unpasteurized milk. Most cases occur in four states (Texas, California, Virginia, Florida). It often causes a chronic granulomatous disease, may cause caseating granulomas, and can affect any tissue. It may be a cause of "sterile" pyuria. Chronic brucellosis may cause chronic fever of undetermined origin. Diagnosis is difficult and is one of exclusion. Calcifications in the spleen may be an indication of the presence of infection (although histoplasmosis also causes splenic calcifications). Serology testing, blood cultures, and bone marrow cultures are helpful in making the diagnosis. Treatment is with doxycycline and streptomycin or rifampin. Cotrimoxazole is sometimes also useful.

- Brucellosis is a chronic granulomatous disease and may cause fever of unknown origin.

Legionnaires' Disease

This disease is caused by fastidious gram-negative bacillus. A significant amount of sporadic community-acquired legionellosis may be due to contaminated potable water. Most nosocomial legionellosis is also due to contaminated water supplies. Clinical features include weakness, malaise, fever, dry cough progressing to slightly productive cough, diarrhea (a very important part of symptom complex and often precedes other symptoms), pleuritic chest pain, relative bradycardia, diffuse rales bilaterally, and patchy infiltrates on chest radiography, usually bilaterally.

Characteristic laboratory features are decreased sodium and phosphorus values, increased leukocyte level, and abnormal liver function tests. The diagnosis must be suspected clinically. The clinical picture of unexplained pneumonitis often accompanied by diarrhea and the other clinical findings described above in association with hyponatremia and decreased serum phosphorus level is sufficient to suspect legionnaires' disease and to begin treatment pending results of serologic and other tests. However, pneumococcal pneumonia can cause identical symptoms. In suspected cases, do not wait for serologic results before initiating treatment. A fourfold increase or decrease in titer requires 2-6 weeks. A single titer ≥1:256 is suggestive of active infection but not diagnostic. The best means of diagnosis is by culture and a fluorescent antibody test of sputum, bronchoalveolar lavage fluid, or an open lung biopsy specimen. Urine antigen detection may be more sensitive but is not yet widely available.

Treatment includes erythromycin with or without rifampin orally or intravenously for 2-3 weeks. If the patient is allergic to erythromycin, doxycycline or ciprofloxacin can be used.

- In legionnaires' disease, diarrhea is an important part of the symptom complex and often precedes other symptoms.
- Lab features are decreased sodium and phosphorus values, increased leukocyte level, and abnormal liver function tests.
- The best means of diagnosis is by culture and a fluorescent antibody test of sputum, bronchoalveolar lavage fluid, or open lung biopsy specimen.

Legionella micdadei

This gram-negative bacillus causes infection in hospitalized immunosuppressed patients receiving high-dose corticosteroid therapy. Diagnosis is based on stains and culture of open lung biopsy tissue or bronchoalveolar lavage fluid. Serologic studies may be helpful retrospectively. The organism is moderately resistant to erythromycin, but it is still the drug of choice. Cotrimoxazole plus rifampin may also be effective.

Tularemia

Francisella tularensis is spread by the bite of an arthropod or direct contact with tissues of infected animals (rabbits, muskrat, squirrels, beaver). Airborne transmission is also possible. If ulceroglandular fever develops, an ulcer or eschar is usually present at the site of inoculation. Pneumonia can also occur. Treatment is with streptomycin.

- *F. tularensis* is spread by arthropod bite and direct contact with tissues of infected animals.

Plague: *Yersinia pestis*

From 1950-1991, there were 336 cases in the United States; >50% of these occurred after 1980. It is enzootic in the southwestern United States; New Mexico has 56% of cases, and 29% of cases are among American Indians. Rats and fleas are vectors. Clinical presentations include 1) lymphadenopathy with septicemia--the most common form, and 2) the pneumonic form (high case fatality rate). Treatment is with streptomycin or tetracycline.

Pasteurella multocida

A cat bite is the most common mode of acquisition. It causes rapidly progressing cellulitis, bacteremia, and, rarely, infective endocarditis. It is sensitive to penicillins and cephalosporins.

Capnocytophaga (Formerly DF-2)

These gram-negative bacilli have difficulty growing in routine media. They are found in oral flora in domestic animals and humans. They cause bacteremia in immunosuppressed patients, patients who have had splenectomy, and alcoholics (may be seen on Gram stain of buffy coat). Fulminant sepsis

and disseminated intravascular coagulation are also associated with infection. Dog and cat bites are associated with 50% of cases. Treatment includes penicillin or a cephalosporin.

- *Capnocytophaga* organisms cause bacteremia in immunosuppressed patients, patients who have had splenectomy, and alcoholics.
- Dog and cat bites are associated with 50% of cases.

GRAM-POSITIVE BACILLI

Anthrax

Bacillus anthracis is an aerobic gram-positive bacillus. Human cases are due to contact with infected animals, bites of contaminated flies, consumption of contaminated meat (rare), and exposure to contaminated animal hides (e.g., imported drums from Haiti, goat hair [yarn]).

- *B. anthracis* due to exposure to contaminated animal hides.

Cutaneous manifestations occur in 95% of cases. The most common presentation is a large, black, chronic skin ulcer, which is frequently a nontender "malignant pustule." Pneumonia ("wool sorter's pneumonia"), bacteremia, meningitis, and gastrointestinal disease are much less common. Treatment is with penicillin G. Alternatives are erythromycin, tetracycline, and chloramphenicol.

- Cutaneous manifestations occur in 95% of cases.

Listeria monocytogenes

This is a gram-positive, small, motile rod. It causes infection in immunosuppressed (T-cell) patients, neonates, and pregnant women. Epidemics have been associated with consumption of contaminated milk and ice cream and undercooked hot dogs. Sporadic listeriosis is associated with contaminated food in approximately 34% of cases. Diarrhea is not a feature of epidemic listeriosis.

- *L. monocytogenes* causes infection in immunosuppressed (T-cell) patients, neonates, and pregnant women.
- Epidemics have been associated with consumption of contaminated milk and ice cream and undercooked hot dogs.
- Diarrhea is not a feature of epidemic listeriosis.

Meningitis and bacteremia are common clinical manifestations in adults.

The approach to treatment is penicillin or ampicillin with or without gentamicin. Cephalosporins are *not* effective. Alternatives are cotrimoxazole and chloramphenicol. Treatment duration is 2-4 weeks.

Corynebacterium diphtheriae

Diphtheria

Clinically, this is usually a focal infection of the respiratory tract (pharynx in 60%-70% of cases, larynx, nasal passages, or tracheobronchial tree). A tightly adherent gray pseudomembrane is the hallmark of the disease, but disease can occur without pseudomembrane formation. Manifestations depend on the extent of involvement of the upper airway and the presence or absence of systemic complications due to toxin. A local complication is respiratory tract obstruction. Toxin-mediated complications include myocarditis (10%-25%), which causes congestive heart failure and dysrhythmias, and polyneuritis (bulbar dysfunction followed by peripheral neuropathy). Respiratory muscles may be paralyzed.

- In diphtheria, toxin-mediated complications include myocarditis (10%-25%), which causes congestive heart failure and dysrhythmias, and polyneuritis.
- Respiratory muscles may be paralyzed.

Diagnosis is definitively established by culture with Löffler's medium. Rapid diagnosis can sometimes be made by methylene blue stain or fluorescent antibody staining of pharyngeal swab specimens. Patients need to be isolated immediately. Antitoxin should be used. Although there is no evidence that antimicrobial agents alter the course of disease, they prevent transmission to susceptible hosts. Erythromycin and penicillin G are effective. Close contacts should be evaluated and treated with erythromycin or penicillin G if culture results are positive. The diphtheria-tetanus toxoid should be given.

- Close contacts should be evaluated and treated with erythromycin or penicillin G if culture results are positive.

Cutaneous Diphtheria

This is reported in indigent patients and alcoholics. It occurs most often in patients with preexisting dermatologic disease and most often in the lower extremities. Patients can have punched-out lesions with membrane, but they may be indistinguishable from other infected ulcers. Toxin-mediated complications (i.e., myocarditis, neuropathy) are uncommon. Diagnosis is established with methylene blue staining and culture in Löffler's medium.

Erythromycin or penicillin is used for therapy. Antitoxin should also be administered, and an immunization series with diphtheria-tetanus toxoid should be given.

- Cutaneous diphtheria is reported in indigent patients and alcoholics.

Erysipelothrix rhusiopathiae

This nonmotile gram-positive rod is a saprophyte. Infection occurs with traumatic inoculation of organism as a result of direct cutaneous contact from animals to humans. Most human cases are related to occupational exposure and occur in fish handlers, slaughterhouse workers, veterinarians, and butchers. Localized cellulitis around a purple-red papule occurs at the site of inoculation, often a finger or upper extremity in a person who has occupational exposure to these products (veterinarians, fish handlers). This is the most common presentation (erysipeloid). If untreated, dissemination with subsequent bacteremia, endocarditis, and septic arthritis can occur. Penicillin G is the drug of choice. Erythromycin is an alternative. *E. rhusiopathiae* is resistant to vancomycin.

- *E. rhusiopathiae* infection occurs with traumatic inoculation of organism after a person comes in contact with dead animals and fish.

Bacillus Species

These are increasingly recognized as a cause of bacteremia in patients with indwelling catheters or prosthetic devices and in injection drug users. Other syndromes include ocular infections (posttraumatic endophthalmitis) and gastroenteritis. Vancomycin or clindamycin with or without gentamicin is used for therapy.

Rhodococcus equi (Corynebacterium equi)

This organism causes necrotizing pneumonia in immunocompromised hosts, such as those with acquired immunodeficiency syndrome (AIDS) or those taking corticosteroids. Mortality rate is 30%. Clinical features include fever, nonproductive cough, and cavity or nodular infiltrates on chest radiography (concomitant brain abscesses have been reported). Bronchoscopy or open lung biopsy is usually required for diagnosis. Treatment is with vancomycin, erythromycin, aminoglycosides, or chloramphenicol.

GRAM-NEGATIVE COCCI

Moraxella catarrhalis (Branhamella catarrhalis) is a respiratory tract pathogen in immunosuppressed, hospitalized patients and those with chronic obstructive pulmonary disease. It causes otitis media, sinusitis, meningitis, bacteremia, and endocarditis in immunosuppressed patients. β-Lactamase production is prevalent. Trimethoprim-sulfamethoxazole, ciprofloxacin, and ampicillin-clavulanate are useful for therapy.

- *M. catarrhalis* causes otitis media, sinusitis, meningitis, bacteremia, and endocarditis in immunosuppressed patients.

ANAEROBIC BACTERIA

Bacteroides Infections

Bacteroides species reside in the oral cavity (*B. melaninogenicus* group) and are also normal colonic flora (*B. fragilis* group, now renamed *Prevotella melaninogenicus*). They often are part of a polymicrobial infection. Any pus described as "foul-smelling" is often caused by anaerobic infection. Clinical syndromes commonly associated with *Bacteroides* species include intra-abdominal infection. Abscesses, for example, are associated with disruption of colonic mucosa resulting from appendicitis, cancer, diverticulitis, and other disorders. *Bacteroides* species are also associated with pelvic infections, particularly in females (e.g., septic abortion, tubo-ovarian abscess, endometritis). These are frequently polymicrobial infections. Bacteremia is usually associated with focal infection elsewhere (e.g., intra-abdominal abscess) or with gastrointestinal surgery. *B. fragilis* is the most common isolate. Osteomyelitis usually results from a contiguous source and is often polymicrobial (e.g., diabetic foot ulcer or osteomyelitis of the maxilla or mandible after dental infection). Pleuropulmonary infections include aspiration pneumonia and lung abscess. *P. melaninogenicus* organisms are major pathogens, as are other oral anaerobes. Skin and soft tissue infections caused by anaerobes include diabetic soft tissue infections of the feet, bite wounds, and gangrene.

- *Bacteroides* species are also associated with intra-abdominal and pelvic infections.
- Bacteremia is usually associated with *B. fragilis*.
- Pleuropulmonary infections include aspiration pneumonia and lung abscess.

Many strains of *Bacteroides* produce penicillinase and thus are resistant to penicillin. Because of increased resistance to penicillin of mouth anaerobes, penicillin is no longer the drug of choice for treatment of putrid lung abscess. In one study, clindamycin was more effective than penicillin or metronidazole for curing lung abscess.

B. fragilis produces penicillinase and is usually resistant to penicillin. Metronidazole, clindamycin (increasing resistance), ampicillin/sulbactam, chloramphenicol, and imipenem are active. Some cephalosporins (cefoxitin) are active in vitro against some *B. fragilis* organisms but should not be considered the drug of choice. Third-generation cephalosporins have little activity against *B. fragilis*.

Peptococcus

These anaerobic streptococci are often involved in polymicrobial infection. They are part of the normal flora of the oral cavity and colon. They are associated with anaerobic pleuropulmonary infection and intra-abdominal abscess. *Peptostreptococcus* can be a part of the polymicrobial flora of anaerobic cellulitis.

Peptococcus is exquisitely sensitive to penicillin G. In patients allergic to penicillin, the alternatives are clindamycin, chloramphenicol, vancomycin, and cephalosporins. The organism is often resistant to metronidazole.

- *Peptococcus* is often resistant to metronidazole.

Tetanus: *Clostridium tetani*

This is a strictly anaerobic gram-positive rod that produces neurotoxin (tetanospasmin). The neurotoxin produced by organisms in contaminated wounds is responsible for the clinical manifestations of disease. Most patients now are women >50 years old (not immunized). Men are usually immunized because of military service and repeated exposure to trauma.

- Most patients with tetanus now are women >50 years old (not immunized).

In generalized tetanus, the first muscles involved are controlled by cranial nerves (trismus, lockjaw, risus sardonicus). Eye muscles (cranial nerves III, IV) are rarely involved. Other muscles are soon involved (generalized rigidity, spasms, opisthotonos). Sympathetic overactivity is common (labile hypertension, hyperpyrexia, arrhythmias). In wound tetanus, manifestations are restricted to muscles near the wound. Diagnosis is based on clinical findings.

- Diagnosis of tetanus is based on clinical findings.

Treatment includes supportive care, proper wound management, and administration of antiserum (human tetanus immune globulin). Hypersensitivity reactions to tetanus immune globulin are very rare. Penicillin G should be administered to eradicate vegetative organisms in the wound. Metronidazole is an alternative agent. Immunization after recovery should also be provided.

- Penicillin G should be administered to eradicate vegetative organisms in the wound.

Clostridium botulinum

This anaerobic gram-positive rod produces a heat-labile neurotoxin that inhibits acetylcholine release from cholinergic terminals at the motor end plate. Major modes of acquisition in adults include ingestion of contaminated food (home canned products and improperly prepared or handled commercial foods) and wound botulism (contaminated traumatic wounds, injection drug users).

- Neurotoxin of *C. botulinum* inhibits acetylcholine release from cholinergic terminals at the motor end plate.

Clinical manifestations can be mild or severe. The diagnosis is considered in patients with unexplained diplopia; fixed, dilated pupils; dry mouth; and descending flaccid paralysis with normal sensation. Patients are usually alert and oriented and have intact deep tendon reflexes. Fever is rare.

● Diagnosis of *C. botulinum* infection is considered in patients with unexplained diplopia; fixed, dilated pupils; dry mouth; and descending flaccid paralysis with normal sensation.

For diagnosis, other compatible clinical syndromes need to be ruled out--myasthenia gravis and atypical Guillain-Barré (ascending paralysis, sensory abnormalities). Electromyography may be helpful. One can also check the suspected contaminated food source for toxin.

Treatment is primarily supportive. Equine antitoxin is available, and its use is now recommended by most experts. In food-borne cases, purging the gut with cathartics, enemas, and emetics to remove unabsorbed toxin may also be of value. Antibiotic therapy is not generally recommended.

Other Clostridial Infections

C. perfringens may cause a food-associated illness. *C. difficile* causes antibiotic-associated diarrhea. Among patients with bacteremia caused by *C. septicum* who have no apparent portal of entry, many have occult bowel carcinoma, especially colon or other malignancies. Clostridial bacteremia often is a transient bacteremia unrelated to a typical clinical syndrome (no identifiable genitourinary or gastrointestinal source). These isolates may not require specific therapy. Clostridial bacteremia with an identifiable source or associated with sepsis syndrome does require therapy. *C. perfringens* is the most common isolate in either case. Penicillin G is the drug of choice.

● *C. perfringens* may cause a food-associated illness.
● *C. difficile* causes antibiotic-associated diarrhea.
● In patients with *C. septicum* bacteremia, occult bowel carcinoma should be suspected.

MYCOBACTERIAL DISEASES

Mycobacterium tuberculosis

Epidemiology

The number of cases of infection with this organism increased in the United States from 1985 through 1992 from 9.3 per 100,000 persons to 10.5 (increase of 13%), and there was an estimated 52,100 excess cases during this time. The increase is largely due to an increase in cases among persons with human immunodeficiency virus (HIV) and other high-risk groups. The incidence of disease due to drug-resistant strains is also increasing. These strains often are resistant to multiple drugs (i.e., multiple drug-resistant tuberculosis, MDR-TB), including isoniazid (INH), rifampin, and other drugs. In a recent national survey, 14.4% of strains were resistant to one drug and 3.3% were resistant to both INH and rifampin. In the past several years, there have been multiple reports of nosocomial transmission of MDR-TB, resulting in more than 50 deaths among health care workers and a purified protein derivative (PPD) conversion rate of 10%-30%.

● In cases of *M. tuberculosis*, 14.4% of strains were resistant to one drug and 3.3% were resistant to both INH and rifampin.

These outbreaks have been related to delay in diagnosis, failure to sterilize secretions because of drug resistance or patient noncompliance, and ineffective isolation practices.

All patients suspected of having tuberculosis should be placed in respiratory isolation when they are hospitalized. These patients include those suspected of having skin lesions due to tuberculosis, because this was recently reported to be a cause of nosocomial transmission of disease.

Transmission is by droplet infection. Infectious droplets are 1-5 μm in diameter. Droplets remain suspended in room atmosphere for 30 minutes-2 hours.

● Transmission is by droplet infection.

Clinical Disease

Most clinically apparent pulmonary and extrapulmonary *M. tuberculosis* infections in adults are due to reactivation, not reinfection. Common sites of reactivation (high Po_2 favors reactivation) are apices of lung ($Po_2 = 120$ mm Hg), vertebra ($Po_2 = 100$ mm Hg), and kidney ($Po_2 = 100$ mm Hg). Tuberculosis should be suspected in young persons with an idiopathic pleural effusion. Diagnosis is made by thoracentesis with culture of pleural fluid and pleural biopsy with special stains and culture. Extrapulmonary manifestations are protean. Common sites include spine, kidneys, large joints, and meninges.

● Most pulmonary and extrapulmonary *M. tuberculosis* infections in adults are due to reactivation.
● Tuberculosis should be suspected in young persons with idiopathic pleural effusion.

Screening

An intermediate-strength PPD test should be performed in patients at high risk of infection with *M. tuberculosis*. These groups include those with HIV infection, the foreign born, close contacts (household) of persons known to have or suspected of having tuberculosis, medically underserved, low-income populations (including high-risk minority populations–blacks, Hispanics, Native Americans), the homeless, alcoholics and injection drug users, residents of institutions (e.g., nursing homes, prisons), and persons with medical conditions that predispose to infection with tuberculosis (Table 14-5).

Prevention

INH prophylaxis reduces the incidence of disease significantly. Lack of compliance is a major source of failure. Treatment is with INH 300 mg/day for 1 year (6 months minimum) or 15 mg/kg twice a week under direct supervision. Optimal prophylaxis for exposure to INH-resistant strain or exposure to MDR-TB is unknown. An outline for preventive therapy with positive PPD results is given in Table 14-6.

Table 14-5.--Medical Conditions That Predispose Patients to *Mycobacterium tuberculosis* Infection

Silicosis	Immunosuppression (T-cell)
Gastrectomy	Hematologic malignancy
Jejunoileal bypass	Other malignancies
Weight 10% or more below ideal body weight	Person with chest radiograph compatible with old tuberculosis
Chronic renal failure	
Diabetes mellitus	

- INH prophylaxis significantly reduces incidence of disease.

Treatment (Table 14-7)

General principles:

- INH and rifampin should be a part of all regimens, unless there are contraindications or the organism is resistant.
- Consider directly observed therapy in all patients.
- For extrapulmonary tuberculosis and tuberculosis in HIV-infected patients, use the same regimens as for pulmonary disease.
- Manage children similar to adults with appropriate adjustment of drug doses.
- For compliant patients with susceptible organisms, a 6-month regimen consisting of INH, rifampin, and pyrazinamide given for 2 months followed by INH and rifampin for an additional 4 months is recommended. For alternative regimens, see Table 14-7.
- Start at least three drugs until drug susceptibility results are known, and include either ethambutol or streptomycin as the fourth drug if INH resistance is suspected or the prevalence of INH resistance in the area is >4%.
- Treatment of MDR-TB should be individualized based on in vitro susceptibility testing, and the duration of therapy is extended to 18 to 24 months or longer.

The initial cure rate in a recent study of MDR-TB in persons without acquired immunodeficiency syndrome (AIDS) (three consecutive sputum cultures with negative results) was 65%.

Table 14-6.--Criteria for Determining Need for Preventive Therapy for Persons With Positive Tuberculin Reactions by Category and Age Group

Category	Age	
	<35 yr	≥35 yr
With risk factor*	Treat at all ages if PPD ≥10 mm (if PPD >5 mm in HIV positive, recent contact, chest radiographic evidence of old not active TB)	Treat at all ages if PPD ≥10 mm (if PPD >5 mm in HIV positive, recent contact, chest radiographic evidence of old not active TB)
No risk factor (high incidence group)†	Treat if PPD ≥10 mm	No treatment
No risk factor (low incidence group)	Treat if PPD ≥15 mm‡	No treatment

*1) Persons with HIV infection or with multiple HIV risk factors, 2) intravenous drug users, 3) recent contact with infected person, 4) recent PPD converters, 5) persons with abnormal chest radiographic finding likely to represent old tuberculosis, 6) persons with certain medical conditions (see Table 14-5).

†1) Foreign-born persons, 2) medically underserved, low-income populations, 3) residents of long-term-care facilities.

‡Controversial; some investigators use cutoff of 10 mm. Depends on relative prevalence of cross-reactivity with other mycobacterial organisms in the population.

PPD, purified protein derivative; TB, tuberculosis.

From Centers for Disease Control: Screening for tuberculosis and tuberculous infection in high-risk populations, and The use of preventive therapy for tuberculous infection in the United States. MMWR 39 (no. RR-8):1-12, 1990.

Table 14-7.--Treatment Options for Tuberculosis Infections*

Option 1	Option 2	Option 3
INH, RIF, and PZA daily for 8 weeks, followed by INH + RIF daily or 2-3 times/week for 16 weeks†	INH, RIF, PZA, and STM or EMB daily for 2 weeks, followed by twice weekly administration of same drugs for 6 weeks, then followed by twice weekly administration of INH and RIF for 16 weeks	INH, RIF, PZA, and EMB or STM three times weekly for 6 months

*Based on the joint statement of the American Thoracic Society and the Centers for Disease Control and Prevention (MMWR 42[no. RR-7]:1-8, 1993).
†All twice and thrice weekly regimens should be monitored by directly observed therapy for the duration of treatment.
INH, isoniazid; RIF, rifampin; PZA, pyrazinamide; STM, streptomycin; EMB, ethambutol.

Among these initial responders, 14% had relapse, most within 2 years. Relapse and treatment failure were associated with a 46% mortality rate. In many of the MDR-TB outbreaks (70%-80% HIV-infected persons), the mortality rate has been 70%-80%. Patients in whom treatment is unsuccessful but who survive pose a major public health problem and must be isolated.

Antituberculosis Drugs: Toxicities

Isoniazid
Peripheral neuritis can be prevented with simultaneous use of pyridoxine. Hepatotoxicity is also common and occurs in 1%-2% of patients. In patients taking INH, the approach for following them for possible hepatotoxicity is controversial. It is more likely to occur in older patients. Slow acetylators are more likely to have hepatotoxicity. Most patients will have transient increase in aspartate aminotransferase value.

- With isoniazid, peripheral neuritis can be prevented with simultaneous use of pyridoxine.
- Hepatotoxicity is common.
- Slow acetylators are more likely to have hepatotoxicity.

Risk of hepatotoxicity is 0.3% in patients 20-34 years old, 1.2% in those 35-49 years, 2.3% in those 50-64 years, and 4% in those older than 64 years.

Ethambutol
Toxicity is rare with this agent. If optic neuritis develops, red-green color vision may be lost first.

Rifampin
Toxic effects include neutropenia, thrombocytopenia, and hepatotoxicity. Hepatotoxicity may be identical to that caused by INH. Rifampin is also a hepatic enzyme inducer and thus has interactions with warfarin and birth control pills, among other medications. Fever with flu-like syndrome is also a common toxic manifestation of rifampin. Body fluids are turned orange with administration of rifampin.

Pyrazinamide
Hepatotoxicity is similar to that with INH. Hyperuricemia may also occur.

Mycobacterial Diseases Other Than Tuberculosis (Atypical Mycobacteria)
Mycobacterium marinum causes swimming pool granuloma and is common in people who have aquariums. Infection occurs while cleaning aquariums. It presents with a chronic, indurated nodule on the finger or hand. Treatment is excision of the nodule. Rifampin plus ethambutol, doxycycline, or trimethoprim-sulfamethoxazole may be effective.

- *M. marinum* causes swimming pool granuloma.

Mycobacterium kansasii is indistinguishable from *M. tuberculosis* clinically; it is more resistant to antituberculosis drugs than is *M. tuberculosis*. Standard regimen includes INH, rifampin, and ethambutol. Treatment is for 12-24 months.

- *M. kansasii* is indistinguishable from *M. tuberculosis* clinically.

Mycobacterium avium-intracellulare is an important cause of infection in patients with AIDS. Treatment is usually difficult because the organism is resistant to the usual antituberculosis agents. Usually 3- to 4-drug regimens are used. Rifampin, ethambutol, clarithromycin, clofazimine, ciprofloxacin, and amikacin are the most commonly used agents. Prophylaxis with rifabutin may prevent infection in patients with AIDS.

- *M. avium-intracellulare* is an important cause of infection

in patients with AIDS.
- Usually 3- to 4-drug regimens are used.

M. avium-intracellulare has also been reported in patients without AIDS. Most patients have chronic lung disease. There seem to be four characteristic chest radiographic appearances: multiple discrete nodules (71% of patients), bronchiectasis, upper lobe infiltrates, and diffuse infiltrates.

Rapid-growing mycobacteria include *Mycobacterium fortuitum* and *Mycobacterium chelonei*. They are associated with subcutaneous abscesses, osteomyelitis, and nosocomial infection (sternal osteomyelitis after cardiac surgery, intramuscular injection). Treatment often requires incision and drainage. They are resistant to antituberculosis drugs. Initial therapy is cefoxitin plus amikacin. Other antimicrobials are used according to results of in vitro susceptibility testing. Clarithromycin is also useful.

SPIROCHETES

Leptospirosis

Person-to-person transmission does not occur. Humans acquire disease from contact with urine from infected animals (rats, dogs). It is a biphasic disease. The *leptospiremic phase* is characterized by abrupt-onset headache (98%), fever, chills, conjunctivitis, severe muscle aching, gastrointestinal symptoms (50%), changes in sensorium (25%), rash (7%), and hypotension. This phase lasts 3-7 days. Improvement in symptoms coincides with disappearance of *Leptospira* organisms from blood and cerebrospinal fluid. The *second phase* (immune stage) occurs after a relatively asymptomatic period of 1-3 days, when fever and earlier symptoms recur. Meningeal symptoms often develop during this period. The second phase is characterized by the appearance of IgM antibodies. Most patients recover after 1-3 days. However, in serious cases, hepatic dysfunction and renal failure may develop. Death in patients with leptospirosis usually occurs in the second phase as a result of hepatic and renal failure. Myocarditis may occur during the second phase.

- In leptospirosis, person-to-person transmission does not occur.
- Humans acquire disease from contact with urine from infected animals (rats, dogs).
- Death usually occurs in the second phase as a result of hepatic and renal failure.

Gastrointestinal complaints, pneumonitis, and aseptic meningitis are common components of leptospirosis and are frequently overlooked. Diagnosis is made with cultures of blood and, rarely, cerebrospinal fluid in the first 7-10 days of infection. Urine cultures become positive after the second week of

illness. Serologic testing is not helpful until the second phase of disease; it must demonstrate a fourfold increase in titer for the diagnosis to be established. Treatment is with penicillin G. Penicillin is effective *only* if given within the first 1-5 days from onset of symptoms; otherwise, antibiotics are of no help.

- Gastrointestinal complaints, pneumonitis, and aseptic meningitis are common in leptospirosis.

Lyme Disease

Epidemiology

Borrelia burgdorferi is the etiologic agent. It is the most common vector-borne (*Ixodes* ticks) disease reported in the United States. It occurs in summer and fall and is reported in most states. It is most common in coastal New England, the mid-Atlantic states, Oregon, Northern California, and the Upper Midwest.

- *B. burgdorferi* is the etiologic agent of Lyme disease.
- It occurs in summer and fall.

Clinical Syndromes

Stage 1 (early) occurs 3-32 days after the tick bite. It presents with a flu-like illness and erythema migrans (60%). Adenopathy and meningismus may also be present. The rash usually enlarges and resolves over 3-4 weeks.

- *Stage 1* presents with a flu-like illness and erythema migrans.

Stage 2 occurs weeks to months after stage 1. In 10%-15% of cases, neurologic abnormalities develop (facial nerve palsy, lymphocytic meningitis, encephalitis, chorea, myelitis, radiculitis, peripheral neuropathy). Carditis (reversible atrioventricular block) occurs in 10% of patients. Dilated cardiomyopathy has been reported, and conjunctivitis and iritis also occur.

- During stage 2, 10%-15% of cases have neurologic abnormalities.
- Carditis occurs in 10% of patients.

Stage 3 occurs months to years after initial infection. Monoarticular or oligoarticular arthritis occurs in 50% of patients who do not receive effective therapy. It becomes chronic in 10%-20%. Chronic arthritis is related to HLA-DR2 and HLA-DR4. Other manifestations are acrodermatitis chronica atrophicans, progressive, chronic encephalitis, and dementia (diagnosed by the presence of locally produced antibodies against *B. burgdorferi* in the spinal fluid or detection of borrelial DNA by polymerase chain reaction); 30%-40% of patients will have arthritis. Most will have positive serum antibodies. Magnetic resonance imaging may show demyelination.

- In stage 3, monoarticular or oligoarticular arthritis occurs in 50% of patients.

Diagnosis

Results of enzyme-linked immunosorbent assay are positive after the first 2-6 weeks of illness. Response may be diminished by antimicrobial therapy early in the course. Tests are not standardized. False-positive results occur with infectious mononucleosis, rheumatoid arthritis, systemic lupus erythematosus, echovirus infection, and other spirochetal disease. Western blot test is an adjunct in diagnosis when antibody response is equivocal or when false-positive result is suspected. It is particularly useful in first few months of illness.

Treatment

For stage 1 (early) Lyme disease, agents used are doxycycline (100 mg twice a day for 10-21 days), amoxicillin (500 mg three times a day for 10-21 days), or cefuroxime axetil (500 mg twice a day for 10-21 days). Erythromycin is less effective than doxycycline or amoxicillin. Amoxicillin is used for children and pregnant women.

In Lyme carditis, the outcome is usually favorable. If first-degree atrioventricular block is present or P-R interval is >0.30 second, ceftriaxone, 2 g a day for 14-21 days, or penicillin G, 20 million units a day for 14-21 days, is recommended.

- In Lyme carditis, the outcome is usually favorable.

The outcome in patients with facial palsy is usually favorable; in one study, 105 of 122 patients had complete recovery. Corticosteroids have no role. If only facial nerve palsy is present (no symptoms of meningitis, radiculoneuritis), use oral therapy with doxycycline or amoxicillin. The treatment applied if other neurologic manifestations are present is described below.

- The outcome in patients with facial palsy is usually favorable.

If meningitis is present, ceftriaxone, 2 g a day for 14-21 days, or penicillin G, 20 million units a day for 14-21 days, should be given. Radiculoneuritis and peripheral neuropathy may have a greater tendency for chronicity and often occur with meningitis. Treatment is the same as that for Lyme-associated meningitis. The regimens for encephalopathy and encephalomyelitis are identical to those for meningitis.

- Radiculoneuritis and peripheral neuropathy may have a greater tendency for chronicity and often occur with meningitis.

Optimal regimens for Lyme arthritis (oral vs. intravenous) are not established. Intra-articular corticosteroids may cause treatment failures. Joint rest and aspiration of reaccumulated joint fluid are often needed. Response to antibiotics may be delayed. If no neurologic disease is present, doxycycline is given (100 mg orally twice a day for 30 days). An alternative regimen is amoxicillin and probenecid (500 mg each four times a day for 30 days) or ceftriaxone (2 g per day intravenously for 14 days).

Prevention

Because of the risk of vertical transmission, all pregnant women with active Lyme disease should be treated. Recent cost-benefit analysis suggested that if probability of infection was ≥3.6% after a tick bite, empiric therapy with oral doxycycline was warranted; if probability of infection was ≤1.0%, treatment was not recommended. However, a subsequent placebo-controlled trial showed no difference in the incidence of late manifestations of Lyme disease in treated (amoxicillin) or untreated patients. Furthermore, the risk of late manifestations after a recognized deer tick bite was estimated to be less than 1% in untreated patients. Currently, routine empiric therapy after a tick bite is not recommended. Appropriate use of repellents and protective clothing are recommended.

- All pregnant women with active Lyme disease should be treated aggressively.
- Routine empiric therapy after a tick bite is not recommended.

ACTINOMYCOSIS

This disorder is caused by *Actinomyces israelii*, an anaerobic, gram-positive, branching, filamentous organism. *A. israelii* probably causes infection in only humans and is the only known species to cause human infection. The most frequent preceding event is dental extraction. Infections are associated with any condition that creates an anaerobic environment (e.g., trauma with tissue necrosis, pus). The pathologic characteristic is formation of "sulfur granules," which are clumps of filaments. Lesions often contain pus. Infection is not characterized by granuloma formation.

- In actinomycosis, most frequent preceding event is dental extraction.
- Pathologic characteristic is "sulfur granules" (clumps of filaments).

Manifestations of the disease include "lumpy jaw" caused by a paramandibular infection with a chronic draining sinus, most often after dental extraction. It takes weeks to develop. Pulmonary disease develops from *A. israelii* aspirated from the mouth into an area of lung with decreased oxygenation (e.g., atelectasis, infection). Chronic suppurative pneumonitis may develop with cavitation, empyema, and, finally, a draining sinus through the chest wall. It may perforate into the esophagus, pericardium, ribs, and vertebrae. There may be spread into the bloodstream (e.g., brain), in which case the prognosis is very poor. Gastrointestinal effects probably result from *A. israelii* being swallowed, and infection occurs through small defects in bowel mucosa. The most common site is the ileocecal area. Appendicitis may be a predisposing factor. Cutaneous fistula (e.g., anorectal or anovaginal) may develop.

● Manifestations include "lumpy jaw" caused by a paramandibular infection with a chronic draining sinus, most often after dental extraction.

Unusual forms of infection include brain abscess, which results from bacteremia (often mixed infection). Bone infection most often involves the mandible or vertebrae. Vertebral infection has a characteristic sieve-like appearance on lateral radiographs because it attacks bodies of vertebrae and not intervertebral spaces; slow progression allows bone to be formed as fast as it is destroyed. Therefore, vertebral collapse is rare; this is an important differentiating characteristic from tuberculosis, malignancy, and other infection. Infection of female pelvic organs may simulate chronic pelvic inflammatory disease and include chronic draining sinuses. It is related to use of intrauterine devices.

● Unusual forms of infection include brain abscess, which results from bacteremia.

Diagnosis involves suspicion of the organism. It must be differentiated from *Nocardia* (which is a gram-positive, filamentous, branching organism that is *aerobic* and partially acid-fast). Anaerobic culture is necessary. The organism has special growth requirements, and *Actinomyces* culture must be specifically requested because the organism may not grow on routine anaerobic cultures.

● Anaerobic culture is necessary for diagnosis.

The prognosis is usually good if the infection is recognized and treated with a combined surgical and medical approach. Brain abscess or hematogenous spread is associated with a poor prognosis.

Therapy is with penicillin for long periods and surgical management. Treatment may be needed for ≥1 year. If patient is allergic to penicillin, tetracycline or erythromycin is used.

NOCARDIOSIS

Nocardia is an aerobic, gram-positive, filamentous, branching organism that is weakly acid-fast. *N. asteroides* is the cause of most human infections in the United States (color plate 14-3). *N. brasiliensis* and *N. madurae* cause mycetomas. There is no proof of human-to-human or animal-to-human

transmission of *N. asteroides*. Infections are most often opportunistic, occurring in immunosuppressed patients, but they can occur in nonimmunosuppressed patients also.

● In nocardiosis, there is no proof of human-to-human or animal-to-human transmission.

● Infections are most often opportunistic, occurring in immunosuppressed patients.

The respiratory tract is probably the portal of entry. Chronic pneumonitis and lung abscess are the most common findings. Bacteremia may occur. In patients with chronic pneumonia who have neurologic symptoms or signs, *Nocardia* brain abscess should be considered. Any organ may be infected.

● In patients with chronic pneumonia who have neurologic symptoms, *Nocardia* brain abscess should be considered.

Manifestations are as described in the preceding paragraph. Findings depend on the organ involved, but almost all patients have pneumonia; other organs are involved if there is hematogenous spread (±25% of patients). The infection is diagnosed at autopsy in ±40% of cases. The diagnosis depends on a suspicion of the infection and on culture. Cultures of sputum are not very sensitive. Bronchoscopically obtained specimens or open lung biopsy with stains of tissue and culture of pus may be needed to confirm the diagnosis. The disease must be differentiated from other chronic pneumonias (i.e., bacterial, actinomycosis, tuberculosis, fungal infections).

The prognosis is poor in immunosuppressed patients and very poor in those with brain abscess. If the patient has no underlying disease, prognosis is usually good if there is no hematogenous spread.

Therapy involves drainage and cotrimoxazole (probably drug of choice); imipenem is also effective.

● Nocardiosis is diagnosed at autopsy in ±40% of cases.

FUNGAL INFECTIONS

Coccidioidomycosis

Coccidioides immitis is dimorphic; in tissue it is a spherule, and in culture it is mycelial (filamentous). It forms arthrospores that are highly infectious to laboratory personnel. It is endemic in the southwestern United States, especially the San Joaquin Valley of California and central Arizona. Currently, a major epidemic is under way in California. Arthrospores are inhaled. Dissemination is most likely to occur in males (especially Filipino and black) and in pregnant females. Nonpregnant white females seem to be more resistant than white males.

- *C. immitis* is endemic in the southwestern United States.
- Dissemination is most likely to occur in males (especially Filipino and black) and in pregnant females.

Primary infection is pneumonitis. Hilar adenopathy is common; pleural effusion occurs in 12% of cases and cavities in ±5% (typically thin-walled). Solid coin lesions may form. If the infection disseminates, it can affect any organ system. The disease rarely, if ever, reactivates after years (unlike tuberculosis). Caseous necrosis often occurs; on silver stain, spherules can be seen.

- In coccidioidomycosis, hilar adenopathy is common; pleural effusion occurs in 12% of cases and cavities in ±5% (typically thin-walled).

Pulmonary disease involves dry cough, fever, and pleural effusion. Erythema nodosum may occur and, if present, is usually a sign of active delayed hypersensitivity and an indication infection will not be disseminated. Erythema nodosum is more common in females and is often associated with arthralgias, especially of the knees and ankles. Disseminated disease (1% of cases) is extrapulmonary, and every organ system can be involved. Affected sites are meninges (most severe manifestation), skin (most common), joints (arthritis), and bones (osteomyelitis).

- Erythema nodosum may occur in coccidioidomycosis.

Diagnosis is based on suspicion of the disease, positive sputum culture, or biopsy with silver stains. On fungal serology (complement fixation), a titer ≥1:4 indicates the infection. Skin test is of epidemiologic value only.

Fluconazole and amphotericin B are used for therapy (*Coccidioides* is one of the more resistant fungi to amphotericin). The acute pulmonary form is usually self-limited and usually requires only symptomatic therapy. It may require therapy if patient is pregnant, has human immunodeficiency virus (HIV) infection, has received a transplant, or has worsening infection without therapy. Ketoconazole is effective for non-life-threatening, nonmeningeal disease in a dosage of 400-800 mg per day for 6 months. If meningitis develops, prognosis is poor and therapy is with fluconazole or intrathecal amphotericin B. The Ommaya reservoir is best means of administering amphotericin. Chronic long-term suppressive therapy is necessary, and there is a high frequency of adhesive arachnoiditis. Fluconazole is effective for long-term suppressive therapy of meningitis.

Histoplasmosis

Histoplasma capsulatum is dimorphic; in tissue it is a small (3 mm in diameter) yeast, and in culture it has a mycelial form.

It is especially prevalent in the Ohio and Mississippi River valleys. Outbreaks have been associated with cleaning chicken coops and bird nesting areas, where exposure to bird droppings occurs. It is acquired by inhalation of spores; granulomas form which may caseate. Histoplasmosis is only rarely an "opportunistic" infection. It usually occurs in previously normal persons but causes fulminant disease in patients with acquired immunodeficiency syndrome (AIDS).

- Histoplasmosis has been associated with cleaning chicken coops and bird nesting areas, where exposure to bird droppings occurs.
- It usually occurs in previously normal persons.

In endemic areas, the *primary (acute)* form may be indistinguishable from influenza or other upper respiratory tract infections. Multiple small, calcified lesions are found on chest radiography with healing. The *progressive (disseminated)* form is rare. It is most likely to occur in infants and elderly men. Manifestations may resemble those of lymphoma: e.g., weight loss, fever of undetermined origin, anemia, increased erythrocyte sedimentation rate, and splenomegaly. Gastrointestinal ulcerations, especially in oral cavity, are common. The infection may also cause endocarditis and meningitis. Addison's disease can occur and may be insidious; adrenal function must be checked periodically. The infection occurs in patients with AIDS; the severe form may present as septic shock. *Chronic cavity disease* is indistinguishable from tuberculosis, usually bilateral upper lung involvement.

- *Primary (acute)* form may be indistinguishable from influenza or other upper respiratory tract infections.
- *Chronic cavity disease* is indistinguishable from tuberculosis, usually bilateral upper lung involvement.

Serologic testing is of limited help and plays little role in diagnosis. Biopsy, silver staining, and cultures are best means of diagnosis. Bone marrow stains and cultures and fungal blood cultures are frequently helpful. Biopsy specimens of mouth lesions can be helpful. Detection of *Histoplasma* antigen in urine or serum is promising as a diagnostic test but is not yet widely available.

The mild, acute forms are usually self-limited and do not require therapy. Amphotericin B in a total dosage of 25-35 mg/kg is the drug of choice for all severe, life-threatening cases. Itraconazole is the drug of choice in most nonmeningeal, non-life-threatening cases and has replaced ketoconazole. Dosage is 200-400 mg per day for 6-12 months. Patients with AIDS need chronic maintenance therapy.

Blastomycosis

Blastomyces dermatitidis is dimorphic. In tissue, the yeast forms are thick-walled and have broad-based buds; they are larger than *Histoplasma* organisms (±10 µm diameter) (color plate 14-4). In culture, a mycelial form is found. The means of transmission is unknown. It may be related to contact with soil. The probable entry is through inhalation. Lung infection may be inapparent and may disseminate hematogenously to bone, skin, or prostate. Granulomas occur, but calcification is less frequent than with histoplasmosis or tuberculosis.

Blastomycosis affects lung, skin, bone, and internal genitalia (prostate, epididymis, testis). The pulmonary form has no characteristic findings: pleural effusion is rare, hilar adenopathy develops occasionally, and cavitation is infrequent. It often mimics carcinoma of the lung. The most common clinical form of blastomycosis is cutaneous. Lesions, especially on the face, are suggestive of blastomycosis. They are characteristically painless and nonpruritic and have a sharp, spreading border. Chronic, crusty lesions are noted. In bone, vertebral involvement is most common. Infection of internal genitalia manifests as painful swelling of the testes and dysuria.

- Blastomycosis affects lungs, skin, bone, and internal genitalia (prostate, epididymis, testis).
- Most common clinical form of blastomycosis is cutaneous.
- In bone, vertebral involvement is most common.

Diagnosis is based on the clinical picture, biopsy, stains, and cultures. Serology is of minimal help, and skin testing is of no help. Thick-walled, broad-based budding yeast is found on stains.

- In blastomycosis, thick-walled, broad-based budding yeast is found on stains.

Therapy involves amphotericin B (organism is usually susceptible; total dosage is 20-25 mg/kg, and this is used for all severe infections). Itraconazole is also effective (dosage, 200-400 mg per day for 6 months) and is the drug of choice for all non-life-threatening disease in immunocompetent persons; it has replaced ketoconazole.

Aspergillosis

There are many species of *Aspergillus*. *A. fumigatus* is one of the most common pathogens in humans. The pulmonary form of the infection is opportunistic in immunosuppressed hosts and is probably acquired by respiratory route. On tissue section, the organisms have large, branching, septate hyphae (phycomycetes are nonseptate) at 45° angle (color plate 14-5). They may invade blood vessels, producing a striking thrombotic angiitis similar to phycomycosis. Metastatic foci may cause suppurative abscess formation.

- *Aspergillus* organisms may invade blood vessels, producing a striking thrombotic angiitis.

A form of aspergillosis is invasive bronchopulmonary disease, which should be considered in any immunosuppressed (neutropenic) host with acute progressive pneumonitis. It is especially common in patients with acute myelomonocytic leukemia, Hodgkin's disease, and chronic lymphocytic leukemia and in patients who have had organ transplantation. Chronic necrotizing aspergillosis is different from invasive disease in granulocytopenic patients. It occurs in patients with chronic lung disease. The chronic progressive infiltrates of this condition often require invasive techniques for diagnosis. Fungus ball may develop in preexisting lung bullae of immunocompetent or immunosuppressed patients (e.g., ankylosing spondylitis, previous tuberculosis). A fungus ball must be surgically excised because it can erode a pulmonary blood vessel and cause hemorrhage. Disseminated disease can involve any organ. Patients usually die quickly. Kidney and brain are most often involved. In otitis externa, *Aspergillus* is part of usual flora and is opportunistic. Allergic bronchopulmonary aspergillosis presents as asthma with colonization of the respiratory tract. It is characterized by migratory pulmonary infiltrates; thick, brown, tenacious mucous plugs in the sputum; eosinophilia; and positive serologic results. Endophthalmitis usually occurs after operation or trauma and often causes blindness. In patients with intact immune defenses, *Aspergillus* is a frequent colonizer of the respiratory tract; therefore, its isolation from sputum culture cannot be relied on as an indication of invasive disease. Cutaneous manifestations of aspergillosis can develop with use of Hickman catheter. Localized black necrotic lesion develops at site of catheter insertion. The catheter is removed and amphotericin B is administered.

- A form of aspergillosis is invasive bronchopulmonary disease, which should be considered in any immunosuppressed (neutropenic) host.
- Chronic necrotizing aspergillosis occurs in patients with chronic lung disease.
- Cutaneous manifestations of aspergillosis can develop with use of Hickman catheter.

Prolonged granulocytopenia is a major risk factor for invasive pulmonary aspergillosis. Serologic and skin tests are of no help for diagnosing invasive disease. In patients with granulocytopenia, a positive sputum culture should raise suspicion for the disease, but histologic examination of tissue is necessary to confirm the diagnosis.

- Prolonged granulocytopenia is the major risk factor for invasive pulmonary aspergillosis.

Therapy is with amphotericin B. A combination of flucytosine or rifampin with amphotericin B for severe disease has been suggested but has not yet been proved to be better than amphotericin B alone. The role of itraconazole is still unclear. For fungus ball, excision is standard approach. For allergic bronchopulmonary aspergillosis, amphotericin B is usually of no help; corticosteroids are used in severe cases.

Cryptococcosis

Cryptococcus neoformans is the only species of *Cryptococcus* that is pathogenic for humans. It is a yeast in both tissue and culture, is 4-7 μm in diameter, has thin-walled buds, and a capsule (color plate 14-6). It is an opportunistic pathogen. Most infections occur in immunosuppressed hosts, especially patients with Hodgkin's disease, hematologic malignancy, organ transplantation, and AIDS. Occasional patients are apparently normal before infections, but they may have some preexisting subtle T-cell dysfunction. Pigeon droppings may play a role in transmission. The respiratory tract is the probable portal of entry. The infection does not incite much inflammatory reaction, there is little necrosis, and calcification is rare.

- *C. neoformans* is an opportunistic pathogen.
- Pigeon droppings may play a role in transmission.

Meningitis is the most common form of infection. It may have an insidious onset, involve cranial nerves, and cause blindness with involvement of the optic nerve. Transient maculopapular rash or subcutaneous masses occur in ±10% of cases.

- Meningitis is the most common form of *C. neoformans* infection.

Isolation of *Cryptococcus* in sputum or bronchial washings in immunosuppressed hosts has a high incidence of dissemination. Patients should have cerebrospinal fluid examination and cultures on specimens from other sites, and they should receive antifungal therapy. Normal hosts with isolation of *Cryptococcus* from sputum or bronchial washings usually do not require antifungal therapy. Cryptococcal infection in bone presents as punched-out lesions with little surrounding inflammatory reaction.

The diagnosis is based on demonstration of the organism in tissue or cultures. The cryptococcal antigen test is the most helpful of all fungal serologic tests. It measures capsular *antigen*; all other fungal serologic tests measure antibody. If antigen is present in cerebrospinal fluid, consider infection present until proved otherwise. If *C. neoformans* is isolated from any source (e.g., sputum, urine, blood) in a susceptible patient, *always* examine cerebrospinal fluid to detect meningitis.

- If *C. neoformans* is isolated from any source, always examine cerebrospinal fluid to detect meningitis.

Amphotericin B and flucytosine are the preferred therapeutic agents. One successful form of therapy with fewer side effects is flucytosine, 100-150 mg/kg per day, plus amphotericin B, 0.3 mg/kg per day, administered for 6 weeks. However, relapse rates are high in compromised hosts.

Patients with AIDS respond poorly to treatment and usually have persistence of infection despite treatment. (Patients with abnormal mental status, hyponatremia, and *Cryptococcus* found on culture of an extraneural site are at increased risk.) Flucytosine has increased hematologic toxicity in patients with AIDS, particularly when levels are not monitored. In a recent study comparing fluconazole (200 mg/day) with amphotericin B for 10 weeks, fluconazole was as effective as amphotericin B (effective is defined as clinical improvement or resolution of symptoms with negative culture results for cerebrospinal fluid), but mortality in the first 2 weeks of therapy was higher with fluconazole (15% vs. 8%). We still recommend initial therapy with amphotericin B with or without flucytosine until culture results of cerebrospinal fluid are negative or there is a need to switch to fluconazole for other reasons. For chronic maintenance, fluconazole is more effective than weekly administration of amphotericin B.

Candidiasis

There are many species of *Candida*. In tissue, it can be either yeast form or mycelial. In culture, it is yeast and mycelial. It is opportunistic and can infect virtually any site in the body.

Cutaneous infection manifests as diaper rash and intertrigo; in the disseminated form, maculopapular rash and subcutaneous nodules may be present.

Fungemia develops from infected intravenous catheters, one of the most common portals of entry, especially in the immunosuppressed host who is receiving broad-spectrum antimicrobials. It represents 5%-10% of nosocomial bloodstream infections. Risk factors include previous antibacterial therapy, cytotoxic or corticosteroid therapy, and parenteral nutrition. Suspect fungemia in a patient with these risk factors who suddenly becomes febrile while receiving antibacterials. Mouth, gastrointestinal tract, or rectum-anus may be the portal of entry. *C. tropicalis* and *C. parapsilosis* most often are found in immunocompromised patients. Endocarditis occurs most often in intravenous drug users. It is often caused by species other than *C. albicans*. Blood culture results are usually positive. Endophthalmitis may occur as long as 1 month after initial fungemia. Therefore, it is necessary to do periodic funduscopic examinations after fungemia occurs.

- Fungemia develops from infected intravenous catheters, especially in the immunosuppressed host.

include previous antibacterial therapy, cyto-
...ticosteroid therapy, and parenteral nutrition.
...itis occurs most often in intravenous drug users.
- En......ditis is often caused by species other than *C.
albicans.*

Metastatic abscesses can occur in any site after an episode
of *Candida* fungemia. Cystitis and nephritis can occur in
patients with chronic indwelling urinary catheters, urinary tract
infection, and immunosuppression. Diagnosis is based on positive culture results, symptoms, and absence of other diagnosis. *Candida* pneumonitis is very rare; *Candida* in respiratory secretions almost always is due to asymptomatic colonization. Osteomyelitis and joint infections are rare; they are complications in immunosuppressed patients or after fungemia.
Hepatosplenic candidiasis typically occurs in neutropenic
patients as the bone marrow recovers and is associated with
typical "bull's-eye lesions" on ultrasonography or computed
tomography. Diagnosis is made from biopsy of the liver.
Treatment is at least 2 g of amphotericin. Fluconazole or lipo-
somal amphotericin B may also be effective. Esophagitis is
common in immunosuppressed patients and those with AIDS.
Diagnosis is made with endoscopy. It must be distinguished
from cytomegalovirus and herpes simplex virus infection.

- Hepatosplenic candidiasis typically occurs in neutropenic
  patients as the bone marrow recovers.
- Esophagitis is common in immunosuppressed patients and
  those with AIDS.

Therapy is described on pages 525 and 526. Need for treating patients with fungemia should be individualized. For central venous catheter-related candidemias, catheter removal followed by amphotericin B (250-500 mg) is indicated. High-
dose fluconazole is equally effective in nonneutropenic patients.
Fluconazole is effective for oral or esophageal candidiasis in
patients with AIDS. Be aware that *C. kruzel* and *C. glabrata*
are often resistant to fluconazole.

Sporotrichosis

Sporothrix schenckii in tissue is a round, cigar-shaped yeast.
In culture, it is mycelial. It is transmitted through accidental
inoculation into skin ("rose gardener's disease") and rarely
through inhalation. It manifests as a suppurative and granulomatous reaction; occasional giant cells are found.
Cutaneous infection has characteristic, almost diagnostic,
crusty lesions ascending the lymphatics in the extremities.
Pulmonary infection is possibly acquired through inhalation. It
may cause chronic pneumonitis, cavities, and empyema. Joint
spaces are rarely involved. Chronic meningitis may also occur.

- In sporotrichosis, crusty, cutaneous lesions ascend the lymphatics in the extremities.

- Pulmonary infection may cause chronic pneumonitis, cavities, and empyema.

The diagnosis is based on suspicion of the infection and on
biopsy and culture results. Serologic testing is occasionally
helpful.
For the cutaneous form, itraconazole or supersaturated solution of potassium iodine is used. For disseminated disease
(pulmonary, joint), amphotericin B is used; itraconazole is an
alternative agent.

Mucor (*Rhizopus*, **Zygomycetes**)

Rhinocerebral infections are the most common. They occur
in patients with diabetes who have ketoacidosis and in immunosuppressed patients, especially those with neutropenia. Infection
has been reported in patients on hemodialysis who are receiving deferoxamine therapy.

- In mucormycosis, rhinocerebral infections occur in patients
  with diabetes who have ketoacidosis and in immunosuppressed patients.

The diagnosis is based on findings of typical black necrotic lesions around the eye or on the soft and hard palates. It is
confirmed by biopsy of skin, mucous membrane, or lung. It
is especially important to consider this diagnosis in patients
who are neutropenic. Organism is nonseptate hyphae.
Aspergillus is *septate* and branches at 45° angle.

- Diagnosis is based on findings of typical black necrotic
  lesions around the eye or on the soft and hard palates in the
  appropriate host.

Treatment usually includes amphotericin B and surgical
debridement. Most patients respond very poorly. Only hope
for recovery is if the neutrophil value increases.

RICKETTSIAL INFECTIONS

Weil-Felix reactions are no longer considered diagnostic
for rickettsial infections. All rickettsial infections have insect
vector except Q fever (respiratory spread), and all are associated with a rash except Q fever and ehrlichiosis. The rash of
Rocky Mountain spotted fever (RMSF) may be indistinguishable from that of meningococcal meningitis. RMSF rash
begins on extremities and moves centrally. Typhus fever
(murine or endemic typhus) rash begins centrally and moves
toward the extremities. RMSF is most common in the mid-
Atlantic states and Oklahoma, not the Rocky Mountain states.
Pathophysiology of all rickettsial infections includes vasculitis and disseminated intravascular coagulation. Rickettsial
pox is a common rickettsial disease in the United States. It is
usually unrecognized. It is an urban disease and is the only

rickettsial disease characterized by vesicular rash. Eschar is present at the site of bite on the extremities in 95% of patients, but one needs to look for it. Rickettsial pox is spread by bite of the mouse mite.

- All rickettsial infections have insect vector except Q fever.
- All are associated with a rash except Q fever and ehrlichiosis.
- RMSF rash begins on the extremities and moves centrally.
- RMSF is most common in the mid-Atlantic states and Oklahoma, not the Rocky Mountain states.

Among persons with Q fever, ±100% have pneumonitis, 15% have hepatitis (granulomatous), and 1% have endocarditis. It is associated with exposure to animal products, especially infected placenta. It can occur in meat packing workers. A mini-epidemic occurred in a group exposed to parturient cats.

- Among persons with Q fever, ±100% have pneumonitis, 15% have hepatitis.
- Can occur in meat packing workers.

The diagnosis is determined with serologic testing. Treatment is with tetracycline or chloramphenicol.

Rickettsia conorii infection has been termed Mediterranean spotted fever, boutonneuse fever, Marseilles fever, and South African tick bite fever. The *R. conorii* organism is common in the Far East, Israel, eastern and southern Africa, and the southern Mediterranean. The vector is the tick *Rhipicephalus sanguineus*. The infection occurs in summer months. It has an incubation period of 1 week. It resembles RMSF, except the rash begins on the trunk rather than the extremities. A "tache noire" lesion (cigarette burn) should be sought at the site of tick bite. Severe disease occurs in patients with underlying illness. The diagnosis is based on immunofluorescent demonstration of organisms in skin biopsy or serologic tests. Treatment is with tetracycline, chloramphenicol, or ciprofloxacin.

MYCOPLASMA PNEUMONIAE

This is one of the smallest microorganisms capable of extracellular replication. It lacks a cell wall; therefore, cell-wall-active antibiotics such as penicillin are not effective treatment. It is spread by droplet inhalation. It occurs in young, previously healthy persons and presents with sudden onset of headache, dry cough, and fever. Results of physical examination are unremarkable with the possible exception of bullous myringitis. Chest radiography usually shows bilateral patchy pneumonitis. The chest radiographic findings are out of proportion to the physical findings. Pleural effusion is present in 15%-20% of cases. Neurologic complications include Guillain-Barré syndrome, cerebellar peripheral neuropathy, aseptic meningitis, and mononeuritis multiplex. Hemolytic anemia may occur late in the illness as a result of circulating cold hemagglutinins. The central nervous system manifestations and hemolytic anemia suggest *Mycoplasma*.

- *M. pneumoniae* is spread by droplet inhalation.
- Chest radiography usually shows bilateral patchy pneumonitis.
- Pleural effusion is present in 15%-20% of cases.
- Neurologic complications include Guillain-Barré syndrome, cerebellar peripheral neuropathy, aseptic meningitis, and mononeuritis multiplex.

The diagnosis is established by specific complement fixation test. Cold agglutinins are nonspecific for *Mycoplasma* infections. Erythromycin is the drug of choice for therapy. Tetracycline is an alternative. In a young person with fever, dry cough, patchy pneumonitis, and few physical findings, the initial drug of choice is erythromycin, *not* penicillin. Immunity is transient; therefore, reinfection may occur. Clinical relapse of pneumonia occurs in up to 10% of cases of *Mycoplasma* pneumonia.

CHLAMYDIA PNEUMONIAE (TWAR AGENT)

This is a new agent, distinct from *C. trachomatis* and *C. psittaci*. In young adults, it causes 10% of cases of pneumonia and 5% of cases of bronchitis. It has been a cause of community outbreaks, and nosocomial transmission has occurred; 50% of adults are seropositive. The mode of transmission is unknown (not birds). Clinical manifestations are usually mild; the symptoms resemble those caused by *M. pneumoniae*. Pharyngitis may occur 1-3 weeks before onset of pulmonary symptoms, and cough may last for weeks. The diagnosis is based on serologic tests (not routinely available). Treatment is with tetracycline or erythromycin.

- In young adults, *C. pneumoniae* causes 10% of cases of pneumonia and 5% of cases of bronchitis.
- It has been a cause of community outbreaks, and nosocomial transmission has occurred.

VIRAL DISEASES

Influenza

Type A is the most common. Epidemics occur every 2-4 years; pandemics occur every 20-30 years. Epidemics and pandemics are a result of major antigenic shift in the influenza virus. About 80%-90% of deaths due to influenza occur in persons ≥65 years old. Complications include 1) primary influenza pneumonia (interstitial desquamative pneumonia) and 2) secondary bacterial infection, which is usually caused by *Streptococcus pneumoniae, Haemophilus,* or *Staphylococcus aureus.* A typical history is as follows: an elderly patient, often with chronic obstructive lung disease, develops influenza, which may or may not improve; then, the severity of symptoms increases substantially, with high fever, marked leukocytosis, and often respiratory failure. This is a medical emergency and must be treated as *S. aureus* pneumonia (although pneumococcal pneumonia is more common in this setting). One needs to be alert to the possibility of toxic shock syndrome related to *S. aureus* infection.

- About 80%-90% of deaths due to influenza occur in persons ≥65 years old.
- Secondary infection is usually caused by *Streptococcus pneumoniae* or *Staphylococcus aureus*.

Amantadine and rimantadine are effective against only influenza A virus. Vaccine, together with amantadine, can give ±95% protection against influenza A infection.

Recommendations for prevention of influenza in patients at risk include vaccination each autumn. Vaccine is given as follows: 6-35 months of age, split virus (chemically treated to prevent febrile reaction); 3-12 years of age, split virus; >12 years of age, whole or split virus. The vaccine can be given simultaneously with pneumococcal vaccine (Pneumovax). Reactions include fever, myalgias, and hypersensitivity. Target groups are persons ≥65 years old, residents of chronic care facilities, persons with cardiopulmonary disorders, children 6 months to 18 years old receiving long-term aspirin therapy (Reye's syndrome), health care personnel, employees of chronic care facilities, providers of home health care, and household members of high-risk persons. Amantadine is also used prophylactically: 200 mg/day; if >65 years old, 100 mg/day. The dosage is decreased in patients with impaired renal function (100 mg/day) or seizure disorders (100 mg/day). Toxicity manifests as dizziness, restlessness, and insomnia.

- Influenza vaccine can be given simultaneously with pneumococcal vaccine.
- Target groups are persons ≥65 years old, residents of chronic care facilities, persons with cardiopulmonary disorders, health care personnel, employees of chronic care facilities, providers of home health care, and household members of high-risk persons.

Influenza A is treated with amantadine. It is effective if given within 48 hours after onset of symptoms. After 48 hours, it has no effect.

Poliovirus

There was a recent outbreak in the Netherlands among members of religious groups who were not vaccinated. The Centers for Disease Control recommend evaluation of a traveler's immunity before extensive travel in the Netherlands. The frequency and severity of disease are increased during pregnancy. It is most often an asymptomatic infection. The virus affects the nuclei of cranial nerves and anterior motor neurons of the spinal cord; therefore, paralysis is flaccid and not spastic. When paralysis develops, it is usually asymmetric. Wild type polio has been eliminated from the Western Hemisphere, but it remains epidemic in parts of Asia and Africa. Vaccine-related polio still occurs only rarely.

Rabies

This infection is difficult to diagnose antemortem. Manifestations are hydrophobia and copious salivation. It should be considered in any case of encephalitis or myelitis of unknown cause, especially in persons who have recently traveled outside the United States. The virus spreads along peripheral nerves to the central nervous system. The most common sources of exposure are dogs, cats, skunks, foxes, raccoons (Florida, Connecticut), wolves, and bats. Spread by other animals is *very rare*. Rodents rarely, if ever, transmit rabies. From 1980-1989, 9 of 13 cases in the United States were due to exposure to rabid animals outside the country. Rabies has also been reported to occur in patients after corneal transplantation. Aerosol spread is possible; it is most often due to exposure to bats during spelunking or in medical laboratories. The risk of nosocomial transmission is low. Definitive diagnosis is established by the presence of Negri bodies on biopsy of the hippocampus. Clinically, serum and cerebrospinal fluid are tested for rabies antibodies. Direct fluorescent antibody testing of a skin biopsy specimen from the nape of the neck is used to detect rabies antigen.

- Rabies should be considered in any case of encephalitis or myelitis of unknown cause.
- Most common sources of exposure are dogs, cats, skunks, foxes, raccoons, wolves, and bats.
- Definitive diagnosis is established by the presence of Negri bodies on biopsy of the hippocampus.

Human diploid vaccine is the most effective and least toxic; it has largely replaced duck embryo vaccine. Human rabies immune globulin (HRIG) is widely available now. Do not use horse serum globulin unless human immune globulin is unavailable. HRIG and vaccine are not of benefit after onset of clinical disease.

Slow Viruses

Progressive Multifocal Leukoencephalopathy (PML)

This is associated with acquired immunodeficiency syndrome (AIDS), leukemia, lymphoma, and carcinomatosis. It is caused by a papovavirus (JC virus). Clinically, diffuse or focal central nervous system abnormalities are present. Despite its name, PML usually presents as a solitary lesion on computed tomography or magnetic resonance imaging. Cerebrospinal fluid is normal in most cases. It is now recognized with increased frequency in patients with AIDS. The diagnosis is based on brain biopsy. There is no proven therapy.

- PML is associated with AIDS, leukemia, lymphoma, and carcinomatosis.
- PML is caused by a papovavirus (JC virus).
- PML is now recognized with increased frequency in patients with AIDS.

Subacute Sclerosing Panencephalitis (Inclusion Body Encephalitis)

This is a progressively fatal disease of children and adolescents. It is thought to be due to previous measles infection. Patients are <11 years old in 80% of cases. Onset is insidious; mental deterioration is characteristic. Later, myoclonic jerks and diffuse abnormalities occur. Measles antibody levels in sera and cerebrospinal fluid are among the highest found in any condition. Brain biopsy is necessary for diagnosis (inclusion body encephalitis). There is no treatment. The disease is uniformly fatal.

Creutzfeldt-Jakob Disease

This is a rare, fatal, degenerative disease of the central nervous system. It occurs equally in both sexes; the median age of patients is in the seventh decade. There are both familial and sporadic forms of the disease. It usually presents as rapidly evolving dementia with myoclonic seizures. Prions (small proteinaceous infectious particles without nucleic acid) are the cause of infection. It has been reported to occur through nosocomial transmission (e.g., corneal transplant recipients, exposure to cerebrospinal fluid). There is no treatment.

- Creutzfeldt-Jakob disease presents as rapidly evolving dementia with myoclonic seizures.

Measles (Rubeola)

There has been a substantial increase in measles cases recently in unvaccinated preschool children and vaccinated high school and college students (1990, 27,786 cases). Prodromal upper respiratory symptoms are prominent. Oral Koplik's spots precede the rash. The disorder has been associated with temporary cutaneous anergy. *Cases of reactivation of previous* Mycobacterium tuberculosis *infection have been reported in patients with measles.* Measles vaccine may also cause temporary cutaneous anergy. Therefore, a tuberculin skin test should be done before measles vaccinations.

- In measles, oral Koplik's spots precede the rash.
- Measles vaccine may also cause temporary cutaneous anergy.

Complications of measles include encephalitis and pneu-

monia. Encephalitis is often severe. It usually occurs after a period of apparent improvement of measles infection. In primary measles pneumonia there are large multinucleated cells (Warthin-Finkeldey cells) found in lung biopsy. Secondary bacterial infection is more common than primary measles pneumonia. *S. aureus* and *Haemophilus influenzae* are the most common bacterial pathogens.

- Complications of measles include encephalitis.
- Secondary bacterial infection is more common than primary measles pneumonia.

Atypical measles occurs in patients vaccinated before 1968. After exposure, atypical rash, fever, arthralgias, and headache (aseptic meningitis) may develop. It can be diagnosed by the presence of a high titer of measles antibody in serum.

Rubella

The prodromal symptoms of rubella are mild (unlike those of rubeola). Posterior cervical lymphadenopathy, arthralgia (70% in adults), transient erythematous rash, and fever are characteristic. Infection is subclinical in many cases. Central nervous system complications and thrombocytopenia are rare.

- Characteristics of rubella: posterior cervical lymphadenopathy, arthralgia (70% in adults), transient erythematous rash, and fever.

For a pregnant female exposed to rubella, the serum titer should be checked. If titer indicates immunity, no treatment is needed. If titer indicates non-immunity, the patient should be followed for evidence of clinical rubella. The serum titer should be checked again in 2-3 weeks to determine whether it is increased. If titer is not increased and there is no evidence of clinical rubella, no treatment is needed. In cases of clinical rubella or seroconversion, abortion counseling should be offered, depending on clinical circumstances. Do *not* give gamma globulin to pregnant non-immune female exposed to rubella. It may mask symptoms of rubella but it does not protect the fetus.

- In cases of clinical rubella or seroconversion, consider therapeutic abortion.

From 6%-11% of young adults remain susceptible to rubella after receiving rubella vaccine. A pregnant female should not be given rubella vaccine because it causes congenital abnormalities. Females of childbearing age should be warned not to become pregnant within 2-3 months from time of immunization. Transient arthralgias will develop in 25% of immunized women. They may also develop fever, rash, and lymphadenopathy. Symptoms may occur as long as 2 months after vaccination. They may be confused with other forms of arthritis.

Viral Meningoencephalitis

Viral infections with low cerebrospinal fluid glucose levels may be confused with bacterial, partially treated bacterial, or tuberculous meningitis. Etiologic agents include mumps, enteroviruses, herpes simplex, and, in summer months, the equine encephalitis viruses. Lymphocytic choriomeningitis is acquired by exposure to rodent urine. It causes profound lymphocytosis in the cerebrospinal fluid. Lactate levels in cerebrospinal fluid are normal in viral meningitis. The lactate level is usually increased in bacterial meningitis.

Herpesvirus

There are now seven known types of herpes simplex virus (HSV): type 1, type 2, Epstein-Barr virus (EBV), cytomegalovirus (CMV), varicella-zoster virus (VZV), human herpesvirus 6 (HHV-6), and HHV-7. HHV-6 caused roseola (exanthem subitum) and up to 14% of acute self-limited febrile illnesses in children ≤2 years old who presented to one emergency room. HHV-7 has yet to be associated with disease.

Serologic evidence of infection is common by the time students enter college: HSV-1, 87%; HSV-2, 5%; EBV, 75%; CMV, 50%; VZV, 80%. The rate of infection increases in populations of lower socioeconomic status.

Herpes Simplex

In cases of genital HSV, infection is caused by HSV-2 in 75% and by HSV-1 in 25%. The reverse is true for oral HSV. Use of sunscreen in patients exposed to significant amounts of sunlight may decrease the incidence of recurrence on lips. *Disseminated infection* is most often due to HSV-1 and occurs in immunocompromised hosts with impaired cell-mediated immunity. In cases of herpes simplex encephalitis, patients may mistakenly be thought to be intoxicated. They appear confused and may have seizures. Simultaneous herpes labialis is present in 10%-15%. Antemortem diagnosis is difficult. HSV is rarely cultured from cerebrospinal fluid. The definitive diagnosis is made with brain biopsy. Recently, new techniques such as magnetic resonance imaging and DNA amplification have shown promise. Electroencephalography shows periodic lateralized epileptiform discharges (PLEDs). Abnormalities are located in temporal areas. Poor neurologic status, age >30 years, and encephalitis of more than 4 days in duration are associated with a poor outcome.

- In herpes simplex, disseminated infection is most often due to HSV-1 and occurs in immunocompromised hosts.
- In cases of herpes simplex encephalitis, patients may mistakenly be thought to be intoxicated.
- Simultaneous herpes labialis is present in 10%-15%.

HSV pneumonia usually occurs in immunosuppressed patients and is a serious disease. HSV also is associated with mucocutaneous disease (e.g., esophagitis, stomatitis). HSV esophagitis must be distinguished from CMV and *Candida* esophagitis. Diagnosis is made with endoscopic biopsy. *Eczema herpeticum* (Kaposi's varicelliform eruption) occurs in areas of eczema. Large areas of skin are involved. *Herpetic whitlow* is painful infection of a finger, often from a contaminated needle. Although nosocomial transmission of HSV-1 is rare, recent reports have stressed the importance of mucous membrane precautions in all patients with HSV, particularly those with respiratory infection who are undergoing invasive procedures.

- *Herpetic whitlow* is painful infection of a finger, often from a contaminated needle.

HSV can cause outbreaks among participants in contact sports (wrestlers, herpes gladiatorum). The infection is transmitted by skin-to-skin contact. Lesions appear on the head (78%), trunk (28%), and extremities (42%). Rash may be atypical. Large ulcerative lesions can develop in patients with AIDS. Some of the lesions are mistaken for decubitus ulcers. Perianal ulcers can present with pain on defecation or pruritus. Treatment for HSV is outlined in Table 14-8.

- HSV can cause outbreaks among participants in contact sports.
- Large ulcerative lesions can develop in patients with AIDS.

Cytomegalovirus

Primary cytomegalovirus (CMV) infection is usually asymptomatic in immunocompetent patients, although it can cause heterophile-negative mononucleosis syndrome. Perinatal infection occurs in utero, intrapartum, or post partum. It can cause congenital malformations. Children commonly excrete CMV in urine.

- CMV can cause heterophile-negative mononucleosis syndrome.

CMV can be transmitted by blood transfusion; the virus is transmitted by granulocytes, most often in fresh blood. Survival of the virus is greatly reduced in stored blood products. Fever and infectious mononucleosis-like picture on peripheral smear are characteristics in postoperative patients who have received blood transfusions. The typical patient has had cardiac bypass 4 weeks previously or has been pregnant and had a large blood loss. Diagnosis is made by detection of seroconversion. CMV causes serious infections (retinitis, pneumonia, gastrointestinal ulcerations, encephalitis, adrenalitis) in patients who have had transplantation (solid organ and bone marrow) and patients with AIDS. The diagnosis is most often established from clinical findings alone (CMV retinitis), by isolation of CMV from

Table 14-8.--Treatment for Herpes Simplex Virus

Infection	Treatment
Genital herpes	
First episode	Acyclovir, 200 mg orally 5 times/day for 7-10 days
	Acyclovir, 5 mg/kg intravenously every 8 hours for 5 days (severe cases)
Recurrence	Acyclovir, 200 mg orally 5 times/day for 5 days
Frequent recurrence	Acyclovir, 400 mg orally twice a day up to 1 year
Encephalitis	Acyclovir, 10 mg/kg intravenously every 8 hours for 10-14 days (vidarabine [ara-A] is less effective alternative)
Mucocutaneous disease in immunocompromised patient	
Initial episode	Acyclovir, 5 mg/kg intravenously every 8 hours or 200-400 mg orally 5 times/day for 7-10 days
Recurrence	Intravenous or oral acyclovir taken daily prevents recurrence during high-risk periods (immediately after bone marrow transplantation); lesion will likely recur when therapy is discontinued
Orolabial disease	
First occurrence	Limited data; acyclovir probably effective, 200 mg orally 5 times/day for 5 days
Frequent recurrence (>6/yr)	Acyclovir, 400 mg twice/day
Acyclovir-resistant strains	Foscarnet, vidarabine

sterile body site (blood), or from culture and histopathologic evidence of CMV infection in involved tissue (e.g., liver, lung, gastrointestinal tract).

- CMV can be transmitted by blood transfusion; the virus is transmitted by granulocytes.
- Fever and infectious mononucleosis-like picture on peripheral smear are characteristics in postoperative patients who have received blood transfusions.
- CMV causes serious infections (retinitis, pneumonia, gastrointestinal ulcerations, encephalitis, adrenalitis) in patients who have had transplantation and patients with AIDS.

Positive blood cultures for CMV in patients with AIDS do not predict subsequent end-organ disease (i.e., low positive predictive value) in the subsequent 6 months of follow-up. This course is in contradistinction to that of patients after solid organ transplantation. Furthermore, only approximately 50% of patients with AIDS and CMV end-organ disease will have positive results of CMV blood culture. In 75% of CMV-negative transplant recipients who receive CMV-positive organs, primary CMV disease will develop. In many of these, end-organ complications will develop. Others will have mononucleosis-like syndrome. This causes enhanced immunosuppression, and patients are more likely to develop other infection (e.g., *Pneumocystis carinii* pneumonia).

CMV retinitis occurs in 20%-30% of patients with advanced AIDS. Diagnosis is based on ophthalmologic examination. CMV esophagitis is third most frequent cause of esophagitis in patients with AIDS. CMV pneumonia is much more common in patients who have had transplantation (bone marrow) than in patients with AIDS. Diagnosis requires tissue confirmation of infection (CMV inclusions in biopsy specimens) because frequently patients can excrete CMV in bronchoalveolar lavage specimens without having active disease. CMV pneumonia can be particularly severe and life-threatening in patients who have had bone marrow transplantation.

- CMV retinitis occurs in 20%-30% of patients with advanced AIDS.
- CMV esophagitis is third most frequent cause of esophagitis in patients with AIDS.
- CMV pneumonia is much more common in patients who have had transplantation (bone marrow) than in patients with AIDS.

Ganciclovir has been the treatment of choice for most CMV infections. A recent randomized, placebo-controlled trial found that foscarnet and ganciclovir are equally efficacious in halting progression of CMV retinitis in patients with AIDS but that patients taking foscarnet lived longer (12 vs. 8 months).

Both drugs are now approved for this indication. The choice of one over the other should be made on an individual basis. All patients with AIDS who have CMV retinitis need chronic suppressive therapy. In patients with CMV pneumonia after bone marrow transplantation, ganciclovir and immunoglobulin containing high titers of CMV antibodies are more effective than ganciclovir alone. Non-immunocompromised patients with CMV do not require treatment.

- Ganciclovir and foscarnet are the treatments of choice for most CMV infections.

Varicella-Zoster

In primary varicella infection (chickenpox), the lesions are in various stages of development in different areas of the body. It differs from smallpox in that lesions are all at the same level of development. Varicella pneumonia occurs in 5%-50% of adults with chickenpox. It occurs 1-6 days after onset of rash and is a serious disease. Pneumonia begins to improve with disappearance of rash, but, in serious cases, pneumonia may persist. Encephalomyelitis is also a serious complication of varicella infection. It occurs predominantly in children. Onset is 3-14 days after appearance of rash.

- Varicella pneumonia occurs in 5%-50% of adults with chickenpox.
- Pneumonia begins to improve with disappearance of rash.

Herpes zoster infection is considered a reactivation of latent varicella infection. It often involves the fifth cranial nerve, especially the ophthalmic branch. Nonimmune patients exposed to zoster may develop varicella, but patients exposed to varicella rarely, if ever, develop zoster.

- Herpes zoster infection often involves the fifth cranial nerve, especially the ophthalmic branch.

Neurologic complications of herpes zoster include motor paralysis (most common). It usually involves the same dermatome and may involve cranial nerves. Encephalitis also occurs. Myelitis is the least common neurologic complication.

Varicella immune globulin is indicated for 1) VZV-seronegative immunocompromised hosts who have had close contact with a person with chickenpox and 2) newborns of mothers with varicella infection that occurs 5 days before or 2 days after delivery.

Among mothers with varicella-zoster, 10% transmit the infection to the fetus. During the first trimester, limb hypoplasia, cortical atrophy, and chorioretinitis develop. During the third trimester, multiple visceral involvement develops, including pneumonia. Mortality rate is 31%. Highest risk period is 5 days before and 2 days after delivery.

- Among mothers with varicella-zoster, 10% transmit the infection to the fetus.

Treatment for *varicella (primary varicella-zoster) infection* is based on whether the patient is immunocompetent. Two recent randomized clinical trials showed that acyclovir (800 mg 5 times/day or equivalent) reduced duration of skin lesions and viral shedding in adults and children. Its efficacy for reducing visceral complications (i.e., pneumonia) remains unknown. Early treatment (<24 hours) is necessary. The cost of therapy may limit its usefulness. In immunosuppressed patients, acyclovir or vidarabine reduces complications. Acyclovir is less toxic and so is the preferred therapy. Acyclovir may reduce the risk of dissemination and of complications in immunocompromised patients. Treatment of zoster ophthalmicus reduces the incidence of uveitis and keratitis. In immunocompetent patients, acyclovir speeds healing and reduces pain. There is no effect on postherpetic neuralgia. Preliminary data suggest that the new antiviral agent famciclovir might decrease the duration of postherpetic neuralgia. For disseminated infections (encephalitis, cranial neuritis), a recent controlled trial showed that high-dose intravenous acyclovir was equivalent to vidarabine. Treatment with acyclovir was associated with 3 fewer days of hospitalization than when vidarabine was used. For acyclovir-resistant varicella-zoster infection, intravenous foscarnet is used.

Epstein-Barr Virus (EBV)

Infectious mononucleosis has the clinical triad of fever, pharyngitis, and adenopathy. Pharyngitis is common (±80%). Splenomegaly occurs in 50% of cases. One of the most serious complications is ruptured spleen, in which case the patient has the sudden onset of severe abdominal pain. Other serious complications include hemolytic anemia and airway obstruction; encephalitis and transverse myelitis also occur but are uncommon. Corticosteroids may be beneficial for treatment of hemolytic anemia and acute airway obstruction. The infection may be transmitted by blood transfusion. If ampicillin is given, a rash often develops.

- Infectious mononucleosis has the clinical triad of fever, pharyngitis, and adenopathy.
- Pharyngitis is common (±80%).
- Splenomegaly occurs in 50% of cases.
- One of the most serious complications is ruptured spleen.
- If ampicillin is given, a rash often develops.

Uncomplicated cases require symptomatic care only. The patient should not participate in contact sports for several months. Corticosteroids are not indicated for uncomplicated infection. Acyclovir therapy is not effective.

Table 14-9 differentiates EBV from other causes of mononucleosis.

Chronic fatigue syndrome is a vague syndrome characterized by low-grade fever, constitutional symptoms, and fatigue; lymphadenopathy, splenomegaly, and abnormal results of liver function tests may be noted. Studies have shown that elevated titers of antibody to early antigen and viral capsid antigen are no more frequent in cases than in controls. Acyclovir is also not effective. Chronic fatigue syndrome is not caused by EBV.

- Chronic fatigue syndrome is characterized by low-grade fever, constitutional symptoms, and fatigue.
- Lymphadenopathy, splenomegaly, and abnormal results of liver function tests may be noted.
- Chronic fatigue syndrome is not caused by EBV.

EBV infection in males with X-linked lymphoproliferative syndrome is a rare disorder of young boys. Fulminant EBV infections develop; 57% die of the infection. Complications include severe EBV hepatitis with liver failure and hemophagocytic syndrome with bleeding. Survivors develop hypogammaglobulinemia, malignant lymphoma, aplastic anemia, and opportunistic infections. Death occurs by age 40 years in all cases. Acyclovir and corticosteroids do not seem to be beneficial.

In EBV-associated Burkitt's lymphoma and nasopharyngeal carcinoma, patients have high titers of antibody to early antigen. *Polyclonal and monoclonal B-cell lymphoproliferative syndromes* have been associated with EBV in patients who have had organ transplantation and are receiving cyclosporine and in patients with AIDS. Oral hairy leukoplakia in patients with AIDS is associated with EBV infection and responds to acyclovir therapy. EBV has recently been associated with leiomyosarcomas in transplant recipients.

- Polyclonal and monoclonal B-cell lymphoproliferative syndromes have been associated with EBV.

Epidemic Keratoconjunctivitis

This is caused by adenovirus type 8. It is now most common in epidemics occurring in ophthalmology clinics (caused by contaminated fluids or instruments).

Mumps

Orchitis occurs in 20% of males; it is unilateral in approximately 75%. Orchitis is characterized by recrudescence of malaise and appearance of chills, fever, headache, nausea, vomiting, and testicular pain. Sterility is *uncommon* even after bilateral infection.

Mumps meningoencephalitis is one of the most common viral meningitides. Patients may have low cerebrospinal fluid glucose values. Pancreatitis can occur.

- Mumps meningoencephalitis is one of the most common viral meningitides.

Mumps polyarthritis is most common in men between the ages of 20 and 30 years. Joint symptoms begin 1-2 weeks after subsidence of parotitis. Large joints are involved. It lasts approximately 6 weeks, and complete recovery is usual. This condition may be confused with other forms of arthritis.

- Mumps polyarthritis is most common in men between the ages of 20 and 30 years.
- Large joints are involved.

Deafness is a rare complication of mumps.

Human T-Cell Leukemia Viruses (HTLV)

Infection with these retroviruses is usually asymptomatic. HTLV-I is endemic in parts of Japan, the Caribbean basin, Melanesia, and Africa. It may be transmitted by sexual contact, infected blood products, and injection drug use. Vertical transmission (breast feeding) also occurs. HTLV-I is associated with human T-cell leukemia and chronic myelopathy (tropical spastic paraparesis). For HTLV-II, no clinical disease is known. The seroprevalence of HTLV-I or -II is as high as 18% in certain high-risk groups (injection drug users, patients attending sexually transmitted disease clinics) (HTLV-II is 2.5 times more prevalent than HTLV-I). Among voluntary blood donors, seroprevalence in the United States is estimated at 0.016%. The risk of transmission of HTLV-I or -II through blood transfusion with current screening practices is estimated to be

Table 14-9.--Infectious Mononucleosis-Like Syndromes

Disease	Pharyngitis	Adenopathy	Splenomegaly	Atypical lymphocytes	Heterophile	Other test
Infectious mononucleosis	++++	++++	+++	+++	+	Specific EBV antibody + (VCA IgM)
CMV	-	-	+++	++	-	CMV IgM
Toxoplasmosis	-	++++	+++	++	-	Toxoserology

-, absent; +, ++, +++, and ++++, present to varying degrees; VCA, viral capsid antigen.

0.0014% (1/70,000 units). Sexual partners of infected persons should be tested for HTLV-I and -II.

- HTLV-I may be transmitted by sexual contact, infected blood products, and injection drug use.
- HTLV-I is associated with human T-cell leukemia and chronic myelopathy.

Parvovirus B19

This is the cause of erythema infectiosum (fifth disease) and transient arthritis. Persistent B19 virus is found in patients with pure red blood cell *aplasia*. This condition has no increase in serum IgG or IgM antibodies and no rash, arthralgias, or other manifestations of fifth disease. Diagnosis is established by demonstration of giant pronormoblasts in bone marrow or identification of viral protein or DNA of parvovirus in bone marrow. Most patients respond to administration of commercial immunoglobulin infusions for 5-10 days.

- Parvovirus B19 is cause of erythema infectiosum (fifth disease) and transient arthritis.
- B19 virus is found in patients with pure red blood cell aplasia.

PARASITIC DISEASES

Amebic Keratitis

The causative organism is *Acanthamoeba*. This condition should be suspected in patients with keratitis as the result of contamination of contact lens solution or in patients who have been swimming in fresh water while wearing contact lenses. The diagnosis is based on microscopic examination of scrapings of the cornea. Treatment is with topical antifungal agents. Patients often respond poorly to therapy and have progressive corneal destruction.

- In amebic keratitis, the causative organism is *Acanthamoeba*.
- Condition is suspected in keratitis caused by contamination of contact lens solution.

Amebic Meningoencephalitis

The causative organism is free-living amebas of the genus *Naegleria*. Many patients have a history of swimming in fresh water lakes, usually in middle Atlantic states or Texas. The presumed portal of entry is through the cribriform plate. Patients have intense hemorrhagic meningoencephalitis. Cerebrospinal fluid findings are like those of bacterial infection--low glucose level, many polymorphonuclear cells, and high erythrocyte count. Motile trophozoites may be found. The infection is almost invariably fatal. Treatment is with amphotericin B (intrathecally and intravenously).

- In amebic meningoencephalitis, the portal of entry is through the cribriform plate.

Amebiasias

Sites of involvement, in decreasing order of frequency, are cecum, ascending colon, rectum, and sigmoid. When symptomatic, the disease causes diarrhea, abdominal pain, fever in ±50% of cases; bloody diarrhea often occurs. Trophozoites are found in stool specimens. Trophozoites do *not* spread disease. Treatment is with metronidazole plus diloxanide furoate or paromomycin. In asymptomatic carriers, amebic cysts are excreted in stool specimens. They are contagious and are responsible for spread of the disease. Treatment is with diloxanide furoate or paromomycin.

- In amebiasis, sites of involvement, in decreasing order of frequency, are cecum, ascending colon, rectum, and sigmoid.
- Bloody diarrhea often occurs.

Patients with hepatic abscess usually have minimal, if any, diarrhea. They may have low-grade fever. Stool specimens are usually negative. Abscess usually is single and is located in the posterior portion of the right lobe of the liver (because this lobe receives most of the blood draining the right colon--site of most frequent involvement with amebiasis). This anatomic location may result in point tenderness in the posterolateral portion of the lower right intercostal space. Jaundice is uncommon. The anatomic location, the fact that it is usually a single abscess, and the absence of other signs of bacterial infection help to distinguish amebic hepatic abscess from bacterial abscess. Serologic tests (complement fixation) are positive in >90% of patients. Hepatic abscess may rupture through the diaphragm into the right pleural cavity. Rarely, *Entamoeba histolytica* may cause brain abscess. Treatment is with metronidazole plus diloxanide furoate or paromomycin.

- Patients with hepatic abscess usually have minimal, if any, diarrhea.
- Serologic tests (complement fixation) are positive in >90% of patients.

Miscellaneous Parasites

Giardia is the most frequently isolated parasite in state laboratories. It characteristically presents with sudden onset of watery diarrhea and malabsorption, bloating, and flatulence. Prolonged disease is particularly common in patients with IgA deficiency. The diagnosis is based on stool examination and duodenal aspirate. Treatment is with metronidazole or quinacrine hydrochloride.

- *Giardia* is the most frequently isolated parasite in state laboratories.

- Presents with sudden onset of watery diarrhea and malabsorption, bloating, and flatulence. Prolonged disease is particularly common in patients with IgA deficiency.

Toxoplasmosis is acquired from eating undercooked meat or exposure to cat feces. Rash, pneumonitis, and generalized lymphadenopathy are characteristics. Toxoplasmosis causes brain lesions and pneumonia in patients with AIDS. The causative organism may result in infectious mononucleosis-like syndrome. Treatment is with pyrimethamine in combination with sulfadiazine or clindamycin.

- Toxoplasmosis is acquired from eating undercooked meat or exposure to cat feces.
- Rash, pneumonitis, and generalized lymphadenopathy are characteristics.
- Causative organism may result in infectious mononucleosis-like syndrome.

Trichinosis is acquired from undercooked meat, especially pork or bear. Features are muscle pain (especially chest and tongue), eosinophilia, and periorbital edema. *Hookworm (Necator americanus)* causes blood loss anemia. *Ascariasis* infection produces intestinal obstruction. *Schistosomiasis* is a tropical disease that causes hepatic cirrhosis, hematuria, and carcinoma of the bladder. Transverse myelitis related to schistosomiasis occurs rarely.

- Trichinosis is acquired from undercooked meat, especially pork or bear.
- Features are muscle pain (especially chest and tongue), eosinophilia, and periorbital edema.

The four main species of *malaria* are *Plasmodium vivax, P. falciparum* (color plate 14-7), *P. malariae, P. ovale.* Malaria is transmitted by bite of the *Anopheles* mosquito. All four species have a primary exoerythrocytic (hepatic) stage. *P. vivax* and *P. ovale* have a secondary exoerythrocytic (hepatic) stage. *P. falciparum* and *P. malariae* do not have this secondary exoerythrocytic stage. The asexual erythrocytic cycle requires 36-48 hours for *P. falciparum*, 48 hours for *P. vivax*, and 72 hours for *P. malariae*. The periodicity of febrile paroxysms caused by the different species coincides with the cyclic discharge of organisms from ruptured erythrocytes. *P. vivax* and *P. malariae* infections may persist for years.

- Malaria is transmitted by bite of *Anopheles* mosquito.

Mosquito-borne malaria occurred in California and Florida in 1990. Self-induced malaria through contaminated blood products, in an attempt to cure Lyme disease, has been reported. Cases in military personnel returning from Somalia have

been reported.

P. vivax invades only immature erythrocytes, *P. malariae* invades only senescent erythrocytes, and *P. falciparum* invades erythrocytes at any age.

The hallmark of the condition is malarial paroxysm. This occurs regularly in all infections by *P. falciparum*. With *P. vivax*, tertian malaria is the most common form. Once synchronization occurs, paroxysms occur on alternate days (48 hours). With *P. malariae*, quartan malaria is most common. Paroxysms occur every third day. *P. malariae* infections may be associated with nephrotic syndrome. With *P. falciparum*, because of the asynchronous cycle of multiplication, the typical paroxysms occur in a minority of patients. *P. falciparum* can multiply in all stages of erythrocyte, so quantity of parasitemia can be large.

The diagnosis of malaria is based on examination of thick and thin blood smears (color plate 14-7).

- Malarial paroxysm occurs regularly in all infections by *P. falciparum*.
- With *P. malariae,* quartan malaria is the most common.
- Paroxysms occur every third day.
- Diagnosis of malaria is based on examination of thick and thin blood smears.

Prophylaxis is increasingly difficult because of resistant *P. falciparum*. Personal protection should always be used (e.g., mosquito nets). For travelers to chloroquine-sensitive areas (Central America [north of Panama], Mexico, Haiti, Dominican Republic, and the Middle East), chloroquine phosphate is taken. For travelers to chloroquine-resistant areas, mefloquine, doxycycline, or sulfadoxine-pyrimethamine (Fansidar) is used. Travelers to the mefloquine-resistant areas of the Thai-Myanmar and Thai-Cambodia borders should use doxycycline. Mefloquine should be avoided in patients taking β-adrenergic blockers. No regimen guarantees 100% prophylaxis. All patients should be advised to seek medical attention if fever develops within 1 year after return from endemic area. Prophylaxis should begin 2 weeks before travel and continue through 4-6 weeks after leaving an endemic area.

For treatment of known susceptible strains of *P. falciparum* and others, chloroquine is used. In cases of chloroquine resistance, therapy is with quinine and sulfadoxine-pyrimethamine or doxycycline. For severe *P. falciparum* infections, quinidine or quinine given intravenously is effective. Primaquine (screen for glucose-6-phosphate dehydrogenase deficiency) is used to eradicate exoerythrocytic phase of *P. ovale* and *P. vivax* infections. Adjunctive therapy may include deferoxamine (iron chelation), which may hasten the clearance of parasitemia and enhance recovery from deep coma in children with cerebral malaria. It also has antimalarial effects in asymptomatic patients with mild parasitemia. Exchange transfusions are used in severe cases with extensive parasitemia.

Pinworms cause anal pruritus. Diagnosis is made by examination for ova on cellophane tape pressed to the anus. A stool specimen is *not* helpful in diagnosis.

Cryptosporidiosis is an important cause of diarrhea in AIDS. It may also be a relatively common cause of self-limited diarrhea in otherwise healthy patients. Waterborne outbreaks (Georgia; Milwaukee, Wisconsin) have been reported. They occur most often in late summer or fall; 35% of patients have another pathogen simultaneously, most often *Giardia*. The diagnosis is based on stool examination or acid-fast stain of stool.

- Cryptosporidiosis is an important cause of diarrhea in AIDS.
- 35% of patients have another pathogen simultaneously, most often *Giardia*.

Leishmaniasis has been reported in soldiers returning from Operation Desert Storm. It is a protozoal disease transmitted by the sand fly. It causes a visceral syndrome (kala-azar; caused by *Leishmania donovani*). Symptoms are fever, hepatosplenomegaly, hypergammaglobulinemia, cachexia, and pancytopenia. The diagnosis is based on bone marrow aspiration (Giemsa stain). Skin test should not be used. Treatment is with stibogluconate sodium. The cutaneous form caused by *L. tropica* is usually self-limited. American cutaneous leishmaniasis is often more destructive and should be treated.

- Leishmaniasis has been reported in soldiers returning from Operation Desert Storm.

Neurocystercercosis is an infection of the central nervous system with a larval stage of the pork tapeworm (*Taenia solium*). It is acquired by ingesting tapeworm eggs from fecally contaminated food. It is endemic in Latin America, Asia, and Africa. Recent cases have been reported among household contacts of foreign-born persons (working as domestic employees); the infected persons had not traveled to an endemic area. Common presentations are seizures and computed tomography scan showing cystic or calcified brain lesions. The diagnosis is based on serum or cerebrospinal fluid serologic testing or brain biopsy. Treatment is with praziquantel or albendazole with or without steroids. Recent evidence suggests that after medical therapy there is usually remission or marked improvement in the seizure disorder.

- Common presentations of neurocystercercosis are seizures and computed tomography scan showing cystic brain lesions.

Babesiosis is a tick-borne (same vector as Lyme disease, *I. dammini*) parasitic disease that affects erythrocytes and causes fever, myalgias, hemolytic anemia, and occasionally splenomegaly. It is a severe disease associated with asplenia.

Rash has not been reported. The disease is endemic in the northeastern United States, especially around Nantucket and Cape Cod. The diagnosis is established with examination of peripheral blood smear. Treatment is with clindamycin and quinine. Simultaneous infection with babesiosis and Lyme disease is especially severe.

The primary pathogen of *visceral larva migrans* is the common dog roundworm, *Toxocara canis*. Humans (usually children) are infected by ingesting eggs found in soil (pica). The clinical syndrome is due to migration of larva to extraintestinal sites (hematogenous spread). Fever, hepatomegaly, eosinophilia, and hypergammaglobulinemia are common. Pulmonary involvement (asthma, pneumonitis) is rare. The diagnosis is presumptive and based on serologic testing. The course is usually self-limited. For severe cases, treatment is with albendazole or mebendazole with or without steroids.

- The pathogen of visceral larva migrans is common dog roundworm, *Toxocara canis*.
- Humans are infected by ingesting eggs found in soil.
- Fever, hepatomegaly, eosinophilia, and hypergammaglobulinemia are common.

Diagnostic tests for detecting various parasitic diseases are listed in Table 14-10.

Table 14-10.--Preferred Diagnostic Tests for Parasitic Infections

Parasite	Means of diagnosis[*]
Ameba: colonic	Stool O & P
Ameba: extracolonic	Serology
Giardia	Duodenal aspirate
Toxoplasma	Serology
Trichinella	Tissue biopsy
Hookworm	Stool O & P
Ascaris	Stool O & P
Schistosoma	Stool O & P or tissue biopsy
Plasmodium (malaria)	Blood smear
Opisthorchis (clonorchiasis)	Stool O & P
Filaria (filariasis)	Blood smear
Trypanosoma	Tissue biopsy
Tapeworm	Stool O & P
Pinworm	Perianal adhesive tape
Babesia	Blood smear
Pneumocystis	Tissue stain

[*]O & P, ova and parasites.

CLINICAL SYNDROMES

INFECTIVE ENDOCARDITIS

Native Valve Infective Endocarditis

Native valve infective endocarditis is more common in males, and the average age of patients is >50 years. It may present with acute (*Staphylococcus aureus*) or subacute (viridans streptococci) manifestations. In 60%-80% of cases there is a predisposing cardiac lesion. Mitral valve involvement is more common than aortic valve involvement. Congenital heart disease is present in 10%-20% of cases. The risk of infective endocarditis from mitral valve prolapse is low, but the prevalence of mitral valve prolapse makes it the underlying cardiac condition in 20%-25% of cases. Antimicrobial prophylaxis is used in patients with mitral valve prolapse who have murmur or echocardiographic evidence of thickening of the mitral valve leaflets and valve redundancy.

- Antimicrobial prophylaxis is used in mitral valve prolapse associated with murmur or thickening of mitral valve leaflets or redundancy.

Microorganisms causing native valve infective endocarditis include viridans streptococci (i.e., *Streptococcus sanguis, S. mutans,* and *S. mitior*), 30%-40% of cases; enterococci (i.e., *Enterococcus faecalis, E. faecium*), 5%-18%; other streptococci (i.e., *S. bovis, S. pneumoniae*), 15%-25%; *S. aureus*, 10%-27%; coagulase-negative staphylococci, 1%-3%; gram-negative bacilli, 1.5%-13%; fungi, 2%-4%; miscellaneous bacteria, <5%; mixed infections, 1%-2%; and "culture-negative," <5%-24% (data from Scheld WM, Sande MA: Cardiovascular infections. *In* Principles and Practice of Infectious Diseases. Third edition. Edited by GL Mandell, RG Douglas Jr, JE Bennett. New York: Churchill Livingstone, 1990, pp 670-706).

- Organisms most commonly involved in native valve infective endocarditis are viridans streptococci.

Treatment of native valve infective endocarditis includes emphasis on short-course therapy in selected cases (i.e., young patients and patients with uncomplicated left-sided native valve infective endocarditis caused by penicillin-susceptible viridans streptococci or *S. bovis*). For enterococcal endocarditis, combination therapy with penicillin G or ampicillin is recommended. Testing for high-level aminoglycoside resistance (gentamicin, >500 µg/mL; streptomycin, >2,000 µg/mL), β-lactamase production, and vancomycin resistance is mandatory.

Table 14-11 shows the recommended and alternative treatment regimens for native valve infective endocarditis.

Table 14-11.--Treatment of Native Valve Infective Endocarditis

Microorganism	Therapy*	Alternative therapy*
Penicillin-sensitive streptococci		
Streptococcus pyogenes, S. pneumoniae, group B streptococci	Aqueous penicillin G, 20 x 10⁶ U/24 hr i.v. for 4 wk	Vancomycin, 30 mg/kg daily for 4 wk, *or* cefazolin,[†] 1 g i.v. every 8 hr for 4 wk
Viridans streptococci or *S. bovis* (MIC, ≤0.1 µg/mL)	Aqueous penicillin G, 20 x 10⁶ U/24 hr i.v. for 2 wk, *plus* streptomycin,[‡] 7.5 mg/kg i.m. every 12 hr for 2 wk, or gentamicin,[‡] 1 mg/kg i.v. every 8 hr for 2 wk, *or* aqueous penicillin G, 20 x 10⁶ U/24 hr i.v. for 4 wk	Vancomycin, 30 mg/kg daily for 4 wk, *or* cefazolin,[†] 1 g i.v. every 8 hr for 4 wk
Nutritional variant or relatively penicillin-resistant viridans streptococci (MIC, >0.1 µg/mL and <0.5 µg/mL)	Aqueous penicillin G, 20 x 10⁶ U/24 hr i.v. for 4 wk, *plus* streptomycin,[‡] 7.5 mg/kg i.m. every 12 hr for 4 wk, or gentamicin,[‡] 1 mg/kg i.v. every 8 hr for 4 wk	Vancomycin, 30 mg/kg daily for 4 wk, *plus* streptomycin,[‡] 7.5 mg/kg i.m. every 12 hr for 4 wk, or gentamicin,[‡] 1 mg/kg i.v. every 8 hr for 4 wk
Enterococci or streptococci with MIC ≥0.5 µg/mL		
Streptomycin-susceptible (MIC, <2,000 µg/mL); organisms must	Aqueous penicillin G, 20 x 10⁶ U/24 hr i.v. for 4-6 wk, *plus*	Vancomycin, 30 mg/kg daily for 4-6 wk, *plus* streptomycin,[‡] 7.5 mg/kg i.m. every 12 hr

Table 14-11 (continued)

Microorganism	Therapy*	Alternative therapy*
be penicillin- or vancomycin-susceptible and not have high-level aminoglycoside resistance (streptomycin MIC <2,000 µg/mL and gentamicin MIC <500 µg/mL)	streptomycin,‡ 7.5 mg/kg i.m. every 12 hr for 4-6 wk, or gentamicin,‡ 1 mg/kg i.v. every 8 hr for 4-6 wk	for 4-6 wk, or gentamicin,‡ 1 mg/kg i.v. every 8 hr for 4-6 wk
Staphylococcus aureus		
Methicillin-sensitive	Nafcillin, 2.0 g i.v. every 4 hr for 4-6 wk, *plus* gentamicin,‡ 1 mg/kg every 8 hr for first 5-7 days	Vancomycin, 30 mg/kg daily for 4-6 wk, *or* cefazolin,† 2 g i.v. every 8 hr for 4-6 wk, *plus* gentamicin,‡ 1 mg/kg every 8 hr for first 5-7 days
Methicillin-resistant	Vancomycin, 30 mg/kg daily for 4-6 wk, *plus* gentamicin,‡ 1 mg/kg i.v. every 8 hr for 5-7 days	Consult infectious diseases specialist
HACEK group	Ampicillin, 1-2 g i.v. every 3 hr for 4 wk or 2nd- or 3rd-generation cephalosporin for 3 wk	Second- or third-generation cephalosporin, 3 wk
Neisseria gonorrhoeae	Ceftriaxone, 1-2 g every 24 hr for 4 wk	Aqueous penicillin G, 20 x 10⁶ U/24 hr i.v. for 4 wk (in β-lactam negative) for penicillin-susceptible isolates
Gram-negative bacilli	Most effective single drug or combination of drugs i.v. for 4-6 wk	
Urgent empiric treatment of culture-negative endocarditis	Vancomycin, 30 mg/kg daily for 6 wk, *plus* gentamicin,‡ 1.0 mg/kg i.v. every 8 hr for 6 wk	
Fungal endocarditis	Amphotericin B *plus* flucytosine, 37.5 mg/kg p.o. every 6 hr, *plus* cardiac valve replacement (flucytosine levels should be monitored)	

*Dosages suggested are for adults with normal renal and hepatic function.
†Other first-generation cephalosporins or cefuroxime may be substituted for cefazolin in equivalent dosages.
‡Gentamicin and streptomycin doses should not exceed 80 mg and 500 mg, respectively. Serum levels should be monitored and peak streptomycin levels of 20 µg/mL and gentamicin levels of 3 µg/mL are acceptable.
i.m., intramuscularly; i.v., intravenously; MIC, minimal inhibitory concentration; p.o., by mouth.
Modified from Steckelberg JM, Giuliani ER, Wilson WR: Infective endocarditis. *In* Cardiology: Fundamentals and Practice. Vol 2. Second edition. Edited by ER Giuliani, V Fuster, BJ Gersh, MD McGoon, DC McGoon. St. Louis, Mosby Year Book, 1991, pp 1739-1772. By permission of Mayo Foundation.

Prosthetic Valve Infective Endocarditis

Prosthetic valve endocarditis is more common in males, and the average age of patients is ≥60 years. The aortic valve is affected more often than the mitral valve. Early-onset endocarditis is defined as infection occurring ≤60 days after implantation, and late-onset endocarditis is infection occurring >60 days postoperatively. Early infection tends to have a more acute presentation. Microorganisms that cause infection are outlined in Table 14-12.

Treatment of prosthetic valve infective endocarditis is given in Table 14-13.

Miscellaneous Information About Infective Endocarditis

● Echocardiography is not a screening tool for detecting endocarditis.
● Endocarditis in injection drug users is caused by *S. aureus*

Table 14-12.--Organisms That Cause Prosthetic Valve Endocarditis

Organism	Onset, %		All, %
	Early	Late	
Coagulase-negative staphylococci	35	12	14
Staphylococcus aureus	17	26	29
Enterococci and group D streptococci	3	9	7
Streptococcus pneumoniae	1	<1	1
Other (i.e., viridans streptococci)	4	25	17
Gram-negative bacilli	16	12	13
Diphtheroids	10	4	7
Other bacteria	1	2	2
Candida	8	4	5
Other fungi	1	<1	1
"Culture negative"	1	4	3

From Threlkeld MG, Cobbs CG: Infectious disorders of prosthetic valves and intravascular devices. *In* Principles and Practice of Infectious Diseases. Third edition. Edited by GL Mandell, RG Douglas Jr, JE Bennett. New York, Churchill Livingstone, 1990, pp 706-715. By permission of the publisher.

(60%), streptococci (16%), gram-negative bacilli (13.5%), polymicrobial organisms (8.1%), and *Corynebacterium* (1.4%). *Candida* endocarditis also occurs in this patient population. *S. aureus* most commonly involves the tricuspid valve.

- Intractable congestive heart failure is the most common indication for operation.
- Culture-negative endocarditis may be the result of previous use of antibiotics (most common) and endocarditis due to the following organisms: HACEK organisms, nutritionally deficient streptococci, *Brucella*, fungi, *Legionella*, *Coxiella burnetii*, and *Chlamydia psittaci*.

Surgical Therapy

If operation is needed it should not be delayed to allow additional days of antimicrobial therapy. Surgical treatment is often indicated in cases with refractory congestive heart failure. Other generally accepted indications for operation include evidence of more than one serious systemic embolic episode, uncontrolled bacteremia despite effective antimicrobial therapy, and inadequate antimicrobial therapy. Other indications include invasive perivalvular infection as manifested by abscess or fistula on echocardiography, new or persistent electrocardiographic changes, persistent unexplained fever, fungal endocarditis, and relapse of appropriately treated prosthetic valve endocarditis due to penicillin-sensitive streptococci.

MENINGITIS

Bacterial Meningitis

The incidence of bacterial meningitis is 4.6-10 cases/100,000 person-years. There are 2,000 deaths per year in the United States, and the case-fatality rate is 14%.

Risk factors for death include age ≥60 years, decreased mental status at admission, and occurrence of seizures within 24 hours of symptom onset. Initial cerebrospinal fluid characteristics include a cell count of 1,000-100,000/μL, a protein value ≥45 mg/dL, and a glucose value ≤40 mg/dL. The leukocyte differential is more likely to show a predominance of polymorphonuclear neutrophils. The Gram stain is positive in 75% of untreated cases. Cerebrospinal fluid bacterial cultures are positive in 70%-80% of cases. Countercurrent immunoelectrophoresis or latex agglutination test is useful for *Haemophilus influenzae* type B, *Streptococcus pneumoniae*, and *Neisseria meningitidis* types A, B, C, and Y.

- Risk factors for death in bacterial meningitis: age ≥60 years, decreased mental status at admission, seizures within 24 hours of symptom onset.
- Cerebrospinal fluid bacterial cultures are positive in 70%-80% of cases.

Among affected patients, 25% present with a fulminant illness over 24 hours, 50% have been ill for 1-7 days (usually with a respiratory illness), and 25% have had symptoms for 1-3 weeks. Organisms most commonly causing community-acquired infection in adults are *S. pneumoniae*, *N. meningitidis*, *H. influenzae*, and *Listeria monocytogenes*.

- 25% of patients with bacterial meningitis present with fulminant illness over 24 hours.
- Organisms most commonly causing community-acquired infection in adults: *S. pneumoniae*, *N. meningitidis*, *H. influenzae*, *L. monocytogenes*.
- Dexamethasone has decreased the incidence of sensorineural hearing loss in children with bacterial meningitis in two controlled trials.
- Dexamethasone treatment in adults remains controversial.

The causative organisms, affected age groups, and predisposing factors in bacterial meningitis are shown in Table 14-14, and treatment is outlined in Table 14-15.

Gram-Negative Meningitis

Gram-negative meningitis that arises spontaneously usually is a result of bacteremia from a focus of infection elsewhere in the body. Gram-negative meningitis also occurs after neurosurgical procedures or head trauma. *Escherichia coli*, *Klebsiella*, and *Pseudomonas* are the most common pathogens.

Table 14-13.--Treatment of Prosthetic Valve Infective Endocarditis

Organism	Therapy*	Therapy for patients allergic to penicillin*
Staphylococcus aureus or *S. epidermidis*		
Penicillin-sensitive (MIC, ≤0.1 µg/mL)	Penicillin G, 20 million U/24 hr i.v. (continuous drip or 6 equal doses) for 4-6 wk	Vancomycin, 30 mg/kg daily for 4-6 wk, *or* cefazolin,[†] 2 g i.v. every 8 hr for 4-6 wk
Penicillin-resistant (MIC, >0.1 µg/mL)	Nafcillin, oxacillin, 2 g i.v. every 4 hr for 4-6 wk	Same as above
Methicillin-resistant	Vancomycin, 30 mg/kg daily, *plus* rifampin,[‡] 300 mg p.o. every 8 hr for 4-6 wk, *plus* gentamicin,[§]1.5 mg/kg i.v. every 8 hr for first 2 wk of therapy	Consult infectious diseases specialist
Streptococci		
Penicillin-sensitive viridans and non-enterococcal group D (MIC, ≤0.1 µg/mL)	Penicillin G, 20 million U/24 hr i.v. (continuous drip or 6 equal doses) for 4 wk, *plus* streptomycin,[§] 7.5 mg/kg i.m. every 12 hr, *or* gentamicin,[§] 1 mg/kg i.v. every 8 hr for first 14 days	Same as for penicillin-sensitive staphylococci
Enterococci and penicillin-resistant (MIC, >0.1 µg/mL)	Penicillin G, 20 million U/24 hr i.v. (continuous drip or 6 equal doses), *plus* streptomycin,[§] 7.5 mg/kg i.m. every 12 hr, *or* gentamicin,[§] 1 mg/kg i.v. every 8 hr for 4-6 wk	Vancomycin, 30 mg/kg daily, *plus* streptomycin,[§] 7.5 mg/kg i.m. every 12 hr, *or* gentamicin,[§] 1 mg/kg i.v. every 8 hr for 4-6 wk, *or* desensitize to penicillin
Diphtheroids	Penicillin G, 20 million U/24 hr i.v. (continuous drip or 6 equal doses), *plus* gentamicin,[§] 1 mg/kg i.v. every 8 hr for 4-6 wk	Vancomycin, 30 mg/kg daily for 4-6 wk
Gram-negative bacilli	Most effective and least toxic agent, i.v. for 4-6 wk (selection should be based on results of in vitro MIC, MBC, and synergy tests)	
Fungi	Amphotericin B *plus* flucytosine *plus* cardiac valve replacement (flucytosine levels should be monitored)	

*Dosages suggested are for adults with normal renal and hepatic function.
[†]Other cephalosporins may be used in equivalent dosage, depending on results of in vitro susceptibility studies.
[‡]Vancomycin alone for methicillin-resistant *S. aureus*; combination therapy for methicillin-resistant *S. epidermidis*.
[§]Streptomycin and gentamicin doses should not exceed 500 mg and 120 mg, respectively.
i.m., intramuscularly; i.v., intravenously; MBC, minimal bactericidal concentration; MIC, minimal inhibitory concentration; p.o., by mouth.
Modified from Steckelberg JM, Giuliani ER, Wilson MR: Infective endocarditis. *In* Cardiology: Fundamentals and Practice. Vol 2. Second edition. Edited by ER Giuliani, V Fuster, BJ Gersh, MD McGoon, DC McGoon. St. Louis, Mosby Year Book, 1991, pp 1739-1772. By permission of Mayo Foundation.

Treatment often includes a third-generation cephalosporin plus an aminoglycoside. Postoperative gram-negative meningitis is usually the result of a wound infection. It is usually caused by nosocomial bacteria. Multidrug resistance is common.

- Spontaneous gram-negative meningitis usually is a result of bacteremia from a focus of infection elsewhere.
- Postoperative gram-negative meningitis is usually the result of wound infection.

Meningococcal Meningitis

Meningitis often occurs in patients who are carriers of meningococci in the nasopharynx. Terminal component complement deficiencies predispose to repeated episodes of infection. Serotypes A, B, C, and Y cause most disease. Meningitis and meningococcemia are the most common presentations. Many patients have a petechial rash. In severe disease, large purpuric areas may develop. Waterhouse-Friderichsen syndrome is not related to adrenal failure; its pathogenesis is prob-

Table 14-14.--Organisms Involved, Affected Age Groups, and Predisposing Factors in Bacterial Meningitis

Organism	Age group	Predisposing factors
Pneumococci	Any age, but often elderly--recurrent meningitis	Cerebrospinal fluid rhinorrhea, alcoholism, splenectomy, multiple myeloma, Hodgkin's disease, HIV
Meningococci	Infants-40 yr	Crowding, military recruits
Haemophilus influenzae	>neonate to 6 yr	Hypogammaglobulinemia in adults, HIV, splenectomy
Escherichia coli, group B streptococci	Neonates	
Listeria monocytogenes	Neonates; immunosuppressed	

HIV, human immunodeficiency virus.

Table 14-15.--Treatment of Bacterial Meningitis

Organism	Therapy	Alternative therapy
Pneumococci	Penicillin (check in vitro susceptibilities)	Cefotaxime, chloramphenicol, ceftriaxone, vancomycin
Meningococci	Penicillin	Same as pneumococci, except do not use vancomycin
Haemophilus influenzae	Cefotaxime, ceftriaxone	Chloramphenicol, ampicillin
Group B streptococci	Penicillin *plus* gentamicin	Same as pneumococci
Listeria	Ampicillin *plus* gentamicin	Cotrimoxazole or chloramphenicol; cephalosporins *not* effective
Gram-negative	Ceftazidime *plus* aminoglycoside	
Empiric therapy to 6 yr	Cefotaxime, ceftriaxone (add ampicillin if *L. monocytogenes* suspected)	

ably related to disseminated intravascular coagulation. Treatment is with penicillin G. If patient is allergic to penicillin, chloramphenicol, cefuroxime, or third-generation cephalosporin is used. If the risk of the carrier state is high (household contacts), rifampin or minocycline should be used for prophylaxis. The carrier state is not eliminated by penicillin. Immunization for certain populations (i.e., military recruits) is also of benefit.

- In meningococcal meningitis, terminal component complement deficiencies predispose to repeated episodes of infection.
- Meningitis and meningococcemia are most common presentations.
- Treatment is with penicillin G.

Aseptic Meningitis

This is a syndrome characterized by an acute onset of meningeal symptoms, fever, cerebrospinal fluid pleocytosis, and negative bacterial cultures from the cerebrospinal fluid. There are many infectious and noninfectious causes, but most often the cause is viral. Viral meningitis is usually a self-limited illness. Common causes include coxsackievirus, echovirus (summer), mumps virus (winter, spring), and others, including arboviruses, lymphocytic choriomeningitis virus, herpes simplex virus types 1 and 2, cytomegalovirus, human immunodeficiency virus, varicella-zoster virus, Epstein-Barr virus, and Colorado tick fever virus.

- Characteristics of aseptic meningitis: meningeal symptoms, fever, cerebrospinal fluid pleocytosis, negative bac-

terial cultures.
- Cause is often viral.
- Viral meningitis usually self-limited.

SEXUALLY TRANSMITTED DISEASES

Neisseria gonorrhoeae

Uncomplicated infection causes urethritis, cervicitis, and pharyngitis. Symptoms are indistinguishable from those of nongonococcal disease. Gram stain and culture are required for diagnosis. Asymptomatic carrier rate is high in both males and females, and these persons are primarily responsible for continued transmission of the infection. In females, concomitant proctitis is common (rectal cultures should be done in all women). Gonococcal pharyngitis is often asymptomatic. Coexistence of chlamydial infection is common (both conditions should be treated). For diagnosis, Gram stain of urethral exudate showing intracellular diplococci has high sensitivity and specificity. Cervical exudate has sensitivity of only 50% but specificity is high. Definitive diagnosis requires culture on modified Thayer-Martin medium.

- Uncomplicated *N. gonorrhoeae* infection causes urethritis, cervicitis, pharyngitis.
- Asymptomatic carrier rate is high in both males and females.

The prevalence of multiply resistant gonococcal strains is increasing (penicillin and tetracycline resistance). Thus, there have been recent changes in antimicrobial regimens. Primary treatment is ceftriaxone (125 mg intramuscularly) plus doxycycline (100 mg orally twice a day for 7 days). Alternative drugs are cefixime, ciprofloxacin, ofloxacin, and spectinomycin. All alternative agents treat urethral, cervical, rectal, and pharyngeal infection, except spectinomycin. Spectinomycin, cefixime, ciprofloxacin, and ofloxacin may not be active against incubating syphilis. Therapy in pregnant patients involves ceftriaxone (125 mg intramuscularly) plus erythromycin (500 mg orally four times a day for 7 days). If patient is allergic to cephalosporin, treatment is with ciprofloxacin or spectinomycin (2 g intramuscularly) and erythromycin (500 mg orally for 7 days). Follow-up gonococcal cultures need to be performed only if nonstandard regimens are used. All patients with sexually transmitted diseases should be considered at risk for human immunodeficiency virus (HIV) infection and testing should be offered.

- Primary treatment of *N. gonorrhoeae*: ceftriaxone (125 mg intramuscularly) plus doxycycline (100 mg orally twice a day for 7 days).

Disseminated gonococcemia is most likely to occur in females during menstruation (sloughing of endometrium allows access to blood supply, enhanced growth of gonococci due to necrotic tissue, and change in pH). There are two distinct phases. The bacteremic phase may manifest by tenosynovitis (±100%), skin lesions (±50%), and polyarthralgias. Joint culture results are usually negative. The nonbacteremic phase may present as monoarticuloarthritis of knee, wrist, and ankle; joint culture results are positive in ±50%.

- Disseminated gonococcemia is most likely to occur in females during menstruation.
- Bacteremic phase may manifest by tenosynovitis (±100%) and skin lesions (±50%); joint cultures usually negative.
- Nonbacteremic phase may present as monoarticuloarthritis of knee, wrist, ankle; joint cultures positive in ±50%.

Treatment is with ceftriaxone (1 g intravenously daily for 7-10 days); alternatives include ceftriaxone (for 3-4 days or until improvement noted) followed by cefixime or ciprofloxacin to complete a course of 7-10 days. If strain is tested and found to be penicillin-susceptible, treatment includes penicillin G (10 million units intravenously daily) for 7-10 days, or it is given for 3-4 days and then oral amoxicillin is used to finish 10-day course. If patient is allergic to cephalosporin, spectinomycin (2 g intramuscularly twice a day for 3 days) is given. Chlamydial infection can coexist with gonococcal infection and should be treated.

- Treatment: ceftriaxone (1 g intravenously daily for 7-10 days).
- Chlamydial infections can coexist with gonococcal infection and should be treated.

For meningitis, treatment includes ceftriaxone (1-2 g intravenously every 12 hours for at least 10-14 days). Alternative drugs are penicillin, if strain is susceptible, or chloramphenicol. For endocarditis, ceftriaxone or penicillin is used for at least 28 days.

Nongonococcal Urethritis and Cervicitis

The most common etiologic agent is *Chlamydia trachomatis*. Doxycycline (100 mg twice a day for 7 days) is standard treatment. Azithromycin as a 1-g single dose and ofloxacin may also be effective. If urethritis does not resolve with a tetracycline, consider tetracycline-resistant *Ureaplasma urealyticum* or *Trichomonas*.

- Nongonococcal urethritis and cervicitis are more commonly caused by *C. trachomatis*.

Herpes Genitalis

For the first episode, therapy with acyclovir (400 mg orally three times a day or 200 mg orally five times a day for 7-10 days) shortens the duration of pain, viral shedding, and systemic symptoms. If symptoms are severe, acyclovir at a dosage of 5 mg/kg intravenously every 8 hours for 5-7 days is used. Topical acyclovir has marginal benefit for decreasing viral shedding and has no effect on symptoms or healing time. For recurrent episodes with severe symptoms, therapy is started at prodrome or within 2 days of onset of symptoms (acyclovir, 400 mg orally three times a day for 5 days). Recurrence after therapy is not related to development of in vitro resistance of herpes simplex to acyclovir. For suppression, in selected patients with more than six recurrences a year, acyclovir, 400 mg twice a day, is used for up to 1 year.

Syphilis

In 1990, the incidence of primary and secondary syphilis was 20/100,000. It is estimated that half of cases are not reported. Incidence has been increasing among heterosexuals since 1985, particularly among inner-city minority populations.

The fluorescent treponemal antibody absorption (FTA-ABS) test is the most helpful serologic test for the diagnosis of syphilis (Table 14-16). Results of this test will be positive before those on VDRL testing and thus may be positive without a positive VDRL result in primary syphilis.

- FTA-ABS is most helpful serologic test for diagnosis of syphilis.
- VDRL results may be negative in 30% of patients with primary syphilis.

A chancre (clean, indurated ulcer) is the main manifestation of *primary syphilis*. It occurs at the site of inoculation and is usually painless. The incubation period is 3-90 days. It should be distinguished from herpes simplex virus and chancroid (painful exudative ulcer, *Haemophilus ducreyi*). Diagnosis is made by dark field examination.

The manifestations of *secondary syphilis* result from hematogenous dissemination and usually occur 2-8 weeks after appearance of the chancre. Constitutional symptoms occur, in addition to rash, alopecia, condylomata lata, and various other symptoms and signs. The diagnosis is based on the

Table 14-16.--Laboratory Diagnosis of Syphilis

Syphilis	Test, % positive	
	FTA-ABS	VDRL
Primary	85	70
Secondary	100	99
Tertiary	98	1[*]

[*]Treated late syphilis.
FTA-ABS, fluorescent treponemal antibody absorption.
Modified from Tramont EC: *Treponema pallidum* (syphilis). *In* Principles and Practice of Infectious Diseases. Third edition. Edited by GL Mandell, RG Douglas Jr, JE Bennett. New York, Churchill Livingstone, 1990, pp 1794-1808. By permission of publisher.

clinical picture and serologic testing. The condition resolves spontaneously without treatment.

Latent syphilis is the asymptomatic stage after symptoms of secondary syphilis subside. Those that occur after 1 year are classified as late. The diagnosis is based on serologic testing.

Tertiary syphilis can involve all body systems (i.e., cardiovascular--aortitis involving ascending aorta, which can cause aneurysms and aortic regurgitation; gummatous osteomyelitis; hepatitis). However, neurosyphilis is the most common manifestation in the United States.

Neurosyphilis is often asymptomatic. Symptomatic disease is divided into several clinical syndromes that may overlap and occur at any time after primary infection. The diagnosis is made by cerebrospinal fluid examination. Abnormalities include mononuclear pleocytosis and elevated protein value. VDRL testing of cerebrospinal fluid is only 30%-70% sensitive. Any cerebrospinal fluid abnormality in a patient who is seropositive for syphilis must be investigated. Syndromes include 1) meningovascular syphilis (occurs 4-7 years after infection and presents with focal central nervous system deficits such as stroke) and 2) parenchymatous syphilis (general paresis or tabes dorsalis). Parenchymatous syphilis occurs decades after infection and may present as general paresis (chronic progressive dementia) or as tabes dorsalis (sensory ataxia, lightning pains, autonomic dysfunction, optic atrophy). A cerebrospinal fluid examination in patients with syphilis is indicated in those with neurologic abnormalities, before re-treatment of relapses, in infants with congenital syphilis, and as a baseline study in all patients to be treated with a nonpenicillin regimen.

- Neurosyphilis is most common manifestation (in tertiary disease) in the United States.
- Diagnosis is made with cerebrospinal fluid examination.
- VDRL testing of cerebrospinal fluid is only 30%-70% sensitive.

Treatment of syphilis is based on whether the disease is early or late. For early syphilis (primary, secondary, or early latent [<1 year]), benzathine penicillin is used--2.4 million units intramuscularly; follow-up serologic testing is done. (Some experts recommend a second dose in 7 days in patients with HIV infection.) Alternatives are doxycycline, 100 mg twice a day for 14 days, and erythromycin, 500 mg four times a day for 14 days. Follow-up serologic testing is important. Treatment for late disease (>1 year in duration, cardiovascular disease, gumma, late latent syphilis) is with benzathine penicillin, 2.4 million units intramuscularly weekly for 3 weeks. Alternatives are doxycycline, 100 mg orally twice a day for 4 weeks. Follow-up serologic tests are recommended.

Treatment for neurosyphilis is with aqueous penicillin G, 12-24 million units intravenously per day for 10-14 days, or procaine penicillin, 2.4 million units intramuscularly per day, plus probenecid, 500 mg four times a day for 10-14 days.

For early and secondary syphilis, follow-up clinical and serologic testing should be performed at 3 and 6 months. Re-treatment with three weekly injections with 2.4 million units of benzathine penicillin G should be given to patients with signs or symptoms that persist or whose VDRL result has a sustained fourfold increase in titer. If VDRL does not decrease fourfold by 3 months, consideration should also be given to re-treatment. Patients with latent syphilis should have follow-up at 6 and 12 months. If titers of VDRL test increase fourfold, if high titer >1:32 fails to decrease fourfold within 12-24 months, or if signs or symptoms attributable to syphilis occur, the patient should be examined for neurosyphilis and re-treated. Follow-up of neurosyphilis should include testing of cerebrospinal fluid every 6 months if cerebrospinal fluid pleocytosis was present initially; this testing is done until results are normal. If the cell count is not decreased at 6 months or if cerebrospinal fluid is not entirely normal at 2 years, re-treatment should be considered.

Pelvic Inflammatory Disease

In this condition, proximal spread of infection from the endocervix causes endometritis, salpingitis, tubo-ovarian abscess, or pelvic peritonitis in various combinations. Organisms responsible are *N. gonorrhoeae, C. trachomatis, Mycoplasma hominis,* and various aerobic gram-negative rods and anaerobes. *Actinomyces israelii* can be a pathogen in patients with an intrauterine device. Tuberculosis in older women, including postmenopausal women, should be considered. Clinical signs and symptoms include lower abdominal tenderness, adnexal tenderness, cervical motion tenderness, oral temperature ≥38.3°C, abnormal cervical discharge, increased erythrocyte sedimentation rate, and evidence of *N. gonorrhoeae* or *C. trachomatis* infection. Laboratory evidence includes laparoscopic or ultrasound documentation.

- In pelvic inflammatory disease, responsible organisms are *N. gonorrhoeae, C. trachomatis,* and anaerobes.

Treatment for inpatients includes cefoxitin, 2 g intravenously every 6 hours, cefotetan, 2 g intravenously every 12 hours, or clindamycin and gentamicin plus doxycycline, 100 mg intravenously every 12 hours, followed by doxycycline, 100 mg orally twice a day for 14 days. For outpatients, treatment is with ceftriaxone, 250 mg intramuscularly once, or cefoxitin, 2 g intramuscularly once, plus doxycycline, 100 mg orally twice a day for 14 days. Hospitalization is indicated when the diagnosis is uncertain, pelvic abscess or peritonitis is present, patient is pregnant, patient is adolescent, HIV infection is present, or noncompliance is suspected. Tubo-ovarian abscess may be characterized by adnexal mass on physical examination or radiographic examination or by failure of antimicrobial therapy. Medical treatment is successful in 50% of cases. Careful follow-up is required.

- Tubo-ovarian abscess is characterized by adnexal mass on physical examination or radiographic examination or by failure of antimicrobial therapy.

Trichomonas vaginalis

Infection with this organism produces a yellow, purulent discharge in 5%-40% of cases. Dysuria and dyspareunia occur in 30%-50% of cases. Petechial lesions on the cervix are noted with colposcopy (strawberry cervix) in 50% of cases. The vaginal pH is usually ≥4.5. The diagnosis is established by wet mount preparation of vaginal secretion (80% sensitive). Culture is done in difficult cases. Treatment is with metronidazole, 500 mg twice a day for 7 days. All partners should be examined and treated if necessary.

- *T. vaginalis* infection is often characterized by yellow, purulent discharge.
- Diagnosis is established with wet mount of vaginal secretion.
- Treatment: metronidazole orally.

Gardnerella vaginalis (Bacterial Vaginosis)

This condition is characterized by a malodorous "fishy" smell and a grayish discharge that is homogeneous and coats the vaginal walls. Dysuria and pain are relatively uncommon. Other organisms associated with the syndrome are *Mobiluncus* and *M. hominis.* The diagnosis is determined by excluding *Candida* and *Trichomonas* infections and other sexually transmitted diseases. The following are characteristics of the vaginal secretion: demonstration of "clue" cells on wet mount examination, pH >4.5 and often ≥6.0, and a "fishy" smell when secretion is mixed with KOH. Metronidazole, 500 mg twice a day, is standard therapy. Topical clindamycin or metronidazole may also be effective. Treatment of asymptomatic carriers is not recommended.

- Diagnosis of *G. vaginalis* is established by excluding *Candida, Trichomonas,* other sexually transmitted diseases.
- Vaginal discharge has "clue" cells and a "fishy" smell when mixed with 10% KOH and has pH >4.5.

Vulvovaginal Candidiasis

The predominant symptom of this condition is pruritus. Usually there is no odor, and discharge is scant, watery, and white. "Cottage cheese curds" may adhere to the vaginal wall. The diagnosis is made by addition of 10% KOH to discharge to demonstrate pseudohyphae. Culture may detect an asymptomatic carrier. Treatment is with topical miconazole, clotrimazole, butoconazole, terconazole, or tioconazole. Oral azoles (ketoconazole, fluconazole) are used only for severe, refractory cases. In severe or recurrent cases, consider HIV infection.

- In vulvovaginal candidiasis, "cottage cheese curds" may adhere to the vaginal wall.
- In severe or recurrent cases, consider HIV infection.

Epididymitis

This condition is usually unilateral. It should be distinguished from testicular torsion. In young, sexually active men, *C. trachomatis* and *N. gonorrhoeae* are the common pathogens. In older men, aerobic gram-negative rods and enterococci predominate. Urologic abnormality is more common in this population than in younger men. Doxycycline, 100 mg orally twice a day for 7 days, plus ceftriaxone, 250 mg intramuscularly, is the treatment of choice in young males. In older men, treatment is individualized on the basis of results of urine Gram stain, results of culture, local susceptibility patterns, and presence of recent instrumentation.

- Epididymitis is usually unilateral; should be distinguished from testicular torsion.
- In young, sexually active men, *C. trachomatis* and *N. gonorrhoeae* are the common pathogens.

GASTROINTESTINAL INFECTION

Bacterial Diarrhea

The principal causes of toxigenic diarrhea are listed in Table 14-17, and those of invasive diarrhea are listed in Table 14-18. Fecal leukocytes are usually absent in toxigenic diarrhea. In invasive diarrhea, fecal leukocytes are usually present.

Campylobacter jejuni is being recognized with increasing frequency as a common cause of bacterial diarrhea. Outbreaks are associated with consumption of unpasteurized milk and undercooked poultry. The incidence of disease peaks in summer and early fall. Diarrhea may be bloody. Fever is usually present. The diagnosis is established by isolation of the organism from stool; a special medium is required. Treatment is with erythromycin. Alternatives are ciprofloxacin and norfloxacin (emergence of resistance to fluoroquinolones has been reported). Supportive care is also needed.

- Outbreaks of bacterial diarrhea caused by *C. jejuni* are associated with consumption of unpasteurized milk and undercooked poultry.

Table 14-17.--Bacterial Diarrhea: Toxigenic

Organism	Onset after ingestion, hr	Preformed toxin	Fever present	Vomiting predominates
Staphylococcus aureus	2-6	Yes	No	Yes
Clostridium perfringens	8-16	No	No	No
Escherichia coli	12	No	No	No
Vibrio cholerae	12	No	Secondary to dehydration	No
Bacillus cereus				
a.	1-6	Yes	No	Yes
b.	8-16	No	No	No

Table 14-18.--Bacterial Diarrhea: Invasive

Organism	Fever present	Bloody diarrhea present	Antibiotics effective
Shigella species	Yes	Yes	Yes
Salmonella (non-*typhi*)	Yes	No	No
Vibrio parahaemolyticus	Yes	Yes (occasional)	No
Escherichia coli 0157:H7	Yes	Yes	No
Campylobacter	Yes	Yes	Yes
Yersinia	Yes	Yes (occasional)	±

In bacterial diarrhea caused by *Staphylococcus aureus*, preformed toxin is ingested in contaminated food. Onset is abrupt, with severe vomiting (often predominates), diarrhea, and abdominal cramps. The duration of infection is 8-24 hours. Diagnosis is based on *rapid onset*, absence of fever, and history. Treatment is supportive.

- Bacterial diarrhea caused by *S. aureus* is caused by ingestion of preformed toxin in contaminated food.

Bacterial diarrhea caused by *Clostridium perfringens* is associated with ingestion of bacteria that produce toxin in vivo in precooked foods (meat and poultry products). Food is precooked and toxin is destroyed but spores survive; when food is rewarmed, spores germinate. When food is ingested, toxin is produced. Diarrhea is worse than vomiting, and abdominal cramping is prominent. Onset of symptoms is later than with *S. aureus* infection. Duration of illness is 24 hours. The diagnosis is based on the later onset of symptoms and a typical history. Treatment is supportive.

- In diarrhea caused by *C. perfringens*, ingested bacteria produce toxin in vivo in precooked food.
- Diarrhea worse than vomiting; abdominal cramping prominent.

Two types of food poisoning are associated with *Bacillus cereus* infection. A short incubation period (1-6 hours) is followed by profuse vomiting; this is associated with the ingestion of a preformed toxin (usually in fried rice). A disease with a longer incubation occurs 8-16 hours after consumption; profound diarrhea develops and is usually associated with eating meat or vegetables. The diagnosis is confirmed by isolation of the organism from contaminated food. The illness is self-limited and treatment is supportive.

Diarrhea caused by *Escherichia coli* can be either enterotoxigenic or enterohemorrhagic. Enterotoxigenic *E. coli* is the most common etiologic agent in traveler's diarrhea. Treatment consists of fluid and electrolyte replacement along with loperamide plus trimethoprim-sulfamethoxazole, ciprofloxacin, or norfloxacin. Medical evaluation should be sought if fever and bloody diarrhea occur. For prophylaxis, water, fruits, and vegetables need to be chosen carefully. Routine use of trimethoprim-sulfamethoxazole, ciprofloxacin, and doxycycline is not recommended because the risks outweigh the benefits in most travelers. Bismuth subsalicylate reduces the incidence of enterotoxigen *E. coli*-associated diarrhea by up to 60%. Patients who are allergic to salicylates or who are taking therapeutic doses of salicylates or anticoagulants should not use bismuth subsalicylate.

- Enterotoxigenic *E. coli* is the most common etiologic agent in traveler's diarrhea.

A relatively uncommon form of bloody diarrhea is caused by *E. coli* 0157:H7. This agent has been identified as the cause of waterborne illness (Missouri), outbreaks in nursing homes and child care centers, and sporadic cases. It has also been transmitted by eating undercooked beef. This mode of transmission was recently the cause of an outbreak in patrons of a fast-food restaurant chain in the state of Washington. This enterohemorrhagic illness is characterized by bloody diarrhea, severe abdominal cramps, fever, and profound toxicity. It may resemble ischemic colitis. At extremes of age (old and young), the infection may produce hemolytic-uremic syndrome, thrombocytopenic purpura, and death. This organism should be considered in all patients with hemolytic-uremic syndrome. Antibiotics are not known to be effective.

- *E. coli* 0157:H7 has been identified as the cause of waterborne illness, outbreaks in nursing homes and child care centers, and sporadic cases.
- Also transmitted by eating undercooked beef.
- Characterized by bloody diarrhea, severe abdominal cramps, profound toxicity; may resemble ischemic colitis.
- Organism should be considered in all patients in age group with hemolytic-uremic syndrome.

Vibrio cholerae causes the only toxigenic bacterial diarrheal disease in which antibiotics (tetracycline) clearly shorten the duration of disease. However, fluid replacement therapy is the mainstay of management. It is associated with consumption of undercooked shellfish. Recently, there was an epidemic in Peru and other parts of South America, and cases in the United States have occurred because of this epidemic.

Diarrhea caused by *Shigella* species is often acquired outside the United States. It is often spread by person-to-person transmission but has also been associated with eating contaminated food or water. A recent outbreak was due to contaminated sandwiches on an airliner. Bloody diarrhea is characteristic, bacteremia may occur, and fever is present. The diagnosis is based on results of stool culture and blood culture (occasionally positive). Treatment is with ampicillin; however, *ampicillin-resistant strains are emerging.* Trimethoprim-sulfamethoxazole is also effective, but in some countries increasing resistance is being reported. Norfloxacin and ciprofloxacin are alternatives. The illness may precede the onset of Reiter's syndrome. Neurotoxin may cause seizures in pediatric patients.

- Diarrhea caused by *Shigella* species is associated with person-to-person transmission and the consumption of contaminated food or water.
- Bloody diarrhea is characteristic, bacteremia may occur, and fever is present.
- Illness may precede onset of Reiter's syndrome.

Salmonella (non-*typhi*)-associated illness is most commonly caused by *S. enteritidis* and *S. typhimurium* in the United States. It is associated with consumption of dehydrated foods or poultry products or with exposure to pet turtles, ducklings, and iguanas. *S. javiana* and *S. oranienburg* are found in contaminated cheese. *Salmonella* infection is a common cause of severe diarrhea and may cause septicemia in patients with acquired immunodeficiency syndrome (AIDS). Fever is present, and bloody diarrhea is absent (main characteristic distinguishing it from *Shigella* infection). The diagnosis is based on stool culture. Treatment is supportive. Antibiotics only prolong the carrier state and do not affect the course of the disease. Antibiotics are used if blood culture results are positive. This illness may precede onset of Reiter's syndrome.

- *Salmonella* infection is common cause of severe diarrhea.
- May cause septicemia in patients with AIDS.
- Bloody diarrhea is absent (feature distinguishing it from *Shigella* infection).

Vibrio parahaemolyticus infection is acquired by eating undercooked shellfish. It is a common bacterial cause of acute food-borne illness in Japan and is appearing with increasing frequency in the United States (Atlantic Gulf Coast and on cruise ships). Acute onset of explosive watery diarrhea and fever are characteristic. The diagnosis is determined with stool culture. Antibiotic therapy is not required.

- *V. parahaemolyticus* infection is acquired by eating undercooked shellfish.
- Acute onset of watery diarrhea and fever are characteristic.
- Antibiotic therapy is not required.

Clinical syndromes associated with *Vibrio vulnificus* include bacteremia, gastroenteritis, and cellulitis. Most patients with bacteremia have distinctive bullous skin lesions and underlying hepatic disease (cirrhosis). The condition is associated with consumption of raw oysters. The mortality rate is high. Wound infections occur in patients who have had contact with sea water, such as with fishing injuries or contamination of wound with sea water. Affected patients have intense pain and cellulitis in the extremities. Gastrointestinal illness is associated with consumption of raw oysters. The incubation period is 18 hours. Vomiting, diarrhea, and severe abdominal cramps are features. Treatment is with tetracycline or chloramphenicol.

- *V. vulnificus* bacteremia can cause distinctive bullous skin lesions and occur in patients who are immunocompromised or have cirrhosis.
- Associated with consumption of raw oysters.

Yersinia enterocolitica is the etiologic agent of four major clinical syndromes. Acquisition of infection is associated with eating contaminated food products. Pigs are a common reservoir, and the infection may be associated with eating pork. Recently, the illness was associated with transfusion-related bacteremia.

The four syndromes that result from *Y. enterocolitica* infection are as follows.
1. Enterocolitis is the most common, especially in young children. Diarrhea is bloody in 25% of cases. Infection itself is limited. Antibiotic therapy is not necessary. 2. Mesenteric adenitis (pseudoappendicitis syndrome) develops in older children and young adults. Antibiotic therapy is not helpful. 3. Postinfectious syndromes usually occur in adults; these include erythema nodosum, polyarthritis, and Reiter's syndrome. Postinfectious syndromes usually begin 1 to 2 weeks after gastrointestinal symptoms. The polyarthritis often includes weight-bearing joints (knees and ankles). Symptoms may last 1 to 4 months or longer. HLA-B27 antigen may be positive in patients with polyarthritis or Reiter's syndrome but is not associated with erythema nodosum. Cultures of synovial fluid are negative. Diagnosis is by stool culture or serologic testing. 4. Bacteremia is associated with contaminated blood products and alcoholism. Many patients have underlying disease such as cirrhosis. Treatment with trimethoprim-sulfamethoxazole, tetracycline, and gentamicin has been effective.

- Adults with *Y. enterocolitica* infection can develop erythema nodosum, polyarthritis, and Reiter's syndrome.

Colitis caused by *Clostridium difficile* should be distinguished from other forms of antibiotic-associated diarrhea (watery stools, no systemic symptoms, negative tests for *C. difficile* toxin). Symptoms often occur 2-4 weeks after stopping use of antibiotics. The illness is associated with antibiotic exposure in 99% of cases (any antibiotic can cause it). Nosocomial spread has been documented. Typical features are profuse, watery stools, crampy abdominal pain, constitutional illness, fecal leukocyte value >50%, positive for *C. difficile* toxin. In toxin-negative disease, proctoscopy or flexible sigmoidoscopy can be used to look for pseudomembranes. Disease can be localized to cecum (postoperative patient with ileus) and can present as fever of unknown origin. Treatment consists of vancomycin (125 mg orally four times a day for 7-10 days) or metronidazole (250-500 mg orally three to four times a day for 7-10 days). Cost differences favor metronidazole. Antiperistalsis drugs should not be used. If patient is unable to take drugs orally, intravenous metronidazole (not vancomycin) or vancomycin enemas can be used. Relapse is frequent and requires re-treatment. Treatment of asymptomatic carriers to decrease nosocomial spread of infection or to reduce risk of pseudomembranous colitis is not recommended.

- Colitis caused by *C. difficile* often occurs 2-4 weeks after stopping use of antibiotics.

- Illness is associated with antibiotic exposure in 99% of cases (any antibiotic can cause it).
- Features: profuse watery stools, crampy abdominal pain, constitutional illness, fecal leukocyte >50%, positive for *C. difficile* toxin.
- Treatment: vancomycin (125 mg orally four times a day for 7-10 days) or metronidazole (250-500 mg orally three to four times a day for 7-10 days).
- Relapse is frequent (about 15% of cases).

Viral Diarrhea

Rotavirus infection is the most common cause of sporadic mild diarrhea illness in children. It may be spread from children to adults. It usually occurs during the winter. Vomiting is a more common early manifestation than watery diarrhea. Hospitalization for dehydration is common in young children. Diagnosis is made by detection of antigen in stool (enzyme-linked immunosorbent assay). Treatment is symptomatic.

Norwalk virus is a common cause of epidemic diarrhea and "winter vomiting disease" in older children and adults. It occurs in families, communities, and institutions. Outbreaks have been associated with eating shellfish, undercooked fish, cake frosting, and salads and with drinking contaminated water. It is the cause of up to 10% of gastroenteritis outbreaks. Illness is characterized by nausea, vomiting, and watery diarrhea. It is a mild, self-limited (<36 hours) illness. Currently, no diagnostic test is available. Treatment is symptomatic.

- Outbreaks of Norwalk virus are associated with eating shellfish, undercooked fish, cake frosting, and salads and with drinking contaminated water.
- Illness is mild, self-limited (<36 hours).

SEPTIC SHOCK

This clinical syndrome is characterized by impaired tissue perfusion, hypotension, and multiorgan dysfunction in the setting of infection (blood cultures positive in 50%-60% of cases). Causative organism is gram-negative aerobic bacilli in 70% of cases, gram-positive aerobic cocci in 20%-30%, and other organisms in 2%-3% (i.e., *Candida* species). In septic shock, most frequent blood isolates are *Escherichia coli, Klebsiella-Enterobacter, Proteus, Pseudomonas, Staphylococcus aureus*, and *Streptococcus pneumoniae*. Frequency of any one organism depends on the host (i.e., neutropenia is associated with *P. aeruginosa*, central lines are associated with coagulase-negative staphylococci, *S. aureus*, and *Candida* species). Overall mortality rate is 20%-30%. Endotoxin activates endogenous mediators of inflammation with catastrophic consequences. Result can be increased vascular permeability, a decrease in peripheral vascular resistance, profound hypotension with progressive lactic acidosis, and death. Management involves maintaining intravascular volume, administering appropriate bactericidal antimicrobials, and correcting any problems that lead to infection (e.g., draining abscesses). Steroids are of no benefit and may be harmful.

- In septic shock, blood cultures positive in 50%-60% of cases.
- Most frequent blood isolates: *E. coli, Klebsiella-Enterobacter, Proteus, Pseudomonas, S. aureus, S. pneumoniae*.
- Endotoxin activates endogenous mediators of inflammation with catastrophic consequences.

GRANULOCYTOPENIA

This condition is characterized by an absolute polymorphonuclear neutrophil value ≤500/mm^3. If ecthyma gangrenosum is present, *Pseudomonas* infection should be considered. Other gram-negative aerobic rods (i.e., *Escherichia coli*) also cause bacteremia. Aerobic gram-positive cocci (*Staphylococcus aureus*, coagulase-negative staphylococci, enterococci, viridans streptococci, *C. jeikeium*) are often associated with infection in neutropenic patients with central venous catheters. *Candida* species should be considered in cases associated with nodular skin lesions, fluffy white chorioretinal exudates, and fever unresponsive to empiric antibacterial agents. Anaerobic organisms are uncommon, except in cases of perirectal abscess and gingivitis. Empiric antimicrobial therapy is required. Ceftazidime alone is the preferred initial empiric antibacterial regimen. Alternative therapy is an aminoglycoside plus an antipseudomonal penicillin. There is no need to use vancomycin empirically. If subsequent cultures show presence of staphylococci, vancomycin can be added to the regimen. If there is no response after 4-7 days of treatment, amphotericin B therapy is often recommended.

URINARY TRACT INFECTION

In Females

Table 14-19 outlines the categories of acute dysuria.

Because urethritis or cystitis can occur with low colony counts of bacteria, routine urine cultures in young women with dysuria are not recommended. Urinalysis should be done with or without a Gram stain. If pyuria and uncomplicated urinary tract infection (UTI) are present, short-course treatment should be initiated. (Only if occult upper tract disease, a complicated UTI, or sexually transmitted disease is suspected should appropriate culture and sensitivity testing be performed.) Risk factors for occult infection and complications include emergency room presentation, low socioeconomic status, hospital-acquired infection, pregnancy, use of Foley catheter, recent instrumentation, known urologic abnormality, previous relapse, UTI at

Table 14-19.--Categorization of Acute Dysuria

Category	Site affected			Colony count	Pyuria present	Antimicrobial treatment effective
	Upper tract	Bladder	Urethra			
Subclinical pyelo-nephritis	Yes	Yes	Yes	>100,000	Yes	Yes
Lower UTI--urethritis or cystitis	No	Yes	Yes	>100	Yes	Yes
Chlamydia, HSV, Neisseria gonorrhoeae	No	No	Yes	0-100	Yes	Yes
No recognized pathogen	No	?	Yes	0-100	No	No
Vaginitis	No	No	No	0-100	No	Yes

HSV, herpes simplex virus; UTI, urinary tract infection.

age <12 years, acute pyelonephritis or three or more UTIs in 1 year, symptoms ≥7 days, recent antibiotic use, diabetes mellitus, and immunosuppression. Causative organisms include *Escherichia coli* and *Staphylococcus saprophyticus* (susceptible to ampicillin and trimethoprim-sulfamethoxazole).

- Routine urine cultures are not recommended in young women with dysuria.
- Associated organisms: *E. coli, S. saprophyticus* (susceptible to trimethoprim-sulfamethoxazole).

For first episode of cystitis or urethritis, treatment is given but no investigation is needed. Trimethoprim-sulfamethoxazole is more effective than ampicillin. Short-course treatment (single-dose) has fewer side effects than standard (7-10 days) therapy, but the risk of relapse (due to retention of viable organisms in vaginal or perivaginal area) is higher. Three-day therapy may be associated with relapse rates equal to those with treatment for 7-10 days with less toxicity. If recurrence develops after 3-day therapy, subclinical pyelonephritis is likely and treatment is then given for 14 days. Urologic evaluation is usually not necessary. It should be performed in patients with multiple relapses, painless hematuria, a history of childhood UTI, renal lithiasis, and recurrent pyelonephritis.

- For first episode of cystitis or urethritis, trimethoprim-sulfamethoxazole is more effective than ampicillin.
- Short-course treatment (3 days) has fewer side effects than standard (7-10 days) therapy, and risk of relapse of infection may be the same.
- Urologic evaluation should be done in patients with multiple relapses, painless hematuria, history of childhood UTI, renal lithiasis, and recurrent pyelonephritis.

For acute pyelonephritis, 2 weeks of therapy is equal in effi-

cacy to 6 weeks of therapy. Most patients are sufficiently ill to require hospitalization. Many are bacteremic. Unless gram-positive cocci are seen on Gram stain (?enterococci), a third-generation cephalosporin can be used as empiric therapy. If enterococci are suspected, use ampicillin or mezlocillin with or without gentamicin. Oral regimens can be quickly substituted as the patient improves. A urine culture is recommended at the completion of therapy. If relapse occurs, treatment is given for 6 weeks and a urologic evaluation is done. For recurrent lower UTI (more than two episodes per year), single-dose therapy, 3-day therapy, or 6-week therapy is used. For treatment failure, chronic suppressive therapy may be used; however, the risk of resistant organisms must be weighed.

- For acute pyelonephritis, 2 weeks of therapy is equal in efficacy to 6 weeks of therapy.
- Urine culture is recommended at 2 weeks after therapy.

In Males

UTI is less common in males than females. Urologic abnormalities (e.g., benign prostatic hyperplasia) are common. Symptoms are unreliable for localization. Physical examination should include prostate examination, retraction of the foreskin to look for discharge, and palpation of the testicles and epididymides. When a UTI is suspected, urine culture and sensitivity testing should always be done. Causative organisms include *E. coli* in 50% of cases, other gram-negative organisms in 25%, enterococci in 20%, and others in 5%. If signs and symptoms of epididymitis, acute prostatitis, and pyelonephritis are present, treat accordingly. If uncomplicated lower UTI is present, treat for 10-14 days. If symptoms persist or relapse, repeat the urine culture. If results are positive, treat for a minimum of 6 weeks. If culture results are negative, consider chronic prostatitis or nonbacterial or noninfectious diseases and treat accordingly.

- Causes of UTI in males: *E. coli* in 50%, other gram-negative organisms in 25%, enterococci in 20%, others in 5%.

ANAEROBIC SOFT TISSUE INFECTIONS

These may be caused by various aerobic and anaerobic organisms. Findings and treatments for these are outlined in Table 14-20.

BONE AND JOINT INFECTIONS

Acute Bacterial Arthritis (Nongonococcal)

This is most commonly due to hematogenous spread of bacteria. The hip and knee joints are commonly involved. Bacteria involved are gram-positive aerobic cocci (about 75% of cases): *Staphylococcus aureus* (most common), β-hemolytic streptococci, and *Streptococcus pneumoniae*. Gram-negative aerobic bacilli can also cause infection (about 20% of cases); *Pseudomonas aeruginosa* is a common cause in injection drug users. Anaerobes, fungi, and mycobacteria are unusual causes. Clinical features include involvement usually of monoarticular, large joints. Fever, pain, swelling, and restriction of motion are the most frequent signs and symptoms. The synovial fluid is usually turbid, and the leukocyte count is 10,000-300,000/μL (predominantly polymorphonuclear neutrophils). The condition may overlap with other inflammatory arthropathies. Gram stain is 50%-95% sensitive. Culture results are positive unless antibiotics have been used previously or the pathogen is unusual. Blood culture results are often positive. Radiographs are not helpful in routine cases because destructive changes have not had time to occur. Specific antimicrobial therapy is based on results of Gram stain, culture, and sensitivity testing. The duration of therapy is dependent on individual circumstances, such as the presence of complicating osteomyelitis. Usually, treatment is given for 2-6 weeks. Empiric therapy should include agents directed against *S. aureus* and gram-negative bacilli. Drainage is essential. Percutaneous, arthroscopic, or open procedures are used. Hip, shoulder, and sternoclavicular joint involvement, development of loculations, and persistently positive culture results (not due to resistant organisms) are standard indications for arthroscopy or open debridement.

- Acute bacterial arthritis (nongonococcal) is most commonly due to hematogenous spread of bacteria.
- Bacteria involved are gram-positive aerobic cocci (about 75% of cases): *S. aureus* is most common.
- Monoarticular, large joints are usually involved.
- Fever, pain, swelling, and restriction of motion are frequent.
- Synovial fluid is turbid; leukocyte count is 10,000-300,000/μL.
- Blood culture results are positive in 50% of cases.
- Drainage is essential.

Viral Arthritis

This is usually transient, self-limited polyarthritis. It may be caused by rubella (may also occur after vaccination), hepatitis B, mumps, coxsackievirus, adenovirus, and parvovirus B19.

Chronic Monoarticular Arthritis

Organisms involved include *Mycobacteria* (*M. tuberculosis* is more common than *M. avium-intercellulare*, *M. kansasii*, *M. marinum*), fungi (*Coccidioides immitis* and *Sporothrix schenckii* are more common than *Histoplasma capsulatum*--rare, *Blastomyces dermatitidis*--acute, and *Candida* species--acute), and others (*Brucella*, *Nocardia*).

Table 14-20.--Findings and Treatment in Anaerobic Soft Tissue Infections

	Gas gangrene (organism: *Clostridium perfringens*)	Anaerobic cellulitis (polymicrobial)
Clinical finding		
Gas in tissues	1+	4+
Muscle necrosis	Present by definition	Absent by definition
Pain	4+	1+
Appearance	Skin is taut, swollen, edematous, pale; minimal crepitation	4+ crepitation
Treatment	Immediate wide debridement or amputation, antibiotics, ± hyperbaric oxygen treatment	Antibiotics alone, local wound care, incision and drainage

- *M. tuberculosis, Coccidioides,* and *Blastomyces* are involved in chronic monoarticular arthritis.

Osteomyelitis

Acute hematogenous osteomyelitis is more common in infants and children than adults. Metaphysis of long bones (femur, tibia) is most commonly affected. *S. aureus* is the most common organism. Acute onset of pain and fever are typical features. The illness can present with pain only. Compatible radiographic changes and bone biopsy for culture and pathologic examination are used to establish the diagnosis. Blood culture results may be positive. Specific parenteral antibiotic therapy is used for 3-6 weeks on basis of culture and sensitivity test results. Debridement is usually not necessary unless sequestrum is present.

- *S. aureus* is the most common organism in acute hematogenous osteomyelitis.
- Acute onset of pain and fever are typical features.

Chronic osteomyelitis is more common in adults. It results from direct inoculation caused by trauma or adjacent soft tissue infection, for example. Open fractures and diabetic foot ulcers are common predisposing factors. *S. aureus* is the most common organism. Coagulase-negative staphylococci are often pathogens if a foreign body (e.g., plate, screws) is present. Often, osteomyelitis complicating a foot ulcer is polymicrobial, including aerobic gram-positive and gram-negative organisms and anaerobes. Local pain, tenderness, erythema, and draining sinuses are common. Fever is atypical unless there is concurrent cellulitis. The condition can present with pain only. Compatible radiographic changes (often vague) and bone biopsy for culture and pathologic examination are used to establish the diagnosis. Blood culture results are rarely positive. Adequate debridement, removal of dead space, soft tissue coverage, and fixation of infected fractures are essential. Specific parenteral antibiotic therapy is given for 4-6 weeks on basis of culture and sensitivity test results.

- *S. aureus* is the most common organism in chronic osteomyelitis.
- Coagulase-negative staphylococci is a common pathogen if foreign body is present.
- Local pain, tenderness, erythema, and draining sinuses are common.
- Specific parenteral antibiotic therapy is given for 4-6 weeks.

Vertebral Osteomyelitis

This condition often results from hematogenous dissemination from focal source of infection (e.g., urinary tract, pneumonia). *S. aureus* and gram-negative bacilli are the major pathogens. Only 10% of cases have positive blood culture results. Symptoms include pain and local tenderness. Fever may be present. Leukocyte count may be normal or elevated. Sedimentation rate is often increased. Plain radiographs do not show destruction early in the course of disease. Gallium scan is approximately 80% sensitive. Magnetic resonance imaging is diagnostic test of choice because it is sensitive and specific and shows anatomic detail (coexistent epidural abscess). Percutaneous needle biopsy (computed tomography-guided) or open biopsy of bone or disc tissue may be needed. Treatment includes appropriate parenteral antimicrobial therapy for 4-6 weeks. Drainage may be necessary if a concomitant epidural abscess is present.

- In vertebral osteomyelitis, *S. aureus* and gram-negative bacilli are major pathogens.
- Gallium scan is about 80% sensitive; magnetic resonance imaging is diagnostic test of choice.

SINUSITIS IN ADULTS

The physician's overall impression as to the presence or absence of sinusitis is the best clinical predictor of disease. Independent clinical predictors of disease are maxillary toothache, poor transillumination, poor response to decongestants, and a history or examination finding of purulent discharge. Pertinent sinus radiographic findings include membrane thickening ≥6 mm (maxillary sinus), opaque sinuses, or air-fluid level. Organisms involved are *Haemophilus influenzae, Streptococcus pneumoniae,* and oral anaerobes. Treatment is with oral trimethoprim-sulfamethoxazole, amoxicillin/clavulanate, or cefuroxime axetil.

- Organisms involved in sinusitis in adults are *H. influenzae, S. pneumoniae,* oral anaerobes.

HEPATIC (BACTERIAL) ABSCESS

Mechanisms of bacterial abscess include portal vein bacteremia resulting from, for example, appendicitis and diverticulitis, bacteremia caused by a primary focus elsewhere in the body, ascending cholangitis, direct extension (subphrenic abscess), or trauma. Fever is common. Right upper quadrant pain, tenderness on percussion, and increased values on liver function tests may or may not be present. Computed tomography and ultrasonography are very helpful in diagnosis. Bacteriology depends on the mechanism of abscess formation. Intra-abdominal infection is often caused by polymicrobial aerobic gram-negative rods, anaerobic streptococci, and *Bacteroides* species. Treatment is individualized and depends on suspected and isolated organisms. Empiric therapy with clindamycin or metronidazole plus a third-generation cephalosporin or aminoglycoside is appropriate. If hematogenous route is suspected, an antistaphylococcal agent should be used in the regimen. Drainage (surgical or percutaneous) is of primary importance.

TOXIC SHOCK SYNDROME

This syndrome is caused by the establishment or growth of a toxin-producing strain of *Staphylococcus aureus* in a non-immune person. Clinical scenarios associated with this syndrome include young menstruating women with prolonged, continuous use of tampons, postoperative and nonoperative wound infections, localized abscesses, and *S. aureus* pneumonia developing after influenza. It is a multisystem disease. Clinical criteria include fever, hypotension, erythroderma (often leads to desquamation, particularly on palms and soles), and involvement in three or more organ systems. Onset is acute; blood culture results are usually negative. Condition is caused by production of staphylococcal toxin (TSST-1). Treatment is supportive; subsequent episodes are treated with β-lactam antibiotic, which decreases frequency and severity of subsequent attacks. Relapse rate may be as high as 30%-40% (menstruation-related disease). Mortality rate is 5%-10%.

- Toxic shock syndrome caused by toxin-producing strain of *S. aureus* in non-immune person.
- Multisystem disease: fever, hypotension, erythroderma (often leads to desquamation, particularly on palms and soles).
- Onset is acute; blood culture results usually negative.
- Condition is caused by production of staphylococcal toxin (TSST-1).

TOXIC STREPTOCOCCAL SYNDROME

This is similar to toxic shock syndrome. Patients have invasive group A streptococcal infections with associated hypotension and two of the following: renal impairment, coagulopathy, liver impairment, adult respiratory distress syndrome, rash (may desquamate), or soft tissue necrosis. It is caused by group A streptococci. Symptoms are caused by production of streptococcal toxin (pyrogenic exotoxin A). Most patients have skin or soft tissue infection, are <50 years old, and are otherwise healthy compared with patients with invasive group A streptococcal infections without the toxic streptococcal syndrome. Most are bacteremic (different from toxic shock syndrome due to *Staphylococcus aureus*). Treatment is with appropriate antibiotics, supportive care, and surgical debridement in some cases. Case-fatality rate is 30%.

- Toxic streptococcal syndrome is caused by group A streptococci.
- Symptoms caused by production of streptococcal toxin.

- Most patients are bacteremic (different from toxic shock syndrome due to *S. aureus*).

INFECTIONS IN SOLID ORGAN TRANSPLANTATION

Spectrum of potential pathogens in patients after solid organ transplantation is diverse. Individual risk of specific infection can be classified according to the following: symptoms and signs of illness at presentation (i.e., meningitis vs. pneumonia), posttransplantation time course, serostatus of recipient and donor for certain infections (e.g., cytomegalovirus, toxoplasmosis), type of organ transplantation, type and duration of immunosuppression, type of antimicrobial prophylaxis patient has received, and travel history and previous exposure to pathogens (e.g., tuberculosis, cocci). The time of occurrence of opportunistic infections in solid organ transplantation is given in Table 14-21.

ANTIMICROBIALS

The mechanisms of action, spectrum of activity, route of excretion, and toxicities of various antimicrobial agents are emphasized. Some of this information is given in Tables 14-22 through 14-26.

SPECIFIC ANTIBACTERIAL AGENTS

Penicillins

Natural Penicillins

These *agents* are penicillin G (intravenous, i.v.), penicillin VK (oral), procaine penicillin (intramuscular, i.m.), and benzathine penicillin (i.m., repository formulation).

Table 14-21.--Opportunistic Infections in Solid Organ Transplantation

Month	Type of infection after transplantation
1	Bacterial infections: related to wound, intravenous lines, urinary tract
	Herpes simplex virus; hepatitis B
1-4	Cytomegalovirus, *Pneumocystic carinii*, *Listeria monocytogenes*, *Mycobacterium tuberculosis*, *Aspergillus*, *Nocardia*, *Toxoplasma*, hepatitis B, *Legionella*
2-6	Epstein-Barr virus, varicella-zoster virus, hepatitis C, *Legionella*
>6	*Cryptococcus neoformans*, *Legionella*

Table 14-22.--Routes of Excretion of Antimicrobial Agents

Antibiotic	Major route of excretion
Penicillins*	Kidney
Cephalosporins†	Kidney
Aztreonam	Kidney
Imipenem	Kidney
Aminoglycosides	Kidney
Vancomycin	Kidney
Erythromycin	Liver
Clindamycin	Liver
Chloramphenicol	Liver
Tetracycline‡	Kidney
Flucytosine	Kidney
Rifampin	Liver
Cotrimoxazole	Kidney
Metronidazole	Liver
Fluoroquinolones	Kidney

*Nafcillin and oxacillin are excreted by the liver.
†Cefoperazone and ceftriaxone are excreted primarily in bile.
‡Metabolism in liver, excretion by kidneys. Doxycycline is eliminated by the liver.

Their *spectrum of activity* includes nonpenicillinase-producing staphylococci, β-hemolytic streptococci (group A, B, C, G), viridans streptococci, group D streptococci, penicillin-susceptible *Streptococcus pneumoniae, Neisseria gonorrhoeae, N. meningitidis*, and susceptible anaerobes (*Clostridium* species, oral *Bacteroides* species, *Peptostreptococcus,* and *Fusobacterium*). Enterococci are inhibited but not killed by the natural penicillins. Less common microbes that these agents are active against include *Erysipelothrix, Listeria monocytogenes, Pasteurella multocida, Streptobacillus, Spirillum, Treponema pallidum, Borrelia burgdorferi*, and *Actinomyces israelii*.

Toxicity to these agents includes hypersensitivity reactions. These are the most common adverse reactions (3%-10% of cases). These reactions include maculopapular rash, urticaria, angioedema, serum sickness, and anaphylaxis. True anaphylaxis occurs in 0.004%-0.015% of patients receiving penicillin.

Intravenous preparations cause more frequent allergic reactions than oral agents. Skin testing in difficult cases can be used to predict subsequent severe (type I) penicillin allergy but will not predict maculopapular drug eruptions. Patients allergic to one penicillin should be considered allergic to all penicillins. Furthermore, there is a cross-allergenicity rate of 3%-7% with cephalosporin compounds. Cephalosporins should be avoided when possible in patients who have had a severe, immediate penicillin allergy (type I anaphylaxis or urticarial eruption). An intestinal side effect is diarrhea, including *Clostridium difficile* colitis. Hematologic side effects are neutropenia, platelet dysfunction, and hemolytic anemia. Drug fever can also occur. Central nervous system side effects with penicillin G, when given in high doses, may involve tremors, lowered seizure threshold, and neuromuscular irritability.

- With natural penicillins, intravenous preparations cause more frequent allergic reactions than oral agents.
- There is a cross-allergenicity rate of 3%-7% with cephalosporin compounds.

Aminopenicillins
The *agents* are ampicillin and amoxicillin. The advantages of amoxicillin over oral ampicillin are increased gastrointestinal absorption, decreased incidence of diarrhea, and dosing three times a day.

Their *spectrum of activity* extends the antibacterial spectrum of the natural penicillins to include certain strains of *Escherichia coli, Proteus mirabilis, Salmonella, Shigella* (amoxicillin is less active than ampicillin), and β-lactamase-negative *Haemophilus influenzae* and *Moraxella catarrhalis*.

Toxicity is the same as outlined under Natural Penicillins (page 516). Rash is common when these agents are given to patients with infectious mononucleosis.

Penicillinase-Resistant Penicillins
Agents include methicillin (i.v.), oxacillin (i.v.), nafcillin (i.v.), dicloxacillin (oral), and cloxacillin (oral).

Spectrum of activity includes methicillin-susceptible *Staphylococcus aureus*. Treatment of serious infections caused by methicillin-susceptible coagulase-negative staphylococci

Table 14-23.--Mechanisms of Action of Antibiotics

Cell wall	Protein synthesis	Cell membrane	Cell synthesis	RNA synthesis
Penicillins	Aminoglycosides	Amphotericin B	Naladixic acid	Rifampin
Cephalosporins	Tetracycline	Azoles	Quinolones	
Vancomycin	Clindamycin		Flucytosine	
Imipenem	Chloramphenicol			
Aztreonam	Erythromycin			
	Metronidazole			

Table14-24.--Antimicrobials and Renal Failure

Antibiotics that do not require reduction of dosage in renal failure
Nafcillin, oxacillin
Cefoperazone, ceftriaxone
Erythromycin*
Clindamycin
Chloramphenicol
Metronidazole
Rifampin
Doxycycline

*May accumulate in patients on hemodialysis and cause reversible deafness.

with these agents is controversial because of the difficulty of detecting resistance in the laboratory. Penicillinase-resistant penicillins have no gram-negative or anaerobic activity but are active against most nonenterococcal streptococci.

Their *toxicities* are the same as outlined under Natural Penicillins (page 516). Nephritis (methicillin), phlebitis (nafcillin), and hepatitis (oxacillin) can occur.

● Penicillinase-resistant penicillins are primarily used for treatment of methicillin-susceptible *S. aureus*.

Carboxypenicillins
Agents include carbenicillin and ticarcillin.
The carboxypenicillins have a broader gram-negative *spectrum of activity* than ampicillin. When used as antipseudomonal agents, they are used in combination with an aminoglycoside to provide synergism and to prevent the emergence of resistant organisms. They have little or no activity against staphylococci, streptococci, enterococci, or *Klebsiella* species. Because ticarcillin has more (2-4 times) antipseudomonal activity in vitro, it is more effective in smaller quantities than carbenicillin against *Pseudomonas aeruginosa*; thus, the adverse effects of large quantities of carbenicillin can be avoided.

Toxicity is the same as described under Natural Penicillins (page 516). Sodium overload, hypokalemia, and platelet dysfunction can occur.

● Carboxypenicillins have little or no activity against staphylococci, streptococci, enterococci, or *Klebsiella* species.

Ureidopenicillins
Agents include mezlocillin, piperacillin, and azlocillin.

These agents have a wide *spectrum of activity* against gram-negative bacteria. Compared with carbenicillin and ticarcillin, they have a lower sodium content per gram, less associated hypokalemia, less platelet inhibition, and greater hepatic excretion. Compared with penicillin G and ampicillin, they are slightly less active against streptococci and enterococci (except mezlocillin), but they are more active against *H. influenzae*. Mezlocillin is more active than carbenicillin and ticarcillin against Enterobacteriaceae, including most strains of *Klebsiella*. It is also more active than ticarcillin against *Bacteroides fragilis*. Its activity against *Pseudomonas* is similar to that of ticarcillin. Azlocillin is more active than ticarcillin against *Pseudomonas* species; however, piperacillin is the most active

Table 14-25.--Cerebrospinal Fluid Penetration of Antibiotics

Excellent without inflammation	Good with inflammation	Fair	Poor or none
Chloramphenicol	Penicillin G	Aminoglycosides	Clindamycin
Flucytosine	Carbenicillin	Amphotericin B	Erythromycin
Rifampin	Nafcillin,	Ketoconazole	Cefazolin
Metronidazole	oxacillin	Itraconazole	
Fluconazole	Ampicillin		
	Cefuroxime		
	Cefotaxime		
	Ceftizoxime		
	Ceftazidime		
	Ceftriaxone		
	Cotrimoxazole (trimethoprim-sulfamethoxazole)		
	Imipenem		
	Ciprofloxacin		

Table 14-26.--Mechanisms of Resistance to Antibiotics

Mechanism	Antibiotic
β-Lactamase production: hydrolyze β-lactam ring so molecule cannot bind to pencillin-binding proteins	Penicillins Cephalosporins Monobactams
Mutation with altered affinity for penicillin-binding protein (penicillin-resistant pneumococci, methicillin-resistant staphylococci)	Penicillins Cephalosporins Monobactams Carbapenems
Modifying enzymes, plasmid mediated: acetyltransferases, phosphotransferases, adenyltransferases	Aminoglycosides (amikacin and netilmicin resistant to some of these enzymes) Chloramphenicol
Alteration ribosomal target site	Streptomycin
Acquired changes in permeability	Aminoglycosides, imipenem
Prevention of binding with ribosomes	Clindamycin Erythromycin
Alteration of active transport system	Tetracycline
Single-step mutation	Rifampin
Plasmid-mediated production of enzymes used in folic acid production	Trimethoprim-sulfamethoxazole
Alterations in DNA gyrase	Quinolones

penicillin against this organism. Like carboxypenicillins, combination therapy with an aminoglycoside may forestall the frequent emergence of resistance by *Pseudomonas* and *Enterobacter* species. Because of the cost of ureidopenicillins, the need for frequent dosing, and frequency of primary resistance (20%-40%) among certain Enterobacteriaceae, their use is becoming less common.

Toxicity is the same as detailed under Natural Penicillins (page 516). Other effects are hypokalemia (less common than with carbenicillin and ticarcillin), bleeding (less than with carbenicillin and ticarcillin), and hepatitis (similar to that with carbenicillin and ticarcillin).

β-*Lactamase Inhibitors*

Agents in this group are amoxicillin/clavulanate, ampicillin/sulbactam, ticarcillin/clavulanate, and piperacillin/tazobactam.

The *spectrum of activity* is increased by the addition of β-lactamase inhibitors; this results in activity against β-lactamase-producing organisms such as *S. aureus, B. fragilis, Klebsiella pneumoniae, H. influenzae,* and *M. catarrhalis.* These agents are not active against methicillin-resistant *S. aureus* and do not change the activity of the parent compound against most strains of *Pseudomonas* or *Enterobacter.*

Toxicity is the same as discussed under Natural Penicillins (page 516) and the parent compounds. Clavulanate may rarely

cause hepatitis.

- β-Lactamase inhibitors are not active against methicillin-resistant *S. aureus.*

Cephalosporins

First-Generation Cephalosporins

Representative agents are cefazolin (long serum half-life allows dosing every 8 hours), cephalothin, and cephalexin.

The *spectrum of activity* of the first-generation agents includes being active against staphylococci, β-hemolytic streptococci, penicillin-susceptible (minimal inhibitory concentration <0.12) pneumococci, and many strains of *P. mirabilis, E. coli,* and *Klebsiella* species. They are not active, as are all cephalosporins, against methicillin-resistant staphylococci, enterococci, *L. monocytogenes, Legionella* species, *Chlamydia pneumoniae, Mycoplasma pneumoniae,* and *C. difficile.*

Cephalosporins are usually well tolerated. *Toxicity* can include adverse reactions related to the gastrointestinal tract (e.g., nausea, vomiting, diarrhea); these are the most common. Hypersensitivity reactions, primarily rashes, occur in 1%-3% of patients taking cephalosporins. Anaphylaxis is extremely rare. Cross-allergenicity may occur with penicillins. Other adverse reactions associated with cephalosporins include drug fever and *C. difficile* colitis.

...ins are not active against
...occi.

...orins

...andole, cefoxitin, cefurox-
...ese agents is similar to that
...orins unless specified.

...tage over cefazolin and is
...ure expensive. It has some increase in activity against *E. coli*, *Klebsiella*, indole-positive *Proteus*, *Enterobacter*, and non-β-lactamase-producing *H. influenzae*. The methyl-thiotetrazole (MTT) side chain causes bleeding problems and a disulfiram-like reaction. Dosing is every 4-6 hours.

Cefoxitin has some increase in activity over first-generation agents against *E. coli*, *Klebsiella*, indole-positive *Proteus*, and *Serratia*. It is less active against *S. aureus* than first-generation cephalosporins. It is active against most strains of *B. fragilis*. It is used for treatment of intra-abdominal infections and pelvic inflammatory disease (in combination with doxycycline). Dosing is every 4-6 hours.

Cefuroxime has good activity against *S. aureus* and β-lactamase-producing *H. influenzae*. It is the only second-generation agent with good penetration of the central nervous system. It is used to treat community-acquired pneumonia and meningitis (except *Listeria*). Dosing is every 8 hours.

Cefotetan is similar to cefoxitin in activity against gram-positive cocci and *B. fragilis*, but it has better activity than cefoxitin against aerobic gram-negative rods. It has the MTT side chain with the associated toxicities described for cefamandole.

Third-Generation Cephalosporins

Representative agents are cefotaxime, ceftizoxime, ceftriaxone, cefoperazone, and ceftazidime. Their *toxicity* is similar to that with the first-generation cephalosporins unless specified.

Cefotaxime is less active against *Pseudomonas* than ceftazidime or cefoperazone. It has better activity against staphylococci and streptococci than ceftazidime and cefoperazone. It has good cerebrospinal fluid penetration. It is the drug of choice along with ceftriaxone for community-acquired meningitis (except *Listeria*). It is more effective than cefuroxime in *H. influenzae* meningitis. Desacetyl metabolite may allow dosing every 8 hours except in life-threatening infections.

Ceftizoxime is less active against *P. aeruginosa* than ceftazidime and cefoperazone. Activity against anaerobes is limited. It is essentially the same as cefotaxime.

Ceftriaxone has activity similar to that of other third-generation cephalosporins but is less active against *Pseudomonas* than ceftazidime and cefoperazone. It is less active against *S. aureus* than cefotaxime. One of its advantages is the long half-life (8 hours); thus, it can be given in a single daily dose. It

has good cerebrospinal fluid penetration. It has been reported to cause pseudocholelithiasis, cholelithiasis, biliary colic, and cholecystitis as a result of biliary precipitation of ceftriaxone as the calcium salt in up to 2% of cases, especially in children. This effect usually resolves with discontinuation of therapy.

Cefoperazone is somewhat active against *Pseudomonas*. Penetration into cerebrospinal fluid is less than that of other available third-generation cephalosporins. Advantages include its excretion primarily in the bile; therefore, there is no change in dose with abnormal renal function. Cefoperazone has the MTT side chain with the associated toxicities described for cefamandole.

In regard to its spectrum of activity, ceftazidime is much more active than any other third-generation cephalosporin against *Pseudomonas*. It is less active against *S. aureus* and streptococci than most other third-generation cephalosporins. Pseudomonads may acquire resistance if the drug is used alone. It is often used empirically in patients with neutropenic fever. It penetrates into cerebrospinal fluid as well as cefotaxime and ceftriaxone.

- Ceftazidime is more active than any other third-generation cephalosporin against *Pseudomonas*.

Imipenem

Imipenem is a new, broad-spectrum β-lactam. Its mechanism of action is similar to that of other β-lactam congeners (i.e., inhibition of cell wall synthesis). Bacterial resistance, particularly among *P. aeruginosa*, is increasing and is mediated by various mechanisms. Imipenem is administered intravenously and is hydrolyzed in the kidney by a peptidase located in the brush border of renal tubular cells. Administration with cilastatin, a dihydropeptidase inhibitor, solves this problem.

Imipenem has the broadest antibacterial activity of any antibiotic currently available. Its *spectrum of activity* includes excellent activity against *Pseudomonas*, anaerobes including *B. fragilis*, β-hemolytic streptococci, pneumococci, methicillin-susceptible *S. aureus*, enterococci (inhibited only), Enterobacteriaceae, *H. influenzae*, and *Nocardia*. The agent is not active against methicillin-resistant *S. aureus*, *Enterococcus faecium*, *Legionella*, *Chlamydia* species, *Mycoplasma* species, *Pseudomonas cepacia*, and *Xanthomonas maltophilia*. Toxic effects include nausea and vomiting (particularly during drug infusion) (1% of cases), diarrhea (3%), rash or drug fever (2.7%), and dysgeusia. Seizures occur in 1.5% of patients, particularly those with a history of previous seizure, renal insufficiency, or structural central nervous system defects. Meropenem is a new agent that is virtually identical to imipenem. However, it does not require co-administration with cilastatin.

Aztreonam

The monobactam antibacterial agents, of which aztreonam is the only one commercially available, are derivatives of naturally occurring monocyclic β-lactam compounds. The mechanism of action of aztreonam, like that of other β-lactam antimicrobials, is the inhibition of cell wall synthesis. Aztreonam is administered intravenously and is excreted by the kidneys.

Its *spectrum of activity* involves only aerobic gram-negative bacteria, including many *P. aeruginosa*. It has minimal activity against *Acinetobacter, Alcaligenes, Flavobacterium, Pseudomonas fluorescens*, and *X. maltophilia*. Furthermore, it has no activity against gram-positive aerobic or anaerobic bacteria, and it is not synergistic with penicillins against the enterococci, as are gentamicin and streptomycin.

The *toxicity* of aztreonam is similar to that of other β-lactams. Patients with a penicillin allergy may tolerate aztreonam because cross-reactivity is uncommon.

Aminoglycosides

Agents in this group are gentamicin, tobramycin, amikacin, netilmicin, streptomycin, kanamycin, and neomycin.

The *spectrum of activity* of these agents includes aerobic gram-negative bacilli, mycobacteria (*Mycobacterium tuberculosis*, streptomycin; *Mycobacterium avium-intracellulare*, amikacin; *Mycobacterium chelonei*, amikacin), *Brucella* (streptomycin), *Nocardia* (amikacin), *Francisella tularensis* (streptomycin), and *Yersinia pestis* (streptomycin). They are synergistic with certain β-lactams in the treatment of serious infections due to susceptible enterococci (gentamicin, streptomycin), staphylococci, and several aerobic gram-negative species.

The major *adverse reactions* to aminoglycosides include nephrotoxicity and auditory or vestibular toxicity. Neuromuscular blockade, drug fever, and hypersensitivity reactions are much less common. The risk of nephrotoxicity varies among the different aminoglycosides; neomycin is the most nephrotoxic, and streptomycin is the least nephrotoxic. Gentamicin, tobramycin, and amikacin have intermediate nephrotoxicity. Risk factors include old age, hypotension, concomitant use of other nephrotoxic drugs, and liver disease. Aminoglycoside nephrotoxicity is almost always reversible with discontinuation of use of the drug, and it can be minimized or avoided if dosages are adjusted to achieve therapeutic serum concentrations and if renal function is carefully monitored. Nephrotoxicity is potentiated by cisplatin, amphotericin B, vancomycin, and cyclosporine. Ototoxicity is almost always irreversible. Streptomycin, gentamicin, and tobramycin are preferentially toxic to the vestibular system, whereas amikacin and neomycin are toxic to the auditory nerve. Advanced age and concomitant use of ethacrynic acid or furosemide seem to be risk factors for ototoxicity. Because of the imprecision of bedside testing for auditory and vestibular toxicity, routine audiographic and vestibular function evaluation should be con-

sidered when prolonged administration is anticipated and in patients predisposed to ototoxicity.

- Major adverse reactions to aminoglycosides are nephrotoxicity and auditory or vestibular toxicity.
- Neomycin is most nephrotoxic, and streptomycin is least nephrotoxic.
- Aminoglycoside nephrotoxicity is almost always reversible with discontinuation of use of drug.
- Ototoxicity is almost always irreversible.

Tetracycline

Agents are short-acting (tetracycline, chlorotetracycline, oxytetracycline), intermediate-acting (demeclocycline, methacycline), and long-acting (doxycycline, minocycline).

These agents are the drugs of choice for *Rickettsia, Chlamydia* species (includes pelvic inflammatory disease), *M. pneumoniae, Vibrio cholerae, Vibrio vulnificus, Brucella* species (with streptomycin or rifampin), *B. burgdorferi* (early stages), and *B. recurrentis*. These agents are also *effective therapy* or *alternatives* for *Actinomyces*, anthrax, *Campylobacter, Pasteurella multocida, Spirillum minus, Streptobacillus moniliformis, Treponema pallidum, F. tularensis*, Whipple's disease, *Y. pestis, Nocardia* (minocycline), and *Mycobacterium marinum*. Minocycline may be active against methicillin-resistant *S. aureus* (patients who cannot tolerate vancomycin). The tetracyclines are used as *prophylaxis* for traveler's diarrhea and meningococcal disease (minocycline only; rifampin is drug of choice). Although the tetracyclines are active in vitro against many aerobic gram-positive and gram-negative organisms as well as some anaerobes, they are not the drugs of choice to treat the infections caused by these organisms because of the presence or emergence of resistant strains.

Toxicity includes gastrointestinal upset, rash, and photosensitivity. Uremia is increased in patients with renal failure (i.e., catabolic), acute fatty liver of pregnancy, Fanconi's syndrome (old tetracycline), or pseudotumor cerebri. The tetracyclines are not used in pregnant females or in children; they impair bone growth of the fetus and stain the teeth of children. Minocycline is associated with vestibular toxicity, and recently cell-mediated hypersensitivity pneumonitis was reported.

Chloramphenicol

The *spectrum of activity* of this agent includes inhibition of most strains of clinically important aerobic and anaerobic bacteria. Exceptions include enterococci, methicillin-resistant *S. aureus*, many *Klebsiella* isolates, *Enterobacter, Serratia*, indole-positive *Proteus*, and *P. aeruginosa*. It is active against *Rickettsia* organisms and has bactericidal activity against *S. pneumoniae, H. influenzae*, and *N. meningitidis*. Major indications are few because of the availability of alternative therapies (severe *Salmonella typhi* infection, bacterial meningitis due to susceptible organisms in patients who cannot tolerate penicillin or cephalosporins, and rickettsial infections in patients who cannot take tetracyclines).

Toxicity includes two types of hematologic manifestations: idiosyncratic aplastic anemia (not dose-related; severe, usually fatal; incidence approximately 1/24,000-1/40,000) and dose-related bone marrow suppression (much more common with a dose >4 g/day). Gray baby syndrome (abdominal distention, cyanosis, vasomotor collapse) occurs in premature infants who cannot conjugate chloramphenicol and who have high serum levels. Rare toxic effects are hemolytic anemia, retrobulbar neuritis, peripheral neuritis, and potentiation action of oral hypoglycemics.

Clindamycin

Clindamycin has an excellent anaerobic *activity*, although 10%-20% of *B. fragilis* organisms, 10%-20% of non-*Clostridium perfringens* organisms, and 10% of peptostreptococci organisms are resistant to clindamycin. It also is active against many strains of staphylococci and streptococci. However, emergence of resistance by staphylococci is common during treatment. Gram-negative aerobic bacteria and enterococci are resistant to clindamycin.

Toxicity includes antibiotic-associated diarrhea (20%), including *C. difficile* colitis (1%-10%); these are the most common side effects. Minor elevations of transaminase level, reversible neutropenia, thrombocytopenia, and neuromuscular blockade when given concurrently with neuromuscular blocking agents are much less common.

- Emergence of resistance to clindamycin by staphylococci is common during treatment.
- Toxic effects: antibiotic-associated diarrhea (20%), including *C. difficile* colitis (1%-10%).

Metronidazole

Metronidazole has antimicrobial *activity* against most anaerobic microorganisms. The exceptions include some anaerobic gram-positive non-spore-forming bacilli and peptostreptococci, *Actinomyces*, and *Propionibacterium acnes*. The agent is also effective in infections due to *Entamoeba histolytica*, *Giardia lamblia*, and *Gardnerella vaginalis*.

Toxicity includes side effects such as nausea, vomiting, reversible neutropenia, metallic taste, a disulfiram reaction when coadministered with alcohol, and potentiation of the effects of oral anticoagulants. Major adverse reactions are rare; they usually include central nervous system effects (seizure, cerebellar ataxia, peripheral neuropathy).

Macrolides

Erythromycin

Indications for this agent are infections caused by *Legionella* species, *M. pneumoniae*, and *Campylobacter jejuni*. It is an effective or alternative agent for *Chlamydia* species, group A hemolytic streptococci, *S. pneumoniae*, *S. aureus* (methicillin sensitive) (mild skin and soft tissue infections), *N. gonorrhoeae*, and *T. pallidum*. It may eradicate the carrier state of *Corynebacterium diphtheriae* and shorten the duration of *Bordetella pertussis* disease (whooping cough).

Toxicity may include gastrointestinal upset (dose-related), cholestatic jaundice (erythromycin estolate compound), increased theophylline or cyclosporine concentration, increased serum concentrations of terfenadine (may cause ventricular arrhythmias), and transitory deafness, especially with large doses (≥4 g/day).

Clarithromycin

This agent provides excellent *activity* against *S. pneumoniae*, β-hemolytic streptococci, viridans streptococci, *S. aureus* (methicillin-sensitive), *M. catarrhalis*, *Legionella pneumophila*, *M. pneumoniae*, *C. pneumoniae*, *Chlamydia trachomatis*, *B. burgdorferi*, *M. avium-intracellulare*, and *M. chelonei*. It is superior to erythromycin for *S. pneumoniae* and β-hemolytic streptococci. It is moderately effective against *H. influenzae* and *N. gonorrhoeae*. It provides poor activity against *S. aureus* (methicillin-resistant).

In regard to *bioavailability*, excellent concentrations are achieved in many body fluids. The drug penetrates macrophages and polymorphonuclear neutrophils. Food has no effect on absorption. Half-life is 4-6 hours, which allows twice-daily dosing. Excretion is through liver and kidney.

Adverse effects include nausea (3%) and other gastrointestinal complaints; these occur less often than with erythromycin, but they are the most common adverse reactions. As with erythromycin, reversible hearing loss may occur at high dosages. Theophylline and carbamazepine concentrations increase, and levels of terfenadine may increase (cause of arrhythmias).

Clinical uses include mild to moderate upper and lower respiratory tract infection (may not be appropriate initial therapy if *H. influenzae* is expected pathogen). Others are pharyngitis, skin and soft tissue infection, and *M. avium-intracellulare* and other atypical mycobacterial infections.

Azithromycin

The *spectrum of activity* is the same as that of clarithromycin. It is twofold to fourfold less active against streptococci, including pneumococci, than erythromycin. It is more active against *H. influenzae* than clarithromycin.

In regard to *bioavailability*, excellent concentrations are achieved in many body fluids. The agent penetrates macrophages and polymorphonuclear neutrophils. Food decreases absorption. Half-life is 68 hours, which allows once-daily dosing. Excretion is hepatic. *Adverse effects* are the same as those for clarithromycin.

Clinical uses include treatment of mild to moderate upper and lower respiratory tract infection (may not be appropriate initial therapy if *H. influenzae* is expected pathogen), pharyngitis, skin and soft tissue infection, nongonococcal urethritis and cervicitis (single 1-g dose), *M. avium-intracellulare*, other atypical mycobacteria, and *Toxoplasma gondii*.

Vancomycin

Vancomycin, a glycopeptide antibiotic, has a *spectrum of activity* against most aerobic and anaerobic gram-positive organisms, with the exception of certain strains of *Lactobacillus*, *Leukonostoc*, *Actinomyces*, and enterococci (vancomycin-resistant strains). Vancomycin is the drug of choice for infections caused by methicillin-resistant *S. aureus*, methicillin-resistant coagulase-negative staphylococci, *Bacillus* species, *Rhodococcus equi*, and other multiply resistant gram-positive organisms such as *Corynebacterium jeikium*. It is also an alternative agent for infections caused by staphylococci, enterococci (synergistic with aminoglycosides), or streptococci in patients intolerant of β-lactam antimicrobials, although recent data suggest that vancomycin may be less effective than antistaphylococcal β-lactams for methicillin-susceptible *S. aureus* infections. Oral vancomycin is not absorbed and is used to treat only *C. difficile* colitis.

Although rare, the major *toxicity* with vancomycin is ototoxicity. This side effect is more common in the elderly and when vancomycin and aminoglycosides are administered concurrently. Infusion-related pruritus and the production of an erythematous rash involving the face, neck, and upper body ("red man" syndrome) are due to nonimmunologic-related release of histamine. Its frequency can be reduced by slowing the rate of infusion and by the administration of antihistamines before vancomycin infusion. Nephrotoxicity is rare with the newer preparations of vancomycin, except when vancomycin and aminoglycosides are administered concurrently. Chemical thrombophlebitis (13%) and reversible neutropenia (2%) are also known side effects.

- Vancomycin is bactericidal against most aerobic and anaerobic gram-positive organisms.
- Vancomycin is drug of choice for infections caused by methicillin-resistant *S. aureus*, methicillin-resistant coagulase-negative staphylococci, *Bacillus* species.
- Major toxic effect is ototoxicity.
- "Red man" syndrome is due to nonimmunologic-related release of histamine.

Cotrimoxazole (Trimethoprim-Sulfamethoxazole)

Cotrimoxazole consists of two separate antimicrobials, trimethoprim and sulfamethoxazole, combined in a fixed (1:5) ratio. Both trimethoprim and sulfamethoxazole inhibit microbial folic acid synthesis, and when combined they have a synergistic effect.

The *spectrum of activity* of cotrimoxazole includes a wide variety of aerobic gram-positive cocci and gram-negative bacilli, including *S. aureus* (moderate activity), coagulase-negative staphylococci, *S. pneumoniae*, *H. influenzae*, *L. monocytogenes*, and many Enterobacteriaceae. It is not active against anaerobic bacteria and many strains of *Citrobacter freundii*, *Proteus vulgaris*, and *Providencia*. It is inactive against *P. aeruginosa* and enterococci. It is active against *Pneumocystis carinii*, *Isospora belli*, and *Nocardia asteroides*.

Toxicity with the agent can include the common adverse reactions of nausea and vomiting (3.2%) and rash (3.4%). Hypersensitivity reactions are common in patients with acquired immunodeficiency syndrome (AIDS; 60%). Diarrhea, nephrotoxicity, neutropenia, drug fever, and cholestatic hepatitis are less common. Its use is contraindicated during the last month of pregnancy and in patients with known glucose-6-phosphatase dehydrogenase deficiency. In 20%-53% of patients with AIDS treated for *Pneumocystis carinii* pneumonia (PCP), hyperkalemia due to trimethoprim component develops. Cotrimoxazole has several known drug interactions, including increasing the activity of oral anticoagulants, increasing plasma phenytoin concentrations, enhancing hypoglycemia in patients on oral hypoglycemics, and contributing to pancytopenia when coadministered with methotrexate.

- With cotrimoxazole, hypersensitivity reactions are common in patients with AIDS.

Fluoroquinolones

Agents are norfloxacin, ciprofloxacin, ofloxacin, lomefloxacin, and enoxacin.

Fluoroquinolones are derivatives of naladixic acid, the first quinolone. They are bactericidal against a wide variety of microorganisms because of their ability to inhibit DNA gyrase, an essential enzyme involved in the supercoiling of bacterial DNA.

Although the *spectrum of activity* of fluoroquinolones varies from drug to drug, they are generally extremely active against selected Enterobacteriaceae (including most strains that cause bacterial gastroenteritis) and *P. aeruginosa*. *S. aureus* (including methicillin-resistant), coagulase-negative staphylococci, and enterococci (urinary tract isolates only, because of high drug levels achieved in the urine) are less susceptible to all currently available fluoroquinolones, and none of these agents are active against anaerobes. *S. pneumoniae* is generally resistant to quinolones. Bacterial resistance to fluoroquinolones is increasing, particularly among *P. aeruginosa* and staphylococci.

Fluoroquinolones are generally safe. The most common types of *toxicity* are nausea, vomiting, abdominal pain, and diarrhea (1%-5%). *C. difficile* colitis is uncommon. Patients can also experience headache, confusion, restlessness, tremors, and seizures. Patients who have seizures usually have a previous history of a seizure disorder or a central nervous system structural defect. Hypersensitivity reactions, nephrotoxicity, and serum sickness are uncommon. Gastrointestinal absorption of the quinolones may be decreased by coadministration of aluminum- and magnesium-containing antacids, multivitamin preparations that include zinc, oral iron preparations, and high-calcium supplements. Concurrent administration of sucralfate also inhibits ciprofloxacin absorption. Ciprofloxacin increases serum theophylline and caffeine concentrations. Ciprofloxacin can cause erosions in cartilage in animals and thus is not recommended in pregnant women or in patients <18 years old.

- Fluoroquinolones are active against selected Enterobacteriaceae and *P. aeruginosa*.
- Bacterial resistance to fluoroquinolones is increasing, particularly among *P. aeruginosa* and staphylococci.
- *C. difficile* colitis uncommon.
- Gastrointestinal absorption of quinolones may be decreased by coadministration of aluminum- and magnesium-containing antacids and of multivitamin preparations.

Norfloxacin

Excellent concentrations of this agent are achieved in urine, kidney tissue, bile, and feces. Levels are poor in other sites. Food may decrease absorption. It is used for treatment of complicated and uncomplicated urinary tract infection, prostatitis, and bacterial diarrhea. More cost-effective agents are often available. It is also used for bowel decontamination (neutropenic patients).

Ciprofloxacin

Spectrum of activity of this agent is the same as that of other quinolones. In addition, it is active against *N. gonorrhoeae* (including penicillin-resistant strains), *H. influenzae* (including penicillin-resistant strains), *M. catarrhalis* (including penicillin-resistant strains), *M. tuberculosis*, *L. pneumophila*, and *Brucella*. Excellent concentrations are achieved in most body fluids. An adverse effect is more of an increase in theophylline levels than with norfloxacin.

Clinical uses include complicated and uncomplicated urinary tract infection (cure rates are less in infections due to enterococci or in complicated infection) and chronic prostatitis. In many cases, more cost-effective agents are often available. Ciprofloxacin is also used for treatment of infectious diarrhea (recurrence of *Salmonella* and resistance to *C. jejuni* have been reported) and for treatment and prophylaxis of traveler's diarrhea. It may eradicate the *S. typhi* carrier state. When utilized in cases of upper and lower respiratory tract infection, failures against pneumococci have been reported, and it is not drug of choice for empiric therapy of community-acquired pneumo-

nia. Other conditions for which it is used are malignant external otitis due to *P. aeruginosa*, skin and soft tissue infection (avoid in streptococcal cellulitis), bone and joint infection (aerobic gram-negative), *M. avium-intracellulare* and multiple drug-resistant tuberculosis, and uncomplicated gonococcal urethritis or cervicitis; it is also an alternative agent for prophylaxis of meningococci.

Ofloxacin

The *spectrum of activity* is similar to that of ciprofloxacin; it is less active against *P. aeruginosa* and Enterobacteriaceae. This drug increases theophylline levels, but less so than with ciprofloxacin.

Clinical uses are complicated and uncomplicated urinary tract infection (cure rates are lower in infections due to enterococci or in complicated infection) and chronic prostatitis. More cost-effective agents are available in many such cases. Ofloxacin is also used for lower respiratory tract infection (see Ciprofloxacin, this page), skin and soft tissue infection (see Ciprofloxacin, this page), and gonococcal and nongonococcal urethritis and cervicitis.

Lomefloxacin

The *spectrum of activity* of this agent is similar to that of ciprofloxacin. It is not active against *M. tuberculosis, C. trachomatis, C. pneumoniae, L. pneumophila, M. pneumoniae,* or *Brucella*. Theophylline levels are not increased with this drug. Photosensitivity reaction may be more common than with ciprofloxacin.

Clinical uses include complicated and uncomplicated urinary tract infection (cure rates are lower in infections due to enterococci or in complicated infection) and chronic prostatitis. More cost-effective agents are available in many of these cases. It is also used for prophylaxis for transurethral surgical procedures.

Enoxacin

The *spectrum of activity* is similar to that for ciprofloxacin. It is less active against *P. aeruginosa*. It has only moderate activity against staphylococci and enterococci. It is not active against pneumococci, group A streptococci, *M. tuberculosis, C. trachomatis, C. pneumoniae, L. pneumophila, M. pneumoniae,* or *Brucella*. Adverse effects include increased theophylline and caffeine levels (more than with the other quinolones). Ranitidine and other agents may inhibit absorption. Reports from Japan have described convulsions in several patients taking fenbufen (nonsteroidal anti-inflammatory drug) concurrently. Digoxin levels may also increase.

Clinical uses include complicated and uncomplicated urinary tract infection, prostatitis, and gonococcal urethritis and cervicitis.

ANTIFUNGAL THERAPY

Amphotericin B

The *mode of action* of this agent is binding of ergosterol in cell walls and increasing cell wall permeability. Its indications are for most serious or life-threatening fungal infections. Exceptions include *Pseudallescheria boydii* (azoles) and chromoblastomycosis (flucytosine).

Toxicity can include fever, phlebitis, and nephrotoxicity (increased intravascular volume, salt loading may decrease risk of nephrotoxicity). Nephrotoxicity is increased with concomitant use of cyclosporine. In patients with acquired immunodeficiency syndrome (AIDS), acute renal failure has occurred with concomitant use of pentamidine intravenously. Other effects are bone marrow suppression, hypokalemia (may exacerbate digitalis toxicity), hypomagnesemia, and, when given to patients who have had leukocyte transfusion, pulmonary infiltrates.

Flucytosine

The *mode of action* of this agent involves conversion to 5-fluorouracil intracellularly. Resistance develops rapidly when it is used alone. It has *activity* against cryptococci, *Candida* species, and chromoblastomycosis. *Indications* are cryptococcal meningitis (used in combination with amphotericin B), *Candida* meningitis (good cerebrospinal fluid penetration; in combination with amphotericin B), *Candida* cystitis (urinary levels are high), and chromoblastomycosis.

Toxicity is associated with high serum levels. Neutropenia, thrombocytopenia, diarrhea, nausea, gastrointestinal upset, colitis, and hepatotoxicity (idiosyncratic, uncommon) are possible side effects.

Azoles

Pharmacologic properties of the azoles are outlined in Table 14-27.

Ketoconazole

This is a bis-triazole compound that inhibits production of ergosterol, a major constituent of fungal cell membranes, by inhibiting the cytochrome P450 enzyme responsible for conversion of lanosterol to ergosterol. It requires gastric acid for absorption. The presence of low gastric pH should always be determined to ensure the adequate absorption of ketoconazole. Coadministration of isoniazid and rifampin can decrease drug levels. Ketoconazole can elevate cyclosporine levels and potentiate the effect of warfarin.

Ketoconazole is second-line therapy (itraconazole is drug of choice) for nonmeningeal and non-life-threatening *Histoplasmosis* and *Blastomycosis* in immunocompetent patients. It has poor cerebrospinal fluid penetration and should not be used to treat central nervous system fungal infections. The drug is also used for chronic mucocutaneous candidiasis, paracoccidioidomycosis, and *P. boydii*.

The most common *toxic effect* of ketoconazole is dose-related gastrointestinal upset. Decreased synthesis of adrenal corticosteroids, most notably androgenic steroids, has been reported. Patients may have gynecomastia and loss of libido with impotence, especially with higher dosages of ketoconazole. Arterial hypertension has also been reported. Acute hepatitis, which can be fatal, occurs rarely.

- Ketoconazole requires gastric acid for absorption.
- Potentiates the effect of warfarin.
- Gynecomastia is fairly common side effect.

Table 14-27.--Selected Pharmacologic Properties of Azole Drugs

Factor	Ketoconazole	Fluconazole	Itraconazole
Route of administration	Oral	Oral, parenteral	Oral
Requires acid for GI absorption	Yes	No	Yes
Protein binding	99%	12%	99%
CSF concentrations	Nil	≈80%	Nil
Half-life, hr	9	25	15-42
Clearance	Hepatic	Renal	Hepatic
Urinary levels of active drug	Low	High	Low
Dose reduction in renal failure	No	Yes	No

CSF, cerebrospinal fluid; GI, gastrointestinal.

Modified from Terrell CL, Hughes CE: Antifungal agents used for deep-seated mycotic infections. Mayo Clin Proc 67:69-91, 1992. By permission of Mayo Foundation for Medical Education and Research.

Fluconazole

This is a bis-triazole compound that inhibits ergosterol, a major constituent of fungal cell membranes, by inhibiting the cytochrome P450 enzyme responsible for conversion of lanosterol to ergosterol. It has a broad spectrum of antifungal activity in vivo in animal models. Activity has been demonstrated against *Candida, Cryptococcus neoformans, Coccidioides immitis, Histoplasma capsulatum, Blastomyces dermatitidis,* and paracoccidioidomycosis. Food hinders absorption of the drug.

Adverse effects occur in 16% of patients. Discontinuation of therapy is necessary in 1%-2% of patients. Most common effects are gastrointestinal (1.5%-3.5%), rash (1.8%), and headache (1.9%). Fatal hepatic necrosis and exfoliative rash have also been reported. There is no interference with adrenocortical function or synthesis of testosterone, which can occur with ketoconazole.

Fluconazole inhibits metabolism and increases serum levels of phenytoin, oral hyoglycemic agents, carbamazepine, and warfarin. Increases in cyclosporine levels due to fluconazole have been reported. Coadministration with rifampin and isoniazid decreases serum concentrations of fluconazole.

Clinical uses include candidal infection and cryptococcal meningitis. In candidal infection, oropharyngeal and esophageal candidiasis are effectively treated, both in patients with AIDS and in patients with neutropenia. Hepatosplenic candidiasis and vaginitis (topical agents may be more cost-effective) are also treated with fluconazole. For urinary tract infection, no trials have compared the drug with amphotericin B bladder washes. For candidemia, amphotericin B and fluconazole have not been compared. Failures with fluconazole have been reported. The drug is also used for prophylaxis of candidal infection in neutropenic patients and in patients undergoing bone marrow transplantation. A concern is emergence of resistant fungi (*C. krusei*). Fluconazole is also used as initial therapy for cryptococcal meningitis. A recent randomized study of 194 patients who had AIDS with acute cryptococcal meningitis found no difference in clinical cure or overall survival between groups receiving amphotericin B and fluconazole, but time to cerebrospinal fluid sterilization was less with amphotericin B, and there were more early deaths in the fluconazole group. Most experts still recommend initial therapy with amphotericin B. Maintenance therapy with fluconazole is more efficacious and less toxic than weekly administration of amphotericin B. The role of the drug in treatment of patients without AIDS remains undefined.

Itraconazole

The *mechanism of action* of this drug is similar to that for fluconazole. A major advantage over fluconazole is its greater activity against *Aspergillus, Sporothrix schenckii, H. capsulatum,* and *B. dermatitidis*. Food enhances its absorption.

Minor *side effects* occur in 2%-20% of patients if doses <400 mg/day are used. Most common side effects involve gastrointestinal tract: nausea, 10.6%; vomiting, 5.1%; and abdominal pain, 1.5%. Rash occurs in 8.6% of patients. Hepatitis can occur but is rare. If dose is <400 mg/day, there is no effect on glucocorticoid or testosterone synthesis. At doses >400 mg/day, edema, hypokalemia, nausea, and vomiting can occur.

Itraconazole inhibits metabolism and increases serum levels of cyclosporine, digoxin, and terfenadine. Cyclosporine and digoxin levels should be monitored, and terfenadine should not be administered concurrently because of potentially fatal ventricular arrhythmias. Astemizole coadministration is also contraindicated. Coadministration with rifampin, isoniazid, and H2 blockers decreases serum concentrations of itraconazole. Failures in therapy have also been reported when phenytoin and carbamazepine have been administered concurrently.

Clinical uses include histoplasmosis: chronic cavitary pulmonary disease and disseminated non-life-threatening, nonmeningeal disease. Itraconazole is also effective maintenance therapy in patients with AIDS. A recent study also demonstrated its effectiveness in pulmonary and nonpulmonary (bone, joint, skin) blastomycosis. It is now the drug of choice for this condition. For coccidioidomycosis (pulmonary, bone, and joint), the efficacy rate is 57%-72%. A small number of patients with coccidioidal meningitis have also been effectively treated. When used for sporotrichosis, itraconazole is effective in lymphocutaneous and bone and joint disease, although relapse may occur in disseminated disease. An ongoing trial is comparing fluconazole and itraconazole for treatment of cryptococcal meningitis in patients with AIDS. As therapy for *Aspergillus*, success rates of 44%-77% have been reported for invasive pulmonary and sinus disease. No studies comparing itraconazole with amphotericin B have been reported, and amphotericin B remains the drug of choice for these diseases unless contraindications to its use exist.

ANTIVIRAL AGENTS

Current agents are virustatic and have no activity against nonreplicating or latent viruses.

Acyclovir

This is a nucleoside analog of guanosine. After phosphorylation by virus-specific thymidine kinase to monophosphate and further phosphorylation to triphosphate by cellular enzymes, it inhibits DNA polymerase. In vitro activity and clinical efficacy correlate with the amount of viral-specific thymidine kinase produced (herpes simplex virus type 1 > herpes simplex virus type 2 > varicella-zoster virus > Epstein-Barr virus). Cytomegalovirus does not produce thymidine kinase and is resistant. Oral and intravenous forms are available. Mutations of either viral thymidine kinase or DNA polymerase cause resistance. Most acyclovir-resistant isolates (herpes simplex virus, varicella-zoster virus) have been isolated in patients with acquired immunodeficiency syndrome (AIDS) and in recipients of bone marrow transplantation. Drug of choice is then foscarnet.

Acyclovir is generally well tolerated. *Toxicity* includes gastrointestinal distress and headaches (oral form), phlebitis (intravenous form), and crystalline nephropathy (increased risk with high dose, bolus infusion, dehydration, and preexisting renal impairment). Confusion, delirium, lethargy, and seizures can occur (<1% of cases, higher rate with serum concentration >25 µg/mL). Use of the drug is avoided during pregnancy.

Indications for the drug include herpes simplex virus infections. It is effective for treatment of primary and recurrent episodes of herpes genitalis and suppression of frequent recurrences. Topical acyclovir is also effective in primary genital herpes simplex virus infection, but the oral form is more effective. Intravenous therapy should be considered in serious disease. If chronic suppression is used, reassess after 1 year. Oral-labial disease may respond to oral acyclovir, but it is not recommended for routine use. In immunocompromised patients, however, oral or intravenous acyclovir is highly effective in the prophylaxis and treatment of oral-labial disease. Acyclovir is the drug of choice for herpes simplex virus encephalitis; a high dose is used (10 mg/kg every 8 hours). Acyclovir is also used for varicella-zoster virus. Intravenous form in immunocompromised patients halts progression and prevents dissemination of herpes zoster. It is also effective for decreasing viral shedding, decreasing the number of new lesions, and increasing healing in primary varicella in immunocompetent children and adults if it is given within the first 24 hours of rash or in immunocompromised hosts. There is no good evidence that treating primary varicella in immunocompetent adults decreases the risk of visceral dissemination. Oral therapy is effective against herpes zoster ophthalmicus (most effective within 72 hours; 600-800 mg five times a day). Herpes zoster in immunocompetent host responds to acyclovir, 800 mg five times a day (decreased viral shedding, time to healing). There is no effect on postherpetic neuralgia. It should be used only if given within 72 hours after onset of symptoms.

- With acyclovir, crystalline nephropathy increased with high dose, bolus infusion, dehydration, preexisting renal impairment.
- Acyclovir is drug of choice for herpes simplex encephalitis.

Ganciclovir

This agent inhibits DNA polymerase, but it is not dependent on phosphorylation by viral thymidine kinase. Thus, it is active against cytomegalovirus. No oral form is available. *Indications* for ganciclovir include treatment of cytomegalo-

virus retinitis in patients with AIDS. Studies have shown beneficial results in other cytomegalovirus infections (colitis, esophagitis, gastritis, and pneumonia) in patients with AIDS and in immunocompromised hosts. In patients with AIDS, maintenance therapy may be necessary to prevent relapse. Used in combination with hyperimmune globulin, ganciclovir reduces mortality from cytomegalovirus pneumonitis in patients who have had allogeneic bone marrow transplantation. Several recent studies suggest that ganciclovir therapy before the development of cytomegalovirus disease in patients who have had heart or bone marrow transplantation may decrease the incidence of cytomegalovirus infection.

Toxicity may manifest as neutropenia and thrombocytopenia. The incidence of neutropenia is increased when ganciclovir is used in combination with zidovudine in patients with AIDS. Cytopenias are reversible after use of the drug is stopped. It is teratogenic, carcinogenic, and mutagenic in animals. Less common are fever, rash, anemia, and increased values on liver function tests.

Ganciclovir *resistance* is associated with persistent viremia and progressive disease. Mechanism of resistance is postulated to be decreased cellular phosphorylation.

Oral ganciclovir has recently been approved for maintenance therapy in cytomegalovirus retinitis.

- Ganciclovir, used in combination with hyperimmune globulin, reduces mortality from cytomegalovirus pneumonitis in patients after bone marrow transplantation.
- Incidence of neutropenia is increased when ganciclovir is used in combination with zidovudine in patients with AIDS.

Famciclovir

Famciclovir is a recently released new antiviral agent. Available only as an oral drug, it is converted to its active form penciclovir through tissue and hepatic enzymatic processes. A prolonged intracellular half-life allows for dosing three times daily. It has good bioavailability, is well tolerated, and has no significant toxicities. Unlike acyclovir, preliminary studies show that it reduces the duration of postherpetic neuralgia.

Foscarnet

This is a noncompetitive inhibitor of viral DNA polymerase and reverse transcriptase. It does not require phosphorylation. It has in vitro activity against human immunodeficiency virus (HIV), all human herpes viruses, and hepatitis B.

Indications include cytomegalovirus retinitis, including disease that is due to ganciclovir-resistant strains. It also may be effective in gastrointestinal disease in patients with AIDS. It is more expensive and less well tolerated than ganciclovir. It requires controlled rates of infusions and large volumes of fluid. Controlled trials in patients with AIDS and cytomegalovirus retinitis showed no difference in the progression of the retinitis between foscarnet-treated and ganciclovir-treated patients. However, there was an unexplained increased mortality in the ganciclovir group.

Foscarnet is less well tolerated than ganciclovir. *Toxicity* involves nephrotoxicity, which usually develops during the second week and is reversible. Risk of nephrotoxicity is increased with concurrent use of nephrotoxic drugs (e.g., amphotericin B, aminoglycosides). Hydration may decrease the risk of nephrotoxicity. Electrolyte disturbances, such as hypocalcemia, hyperphosphatemia or hypophosphatemia, hypokalemia, and hypomagnesemia, also occur. Risk of hypocalcemia is increased with concomitant use of pentamidine intravenously. Fever, nausea, vomiting, anemia, fatigue, headache, leukopenia, pancreatitis, and genital ulceration also have been reported.

Resistance has occurred in strains of herpes simplex virus, varicella-zoster virus, and cytomegalovirus, but in vitro resistance has not been correlated with decreased clinical response.

- Foscarnet is effective for cytomegalovirus retinitis, including disease due to ganciclovir-resistant strains.
- With foscarnet, nephrotoxicity may occur; usually develops during second week and is reversible.

Antiretroviral Therapy

Zidovudine (AZT)

This is a dideoxynucleoside (thymidine analog) that must be phosphorylated to active triphosphate form by cellular enzymes. Its *mechanism of action* is to inhibit reverse transcriptase and terminate HIV nucleic acid chain elongation. In regard to its *clinical pharmacology*, its rate of absorption is 60%-65%. Central nervous system concentrations are 0.1-1.35 times the serum concentrations. Serum half-life is 1 hour, and intracellular half-life is 3-4 hours. It is eliminated through hepatic metabolism and renal excretion. Elimination is reduced in patients with uremia and cirrhosis (dosing every 8 hours may be appropriate). *Drug interactions* include an increased half-life of AZT when used with probenecid; ganciclovir and AZT are additive in their myelosuppressive properties.

Clinical indications are HIV infection in adults and children, in which case it is the drug of choice for initial treatment. In patients with AIDS, it decreases the frequency of opportunistic infection, increases survival, increases body weight and CD4 cell counts (for 4-6 months), and decreases p24 antigenemia. Studies have shown that 500 mg/day is as effective as 1,500 mg/day in patients with AIDS, but toxicity (neutropenia, anemia) is significantly decreased and survival is prolonged. AZT is effective in the treatment of HIV neurologic disease (1,200-1,500 mg/day) and thrombocytopenia. In asymptomatic HIV infection, AZT delays progression of disease in HIV-infected persons with CD4 counts of 200-

500/μL (may or may not increase survival).

Table 14-28 outlines a treatment schedule based on the CD4 cell count.

Adverse effects include anemia and neutropenia, which are dose-limiting toxicities. They are less common with low doses (500-600 mg/day). Granulocyte-macrophage colony-stimulating factor and granulocyte colony-stimulating factor may increase neutrophils, and recombinant erythropoietin in patients with low erythropoietin levels (<500 IU/L) may decrease transfusion requirements. Risk factors for developing anemia include low pretreatment CD4 cell count and hemoglobin value, more advanced HIV disease, and vitamin B_{12} deficiency. Concomitant use of ganciclovir and AZT exacerbates the risk of neutropenia. Asthenia, headache, dizziness, insomnia, anorexia, nausea, vomiting, malaise, and myalgia are common initial events after initiation of therapy, but they usually diminish with continued therapy and seldom require stopping use of the drug. Esophageal ulceration and hyperpigmentation of skin have also been reported. Myopathy occurs in 6%-18% of patients who receive therapy for >6 months. It is difficult to distinguish from HIV-associated myopathy. It occurs 6-12 months after initiation of therapy. Mitochondrial abnormalities are noted on electron microscopy. Most patients (70%-100%) are asymptomatic 6-8 weeks after stopping use of AZT.

Primary infection with AZT-resistant HIV has been reported. The frequency of this finding is unknown. Most reports of in vitro resistance have been in patients treated for at least 6-9 months. Appearance of resistance is related to stage of disease and CD4 cell count. Clinical significance of resistance is unknown. Studies to address this issue are ongoing.

- With AZT, anemia and neutropenia are dose-limiting toxicities.
- Concomitant use of ganciclovir and AZT exacerbates risk of neutropenia.
- Myopathy occurs in 6%-18% of patients who receive AZT for >6 months.

Didanosine (ddI)

This dideoxynucleoside is similar to AZT. It also must be phosphorylated to be active. Its *mechanism of action* is identical to that of AZT. In regard to its *clinical pharmacology*, its rate of absorption is 37%, and absorption is decreased with food. Central nervous system concentrations are 0.1-0.85 times the serum concentrations. Serum half-life is 1.4 hours, and intracellular half-life is 8-24 hours. It is eliminated through hepatic metabolism and renal excretion.

Adverse reactions can occur with concomitant use of intravenous pentamidine (pancreatitis). Because ddI tablets contain antacid to enhance absorption, drugs that require gastric acidity (ketoconazole) should be administered 2 hours before ddI. Similarly, quinolones should not be coadministered with ddI.

Table 14-28.--Strategies for Antiretroviral Therapy in Adults Infected With Human Immunodeficiency Virus*

	CD4 count, cells/μL	Symptoms	Treatment
No prior zidovudine (AZT)	>500	None	None
	200-500	None	1) Observe, monitor CD4
			2) AZT 200 mg three times daily
	200-500	Present, or rapidly ↓ CD4 (>50 cells/μL in 6 mo)	AZT 200 mg three times daily
	<200 cells	None or present	AZT 200 mg three times daily
	<50		AZT 200 mg three times daily[†]
Prior zidovudine (AZT)	>300	Clinically stable, tolerating AZT	Continue AZT 200 mg three times daily
	<300	Clinically stable, tolerating AZT	Continue AZT 200 mg three times daily OR ddI monotherapy OR combination (AZT:ddI, AZT:ddC)
	Any level	Clinical and immuno-logic (CD4 count) deterioration	ddI monotherapy OR combination (AZT:ddI, AZT:ddC)
Zidovudine (AZT) intolerance	...	...	↓ AZT to 300 mg/day Consider erythropoietin or GCSF if hematologic toxicity and appropriate Monotherapy: ddI, ddC, d4T Combination with lower-dose AZT (AZT:ddI, AZT:ddC)

*These are current published recommendations, but thinking is shifting toward early and aggressive therapy with combinations including nucleoside analogs and protease inhibitors.
[†]But prophylaxis of opportunistic infections and minimization of drug side effects should be emphasized over antiretroviral therapy.
ddC, zalcitabine; ddI, didanosine; d4T (stavudine), a nucleoside analog that inhibits human immunodeficiency virus replication by interfering with viral reverse transcriptase and elongation of viral DNA; GCSF, granulocyte colony-stimulating factor.

Clinical indications are advanced HIV infection in patients intolerant of AZT or those in whom AZT is failing. Administration of ddI results in increased CD4 cell count, decreased p24 antigenemia, and decreased symptoms in patients with AIDS.

Toxicity with ddI includes painful peripheral neuropathy. Pancreatitis can develop (7% in one study); risk is increased with high dosage, history of pancreatitis, alcohol abuse, advanced HIV disease, or concomitant use of intravenous pentamidine. Optic neuritis and fulminant hepatitis have also been reported. Anemia and neutropenia significantly less common than in patients administered AZT.

Cross-resistance with AZT has not been reported. Strains resistant to ddI may be resistant to ddC. Patients switched to ddI therapy from AZT therapy may regain AZT sensitivity.

Zalcitabine (ddC)

This is a dideoxynucleoside similar to zidovudine. It also must be phosphorylated to be active. *Mechanism of action* is identical to that of AZT. In regard to its *clinical pharmacology*, its absorption rate is 80%. Absorption is decreased with food. Central nervous system concentrations are 0.1-0.37 times serum concentrations. Serum half-life is 1-3 hours, and intracellular half-life is 8-24 hours. Elimination is through renal excretion. Dose is decreased with renal failure.

Drug interactions occur with concomitant use of drugs that have potential to cause peripheral neuropathy either through direct neurotoxicity or by decreasing renal clearance of ddC. The drug should not be used concomitantly with intravenous pentamidine because of the risk of pancreatitis.

Clinical indications include patients with advanced HIV

infection in whom AZT monotherapy is failing; in these cases, ddC is used in combination with AZT. Increased p24 antigenemia, symptoms in patients with AIDS or AIDS-related complex, and CD4 cell counts <300/μL have been cited as indications in small preliminary studies.

Toxicity includes painful distal sensorimotor peripheral neuropathy (17%-31% of cases in monotherapy studies). This is usually reversible with discontinuation of use of the drug. There are no data on use in patients with preexisting neuropathy. Pancreatitis has been reported (<1% of cases) in monotherapy studies. It is assumed that risk factors for pancreatitis due to ddI are also factors with ddC, but no data are available. Esophageal ulcers have been reported. Anemia and neutropenia significantly less common than in patients administered AZT.

Cross-resistance with AZT has not been reported; ddI cross-resistance has been reported.

- AZT should be used in all previously untreated patients with HIV (i.e., first-line therapy), although patients with AZT-resistant strains have been described.
- If clinical failure or toxicity develops with AZT, switching to ddI monotherapy is appropriate if there are no contraindications.
- All patients receiving antiretroviral therapy should be monitored for drug toxicity, which is common and can be life-threatening.

Ribavirin

This is a purine analog. *Indication* for aerosolized ribavirin is respiratory syncytial virus bronchiolitis in children, in whom treatment decreases morbidity. *Adverse teratogenic and embryotoxic effects* have been noted in animals. The drug is contraindicated in pregnancy, and precautions must be taken when aerosolized ribavirin is used in the hospital.

IMMUNIZATIONS

Tables 14-29 through 14-32 provide basic information about immunizations.

HUMAN IMMUNODEFICIENCY VIRUS (HIV)

Human immunodeficiency virus (HIV) belongs to the family of Retroviridae, subfamily Lentivirinae.

The viruses share a distinct biologic characteristic, which consists of an initial stage of primary infection followed by a relatively asymptomatic period of months to years, culminating in a final and generally fatal stage of overt disease.

There are two types of HIV: HIV-1 and HIV-2. Most reported cases of HIV disease around the world are caused by HIV-1. HIV-2 is found predominantly in Western Africa. HIV-1 and

Table 14-29.--Vaccines Containing Live Viruses

Live viruses	
Smallpox	Mumps
Polio	Rubella
Yellow fever	Rubeola

Table 14-30.--Vaccination Schedules in Adults

Vaccine	Age, yr		
	18-24	25-64	≥65
Tetanus, diphtheria	x	x	x
Measles	x	x*	
Mumps	x	x	
Rubella	x	x	
Influenza			x
Pneumococcal			x[†]

*Indicated for persons born after 1956.
[†]Persons at high risk of fatal disease (e.g., those who have had transplantation, those with asplenia, those who are nephrotoxic) should be revaccinated after 6 years.
Modified from Centers for Disease Control: Update on adult immunization: recommendations of the Immunization Practices Advisory Committee (ACIP). MMWR 40 (no. RR-12):1-71, 1991.

HIV-2 are clinically indistinguishable with identical modes of transmission and pathogenicity.

EPIDEMIOLOGY

HIV infection is a global epidemic affecting more than 15 million people. Worldwide, 40 to 120 million people will be infected by the year 2000. Most of these will be women and children. Seventy percent of all cases of acquired immunodeficiency syndrome (AIDS) are thought to occur in Africa. One to two million Americans are now infected with HIV, more than 400,000 Americans have AIDS, and more than 200,000 deaths have resulted. In 1994, 80,691 new cases of AIDS were reported in the United States.

In recent years, heterosexual transmission has continued to increase as a proportion of all cases (from 17% in 1986 to 24% in 1992), although most new cases still occur in homosexual men. This increase in heterosexual transmission accounts for the dramatic increase in HIV infection in women. In 1992, HIV was the fifth leading cause of death in women of reproductive age and the second leading cause of death among men ages 25 to 44 years. The prevalence of HIV infection is disproportionately high in racial and ethnic minorities. As of

Table 14-31.--Vaccines Specifically Indicated or Contraindicated, According to Special Health Status or Occupation (United States)

Health status or occupation	Vaccine indicated	Vaccine contraindicated
Pregnant	Tetanus, diphtheria (except first trimester)	Live virus vaccine *Bacille Calmette-Guérin* (BCG), oral typhoid
Immunocompromised	Influenza, pneumococcal, HbCV*	Live virus vaccine *Bacille Calmette-Guérin* (BCG), oral typhoid
Splenic dysfunction	Influenza, pneumococcal, HbCV,* meningococcal	
Hemodialysis/transplant	Hepatitis B, influenza, pneumococcal	
Factor VIII, IX	Hepatitis B†	
Chronic alcoholism	Pneumococcal, influenza	
Nursing home resident, age ≥65 yr, diabetes, CHF, COPD, malignancy, CRF	Pneumococcal, influenza	
Homeless/immigrants	Review all vaccines	
Prison inmates	Hepatitis B	
Health care workers	Hepatitis B, influenza, MMR	

*May be considered.
†May need increased dose.
CHF, congestive heart failure; COPD, chronic obstructive pulmonary disease; CRF, chronic renal failure; HbCV, *Haemophilus influenzae* B conjugate vaccine; MMR, measles, mumps, rubella.
Modified from Centers for Disease Control: Update on adult immunization: recommendations of the Immunization Practices Advisory Committee (ACIP). MMWR 40 (no. RR-12):1-71, 1991.

Table 14-32.--Indicated Vaccines in Human Immunodeficiency Virus (HIV) Infection

Vaccine	Asymptomatic HIV	Symptomatic HIV
DTP/Td	Yes	Yes
OPV	No	No
Enhanced-potency inactivated poliovirus*	Yes	Yes
MMR	Yes	Yes†
HbCV†	Yes	Yes
Pneumococcal	Yes	Yes
Influenza	Yes†	Yes

*For adults ≥18 years of age, use only if indicated.
†Should be considered.
DTP/Td, diphtheria, tetanus, pertussis/tetanus, diphtheria; HbCV, *Haemophilus influenzae* B conjugate vaccine; OPV, oral poliovirus; MMR, measles, mumps, rubella.
Modified from Centers for Disease Control: Update on adult immunization: recommendations of the Immunization Practices Advisory Committee (ACIP). MMWR 40 (no. RR-12):1-71, 1991.

Jan. 1, 1993, 53% of HIV-infected persons were white, 30% black, 16.5% Hispanic, and 0.8% other racial groups.

TRANSMISSION

HIV is transmitted sexually, perinatally, by parenteral inoculation (intravenous drug injection, occupational exposure), through blood products, and, less commonly, through organ transplantation. Sexual transmission is the most common means of infection. Female-to-male sexual transmission of HIV is less efficient than male-to-female, as is true for other sexually transmitted diseases. Some of the conditions that may increase the risk of sexually acquiring HIV infection are traumatic intercourse (e.g., receptive anal), ulcerative genital infections such as syphilis, herpes simplex, and chancroid, and lack of circumcision. The use of latex condoms, especially if used properly, reduces the risk of HIV transmission.

HIV infection develops in 16%-30% of infants born to HIV-infected mothers. Infection can also be transmitted through breast milk. Recently, zidovudine treatment of HIV-infected pregnant women in the second and third trimesters and zidovudine treatment of their infants in the first six weeks of life resulted in a significant reduction of maternal-infant transmission of HIV (zidovudine group 8.3% and placebo group 25.5%, $P < 0.00006$).

In the United States, all blood donations have been routinely tested for HIV-1 antibody since early 1985. As of June 1, 1992, all U.S. blood centers test for antibodies to both HIV-1 and HIV-2. Today, the estimated risk of acquiring HIV through blood transfusion is 1 in 225,000. No cases of transfusion-associated HIV-2 infection have been reported in the United States.

Occupational exposure occurs through needle sticks. The risk associated with needle injury is approximately 0.32%. Factors that influence transmission include stage of HIV infection in the source case (this relates to virus titer in the specimen) and size and type of needle (hollow needle or suture needle). The risk associated with mucous membrane and nonintact skin contact is low but is not zero.

NATURAL HISTORY OF HIV DISEASE

Despite clinical latency, HIV replication and immune system destruction continue to occur through all stages of the disease. Most of this active replication occurs in lymphoid tissues.

In *early disease*, the CD4 count is more than 500 cells/μL. The patient is generally asymptomatic. Antiretroviral treatment is not recommended.

In *intermediate disease*, the CD4 count is 200-500 cells/μL. Antiretroviral therapy usually is indicated. Symptoms include headache, fatigue, fever, and weight loss. Related disorders include oral hairy leukoplakia, thrush, seborrheic dermatitis, recurrent vaginal candidiasis, herpes zoster and herpes simplex infections, skin and nail infections, bacterial infections, Kaposi's sarcoma, peripheral non-Hodgkin's lymphoma, and tuberculosis.

In *advanced HIV disease*, the CD4 count is less than 200 cells/μL. The 1993 revised Centers for Disease Control AIDS case definition designated a CD4 count of less than 200 cells/μL and invasive cervical cancer, pulmonary tuberculosis, and recurrent pneumonia as additional AIDS-defining conditions. Opportunistic infections commonly occur. *Pneumocystic carinii* pneumonia prophylaxis is recommended. Antiretroviral treatment is recommended.

In *late-stage HIV disease*, the CD4 count is less than 50 cells/μL. *Mycobacterium avium* complex, toxoplasmosis, central nervous system non-Hodgkin's lymphoma, cryptococcal meningitis, cytomegalovirus disease, progressive disseminated histoplasmosis, and progressive multifocal leukoencephalopathy occur in this stage. Anti-*Pneumocystis carinii* pneumonia and anti-*Mycobacterium avium* complex prophylaxis and antiretroviral treatment are recommended.

LABORATORY DIAGNOSIS

Routine Tests

The enzyme-linked immunosorbent assay (ELISA) is a screening test that detects specific HIV antibodies (primarily gp41 and p24 antibodies). It is 99% sensitive and specific, but its positive predictive value is low in low-prevalence populations. False-positive results occur because of the presence of cross-reacting antibodies in certain patients (e.g., multiparous women, patients with multiple transfusions). False-negative results are caused by testing patients before seroconversion, patients who have undergone replacement transfusions or bone marrow transplantation, or by poorly manufactured testing equipment.

The Western blot test (confirmatory test) detects antibodies directed against gag (p18, p24, p55), pol (p31, p51, p66), and env (gp41, gp120-160). The Centers for Disease Control guidelines for interpretation of the Western blot are as follows: any 2 of p24, gp41, or gp120-160 = positive, 1 only = indeterminate, and no bands = negative. If results are indeterminate, the clinician should assess risk of HIV infection in the individual patient and retest at 3-6 months. The risk of HIV infection is extremely low in patients with an indeterminate Western blot.

Other Tests

These tests include peripheral blood mononuclear cell co-culture (95%-99% sensitive), HIV p24 antigen test (most prevalent in early and end-stage disease), and polymerase chain reaction (false-positive results can be due to laboratory contamination). These tests may be useful in certain situations (acute infection, indeterminate results of Western blot test, infants of seropositive mothers, prognostic markers). These tests are more expensive than routine tests.

CLINICAL SYNDROMES

Acute HIV Infection

Synonyms for this syndrome are primary HIV infection and acute retroviral syndrome. Acute infection is symptomatic in 53%-93% of cases. The incubation period is 2-4 weeks, and clinical illness usually lasts 1-2 weeks. Clinical manifestations are protean (Table 14-33). An atypical lymphocytosis is present in approximately 50% of patients. ELISA results may be negative (usually positive at 6-12 weeks); p24 antigen, HIV culture, or polymerase chain reaction results may be positive. The differential diagnosis includes infection due to Epstein-Barr virus, cytomegalovirus, primary herpes simplex virus, toxoplasmosis, rubella, viral hepatitis, secondary syphilis, and drug reactions. There are few data supporting the concept that antiretroviral therapy hastens resolution of symptoms or prevents development of persistent infection.

Asymptomatic Illness

Asymptomatic illness lasts from months to years. The cumulative incidence of AIDS varies among different patient populations, but, in general approximately 50% of patients will develop AIDS (1987 definition) within 7-11 years after seroconversion. It is presumed that immunodeficiency and AIDS will eventually develop in almost all patients. The most reliable clinical predictors of HIV disease progression are development of thrush or unexplained fever, weight loss, or diarrhea. Commonly used laboratory markers for disease progression are listed in Table 14-34. The most experience is with CD4 cells (e.g., the risk of developing *Pneumocystis carinii* pneumonia [PCP] is 4.9-fold more in patients with CD4 cell counts <200/μL, and the median survival time is 1 year if CD4 count is <50/μL). CD4 cell counts are also useful for defining when to start antiretroviral therapy and PCP prophylaxis.

INFECTIONS ASSOCIATED WITH HIV INFECTION

Syndromes associated with HIV, by CD4 cell count, are listed in Table 14-35.

Pneumocystis carinii Pneumonia

PCP is one of the most common opportunistic infections in patients with AIDS (color plate 14-8). It occurs in approx-

imately 80% of patients who do not receive primary prophylaxis. Onset is insidious with several weeks of fever, weight loss, malaise, and night sweats. The chest radiograph typically shows bilateral interstitial pulmonary infiltrates, but a lobar distribution and spontaneous pneumothoraces may occur. The arterial blood gas analysis usually reveals hypoxia and respiratory alkalosis. A wide A-a gradient (>35 mm Hg) and low Po_2 (<70 mm Hg) are associated with increased mortality. Several methods are used for the diagnosis of PCP. Staining for PCP in hypertonic saline-induced expectorated sputum is 30%-85% sensitive. The sensitivity improves with liquefaction and the use of monoclonal antibody staining, and it decreases with use of PCP prophylaxis. Bronchoalveolar lavage is 85%-90% sensitive. If the patient is receiving PCP prophylaxis, transbronchial lung biopsy may be needed to make the diagnosis. Open lung biopsy is rarely needed.

The treatment of choice for severe disease is cotrimoxazole, 15-20 mg/kg per day (trimethoprim component) for 21 days. Adverse reactions develop in 76% of cases and include fever, rash, neutropenia, thrombocytopenia, elevated results of liver function tests, and renal dysfunction. Intravenous pentamidine is an alternative to cotrimoxazole (3-4 mg/kg per day for 21 days). The adverse reaction rate is >60%; reactions include hypotension, nephrotoxicity, hypoglycemia, and pancreatitis. If there is no improvement 5-7 days after beginning treatment, switching to or adding an alternative agent should

Table 14-33.--Clinical Manifestations of Primary Human Immunodeficiency Virus Infection

General	Neuropathic	Dermatologic	Gastrointestinal
Fever	Headache, retro-orbital pain	Maculopapular rash	Oral candidiasis
Pharyngitis	Meningoencephalitis	Roseola-like rash	Nausea, vomiting
Lymphadenopathy	Peripheral neuropathy	Diffuse urticaria	Diarrhea
Myalgia	Radiculopathy	Desquamation	
Lethargy	Guillain-Barré syndrome	Alopecia	
Anorexia, weight loss	Cognitive impairment	Mucocutaneous ulceration	

From Tindall B, Imrie A, Donovan B, Penny R, Cooper DA: Primary HIV infection. *In* The Medical Management of AIDS. Third edition. Edited by MA Sande, PA Volberding. Philadelphia, WB Saunders Company, 1992, pp 67-86. By permission of publisher.

Table 14-34.--Laboratory Markers of Progression of Human Immunodeficiency Virus (HIV) Disease

Nonspecific markers	Immunologic markers	HIV specific markers
Anemia	Decreased CD4 (or CD4%)	p24 antigenemia
Thrombocytopenia	Decreased CD4:CD8 ratio	Quantitative HIV culture
Elevated erythrocyte sedimentation rate	Elevated β$_2$-microglobulin	
	Elevated neopterin	
	Absent or decreased anti-p24 antibody	
	Elevated acid labile interferon	

From Clement M, Hollander H: Natural history and management of the seropositive patient. *In* The Medical Management of AIDS. Third edition. Edited by MA Sande, PA Volberding. Philadelphia, WB Saunders Company, 1992, pp 87-96. By permission of publisher.

Table 14-35.--General Relationship of Clinical Syndromes to CD4 Cell Count in Human Immunodeficiency Virus-Infected Patients

Clinical syndrome	CD4 cell count			
	>500	500-200	<200	<50
Asymptomatic	x			
Kaposi sarcoma	x			
Fever, sweats, weight loss		x		
Hairy leukoplakia		x		
Oral, esophageal *Candida*		x		
Tuberculosis		x		
PCP			x	
Cryptococcosis			x	
Dementia			x	
Toxoplasmosis				x
MAI				x
CMV				x
Lymphoma				x

CMV, cytomegalovirus; MAI, *Mycobacterium avium-intracellulare*; PCP, *Pneumocystis carinii* pneumonia.

From Shelhamer JH, Toews GB, Masur H, Suffredini AF, Pizzo PA, Walsh TJ, Henderson DK: Respiratory disease in the immunosuppressed patient. Ann Intern Med 117:415-431, 1992. By permission of the American College of Physicians.

be considered.

For mild to moderate disease, treatment regimens include oral trimethoprim-sulfamethoxazole for 21 days, oral trimethoprim-dapsone (patient should be checked for glucose-6-phosphatase deficiency) for 21 days (mild hyperkalemia and methemoglobinemia can occur), oral primaquine plus clindamycin (methemoglobinemia has been reported with primaquine), aerosolized pentamidine (two studies have found that intravenous administration is more effective than aerosolized pentamidine), trimetrexate plus folinic acid, and atovaquone (for patients intolerant of trimethoprim-sulfamethoxazole).

Controlled studies have shown that adjunctive corticosteroids in patients with moderate to severe disease increase survival in patients with AIDS. Benefit was shown when PaO_2 with patient breathing room air was <70 mm Hg or A-a gradient was >35 mm Hg. Recommended dosages of prednisone are 40 mg orally twice a day on days 1-5, 20 mg orally twice a day on days 6-10, and 20 mg orally each day on days 11-21.

Primary prophylaxis of PCP is indicated in all HIV-infected patients with a CD4 count < 200 cells/µL and in HIV-infected persons with higher CD4 cell counts but with symptoms of fever, weight loss, night sweats, or oral candidiasis. Treatment options are as follows: 1) trimethoprim-sulfamethoxazole is the drug of choice (1 double-strength tablet orally each day or 1 double-strength tablet 3 times per week); 2) dapsone, 50 mg; 3) aerosolized pentamidine, 300 mg inhaled monthly via Respigard II nebulizer; 4) dapsone, 50 mg orally each day or 100 mg orally twice a week.

Recent trials of trimethoprim-sulfamethoxazole compared with inhaled pentamidine for primary and secondary prophylaxis showed conclusively that trimethoprim-sulfamethoxazole was more effective than inhaled pentamidine. Also, it may add prophylaxis against other infectious agents (*Nocardia, Toxoplasma gondii, Streptococcus pneumoniae, Haemophilus influenzae, Listeria monocytogenes, Isospora belli*) and prevent extrapulmonary pneumocytosis. As expected, there are many more side effects with trimethoprim-sulfamethoxazole.

Mycobacterial Infections

Mycobacterium tuberculosis is increased in frequency in injection drug users, minorities, and foreign-born persons with AIDS. HIV-infected patients have an increased frequency of extrapulmonary disease and atypical chest radiographic appearance. Extrapulmonary disease, however, presents similarly in HIV- and non-HIV-infected patients. HIV-infected patients may have accelerated primary disease if exposed to patients with active disease.

The incidence of multiple drug-resistant (MDR) tuberculosis is increasing. Patients with newly acquired infection may have a fulminant course. Unlike patients with AIDS who are infected with other strains of tuberculosis, patients infected with MDR tuberculosis more commonly have alveolar or reticulonodular infiltrates or cavitation. Mortality rate is 70%-80%. Average duration of survival is 2-3 months.

For treatment of tuberculosis in patients with AIDS, drugs are the same as used for normal hosts, but drug resistance must be suspected. In initial regimens, if drug resistance is suspected, isoniazid, rifampin, pyrazinamide, and ethambutol are used until drug sensitivity results are available; otherwise, isoniazid, rifampin, and pyrazinamide are used. For drug-susceptible organisms, isoniazid, rifampin, and pyrazinamide are used for 2 months, and isoniazid and rifampin are used for 7 months, or for 6 months after cultures are negative, whichever is longer. For isoniazid-resistant organisms, rifampin and ethambutol with or without pyrazinamide are used for 18 months, or for 12 months after cultures are negative, whichever is longer. Optimal regimens for MDR tuberculosis are unknown. Prophylaxis is used for all patients who are HIV positive with positive results of purified protein derivative testing (≥5 mm).

Mycobacterium avium complex (MAC) causes infection when immunosuppression is severe (CD4 cell count <50/µL). Disseminated MAC infection is the most common systemic bacterial infection in HIV-infected patients. Common presentations include low-grade fever, night sweats, weight loss, and diarrhea. Organisms can be isolated from blood, bone marrow, stool, and respiratory tract secretions. The organism is resistant to conventional antimycobacterial agents. Treatment involves multiple drugs with multiple side effects. Some studies have shown an increase in survival with treatment, but symptoms can often be ameliorated. The current recommended treatment regimen includes one of the newer macrolides (clarithromycin, azithromycin), ethambutol, and one or two additional drugs with activity against MAC. These include clofazimine, ciprofloxacin, amikacin, rifabutin, and rifampin. Recently, clarithromycin and rifampin/rifabutin were shown to reduce each other's bioavailability significantly when given together. Prophylaxis with rifabutin has been approved by the Food and Drug Administration for patients with AIDS whose CD4 cell count is less than 100 cells/µL.

Treponema pallidum

There are rare reports of seronegative secondary syphilis in patients with AIDS. Neurosyphilis has been reported to occur earlier in patients with AIDS than in HIV-negative patients. Patients with AIDS have also been reported to have unusually severe manifestations of all stages of syphilis. Recent studies, however, suggest that these phenomena are rare. However, because of these concerns, some physicians advocate cerebrospinal fluid examination in patients with primary or secondary syphilis and AIDS before initiating treatment.

Serologic response to standard treatment regimens was the same in HIV-positive and HIV-negative persons in a recent study of 50 injection drug users. However, because of reports of patients with primary, secondary, and latent syphilis failing to respond to intramuscular benzathine or procaine penicillin therapy, some investigators have suggested treating patients with AIDS and syphilis more aggressively (additional dose of benzathine penicillin or intravenous penicillin therapy for 5-10 days). However, data on the frequency of this problem are not available, and these practices remain controversial.

Ceftriaxone has been advocated as an alternative therapy for patients with AIDS who have neurosyphilis because it attains treponemacidal cerebrospinal fluid levels and is easy to administer. In a recent small study, however, the use of ceftriaxone in patients with latent and presumed latent syphilis (no cerebrospinal fluid examination) and asymptomatic neurosyphilis had a 23% failure rate within 1-2 years of initiation of therapy. For patients with latent or presumed latent disease, the efficacies of the standard penicillin regimen and ceftriaxone were equivalent.

Fungal Infections

Cryptococcus neoformans

Meningitis and disseminated disease occur in 10% of patients with AIDS and are common initial manifestations. Subtle presentations may occur. Meningismus may not be present. Poor prognostic factors include hyponatremia and positive culture results from a source other than cerebrospinal fluid. The diagnosis of cryptococcal disease relies on assays of serum and cerebrospinal fluid cryptococcal antigen and fungal blood and spinal fluid cultures. Initial therapy includes amphotericin B with or without flucytosine for 2-4 weeks, followed by fluconazole 400 mg daily for a total of 10-12 weeks. Flucytosine may be associated with increased hematologic toxicity in patients with AIDS, particularly if levels are not measured. Fluconazole (400 mg daily) is an alternative agent in patients with less severe disease (i.e., patients with no alteration of mental status at baseline and low cerebrospinal fluid cryptococcal antigen titers). Fluconazole (200 mg daily) is more effective than amphotericin B (1 mg/kg weekly) for chronic suppression. Persistence of infection in the prostate may be a cause of relapse of infection.

Dimorphic Fungi (Histoplasma capsulatum, Coccidioides immitis, Blastomyces dermatitidis)

Coccidioidomycosis and histoplasmosis are reported more often than blastomycosis. Disease with all three pathogens usually presents as disseminated infection and can even present as septic shock (histoplasmosis). Localized pulmonary involvement occurs but is much less common, except with blastomycosis (50% of cases). Disseminated disease often involves the central nervous system (blastomycosis, coccidioidomycosis). Organisms may be seen in buffy coat of blood (histoplasmosis) in some cases. Travel history and geographic location are important clues to the diagnosis. Initial therapy is with amphotericin B for all three pathogens. For nonmeningitic and nonseptic histoplasmosis, itraconazole (200 mg twice daily) can be used as initial treatment. For chronic suppression, itraconazole or amphotericin B is effective for histoplasmosis. For coccidioidomycosis, amphotericin B or fluconazole is used. Treatment of blastomycosis is the same as that of histoplasmosis. An acid environment is required for optimal absorption of itraconazole and drug-drug interactions with H_2 receptor antagonists, antacids, phenobarbital, and rifampin.

Candida albicans

Mucocutaneous disease (e.g., oral thrush or recurrent vaginitis) is common. Esophagitis is also frequent and is a common cause of dysphagia. Systemic candidal infection, including candidemia, is rare unless additional risk factors for disseminated fungal infection such as severe neutropenia and indwelling catheters are involved. Treatment is with clotrimoxazole troches or nystatin initially for mucocutaneous disease. Fluconazole or ketoconazole is used for treatment of topical treatment failures. In a recent study, fluconazole was more effective than ketoconazole for esophagitis in patients with AIDS. Amphotericin B is used for azole failures.

Aspergillus

Aspergillosis is rare except in the setting of neutropenia.

Viral Infections

Cytomegalovirus disease usually affects persons with advanced HIV disease (CD4 cell count <100/μL). Chorioretinitis is the most common clinical manifestation of CMV disease, occurring in approximately 20% of patients with AIDS. The usual symptoms are floaters, visual field deficits, and painless loss of vision. Funduscopic examination reveals yellowish white granules with perivascular exudates and hemorrhages. Cytomegalovirus gastrointestinal disease may manifest as abdominal pain, dysphagia, and bloody diarrhea. It most commonly involves the esophagus and colon. Cytomegalovirus can also cause hepatitis, pneumonitis, sclerosing cholangitis, encephalitis, adrenalitis, polyradiculopathy, and myelopathy. Treatment is with ganciclovir or foscarnet. The limiting side effect of ganciclovir is bone marrow suppression, and the major effect of foscarnet is renal toxicity.

With herpes simplex virus, severe mucocutaneous ulceration may occur, and the frequency of recurrent oral-labial and genital disease may increase.

Prolonged or severe herpes zoster infection may herald the diagnosis of HIV infection. Central nervous system infection can occur weeks to months after the diagnosis of herpes zoster.

Enteric Infections

Differential diagnoses for various clinical syndromes are outlined in Table 14-36.

Initial evaluation of patients with AIDS who have abdominal pain, large-volume diarrhea, and weight loss should include stool cultures for bacteria, three separate stool specimens for ova and parasites, specific examination for cryptosporidiosis, and *Clostridium difficile* toxin. In cases of persistent diarrhea despite routine studies, cytomegalovirus or *M. avium-intracellulare* should be considered. If no diagnosis is made, upper and lower gastrointestinal endoscopy and biopsy may yield pathogens that are treatable.

Salmonellosis presents with fever, severe diarrhea, abdominal pain, or typhoidal illness without diarrhea. Bacteremia is common. Ciprofloxacin is used for treatment for 10-14 days. Recurrence is common; maintenance therapy may be needed.

Cryptosporidiosis and *I. belli* infection often cause massive, watery diarrhea, crampy abdominal pain, anorexia, flatulence, and malaise. Fever and bloody diarrhea are uncom-

Table 14-36.--Differential Diagnoses of Enteric Infections in Association With Human Immunodeficiency Virus

Proctitis	Proctocolitis	Enteritis
Neisseria gonorrhoeae	*Campylobacter*	*Giardia*
Herpes simplex	*Shigella*	Cryptosporidiosis
Chlamydia	*Chlamydia*	*Isospora*
Treponema pallidum	*Entamoeba histolytica*	Microsporidia
Cytomegalovirus	*Clostridium difficile*	
	Salmonella typhimurium	
	Cytomegalovirus	

mon. Malabsorption and dehydration are common. Biliary tract involvement may occur with cryptosporidiosis infection. Acid-fast bacilli smear of stool or cryptosporidium-specific stain of stool is diagnostic. If CD4 cell count is >180/μL, cryptosporidium infection is usually self-limited (<4 weeks); if it is <140/μL, persistent disease will develop in 80%-90%. There are no proven regimens for the treatment of cryptosporidiosis, but paromomycin, a nonabsorbable aminoglycoside used for the treatment of *Entamoeba histolytica*, has been effective in some patients. For *Isospora*, trimethoprim-sulfamethoxazole is used.

Central Nervous System Infections

HIV encephalopathy may begin early in the course of HIV disease and is slowly progressive. Subtle cognitive impairment is common; it can progress to severe dementia and marked motor dysfunction. Computed tomography and magnetic resonance imaging show diffuse atrophy. No therapy is proved to be effective. Antiretroviral therapy may be helpful (dosage of zidovudine may need to be increased--1,200 mg/day).

Progressive multifocal leukoencephalopathy is a demyelinating disease caused by papovavirus (JC virus). Symptoms and signs are variable. Magnetic resonance imaging shows characteristic white matter changes. Prognosis is poor, and there is no proven treatment.

Toxoplasma gondii, a protozoan, is the most common cause of focal central nervous system lesions in patients with AIDS. The most common symptoms of *Toxoplasma encephalitis* include headache, confusion, and fever. Focal neurologic deficits occur in 69% of cases. Median CD4 cell count at diagnosis is 50/μL. Multiple mass lesions develop in central nervous system in patients with AIDS, typically either toxoplasmosis or lymphoma. Magnetic resonance imaging is more sensitive than computed tomography with contrast (ring-enhancing lesions are characteristic). Single mass lesions are found in up to 40% of patients evaluated by computed tomography and in 20% by magnetic resonance imaging. If serum toxoplasmosis antibody is positive (10%-40% of individuals in United States), treatment should be empiric with pyrimethamine and sulfadiazine plus leucovorin. However, 15%-20% of patients in a recent study were seronegative at presentation. Immunofluorescence assay is less sensitive than enzyme-linked immunosorbent assay. If patient is seronegative, has a single mass lesion, or has no response to empiric therapy (2 weeks), brain biopsy is indicated. Long-term suppressive therapy (secondary prophylaxis) is necessary to prevent relapse, although even with suppressive therapy 20%-25% of patients will have relapse. Primary prophylaxis in seropositive individuals (trimethoprim-sulfamethoxazole) or other regimens is controversial. Alternative therapy is clindamycin and pyrimethamine.

The differential diagnosis of *central nervous system mass lesions* in patients with AIDS includes *T. gondii*, neoplasm (lymphoma or Kaposi's sarcoma), *Cryptococcus neoformans, Coccidioides immitis, Candida albicans, Mycobacterium tuberculosis*, and *Nocardia asteroides*, among others.

Neoplastic Diseases

Kaposi's sarcoma is a tumor of uncertain origin, with vascular proliferation being its most prominent feature. Clinical manifestations include nodules, plaques, lymph node enlargement, and signs and symptoms of visceral involvement. Skin, lung, and gastrointestinal tract are the commonly affected organs. Lung involvement may mimic infection. Bloody pleural effusions suggest Kaposi's sarcoma. It is most common in the homosexual population with AIDS. Treatment options include local therapy (radiotherapy, intralesional chemotherapy, cryotherapy) and systemic therapy (chemotherapy, interferon-α). There is some speculation that an as yet unidentified sexually transmitted agent might be responsible for Kaposi's sarcoma.

Non-Hodgkin's lymphoma is a complication of advanced HIV disease. Usually it is B cell in origin. As patients with AIDS live longer, this complication will become more frequent. Central nervous system involvement is common, and it can be the only anatomic site of disease. Treatment options include combination chemotherapy and whole-brain radiotherapy. Treatment can often improve quality of life, but duration of remission is usually measured in months. Recent reports suggest a link between Hodgkin's disease and HIV, particularly in patients with advanced disease at presentation and with mixed cellular and lymphocyte depletion on pathologic examination.

Miscellaneous Infections and Clinical Syndromes

Idiopathic thrombocytopenic purpura should be suspected in patients with HIV infection in whom purpura or ecchymotic skin lesions develop. Treatment is with antiretroviral therapy; if this fails, prednisone, plasmapheresis, splenic irradiation, or splenectomy can be tried.

Bacillary angiomatosis is a clinical syndrome consisting of constitutional symptoms in conjunction with angiomatous nodules of skin or bone and occasionally peliosis hepatis. Central nervous system mass lesions have also been reported. Diagnosis is established by biopsy, demonstration of organism on Warthin-Starry (Steiner) stain, and cultivation of the causative organisms (*Bartonella quintana, B. henselae*). Results of blood culture (lysis centrifugation technique) may also be positive if incubation is prolonged. Treatment is with erythromycin or doxycycline.

Bacterial pneumonia in patients with AIDS may be as common as PCP. In injection drug users, it is particularly common and occurs before and after the onset of HIV infection. Common causes are *S. pneumoniae* and *H. influenzae*. It should be suspected in patients with purulent sputum and lobar infiltrates. Remember that recurrent pneumonia is an AIDS-defining illness. *Rhodococcus equi* (formerly *Corynebacterium equi*) causes necrotizing pneumonia in patients with HIV which resembles tuberculosis and nocardiosis.

Endocrine abnormalities in HIV infection can affect the adrenal glands, which are involved by infections, tumor, and medications. Infection is caused by cytomegalovirus, *Mycobacterium tuberculosis* and atypical *Mycobacteria, C. neoformans, H. capsulatum, T. gondii*, and *P. carinii*. Adrenal insufficiency is rare. Noninfectious diseases that involve the adrenal glands include lymphoma, Kaposi's sarcoma, and hemorrhage. Adrenal insufficiency is rare. Hyponatremia should instigate a workup for adrenal insufficiency. Ketoconazole inhibits adrenal steroidogenesis. Rifampin, phenytoin, and opiates accelerate degradation of cortisol.

Most asymptomatic patients have normal thyroid function. Increased thyroxine-binding globulin can cause increased thyroxine level with normal thyroid-stimulating hormone value. Thyroxine and triiodothyronine levels decline with advancing illness. Triiodothyronine level is less than in other chronic illnesses. Persistence of relatively normal triiodothyronine value despite progressive HIV infection may contribute to weight loss. *P. carinii* infection of thyroid has been described.

Common causes of hyponatremia include diarrhea, syndrome of inappropriate secretion of antidiuretic hormone (most common cause if hyponatremia developed while patient hospitalized), and renal insufficiency.

Hypercalcemia can be caused by lymphoma and human T-cell leukemia virus-I coinfection. Hypocalcemia is also caused by ketoconazole and foscarnet.

In regard to gonadal function, testosterone levels are normal in asymptomatic HIV. In advanced disease, gonadal, pituitary, or hypothalamic failure may occur.

Pancreatitis can be caused by cytomegalovirus, trimethoprim-sulfamethoxazole, intravenous pentamidine, didanosine (ddI), and zalcitabine (ddC).

The most common *rheumatologic manifestations* in HIV are Reiter's syndrome, reactive arthritis, polymyositis and polymyalgia, and sicca syndrome. All of these are associated with the onset of active AIDS complications and infections.

Cholangitis and *acalculous cholecystitis* are associated with cytomegalovirus, cryptosporidiosis, and Microsporidia (*Enterocytozoon bieneusi*). Most common syndrome associated with Microsporidia, however, is chronic diarrhea; it can also cause keratoconjunctivitis, hepatitis, and peritonitis.

Renal abnormalities include almost any type of chronic nephropathy, but HIV-associated nephropathy is most common. About 85% of cases have occurred in blacks. Pathologic feature is focal and segmental glomerulosclerosis, which may cause nephrotic syndrome, and this leads rapidly to end-stage renal failure. Peripheral edema and hypertension are usually absent. Renal abnormalities occur in any stage of HIV disease. IgA nephropathy was recently reported.

Common dermatologic diseases that are associated with HIV disease include prurigo xerosis, ichthyosis, seborrheic dermatitis, psoriasis, and neoplasms (Kaposi's sarcoma, lymphoma).

Oral disease is common and can occur at any stage of HIV disease. The clinical manifestation of oral candidiasis is varied and includes pseudomembranous candidiasis, erythematous candidiasis, and angular cheilitis. Treatment is either local (clotrimazole, nystatin) or systemic (fluconazole). Periodontal disease is also common, causing linear gingival erythema and necrotizing periodontitis. The causative oral flora are similar to those in non-HIV-infected persons. Treatment includes local debridement, daily chlorhexidine mouth rinses, and, in cases of necrotizing periodontitis, the addition of metronidazole, amoxicillin/clavulanate, or clindamycin. The etiologic agent of *oral hairy leukoplakia* is Epstein-Barr virus. It usually responds to acyclovir therapy.

Gynecologic complications in women with HIV infection include recurrent or chronic genital infections (vulvovaginal candidiasis, trichomoniasis, HSV-2), anogenital infections with human papilloma virus, and invasive cervical cancer. Note that, as of January 1993, invasive cervical cancer is an AIDS-defining condition. *HIV-2* is a human retrovirus with significant antigenic differences from HIV-1. This infection is prevalent in Western Africa. In certain urban centers, 15%-64% of prostitutes are infected. Seroprevalence increases with age; 100% of prostitutes >50 years are infected. By April 1992, 32 cases had been reported in the United States. In all 32 cases, the patient either had lived in Western Africa or had sexual partners who had lived there. No cases of transfusion-related disease have been reported. Since June 1992, the blood supply has been screened for HIV-2. Transmission is through sexual contact or blood products. Vertical transmission is less common than with HIV-1. HIV-2 can cause AIDS. Rate of progression to severe immunosuppression and AIDS is 12-13 times slower than with HIV-1. Asymptomatic period is likely much longer. Clinical manifestations of AIDS are similar between HIV-1 and HIV-2. Diagnosis should be considered in patients from endemic areas or patients who have sexual partners who reside in endemic areas. In 80% of HIV-2-infected patients, results of enzyme-linked immunosorbent assay designed to detect HIV-1 will be positive. An HIV-2-specific assay is available. Western blot test results may be indeterminate. The length of seronegative interval after infection is unknown. A polymerase chain reaction test is also available. Antiretroviral therapy is used according to protocols used for HIV-1. However, because of long asymptomatic interval, instituting therapy when the CD4 cell count is beween 200-500/μL is controversial. Treatment strategies for opportunistic infections are identical.

ACKNOWLEDGMENT

The authors gratefully acknowledge the contributions by Walter R. Wilson, M.D., to the earlier versions of this chapter and thank Franklin R. Cockerill, M.D., John G. Hughes, and Jon E. Rosenblatt, M.D., from the Division of Clinical Microbiology for providing the slides.

Color plate 14-1. ß-Hemolytic *Streptococcus* in cerebrospinal fluid. (Gram stain.)

Color plate 14-2. *Streptococcus pneumoniae* in sputum. (Gram stain.)

Color plate 14-3. *Nocardia asteroides*. (Modified acid-fast stain.)

Color plate 14-4. *Blastomyces dermatitidis* in bronchoalveolar lavage. (x100.)

Color plate 14-5. *Aspergillus fumigatus* in bronchoalveolar lavage. (x100.)

Color plate 14-6. *Cryptococcus neoformans* in cerebrospinal fluid. (x100.)

Color plate 14-7. Thin blood smear showing banana-shaped gametocyte of *Plasmodium falciparum*.

Color plate 14-8. *Pneumocystis carinii* in induced sputum from a patient infected with human immunodeficiency virus.

QUESTIONS

Multiple Choice (choose the one best answer)

1. Which of the following is *not* characteristic of diphtheria in indigent patients with chronic alcoholism?
   a. Pneumonitis
   b. Cutaneous lesions
   c. Pharyngitis
   d. Conjunctivitis
   e. Clinical response to erythromycin

2. Gram-negative aerobic rods are the most common cause of urinary tract infections. Which of the following gram-negative bacteria is associated with nephrolithiasis and alkaline urine?
   a. *Proteus mirabilis*
   b. *Hafnia alvei*
   c. *Pseudomonas aeruginosa*
   d. *Klebsiella pneumoniae*
   e. *Citrobacter freundii*

3. Pneumonia develops in a patient who is on a ventilator in the intensive care unit. *Enterobacter cloacae* grows from the sputum and blood. Although the organism is susceptible to cefotaxime, you recommend treatment with mezlocillin and gentamicin because:
   a. *Enterobacter* often has an inducible β-lactamase that causes it to become resistant to cephalosporins
   b. There are likely uncultured organisms present which can better be treated with the combination

   c. Cefotaxime will not reliably treat pneumonia
   d. The laboratory probably misidentified the organism and it is actually a *Pseudomonas*
   e. Two drugs are better than one

4. You are caring for a 43-year-old woman undergoing chronic hemodialysis. On three occasions during the past 4 months, *Staphylococcus aureus* bacteremia has developed. Each time, she clinically improved and the bacteremia cleared during a 2-week course of intravenous nafcillin, but then relapse developed. The most likely explanation for these relapses is:
   a. The *Staphylococcus aureus* is resistant to nafcillin
   b. The patient has inadequately treated endocarditis
   c. The patient's vascular access graft is infected
   d. The dose of nafcillin is inadequate because of the dialysis
   e. The infections are self-induced

5. Which one of the following statements about tetanus is true?
   a. After tetanus, a patient will not require further immunization
   b. Allergic reactions to tetanus immunoglobulin are common
   c. Tetanus begins in the extremities and affects cranial nerves only in severe cases
   d. The causative organism is an obligate anaerobe that produces a neurotoxin known as tetanospasmin
   e. Most patients in the United States with tetanus are children

6. *Enterococcus faecalis* endocarditis should be treated with which of the following antibiotic regimens?
   a. Cefazolin and amikacin
   b. Imipenem-cilastatin
   c. Nafcillin
   d. Vancomycin and rifampin
   e. Ampicillin and gentamicin

7. Which one of the following is *not* a symptom associated with Lyme disease?
   a. Transient cardiac dysrhythmias
   b. Bell's palsy
   c. Chronic meningitis
   d. Arthritis
   e. Erythema infectiosum

8. Which one of the following is *not* a common manifestation of nosocomial infection with *Candida albicans*?
   a. Endophthalmitis after removal of an infected central venous catheter
   b. Pneumonitis
   c. Asymptomatic urinary colonization
   d. Fever in a neutropenic host
   e. Rising liver enzyme values and fever after recovery from neutropenia

9. Which of the following is a risk factor for acquiring toxoplasmosis?
   a. Receiving a heart transplant
   b. Multiple blood transfusions
   c. Walking barefoot on Nantucket Island
   d. Drinking unpasteurized milk
   e. Tick bites

10. Which one of the following infections cannot be transmitted by tick bites?
    a. Rocky Mountain spotted fever
    b. Lyme disease
    c. Leptospirosis
    d. Colorado tick fever
    e. Ehrlichiosis

11. A previously healthy 32-year-old man presents with multiple raised, crusting nodules on his right hand which extend up the forearm. They have slowly progressed during 1 month and are not associated with systemic symptoms. Two weeks before noting the initial lesion, he sustained several scratches while planting rose bushes. You correctly initiate which one of the following therapies?
    a. Cephalexin
    b. Itraconazole
    c. Topical triamcinolone cream

    d. Trimethoprim-sulfamethoxazole
    e. Surgical consultation for debridement

12. An 18-year-old female college student presents with a 1-week history of fever, sore throat, and malaise. Oral ampicillin was prescribed. She has a new macular rash. On examination, you find multiple enlarged lymph nodes. The most likely diagnosis is:
    a. Rubella
    b. Infectious mononucleosis
    c. Atypical measles
    d. Toxic strep syndrome
    e. Disseminated gonococcal infection

13. A 25-year-old previously healthy white man taking prednisone (30 mg) for rheumatoid arthritis presents to the emergency room with a 24-hour history of fever (temperature 40°C), chills, and a severe headache. On physical examination, meningismus is the only abnormal finding. Cerebrospinal fluid examination reveals a leukocyte count of 20,000 (50% polymorphonuclear leukocytes, 50% lymphocytes). The cerebrospinal fluid Gram stain reveals gram-positive rods. The most likely cause of the acute meningitis is:
    a. *Haemophilus influenzae*
    b. *Neisseria meningitidis*
    c. *Streptococcus pneumoniae*
    d. *Listeria monocytogenes*
    e. *Mycobacterium tuberculosis*

14. A 60-year-old previously healthy man is admitted to the hospital with a 2-week history of fever, chills, and malaise. On physical examination, abnormal findings include bilateral conjunctival hemorrhages, splenomegaly, and a 2/4 holosystolic murmur consistent with mitral regurgitation. He has no known antimicrobial allergies. Four separate blood cultures 48 hours after admission are positive for *Enterococcus faecalis* (penicillin minimal inhibitory concentration 2 g/mL; gentamicin minimal inhibitory concentration ≤500). The best therapeutic regimen for this patient is:
    a. Aqueous penicillin G (intravenously) for 4-6 weeks
    b. Aqueous penicillin G (intravenously) *plus* gentamicin for 4-6 weeks
    c. Vancomycin (intravenously) for 4-6 weeks
    d. Aqueous penicillin G (intravenously) *plus* gentamicin for 2 weeks
    e. Cefazolin (intravenously) for 4-6 weeks

15. A 45-year-old woman with degenerative joint disease presents to the emergency room with a painful left knee. There is no history of tick exposure or family history of

rheumatologic disease. On physical examination, her temperature is 38.5°C, the knee is erythematous and warm, and there is marked limitation of motion. A large effusion is also present. Arthrocentesis reveals a synovial leukocyte count of 45,000/mm³. The Gram stain and bacterial culture results are negative. The most likely cause of this acute arthritis is:
a. Rheumatoid arthritis
b. *Staphylococcus aureus*
c. *Borrelia burgdorferi*
d. *Neisseria gonorrhoeae*
e. Coagulase-negative staphylococci

16. The treatment of choice for late latent syphilis is:
a. Doxycycline 100 mg orally twice a day for 14 days
b. Benzathine penicillin 2.4 million U intramuscularly, 1 dose
c. Benzathine penicillin 2.4 million U intramuscularly weekly for 3 weeks
d. Erythromycin 500 mg three times a day for 14 days
e. Aqueous penicillin G 12-24 million U intravenously/day for 10 days

17. The organism that has been associated with infectious diarrhea and the hemolytic uremic syndrome is:
a. *Escherichia coli* 0157:H7
b. *Clostridium perfringens*
c. *Vibrio parahaemolyticus*
d. *Salmonella typhimurium*
e. Norwalk virus

18. Which of the following is not a risk factor for occult upper urinary tract infection in women?
a. Symptoms ≤24 hours
b. Emergency room presentation
c. Recent urinary tract instrumentation
d. Acute pyelonephritis or ≥3 urinary tract infections in 1 year
e. Pregnancy

19. Which one of the following antimicrobial drugs is not excreted primarily by the kidneys?
a. Penicillin G
b. Ciprofloxacin
c. Erythromycin
d. Cefazolin
e. Gentamicin

20. Fever in the patient with neutropenia (absolute neutrophil count <0.5 x 10⁹/L) generally requires empiric antimicrobial therapy before culture results are known. Which one of the following is not an acceptable choice for that empiric therapy?
a. Ceftriaxone and amikacin
b. Ceftazidime
c. Ceftazidime and gentamicin
d. Cefotaxime and vancomycin
e. Vancomycin and ceftazidime

21. Which one of the following does not affect the absorption of ciprofloxacin?
a. Sucralfate
b. Oral iron preparations
c. Aluminum-containing antacids
d. Zinc-containing supplements
e. Cimetidine

22. Which one of the following antibiotics has as its mechanism of action inhibition of DNA gyrase?
a. Penicillin G
b. Tetracycline
c. Rifampin
d. Chloramphenicol
e. Ciprofloxacin

23. Which one of the following antibacterial agents is active against *Streptococcus pneumoniae* (penicillin minimal inhibitory concentration ≥2 µg/mL):
a. Ciprofloxacin
b. Ampicillin/sulbactam
c. Vancomycin
d. Cefuroxime
e. Penicillin G

24. Which one of the following antibiotics does not reach therapeutic levels in cerebrospinal fluid?
a. Fluconazole
b. Cefotaxime
c. Cefazolin
d. Ceftriaxone
e. Penicillin G

25. A 37-year-old man from Minneapolis with human immunodeficiency virus (HIV) infection (CD4 cell count, 150 µL) is admitted to the hospital with a 10-day history of fever (temperature 38.3°C) and a dry, nonproductive cough. There is no history of previous tuberculosis or exposure to persons with tuberculosis. His current medications include zidovudine and inhaled pentamidine. Physical examination reveals crackles in the upper lung fields. Chest radiography reveals bilateral upper lobe infiltrates. Initial results of his induced sputum examination include negative Gram stain, fungal stain, acid-fast stain, and stain for *Pneumocystis carinii* pneumonia. Which treatment

regimen would be most effective against the likely cause of this man's symptoms?

a. Isoniazid plus rifampin

b. Itraconazole

c. Trimethoprim-sulfamethoxazole

d. Ganciclovir

e. Clarithromycin, rifabutin, and ethambutol

26. Which of the following is not a recognized cause of anemia in patients with acquired immunodeficiency syndrome (AIDS)?

a. Zidovudine therapy

b. *Mycobacterium avium-intracellulare*

c. Parvovirus B19

d. HIV infection

e. Didanosine (ddI) therapy

27. Which of the following antimicrobial agents is not used for the treatment of *Pneumocystis carinii* pneumonia?

a. Trimethoprim-sulfamethoxazole

b. Pentamidine intravenously

c. Atovaquone

d. Doxycycline

e. Trimetrexate

28. A 28-year old white man with newly diagnosed HIV infection develops *Pneumocystis carinii* pneumonia. His initial A-a gradient on room air is >40 mm Hg. In the past, he has had Stevens-Johnson syndrome during treatment with trimethoprim-sulfamethoxazole. The most appropriate therapy for this infection at this time is:

a. Trimethoprim-sulfamethoxazole intravenously

b. Pentamidine intravenously *plus* corticosteroids

c. Trimethoprim-sulfamethoxazole intravenously *plus* steroids

d. Pentamidine intravenously

e. Trimethoprim-sulfamethoxazole orally

29. A 34-year-old foreign-born man who is HIV-antibody positive (CD4 cell count, 50/μL) develops cryptococcal meningitis. On presentation he is comatose. The most appropriate *initial* therapy for this patient is:

a. Fluconazole

b. Itraconazole

c. Amphotericin B

d. Miconazole

e. Amphotericin B plus rifampin

30. A 26-year-old man with AIDS (CD4 cell count, 32/μL) presents with headache, fever, and confusion. Computed tomography of the brain shows multiple, hypodense, ring-enhancing lesions. At the time of the initial diagnosis of

HIV infection 9 years previously, his IgG *Toxoplasma* antibody was positive. What is the next step in the management of this patient?

a. Repeat determination of serum *Toxoplasma* antibody titer

b. Obtain cerebrospinal fluid for measurement of intrathecal production of antibody to *T. gondii*

c. Start empiric therapy with pyrimethamine and sulfadiazine

d. Magnetic resonance imaging for better definition of intracranial lesions

e. Brain biopsy

31. The most common systemic bacterial infection in HIV-infected patients is

a. *Pneumocystis carinii* pneumonia

b. Toxoplasmosis

c. Tuberculosis

d. *Mycobacterium avium* complex (MAC) infection

e. Bacillary angiomatosis

32. Chronic suppressive treatment is not indicated in which one of the following infections?

a. Cryptococcal meningitis

b. Cytomegalovirus retinitis

c. *Mycobacterium avium* complex (MAC)

d. *Pneumocystitis carinii* pneumonia

e. Tuberculosis

33. A 37-year-old intravenous drug user, not receiving any medication, presents with fever, dyspnea, and nonproductive cough of several weeks in duration. He has dry rales on physical examination, and chest radiography reveals diffuse interstitial infiltrates. On further investigation, he is found to be HIV-positive, and the CD4 cell count is 106/μL. Induced sputum is negative for *Pneumocystis carinii*. What is the next step?

a. Pulmonary function test

b. Gallium scanning

c. Transbronchial biopsy

d. Bronchoalveolar lavage

e. Open lung biopsy

34. Isoniazid chemoprophylaxis for tuberculosis is not indicated in which one of the following patients?

a. A 46-year-old intravenous drug user with a tuberculin reaction of 12 mm

b. A 38-year-old HIV-infected woman with a tuberculin reaction of 6 mm

c. A 56-year-old man with tuberculin reaction of 14 mm

d. A 28-year-old recent immigrant from Somalia who is HIV-negative and has a history of Bacille Calmette-

Guérin vaccination in childhood but now has a positive tuberculin reaction of 12 mm
   e. A 46-year-old wife of a man in whom pulmonary tuberculosis was diagnosed 2 weeks ago; she has a positive tuberculin reaction of 7 mm

35. Which one of the following is not thought to be a possible explanation for the resurgence of invasive group A streptococcal infections?
   a. Presence of virulent strains
   b. Increased resistance to antibiotics
   c. Presence of virulence factors such as streptococcal pyrogenic exotoxin
   d. Relative lack of immunity in affected patients to the virulent strains
   e. Protease production

36. A 24-year-old man has fever, pharyngitis, oral ulcers, and lymphadenopathy and is concerned about his HIV status because he had an unprotected sexual encounter with a sex worker 2 weeks ago. The HIV antibody test (enzyme-linked immunosorbent assay) is negative. Which of the following is not an option for the diagnosis of HIV infection in this case?
   a. Measure the CD4 cell count
   b. HIV culture
   c. Polymerase chain reaction
   d. Repeat HIV antibody testing in 3-6 months
   e. P24 antigen determination

True/False (indicate whether each answer is true or false)
37. Group A β-hemolytic streptococci cause various non-suppurative complications of infection. Each of the following describes one of these complications.
   a. Myocarditis
   b. Relapsing pharyngitis
   c. Subcutaneous nodules
   d. Rising creatinine with red cell casts in the urine
   e. Arthritis
   f. Chorea

38. Evaluate each of the following statements concerning the treatment of tuberculosis.
   a. Never add a single drug to a failing antituberculosis regimen
   b. Multidrug-resistant tuberculosis infection has a higher mortality rate than infection with susceptible tuberculosis
   c. Steroids are an important adjunct to the therapy of tuberculosis meningitis
   d. Patients with active pulmonary tuberculosis should be

in respiratory isolation for at least 1 month after initiating therapy
   e. Six months is the shortest course of therapy that reliably cures tuberculosis
   f. Treatment for extrapulmonary tuberculosis is different from that for pulmonary tuberculosis

39. Each of the following is an epidemiologic factor associated with *Listeria monocytogenes* meningitis
   a. Patient receiving chronic corticosteroids
   b. Consumption of unpasteurized milk products
   c. Travel to South America
   d. Pregnancy
   e. Consumption of undercooked chicken
   f. Diarrhea associated with epidemics of listeriosis

40. Each of the following describes a clinical syndrome associated with *Aspergillus* infections.
   a. Invasive bronchopulmonary disease in an immunocompromised host
   b. A noninvasive "fungus ball" in a pulmonary cavity
   c. Asthma, productive cough, and eosinophilia
   d. Asymptomatic colonization of the respiratory tract
   e. Otitis externa
   f. Disease cured by therapy with fluconazole

41. The following statements describe characteristics of infection with *Histoplasma capsulatum* (histoplasmosis).
   a. Highest incidence is in the Midwest
   b. Acute infection is usually self-limited
   c. Biopsy of infected tissue reveals angioinvasive hyphae
   d. Ketoconazole and itraconazole are effective therapeutic agents
   e. Oral mucosal lesions are common with disseminated histoplasmosis
   f. Adrenal glands are rarely affected by disseminated histoplasmosis

42. The following statements describe characteristics of rickettsial infections.
   a. All are transmitted by an insect vector
   b. Rocky Mountain spotted fever is most common in Colorado and Wyoming
   c. Low platelet counts are common during rickettsial infection
   d. *Ehrlichia chafeensis* causes a rash indistinguishable from that of rickettsial pox
   e. Colorado tick fever is most reliably cured with tetracycline
   f. Chloramphenicol is active against most rickettsial organisms

43. True statements concerning toxic shock syndrome (TSS) include:
   a. 90% of cases of TSS due to *Staphylococcus aureus* are related to a cellulitis
   b. TSS can occur after a postoperative wound infection
   c. Most patients with TSS due to *Streptococcus pyogenes* are bacteremic
   d. TSS due to *S. pyogenes* is often associated with cellulitis or fasciitis
   e. The relapse rate for menstruation-related TSS is <10%
   f. The diagnosis of TSS is based on clinical criteria and not isolation of *S. aureus* or *S. pyogenes* from a normally sterile site

44. True statements concerning infections after solid organ transplantation include:
   a. Bacterial infections are the most common type of infection 2 to 6 months after transplantation
   b. *Cryptococcus neoformans* causes meningitis usually within the first month after transplantation
   c. The risk of cytomegalovirus infection in the post-transplant period is not related to the serostatus of the recipient and donor
   d. *Pneumocystis carinii* pneumonia usually presents within 4 months of transplantation
   e. Wound infections occur 1-4 months after solid organ transplantation
   f. Type and duration of immunosuppression are related to the incidence of infection after transplantation

45. Which of the following statements are true regarding infective endocarditis?
   a. Coagulase-negative staphylococci are the most common cause of early prosthetic valve endocarditis
   b. If surgical intervention in infective endocarditis is needed, it should be delayed to allow additional days of antimicrobial therapy
   c. The most common cause of culture-negative endocarditis is infection due to *Candida albicans*
   d. Colonic neoplasms have been associated with enterococcal infective endocarditis
   e. The treatment of choice for urgent empiric treatment of culture-negative endocarditis is vancomycin and gentamicin
   f. Gram-negative bacilli and *Candida* species are the agents that most commonly cause infective endocarditis in young healthy adults

46. The following antimicrobial agents are primarily metabolized by the liver.
   a. Rifampin
   b. Ganciclovir
   c. Amoxicillin-clavulanic acid
   d. Erythromycin
   e. Itraconazole
   f. Amikacin

47. β-Lactamase inhibitors such as clavulanate and sulbactam expand the antibacterial spectrum of the penicillins to include each of the following:
   a. *Enterobacter aerogenes*
   b. *Prevotella melaninogenicus*
   c. Methicillin-resistant *Staphylococcus aureus*
   d. Methicillin-susceptible *Staphylococcus aureus*
   e. Penicillin-resistant *Pneumococcus*
   f. Ampicillin-resistant *Moraxella catarrhalis*

48. The following statements describe a characteristic of the antifungal drug ketoconazole.
   a. It is effective therapy for meningitis due to *Coccidioides immitis*
   b. Gastric acid does not need to be present to absorb the medication
   c. It is effective therapy for nonmeningeal blastomycosis
   d. It potentiates the effect of warfarin
   e. It is effective as maintenance therapy for cryptococcal meningitis in patients with AIDS
   f. The mechanism of action is the binding of ergosterol in cell walls and increasing cell wall permeability

49. Which of the following statements are true concerning infections with *Mycobacterium avium-intracellulare* in patients with AIDS?
   a. They usually present late in the course of HIV infection when immunosuppression is severe
   b. Pneumonia is the most common presentation
   c. They are susceptible to conventional antimycobacterial agents
   d. They are a cause of fever of unknown origin in patients with AIDS
   e. Rifabutin is an effective agent for prophylaxis
   f. Diagnosis is often made by isolation of the organism from blood and bone marrow specimens

50. Which of the following statements are true concerning infection with HIV?
   a. Most patients infected with HIV have seroconversion within 6-12 weeks of infection
   b. The incidence of HIV infection in adolescents is decreasing
   c. Encephalitis is the most common presentation of primary HIV infection

d. HIV infection can cause a self-limited aseptic meningitis

e. The enzyme-linked immunosorbent assay for the detection of HIV infection has a high positive predictive value in populations in which the prevalence of HIV infection is high

f. The mean time to the development of AIDS after infection with HIV is 7-11 years

51. The following clinical syndromes are associated with HIV infection.
   a. Refractory vaginal candidiasis
   b. Seborrheic dermatitis
   c. Psoriasis
   d. Polymyositis
   e. Nephrotic syndrome due to glomerulosclerosis
   f. Immune thrombocytopenia

ANSWERS

1. Answer a.

Corynebacterium diphtheriae is a gram-positive bacillus that causes focal infection, usually in the upper respiratory tract: pharynx, larynx, nasal passages, and tracheobronchial tree. It can also cause skin infections (cutaneous diphtheria), which primarily occur in the tropics but have also been reported in homeless alcoholic men and impoverished indigent groups such as Native Americans. Unusual sites of infection include ear, conjunctiva, and vagina. *C. diphtheriae* does not cause pneumonitis.

2. Answer a.

Proteus mirabilis is a gram-negative bacillus that, through its enzyme urease, splits urea into ammonium hydroxide, thus raising the urinary pH level and promoting struvite stone formation.

3. Answer a.

Enterobacter organisms (e.g., *Enterobacter cloacae*) develop antibiotic resistance to cephalosporins because of the presence of an inducible β-lactamase. For this reason, the combination of an antipseudomonal penicillin (e.g., piperacillin, mezlocillin) with an aminoglycoside has been recommended for treatment of infections with these organisms.

4. Answer c.

Management of *Staphylococcus aureus* bacteremia and distinguishing endocarditis from "simple" septicemia is a well-recognized clinical dilemma. In general, patients in whom bacteremia develops while hospitalized and who have a recognizable primary site of infection (e.g., vascular access graft, intravenous catheter) do not, for the most part, go on to have clinical endocarditis, and they should be treated with removal of the primary site of infection and 2 weeks of antistaphylococcal antibiotic. Nafcillin is excreted primarily by the liver and does not require adjustment of dosage with decreasing renal function

5. Answer d.

Tetanus is caused by *Clostridium tetani*, a gram-positive obligate anaerobe that produces a neurotoxin, tetanospasmin. Tetanospasmin acts on the nervous system by preventing neuromuscular transmission from GABAergic neurons, leading to muscular rigidity and spasms. Both the central nervous system, including the cranial nerves, and the autonomic nervous system are involved. Most patients in the United States are older than 60 years. Management of tetanus includes administration of human tetanus immune globulin (HTIG), tetanus toxoid, debridement of wound, and antibiotics (metronidazole). The tetanus toxoid series should be completed during the convalescent period. Allergic reactions to HTIG are not common.

6. Answer e.

Treatment for enterococcal endocarditis is with a combination of penicillin or ampicillin with an aminoglycoside. Vancomycin is an alternative agent in patients who are allergic to penicillin or for organisms that are penicillin-resistant.

7. Answer e.

Erythema infectiosum, also known as fifth disease, is a childhood exanthem caused by parvovirus B19. It is characterized by fever and a lacy pink rash that starts on the face (slapped-cheek appearance) and spreads to the extremities.

8. Answer b.

Although *Candida albicans* is a relatively common colonizer of the respiratory tract in ill patients, it rarely causes a pneumonitis.

9. Answer a.

The major routes of transmission of toxoplasmosis are oral (undercooked meat, unpasteurized goat milk, vegetables) and congenital. Transmission by organ transplantation (e.g., heart) also occurs.

10. Answer c.

Leptospirosis is an acute, generalized infection caused by species of the spirochete genus *Leptospira*. Humans acquire the infection through contact with animals such as rats (most common), other rodents, dogs, cats, and livestock. The human-animal contact can be indirect or direct (e.g., urine).

11. Answer b.

The patient has cutaneous sporotrichosis. This usually occurs at the site of minor trauma or inoculation (e.g., exposure to thorned plants). The primary papulonodular erythematous lesion may be followed by development of secondary lesions proximally along lymphatic channels. Treatment is with a saturated solution of potassium iodide (SSKI) or itraconazole. Extracutaneous sporotrichosis may require treatment with intravenous amphotericin B.

12. Answer b.

Infectious mononucleosis is an acute illness that usually occurs in adolescents and young adults. It is characterized by sore throat, fever, and lymphadenopathy. The administration of ampicillin produces a maculopapular pruritic rash in 90%-100% of patients. Rash is a feature in the other choices presented, but the whole clinical picture is typical for infectious mononucleosis. Atypical measles is a syndrome that develops in persons who have received killed measles vaccine and were later exposed to wild measles virus. Unlike classic measles, the rash begins peripherally, and the disease is severe and has a more prolonged course.

13. Answer d.

Listeria monocytogenes is a diphtheroid-like gram-positive rod that causes meningitis in neonates and in immunocompromised adults, such as patients with underlying neoplastic disease or cirrhosis or those receiving corticosteroid treatment. *Haemophilus influenzae* and *Neisseria meningitidis* are gram-negative bacteria, and *Streptococcus pneumoniae* is a gram-positive diplococcus. *Mycobacterium tuberculosis* causes chronic meningitis and does not stain with Gram stain.

14. Answer b.

The patient has endocarditis due to *Enterococcus faecalis* that is susceptible to penicillin and does not have high-level resistance to gentamicin; thus, a synergistic combination of those two antibiotics is possible. Duration of treatment is 4-6 weeks, depending on the duration of symptoms before diagnosis and on clinical progress.

15. Answer b.

Staphylococcus aureus is the most common cause of bacterial arthritis in adults. Both rheumatoid arthritis and osteoarthritis predispose to bacterial arthritis. The Gram stain of the joint fluid is positive only in one-third of cases. *Neisseria gonorrhoeae* is a common cause of bacterial arthritis in adults younger than 30 years. Coagulase-negative staphylococci commonly cause infection in prosthetic joints. Arthritis can be a feature of Lyme disease (*Borrelia burgdorferi*). When seen early, it is migratory. Frank arthritis usually occurs months after the onset of disease.

16. Answer c.

Latent syphilis is the period after infection with *Treponema pallidum* when patients are seroreactive but show no other evidence of disease. Those who have or can be demonstrated to have acquired syphilis within the preceding year are designated as having early latent syphilis. All the others are classified as having late latent syphilis. The treatment of choice for late latent syphilis is benzathine penicillin 7.2 million units administered as 3 doses of 2.4 million units intramuscularly each, at 1-week intervals.

17. Answer a.

Escherichia coli 0157:H7, also known as enterohemorrhagic *E. coli* (EHEC), has caused outbreaks of hemorrhagic colitis associated with eating undercooked hamburger. Hemolytic uremic syndrome develops in 8% of EHEC infections. Alternatively, EHEC is associated with 75%-80% of all cases of hemolytic uremic syndrome in North America.

18. Answer a.

Occult urinary tract infection in women has a subacute course with a duration of symptoms usually >7 days.

19. Answer c.

Erythromycin is primarily excreted by the liver.

20. Answer d.

The initial empiric treatment of neutropenic fever should be with broad-spectrum antibiotics that also provide adequate coverage of *Pseudomonas aeruginosa*. Neither cefotaxime nor vancomycin has activity against *Pseudomonas aeruginosa*.

21. Answer e.

Quinolones have decreased bioavailability when coadministered with aluminum-, magnesium-, and calcium-containing antacids, as well as sucralfate, iron sulfate, zinc-containing supplements, and buffered formulations of didanosine (ddI). Histamine receptor antagonists (e.g., cimetidine, ranitidine) may delay absorption but do not affect the completeness of absorption.

22. Answer e.

The mechanism of action of quinolones is through inhibition of bacterial DNA gyrase, an enzyme essential for DNA synthesis.

23. Answer c.

Streptococcus pneumoniae has increasingly become more resistant to penicillin during the past few years. Susceptible strains have minimal inhibitory concentration (MIC) to penicillin of <0.1 μg/mL, strains with intermediate resistance have MIC 0.1-1.0 μg/mL, and highly resistant strains have MIC > 2.0 μg/mL. Strains with intermediate resistance can be treated with third-generation cephalosporins. Highly resistant strains should be treated with vancomycin.

24. Answer c.

First-generation cephalosporins, such as cefazolin, do not cross the blood-brain barrier and thus do not reach therapeutic levels in the cerebrospinal fluid.

25. Answer c.

The clinical presentation of this patient is compatible with *Pneumocystis carinii* pneumonia (PCP). Inhaled pentamidine is not as effective as trimethoprim-sulfamethoxazole in preventing PCP. Focal upper lobe infiltrates are more common in patients who have been receiving aerosol pentamidine prophylaxis. The sensitivity of induced sputum for PCP might be decreased in patients receiving pentamidine prophylaxis. This patient requires bronchoscopy with bronchoalveolar lavage for diagnosis, and unless he has allergy to trimethoprim-sulfamethoxazole, it is the drug of choice for treatment.

26. Answer e.

Neuropathy, pancreatitis, gastrointestinal complaints, and hyperuricemia are the common side effects of didanosine (ddI) therapy. Anemia is not a side effect of didanosine (ddI) therapy.

27. Answer d.

Drugs used for treatment of *Pneumocystis carinii* pneumonia include trimethoprim-sulfamethoxazole, intravenous pentamidine, trimethoprim-dapsone, trimetrexate, clindamycin with primaquine, and atovaquone. Doxycycline is not effective against *Pneumocystis carinii* pneumonia.

28. Answer b.

AIDS patients with *Pneumocystis carinii* pneumonia with A-a gradient >35 mm Hg and Po_2 <70 mm Hg are at increased risk for fatal outcome and may benefit from adjunctive corticosteroid therapy. Intravenous pentamidine is the alternative agent of choice to trimethoprim-sulfamethoxazole in severe *Pneumocystis carinii* pneumonia.

29. Answer c.

Amphotericin B is the drug of choice for initial treatment of cryptococcal meningitis. After 2 weeks of treatment and clinical improvement, one can switch to fluconazole. Some clinicians suggest that fluconazole can be used as initial treatment in patients without mental status changes and with low cryptococcal antigen titers.

30. Answer c.

AIDS patients with multiple focal lesions on neuroimaging studies and history of positive *Toxoplasma* antibody titer should be treated for presumptive toxoplasmic encephalitis. Brain biopsy would be a consideration if there was no clinical or radiologic improvement after 14 days of therapy. Repeat determination of serum *Toxoplasma* antibody titer is not necessary, and lumbar puncture is usually contraindicated in the presence of intracranial mass lesions. All persons with HIV infection should be tested for *Toxoplasma* IgG antibody at the time of diagnosis of HIV.

31. Answer d.

Mycobacterium avium complex (MAC) is the most common systemic bacterial infection in HIV-infected patients. *Pneumocystis carinii* pneumonia is the most common opportunistic infection in HIV-infected patients but is not a bacterium. There is an ongoing debate whether it is a fungus or a protozoan. Tuberculosis is the most common opportunistic infection in HIV-infected persons in some third-world regions. *Toxoplasma gondii*, a protozoan, is the most common cause of focal central nervous system lesions in AIDS patients.

32. Answer e.

All, except tuberculosis, require chronic, lifelong suppressive treatment to prevent recurrence.

33. Answer d.

This patient's presentation and immune status (CD4 count) suggest *Pneumocystis carinii* pneumonia. Induced sputum is a relatively sensitive test for its diagnosis in HIV-infected patients (sensitivity, around 70%), but its success is dependent on the adequacy of the sample and processing. Pulmonary function test (low DLCO) and gallium scan (increased uptake) can be useful as additional measures to assist in the diagnosis, especially in a symptomatic patient with a normal chest radiograph, but they are nonspecific and are not indicated in this case. The next step in management of patients in which *Pneumocystis carinii* pneumonia is not found in induced sputum is bronchoalveolar lavage, which has a sensitivity of 94%. If it is negative, one should perform transbronchial biopsy to look for other diagnosis (e.g., tuberculosis, histoplasmosis).

34. Answer c.

Please refer to Table 14-6 for current recommendations regarding tuberculosis chemoprophylaxis.

35. Answer b.

Streptococcal strains causing invasive disease are not more resistant to antibiotics than the less virulent strains. The other choices relate to some of the possible pathogenic mechanisms for the resurgence of invasive group A streptococcal infections.

36. Answer a.

This patient has a symptom complex compatible with acute HIV infection. It takes 6-12 weeks from the time of infection for the HIV antibody test to be positive. In such cases, determination of p24 antigen, HIV culture, and polymerase chain reaction are useful to establish the diagnosis of HIV infection. It is important to exclude other infections such as Epstein-Barr virus, cytomegalovirus, toxoplasmosis, and herpes simplex virus. Although useful as a surrogate marker for a patient's immune status, CD4 count is nonspecific and variable and does not establish the diagnosis of HIV.

37. a, true; b, false; c, true; d, true; e, true; f, true.

Acute rheumatic fever (ARF) and acute glomerulonephritis (AGN) are the nonsuppurative complications of group A β-hemolytic streptococcal infections. ARF is a clinical syndrome with major manifestations that include carditis, polyarthritis, subcutaneous nodules, chorea, and erythema marginatum. AGN is clinically characterized by edema, hypertension, hematuria, and proteinuria. Laboratory findings include normocytic normochromic anemia, elevated erythrocyte sedimentation rate, elevated serum creatinine level and blood urea nitrogen, reduced serum total complement and C3 complement, and a urine sediment with hyaline, granular, and red blood cell casts.

38. a, true; b, true; c, true; d, false; e, true; f, false.

A patient with active pulmonary tuberculosis should not be considered noninfectious until he or she has received adequate treatment and demonstrated good clinical response as well as three daily negative sputum smears. Treatment of extrapulmonary tuberculosis should be similar to that of pulmonary tuberculosis.

39. a, true; b, true; c, false; d, true; e, true; f, false.

Listeria monocytogenes is a gram-positive aerobic bacillus that causes various human diseases. Predisposing factors include immunosuppression (malignancy, organ transplant, corticosteroid therapy), pregnancy, and neonatal period. Several foods, such as cole slaw, vegetables, dairy products, undercooked chicken, and raw hot dogs, have also been implicated. Diarrhea is not a feature of *Listeria monocytogenes* infections.

40. a, true; b, true; c, true; d, true; e, true; f, false.

Fluconazole is an ineffective treatment for infections caused by *Aspergillus* species. Amphotericin B is the drug of choice in serious and invasive aspergillosis. Itraconazole is an alternative agent.

41. a, true; b, true; c, false; d, true; e, true; f, false.

Angioinvasive hyphae in biopsy material are a feature of *Aspergillus* infections. Studies involving autopsied patients have confirmed the very common (>80%) involvement of the adrenal glands by disseminated histoplasmosis.

42. a, false; b, false; c, true; d, false; e, false; f, true.

Among rickettsial infections, Q fever and Brill-Zinsser disease are not transmitted by insect vectors. Rocky Mountain spotted fever is most common in the south Atlantic states. Fewer than 50% of patients with ehrlichiosis have a rash. Colorado tick fever is not a rickettsial infection. It is caused by the Colorado tick fever virus, belonging to the family Reoviridae. Treatment is mainly supportive. Ribavirin can be considered in severe cases.

43. a, false; b, true; c, true; d, true; e, false; f, true.

Most TSS cases due to *Staphylococcus* occur in menstruating women. The relapse rate of menstruation-related disease can be as high as 30%-40%. Prevention consists of antibiotic treatment of the first episode, education of the patient, and avoidance of tampon use.

44. a, false; b, false; c, false; d, true; e, false; f, true.

Bacterial infections occur early (in the first month) in the posttransplantation period. They are usually associated with wound infections, infection of intravenous lines, and urinary tract infections. *Cryptococcus* meningitis usually occurs 6 months after transplantation. Patients who were seronegative before transplantation are at increased risk for cytomegalovirus infection, especially if they receive a cytomegalovirus seropositive organ or blood transfusion.

45. a, true; b, false; c, false; d, false; e, true; f, false.

Early prosthetic valve endocarditis (<60 days after implantation) is most commonly caused by coagulase-negative *Staphylococcus*. If operation is needed, it should not be delayed for additional days of antimicrobial treatment. The most common cause of culture-negative endocarditis is prior use of antimicrobials. Colonic neoplasms have been associated with *Streptococcus bovis* endocarditis. Gram-negative bacilli and *Candida* species cause endocarditis in injection drug users.

46. a, true; b, false; c, false; d, true; e, true; f, false.

Rifampin, erythromycin, and itraconazole are primarily excreted by the liver.

47. a, false; b, true; c, false; d, true; e, false; f, true.

β-Lactamase inhibitors such as clavulanic acid and sulbactam are active mostly against plasmid-encoded β-lactamases produced by organisms such as *Haemophilus influenzae, Moraxella catarrhalis, Prevotella melaninogenica,* and methicillin-susceptible *Staphylococcus aureus. Enterobacter* species produce an inducible chromosomal β-lactamase not inhibited by therapeutically achievable concentrations of β-lactamase inhibitors. Penicillin-resistant strains of *Streptococcus pneumoniae* and methicillin-resistant *Staphylococcus aureus* have penicillin-binding proteins with decreased affinity to penicillin, and the mechanism of their resistance is not through β-lactamase production.

48. a, false; b, false; c, true; d, true; e, false; f, false.

Ketoconazole is an imidazole that exhibits its antifungal activity through inhibition of synthesis of ergosterol, a sterol necessary for a normal fungal cytoplasmic membrane. It requires an acidic gastric medium for adequate absorption. Its

penetration into the cerebrospinal fluid, even in the presence of inflamed meninges, is very poor, and therefore it should not be used for the treatment of meningitis. It is effective in nonmeningeal histoplasmosis, blastomycosis, paracoccidioidomycosis, and coccidioidomycosis. It has no activity against cryptococcosis. It inhibits the cytoplasmic P-450 system and thus decreases the metabolism of warfarin and dilantin (thus potentiating their effects) and decreases the synthesis of testosterone and cortisol. Amphotericin B, another antifungal agent, binds to ergosterol in fungal cell walls and increases cell wall permeability.

49. a, true; b, false; c, false; d, true; e, true; f, true.

Mycobacterium avium-intracellulare (MAI) is the most common cause of systemic bacterial infection in AIDS patients. It presents with nonspecific symptoms: generalized wasting, fever, night sweats, and chronic diarrhea. Pneumonia is not a common feature. Blood culture is a sensitive and easy means of diagnosis. Diagnosis can also be made by culture of biopsy specimens from bone marrow, liver, and lymph nodes. Two controlled clinical trials have shown rifabutin to be effective in preventing or delaying MAI bacteremia. MAI is resistant to conventional antimycobacterial agents. A multiple-drug regimen with clarithromycin and ethambutol as the mainstay and one or two additional agents (rifabutin, rifampin, clofazimine, ciprofloxacin, amikacin) is recommended.

50. a, true; b, false; c, false; d, true; e, true; f, true.

A mononucleosis-like syndrome is the most common presentation of primary HIV infection. The incidence of HIV infection is increasing in heterosexuals, minorities, women, and children.

51. a, true; b, true; c, true; d, true; e, true; f, true.

All the conditions presented have been associated with HIV infection.

CHAPTER 15

MEDICAL ETHICS

Udaya B. S. Prakash, M.D.
William F. Dunn, M.D.

DEFINITION

Medical ethics is a set of principles that attempts to guide physicians in their relationships with patients and others. These principles are based on moral values shared by both the lay society (may vary from culture to culture) and the medical profession. Several oaths reflect physicians' beliefs and principles, including the Declaration of Geneva (1983), World Medical Association International Code of Medical Ethics (1983), American Medical Association Principles of Medical Ethics (1973), and the American College of Physicians Ethics Manual (1989). The Hippocratic oath is of major historical significance. Its principles form the framework for many of our current ethical standards, including beneficence, nonmaleficence, confidentiality, and active euthanasia. From its model come oaths sworn by many graduating physicians today.

ETHICAL DILEMMAS

Ethical issues in medicine are as dynamic as the scientific and technical progresses in medicine. In fact, the relentless advances in medical science are greatly responsible for the dynamism in medical ethics. These factors are partly responsible for ethical dilemmas. Furthermore, changes in societal mores and laws also have an impact on the ethical issues in medicine. An ethical dilemma can be defined as a predicament in which there is no clear course to resolve the problem of conflicting moral principles because of credible evidence both for and against a certain action. Increasing emphasis is being placed on medical ethics in the certifying and licensing examinations for physicians.

- Ethical dilemma: predicament in which there is no clear course to resolve the problem of conflicting moral principles because of credible evidence both for and against a certain action.
- Ethical issues in medicine are dynamic and will continue to change.

PRINCIPLES OF MEDICAL ETHICS

The four major tenets are 1) autonomy, 2) beneficence, 3) nonmaleficence, and 4) justice.

Autonomy

This tenet involves respecting the patient's right to self-determination and the pursuit of one's own life plan. Autonomy implies "decisional capability" (the term "competence" is avoided here because of its competing legal definition). Decisional capability is the ability to deliberate about the available information and to draw inferences. Clinical evidence of confusion, disorientation, and psychosis resulting from organic diseases, metabolic disturbances, and iatrogenic interference can adversely affect decision-making ability. In clinical practice, the lack of decisional capability should be proved, and not presumed. Decisionally capable patients have the right to refuse medical therapy, even at the risk of death. If a previously decisionally capable patient had indicated, clearly and convincingly, whether life-sustaining therapy should be administered or withheld in the event of permanent unconsciousness, that wish should be respected (see "Living Will," page 552), unless it was subsequently clearly rescinded.

- Autonomy: respecting the patient's right to self-determination and pursuit of one's own life plan.
- Autonomy implies "decisional capability" (the right to refuse medical therapy, even at the risk of death).
- Lack of decisional capability should be proved, and not presumed.

The principle of autonomy, particularly as it affects the right of an individual to die, has been reaffirmed in the recent writings of ethicists and legal judgments. Indeed, the populace of the state of Oregon voted in 1994 to grant immunity to physicians for prescribing drugs to be used by a terminally ill person wishing to die. Nevertheless, a survey of physicians published in 1995 reported that 34% of physicians had, at least once in the preceding 12 months, declined to withdraw life-sustaining mechanical ventilation despite being requested to do so by a capable patient or by the family of a patient lacking decision-making capacity. Nearly 20% of physicians engaged in this practice because of the fear of malpractice litigation. Unfortunately, a significant number of physicians in the United States have either a poor or no understanding of the laws of states regarding the principle of autonomy. The 1995 survey revealed that 46% of the respondents from New York incorrectly believed that withdrawal of mechanical ventilation was illegal.

- Significant number of physicians have poor understanding of the principle of autonomy.

Substituted Judgment

This is the ability of family members or other duly appointed person(s) to make therapeutic decisions on behalf of the patient, on the basis of what they believe the patient, if decisionally capable, would have chosen.

Surrogate Decision Maker

The surrogate represents the patient's interests and previously expressed wishes in the context of the medical issues. The surrogate is optimally designated by the patient before critical illness. One type of surrogate is the durable power of attorney, in which a legally binding proxy directive authorizes a designated individual to speak on behalf of the patient. The second type of surrogate is the patient's family, physician, or the court. The third type is a moral surrogate (usually a family member) who best knows the patient and has the patient's interest at heart. Difficulties may arise when the moral surrogate is not the legal surrogate. Dialogue between the physician and surrogate is important.

- Optimally, surrogate is designated by patient before critical illness.

Living Will

This is a type of "advance directive" or "health-care declaration." This document commonly includes a declaration of "durable power of attorney for health-care matters (proxy)." The living will reflects the patient's autonomy. It can aid greatly in medical decision making, but it becomes ineffective if vaguely written or applied to patients with uncertain prognoses. Legal reliability may vary from state to state, and all clinicians should be aware of state-specific statutes regarding advance directives. Any decisionally capable person 18 years or older can have a living will.

- Living will: a type of "advance directive" or "health-care declaration."
- The living will reflects a patient's autonomy.

- Legal reliability may vary from state to state.

Disclosure

To make the principle of autonomy function, the physician must provide decisionally capable patients with adequate and truthful information on which to base medical decisions. Truth telling on the part of the physician is an integral part of autonomy. Without this, patients cannot make autonomous decisions about their life plans. Severity of illness scoring systems hold promise in assisting the physician in quantifying the risk of mortality, thereby providing the patient more concise input to aid in decision making than has been available in the past. Scoring system data should be interpreted, however, only within the clinical context and cautiously until they are widely validated; these systems remain in evolution. Occasionally, the physician may withhold part or all of the truth if telling the whole truth is likely to cause more harm than good. This action is considered *paternalistic*. In clinical reasoning, the physician must consider ethical issues as well as the patient's values and preferences. For example, even though folklore remedies are without scientific basis for treating advanced malignancies, and are considered unethical as primary therapy by the physician, the patient may not agree. If the patient wants unconventional treatment, the physician cannot simply dismiss the issue without a well-reasoned and convincing discussion with the patient.

A more serious issue is the availability of more than one acceptable form of therapy for a disease. In a patient with a cancer amenable to surgical resection, chemotherapy or radiation may provide a similar long-term outlook, albeit with different complications and side effects. However, the physician may be biased toward one of the three treatments. In this situation, it is the duty of the physician to set aside personal bias and provide detailed information on each treatment and its potential complications and to allow the well-informed patient to express personal preferences. If the physician assumes sole responsibility in the decision making (even though the patient is capable of analyzing the alternatives and coming to a reasoned conclusion), the important aspects to the patient may be overlooked or underestimated, including the impact of various treatments on the patient's quality of personal life, occupation, and social and economic aspects. The final plan should reflect an agreement between a well-informed patient and a well-informed, sympathetic, and unbiased physician.

- Physician must provide decisionally capable patients with adequate and truthful information on which to base medical decisions.
- Physician must consider ethical issues as well as the patient's values and preferences.
- Truth telling is an integral part of autonomy.
- Severity of illness scoring systems may assist in assessment of mortality risk.

Informed Consent

This is voluntary acceptance of physician recommendations by decisionally competent patients or surrogates who have been furnished with ample truthful information regarding risks, benefits, and alternatives and who clearly indicate their comprehension of the information. Informed consent is essential when performing new, innovative, nonstandard surgical procedures and research procedures. Informed consent from surrogates is necessary to perform autopsy (except in specific instances such as coroners' cases, in which the decision is made by outside authorities) or to practice intubation, placement of intravascular lines, or other procedures on the newly dead. The amount of information needed by the patient to give informed consent is not that which the physician feels is adequate (Professional Practice Standard) but that which the average prudent person would need to make a decision (Reasonable Person Standard). In rare exceptions, the physician can treat a patient without truly informed consent (e.g., in an emotionally unstable patient who requires urgent treatment, informing the patient of the details may produce further problems). Many "informed consent" forms in clinical use do not meet the Reasonable Person Standard and are therefore of no value morally or legally.

- Amount of information needed by patient is that which the average prudent person would need to make a decision (Reasonable Person Standard).
- Many "informed consent" forms do not meet Reasonable Person Standard and are therefore of no value morally or legally.

Confidentiality

Patient confidentiality provides the patient the right to keep medical information solely within the realm of the physician-patient relationship. The physician is obliged to maintain the medical information in strict confidence. Exceptions to this include instances when data, if not released to appropriate agencies, have the potential to cause greater societal harm. Typical examples include positive results of the human immunodeficiency virus (HIV) test or a sputum culture that is positive for *Mycobacterium tuberculosis*. Patients who voluntarily request the HIV test should be informed by the physician that the result, if positive, will be automatically reported to the appropriate health agency. Confidentiality may also be breached when patients ask about hereditary diseases in their parents or siblings.

- Physician is obliged to maintain medical information in strict confidence.
- Exceptions include instances when data, if not released to appropriate agencies, may cause greater societal harm (e.g., positive HIV test, positive sputum culture for *Mycobacterium tuberculosis*).

Group-Specific Beliefs

Certain religious practices preclude or compromise accepted medical practices. The principle of autonomy provides that adult patients who refuse life-saving measures (e.g., blood transfusion) should be allowed to maintain their religious practices. However, in cases involving children, the courts have overruled the religious objections.

- Adult patients who refuse life-saving measures (e.g., blood transfusion) should be allowed to maintain their religious practices.

Beneficence

Beneficence is acting to benefit patients by preserving life, restoring health, relieving suffering, and restoring or maintaining function. The physician (acting in good faith) is obligated to help patients attain their own interests and goals as determined by the patient, *not* the physician.

- Beneficence: preservation of life, restoration of health, relief of suffering, and restoration or maintenance of function.

Implied Consent

The principle of implied consent is invoked when true informed consent is not possible because the patient (or surrogate) is unable to express a decision regarding treatment, specifically, in emergency situations in which physicians are compelled to provide medically necessary therapy, without which harm would result. This clarifies that there is a duty to assist a person in urgent need of care. This principle has been legally accepted, and it provides the physician a legal defense against battery (although not negligence).

- Implied consent is invoked when true informed consent is not possible.

Incurable Disease and Death

Probably the most distressing aspect of medical practice is the encounter with a patient who has an incurable disease and in whom premature death is inevitable. The physician and patient (or surrogate) must formulate appropriate goals of therapy, choose what measures should be taken to maintain life, and decide how aggressive these measures ought to be. It is important to remind oneself that the patient is under enormous mental anguish and physical stress and that the ability to make solid decisions may be clouded. Furthermore, the decision(s) made by the patient may be guided by his or her understanding (whether adequate or not) of the medical condition and prognosis; religious beliefs; financial status; and other personal wishes. The patient may seek counsel from family, friends, and clergy as well as the attending physician.

- In incurable disease, recognize that patient is under enormous mental anguish and physical stress.
- Ability of patient to make solid decisions may be clouded.

The following guidelines are suggested in dealing with incurable disease and death. The patient and family (if the patient so desires) must be provided ample opportunity to talk with the physician and ask questions. An unhurried openness and "willing-to-listen" attitude on the part of the physician are critical for a positive outcome. Patients often find it easier to share their feelings about death with their physician, who is likely to be more objective and less emotional, than with family and friends. Nevertheless, the physician should not remain or "appear" completely detached from the patient's feelings and emotions. Even an attempt on the part of the physician to enter the "inner" feelings of the patient will have a soothing, if not therapeutic, effect.

- The patient and family must be provided every opportunity to talk with the physician and ask questions.
- An unhurried openness and "willing-to-listen" attitude on the part of the physician are critical for a positive outcome.

The physician should assume the responsibility to furnish or arrange for physical, emotional, and spiritual support. Adequate control of pain, maintenance of human dignity, and close contact with the family are crucial. The emotional and spiritual support available through local clergy (as appropriate, given the patient's personal beliefs) should not be underestimated. At no other time in life is the reality of human mortality so real as in the terminal phases of disease. It is always preferable to allay the anxiety of the dying patient through adequate emotional and spiritual support rather than by sedation. The physician should constantly remind herself or himself that despite all the medical technology that surrounds the patient, the patient must not be dehumanized.

- Adequate pain control, maintenance of human dignity, and close contact with family are crucial.
- Despite all the technology that surrounds the patient, human-to-human contact should be most important aspect of treatment.
- It is always preferable to allay anxiety by adequate emotional and spiritual support rather than by sedation.

Control of Pain

The principle of beneficence calls for relief of suffering. Adequate analgesia, particularly in patients with incurable disease, is the responsibility of the physician. If death ensues in a terminally ill patient because of respiratory depression from analgesia, the physician has not acted immorally. Patients allowed to die after removal from ventilators are commonly treated in this fashion. Nevertheless, it is necessary to stress that the primary objective of analgesia is relief of pain and not the hastening of death, even in terminally ill patients.

- Beneficence calls for relief of suffering.
- Adequate analgesia, particularly in patients with incurable disease, is the responsibility of the physician.
- Physician has not performed immorally if death in a terminally ill patient is result of respiratory depression from analgesic therapy; euthanasia is not the goal.

Futility

Within the context of medical ethics, futility may be defined as a unilateral decision by the physician to withhold or withdraw medical interventions if, in the opinion of the physician, the intervention has no pathophysiologic rationale, intervention has already failed in the past, maximal therapy is failing or has failed, and the intervention will not achieve the goals of care. *Physiologic futility* is determined by the physician, who needs to decide whether a treatment can achieve its physiologic goal. One of the problems with this definition is that there can be a wide variation in the definition of the "physiologic goal" by various physicians. An example of physiologic futility is when aggressive cardiopulmonary resuscitation (CPR) is performed in a patient with end-stage acquired immunodeficiency syndrome (AIDS) in whom all therapies have failed and death is imminent. The physician can refuse CPR if the treatment options are most likely to be physiologically futile. *Medical futility*, alternatively, is determined by the patient or surrogate(s). Medical futility is the perception by the patient or surrogate(s) of the quality of life during or after therapy. This definition also suffers from the wide variation in the definition or perception of quality of life among patients. If there is no physiologic futility involved from the physician's point of view, then the patient should be permitted to determine what constitutes futile treatment. This step assumes that the patient has been provided all the information necessary to make a decision. Futile therapies can and should be provided in extenuating circumstances. For example, if a terminally ill patient wishes to be kept alive for a day or two because he or she wants to see a friend or relative who is coming from afar, futile therapy should be provided. It is imperative, however, for the physician to recognize that improper institution (i.e., without informing the patient of the futile nature of the treatment) of futile therapy will falsely offer hopes of improvement or cure to the patient and foil the patient's ability for reasoned judgment and autonomy.

- Physiologic futility is determined by the physician.
- Medical futility is determined by the patient or surrogate(s).

Casuistry

Casuistry is the process of resolving specific cases of conscience, duty, or conduct through interpretation of ethical principles or religious doctrine. The lexicon also defines casuistry as rationalization or use of specious argument to solve ethical problems. Casuists reject the notion that the practice of ethics should be based on universal principles of ethics. They believe that ethical judgments should emerge from particular cases or from experience based on several cases that can be compared to one another in various ways. The opponents of case-based analysis contend that decisions formed in this manner are riddled with bias, and the weight given to each factor varies greatly from case to case. In day-to-day caring for very sick and terminally ill patients, most physicians make their ethical decisions by adhering to both the standard principles of medical ethics and the practice of casuistry.

● Casuistry is the tenet that ethical judgments should emerge from particular cases or from experience based on several cases.

Nonabandonment

Within the context of medical ethics, abandonment connotes leaving the patient (for whom the physician has provided health care in the past) without care. This conduct is unacceptable and has been "universally condemned as a serious and punishable infraction of both the legal and ethical obligations that physicians owe patients" (Ann Intern Med 122:377-378, 1995). In contrast, nonabandonment denotes a requisite ethical obligation of physicians once patient and physician mutually concur to enter into an alliance. Some ethicists believe that the practice of nonabandonment is closely related to the principle of beneficence and that nonabandonment is fundamental to the long-term physician-patient relationship. This tenet has several drawbacks and limitations. The degree of physician's involvement in the relationship cannot be measured as to its quantity or quality. Furthermore, the extent of the relationship is dictated by the underlying medical condition. For instance, an annual examination may require a single visit to the physician, whereas a complicated disease process may bring the physician and patient closer to each other over a long period. It would be improper for the physician to force a patient to maintain a long-term physician-patient relationship if the latter is unwilling, for whatever reason. Noncompliance, in terms of taking medications or following a physician's instructions, by the patient is not grounds for abandonment. Physicians should strive to respond to the needs of their patients over time, but they should not trespass their own values in the process.

Conflict of Interest

The principle of beneficence requires that the physician not engage in activities that are not in the patient's best interest. This is considered to be a significant problem in the United States. Some studies have suggested that physicians' prescribing practices are influenced by financial and other significant rewards from drug companies. If the physician does not ardently avoid areas of potential conflict of interest (because of the principle of beneficence), the result may be maleficence.

Nonmaleficence

This principle is based on "do no harm, prevent harm, and remove harm." This principle addresses unprofessional behavior; verbal, physical, and sexual abuse of patients; and uninformed and undisclosed experimentation on patients with drugs and procedures with the potential to cause harmful side effects. Breach of physician-patient confidentiality which results in harm to the patient is another example of maleficence.

● Nonmaleficence: "do no harm, prevent harm, and remove harm."

Justice

Every patient deserves and must be provided optimal care as warranted by the underlying medical condition. Allocation of medical resources fairly and according to medical need is the basis for this principle. The decision to provide optimal medical care should be based on the medical need of each patient and the perceived medical benefit to the patient. The patient's social status, ability to pay, or perceived social worth should not dictate the quality or quantity of medical care. The physician's clear-cut responsibility is to the patient's well-being (beneficence). Physicians should not make decisions about individual care of their patients based on larger societal needs. The bedside is not the place to make general policy decisions.

● Justice: allocation of medical resources fairly and according to medical need.
● Physician should not make decisions about individual care of patients based on larger societal needs.

"DO NOT RESUSCITATE" (DNR)

DNR orders affect administration of CPR only; other therapeutic options should not be influenced by the DNR order. Every person whose medical history is unclear or unavailable should receive CPR in the event of cardiopulmonary arrest. CPR is not recommended when it merely prolongs life in a patient with terminal illness or when the fatal outcome is clinically evident (Table 15-1).

Of paramount importance are the patient's knowledge of the extent of disease and the prognosis, the physician's estimate of the potential efficacy of CPR, and the wishes of the patient (or surrogate) regarding CPR as a therapeutic tool. However, if, in the physician's judgment, CPR would be futile, multiple physician groups, including the American Medical Association's Council on Ethical and Judicial Affairs, have recommended that CPR not be offered; however, the extent of legal support for this recommendation is as yet unclear. The

Table 15-1.--Clinical Situations in Which Cardiopulmonary Resuscitation Is Unlikely to Prolong Life

---

Advanced, progressive, ultimately lethal illness
    Bedfast metastatic cancer
    Child's class C cirrhosis
    Infection by human immunodeficiency virus (with ≥2 episodes of *pneumonia caused by Pneumocystis carinii*)
    Dementia requiring long-term care
Acute, near-fatal illness without evidence of improvement after admission to the intensive-care unit
    Coma (traumatic or nontraumatic) lasting ≥48 hours
    Multiple organ system failure with no improvement after 3 consecutive days in the intensive-care unit
Unsuccessful out-of-hospital cardiopulmonary resuscitation

From Murphy DJ, Finucane TE: New do-not-resuscitate policies: a first step in cost control. Arch Intern Med 153:1641-1648, 1993. By permission of the American Medical Association.

DNR order should be reviewed frequently because clinical circumstances may dictate other measures (e.g., a patient with terminal cardiomyopathy who had initially turned down heart transplantation and wanted to be considered a "DNR candidate" may change her or his mind and now opt for the transplantation). Physicians should discuss the appropriateness of CPR or DNR with patients at high risk for cardiopulmonary arrest and with the terminally ill. The discussion should optimally take place in the outpatient setting, during the initial period of hospitalization, and periodically during hospitalization, if appropriate. DNR orders (and rationale) should be entered in the patient's medical records.

- DNR orders affect CPR only.
- Other therapeutic options should not be influenced by the DNR order.
- Every patient should be considered a candidate for CPR unless clear indications exist otherwise.
- CPR is not recommended when it merely prolongs life in a patient with a terminal illness.
- DNR order should be reviewed frequently.
- DNR orders (and rationale) should be entered in the patient's medical records.

PATIENT SELF-DETERMINATION ACT OF 1990

This federal act requires hospitals, nursing homes, and hospices to advise patients at admission of their right to accept or refuse medical care and to execute an advance directive. Managed care organizations and home health care agencies must provide the same information to each of their members at the time of enrollment. These organizations are required to 1) document whether patients have advance directives, 2) implement advance directive policies, and 3) educate their staffs and communities about advance directives.

- Hospitals, nursing homes, and hospices should advise patients, on admission, of their right to accept or refuse medical care and to execute an advance directive.

WITHHOLDING AND WITHDRAWING LIFE SUPPORT

This decision may be compatible with beneficence, nonmaleficence, and autonomy. The right of a decisionally capable person to refuse lifesaving hydration and nutrition was upheld by the U.S. Supreme Court (Table 15-2), but a surrogate decision maker's right to refuse treatment for decisionally incapable persons can be restricted by states. Brain death is not a necessary requirement for withdrawing or withholding life support. The value of each medical therapy (risk:benefit ratio) should be assessed for each patient. The American Medical Association has issued certain guidelines, and one of them states that a life-sustaining medical intervention can be limited without the consent of the patient or surrogate when the intervention is judged to be futile. The extent to which these guidelines will be upheld by legal authorities is as yet unclear, as evidenced by a recent state court ruling in Minnesota (Table 15-2). When appropriate, the withholding or withdrawal of life support is best accomplished with input from more than one experienced clinician.

- Withholding or withdrawing life support does not conflict with the principles of beneficence, nonmaleficence, and autonomy.
- Brain death is not a necessary requirement for withdrawing or withholding life support.

PERSISTENT VEGETATIVE STATE

This is a chronic state of unconsciousness (loss of self-awareness) lasting for more than a few weeks, characterized by the presence of walk/sleep cycles, but without behavioral or cerebral metabolic evidence of possessing cognitive function or of being able to respond in a learned manner to external events or stimuli. The body retains functions necessary to sustain vegetative survival, if provided nutritional and other supportive measures--note that the U.S. Supreme Court has ruled that there is no distinction between artificial feeding and hydration versus mechanical ventilation (Table 15-2).

Table 15-2.--Pertinent Legal Rulings

Case, yr	Legal issue	Court	Decision
Quinlan, 1976	PVS--discontinuation of mechanical ventilation, previously articulated directive	New Jersey Supreme Court	Discontinuation (based on right to privacy)
Brophy, 1986	PVS--discontinuation of gastrostomy feedings, previously articulated directive	Massachusetts Supreme Court	Discontinue feedings (based on autonomy)
Bouvia, 1986	Severely impaired, refusal of nasogastric tube feedings by a decisionally capable patient	California Court of Appeals	Removal of nasogastric tube (based on autonomy)
Corbett, 1986	PVS--discontinuation of nasogastric tube feedings, no predefined directive(s)	Florida Court of Appeals	Discontinue feedings (based on right to privacy)
Cruzan, 1990	PVS--state of Missouri required "clear and convincing" evidence of individual's wishes before allowing withdrawal of life support	U.S. Supreme Court	States have right to restrict exercise of right to refuse treatment by surrogates; decisionally capable patients may refuse life-sustaining therapy, including hydration, nutrition, and mechanical ventilation
Wanglie, 1991	PVS--family wished continued support despite objections to continued life-sustaining therapy by the physicians and institution	Minnesota Supreme Court	Continuation (based on autonomy, substituted judgment)

PVS, persistent vegetative state.

- Persistent vegetative state: unconsciousness (loss of self-awareness) lasting for more than a few weeks.
- U.S. Supreme Court ruling states that there is no distinction between artificial feeding and hydration versus mechanical ventilation.

DEFINITION OF DEATH

Death is irreversible cessation of circulatory and respiratory function *or* irreversible cessation of all functions of the entire brain, including the brain stem. Clinical criteria (at times substantiated by electroencephalographic testing or assessment of cerebral perfusion) permit the reliable diagnosis of "cerebral death."

The family should be informed of the brain death but should not be asked to decide whether further medical therapy should be continued. One exception is when the patient had earlier directed the family to make certain decisions, such as organ donation, in case of brain death.

Once it is ascertained that the patient is "brain dead" and that no further therapy can be offered, the primary physician, preferably after consultation with another physician involved in the care of the patient, may withdraw supportive measures.

The imminent possibility of harvesting organs for transplantation should in no way affect any of the above-outlined decisions. When organ donation is possible after the determination of brain death, the family should be approached, preferably before cessation of cardiac function, regarding organ donation.

- Death: irreversible cessation of circulatory and respiratory function *or* irreversible cessation of all functions of entire brain, including brain stem.
- Electroencephalography is not necessary to establish death.

AUTHORS' NOTE

Laws concerning ethical issues in medicine continue to evolve, reflecting changing attitudes of society. It is certain that legal decisions will continue to influence the practice of medicine. Many states have no directly applicable statutes or court cases relating to difficult ethical issues in medical practice. Although this review is meant as a guide, for further information regarding state-specific mandates the individual practitioner is referred to the appropriate state medical society.

QUESTIONS

Multiple Choice (choose the one best answer)

1. Your patient, a decisionally capable 54-year-old man, has just undergone extensive medical evaluations. He is clinically determined to have a stage I lung cancer with 5-year survival rate of more than 85% if surgical resection is done. Despite this information, he refuses all forms of therapy. Which one of the following is the most appropriate next step?
   a. Declare the patient mentally incompetent because of his "unreasonable" attitude
   b. Call close family members and tell them to persuade the patient to have resection
   c. Arrange for the patient to discuss his clinical situation with other patients who have a similar problem
   d. Respect the wishes of the patient and record the discussions in the medical record
   e. Obtain psychiatric consultation

2. Which one of the following is incorrect regarding a living will?
   a. It is a type of advance directive or health-care declaration
   b. It reflects the patient's autonomy and aids greatly in medical decision making
   c. A living will is ineffective if applied to patients with an uncertain clinical prognosis
   d. Legal reliability may vary from state to state in the United States
   e. Any decisionally capable person 13 years or older can have a valid living will

3. A psychiatric patient has a history of several suicide attempts after being provided unpleasant medical information. Now you are seeing him for an evaluation of a 6-mm lung nodule. The chance of this being malignant, in your opinion, is small. If you do not inform the patient about the lung nodule, then you are:
   a. Not respecting the patient's autonomy by withholding "truth telling"
   b. Proceeding correctly because you are acting "paternalistically" in the interest of the patient
   c. Liable for legal action for withholding medical information
   d. Taking the responsibility of the psychiatrist
   e. Practicing "bad medicine"

4. Cardiorespiratory arrest develops in a 75-year-old hospitalized patient with metastatic cancer unresponsive to therapy. The patient and family demand cardiopulmonary resuscitation (CPR). As the physician in charge of the CPR team and well aware of the patient's history and clinical situation, which of the following actions should you choose?
   a. Provide CPR for as long as you feel it is necessary
   b. Refuse CPR because it is physiologically futile
   c. Provide a limited (for a few minutes) CPR to satisfy the family
   d. Have your nurse/colleague discuss the futility of CPR with the relative when you are providing the CPR
   e. Contact the patient's personal physician before you refuse CPR

5. A physician (critical care fellow) in charge of bed allocation of a 14-bed medical intensive-care unit (ICU), while on call, notes that all beds are full with critically ill patients. Anticipating potential additional admissions, the fellow prioritizes the need for continued ICU stay based purely on medical necessity in an effort to provide a potential open bed. Which one of the following ethical principles is involved in this decision?
   a. Substituted judgment
   b. Autonomy
   c. Beneficence

d. Nonmaleficence
e. Justice

6. Which one of the following clinical features is not necessary to establish the clinical diagnosis of brain death?
   a. An isoelectric pattern by electroencephalography
   b. Absence of brain stem responses
   c. Absence of hepatic encephalopathy
   d. Absence of barbiturate intoxication
   e. Absence of hypothermia

7. You are a junior partner in a small group practice. You are aware (or strongly suspect) that one of your senior partners is an alcoholic but you are not sure whether anyone else is aware of this information. Which one of the following steps is appropriate for you to take?
   a. Confront your partner and discuss the issue
   b. Send an anonymous letter to your partner and threaten exposure if he or she does not seek treatment
   c. Send an anonymous letter to the state's medical licensing body
   d. Voice your concern to the most senior partner or administrator
   e. Ignore the issue as long as this partner has nothing to do with you or your patients

True/False (indicate whether each answer is true or false)
8. A 55-year-old married male executive undergoes an annual physical examination. As part of the blood tests, he requests a human immunodeficiency (HIV) serologic test and asks you to keep the result confidential. The HIV result is positive. Which of the following procedures are appropriate regarding the reporting of the test result?
   a. Inform the patient

b. Inform the patient's insurance company
c. Inform the patient's children
d. Inform the patient's wife
e. Notify local health agency

9. A 75-year-old demented patient is brought to the emergency room by ambulance from his nursing home because of an acute abdomen. He is found to have a board-like rigidity to his abdomen. There are no family members present or available. He has no living will. Which of the following statements are true regarding this patient?
   a. Operation cannot be performed because of the absence of informed consent
   b. The physician in charge can assume the role of a moral surrogate
   c. A legal guardian must be procured via the court system
   d. The principle of disclosure is in conflict with the principle of beneficence
   e. A hospital ethics committee must make the final decision regarding the need for operation

10. Which of the following statements are true regarding the "do not resuscitate" (DNR) order?
    a. DNR orders affect administration of cardiopulmonary resuscitation (CPR) only
    b. Other treatment options are not influenced by the DNR order
    c. Every patient is a potential candidate for CPR unless clear indications exist otherwise
    d. The DNR order, once written, is permanent
    e. The DNR order and rationale should be recorded in the patient's chart

ANSWERS

1. Answer d.

The principle of autonomy is stressed by this question. It is reasonable to have several discussions with the patient to impress on him the fact that the disease is treatable and perhaps curable. This action should not turn into coercion, nor should the patient perceive it as such.

2. Answer e.

The patient presented here is a minor; therefore, a living will is invalid. Some states have the "mature minor" clause that permits a younger person (<17 years) to establish a living will and to assume autonomy. Please check with your state's laws regarding this.

3. Answer b.

Paternalistic action in the interest of this patient's overall well-being is acceptable. Truth telling on the part of the physician is an integral part of the principle of autonomy. However, in certain situations, as in this case, the physician may withhold part or all of the truth if the physician believes the truth telling will do more harm than good.

4. Answer b.

If the patient's condition is deemed terminal with no hope of recovery despite the most aggressive therapy, the physician in charge can refuse CPR. In the case presented, it would be important to ensure that the patient and family are well aware of the incurable nature of the disease and the terminal state of the patient.

5. Answer e.

The principle of justice is illustrated in this example, in which the physician appropriately serves in the allocation of medical resources fairly and according to medical need, in order to provide the greatest good. Understandably, beneficence and non-maleficence principles play a role in the decision making, but the primary goal in this example is that of justice.

6. Answer a.

Although potentially useful in many situations for diagnostic confirmation or family counseling, electroencephalography is not a necessary tool for establishing the diagnosis of brain death. All the other listed options are necessary to establish the diagnosis.

7. Answer d.

Unless you are very close to the partner suspected of being an alcoholic, personal confrontation is not recommended. The other choices are unacceptable actions on your part.

8. a, true; b, false; c, false; d, false; e, true.

The principle of autonomy should be applied here. The patient should be encouraged to reveal the results to his wife.

9. a, false; b, true; c, false; d, true; e, false.

This example illustrates that conflicts may frequently arise between various ethical principles which must be addressed within the decision-making process--most notable here between the principles of disclosure and beneficence. The medical urgency described precludes the usefulness of a hospital ethics committee. The principle of implied consent should be invoked here to justify proceeding with the life-saving procedure.

10. a, true; b, true; c, true; d, false; e, true.

The DNR order is not permanent and indeed should be renewed on a daily basis, depending on the daily evaluation of the patient's clinical status. A patient can revoke the DNR status at any time.

CHAPTER 16

NEPHROLOGY

Thomas R. Schwab, M.D.

ACUTE RENAL FAILURE–DEFINITIONS

Three important principles in the clinical evaluation of acute renal failure are: 1) It must be determined whether an increase in serum levels of creatinine or urea reflects a *genuine* and *recent* decrease in glomerular filtration rate. Many medications and substances interfere with the measurement of creatinine and urea and its renal handling. 2) If substantial irreversible renal dysfunction is to be avoided, acute renal failure must be recognized early. Remember, an increase in serum creatinine of 0.8 to 1.8 mg/dL reflects as much as a 50% loss of renal function. 3) Appropriate treatment of patients with acute renal failure demands that the cause be pinpointed promptly from the more than 100 potential causes. Currently, acute renal failure is broadly classified into prerenal, renal, and postrenal types.

- Increase in creatinine levels independently of glomerular filtration rate: ketoacidosis (acetoacetate), cefoxitin, cimetidine, trimethoprim, flucytosine, massive rhabdomyolysis, and high intake of meat.
- Increase in urea (BUN) independently of glomerular filtration rate: gastrointestinal tract bleeding, tissue trauma, glucocorticoids, and tetracyclines.
- Anuria <50 mL/day (limited differential diagnosis!): rapidly progressive glomerulonephritis, cortical necrosis, and bilateral renal artery occlusion (e.g., dissection), but not acute tubular necrosis.
- Oliguria is <400 mL/day or < 20 mL/hour: patients with an inability to concentrate urine may be "oliguric" with 1,000+ mL/day.
- Nonoliguric renal failure is >800 mL/day (most cases are nonoliguric).
- Polyuria is >3,000 mL/day (a clue to partial obstruction).

POSTRENAL FAILURE (OBSTRUCTION)

The pathogenesis of an obstructive uropathy is characterized by early vasoconstriction followed by vasodilatation. Obstruction may be anatomical (e.g., methysergide = retroperitoneal fibrosis) or functional (neurogenic bladder). Wide fluctuations in urine volume may be present with partial obstruction.

- Pathogenesis of obstructive uropathy: early vasoconstriction followed by vasodilatation.
- Obstruction: anatomical or functional.

The most useful clinical test is renal ultrasonography. However, 2% of these studies are false negative (usually because of early obstruction or possible retroperitoneal fibrosis). Up to 26% of ultrasonograms are falsely positive. A combination of renal ultrasonography and abdominal computed tomography (CT) without contrast media is 100% diagnostic for obstruction and can pinpoint the cause of obstruction in 84% of cases. Urinalysis results are usually normal in obstructive uropathy. Hyperchloremic normal anion gap hyperkalemic metabolic acidosis is often a clue to obstruction.

- Renal ultrasonography: 2% of studies are false negative and as many as 26% are false positive.
- Ultrasonography plus CT (no contrast agent): 100% diagnostic; can pinpoint the cause in 84% of cases.
- Hyperkalemic metabolic acidosis: often a clue to obstruction.

Treatment

Always irrigate and change urinary catheters in evaluating obstructive uropathy. If the obstruction is relieved, replace 2/3 of the postobstructive diuresis volume. According to animal studies, treatment instituted within 1 week produces 50% recovery of the glomerular filtration rate; treatment in 2 weeks results in 30% recovery, and treatment after 8 weeks produces little, if any, recovery.

PRERENAL FAILURE

Prerenal failure is defined as a rapidly reversible cause of renal insufficiency due to renal hypoperfusion. It accounts for at least 50% of cases of acute renal failure in hospitalized patients. The urine sediment is benign (hyaline and granular casts). Urinary indices of oliguria are helpful in distinguishing prerenal from renal failure. These diagnostic indices are listed in Table 16-1. It is important in treatment to correct the underlying disorder if known and to replace fluids if hypovolemic.

- Prerenal failure: rapidly reversible renal insufficiency due to renal hypoperfusion.
- Urinary indices of oliguria help to distinguish between prerenal and renal failure.

The fractional excretion of sodium is the most helpful urinary index to distinguish prerenal oliguria from oliguria due to acute intrinsic renal failure. It is an index of the quantity of sodium excreted divided by the quantity of sodium filtered times 100. Normally, this value is <1%; it is also <1% in prerenal insufficiency. Patients with tubular dysfunction have >3% of the sodium filtered eventually excreted. There are some causes of acute *intrinsic* renal failure associated with a low fractional excretion of sodium. All these causes have a decrease in renal blood flow. They include renal failure due to nonsteroidal anti-inflammatory drugs (NSAIDs), angiotensin converting enzyme inhibitors, radiocontrast media, hemoglobinomyoglobinuria, early obstruction, acute glomerulonephritis, and hepatorenal failure.

HEPATORENAL SYNDROME

Hepatorenal syndrome is a severe state of prerenal hypoperfusion that occurs in 40%-50% of patients with terminal cirrhosis. It usually occurs in the presence of jaundice, ascites, and stigmata of portal hypertension. This syndrome usually develops in the hospital, triggered by diuretics, gastrointestinal tract bleeding, or paracentesis. Hyponatremia, hypokalemia, and hypoalbuminemia commonly accompany the syndrome. The pathogenesis of this disorder is accompanied by severe vasoconstriction. Endothelin levels are ten times higher than normal. Laboratory findings include urinary sodium <10 mOsm/L, urinary osmolality >500 mOsm/L, and only a transient response to fluids. A transition to acute tubular necrosis is possible, and recovery is only about 10%. Treatment includes liver transplantation, LaVeen shunt, dopamine, and high doses of spironolactone (Aldactone); occasionally, plasma infusions have been beneficial. Other causes of renal failure associated with liver disease include amyloidosis, leptospirosis, methoxyflurane, vasculitis, and acute Wilson's disease.

- Hepatorenal syndrome: severe state of prerenal hypoperfusion.
- Occurs in 40%-50% of patients with terminal cirrhosis.
- Hyponatremia, hypokalemia, and hypoalbuminemia are common.
- Urinary sodium is <10 mOsm/L and urinary osmolality is >500 mOsm/L.
- 10% of patients recover.
- Pathogenesis: accompanied by severe vasoconstriction.
- Endothelin levels are 10x normal.

ACUTE INTRINSIC RENAL FAILURE

Acute Tubular Necrosis

Most patients (60%) with acute tubular necrosis are not oliguric and carry a better prognosis than oliguric patients (40%). The mean incidence of acute tubular necrosis in hospitals is about 5%. It occurs in 50% of emergency abdominal aortic aneurysm repairs, 10% of elective abdominal aortic aneurysm repairs, and in 20% of patients undergoing heart operations or operations related to trauma. The pathogenesis of acute tubular necrosis is usually due to ischemia, which may occur without hypotension, as in 50% of postoperative cases. Acute tubular necrosis has more than one cause in 70% of patients. Important toxins that can cause tubular damage include endogenous toxins (calcium, uric acid, hemoglobinuria, and myoglobinuria) and exogenous toxins (antibiotics, contrast dye, chemotherapeutic agents, cyclosporin A, and acyclovir).

- Acute tubular necrosis: 60% of patients are not oliguric and 40% are.
- It occurs in 50% of emergency abdominal aortic aneurysm repairs.
- Pathogenesis: usually is ischemia.

Ischemia affects the kidney similar to the way it affects the myocardium. We often think of ischemia being a continuum

Table 16-1.--Diagnostic Indices of Oliguria

	Prerenal	Acute tubular necrosis
Urine osmolality, mOsm/L	≥500	≤350
Urine/plasma creatinine ratio	≥40	≤20
BUN/plasma creatinine ratio	>20	<15
Fractional excretion of sodium	<1%	>3%

in the myocardium, going from angina to subendocardial infarction to true transmural infarction. Ischemia can affect the kidney by initially inducing prerenal insufficiency, followed by acute tubular necrosis, and then cortical necrosis. Studies demonstrate that the redistribution of blood flow, medullary ischemia, backleak of filtrate through damaged tubules, intrarenal obstruction by necrotized tubule casts, and glomerular filter damage all have a role in acute tubular necrosis. Sublethal ischemia leads to loss of tubular cell polarity and, therefore, lack of transport. Free radicals of oxygen and high intracellular concentrations of calcium also promote tubule cell injury.

Urinalysis often demonstrates cellular debris, tubular epithelial cell casts, granular casts, and a "muddy brown" appearance. Erythrocyte casts are associated with acute glomerular nephritis and not with acute tubular necrosis. Also, leukocyte casts, leukocytes, and eosinophils accompany acute interstitial nephritis and not acute tubular necrosis.

A stepwise approach to immediate treatment of acute renal failure is outlined in Table 16-2.

Urine alkalinization is helpful in acute tubular necrosis induced by uric acid, myoglobin, or methotrexate.

The typical course of acute renal failure includes an oliguric phase, which lasts 1-2 weeks but not usually more than 4 weeks. If the oliguric phase lasts more than 4 weeks, biopsy should be considered to look for causes of acute renal failure other than acute tubular necrosis. The diuretic phase is characterized by increases in urine flow that are not necessarily associated with improvement in creatinine levels early in the disease. Late in the disease, improvement in the creatinine level occurs as the glomerular filtration rate begins to increase.

Table 16-2.--Stepwise Approach to Immediate Treatment of Acute Renal Failure

---

1. Exclude postrenal and prerenal causes. Try a volume challenge if indicated.

2. Discontinue use of all nephrotoxic agents.

3. Treat with mannitol (12.5-25 g i.v.) and/or furosemide (20 mg i.v.); 25 g of mannitol increases plasma volume 250 mL. Do not exceed total dose of 50 g in renal failure (mannitol intoxication with hyponatremia, extracellular fluid overload).

4. No response (<60 mL/hr), treat with furosemide (400-500 mg i.v.).

5. Response (>60 mL/hr), 20% mannitol (i.v. infusion; no more than 100 g/24 hr) and furosemide (200 mg) to keep urine output >60 mL/hr. Replace urine 1:1.

6. Other--avoid high doses of furosemide, ethacrynic acid (ototoxicity); use dopamine (2-5 μg).

It is during this phase that severe hypercalcemia can occur in rhabdomyolysis-induced renal failure. The third and final phase is the recovery phase of intrinsic renal failure. During this phase, glomerular filtration rate improves over a period of 3-12 months. In general, the condition of 60% of patients stabilizes with reduced glomerular filtration rate, especially if the patients have been oliguric for more than 16 days. Complications of acute renal failure include infection, which is the number one cause of death and occurs in 50%-90% of patients. It is important to note that fever may be absent and that a careful search for pulmonary and urinary tract infections, abscesses, and other sources of infection must be completed. Other complications include gastrointestinal tract bleeding, hypervolemia with congestive heart failure, hyperkalemia, hyponatremia, metabolic acidosis, and uremia.

Management of acute renal failure includes allowing 0.5 lb loss/day for catabolism. Restricting fluid and sodium, in addition to a 100-g carbohydrate diet with limitations of potassium, magnesium, phosphate, and protein, is also recommended. Treatment with thiazide diuretics, magnesium-containing antacids, and NSAIDs must stop, and contrast agent must be avoided if possible. It is also important to adjust drug doses, especially of digoxin, antibiotics, antihypertensive agents, and benzodiazepines. Phosphate binders are also helpful in patients taking oral nutrition. Although patients have low serum levels of calcium, this is rarely treated.

Dialysis can be performed with hemodialysis, continuous hemofiltration, or peritoneal dialysis. It is best to anticipate the patient's course and to maintain the predialysis BUN <100. Other indications include extracellular fluid volume excess, hyperkalemia, severe acidosis, pericarditis, and the need to make space for parenteral nutrition. Dialysis is often necessary daily in hypercatabolic patients.

Patients with aminoglycoside-induced renal failure are often nonoliguric. The renal failure occurs only after 5-7 days of therapy and correlates with the cumulative dose received. Aminoglycosides are freely filtered and absorbed partially in the proximal tubule: the more amino groups on the aminoglycoside, the more toxic the agent (streptomycin is more toxic than gentamicin, which is as toxic as tobramycin). Magnesium and potassium wasting from tubular dysfunction are common accompaniments, and urine myeloid bodies can sometimes be seen with electron microscopic examination of the urine of affected patients. Regular measurement of serum creatinine concentrations is the best way to detect nephrotoxicity.

- Aminoglycoside-induced renal failure: often nonoliguric.
- Occurs after 5-7 days of therapy.
- Urine myeloid bodies are sometimes seen.

Acute renal dysfunction due to amphotericin B occurs after a 2-3-g dose of treatment and is rare if <600 mg. It is also associated with distal tubular dysfunction. Patients also develop nephrogenic diabetes insipidus and a type IV renal tubular acidosis. Some evidence suggests that alkalinizing the urine may be beneficial in these patients.

- Volume depletion is a principal risk factor.
- Amphotericin-B-induced renal failure: occurs with a 2-3-g dose but rarely if the dose is <600 mg.

Up to 30% of the patients receiving cisplatin develop renal failure if the cumulative dose is 50-75 mg/m^2. Renal failure can be avoided with adequate hydration and forced diuresis; it is associated with hypomagnesemia and hypokalemia.

- Cisplatin-induced renal failure: occurs in 30% of patients receiving 50-75 mg/m^2.

Methotrexate is a dose-related (>50 mg/kg) cause of renal failure. It precipitates in the renal tubules, as does acyclovir and some sulfas (treatment with an alkaline diuresis has been helpful).

- Methotrexate-induced renal failure: dose related.
- Methotrexate precipitates in the renal tubules.

Contrast dye-induced nephropathy is likely due to vasoconstriction, obstruction, and direct tubular toxicity of contrast agents. Its incidence is probably less than previously believed, but patients who are at risk can be identified, including those with severe renal insufficiency alone or diabetic patients with mild renal insufficiency. Patients who receive multiple exposures to contrast agent are at increased risk, as are those who receive high doses of contrast agent. The acute renal failure that accompanies radiocontrast dye toxicity is often associated with a low fractional excretion of sodium. The patients usually become oliguric 24-48 hours after exposure, with dense nephrotomograms on radiography; this reverses within 7 days. Low osmolar, low ionic contrast agents cause less allergic reactions and may be helpful in selected patients. Other measures include prevention by normal saline-induced diuresis and decreasing the dose of contrast agent. There is some investigational evidence that calcium channel blockers and atrial natriuretic factor may be helpful in preventing acute contrast-induced nephropathy. Spacing contrast studies for several days is also an important preventive measure. Contrast agent can be removed by dialysis, but this generally is not done clinically.

- Contrast dye-induced renal failure: due to vasoconstriction, obstruction, and direct tubular toxicity.
- Patients at risk: those with severe renal insufficiency and diabetic patients with mild renal insufficiency.
- Prevention: hydration, forced diuresis, low dose of contrast agent.

Heme pigments (Table 16-3) induce renal failure by intrarenal vasoconstriction and obstruction. Rhabdomyolysis can be due to traumatic causes (crush, seizures, alcoholic coma, and ischemia) and to nontraumatic causes (cocaine, clofibrate, lovastatin, heat stroke, sickle cell trait, carbon monoxide poisoning, spider bite, and polydermatomyositis). Hypocalcemia, frequently severe, can often accompany the acute syndrome, followed by severe hypercalcemia in the diuretic phase of recovering renal failure. Treatment includes a forced diuresis and urine alkalinization, with careful attention to the patient's serum levels of calcium and potassium.

- Heme pigment-induced renal failure: due to intrarenal vasoconstriction and obstruction.
- Hypocalcemia can occur in acute phase and hypercalcemia in diuretic phase.

NSAIDs may cause reversible acute renal failure due to intense intrarenal vasoconstriction. Renal blood flow depends on prostaglandins in the setting of extracellular fluid volume contraction (especially with heart failure, cirrhosis, nephrotic syndrome, and chronic renal failure). Inhibition of prostaglandin synthesis results in acute renal failure. NSAIDs also may be associated with hyperkalemia, hyponatremia, aggravation of hypertension, acute interstitial nephritis, and acute nephrotic syndrome.

Angiotensin converting enzyme inhibitors cause acute renal failure in the setting of preexisting decreased renal blood flow. This may be due to large or small vessel renal disease and often is reversed after discontinuation of treatment with the angiotensin converting enzyme inhibitor. Hyperkalemia may also occur.

Cyclosporine induces reversible intrarenal vasoconstriction and aggravates hypertension. This is best treated with a calcium channel blocker. Chronic cyclosporine nephrotoxicity has been associated with hyperkalemia, hyperuricemia, and hyperchloremic metabolic acidosis. Some patients develop chronic interstitial fibrosis.

Table 16-3.--Heme Pigments

	Serum color	Haptoglobin	CPK	Heme dipstick	Urine benzidine
Hemoglobin	Red	Decreased	Normal	+	-
Myoglobin	Clear	Normal	Increased	+	+

Acute renal failure may occur in 25%-35% of patients infected with the HIV virus. Opportunistic infections of the kidney may occur. Hypovolemia due to diarrhea may cause prerenal insufficiency. High doses of acyclovir and sulfa antibiotics may cause intrarenal obstructive renal failure. Rifampin and sulfas may cause acute interstitial nephritis. Pentamidine and amphotericin B have been associated with hyperkalemic metabolic acidosis and acute tubular necrosis.

Acute Renovascular Disease

Atheroembolic-induced renal failure is an increasingly recognized cause of renal failure. It generally occurs, either spontaneously or after an invasive procedure, in older patients. The patients often have livedo reticularis of the extremities and emboli seen on funduscopic examination. Laboratory studies can demonstrate a high erythrocyte sedimentation rate, low level of complement, eosinophilia, eosinophiluria, and thrombocytopenia. Whereas contrast nephropathy is usually reversible, patients with atheroembolic-induced renal failure often have minimal reversibility. Renal biopsy specimens demonstrate cholesterol emboli in medium-sized arteries, with intense tubulointerstitial nephritis. The only treatment is to correct the source of the embolization, looking for atrial fibrillation, cardiac valve disease, endocarditis, etc. Anticoagulation may actually aggravate the tendency for embolization.

- Atheroembolic-induced renal failure: generally in older patients.

- Findings: high erythrocyte sedimentation rate, low levels of complement, eosinophilia, eosinophiluria.

DISORDERS OF WATER BALANCE

The most important principle in understanding disorders of water balance is that the serum level of sodium is the clinical index of total body water. The serum sodium level is not an index of total body sodium. Total body sodium can be determined only by physical examination. The serum sodium level is a useful clinical index to evaluate water balance, not sodium balance, disorders. Water balance is regulated by thirst, antidiuretic hormone, and renal medullary concentration of water.

- Total body sodium can be determined only by physical examination.
- Water balance is regulated by thirst, antidiuretic hormone, and renal medullary concentration of water.

Hyponatremia

Hyponatremia is the number one electrolyte abnormality in hospitalized patients. Its symptoms are protean, including lethargy, cramps, decreased deep tendon reflexes, and seizures. The diagnosis and management of hyponatremia are shown in Figure 16-1.

- Hyponatremia: number one electrolyte abnormality in hospitalized patients.

Fig. 16-1. Diagnosis and management of hyponatremia.

Diagnosis

The first step in evaluating patients with hyponatremia is to measure serum osmolality. Isotonic hyponatremia may be due to severe hypertriglyceridemia (>1,500, lipemia retinalis is always present), severe hyperproteinemia (>8.0, Waldenström's macroglobulinemia, myeloma), or isotonic infusions of glucose, mannitol, or glycine. Hypertonic hyponatremia is due to severe hyperglycemia (sodium decreases 1.6 for each 100 mg/dL increase in glucose) and to hypertonic infusions of glucose, mannitol, or glycine.

The second step is to assess the extracellular fluid volume of the hypotonic hyponatremic patient and to determine whether he or she is hypovolemic, euvolemic, or hypervolemic. 1) Hypotonic hypovolemic hyponatremia: check urine osmolality and sodium concentration; common causes are thiazides and adrenal insufficiency. 2) Hypotonic hypervolemic hyponatremia: check urine osmolality and sodium concentration; edematous states and renal failure are common. 3) Hypotonic euvolemic hyponatremia: check cortisol level, thyroid, urine osmolality, hypothyroidism, Addison's disease, reset osmostat, and psychogenic polydipsia.

The syndrome of inappropriate secretion of antidiuretic hormone is a diagnosis of exclusion. Patients must meet the following criteria: 1) hypotonic plasma, 2) urine less than maximally dilute, 3) urine sodium matches intake, 4) absence of hypoadrenocorticism and hypothyroidism, and 5) improvement with water restriction. An important clinical hint is the presence of a low serum level of uric acid. The BUN also tends to be low.

Acute hyponatremia has been described in several special clinical settings. Hyponatremia may occur in up to 5% of patients after surgery and anesthesia. Plasma vasopressin concentrations are increased because of nonosmolar stimuli. Rarely, profound hyponatremia may occur. During transurethral prostatic resection, isotonic or hypotonic fluids containing glycine, mannitol, or sorbitol can be absorbed and depress the serum level of sodium. Schizophrenic patients with severe compulsive water drinking occasionally have acute hyponatremia. Also, infusions of oxytocin during infusions of cyclophosphamide may induce acute hyponatremia.

Chronic hyponatremia may be induced by the use of thiazides, chlorpropamide, carbamazepine, and NSAIDs.

- Syndrome of inappropriate secretion of antidiuretic hormone: serum level of uric acid and BUN are low.

Patients with acute hyponatremia in the presence of neurologic symptoms generally respond to infusion of isotonic saline and a loop diuretic. Water intake should be restricted. The use of hypertonic saline and loop diuretics may be necessary in patients with severe clinical hyponatremia and should be monitored in an intensive care unit. In symptomatic patients with acute hyponatremia, the serum level of sodium should be increased no faster than 1 to 1.5 mEq/L per hour to 100 or 125 mEq/dL. Generally, hyponatremia should be reversed cautiously at a rate similar to that at which it developed to avoid central pontine myelinolysis. In patients with chronic syndrome of inappropriate secretion of antidiuretic hormone, demeclocycline may be of benefit. Increasing protein intake also facilitates water excretion.

Hypernatremia

As in hyponatremia, the symptoms of hypernatremia are often protean, with irritability, hyperreflexia, ataxia, and seizures. All forms of hypernatremia are associated with hypertonicity, so there is no pseudohypernatremia. Cases are categorized as hypovolemic, hypervolemic, and euvolemic hypernatremia. The diagnosis and management of hypernatremia are shown in Figure 16-2.

- Hypovolemic hypernatremia: check urine sodium; may be caused by osmotic diuresis, excess sweating, and diarrhea.
- Hypervolemic hypernatremia: may be caused by sodium poisoning.
- Euvolemic hypernatremia: loss of water; extrarenal (skin, lung) versus renal; diabetes insipidus, central versus nephrogenic water deprivation test.

Patients with hypovolemic hypernatremia often respond to saline followed by hypotonic solution. Patients with hypervolemic hypernatremia respond to diuretics and may or may not need dialysis. Euvolemic patients should receive free water, either orally or intravenously, to correct the serum level of sodium at approximately 1-2 mEq/hr.

DISORDERS OF SODIUM BALANCE

Disorders of sodium balance can be determined only by clinical examination. Orthostatism implies volume depletion and sodium deficiency. Edema implies volume excess and sodium excess.

DISORDERS OF POTASSIUM BALANCE

Potassium is predominantly an intracellular cation. Total body potassium is approximately equal to 4,200 mEq, with only 60 mEq in the total extracellular fluid volume. Gastric fluid contains 5-10 mEq of potassium/L, and diarrheal fluid contains 10-100 mEq/L. The internal balance of potassium is regulated by endogenous factors such as acidemia, sodium, potassium, ATPase, insulin, catecholamines, and aldosterone. The external balance is regulated primarily by potassium excretion, which in large part is regulated by urinary flow rate, aldosterone, antidiuretic hormone, and sodium delivery to the distal tubule.

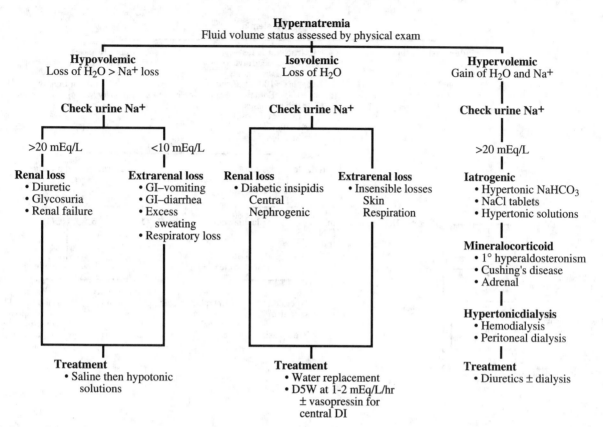

Fig. 16-2. Diagnosis and management of hypernatremia.

Hypokalemia

Symptoms of hypokalemia include weakness, ileus, polyuria, and, sometimes, rhabdomyolysis. Hypokalemia also aggravates digoxin toxicity. A stepwise approach to the diagnosis of hypokalemia is given in Table 16-4 and outlined in Figure 16-3.

● Hypokalemia symptoms: weakness, ileus, and polyuria.

Therapy. If the serum level of potassium is <2 mEq/L, total potassium deficit = 1,000 mEq; if the serum level of potassium is between 2 and 4 mEq/L, then a decrease of 0.3 = 100 to 500 mEq deficit, usually potassium chloride (diabetic ketoacidosis, potassium phosphate; potassium citrate, severe acidosis). Do not exceed 10 mEq/hr i.v. unless using a central catheter and ECG monitoring. Dietary sodium restriction decreases potassium-losing effects of diuretics.

Hyperkalemia

A stepwise approach to the diagnosis of hyperkalemia is given in Table 16-5 and outlined in Figure 16-4.

Therapy: antagonize membrane effects and then redistribute (treat with calcium, then sodium bicarbonate, then insulin), then resins, and finally dialysis. For chronic therapy, use loop diuretics, NaHCO3, resins, fludrocortisone, dialysis.

Table 16-4.--Stepwise Approach to Diagnosis of Hypokalemia

1. Exclude redistribution--β-agonists (albuterol and terbutaline for asthma and ritodrine for labor), acute alkalosis, vitamin B_{12} therapy for pernicious anemia (especially if thrombocytopenic), barium carbonate

2. Determine whether potassium losses are renal or extrarenal--check urine potassium level on high sodium diet, is potassium > or < 20 mEq/day

3. If loss is extrarenal, determine cause (laxative screen)-- usually diarrhea, enemas, laxative abuse, villous adenomas, ureterocolostomy

   If loss is renal, determine if hypertensive or normotensive (diuretic screen)

4. If hypertensive, check plasma renin and aldosterone levels, includes primary aldosteronism or hyperplasia (glycyrrhizic acid in licorice, chewing tobacco), adrenal abnormalities

   If normotensive, check plasma HCO_3 levels and urine chloride, includes renal tubular acidosis, vomiting, diuretic abuse, Bartter's syndrome, magnesium deficiency

   High doses of penicillin, amphotericin B, cisplatin

   Renal loss and metabolic acidosis--diabetic ketoacidosis, renal tubular acidosis, acetazolamide

   Renal loss and metabolic alkalosis--vomiting, diuretics, Bartter's syndrome, excess aldosterone

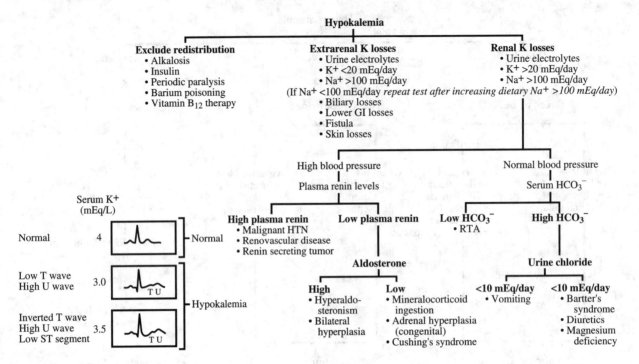

Fig. 16-3. Diagnosis of hypokalemia.

Table 16-5.--Stepwise Approach to Diagnosis of Hyperkalemia

1. Exclude pseudohyperkalemia--ECG is normal, heparinized plasma potassium is normal

   Hemolysis of clotted blood (0.3 increase), tourniquet ischemia, severe leukocytosis or thrombocytosis

2. Determine cause based on redistribution or excess total body potassium (see Fig. 16-4)

ACID-BASE DISORDERS

Clinically, it is absolutely critical that a stepwise approach to acid-base disorders be followed. The six steps listed in Table 16-6 should always be followed before interpreting an acid-base disorder.

Metabolic Acidosis

Metabolic acidosis is defined as a primary disturbance in which retention of acid consumes endogenous alkali stores. This is reflected by a decrease in HCO_3. The secondary response is increased ventilation with a decrease in PCO_2. Metabolic acidosis can be caused by overproduction of endogenous acid (e.g., diabetic ketoacidosis), loss of alkali stores (diarrhea, renal tubular acidosis), or failure of renal acid secretion or base resynthesis (renal failure).

- Metabolic acidosis: primary disturbance is retention of acid.

- Secondary response: increased ventilation with PCO_2.

Some of the signs and symptoms of metabolic acidosis include fatigue, dyspnea, abdominal pain, vomiting, Kussmaul's respiration, myocardial depression, hyperkalemia, leukemoid reaction, insulin resistance, and, when pH is <7.2, arteriolar dilatation and hypotension.

Some formulas for the predicted compensation for pure metabolic acidosis (which will take up to 24 hours) are 1) PCO_2 = last two digits of the pH, 2) PCO_2 decreases by 1-1.3 mm Hg for each mEq/L decrease in HCO_3, and 3) $PCO_2 \pm 2 = 1.5$ (HCO_3) + 8 (this is the best formula).

The metabolic acidoses are classified as either normal anion gap or high anion gap. Normal anion gap metabolic acidosis is defined in terms of serum levels of potassium.

Hypokalemic normal anion gap metabolic acidosis can be associated with diarrhea, ureteral diversion, or the use of carbonic anhydrase inhibitors such as acetazolamide. Renal tubular acidosis type I, or classic renal tubular acidosis, is also a cause. This is associated with nephrocalcinosis and osteomalacia. The causes of type I renal tubular acidosis include toluene sniffing, amphotericin B, lithium, Sjögren's syndrome, hypergammaglobulinemia, and sickle cell disease. Type II renal tubular acidosis is also a hypokalemic anion gap metabolic acidosis. In adults, it is often associated with other proximal tubule defects, including glycosuria, uricosuria, phosphaturia, and aminoaciduria (Fanconi's syndrome). Causes of type II renal tubular acidosis include myeloma, cystinosis (not cystinuria), lead, tetracycline, and acetazolamide.

Fig. 16-4. Diagnosis of hyperkalemia.

Table 16-6.--Six Steps for Interpreting Acid-Base Disorder

1. Note the clinical presentation
2. Always check the anion (hidden acidosis) and osmolar
   gaps if possible
   Normal anion gap Na - (HCO_3 + Cl) = 8 to 12
   Cations = Na, gammaglobulins, Ca, Mg, K
   Anions = Cl, HCO_3, albumin, PO_4, SO_4, organic
   High anion gap >12--K-U-S-S-M-A-U-L
   Low anion gap <8--Bromism, paraproteinemia,
   hypercalcemia/magnesemia, lithium toxicity, severe
   hypernatremia, severe hypoalbuminemia
   Osmolar gap >10 -OLS--methanol, ethanol, ethylene
   glycol, isopropyl alcohol, mannitol
3. Use the Henderson equation to check the validity of the
   arterial blood gases values:

$$H^+ \text{ (nEq/L)} = \frac{24 \times \text{lungs} (P_{CO_2})}{\text{kidneys} (HCO_3)}$$

pH	7.00	7.10	7.20	7.30	7.40	7.50	7.60	7.70
H^+	100	79	63	50	40	32	25	20

4. Is the pH high or low?
5. Is the primary disturbance metabolic (HCO_3) or
   respiratory (P_{CO_2})?
6. Is it simple or mixed?

The causes of hyperkalemic normal anion gap metabolic acidosis include acid loads such as NH_4Cl, arginine chloride, lysine chloride, cholestyramine, total parenteral nutrition, HCl, oral $CaCl_2$, obstructive uropathy, hypoaldosteronism (Addison's disease), 21-hydoxylase deficiency, sulfur toxicity, and type IV renal tubular acidosis. Type IV renal tubular acidosis is associated with hyporenin and hypoaldosteronism, and it may be caused by diabetes mellitus, interstitial nephritis, spirono-lactone, amiloride, triamterene, or cyclosporin A.

High anion gap metabolic acidosis is due to several causes. In chronic renal failure, the anion gap is usually <25. If anion gaps are >25, one should immediately think of an ingestion of a poison. Isopropyl alcohol increases the osmolar gap but not the anion gap (acetone is not an anion).

- In chronic renal failure, the anion gap usually is <25.
- A gap >25 should suggest ingestion of a poison.

Metabolic acidosis is generally corrected by treating the underlying disorder, but the bicarbonate deficit can be determined by the following formula:

Bicarbonate deficit = 0.2 x body weight (kg) x (normal HCO_3 [i.e., 24] - measured HCO_3)

Metabolic Alkalosis

Metabolic alkalosis is defined as a primary disturbance in which plasma bicarbonate is increased. This can be caused by 1) endogenous alkali, 2) acid loss through the gastrointestinal tract or kidney, or 3) loss of nonbicarbonate fluid causing contraction of the remaining fluid around unchanged total body bicarbonate. The kidney must also be stimulated to sustain the high level of plasma bicarbonate. This can occur by 1) extracellular fluid volume contraction, 2) hypercapnia, 3) potassium depletion, 4) steroid excess, 5) hypercalcemia, or 6) hypoparathyroidism. The secondary response is decreased ventilation with an increase in PCO_2. The signs and symptoms of metabolic alkalosis include weakness, muscle cramps, hyperreflexia, alveolar hypoventilation, and dysrhythmias.

- Metabolic alkalosis: primary disturbance is increased plasma bicarbonate.
- The kidney must be stimulated to sustain the high level of plasma bicarbonate.
- Secondary response: decreased ventilation with increased PCO_2.

The predicted compensation for pure renal metabolic alkalosis (which will take up to 24 hours) can be calculated by using the following formulas:
1. $PCO_2 \pm 5 = 0.9(HCO_3) + 15$
2. PCO_2 increases 6 mm Hg for each 10 mEq/L increase in HCO_3

Metabolic alkalosis can be classified in terms of the spot urine chloride.

Mixed Acid-Base Disorders
- HCO_3 <15 usually is caused partly by a metabolic acidosis.
- HCO_3 >45 usually is caused partly by a metabolic alkalosis.
- Arterial blood gas values may be normal but a high anion gap indicates a mixed metabolic alkalosis/acidosis.
- In metabolic acidosis and respiratory alkalosis, the PCO_2 is lower than predicted for the acidosis.
- In metabolic alkalosis and respiratory acidosis, the HCO_3 is higher than predicted for acidosis.
- In mixed metabolic and respiratory alkalosis, HCO_3 is higher and PCO_2 is lower than expected.
- Triple disorders--diabetic/alcoholic (vomiting) + (keto/lactic acidosis) + (sepsis or liver disease).

CLINICAL MANIFESTATIONS OF GLOMERULAR INJURY
The glomerular basement membrane is an important size barrier (MW, 70,000) and negative charge barrier, repulsing albumin and immune globulins. There is also tubular reabsorption of protein in the range of 500-1,500 mg/24 hours by the proximal tubule.

Orthostatic proteinuria is usually benign and remits spontaneously. The diagnosis can be made by obtaining two 12-hour urine collections for protein: one supine and one upright. Significant proteinuria is defined as >75 mg/12 hours.

Tubulointerstitial disease is sometimes associated with proteinuria, but it is usually <1,500 mg/day. Overflow low molecular weight proteinuria is due to increased light chain or lysozyme excretion without nephrosis.

Renal biopsy is indicated to determine the prognosis and diagnosis of patients with >2 g/day non-nephrotic range proteinuria if it is associated with an abnormal sediment or renal insufficiency. Other indications for biopsy include nephrotic range proteinuria, microscopic hematuria with abnormal urine sediment or renal function, progressive renal insufficiency, and acute renal failure lasting >3-4 weeks. Patients with an atypical course of diabetes mellitus and undiagnosed systemic disease such as amyloid, systemic lupus erythematosus, and polyarteritis nodosa should undergo biopsy. Renal biopsy is contraindicated in bleeding disorders, uncontrolled hypertension, urinary tract infections, solitary kidneys other than allografts, and uncooperative patients. Complications include microscopic hematuria, gross hematuria (10%-20%), need for nephrectomy, biopsy of other tissue, and death (0.001%).

- Renal biopsy: to determine the prognosis and diagnosis of patients with >2 g/day non-nephrotic range proteinuria.
- Other indications: nephrotic range proteinuria, microscopic hematuria, progressive renal insufficiency, acute renal failure lasting >3-4 weeks, atypical course of diabetes mellitus, and undiagnosed systemic disease.
- Contraindications: bleeding disorders, uncontrolled hypertension, urinary tract infections, solitary kidneys other than allografts, and uncooperative patients.

Nephrotic Syndrome
Nephrotic syndrome is defined by the presence of urinary protein >3.5 g/1.73 m^2 per day, hypoalbuminemia (<3.0 g/dL), peripheral edema, and hypercholesterolemia (total >200 mg/dL). Urinalysis demonstrates waxy casts, free fat, oval fat bodies, and lipiduria. Other associations include hypogammaglobulinemia (increases infection risk), vitamin D deficiency due to loss of vitamin D-binding protein, and iron deficiency anemia due to hypotransferrinemia. Renal vein thrombosis may occur because of an increased thromboembolic tendency (increased factor V, VIII, fibrinogen, platelets and decreased antithrombin III and antiplasmin). Management includes controlling blood pressure and limiting sodium and lipid intake.

- Nephrotic syndrome: urinary protein >3.5 g/1.73 m^2 daily.
- Hypoalbuminemia, <3 g/dL.
- Peripheral edema.
- Hypercholesterolemia, total >200 mg/dL.

Nephritic Syndrome
Nephritic syndrome is characterized by the presence of erythrocyte casts with variable amounts of proteinuria. Because

of methemoglobin formation in acid urine, it has a "Coca-Cola" or smokey appearance.

- Nephritic syndrome: erythrocyte casts with variable amounts of proteinuria.
- Urine: Coca-Cola or smokey appearance.

GLOMERULAR DISEASE WITH ACUTE REVERSIBLE RENAL FAILURE

Poststreptococcal Glomerulonephritis

Poststreptococcal glomerulonephritis is usually caused by group A β-hemolytic streptococcal infections. The latent period is 6-21 days (type 12 pharyngeal infection) or 14-28 days (type 49 skin infection). The urine sediment is active, with usually <3 g proteinuria/24 hours and a fractional excretion of sodium <1%. Because of activation of the alternative complement pathway, total and C3 complements are low but only up to 8 weeks. Antistreptolysin-O is present in pharyngeal infections and anti-DNase B in skin infections. In renal biopsy specimens, light microscopy demonstrates many polymorphonuclear neutrophils, with proliferation and subepithelial deposits or humps. Immunofluorescence demonstrates a granular "lumpy-bumpy" pattern with IgG and C3. Treatment is supportive alone, with control of blood pressure and edema. Penicillin therapy for the patient and contacts may prevent new cases. The course and prognosis are excellent in children and adults unless crescents or persistent proteinuria is present.

- Poststreptococcal glomerulonephritis: usually due to group A β-hemolytic streptococcal infections.
- Urine sediment: active, <3 g proteinuria/24 hours and fractional excretion of sodium is <1%.
- Total and C3 complement are low.
- Immunofluorescence: granular "lumpy-bumpy" pattern with IgG and C3.

Other forms of postinfectious glomerulonephritis include bacterial endocarditis and infected ventriculoatrial shunts.

CRESCENTIC GLOMERULAR DISEASE WITH PROGRESSIVE RENAL FAILURE

Rapidly progressive glomerulonephritis is defined as an acute (days to weeks to months) deterioration of renal function associated with active urinary sediment and crescentic glomerulonephritis (Fig. 16-5). Usually, adults (mean age, 55 years) are affected. The pulmonary-renal syndrome is frequent, and oliguria is not uncommon. On light microscopy, there is fibrinoid necrosis and >50% crescents. Immunofluorescence demonstrates three patterns: type I, linear IgG (Goodpasture's syndrome or anti-GBM mediated); type II, granular immune complexes (D-penicillamine); and type III,

Fig. 16-5. Algorithm of the serologic and pathologic categorization of rapidly progressive (crescentic) glomerulonephritis. (From MKSAP in the Subspecialty of Nephrology and Hypertension. Book 1 Syllabus and Questions, 1994. American College of Physicians. By permission.)

negative immunofluorescence. Treatment of rapidly progressive glomerulonephritis: pulse methylprednisolone sodium succinate (SoluMedrol), 1 g for 3 days, with or without cytotoxic agents. Plasmapheresis is helpful if there is pulmonary hemorrhage in Goodpasture's syndrome. Prognosis: 35% develop end-stage renal disease, with 25% mortality, and 40% progress to chronic renal insufficiency. Oliguria, a high creatinine level (>7), and old age are poor prognostic signs.

- Rapidly progressive glomerulonephritis: subacute deterioration of renal function.
- Crescentic glomerulonephritis.
- Pulmonary-renal syndrome is common; oliguria is not uncommon.
- 25% mortality.
- 40% progress to chronic renal insufficiency.

GLOMERULAR DISEASE WITH HEMATURIA AND VARIABLE PROTEINURIA AND FUNCTION

IgA Nephropathy

IgA nephropathy is the most common glomerulopathy worldwide. Patients present with synpharyngitic hematuria (microscopic with or without macroscopic hematuria), often with erythrocyte casts. Urine sediment activity may be exacerbated by an upper respiratory tract infection. Pathogenesis may be due partly to exaggerated IgA mucosal production. Secondary causes include advanced chronic liver disease, sprue, dermatitis herpetiformis, and ankylosing spondylitis. Poor prognostic signs are heavy proteinuria, hypertension, and renal insufficiency. Plasma IgA is increased in only 50% of the patients. Skin biopsy for IgA is not helpful. Renal biopsy in IgA demonstrates mesangial proliferation on light microscopy. The immunofluorescence studies are diagnostic and demonstrate IgA within the mesangium. The prognosis is generally good for IgA nephropathy; however, 20% of patients may reach end-stage renal disease in 20 years. Progression to end-stage renal disease in those patients at high risk has been shown to be slowed by administration of fish oil capsules containing omega-3 fatty acids. This disorder often recurs in renal transplant recipients but often is not clinically significant. Poor prognostic signs are diminished renal function, heavy proteinuria, and hypertension.

- IgA nephropathy: most common glomerulopathy worldwide.
- Presents with synpharyngitic hematuria, often with erythrocyte casts.
- Pathogenesis: exaggerated IgA mucosal production or regulation.
- Secondary causes: advanced chronic liver disease, sprue, dermatitis herpetiformis, ankylosing spondylitis.
- Plasma IgA increased in only 50% of patients.

- Prognosis: generally good.

Henoch-Schönlein Purpura

Patients with Henoch-Schönlein purpura present with microscopic and/or macrohematuria along with erythrocyte casts, purpura, and abdominal pain. Renal biopsy findings are similar to those of IgA nephropathy with or without vasculitis. The prognosis generally is good for children and variable for adults. Treatment is supportive only.

Membranoproliferative Glomerulonephritis

Patients with membranoproliferative glomerulonephritis present with nephrotic syndrome (50% of patients), non-nephrotic range proteinuria (30%), or nephritic sediment (20%). Complement values are persistently low (>8 weeks). Antistreptolysin-O may be present, and a C3 nephritic factor is present in many cases. It is an autoantibody to alternative pathway C3 convertase, resulting in persistent C3 breakdown. Secondary causes include chronic infections, "shunt nephritis," malaria, hepatitis B, systemic lupus erythematosus, congenital complement deficiency (C2, C3), mixed cryoglobulinemia, sickle cell disease, partial lipodystrophy (only type II), and α_1-antitrypsin deficiency. The two idiopathic forms are type I and type II (dense-deposit disease).

- Membranoproliferative glomerulonephritis: presents with nephrotic syndrome in 50% of patients, non-nephrotic range proteinuria in 30%, and nephritic sediment in 20%.
- Complements are persistently low.
- C3 nephritic factor is often present.
- Secondary causes: chronic infections, "shunt nephritis," hepatitis B, systemic lupus erythematosus, and sickle cell disease.

In biopsy samples of membranoproliferative glomerulonephritis, light microscopy demonstrates duplication or splitting, tramtracking, or double contouring of the glomerular basement membrane. This proliferation within the glomerulus and capillary loop thickening result in a lobular appearance of the glomeruli. Immunofluorescence demonstrates complex deposition in the mesangium and capillary walls. Electron microscopy demonstrates a distinctive ribboning or sausaging of dense material in type II membranoproliferative glomerulonephritis. Generally, adults receive supportive care; steroids have been helpful in some children. Dipyridamole (225 mg/day) and aspirin (975 mg/day) have been used to slow the progression of adult membranoproliferative glomerulonephritis. The prognosis is worse with hypertension, poor renal function, and heavy proteinuria. This disorder tends to recur in transplants (type I, 30%; type II, 90%).

- Prognosis: worse with hypertension, poor renal function, heavy proteinuria.

GLOMERULAR DISEASE WITH HEAVY PROTEINURIA AND VARIABLE RENAL FAILURE

Minimal Change Nephropathy

Patients with minimal change nephropathy present with abrupt nephrotic syndrome with normal renal function (exceptions, hypovolemia and NSAIDs). This is the number one cause of nephrotic syndrome in children and the cause of 20% of adult cases of idiopathic nephrotic syndrome. Pathogenesis may be due to an attack on the glomerular epithelial cells by T-cell lymphokines, resulting in fusion of the foot processes. The heparin sulfate basement membrane negative charge barrier is lost. Secondary causes include Hodgkin's disease and NSAIDs (with interstitial nephritis). Light microscopic and immunofluorescence findings on renal biopsy specimens in minimal change nephropathy are normal. Electron microscopy shows fusion of the foot processes. A relapsing course is common (60% of patients). Patients are generally responsive, and 90% have complete remission within 4 weeks. Generally, therapy is continued for 4 weeks after remission. Although 80% of adults respond to steroid therapy, 60% have repeated relapses. Cyclophosphamide can prolong remission and may decrease steroid dependence after 8 weeks of therapy; 50% of these patients have prolonged remissions. If patients are unresponsive, another biopsy is indicated to exclude focal segmental glomerulosclerosis.

- Minimal change nephropathy: abrupt nephrotic syndrome with normal renal function.
- Number one cause of nephrotic syndrome in children and cause of 20% of adult cases of idiopathic nephrotic syndrome.
- Secondary causes: Hodgkin's disease and NSAIDs (with interstitial nephritis).
- 80% of adults respond to steroid therapy; 60% have repeated relapses.

Focal Glomerular Sclerosis

Focal glomerular sclerosis accounts for 10% of cases of adult nephrotic syndrome. Mean age at disease onset is 21 years. Patients present with hypertension, renal insufficiency, proteinuria, and gross or microscopic hematuria. Secondary causes include AIDS (more frequent in drug abusers than in homosexuals), heroin abuse, reflux nephropathy, and massive obesity. Light microscopic results of renal biopsy samples demonstrate focal and segmental sclerosis without proliferation. Foam cells are often seen. Immunofluorescence shows IgM and C3 and deposits within the mesangium. Electron microscopy demonstrates fusion of foot processes in all glomeruli. Generally, therapy is supportive, although some patients may respond to a 4-6-month course of corticosteroid treatment. Cyclosporine may also have a role in treating these patients. Angiotensin converting enzyme inhibitors decrease heavy proteinuria independent of their effect on lowering blood pressure. In selected patients with heavy proteinuria, meclofenamate has also decreased complications due to proteinuria. This disorder can recur in renal transplant recipients, and its prognosis is poor if proteinuria is >10 g/day.

HIV nephropathy is characterized by progressive renal insufficiency in patients with heavy proteinuria but often little edema. Large echogenic kidneys are seen on ultrasonography, and renal biopsy demonstrates focal and segmental glomerulosclerosis and glomerular collapse. Visceral epithelial cell swelling in the glomeruli is also present.

This predominates in intravenous drug-using HIV-infected patients. Some patients have had considerable improvement after the administration of corticosteroids.

- Focal glomerular sclerosis: 10% of cases of adult nephrotic syndrome.
- Mean age is 21 years.
- Presents with hypertension, renal insufficiency, proteinuria, and gross or microscopic hematuria.
- Secondary causes: AIDS, heroin abuse, reflux nephropathy, massive obesity.
- Steroid therapy: <10% of patients respond.
- Prognosis is poor if proteinuria is >10 g/day.

Membranous Glomerulopathy

Membranous glomerulopathy is the primary cause of idiopathic nephrotic syndrome in adults (50% of patients). Mean age at disease onset is 35 years. However, 25% of the patients do not have nephrotic range proteinuria. Patients are often hypertensive (40%), with some renal insufficiency. Pathogenesis is due to in situ deposition of cationic antigens in the subepithelial space. Renal vein thrombosis (25%-50%) in some cases may cause sudden loss of renal function. Secondary causes include infections (hepatitis B, quartan malaria, syphilis), multisystem disease (systemic lupus erythematosus, Sjögren's syndrome, sarcoidosis), and neoplasms (1.5% of cases, including carcinoma [lung, colon, stomach, breast] and lymphoma). Malignancies occur at 5x the expected rate in adults with membranous nephropathy. Medications that cause membranous glomerulopathy are gold, D-penicillamine, captopril, and probenecid. Hereditary and metabolic causes include sickle cell disease. Renal biopsy demonstrates "spike and dome" epithelial deposits, with thickened capillary loops seen on light microscopy. Granular IgG and C3 are seen on immunofluorescence. Therapy for membranous nephropathy is generally supportive, although 8 weeks of alternate-day steroids are often recommended. Other measures include the necessity to control hypertension and to treat any underlying disorders. Corticosteroids with or without cyclophosphamide (Cytoxan) may have a role in treatment of heavy proteinuria and worsening renal insufficiency. Without treatment, nearly 25% of the patients have spontaneous complete remission and

50% have partial remission. Approximately 20% of these patients progress to end-stage renal disease; the prognosis is related to the degree of proteinuria.

- Membranous glomerulopathy: primary cause of idiopathic nephrotic syndrome in adults.
- Mean age is 35 years.
- Pathogenesis: in situ deposition of cationic antigens in the subepithelial space.
- Renal vein thrombosis causes sudden loss of renal function in 25%-50% of patients.
- Secondary causes: infections, multisystem disease, neoplasms, and medications.
- Complete remission in 25% of patients and partial remission in 50%.

OTHER GLOMERULAR DISORDERS

Diabetes Mellitus

From 2%-4% of U.S. citizens have diabetes mellitus. Diabetic nephropathy occurs in both insulin-dependent (30%-40%) and noninsulin-dependent (20%-30%) diabetics. More than 30% of patients hospitalized with end-stage renal disease have diabetic nephropathy, the single most common cause of end-stage renal disease in the U.S. Pathogenesis is secondary to glycosylation, renal hemodynamic changes, and hypertension. Microalbuminuria is the primary predictor of renal disease. The stages of diabetic nephropathy are listed in Table 16-7.

- Diabetic nephropathy occurs in insulin-dependent (30%-40%) and noninsulin-dependent (20%-30%) diabetics.
- Diabetes mellitus is the single most common cause of end-stage renal disease in the U.S.
- Microalbuminuria is the primary predictor of renal disease.

Table 16-7.--Stages of Diabetic Nephropathy

Stage I	Hyperfiltration, glomerular filtration rate is 20%-50% above normal, microalbuminuria (>300 mg/24 hours)
Stage II	Normalization of glomerular filtration rate with early structural damage
Stage III	Early hypertension
Stage IV	Progression to proteinuria >0.5 g/day, hypertension, declining glomerular filtration rate (lasts 10-15 years)
Stage V	Progression to end-stage renal disease (5-7 years), heavy proteinuria persists even to end-stage disease

Renal biopsy of diabetic involvement of the kidney demonstrates a nodular and diffuse glomerular scarring or sclerosis. Capsular drop lesions and fibrin cap lesions are also pathognomonic. There is thickening of all basement membranes, with arteriolar hyalinosis and arteriosclerosis. Interstitial fibrosis and tubular atrophy may also be present. Other manifestations of diabetic urinary tract disease include papillary necrosis, perinephric abscess, acute pyelonephritis, neurogenic bladder and hydronephrosis with functional obstruction, bacteriuria, cystitis, and hypertension. Although tight glucose control by all current means available does not reverse diabetic nephropathy, it does tend to slow development of the disease. Patients with end-stage renal disease due to diabetes mellitus are kidney transplant candidates. Hemodialysis and continuous ambulatory peritoneal dialysis are also alternatives. Whether combined kidney/pancreas transplantation will prevent diabetic nephropathy is not clear. However, it is clear that aggressive control of blood pressure and glycemia definitely slows the progression of diabetic nephropathy.

- Other manifestations of diabetic urinary tract disease: papillary necrosis, perinephric abscess, acute pyelonephritis, neurogenic bladder and hydronephrosis with functional obstruction, bacteriuria, cystitis, hypertension.

Although tight control by all means available does not reverse diabetic nephropathy it does tend to slow the development of the disease. Angiotensin converting enzyme inhibitors slow the rate of decline of renal function in insulin-dependent diabetes mellitus, even in the absence of hypertension. Nondihyropteridine calcium channel blockers may have a similar effect.

Aldose reductase inhibitors, nonenzymatic glycosylation inhibitors, and low protein diet may also be beneficial in slowing progressive renal insufficiency.

- Aggressive control of blood pressure and glycemia slows progression.
- Diabetes mellitus is the most common cause of type IV renal tubular acidosis.
- Patients with noninsulin-dependent diabetes mellitus also benefit from aggressive blood sugar and blood pressure control.

Lupus Erythematosus

Of patients with lupus erythematosus, 50% have renal disease at presentation and 90% have renal disease at some time. If renal involvement occurs with lupus, it usually presents early in the course of the disease. The presenting histologic renal lesion is fairly stable except that a focal proliferative lesion progresses to diffuse proliferative lesion in 20% of patients. An active diffuse proliferative lesion is treatable with steroids with or without cytotoxic agents. Membranous systemic lupus erythematosus is usually not treatable with immunosuppressive agents. Kidney biopsy is indicated for active urinary sediment with or without decreased glomerular function to define the renal lesion in lupus erythematosus. The five classes of renal disease that may be present are listed in Table16-8.

- Lupus erythematosus: 50% of patients present with renal disease and 90% have renal disease some time during the course of lupus erythematosus.
- Active diffuse proliferative lesion is treatable with steroids with or without cytotoxic agents.
- Membranous systemic lupus erythematosus usually is not treatable with immunosuppressive agents.

Other manifestations of lupus include acute and chronic tubulointerstital nephritis and vasculitis. Chronic changes include glomerular scarring, tubular atrophy, and interstitial fibrosis, all of which are untreatable. Therapy for lupus nephritis is often limited to treatment of proliferative nephritis. Patients with acute proliferative nephritis and acute renal failure should receive high doses of steroids with or without cytotoxic agents. Diffuse proliferative glomerulonephritis without azotemia is also treated with high doses of steroids for 6-8 weeks. Cyclophosphamide can be added to the therapy if necessary. Aside from proteinuria, membranous lupus involvement often is characterized by weakly positive or negative antinuclear antibody without red cell casts. Generally, therapy is supportive only. It is important to remember that drug-induced lupus rarely involves the kidney. Pregnancy should be delayed until after lupus is inactive for 6 months; 25%-45% of lupus patients have exacerbations usually 8 weeks after delivery. Lupus "burns out" with end-stage renal disease and generally does not recur in transplant recipients.

- Drug-induced lupus rarely involves the kidney.
- Pregnancy should be delayed until after lupus is inactive for 6 months.
- Lupus "burns out" with end-stage renal disease and generally does not occur in transplant recipients.

Table 16-8.--Five Classes of Renal Diseases Present With Lupus

Class I	Normal
Class II	Mild mesangial change (no clinical findings of renal disease in 50% of patients)
Class III	Focal and segmental proliferative glomerulonephritis (20% nephritic with or without nephrotic syndrome)
Class IV	Diffuse proliferative glomerulonephritis (70% nephritic with or without nephrotic syndrome), "wire loop"
Class V	Membranous glomerulonephritis (nephrotic but not active sediment)

Vasculitis

The types of vasculitis are listed in Table 16-9.

Microscopic polyarteritis nodosa presents with hypertension, weight loss, arthralgias, myalgias, mononeuritis multiplex, epididymitis, subcutaneous nodules, gastrointestinal tract bleeding, active urine sediment, and proteinuria. Anemia, azotemia, normal levels of complement, perinuclear ANCA (antimyeloperoxidase antibodies), and erythrocyte sedimentation rate >100 mm/hour are common. Renal biopsy and not angiography is best to determine diagnosis in patients with abnormal urinalysis. Light microscopy of biopsy sample demonstrates a segmental necrotizing glomerulonephritis with or without crescents. Renal granulomas are rarely seen in Wegener's granulomatosis. Prednisone with a slow taper over 6-12 months is often prescribed for therapy. Dialysis-dependent patients have regained renal function after treatment. Remissions are common but vasculitis may recur. Patients with Wegener's granulomatosis often have positive cytoplasmic ANCA (antiproteinase 3 antibodies) and respond to steroids and cyclophosphamide (Cytoxan) given orally.

- Microscopic polyarteritis nodosa: presentation includes hypertension, weight loss, arthralgias, myalgias, mononeuritis multiplex, epididymitis, subcutaneous nodules, gastrointestinal tract bleeding, active urine sediment, proteinuria.
- Common features: anemia, azotemia, normal levels of complement, perinuclear ANCA, erythrocyte sedimentation rate >100 mm/hour.
- Renal biopsy and not angiography is best for determining diagnosis.

MONOCLONAL GAMMOPATHIES

Amyloidosis (primary, AL; secondary, AA), multiple myeloma, light chain nephropathy, and fibrillary and immunotactoid nephropathy are renal manifestations of monoclonal gammopathies. Renal manifestations include proteinuria (λ light chains: amyloid; κ light chains: light chain nephropathy; λ

Table 16-9.--Types of Vasculitis

Microscopic polyarteritis nodosa--overlap (most common form of vasculitis) (p-ANCA)

Wegener's granulomatosis (c-ANCA)

Classic polyarteritis nodosa

Allergic granulomatosis (Churg-Strauss syndrome)

Hypersensitivity vasculitis

Essential mixed cryoglobulinemia

Rheumatoid arthritis, systemic lupus erythematosus-associated vasculitis

Giant cell arteritis (no renal involvement?)

and κ light chains: myeloma), nephrotic syndrome, hematuria, nephritic syndrome, acute renal failure, and tubulointerstitial disease. Patients may also have renal manifestations of myeloma, including normal- or large-sized kidneys, pseudohyponatremia, low anion gap, hypercalcemia, Fanconi's syndrome (low phosphorus, urate, potassium; glycosuria; aminoaciduria; type II and renal tubular acidosis), and Bence Jones proteinuria.

Renal biopsy: diagnostic stains for amyloid are Congo red, thioflavin T, and methyl violet. Light chain nephropathy demonstrates κ light chain deposition, and the nodular glomerulosclerosis often mimics diabetes mellitus. Immunofluorescence generally demonstrates λ light chains in amyloid and κ light chains in light chain nephropathy. Electron microscopy is helpful in further differentiating the type of light chain fibrils. Renal biopsy findings correlate poorly with the clinical course and renal function in patients with monoclonal gammopathies. Treatment is often supportive, but melphalan and prednisone have had some beneficial effect in selected patients. In secondary causes of this disorder, it is necessary to treat the underlying disorder. Colchicine is helpful in the treatment of familial Mediterranean fever.

CRYOGLOBULINEMIAS

Patients with cryoglobulinemia often present with palpable purpura and are either nephritic or nephrotic (Table 16-10). Acute renal failure can occur if the cryocrit is >1 g/dL. Renal biopsy demonstrates characteristic fibrin thrombi within glomeruli. Prednisone, cytotoxic agents, and plasmapheresis are used with variable results in cryoglobulinemia.

HEMOLYTIC UREMIC SYNDROME AND THROMBOCYTOPENIC PURPURA

Patients present with severe hypertension, proteinuria, active sediment, and renal failure. Both hemolytic uremic syndrome and thrombocytopenic purpura are associated with a microhemangiopathic hemolytic anemia and thrombocytopenia. Endothelial cell injury and subendothelial deposits are present on biopsy, "endotheliosis." The glomerular lesion is also seen in malignant hypertension, scleroderma, and postpartum acute renal failure. Secondary causes include mitomycin C, bleomycin, cyclosporin A, quinine, *E. coli* 0157, and radiation. Children with hemolytic uremia syndrome have a good prognosis (90% recover renal function), but adults have a poor prognosis. Thrombocytopenic purpura includes fever, neurologic signs, and purpura in addition to the above. Therapy is plasma infusion and plasmapheresis with or without antiplatelet therapy and corticosteroids. For scleroderma, the therapy includes treating hypertension with angiotensin converting enzyme inhibitors.

- Presentation: severe hypertension, proteinuria, active sediment, renal failure.
- Associated with: microhemangiopathic hemolytic anemia and thrombocytopenia.
- Glomerular lesion also seen in malignant hypertension, scleroderma, postpartum acute renal failure.
- Therapy: plasma infusion plus plasmapheresis with or without antiplatelet therapy/corticosteroids.

ALPORT'S SYNDROME AND THIN GLOMERULAR BASEMENT MEMBRANE DISEASE--DISEASES WITH GLOMERULAR BASEMENT MEMBRANE ABNORMALITIES

Patients present with hematuria, proteinuria, and nephrosis (end-stage renal disease by age 16-30). High-frequency hearing loss and ocular abnormalities (anterior lenticonus and cataracts) are present. Inheritance is X-linked dominant (males have a worse prognosis). Transplant recipients may develop anti-glomerular basement membrane-mediated renal disease. In Alport's syndrome, the lack of the domain of noncollagenous type IV collagen and the absence of Goodpasture's antigen mean that anti-glomerular basement membrane antibodies cannot be bound.

In thin glomerular basement membrane disease, the glomerular basement membrane is 200-nm thick. Patients present with hematuria.

Table 16-10.--Cryoglobulins and Associated Diseases

Cryoglobulin type	Ig class	Associated disease
I, monoclonal immunoglobulins	M>G>A>BJP	Myeloma, Waldenström's macroglobulinemia
II, mixed cryoglobulins with monoclonal immunoglobulins	M/G>>G/G	Sjögren's syndrome, Waldenström's macroglobulinemia, lymphoma
		Essential cryoglobulinemia
III, mixed polyclonal immunoglobulins	M/G	Infection, systemic lupus erythematosus, vasculitis, neoplasia
		Essential cryoglobulinemia

CLINICAL MANIFESTATIONS OF TUBULOINTERSTITIAL RENAL DISEASE

Acute and chronic acute interstitial disease preferentially involves renal tubules. Some of the patterns of renal tubular injury are 1) tubular proteinuria, <1.5-2 g/day; 2) proximal tubule dysfunction (hypokalemia, hypouricemia, hypophosphatemia, acidosis, glycosuria, aminoaciduria); 3) distal tubule dysfunction (hyperchloremic acidosis, hyperkalemia or hypokalemia, salt wasting); 4) medullary concentration dysfunction, nephrogenic diabetes insipidus with decreased urine concentrating ability; 5) urine sediment (pyuria, leukocyte casts, eosinophiluria, hematuria); and 6) azotemia, renal insufficiency.

- Tubular proteinuria, <1.5-2 g/day.
- Proximal tubule dysfunction and distal tubule dysfunction.
- Medullary concentration dysfunction.

ACUTE INTERSTITIAL NEPHRITIS

Patients with acute tubulointerstitial nephritis present with fever of mean onset of 15 days (90% of patients), pyuria (100%), hematuria (95%), proteinuria (75%), renal insufficiency (60%), eosinophilia (50%), arthralgias (25%), and rash (25%). Diagnosis sometimes requires renal biopsy. Gallium or indium scans can also be helpful.

- Acute tubulointerstitial nephritis: 100% have pyuria; 90%, fever; 60%, renal insufficiency; 50%, eosinophilia; and 25%, arthralgias.

Drug-induced acute tubulointerstitial nephritis can be due to several agents:
1. Antibiotics--penicillin, methicillin (anti-tubular basement membrane antibodies), ampicillin, rifampin, sulfa drugs, ciprofloxacin, pentamidine
2. NSAIDs--tubulointerstitial nephritis with nephrotic syndrome and renal insufficiency may have a latent period, not dose-dependent, recurs, possibly T-cell mediated, allergic signs and symptoms are absent
3. Diuretics--thiazides, furosemide, bumetanide (sulfa derivatives)
4. Cimetidine
5. Allopurinol, phenytoin, phenindione--exfoliative dermatitis, hepatitis, and acute tubulointerstitial nephritis
6. Cyclosporin A--acute renal vasoconstriction

Treatment is to discontinue use of the drug and possibly to prescribe a short course of prednisone (60 mg every other day) for 2-4 weeks.

- Methicillin (anti-tubular basement membrane antibodies).
- NSAIDs: tubulointerstitial nephritis with nephrotic syndrome and renal insufficiency.

- Sulfa derivatives.
- Cimetidine.

Acute interstitial nephritis can be caused by infection (streptococcosis, leptospirosis, Rocky Mountain spotted fever, legionnaires' disease, Epstein-Barr virus, cytomegalovirus), lymphoma, leukemic infiltration, lupus, renal transplant rejection, toxic radiation, and acute pyelonephritis.

ANALGESIC CHRONIC INTERSTITIAL NEPHRITIS

Analgesic nephropathy is a good example of chronic interstitial nephritis and is responsible for 20% of cases of tubulointerstitial nephritis, with 3%-10% of patients entering end-stage renal disease. Patients have a chronic pain problem. Other features: arthritis and muscular aches, female (85% of patients), anemia (85%), headache (80%), history of peptic ulcer (40%), hypertension (40%), urinary tract infection with history of dysuria (25%), history of obstruction (10%), and premature aging. Patients generally do not admit to analgesic abuse. Findings include sterile pyuria, small kidneys (50%), papillary necrosis (30%), and normal excretory urogram (10%).

- Analgesic nephropathy: responsible for 20% of cases of chronic tubulointerstitial nephritis (3%-10% have end-stage renal disease).
- Chronic pain problem, headache (80%), arthritis and muscular aches, female (80%), history of peptic ulcer (40%).
- Patients generally do not admit to analgesic abuse.
- Findings: sterile pyuria, small kidneys (50%), papillary necrosis (30%), and normal excretory urogram (10%).

Phenacetin and its metabolites are concentrated in the renal papillae. Renal hydroperoxidases react with these metabolites and produce reactive intermediates that damage the papilla by lipid peroxidation. Aspirin diminishes local renal blood flow and lowers the concentration of glutathione, which normally inactivates phenacetin metabolites. The result is papillary ischemia and eventually necrosis. Amount necessary to cause analgesic nephropathy: total intake of 3 kg of phenacetin or 1 g/day for 3 years. Aspirin or acetaminophen alone *does not* cause this disorder but NSAIDs may. Patients with a history of analgesic ingestion may even continue ingestion after kidney transplantation. Multicentric transitional cell carcinomas of the collecting system, although rare, are more common in patients with analgesic nephropathy. Evidence suggests that these patients have accelerated arteriosclerosis.

- Phenacetin and its metabolites are concentrated in the renal papillae.

- Amount necessary to cause analgesic nephropathy: total intake of 3 kg of phenacetin or 1 g/day for 3 years.

Papillary necrosis is a common accompaniment of analgesic nephropathy. Other causes of papillary necrosis can be remembered by the mnemonic P-O-S-T C-A-R-D (pyelonephritis, obstruction, sickle cell disease or trait, tuberculosis, chronic alcoholism with cirrhosis, analgesics, renal vein thrombosis, and diabetes mellitus).

OTHER RENAL DISEASES PRESENTING WITH INTERSTITIAL NEPHRITIS

Other renal diseases presenting with interstitial nephritis are glomerular injury (lupus, mixed cryoglobulinemia, hypertension, diabetes mellitus, Sjögren's syndrome, Alport's syndrome, myeloma), Balkan nephropathy (as with analgesic nephropathy, increased incidence of uroepithelial cancers), granulomatous nephropathy (tuberculosis, sarcoidosis), and sickle cell trait/disease.

ELECTROLYTE- AND TOXIN-INDUCED INTERSTITIAL NEPHRITIS

Acute uric acid nephropathy is associated with the tumor lysis syndrome after chemotherapy, myeloproliferative disorders, heat stroke, status epilepticus, and Lesch-Nyhan syndrome. In this disorder, intraluminal crystals cause intrarenal obstruction, and serum uric acid is often >15 mg and 24-hour urinary uric acid is >1,000 mg. The spot urinary uric acid divided by spot urinary creatinine is often >1.0. Prevention requires alkaline diuresis, allopurinol, and, sometimes, hemodialysis. Generally, this disorder is completely reversible. Chronic uric acid nephropathy due to saturnine gout (lead from "moonshine" or paint) or chronic tophaceous gout is due to interstitial crystal formation, microtophi present in the renal parenchyma. It has only limited reversibility. Remember that de novo gout in renal failure is rare; in this setting, it should be assumed that the patient has lead nephropathy until proved otherwise.

- Acute uric acid nephropathy associated with tumor lysis syndrome and myeloproliferative disorders.
- Serum uric acid is >15 mg and 24-hour urinary uric acid is >1,000 mg.
- The urine uric acid-to-urine creatinine ratio is >1.
- Prevention: alkaline diuresis and allopurinol.

Early on, hypercalcemia results in mitochondrial deposits of calcium in the proximal and distal tubules as well as in the collecting duct. Later, tubular degeneration with calcium deposition and obstruction occurs. Calcium inhibits sodium transport, induces nephrogenic diabetes insipidus,

and causes intrarenal vasoconstriction. It also stimulates the release of renin and catecholamines, producing increased blood pressure.

Hypokalemia has been associated with vascularization of the proximal and distal tubules and possibly chronic interstitial fibrosis. Nephrogenic diabetes insipidus is also associated with chronic hypokalemia.

Oxalate deposition from primary hyperoxaluria causes renal and extrarenal oxalate deposition. Extrarenal sites include the eye, heart, bone, joint, and vascular system. Oxalate deposition from secondary causes can be due to ethylene glycol, methoxyflurane, high doses of ascorbic acid, vitamin B_6 deficiency, and enteric hyperoxaluria.

Lithium induces a nephrogenic diabetes insipidus and microcystic changes in the renal tubules. Interstitial fibrosis may be present.

Heavy metals such as cadmium, pigments, glass, plastic, metal alloys, electrical equipment manufacturing, and some cigarettes induce a proximal renal tubular acidosis and tubulointerstitial nephritis. Lead intoxication can cause lead nephropathy, as mentioned above. The organic salt of mercury can induce chronic tubulointerstitial nephritis and membranous nephritis or acute tubulonecrosis.

CYSTIC RENAL DISEASE

Autosomal-dominant polycystic kidney disease is the cause of renal failure in 10% of all patients who reach end-stage renal failure. It is the most common hereditary renal disease. Chromosome abnormalities found thus far include mutations of the short arm of chromosome 16 and mutations of chromosome 4. Patients with polycystic kidney disease have cysts that grow from birth and are present in all nephron segments. By age 25, the cysts are usually seen on ultrasonography or CT. Other cysts can form in the liver (more prevalent in females), spleen, and pancreas. Urinary tract infections are common in polycystic kidney disease and can be localized with CT, gallium or indium scans, or MRI. Lipid-soluble antibiotics tend to penetrate the cysts well. Hematuria may also be seen with hemorrhage into a cyst, a stone, or, sometimes, a malignancy. Uric acid and calcium oxalate stones are common. Other associations with adult autosomal-dominant polycystic kidney include diverticulosis, cardiac valve myxomatous degeneration, and intracranial aneurysms. Also, the hematocrit may be higher than expected because of production of renal erythropoietin.

- Autosomal-dominant polycystic kidney disease: cause of 10% of cases of end-stage renal failure.
- By age 25, cysts usually seen with ultrasonography or CT.
- Other cysts in liver, spleen, and pancreas.
- Other associations: diverticulosis, cardiac valve myxmatous degeneration, intracranial aneurysms, and hypertension.

Medullary sponge kidney is due to dilated collecting ducts, seen on excretory urography, and may be unilateral, bilateral, or involve a single papilla. There is no known pattern of inheritance of this disorder, which is associated with nephrolithiasis and some renotubular abnormalities.

Acquired renal cystic disease can affect up to 50% of long-term dialysis patients and may present with hematuria and an increasing hematocrit. Although these cysts sometimes have neoplastic potential, they rarely metastasize.

UROLITHIASIS

The prevalence of urolithiasis is about 5% in the U.S. (there is an increased incidence of urolithiasis in the southeastern U.S.). The annual incidence is about 0.1%. Of patients with urolithiasis who are untreated, 50%-75% have recurrence within 7 years. Urolithiasis is strongly familial and related to diet and urine volume. Most patients have a metabolic disorder that can be demonstrated with further testing, but conservative treatment with diet and increased fluid intake eliminates the stone-forming tendency in 70% of patients. For those who

fail conservative therapy, medications are curative in another 25% (Fig. 16-6 and 16-7).

- Prevalence of urolithiasis in the U.S., about 5%.
- It is strongly familial and related to diet and urine volume.

Urine pH is important in the pathogenesis of some renal stones. Struvite and calcium phosphate stones tend to form in alkaline urine; uric acid and cystine stones form in acid urine. Some anatomical factors predisposing to urolithiasis include medullary sponge kidney, polycystic kidney disease, and chronic obstruction.

- Struvite and calcium phosphate stones form in alkaline urine.
- Uric acid and cystine stones form in acid urine.

An evaluation of patients with urolithiasis is important to classify the patient's activity. Surgical activity: indicated by hydronephrosis, unrelieved pain, decreasing function (stones <5 mm should pass). Metabolic activity: formation of new

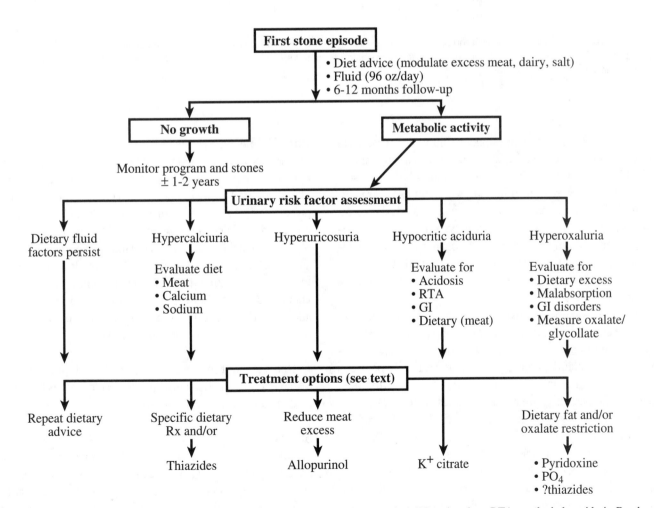

Fig. 16-6. Approach to therapy for idiopathic renal lithiasis. GI, gastrointestinal; K+, potassium; PO₄, phosphate; RTA, renal tubular acidosis; Rx, therapy; ?, possible. (From MKSAP in the Subspecialty of Nephrology and Hypertension. Book 1 Syllabus and Questions, 1994. American College of Physicians. By permission.)

Asymptomatic--no Rx (see text)

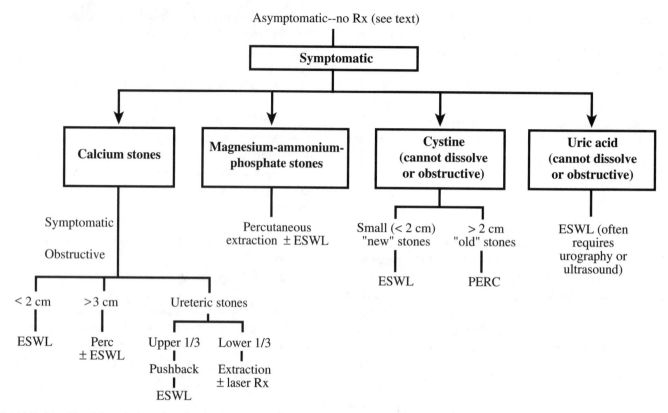

Fig. 16-7. Algorithm for surgical treatment choices for renal stones based on size, location, and type. ESWL, extracorporeal shock-wave lithotripsy; PERC, percutaneous lithotripsy; Rx, therapy. (From MKSAP in the Subspecialty of Nephrology and Hypertension. Book 1 Syllabus and Questions, 1994. American College of Physicians. By permission.)

stone or growth of an existing stone within 1 year. Historical factors include fluid intake, dietary intake, urinary tract infection history, drugs, family history, and other illnesses. Laboratory studies should include reviewing earlier radiographic findings; excretory urography; stone analysis; serum calcium and phosphorus; fasting urinalysis; urine culture; 24-hour urinary volume; and calcium, phosphorus, citrate, creatinine, oxalate, and cystine analysis with usual diet.

Calcium Stones

From 75%-85% of all renal stones contain calcium. Patients may develop calcium oxalate and calcium phosphate stones or, rarely, pure calcium phosphate stones. Causes include idiopathic hypercalciuria, other hypercalciuric states, hypouricosuria, hyperoxaluria, and reduced inhibitor excretion (see below). Conservative treatment includes correcting dietary stresses and increasing urine volume >2.5 L/day. Medications include neutral sodium phosphate for idiopathic calcium urolithiasis (2 g/day, but not in cases of urinary tract infection or renal insufficiency), thiazides for patients with hypercalciuria (sodium must be restricted for urine calcium to decrease 50%), and allopurinol for patients with hyperuricosuria. Patients with primary hyperparathyroidism and urolithiasis generally should have their parathyroid adenomas resected.

Pure Uric Acid Stones

Patients with uric acid urolithiasis often have normal plasma and urinary uric acid. They often have very acidic urine. Of patients with primary gout, 25% form renal stones. Dietary protein excess also can predispose to uric acid stones, as can colectomy and ileostomy because of decreased intestinal ureolysis. Uric acid urolithiasis is treated with preventative measures such as increased intake of fluid and decreased protein intake. Alkalinizing the urine to pH 6.5 not only helps prevent uric acid urolithiasis but dissolves renal stones. Although allopurinol is not as effective as alkalinizing the urine, it can be helpful in patients with hyperuricosuria.

- Renal stones form in 25% of patients with primary gout.
- Colectomy and ileostomy predispose to stones because of decreased intestinal ureolysis.

Struvite Stones

All patients with magnesium ammonium phosphate stones are infected with urease-producing bacteria, which can include *Proteus*, *Staphylococcus*, *Klebsiella*, *Pseudomonas*, and *E. coli*. The urine pH of these patients is alkaline, sometimes >7.8. Also, most of the patients have an underlying stone-forming tendency. Staghorn stones are not uncommon, and

50% are bilateral. Treatment includes antibiotics given preoperatively and then surgical removal of all stone material, followed by an attempt to identify the underlying stone-forming tendency, and treatment of this followed by bactericidal antibiotics for 6-12 months for suppression.

- All patients with magnesium ammonium phosphate stones are infected with urease-producing bacteria.
- Urine pH is very alkaline.
- 50% of staghorn stones are bilateral.
- Treatment: bactericidal antibiotics for 6-12 months for suppression.

Urolithiasis and Bowel Disease

Hyperoxaluria: patients must have an intact colon to absorb free oxalate. Free oxalate is malabsorbed when free fatty acids complex calcium and magnesium (the usual oxalate complexers). Fatty acids and bile acids also increase the colonic permeability to oxalate. Other factors that increase hyperoxaluria and malabsorption include decreased water absorption, decreased bicarbonate absorption, and decreased absorption of magnesium, phosphate, and pyrophosphate (inhibitors). Treatment of this disorder includes correcting the underlying problem, increasing dietary calcium, decreasing dietary oxalate and fat, considering cholestyramine to bind bile acids, and chelating oxalate.

- Absorption of free oxalate requires an intact colon.

Patients with bowel disease may also develop uric acid urolithiasis. Ileostomy patients are frequently susceptible to these stones because of the loss of alkali and water. Treatment includes alkali, fluids, and allopurinol.

Renal Tubular Disorders

Renal tubular disorders associated with urolithiasis include distal renal tubular acidosis type I. These patients can often make pure calcium phosphate stones. They also have nephrocalcinosis, a urine pH that is always >5.3, and a hyperchloremic hypokalemic normal anion gap acidosis with decreased urinary citrate (a stone inhibitor) and high level of urinary calcium. Treatment is to correct the acidosis with alkali and to monitor urinary citrate excretion.

Cystinuria is an autosomal recessive disorder in which homozygotes develop urolithiasis. Cystine crystalluria in routine urine is diagnostic, as are positive findings on the nitroprusside test. These patients have a defect in the renal and intestinal absorption of cystine, ornithine, lysine, and arginine ("COLA"). The stones can be dissolved with urinary alkalinization and high intake of fluid; however, urinary alkalinization must be very intense, with urine pH maintained at about 7. D-Penicillamine is useful in decreasing the solubility of the increased cystine excretion. Remember that D-penicillamine

can be associated with blood dyscrasias, gastrointestinal tract upset, membranous glomerulopathy, and a Goodpasture-like syndrome. Patients with cystinuria often receive pyridoxine (25 mg/day) in addition to the above.

Some medications that increase the tendency for stone formation are listed in Table 16-11.

Enzyme Disorders

Several enzyme disorders can be associated with increased stone formation.

Primary hyperoxaluria is the most aggressive stone disease. Type I, glycolic and oxalic aciduria (glyoxylate carboxylase deficiency); type II, L-glyceric and oxalic aciduria (D-glyceric dehydrogenase deficiency). Treatment includes fluids, pyridoxine (alters glycine metabolism, an oxalate precursor), orthophosphates, and liver transplantation.

Xanthinuria, caused by xanthine oxidase deficiency, is characterized by low serum and urinary levels of uric acid. Xanthine stones are radiolucent. Treatment: fluids, alkalinization of urine, and allopurinol.

2,8-Dihydroxyadenuria is caused by deficient adenine phosphoribosyl transferase. The stones resemble urate stones. Treatment is with allopurinol.

CHRONIC RENAL FAILURE

Chronic renal failure is defined as a decrease in glomerular filtration rate to <25-33 mL/min. End-stage renal failure is generally defined as glomerular filtration rate <8-10 mL/min. Often, patients with chronic renal failure have small kidneys (<10 cm), as seen on KUB with tomograms. The renal size is often preserved in end-stage renal disease in diabetes mellitus, amyloidosis, myeloma, and polycystic kidney disease. Chronic renal insufficiency tends to be progressive because of the persistence of the underlying disorder and possible hyperfiltration by the remaining nephrons. The causes of end-stage renal disease include chronic glomerulonephritis (33%), chronic tubulointerstitial disease (21%), polycystic kidney disease (10%), diabetes mellitus (20%), hypertension (33% blacks, 10% whites), analgesics (5%), familial (5%), and unknown (5%). One should approach chronic renal failure by first exclud-

Table 16-11.--Medications Increasing the Tendency for Stone Formation

Acetazolamide for glaucoma (calcium phosphate stones)
Calcium carbonate (milk alkali)
Allopurinol (xanthine or oxypurinol stones)
Triamterene
Methoxyflurane (oxalate)
Vitamin D, nonthiazide diuretics, steroids (hypercalciuria)
Chemotherapy (increased urate load)

ing any reversible cause such as heart failure, hypertension, infection, hypothyroidism, hypoadrenalism, obstruction, hypercalcemia, medications, and volume loss in salt wasters. After excluding reversible causes, management includes control of blood pressure and early treatment of metabolic acidosis and use of phosphate binders. Late treatment and management include the use of erythropoietin, fluid, sodium, potassium, and protein restrictions; treatment of acidosis; calcium and vitamin D supplements; and use of loop diuretics.

- Chronic renal failure: glomerular filtration rate <25-33 mL/min.
- End-stage renal failure: glomerular filtration rate <8-10 mL/min.
- Small kidneys, <10 cm.
- Kidney size is preserved in diabetes mellitus, amyloidosis, myeloma, and polycystic kidney disease.

UREMIC SIGNS AND SYMPTOMS

Anemia of chronic renal failure is normochromic, normocytic, and multifactorial, i.e., decreased erythropoietin production, hemolysis, and blood loss.

The metabolic acidosis of chronic renal failure is first a normal then a high anion gap due to decreased ammonium secretion, followed by retention of phosphates and sulfates. Always check the anion gap in chronic renal failure; it is rarely >25.

Hypertension is common and is associated with extracellular fluid excess and, in some cases, with excess renin production. Multiple agents are often necessary to control hypertension.

Heart failure is common in chronic renal failure. Thus, use caution with digoxin, long-acting calcium channel blockers, and angiotensin converting enzyme inhibitors.

Pericarditis frequently occurs in two patterns: pattern I is a hemorrhagic pericarditis that often occurs predialysis and for which dialysis is helpful. Pattern II is sometimes hemorrhagic, occasionally with tamponade, and can occur in well-dialyzed patients. Intrapericardial steroids are often necessary. Pattern II may be due to viral pericarditis.

Hyperkalemia occurs in two patterns: pattern I is associated with a glomerular filtration rate of <20 mL/min and oliguria. Pattern II occurs when the glomerular filtration rate is >20 mL/min and often is associated with type IV renal tubular acidosis due to aldosterone deficiency, particularly in diabetics. Other causes of hyperkalemia include NSAIDs, β-blockers, angiotensin converting enzyme inhibitors, and potassium-sparing diuretics. Emergent treatment of hyperkalemia includes the use of calcium infusion to protect the myocardium, followed by bicarbonate and then insulin to redistribute the potassium, then resins and dialysis are used to eliminate potassium.

Bleeding tendency is common in chronic renal failure due to a platelet defect. Thus, use of antiplatelet drugs should be avoided. Treatment with desamino-D-arginine vasopressin is helpful in reversing the bleeding tendency acutely.

Renal osteodystrophy has four components: 1) osteitis fibrosa cystica: hyperparathyroidism, osteoclastic overactivity; 2) osteomalacia due to 1,25-vitamin D deficiency, in which case there is increased osteoid formation within bone; 3) osteoporosis; and 4) growth retardation. Renal disease leads to phosphate retention, which decreases urinary calcium and stimulates parathyroid hormone excretion. Bone is often poorly responsive to parathyroid hormone in chronic renal failure. Also, the 1,25-vitamin D deficiency leads to a vicious cycle of steadily increasing phosphorus and parathyroid hormone. Treatment is to bind phosphorus enterically by giving calcium-containing antacids such as calcium carbonate and calcium acetate to decrease the serum level of phosphorus and to increase calcium. Vitamin D supplements are often necessary. Selected patients who have received aluminum-containing salts for many years become hypercalcemic with low serum levels of parathyroid hormone and 1,25-vitamin D. These patients often have microcytic anemia and frequent fractures and need to have an iliac crest bone biopsy for diagnosis. Aluminum osteodystrophy is treated with deferoxamine chelation.

Endocrine abnormalities in chronic renal failure include low levels of total thyroxine and high levels of growth hormone, luteinizing hormone, and prolactin despite thyroid, adrenal, and pituitary function usually being normal. Hypergastrinemia is present, but peptic ulcer disease is not more common in these patients. Impaired fertility and sexual function and amenorrhea are common. Pregnancy is rare if the creatinine level is >2.0 μg/dL. There is increased resistance to insulin but also decreased insulin degradation associated with an impaired carbohydrate tolerance.

Hyperlipidemia and accelerated atherosclerosis are common. Gastritis, not peptic ulcer disease, is common and usually drug-induced. Constipation is common and aggravated by phosphate binders that contain aluminum. Pseudogout and periarthritis are due to hydroxyapatite deposited in joint spaces.

In peripheral neuropathy of chronic renal failure, sensory fibers are affected more than motor fibers and the lower extremities are involved more than the upper extremities. It is often associated with asterixis and seizures.

DIALYSIS

Indications for dialysis include uremia, pericarditis, neuropathy, hyperkalemia, and intractable metabolic acidosis.

Complications

Hepatitis B--Patients may have mild or no symptoms and may go on to carrier state (also cytomegalovirus, Epstein-Barr virus, hepatitis C, methyldopa, anabolic steroids, azathioprine). Treatment is with vaccine and hepatitis B immune globulin. Hepatitis C is the type of hepatitis that is most common in dialysis patients. Neurologic complications include dialysis disequilibrium (brain edema and osmolar shifts), subdural hematomas, and dialysis dementia (dyspraxia, myoclonus, and gait disturbance due to aluminum overload). Infections: vascular access, peritonitis, tuberculosis (10x the frequency of that in the normal population). Carpal tunnel syndrome and diffuse arthropathy due to β_2 microglobulin amyloid deposition may occur in longer-term dialysis.

Continuous Ambulatory Peritoneal Dialysis

Indications for continuous ambulatory peritoneal dialysis are cardiovascular instability, poor hemodialysis access, and patient preference. Recent abdominal surgery, colostomy, nephrostomy, and adhesions are contraindications. Complications include peritonitis, catheter leak, hyperlipidemia, obesity, hyperglycemia, and protein malnutrition.

Continuous Arteriovenous Hemofiltration or Slow Continuous Ultrafiltration

The indications for these techniques are cardiogenic shock and pulmonary edema, diuretic unresponsive congestive heart failure, and acute renal failure with hemodynamic instability.

Dialysis and Overdoses

Dialysis can be used to treat overdoses of methanol, aspirin, ethylene glycol, lithium, sodium, mannitol, and theophylline. Dialysis is not used for overdoses of tricyclics, benzodiazepines, digoxin, dilantin, and phenothiazines.

Medications in Dialysis

Of the antibiotics, ampicillin and cephalosporins are helpful. **AVOID** using tetracyclines, nitrofurantoin, probenecid, neomycin, bacitracin, methenamine, nalidixic acid, clofibrate, lovastatin, magnesium, oral hypoglycemic agents, and antiplatelet drugs. Be careful when using angiotensin converting enzyme inhibitors, other potassium-sparing agents, metoclopramide, NSAIDs, acyclovir, long-acting calcium channel blockers, and renal-excreted β-blockers.

TRANSPLANTATION

Transplantation is the treatment of choice of eligible patients with end-stage renal disease. Since the time of the first kidney transplantation (performed in 1954), more than 100,000 of these procedures have been performed; 11,000 are performed annually (8,000 cadaveric and 3,000 living related). The main limitation is the limited number of donor kidneys. Lifetime immunosuppression is required. Recipients are from <1 to >50 years old. The recipients must not have cancer; infections (e.g., teeth, sinuses, bladder) have to be eradicated, and cholecystectomy for gallstones has to be performed. Living-related donors must be >18 years old and without systemic or renal disease. Cadaveric donors must be >6 months old and be without infection or malignancy (except for nonmetastasizing brain cancer).

- Transplantation is the treatment of choice for eligible patients with end-stage renal disease.
- Lifetime immunosuppression is required.

Recurrent Allograft Renal Disease

Causes of recurrent allograft renal disease include type II membranoproliferative glomerulonephritis, focal glomerulosclerosis, diabetes mellitus, primary hyperoxaluria, hemolytic-uremic syndrome, and IgA (not clinically significant).

Immunosuppression

Agents for immunosuppression include the following: 1) prednisone, which blocks interleukin-1 production by macrophages and cytokine production (complications include cataracts, psychoses, peptic ulcer disease, infection, diverticulitis, aseptic necrosis); 2) azathioprine, which inhibits proliferation of activated T cells (marrow suppression, cholestasis, infection; never treat with allopurinol); 3) cyclosporine A, which inhibits helper T cell activation and interleukin-2, -3, -4, and -5 production; it is hydrophobic and lipophilic, requiring bile acids for absorption.

Cyclosporine A levels are increased or decreased by the following agents: increased levels with ketoconazole, cimetidine, ranitidine, verapamil, diltiazem, and erythromycin and decreased levels with phenytoin, phenobarbital, ethambutol, sulfamethoxazole, ethanol, and cholestyramine.

Toxicity effects of immunosuppression include gum hyperplasia, hyperkalemia, hypertension, hemolytic-uremic syndrome, and thrombotic thrombocytopenic purpura.

Graft Failure (Chronic Rejection Most Commonly)

Graft failure commonly is due to chronic rejection. Acute tubular necrosis occurs after transplantation in 20%-50% of patients. The stages of rejection are hyperacute (hours), acute (days to years), and chronic (months-years). Treat only acute stages of rejection. Recurrent disease occurs in 1% of cases. Surgical complications include renal artery stenosis, ureteral obstruction-leak, and lymphocele.

Medical complications--Opportunistic infections are the number one cause of death. *Anything is possible.* Cardiovascular problems are the number two cause. Other complications are hyperlipidemia; suicide (9% of patients); cancer (1%, including skin, sarcomas, lymphomas [Epstein-Barr virus-associated], solid tumors); polycythemia; proximal/distal renal tubular acidosis; and kidney stones (1%).

PREGNANCY AND THE KIDNEY

Anatomical changes associated with pregnancy are renal enlargement (1 cm) and dilatation of the calyces, renal pelvis, and ureters. Physiologic changes include 1) a 30%-50% increase in glomerular filtration rate and renal blood flow; 2) mean creatinine level of 0.5 µg/dL and mean urea of 18 (limits: creatinine of 0.8 and urea of 26); 3) intermittent glycosuria independent of plasma glucose (<1 g/day); 4) proteinuria but <300 mg/day (sometimes postural); 5) aminoaciduria <2 g/day (most but not all amino acids); 6) increased uric acid excretion; 7) increased total body water (6-8 L) with osmostat resetting; 8) 50% increases in plasma volume and cardiac output; and 9) increased ureteral peristalsis. Bacterial growth in urine is promoted by the intermittent glycosuria and aminoaciduria. Hormonal effects are 1) increased levels of renin, angiotensin II, aldosterone, cortisol, estrogens, prostaglandins (E_2, I_2), and progesterone; 2) insensitivity to pressor effects of norepinephrine and angiotensin II; and 3) progesterone counteracting the kaliuretic effects of aldosterone.

Urinary Tract Infections

The prevalence of asymptomatic bacteriuria among pregnant women is similar to that among nonpregnant women, except it is higher in those with diabetes mellitus and sickle cell trait. Asymptomatic urinary tract infections progress to pyelonephritis or cystitis in 40% of pregnant women. Screen for asymptomatic bacteriuria monthly, and treat asymptomatic bacteriuria (10-14 days). Symptomatic urinary tract infections relapse and reinfect frequently. Pyelonephritis occurs in 1%-2% of patients. Treat symptomatic urinary tract infection aggressively with antibiotics (ampicillin, cephalosporins) for 6 weeks. Perform follow-up cultures every 2 weeks. Avoid use of sulfa drugs near term and tetracyclines (because of fetal bone and teeth development and maternal liver failure).

Acute Renal Failure in Pregnancy

Conditions predisposing to acute renal failure in pregnancy are sepsis, severe eclampsia, abruptio placenta, intrauterine fetal death, uterine hemorrhage, and nephrotoxins. Cortical necrosis--10%-30% of cases of gestational acute renal failure. Patients become anuric. Although they may have partial recovery, they can have progression to end-stage renal disease years later. Idiopathic postpartum renal failure (retained placenta?) presents at 3-6 weeks post partum. It is characterized by acute oliguria, uremia, severe hypertension, and microhemangiopathic hemolytic anemia. There are disseminated intravascular coagulation and Schwartzman reaction, as in thrombotic thrombocytopenic purpura. Therapy includes dilatation and curettage, support, antiplatelet therapy(?), and plasma infusion. Acute renal failure and acute fatty liver of pregnancy (similar to hepatorenal syndrome) are caused by tetracyclines and possibly disseminated intravascular coagulation. Progressive hepatic failure has a mortality rate of 75%.

Parenchymal Renal Disease in Pregnancy

Lupus erythematosus--Outcome depends on clinical status prepartum. If the disease is quiescent 6 months before birth, 90% of the women have live births. If the disease is active prepartum, 50% have exacerbation and 35% have fetal loss. If the disease is stable prepartum, 30% of the women have reversible exacerbations. Congenital heart block may occur in the newborn. Glucocorticoids and cytotoxic agents have been used without teratogenicity.

Diabetes mellitus--It is associated with increased asymptomatic and symptomatic bacteriuria and increased preeclampsia. Proteinuria and hypertension may worsen, but renal function usually is stable.

Renal transplant recipients--These women should postpone pregnancy for 2 years after transplantation. Increased preeclampsia, infection, and adrenal insufficiency occur. It is usually uncomplicated if the creatinine level is <1.5, blood pressure is normal, and the patient is taking a low dose of immunosuppressive agent. Preeclampsia occurs in 25% of women, prematurity in 7%, and loss of renal function in 7%. Nonobstetrical abdominal pain indicates allograft stone or infection.

Table 16-12.--Causes of Urine Discoloration

Color	Cause
Dark yellow, brown	Bilirubin
Brown-black	Homogentisic acid (ochronosis)
	Melanin (melanoma)
	Metronidazole
	Methyldopa/levodopa
	Phenothiazine
Red	Beets
	Rifampin
	Porphyria
	Hemoglobinuria/myoglobinuria
	Phenazopyridine hydrochloride (Pyridium)
	Urates
Blue-green	Indomethacin
	Amitriptyline
Turbid white	Pyuria
	Chylous fistula
	Crystalluria

EVALUATION OF KIDNEY FUNCTION

Urinalysis

Causes of urine discoloration are listed in Table 16-12.

Urinary sediment: dysmorphic erythrocytes (>80%) indicate upper urinary tract bleeding. Hansel's stain: urine eosinophils.

Osmolality and pH--Urine osmolality is 40-1,200 mOsm/kg and pH is 4-7.5. pH <5.5 excludes renal tubular acidosis type I. pH >7:? infection. Acid urine is indicative of high protein diet, acidosis, and potassium depletion. Alkaline urine is associated with a vegetarian diet, alkalosis (unless potassium depleted), and urease-producing bacteria.

Glucose--Glycosuria in the absence of hyperglycemia suggests proximal tubule dysfunction.

Renal blood flow--Clearance of *p*-aminohippurate is a measure of renal blood flow. Ortho-iodohippurate is used in renal scans.

Glomerular filtration rate--Clearance of inulin, iothalamate, DTPA, and creatinine are measures of glomerular filtration rate. The Cockgroft-Gault Estimate formula for males is

$$GFR = \frac{(140 - \text{age in years}) \times (\text{lean body weight in kg})}{S_{Cr} \times 72}$$

in which GFR is glomerular filtration rate and S_{Cr} is serum level of creatinine. For females, the formula is males x 0.85. Creatinine levels are increased independently of the glomerular filtration rate with ketoacidosis (acetoacetate), cefoxitin, cimetidine, trimethoprim, flucytosine, massive rhabdomyolysis, high meat intake, and probenecid. Urea (BUN) levels are increased independently of glomerular filtration rate with gastrointestinal tract bleeding, tissue trauma, glucocorticoids, and tetracyclines.

Renal Imaging

1. KUB-plain films magnify the kidneys 30%. Normal renal size is 3.5 x height of vertebra L-2 (>11 cm). The left kidney is up to 1.5 cm longer than the right one. An enlarged kidney indicates obstruction, infiltration (amyloid, leukemia, diabetes), acute glomerulonephritis, acute tubulointerstitial nephropathy, renal vein thrombosis, and polycystic kidney disease. Calcifications are associated with stone, tuberculosis, aneurysms, and papillary tip necrosis.

2. Excretory urography provides a detailed definition of the collecting system and can be used to assess renal size and contour and to detect and locate calculi. It is also used to assess qualitative renal function. Poor screen for renovascular hypertension-- rapid sequence excretory urography. Complications: large osmotic load (congestive heart failure), reactions (5%). Premedicate with antihistamines/glucocorticoids, iodine load (hyperthyroidism).

3. Ultrasonography is used to measure renal size (>9 cm) and to screen for obstruction, but the results may be negative early. Ultrasonography can be used to characterize mass lesions (angiomyolipoma, solid versus cystic) and to screen for polycystic kidney disease. Use it to assess for renal vein thrombosis, i.e., presence or absence of blood flow. It is not a screen for renal artery stenosis.

4. Computed tomography shows calcification patterns. It is used to stage neoplasms and as an adjunct to determining the cause of obstruction (no contrast). Computed tomography assesses cysts, abscesses, and hematomas.

5. Magnetic resonance imaging can be used to identify adrenal hemorrhage and to assess a mass in patients sensitive to contrast dyes. MRI angiography is a promising screen for renal artery stenosis.

6. Arteriography and venography are used in cases of arterial stenosis, aneurysm, fistulae, vasculitis, and mass lesions and to assess living-related donor transplants.

7. Gallium/indium scans are used in cases of acute interstitial nephritis, abscess, pyelonephritis, lymphoma, and leukemia.

8. DTPA/hippuran renal scan is used to assess post-transplant kidney, obstruction (pre- and postfurosemide), and infarct (presence or absence of blood flow).

QUESTIONS

Multiple Choice (choose the one best answer)

1. In a 24-year-old woman, acute hypertension and anuria develop 3 weeks after an uncomplicated delivery of twins. Which of the following is the most likely cause of her renal failure?
   a. Acute tubular necrosis
   b. Cortical necrosis
   c. Obstructive uropathy
   d. Acute interstitial nephritis
   e. Eclampsia

2. Acute oliguric renal failure and eosinophilia develop in a 70-year-old man after coronary angiography. Renal biopsy 7 days later demonstrates which of the following?
   a. Acute tubular necrosis
   b. Acute glomerulonephritis
   c. Acute tubulointerstitial nephritis
   d. Glomerulosclerosis
   e. Immune deposits

3. Diabetic ketoacidosis and hyponatremia develop in a 50-year-old woman with a history of diabetes mellitus. The plasma glucose level is 800 mg/dL. The serum sodium value is 129 mEq/L. What is the preferred initial treatment for the hyponatremia?
   a. Hypertonic saline
   b. Normal saline and furosemide
   c. Water restriction
   d. Increased dietary sodium
   e. Insulin

4. A 60-year-old man arrives in the emergency room with a serum sodium level of 110 mEq/L. He recently started taking hydrochlorothiazide. What is the most likely cause of his hyponatremia?
   a. Decreased glomerular filtration rate
   b. Increased sodium loss
   c. Impaired water excretion
   d. Renal failure
   e. Adrenal insufficiency

5. A 20-year-old woman with known hypokalemia, a history of urolithiasis, and a serum bicarbonate value of 15 mEq/L may have a history of which of the following?
   a. Bartter's syndrome
   b. Sjögren's syndrome
   c. Villous adenoma
   d. Diuretic abuse
   e. Multiple myeloma

6. A 65-year-old man with chronic renal failure has a potassium level of 7.8 mEq/L. What is the medication of choice for initial treatment?
   a. Calcium chloride
   b. Sodium bicarbonate
   c. Sodium citrate
   d. Albuterol
   e. Sodium polystyrene sulfonate

7. An 18-year-old man with chronic renal failure presents to the emergency room with a 2-day history of vomiting. The P_{CO_2} is 40 mEq/L, pH 7.4, bicarbonate level 24 mEq/L. What is the most likely acid-base abnormality?
   a. No acid-base problem
   b. Metabolic acidosis
   c. Mixed metabolic acidosis and alkalosis
   d. A triple disorder
   e. Acute respiratory alkalosis

8. A 40-year-old man with diabetes has a creatinine level of 2 mg/dL and hyperkalemia. What is the most likely cause?
   a. Type IV renal tubular acidosis
   b. Type I renal tubular acidosis
   c. Adrenal insufficiency
   d. Renal insufficiency
   e. Excess potassium intake

9. An 18-year-old attempted suicide. The osmolar gap was elevated, but the patient had normal anion gap. What is likely the ingested poison?
   a. Isopropyl alcohol
   b. Methanol
   c. Ethanol
   d. Salicylates
   e. Ethylene glycol

10. Nephrotic syndrome develops in a 30-year-man and he is found to have Hodgkin's disease. Renal biopsy will likely demonstrate which of the following?
    a. Membranous nephropathy
    b. Membranoproliferative glomerulonephritis
    c. IgA nephropathy
    d. Crescenteric nephritis
    e. Minimal change disease

11. A 40-year-old man has nephrotic syndrome without signs or symptoms of a systemic illness. What is the most likely cause of his idiopathic nephrotic syndrome?
    a. Minimal change disease
    b. Membranoproliferative glomerulonephritis
    c. Membranous nephropathy
    d. Amyloid
    e. Focal segmental glomerulosclerosis

12. A 35-year-old woman has a 15-year history of diabetes and known retinopathy with no known renal involvement. What is the best screening for predicting eventual diabetic nephropathy in this patient?
   a. Microalbuminuria determination
   b. 24-Hour urine protein testing
   c. Careful urinalysis
   d. Intravenous pyelography
   e. Fractional excretion of sodium determination

13. A 65-year-old man was admitted to the hospital with a severe exfoliative rash and a creatinine value of 5 mg/dL. What is the most likely cause?
   a. Cimetidine
   b. Allopurinol
   c. Methicillin
   d. Hydrochlorothiazide
   e. Lead intoxication

14. A 40-year-old woman with a history of peptic ulcer disease, back pain, renal colic, and nocturia for many years has a creatinine level of 2 mg/dL. What is the most likely cause?
   a. Vasculitis
   b. Milk-alkali syndrome
   c. Analgesic nephropathy
   d. Lupus
   e. Gout

15. A 20-year-old man with a long history of renal stones was found to have a hexagonal crystal in his urine. What do you recommend?
   a. Allopurinol
   b. Urine alkalinization
   c. Urine acidification
   d. Decreasing dietary oxalate intake
   e. Antibiotic treatment

16. A 42-year-old man is interested in donating a kidney for his brother who has end-stage renal disease due to autosomal dominant polycystic kidney disease. What do you recommend?
   a. No donation because of his family history
   b. No donation because of his age
   c. Donation if kidney ultrasonography is negative
   d. Donation only if his children have no renal cysts
   e. No donation unless he has chromosome studies

17. Hemodialysis can be used in the treatment of an overdose of which of the following?
   a. Tricyclics
   b. Benzodiazepine
   c. Digoxin

   d. Methanol
   e. Phenothiazines

18. End-stage renal dise
   woman being treate
   recommend?
   a. Hemodialysis
   b. Kidney transplantation
   c. Observation
   d. Bilateral nephrectomy
   e. Erythropoietin therapy alone

19. A 40-year-old man with recurrent calcium oxalate urolithiasis has normal serum and urine calcium and oxalate levels. He has failed therapy with high fluid intake. What do you recommend?
   a. Thiazides
   b. D-Penicillamine
   c. Neutral sodium phosphate
   d. Allopurinol
   e. Sodium citrate

20. Which of the following increases the serum creatinine value independent of decreases in the glomerular filtration rate?
   a. Penicillin
   b. Gentamicin
   c. Acetoacetate
   d. Ranitidine
   e. Cefazolin

True/False (indicate whether each answer is true or false)

21. Tumor lysis-induced renal failure is associated with the following.
   a. Hyperphosphatemia
   b. Hyperuricemia
   c. Hemolysis
   d. Improvement with urine acidification
   e. Hypokalemia

22. A 30-year-old woman who is suspected of having psychogenic polydipsia will likely have the following:
   a. Hyponatremia
   b. Polyuria
   c. A decreased ability to concentrate urine after antidiuretic hormone
   d. A high plasma osmolality
   e. Edema

23. A 60-year-old man with chronic obstructive uropathy will likely have the following conditions:
   a. Hyperkalemia
   b. Metabolic acidosis
   c. Hypocalcemia

phosphatemia
e IV renal tubular acidosis

following are associated with hypocomplementemia:
a. Membranoproliferative glomerulonephritis type I
b. Cryoglobulinemia
c. Poststreptococcal glomerulonephritis
d. Polyarteritis nodosa
e. Wegener's granulomatosis

25. Multiple myeloma may be associated with the following:
a. Pseudohyponatremia
b. Fanconi's syndrome
c. Syndrome of inappropriate secretion of antidiuretic hormone
d. A low anion gap
e. Papillary necrosis

26. Diabetes may affect the urinary tract by causing the following:
a. Neurogenic bladder obstruction
b. Papillary necrosis
c. Nephrotic syndrome

d. Type IV renal tubular acidosis
e. Urolithiasis

27. In a 50-year-old man end-stage renal disease develops as a result of IgA nephropathy. The following are true statements concerning his neuropathy.
a. The neuropathy is sensory more than motor
b. Motor involvement is common
c. Asterixis may accompany uremia
d. Lower extremity involvement is more common than upper extremity involvement
e. Seizure precautions should always be taken

28. In a 50-year-old man receiving prednisone and azathioprine immunosuppression for renal transplantation, gout develops and he has normal renal function. You consider beginning therapy with allopurinol. The following statements can be made:
a. This therapy may cause interstitial nephritis
b. The prednisone dose should be increased
c. The allopurinol dose should be decreased
d. The azathioprine dose should be increased
e. Alternatives to allopurinol should be considered

ANSWERS

1. Answer b.
Postpartum acute renal failure associated with anuria 3 weeks after delivery is most likely due to bilateral cortical necrosis. The clinical clue of anuria has a very limited differential diagnosis and is not associated with acute tubular necrosis.

2. Answer c.
Atheroemboli can not only physically occlude intrarenal arteries but also induce an intense acute tubulointerstitial nephritis associated with eosinophilia and eosinophiluria.

3. Answer e.
In the absence of symptoms, hyponatremia associated with severe hyperglycemia is best treated initially with insulin.

4. Answer c.
Thiazide-induced hyponatremia is the result of the impaired capacity of the kidneys to excrete water. Thiazides specifically impair transport in the diluting segment of the distal nephron.

5. Answer b.
Sjögren's syndrome is associated with polyclonal hypergammaglobulinemia and distal renal tubular acidosis. Distal renal tubular acidosis is associated with urolithiasis and hypokalemia.

6. Answer a.
Calcium chloride is the initial treatment of choice in patients with severe hyperkalemia that threatens myocardial contractility. In general, calcium is administered intravenously at least until normalization of the P waves on electrocardiography.

7. Answer c.
To first evaluate an acid-base problem, the clinical history must always be considered. Patients with chronic renal failure are expected to have a metabolic acidosis, and prolonged vomiting induces a metabolic alkalosis. An elevated anion gap invariably would have been present with further testing of this patient. This finding suggests a hidden metabolic acidosis compensated by a hidden metabolic alkalosis.

8. Answer a.
Hyperkalemia is uncommon unless there is a concomitant

abnormality in the renal capacity to excrete potassium. Type IV renal tubular acidosis is associated with an inability to secrete potassium and is common in diabetes.

9. Answer a.

Isopropyl alcohol, methanol, ethanol, and ethylene glycol all are substances that increase the osmolar gap. Only isopropyl alcohol does not increase the anion gap after ingestion.

10. Answer e.

Minimal change disease may be due to an abnormal circulating T-cell lymphokine and has been associated with Hodgkin's disease. Treatment of the Hodgkin's disease results in remission of the nephrotic syndrome due to minimal change disease.

11. Answer c.

Membranous nephropathy remains the single most common cause of idiopathic nephrotic syndrome in adults.

12. Answer a.

The American Diabetes Association recommends that all persons with insulin-dependent diabetes have microalbuminuria determinations annually because they are the best screen for predicting eventual diabetic nephropathy in these patients.

13. Answer b.

Allopurinol may induce an intense, acute tubulointerstitial nephritis that is sometimes associated with a characteristic, severe exfoliative rash.

14. Answer c.

In patients with a significant pain problem, peptic ulcer disease often develops with chronic use of analgesics. Analgesic use decreases the ability of the kidneys to concentrate urine, particulary at night, and sloughed papillae may induce renal colic during passage.

15. Answer b.

The amino acid cystine may be seen as a hexagonal crystal in patients with cystinuria. Urine alkalinization is an important measure to increase the solubility of this amino acid and dissolve the often multiple and fast-growing renal stones.

16. Answer c.

To date, the best screening test for polycystic kidney disease in patients in their mid 20s or older is renal ultrasonography. In the absence of cysts at this age, it is unlikely that the patient will be an affected family member of this autosomally dominant inherited disorder.

17. Answer d.

Hemodialysis is efficient for removing methanol. If it is to

be effective, patients who have ingested methanol must be treated early in their course. The other agents listed are not removed efficiently by hemodialysis.

18. Answer a.

Hemodialysis is useful along with chemotherapy in treating patients with multiple myeloma. Kidney transplantation is relatively contraindicated not only because of recurrent disease but also because of the risk of immunosuppression.

19. Answer c.

Neutral sodium phosphate is an effective inhibitor of crystallization in patients with calcium urolithiasis. Thiazides are reserved for patients with elevated urine calcium level and calcium urolithiasis. Allopurinol is reserved for patients with calcium stones and elevated urine uric acid levels.

20. Answer c.

Acetoacetate can increase the serum creatinine level independent of decreases in the glomerular filtration rate. This often occurs in diabetic ketoacidosis. The other agents have no effect on the serum creatinine value independent of decreases in glomerular filtration rate.

21. a, true; b, true; c, false; d, false; e, false.

Hyperphosphatemia and hyperuricemia are common accompaniments of tumor lysis-induced renal failure. Urine alkalinization improves the course in some patients.

22. a, true; b, true; c, true; d, false; e, false.

In patients with psychogenic polydipsia, polyuria develops as a result of their increased fluid intake. They therefore tend to have excess total body water and have washed out their medullary concentrating gradient. Patients tend to have hyponatremia and therefore a low plasma osmolality. Because they do not have a sodium disorder, edema is not present.

23. a, true; b, true; c, true; d, true; e, true.

Obstructive uropathy is often associated with hyperkalemia because of increased total body sodium and also an inability of the kidney to secrete potassium maximally because of type IV renal tubular acidosis. Hypocalcemia nad hyperphosphatemia are common.

24. a, true; b, true; c, true; d, false; e, false.

Hypocomplementemic nephritis may be associated with lupus, cryoglobulinemia, poststreptococcal glomerulonephritis, and membranoproliferative glomerulonephritis. Polyarteritis nodosa and Wegener's granulomatosis do not depress complement levels.

25. a, true; b, true; c, false; d, true; e, false.

High protein levels may induce pseudohyponatremia in

multiple myeloma. The anion gap is sometimes low because of hypercalcemia, and multiple myeloma is the most common cause of Fanconi's syndrome in adults.

26. a, true; b, true; c, true; d, true; e, false.

Diabetic nephropathy is often associated with nephrotic syndrome and is the most common cause of renal failure in adults. Diabetes also induces type IV renal tubular acidosis, papillary necrosis, and neurogenic bladder obstruction.

27. a, true; b, false; c, true; d, true; e, false.

Uremic neuropathy is characterized by sensory neuropathy that involves the lower extremities. Asterixis accompanies uremia and often points to the need for dialysis.

28. a, true; b, false; c, false; d, false; e, true.

6-Mercaptopurine is the active metabolite of azathioprine. 6-Mercaptopurine depends on xanthine oxidase for its breakdown. The xanthine oxidase inhibitor allopurinol slows the breakdown of 6-mercaptopurine and can induce severe bone marrow suppression. Allopurinol should generally be avoided in patients who need to take azathioprine, but if allopurinol is necessary the azathioprine dose must be drastically decreased.

CHAPTER 17

NEUROLOGY

Frank A. Rubino, M.D.

PART I
GENERAL PRINCIPLES OF THE NEUROLOGICAL EXAMINATION

INTRODUCTION

Neurologic disorders are commonly seen in general clinical practice. In decreasing frequency, disorders that neurologists see are headache, spinal column pain and radiculopathies, cerebrovascular disease, head and spinal cord injury, seizure disorders, dementias, developmental disorders including mental retardation, Parkinson's disease, multiple sclerosis, acquired peripheral neuropathies, genetically determined degenerative disorders, brain tumors, neurologic complications of malignancy, and neurologic complications of HIV infection. Because of the increasing number of older people throughout the world, cerebrovascular disorders, dementias, and Parkinson's disease are assuming increasing importance. Continued spread of HIV infection, development of AIDS in those already infected, and improved methods for achieving longer survival increase the number of HIV-positive patients presenting with encephalopathies, infections, lymphomas, and other neurologic manifestations of AIDS.

- About 10% of patients of primary care physicians in the U.S.A. have nervous system disorders.
- About 25% of inpatients have a nervous system disorder as a primary or secondary problem.
- Primary care physicians should have a good working knowledge of common and emergency neurologic problems.

NEUROLOGIC ASSESSMENT

The best approach to neurologic patients is a thorough history and physical examination. Correlation of clinical examination findings with abnormalities seen on diagnostic testing is important. This is especially important in elderly patients, because most healthy elderly people have spondylitic abnormalities on plain cervical and lumbar radiographs and on magnetic resonance imaging (MRI) and computed tomography (CT) of the same areas, white matter changes on head MRI, mild focal slowing on electroencephalography (EEG), slowing of nerve conduction velocities on electrophysiologic testing, etc.

- Most healthy elderly people have spondylitic abnormalities on plain cervical and lumbar radiographs.

A complete neurologic examination includes description of the items in Table 17-1. Accurately describe the neurologic history and examination in everyday terms. Carefully interpret the signs and symptoms, deciding what is normal and what is abnormal. Signs and symptoms may be bilateral and symmetrical, as in myopathies and certain polyneuropathies. Asymmetrical findings may be a clue to cause (e.g., mononeuropathy multiplex in connective tissue disease). Look for asymmetries on the two sides of the body to detect subtle neurologic abnormalities (e.g., unilateral asterixis in focal cerebral disease versus bilateral asterixis in diffuse systemic encephalopathies).

Next, make as accurate an anatomical diagnosis as possible in terms of the general principles of practical neuroanatomy. In many cases, you should be able to state that the problem is on one side or the other and in the cerebral hemisphere, brain stem, spinal cord, peripheral nerve, muscle, myoneuronal junction, etc. Finally, make an etiologic diagnosis and a fairly uncomplicated differential diagnosis consisting of a few logical choices. If neurologic problems are approached this way, you can make an accurate assessment and plan, including diagnostic procedures, therapeutic options, and patient education.

Neurologic abnormalities occur frequently in healthy, cognitively intact, elderly persons. The following signs alone cannot be considered pathologic:

Table 17-1.--Neurologic Examination

Mental status and state of consciousness evaluation
Gait and station evaluation
Cranial nerve evaluation
Sensory evaluation
Primary sensations
Cortical sensations
Motor evaluation
Strength
Muscle bulk
Muscle tone
Evaluation of reflexes
Muscle stretch reflexes (deep tendon reflexes)
Abnormal reflexes (Babinski's sign, grasping of hand and feet)*
Superficial reflexes (abdominal and cremasteric reflexes)
Evaluation of coordination
Finger-to-nose and heel-to-knee tests
Observation of abnormal movements or tremor

*Note that unusual reflexes such as snouting, sucking, and palmomental reflexes are common in elderly patients and are usually *not* pathologic. However, grasping reflexes and paratonic rigidity (gegenhalten) in *awake* patients are pathologic.

1. Decreased acuity of the special senses--olfaction, audition, and vision
2. Decrease in upward gaze, visual pursuit, and saccadic function
3. Abnormal gait with reduced arm swings, shorter steps, and slow walking speed
4. Difficulty with balance with wider base and unsteady turns
5. Decreased vibratory sensation in the legs
6. Decreased pupillary response to light
7. Atrophy of small muscles of the hand
8. Decreased ankle reflexes

GENERAL PRINCIPLES FROM LEVEL OF CEREBRAL CORTEX THROUGH NEURAXIS TO MUSCLE

Consciousness and Cognition

Consciousness has two dimensions: arousal and cognitive content. Arousal is vegetative function maintained by brain stem/medial diencephalic structures. Cognitive content--learning, memory, self-awareness, and adaptive behavior--depends on the functional integrity of the cerebral cortex and associated subcortical nuclei.

Coma or unconsciousness results from either bilateral dysfunction of the cerebral cortex or dysfunction of the reticular activating system in the upper brain stem (above midpons).

Unconsciousness implies global or total unawareness; coma implies the lack of both wakefulness and awareness.

- Brain death is the absence of cerebral cortex and brain stem function.
- Persistent vegetative state is the absence of cerebral cortex function with normal brain stem function (deafferentated state). This is a state of wakefulness without detectable awareness, even though patients have sleep-wave cycles.
- "Locked-in" syndrome is normal cerebral cortex function with absence of brain stem function (the lesion is usually in the pons, causing quadriplegia and inability to speak, swallow, and move the eyes horizontally--de-efferenated state).
- Acute confusional state is malfunction of the cerebral cortex and reticular activating system.
- Dementia is malfunction of the cerebral cortex but normal function of the brain stem.

Dementia

Dementia is a clinical state characterized by a significant loss of function in multiple cognitive domains, not due to an impaired level of arousal. The presence of dementia does not necessarily imply irreversibility, a progressive course, or any specific disease. Dementia is not a disease but an entity with various causes, which can be categorized as follows:

1. Primary generalized brain disease--Alzheimer's disease, Pick's disease, Huntington's disease, Creutzfeldt-Jakob disease, etc.
2. Focal brain disease that mimics generalized disease--subfrontal meningioma.
3. Systemic disease secondarily affecting the entire brain--hypothyroidism, vitamin B_{12} deficiency.
4. Pseudodementia--not a dementia but a psychologic disorder, such as depression, that mimics dementia.

Reversible causes of dementia are found in a small percentage of patients and include medication-induced encephalopathy, depression, thyroid disease, infections of the central nervous system (CNS), vitamin deficiencies, and structural brain lesions (neoplasms, subdural hematomas, and symptomatic hydrocephalus).

- Dementia is not a disease.

Acute Confusional States

Acute confusional states are abrupt, of recent onset, and often associated with fluctuations in the state of awareness and cognition. They are manifested by confusion, inattention, disorientation, and delirium. Thus, patients may be inattentive, dazed, stuporous, restless, agitated, or excited and may have marked autonomic dysfunction and visual and tactile hallucinations. Abnormal motor manifestations are common, including paratonia, asterixis, tremor, and myoclonus. Usual etiologic factors of acute confusional states are toxic, metabolic, traumatic, infectious, organ failure of any sort, or ictal or postictal encephalopathies. Three large categories of general causes are systemic causes, neurologic causes, and psychophysiologic causes.

- Three large categories of causes of acute confusional states are systemic, neurologic, and psychophysiologic causes.

Stupor and Coma

For one to stay awake, the cerebral hemispheres and reticular activating system must be intact. Patients with dysfunction of only one cerebral hemisphere have focal neurologic deficit but are awake. Most common, important, potentially reversible causes of stupor and coma are toxic, metabolic, and infectious problems affecting both cerebral hemispheres diffusely. Thus, most patients in stupor and coma have an underlying systemic problem. In adults and children, with traumatic brain injury, recovery from unconsciousness is unlikely after 12 months. Recovery is rare after 3 months in adults and children with nontraumatic brain injury.

- Most common reversible causes of stupor and coma are toxic, metabolic, and infectious causes.

Patients with systemic encephalopathies have changes in mental status and awareness before going into stupor and coma, but they have no focal signs. Their corneal reflexes are lost early but pupillary reflexes remain. Also, ocular motility tested by the doll's eye maneuver (oculocephalic reflexes) and the cold caloric response (oculovestibular reflex) are fully intact, at least early in the disease.

- Patients with systemic encephalopathies have no focal signs.
- Their corneal reflexes are lost early but pupillary reflexes remain.

Patients with a large unilateral cerebral lesion may go into stupor and coma if the lesion causes shifting and pressure changes in other parts of the brain, such as the opposite hemisphere or brain stem. These patients have focal neurologic signs. Patients with brain stem lesions affecting the ascending reticular activating system directly are in coma but have focal signs. Finally, people who feign coma have no focal signs, no abnormal reflexes, normal caloric responses, and a normal EEG. They are a small percentage of patients seen in stupor and coma.

- Large unilateral cerebral lesions causing a shift and pressure changes in the other hemisphere or brain stem produce focal neurologic signs together with coma.

- Brain stem lesions causing coma also produce focal signs.
- People feigning coma have no focal signs, no abnormal reflexes, normal caloric response, and normal EEG.

Headache and Facial Pain

Headache

Headache may indicate intracranial or systemic disease, a personality or situational problem, or a combination of these. Some headaches have a readily identified organic cause. Classic migraine and cluster headaches form distinctive, easily recognized clinical entities, but their pathophysiology is not understood. The major challenge is that often neither the location nor the intensity of the pain is a reliable clue to the nature of the problem. Episodic tension headache and migraine can be difficult to distinguish.

- Neither location nor intensity of headache pain is a reliable clue to the nature of the problem.

The vascular theory of migraine and the muscle contraction theory of tension headaches are no longer tenable. Headache pain may be generated centrally and involve serotonergic and adrenergic pain-modulating systems. Neurogenically mediated inflammation may account for some migraine pain (sterile inflammation).

Conditions that alert physicians that a headache may have a serious cause are listed in Table 17-2. Chronic recurrent headaches are rarely, if ever, caused by eye strain, chronic sinusitis, dental problems, food allergies, high blood pressure, or temporal mandibular joint syndrome. Headache without other neurologic signs or symptoms is rarely caused by brain tumor. Serious causes of headache in which neuroimaging findings may be negative and lead to a false sense of security are listed in Table 17-3.

- "Worst or first headache of my life" is serious.
- Headache with abnormal neurologic findings, papilledema, obscuration of vision, or diplopia is serious.
- Most of the signs and symptoms in Table 17-2 can occur with chronic benign headache (tension-migraine headache).
- Headache without other neurologic signs/symptoms is rarely caused by brain tumor.

Trigeminal Neuralgia

Characteristically, trigeminal neuralgia is always on same side and is usually in the second or third division of the trigeminal nerve. The idiopathic variety occurs in middle-aged and elderly patients and is heralded by a sharp, lancinating pain that usually has a trigger point. Chewing often precipitates trigeminal neuralgia pain, whereas swallowing often precipitates glossopharyngeal neuralgia pain.

Table 17-2.--Conditions Indicating That a Headache May Have a Serious Cause

"Worst or first headache of my life"

Headache in person not prone to headache, especially middle-aged and elderly patients

Headache associated with abnormal neurologic findings, papilledema, obscurations of vision, or diplopia

Headaches that change with different positions or increase with exertion, coughing, or sneezing

Changes in headache patterns--character, frequency, severity--in someone who has had chronic recurring headaches previously

Headaches that awaken one from sound sleep

Most of above signs and symptoms may occur in chronic benign headache (e.g., tension migraine)

Table 17-3.--Serious Causes of Headache in Which Neuroimaging Findings May Be Negative

Cranial arteritis

Glaucoma

Trigeminal and glossopharyngeal neuralgia

Lesions around sella turcica

Warning leak of aneurysm

Inflammation, infection, or neoplastic invasion of leptomeninges

Cervical spondylosis

Pseudotumor cerebri

Low intracranial pressure syndromes (cerebrospinal fluid leaks)

The pain in glossopharyngeal neuralgia is similar to that in trigeminal neuralgia, but it is in the throat and neck and often radiates to the ear. Glossopharyngeal neuralgia may cause hypotension and syncope. It is usually idiopathic but has been reported with leptomeningeal metastasis or jugular foramen syndrome (head and neck malignancies). The treatment is the same as for trigeminal neuralgia, i.e., carbamazepine and, occasionally, surgical treatment.

In the elderly, trigeminal neuralgia may be due to an enlarged artery (rarely a vein) compressing the trigeminal nerve. Importantly, in idiopathic trigeminal neuralgia, the results of examining the sensory and motor functions of the trigeminal nerve should be normal when the patient is examined during an asymptomatic period. If there are signs or symptoms except pain, look for other compressive lesions, e.g., neoplasm. Consider the possibility of multiple sclerosis if trigeminal neuralgia is in a young person and the pain is unilateral, bilateral, or switches from side to side.

- Chewing often precipitates pain in trigeminal neuralgia, as does swallowing in glossopharyngeal neuralgia.
- In idiopathic trigeminal neuralgia, there should be no other signs/symptoms when patient is examined in asymptomatic period.
- Consider multiple sclerosis if trigeminal neuralgia is in a young person and pain is unilateral or bilateral or switches sides.
- Glossopharyngeal pain is in the throat and neck and radiates to the ear.

Intracranial Lesions

Leptomeningeal Lesions

Inflammation, infection, or neoplastic invasion of the leptomeninges may present with similar signs and symptoms, as follows:

1. Cerebral--headache, seizures, focal neurologic signs.
2. Cranial nerve--any cranial nerve (CN) can be affected, especially CN III, IV, VI, and VII (the latter is often affected in Lyme disease).
3. Radicular (radiculoneuropathy or radiculomyelopathy)-- neck and back pain as well as radicular pain and spinal cord signs.

- CN VII is often affected in Lyme disease.

Parasagittal Lesions

Because the leg area and cortical control for the urinary bladder are located in the interhemispheric area, parasagittal lesions can cause spastic paraparesis with urinary problems. Meningioma is a common lesion in this area and may also be manifested by seizures and headache.

- Parasagittal lesions may cause paraparesis with urinary problems.
- Meningioma may also be manifested by seizures and headache.

Cortical Lesions

Cortical lesions lead to focal signs. If the lesions are in the dominant hemisphere, they cause language dysfunction, including reading, writing, and speaking. Cortical lesions can also impair higher cortical function, producing apraxias, agnosias, and denial of illness or body parts, and impair cortical sensation. Dense loss of primary sensation (e.g., pinprick and touch) occurs with thalamic lesions.

- Cortical lesions may produce apraxia and agnosia.
- Thalamic lesions cause loss of primary sensation (e.g., touch).

Hydrocephalus

A combination of signs and symptoms--impaired mental status, gait disturbance, urinary problems--suggest hydrocephalus. If it is the obstructive type, signs of increased intracranial pressure may be present, including lethargy, nausea, vomiting, and headache; obscurations of vision are often associated with changes in position.

The following are types of hydrocephalus:

1. Hydrocephalus ex vacuo--due to loss of parenchyma, either gray or white matter, and not associated with the signs listed above (if the hydrocephalus is due to aging, the findings on neurologic examination are normal; if it is due to Alzheimer's disease, then the clinical examination reveals signs of dementia).
2. Normal-pressure hydrocephalus--due to decreased reabsorption of cerebrospinal fluid (CSF).
3. Hydrocephalus due to overproduction of CSF--rare and controversial; supposedly occurs with choroid plexus lesions.
4. Types 1-3 above are called communicating hydrocephalus.
5. Obstructive (noncommunicating) hydrocephalus--due to obstructive lesion anywhere in the ventricular system.

- Hydrocephalus ex vacuo is due to loss of parenchyma and is not necessarily associated with impaired mental status, gait disturbance, and urinary problems.

Brain Stem Lesions

Brain stem lesions can produce crossed syndromes; impairment of ocular motility; medial longitudinal fasciculus (MLF) syndrome (internuclear ophthalmoplegia); rotary, horizontal, and vertical nystagmus (downbeat nystagmus is highly suggestive of a lesion at the cervical-medullary junction); ataxia; dysarthria; diplopia; and dysphagia. Cranial nerve signs are ipsilateral to the lesion, but long-tract signs are usually contralateral (crossed syndrome).

- Downbeat nystagmus is highly suggestive of a lesion at the cervical-medullary junction.
- Cranial nerve signs are ipsilateral to the lesion.
- Long-tract signs are usually contralateral to the lesion.

Cerebellar Lesions

Problems with equilibrium and coordination suggest a cerebellar lesion. Cerebellar hemisphere lesions usually produce ipsilateral ataxia of the arm and leg. Lesions restricted to the anterior superior vermis, as in alcoholism, usually cause ataxia of gait, i.e., wide-based gait and heel-to-shin ataxia with relative sparing of the arms, speech, and ocular motility. Lesions of the flocculonodular lobe cause marked difficulty with equilibrium and walking but not much difficulty with finger-to-nose and heel-to-shin tests if the patient is lying down.

Spinal Cord Lesions

Sensory levels, signs of anterior horn cell involvement (atrophy and fasciculations), and long-tract signs in the posterior columns, corticospinal tract, and spinothalamic tract suggest a spinal cord lesion. Extramedullary cord lesions are usually heralded by radicular pain. Intramedullary cord lesions are usually painless but may have an ill-described nonlocalizable pain and sensory dissociation and sacral sparing. Conus medullaris lesions are often indicated by "saddle anesthesia" and early involvement of the urinary bladder.

- Extramedullary lesions heralded by radicular pain.
- Intramedullary lesions are usually painless.
- Conus medullaris lesions are indicated by saddle anesthesia and early bladder involvement.

Radiculopathy

Nerve root lesions are usually indicated by root pain that is often sharp and lancinating, follows a dermatomal pattern, and is increased by increasing intraspinal pressure (e.g., sneezing and coughing) or by stretching of the nerve root. Pain often follows a myotomal (e.g., C-5, 6 root pain in the deltoid and biceps muscles) rather than a dermatomal pattern, with paresthesias in the dermatomal pattern. Findings are in the root distribution and include weakness, sensory impairment, and decreased muscle stretch reflexes. Radiculopathies have many causes, including compressive lesions (osteophytes, ruptured disks, and neoplasms) and noncompressive ones (postinfectious and inflammatory radiculopathies and metabolic radiculopathies, as in diabetes).

- Nerve root lesions are indicated by sharp, lancinating root pain with a dermatomal pattern.
- Pain is increased by sneezing and coughing.
- Pain often has a myotomal rather than a dermatomal pattern.
- Findings are weakness, sensory impairment, and decreased muscle stretch reflexes.
- Radiculopathies have many causes.

Neuropathy

Peripheral neuropathies are usually indicated by distal weakness and distal sensory changes, usually symmetrical, more often in the legs than in the arms, and often accompanied by loss of or impaired distal muscle stretch reflexes. Neuropathy has many causes (Table 17-4), and an extensive search usually uncovers the cause in 70%-80% of cases. A high percentage of the cases of "idiopathic neuropathy" referred to specialty centers are in fact hereditary neuropathies.

Table 17-4.--Diseases Most Commonly Affecting Peripheral Nerves

---

Diabetes
Alcohol
Nutritional
Guillain-Barré syndrome
Trauma
Hereditary
Environmental toxins and drugs
Rheumatic (collagen vascular)
Amyloid
Paraneoplastic syndrome
Infectious disease
Systemic diseases
Tumors

- Peripheral neuropathy: distal weakness and sensory changes more in the legs than in the arms, usually symmetrical, and absent or impaired distal muscle stretch reflexes.
- Cause of peripheral neuropathy is usually found in 70%-80% of cases.

The pattern of the neuropathy might suggest its cause. Mononeuropathy (impairment of a single nerve) is usually due to compression, as in compressive ulnar neuropathy at the elbow, compressive median neuropathy in the carpal tunnel, and compression of the peroneal nerve as it winds around the fibula. Mononeuropathy multiplex (asymmetrical involvement of several nerves) suggests such causes as trauma or compression, diabetes, vasculitis with or without connective tissue disease, leprosy, Lyme disease, sarcoidosis, tumor infiltration, or hereditary liability to pressure palsies. Neuropathy with autonomic dysfunction (e.g., orthostatic hypertension, urinary bladder and bowel dysfunction, and impotency) suggests amyloidosis, diabetes, Guillain-Barré syndrome, porphyria, or familial neuropathy.

- The pattern of neuropathy suggests its cause.
- Mononeuropathy multiplex: diabetes, vasculitis, leprosy, sarcoidosis, Lyme disease.
- Neuropathy with autonomic dysfunction: amyloidosis, diabetes, Guillain-Barré syndrome, porphyria, familial neuropathy.

Predominantly motor polyneuropathy suggests acute or chronic inflammatory demyelinating polyneuropathy (AIDP or CIDP), hereditary neuropathy, osteosclerotic myeloma, porphyria, lead or organophosphate poisoning, or hypoglycemia. Predominantly sensory polyneuropathy suggests diabetes, cancer, Sjögren's syndrome, dysproteinemias, AIDS, vitamin B_{12} deficiency, cisplatin toxicity, vitamin B_6 excess,

or hereditary neuropathy. Most neuropathies are distal, but occasionally there is predominant proximal weakness, which suggests AIDP, CIDP, porphyria, diabetic proximal motor neuropathy, or idiopathic acute brachial plexopathy.

- Motor polyneuropathy: inflammatory demyelinating polyneuropathy, hereditary neuropathy, osteosclerotic myeloma, porphyria, lead poisoning, organophosphate-toxicity, hypoglycemia.
- Sensory polyneuropathy: diabetes, cancer, Sjögren's syndrome, dysproteinemias, AIDS, vitamin B_{12} deficiency, cisplatin toxicity, vitamin B_6 excess, hereditary neuropathy.

Diabetes causes CN III neuropathy, usually including sudden diplopia, eye pain, impairment of the muscles supplied by CN III, and relative sparing of the pupil. With compressive CN III lesions, the pupil usually is involved early. Painful diabetic neuropathies include CN III neuropathy, acute thoracoabdominal neuropathy (truncal), acute distal sensory neuropathy, acute lumbar radiculoplexopathy, and chronic distal small fiber neuropathy.

- Diabetes causes CN III neuropathy.
- Pupil involved early in compression of CN III.

Acute pandysautonomia is a heterogenous, monophasic, usually self-limiting disease involving both the sympathetic and parasympathetic nervous systems. It may produce orthostatic hypotension, anhidrosis, diarrhea, constipation, urinary bladder atony, and impotence. The syndrome usually evolves over a few days to a few months, with recovery usually being prolonged and partial. This may be an immunologic disorder, but it is indistinguishable from paraneoplastic autonomic neuropathy.

Myoneural Junction Lesions

Lesions of the myoneural junction are often missed clinically. Drugs may cause problems at myoneural junctions, e.g., penicillamine can cause a syndrome that looks like myasthenia gravis. Three major clinical syndromes of the myoneural junction are the following:

1. Botulism. This should be suspected when more than one person has a syndrome that looks like myasthenia gravis or when one person has abdominal and gastrointestinal symptoms preceding a syndrome that looks like myasthenia gravis.
2. Myasthenia gravis. This is usually seen in young women and older men and is often heralded by such cranial nerve findings as diplopia, dysarthria, dysphagia, dyspnea, and also fatigability. However, muscle stretch reflexes, sensation, mentation, and sphincter function are normal. Because of remissions and exacerbations in this disease, patients often are considered "hysterical."

3. Myasthenic syndrome, or the Lambert-Eaton syndrome. There is often proximal weakness in the legs and decreased or absent muscle stretch reflexes (sometimes, reflexes are elicited after brief exercise). This syndrome is usually seen in middle-aged men, who often have such vague complaints as diplopia, impotency, urinary dysfunction, paresthesias, mouth dryness, and other autonomic dysfunctions (orthostatic hypotension). Lambert-Eaton syndrome is often associated with lung small cell carcinoma.

- Myoneural junction lesions are often missed clinically.
- Drugs (penicillamine) cause problems at the myoneural junction.
- Botulism: suspect it if more than one person has a syndrome that looks like myasthenia.
- Myasthenia gravis usually occurs in young women and older men.
- Onset of myasthenia gravis: diplopia, dysarthria, dysphagia, dyspnea, fatigability.
- Patients with myasthenia gravis are often considered hysterical.
- In myasthenic syndrome, there is proximal weakness of the legs and decreased/absent muscle stretch reflexes.
- Myasthenic syndrome occurs in middle-age men, who have vague complaints of diplopia, impotency, urinary dysfunction, and dry mouth.
- Myasthenic syndrome is often associated with small cell carcinoma.

Muscle Disease

Muscle disease is usually indicated by symmetrical proximal weakness (legs more than arms) and weakness of neck flexors and occasionally of smooth muscle and cardiac muscle. Other neurologic findings are normal.

Muscle stretch reflexes are usually normal early in muscle disease.

Muscle disease may be acquired disease or progressive hereditary disease. "Myopathy" is a general term for muscle disease. If the disease is progressive and familial, it is called "dystrophy."

Two exceptions to proximal weakness in myopathy are:

1. Unusual distal myopathy, called "distal myopathy," occurs mainly in Scandinavian countries.
2. Myotonic dystrophy is more common and seen everywhere. Atrophy and weakness begin distally and in the face and especially in the sternocleidomastoid muscles. An interesting feature of this dystrophy is myotonia, which is normal contraction of muscle with slow relaxation. Test for myotonia by striking the thenar eminence with a reflex hammer. Test the myotonia by shaking the patient's hand and noting that the patient cannot let go quickly.

In evaluating acquired myopathy such as inflammatory myopathy, look for the underlying cause, but often it is not found in adults. There probably is an increased incidence of occult carcinomas in patients with dermatomyositis. Other important underlying causes of myopathies include collagen vascular disease, endocrinopathies (especially thyroid disease), sarcoidosis, or remote nonmetastatic effects of cancer.

- In early muscle disease, stretch reflexes are normal.
- Muscle disease is "myopathy."
- If the disease is progressive and familial, it is called "dystrophy."
- Distal myopathy is unusual and mainly in Scandinavia.
- Myotonic dystrophy--atrophy and weakness in the face and sternocleidomastoid muscles.
- Myotonia (normal contraction, slow relaxation) is a feature of myotonic dystrophy.
- With myotonia, patient cannot let go quickly after handshake.
- Acquired myopathy: no underlying cause is found in most adults.
- Increased incidence of occult carcinomas in patients with dermatomyositis.
- Causes of myopathies: collagen vascular disease, endocrinopathy, sarcoidosis, and remote nonmetastatic effects of cancer.

Classification of myopathies is given in Table 17-5.

Acute Muscular Weakness

Physicians may overlook serious underlying diseases in patients whose chief or only complaint is weakness, especially if there are few or no obvious clinical signs. Delayed or missed diagnosis can lead to life-threatening complications such as respiratory failure, irreversible spinal cord dysfunction, and acute renal failure. Respiratory muscles may be affected, although strength in the extremities is relatively

Table 17-5.--Classification of Myopathies

Dystrophies
Nonprogressive or relatively nonprogressive congenital myopathies
Inflammatory myopathies
Infectious--toxoplasmosis, trichinosis
Granulomatous--sarcoidosis
Idiopathic--polymyositis, dermatomyositis
With collagen vascular disease
Metabolic myopathies
Glycogenoses
Endocrine
Periodic paralyses
Toxic--emetine, chloroquine, vincristine
Paroxysmal rhabdomyolysis
Miscellaneous

normal. Patients with early Guillain-Barré syndrome may have distal paresthesias and increased respiratory effort and be the given diagnosis of hysterical hyperventilation.

- Missed diagnosis can lead to life-threatening complications: respiratory failure, irreversible spinal cord function, and acute renal failure.
- Early Guillain-Barré syndrome may be misdiagnosed as hysterical hyperventilation.

Acute muscle weakness can be classified into four groups: disease of the spinal cord, peripheral nerve, myoneural junction, muscle.

Spinal Cord Disease

A compressive or noncompressive spinal cord lesion may cause muscle weakness.

The most common noncompressive lesion is transverse myelitis, usually of unknown cause. Some patients have a history of vaccination or symptoms suggestive of viral disease, usually preceding the neurologic symptoms by a few days to 1-2 weeks.

Compressive myelopathy is commonly due to metastatic epidural neoplasm. Most patients present with local vertebral column pain at the level of the spinal cord lesion. This symptom is present for weeks to months before the gross neurologic deficits, although bony pain occasionally may antedate other symptoms by only a few hours.

- Weakness is due to a compressive or noncompressive lesion.
- Transverse myelitis is the most common noncompressive lesion.

Peripheral Nerve Disease

1. Guillain-Barré syndrome. About 50% of patients typically have mild respiratory or gastrointestinal tract infection 1-3 weeks before neurologic symptoms. In the others, the syndrome may be preceded by surgery, viral exanthems, or vaccinations. Also, the syndrome may develop in patients with autoimmune disease or lymphoreticular malignancies. This syndrome has no particular seasonal, age, or sex predilection.
2. Acute intermittent porphyria. Patients are prone to have severe, rapidly progressive, symmetrical polyneuropathy with or without psychosis, delirium, confusion, and convulsions. In most patients, weakness is most pronounced in the proximal muscles.
3. Tick paralysis. This is a rapid, progressive ascending motor weakness caused by neurotoxin injected by the female wood tick. It occurs endemically in the southeastern and northwestern U.S.A. After an asymptomatic period (about 1 week), symptoms develop, usually with leg weakness.
4. Diabetic neuropathy. Acute or subacute muscle weak-

ness can occur in various forms of diabetic neuropathy. Weakness, atrophy, and pain affect the pelvic girdle and thigh muscles (asymmetrical or unilateral--diabetic amyotrophy). In the second form, elderly diabetics have bilateral proximal and pelvic girdle weakness, wasting, weight loss, and autonomic dysfunction.

- In Guillain-Barré syndrome, 50% of patients have mild respiratory or gastrointestinal tract infection 1-3 weeks before neurologic symptoms.
- Surgery, viral exanthems, or vaccinations may precede Guillain-Barré syndrome.
- Guillain-Barré syndrome may develop in autoimmune disease or lymphoreticular malignancy.
- No predilection for season, age, sex in Guillain-Barré syndrome.
- In acute intermittent porphyria, severe, rapidly progressive, symmetrical polyneuropathy with pronounced proximal muscle weakness develops.
- Tick paralysis, endemic in southeast and northwest U.S.A., is caused by female wood tick neurotoxin.
- After neurotoxin injected, the patient is asymptomatic for about 1 week.
- In diabetic neuropathy: weakness, atrophy, and pain of pelvic girdle and thigh muscles.
- In elderly diabetics: bilateral proximal and pelvic girdle weakness, wasting, weight loss, autonomic dysfunction.

Myoneural Junction Disease

1. Botulism. Occurs after ingestion of improperly canned vegetables, fruit, meat, or fish contaminated by exotoxin of *C. botulinum*. Paralysis is caused by toxin-mediated inhibition of acetylcholine release from axon terminals at the myoneural junction.
2. Organophosphate toxicity. This causes the characteristic combination of miosis, excessive bodily secretions, and fasciculations. A key pathophysiologic factor is decreased acetylcholinesterase activity which causes excessive acetylcholine at the myoneural junction. The onset of symptoms varies from 5 minutes to 12 hours after exposure. Treatment is atropine.

- Ingestion of exotoxin of *C. botulinum* causes botulism.
- Acetylcholine release is inhibited at the myoneural junction.
- In organophosphate toxicity, decreased acetylcholinesterase activity causes excessive acetylcholine at the myoneural junction.
- Atropine is the treatment for organophosphate toxicity.

Muscle Disease

1. Polymyalgia rheumatica. It affects elderly patients with aching or pain and stiffness in the neck, upper back, shoulders, upper arms, and hip girdle. Systemic symptoms include

various degrees of fever, anorexia, weight loss, apathy, and depression. True muscle weakness is not present except when attributed to pain. This syndrome is sometimes associated with cranial arteritis.
2. Acute alcoholic myopathy. There is acute pain, swelling, tenderness, and weakness of mainly proximal muscles. Gross myoglobinuria may cause renal failure.
3. Electrolyte imbalance. Severe hypokalemia (<2.5 mEq/L) or hyperkalemia (>7 mEq/L) produces muscle weakness, as do hyper- and hypocalcemia and hypophosphatemia. Familial periodic paralysis of hypo-, hyper-, or normokalemic type-episodes of acute paralysis last 2-24 hours and can be precipitated by a large carbohydrate meal or strenuous exercise; cranial or respiratory muscle paralysis is rare.
4. Endocrine diseases: hyper- and hypothyroidism, hyper- and hypoadrenalism, acromegaly, and primary and secondary hyperparathyroidism cause muscle weakness.

Causes of acute muscle weakness are summarized in Table 17-6.

● Polymyalgia rheumatica: elderly patient with aching/pain and stiffness of the neck, upper back, shoulders, upper arms, and hip girdle.
● No true muscle weakness, but fever, anorexia, weight loss.
● Gross myoglobinuria often occurs in acute alcoholic myopathy.

GENERAL PRINCIPLES FOR INTERPRETING NEUROLOGIC SYMPTOMS

Neurologic symptoms can be subdivided into four general categories.
1. Ill-defined, nonspecific, nonanatomical, and nonphysiologic regional or generalized symptoms.
2. Diffuse cerebral symptoms.
3. Positive focal symptoms (hyperactivity).
4. Negative focal symptoms (loss of function).

Ill-Defined Symptoms

These include such things as ill-defined dizziness, diffuse or unusual regional pain, diffuse and unusual numbness, vague memory problems, and unusual gait. Generally, no serious underlying problem is found, especially if the symptoms are long-standing. Many cases have serious underlying psychopathology, but the patient often either does not recognize this fact or denies it. However, be careful in making a psychiatric diagnosis, which should be made on the basis of positive psychologic factors and not only because physical examination findings and laboratory studies are normal.

● With ill-defined symptoms, no serious underlying problem is found in most patients.

Table 17-6.--Important Causes of A

Spinal cord disease
　Transverse myelitis
　Epidural abscess
　Extradural tumor
　Epidural hematoma
　Herniated intervertebral disk
　Spinal cord tumor
Peripheral nerve disease
　Guillain-Barré syndrome
　Acute intermittent porphyria
　Arsenic poisoning
　Toxic neuropathies
　Tick paralysis
Myoneural junction disease
　Myasthenia gravis
　Botulism
　Organophosphate poisoning
Muscle disease
　Polymyositis
　Rhabdomyolysis-myoglobinuria
　Acute alcoholic myopathy
　Electrolyte imbalances
　Endocrine disease

From Karkal SS: Rapid accurate appraisal of acute muscular weakness. Updates Neurology 1991; pp 31-39. By permission of American Health Consultants.

● Many of the patients have underlying psychopathology.
● Make psychiatric diagnosis based on positive psychologic factors, not because of normal physical examination or laboratory findings.

Diffuse Cerebral Symptoms

Diffuse cognitive problems occur in dementia and acute confusional states. However, a common diffuse symptom is syncope or presyncope, which usually implies diffuse and *not* focal cerebral ischemia. Vasovagal syncope is the major culprit, especially in the young. Syncope is *not* a transient ischemic attack (TIA). Most causes of syncope are systemic, *not* neurologic, problems. In primary autonomic dysfunction, other neurologic signs and symptoms usually help make the diagnosis (e.g., Shy-Drager syndrome, diabetic and amyloid autonomic neuropathy).

● Diffuse cerebral symptoms imply diffuse, not focal, cerebral ischemia.
● Syncope is not a TIA.
● Systemic, not neurologic, problems usually cause syncope.

Positive Phenomena

An example of a positive sensory phenomenon is marching paresthesia and of a positive motor phenomonic or clonic movement. Lights, flashes, sparkles, and ...ed images are examples of positive visual phenomena. ... example of a positive language phenomenon is unusual vocalization. Positive central phenomena usually indicate seizures or migraine accompaniments. Positive peripheral phenomena occur with nerve damage and repair.

Negative Phenomena

They usually indicate damage to a specific central or peripheral area. TIAs and strokes usually produce negative phenomena; if there is more than one symptom, all the symptoms tend to appear at the same time. Migraine syndromes may have positive and negative phenomena; if there is more than one symptom, the symptoms tend to come on one after another and "build up."

- TIAs and strokes produce negative phenomena.
- Migraine syndromes have positive and negative phenomena.

GENERAL PRINCIPLES OF NEUROLOGIC DIAGNOSTIC TESTING

CT and MRI Imaging

CT is a good initial test in evaluating suspected TIA or stroke and is superior to MRI in identifying acute hemorrhage in brain parenchyma or the subarachnoid space. Subacute and chronic intracerebral hemorrhages are better defined by MRI, which is usually the first neuroimaging test to reveal abnormalities during the evolution of an ischemic cerebral infarct. CT (even with contrast enhancement) often gives equivocal or negative results in the first 24-48 hours after an ischemic cerebral infarct. In subacute and chronic stages of an ischemic cerebral infarct, MRI and CT give equivalent information.

- For acute hemorrhage in the brain and subarachnoid space, CT is better than MRI.
- During an evolving ischemic cerebral infarct, MRI is best.
- CT scan with contrast is not useful in the first 24-48 hours after ischemic cerebral infarct.
- For subacute and chronic stages of ischemic cerebral infarct, CT and MRI are equivalent.

Trauma

MRI is competitive with but not comparable to CT for assessing the brain after craniocerebral trauma. During the first 1-3 days after injury, CT is preferable because the examination time is shorter and hemorrhage at this time is more reliably demonstrated by CT. Standard radiographic examination or CT is necessary to evaluate skull fractures because bone cortex not visualized with MRI.

CT is highly dependable for subdural hematomas, which are also visualized with MRI. Coronal MRI sections are usually best for the size, shape, location, and extent of subdural hematomas.

- For the first 1-3 days after trauma, CT is best because it is more reliable for demonstrating hemorrhage.
- Radiography and CT are needed to evaluate skull fractures.
- CT is very dependable for showing subdural hematomas.

Vasculitic Lesions or Microinfarcts

These lesions, as in such diseases as systemic lupus erythematosus, often seen on MRI but missed on CT.

Intracranial Tumors

A wide spectrum of intracranial tumors is visualized with MRI and CT. MRI often shows more extensive involvement than CT, especially in low-grade gliomas. CT is superior to MRI in detecting meningiomas. MRI is far superior to CT for identifying all types of posterior fossa tumors. It is the study of choice for identifying brain stem gliomas.

- MRI is superior to CT for posterior fossa tumors and brain stem gliomas.

White Matter Lesions

MRI is superior to CT in detecting abnormalities in the white matter. MRI is far superior to CT for identifying multiple sclerosis lesions and for assessing patients with isolated optic neuritis. MRI shows that Binswanger's disease may be a common cause of adult-onset dementia (along with multiinfarct dementia). White matter changes in the elderly must be interpreted carefully because most of them have white matter changes on MRI.

- Most normal elderly people have white matter changes on MRI.

Cervical Cord

A wide spectrum of lesions at the cervical-medullary junction and in the cervical spinal cord can be seen clearly with MRI because of the ability to make direct sagittal and coronal sections. MRI is the study of choice for assessing cervical-medullary and cervical spinal cord regions. Generally, MRI is best for identifying intramedullary and extramedullary lesions of the spinal cord.

- MRI is best for assessing cervical-medullary and cervical spinal cord regions and intra- and extramedullary cord tumors.

Dementia

In assessing dementia, either CT or MRI can be used to demonstrate remedial lesions. MRI shows more lesions than

CT in multi-infarct dementia. MRI has *not* exceeded CT in assessing dementia.

- For dementia, CT and MRI are equivalent.
- In multi-infarct dementia, MRI shows more lesions.

Disk Disease

Protruding disks are seen well on MRI sagittal sections, showing the relationship to the spine and nerve roots. MRI is equal to CT myelography in evaluating herniated disks at cervical and thoracic levels, but at the lumbar level, MRI is better than/equal to CT. In spinal stenosis, MRI and CT are roughly equal and less invasive than myelography.

CT myelography has greatest diagnostic accuracy for cervical radiculopathy due to hypertrophic degenerative changes. Bony spicules impinging on nerve roots are not directly shown by MRI, which may replace myelography for cervical and lumbar disease. Often, CT myelography is needed in defining surgical problems.

- MRI sagittal sections show protruding disks.
- For cervical and thoracic herniated disks, MRI is the same as CT myelography.
- CT myelography is best for cervical radiculopathy due to hypertrophic degenerative changes.
- CT myelography is often needed for defining surgical problems.

Additional Comments

Magnetic resonance angiography (MRA) is not invasive but not yet ready to replace regular angiography.

MRI is best for evaluating seizure disorders.

Cerebral angiography is still the reference standard for evaluating the cerebral vasculature for ischemic cerebrovascular disease and hemorrhagic cerebrovascular disease (aneurysm, vascular malformation).

ELECTROMYOGRAPHIC (EMG) NERVE CONDUCTION VELOCITY STUDIES

EMG studies should be performed by experts familiar with the intricacies of the procedure and who know its value and limitations. EMG tests are excellent for eliciting motor unit problems and, thus, are valuable in diseases of the anterior horn cell, nerve root, peripheral nerve, myoneural junction, and muscle. These tests are an extension of the neurologic examination, helping to localize and better define further diagnostic studies.

- EMG should be performed by experts.
- EMG is valuable for motor unit problems--anterior horn cell, nerve root, myoneural junction, and muscle.

ELECTROENCEPHALOGRAPHY (EEG)

The main use of EEG is study of seizure disorders, but EEG is specific in only a few forms of epilepsy, such as petit mal epilepsy. Seizure disorder is a clinical diagnosis and *not* an EEG diagnosis, and a normal EEG does *not* rule out a seizure disorder. EEG has many nonspecific patterns that should not be over-interpreted.

Ambulatory EEG is available for detecting frequent unusual spells. Telemetered EEG with videomonitoring is good for defining epileptic surgical candidates, nonepileptic spells (pseudoseizures), and unusual seizures. EEG is imperative in diagnosing nonconvulsive status epilepticus.

- EEG specific in only a few forms of epilepsy.
- Seizure disorder is a clinical, not an EEG, diagnosis.
- Normal EEG does not rule out seizure disorder.
- Telemetered EEG is good for defining epileptic surgical candidates, nonepileptic spells, unusual seizures.

EEG is valuable for evaluating various encephalopathies. Many drugs cause an unusual fast pattern, and most metabolic encephalopathies cause a diffuse slow or triphasic pattern. Diffuse slow patterns also are seen in diffuse cerebral disease (Alzheimer's disease). Unusual high-amplitude slow and spike activity helps define Creutzfeldt-Jakob disease and subacute sclerosing panencephalitis. EEG is often valuable in infectious encephalopathies (herpes simplex encephalitis).

EEG is essential for diagnosing various sleep disorders and is an *adjuvant* tool in diagnosing brain death. Remember, brain death is a clinical diagnosis. EEG is a monitoring device in surgery (during carotid endarterectomy).

At 6 hours or more after a hypoxic insult, the EEG indicates the likelihood of neurologic recovery. Poor outcome is seen with "alpha" coma, burst suppression, periodic patterns, and electrocerebral silence.

- EEG is valuable in infectious encephalopathies (herpes simplex encephalitis).
- EEG is an adjuvant tool in diagnosing brain death.
- Brain death is a clinical diagnosis.

EVOKED POTENTIALS

Evoked potentials indicate the intactness of various pathways: visual evoked potentials, somatosensory evoked potentials, brain stem auditory evoked potentials, and motor evoked potentials. Generally, these tests are not a practical clinical tool. They are excellent monitoring devices for spinal surgery and posterior fossa surgery (monitoring cranial nerve function intraoperatively). Also, they may help substantiate nonorganic disease, e.g., hysterical paraplegia or hysterical blindness.

- Evoked potentials help substantiate nonorganic disease (hysterical paraplegia, hysterical blindness).

ANTICONVULSANT BLOOD LEVELS

Anticonvulsant blood levels are readily available and help attain best seizure control. It is extremely important to remember that therapeutic levels represent an average bell-shaped curve and that patients with well-controlled seizures are included under the bell-shaped curve. Many patients with levels below or above the therapeutic levels do well. The anticonvulsant dose should *never* be changed based on blood levels alone. Remember, toxicity is a clinical, *not* a laboratory, phenomenon.

- Therapeutic levels represent an average bell-shaped curve.
- Anticonvulsant dose should never be changed based on blood levels alone.
- Toxicity is a clinical, not a laboratory, phenomenon.

LUMBAR PUNCTURE AND CSF ANALYSIS

Perform lumbar puncture only after a thorough clinical evaluation and serious consideration of the potential value versus the hazards of the procedure.

Indications for Lumbar Puncture

Urgent lumbar puncture is performed for suspected acute meningitis, encephalitis, or subarachnoid hemorrhage (unless preceding CT indicates otherwise) and for fever (even without meningeal signs) in infancy, acute confusional states, and immunocompromised patients. Another indication for lumbar puncture is unexplained dementia.

Multiple sclerosis is also an indication for lumbar puncture. If the cell count is >100, look for another disease (e.g., sarcoid). Although IgG synthesis is increased, this is nonspecific. The demonstration of oligoclonal bands is useful, but they occur in other inflammatory diseases of the CNS. Myelin basic protein is not clinically useful.

Lumbar puncture is used to record CSF pressure. High pressure is seen in pseudotumor cerebri. Low pressure is seen in positional headache and CSF leak.

Lumbar puncture is indicated in infectious disease: AIDS, Lyme disease, and any suspected acute, subacute, or chronic infection (viral, bacterial, fungal). It is also indicated in paraneoplastic syndromes: 1) Hu and Yo antibodies to cerebellar Purkinje cells in paraneoplastic cerebellar degeneration, 2) neuronal antinuclear antibodies in subacute sensory neuronopathy and sensory neuropathy, and 3) retinal antibodies in paraneoplastic retinopathy.

Other indications for lumbar puncture are meningeal carcinomatosis, certain neuropathies (Guillain-Barré syndrome, AIDP, and CIDP), and gliomatosis cerebri.

There is *no* difference in headache frequency after immediate mobilization as compared with 4 hours of bed rest after lumbar puncture; post-spinal headache is dependent on the size of the needle used and the leakage of CSF through a dural rent.

Contraindications for Lumbar Puncture

Suppuration in the skin and deeper tissues overlying the spinal canal and anticoagulation therapy or bleeding diathesis are contraindications. Minimum of 1-2 hours should elapse after lumbar puncture before beginning heparin therapy. If platelet count is <20,000, transfuse platelets before the procedure.

Increased intracranial pressure is a contraindication. Lumbar puncture is dangerous when papilledema is due to an intracranial mass, but it is safe (and has been used therapeutically) in pseudotumor cerebri. In complete spinal block, lumbar puncture may aggravate the signs of spinal cord disease.

- Perform lumbar puncture only after a thorough clinical evaluation.
- Increased IgG synthesis is nonspecific.
- High CSF pressure in pseudotumor cerebri.
- Low CSF pressure in positional headache and CSF leak.
- In paraneoplastic cerebellar degeneration, Hu and Yo antibodies to cerebellar Purkinje cells.
- In paraneoplastic retinopathy, retinal antibodies.
- Lumbar puncture is dangerous when an intracranial mass is present with or without papilledema.
- Lumbar puncture is safe in pseudotumor cerebri.
- Lumbar puncture aggravates the signs of spinal cord disease in complete spinal block.

PART II
SPECIFIC ENTITIES

SEIZURE DISORDERS

- "Seizures" refer to electroclinical events, and "epilepsy" indicates a tendency for recurrent seizures.

Classification of seizures is given in Table 17-7.

The proper treatment of epilepsy includes accurate diagnosis of the seizure type, identification of the cause (if possible), and management of psychosocial problems. The EEG can be important in deciding whether to treat a first unprovoked seizure. There is a high risk of recurrent seizures if the initial EEG shows epileptiform activity, and there is a low risk of recurrent seizures if two EEGs (1 sleep-deprived) are normal.

Causes

Seizures occur at any age, but 70%-90% of all epileptic patients have their first seizure before age 20. Both the cause

Table 17-7.--Classification of Seizures

Partial (focal) seizures
   Simple partial seizures
      Partial simple sensory
      Partial simple motor
      Partial simple special sensory (unusual smells or tastes)
      Speech arrest or unusual vocalizations
   Complex partial seizures
      Consciousness impaired at onset
      Simple partial onset followed by impaired
        consciousness
   Evolving to generalized tonic-clonic convulsions
     (secondary generalized tonic-clonic seizures)
      Simple evolving to generalized tonic-clonic
      Complex evolving to generalized tonic-clonic
        (including those with simple partial onset)
   True auras--are actually simple partial seizures
Generalized seizures--convulsive or nonconvulsive (primary
  generalized seizures--generalized from onset)
   Absence and atypical absence
   Myoclonic
   Clonic
   Tonic
   Tonic-clonic
   Atonic
Unclassified epileptic seizures (includes some neonatal
  seizures)

and the type of epilepsy are related to age at onset. However, the cause may not be found in many patients. Neonatal seizures are often due to congenital defects or prenatal injury, and head trauma is often the cause of focal seizures in young adults. Brain tumors and vascular disease are major known causes of seizures in later life. Seizures often occur during withdrawal from alcohol, barbiturates, and benzodiazepines in young and old adults. Also, seizures occur during the acute use of such drugs as cocaine, usually in young adults. Metabolic derangements (e.g., hypoglycemia, hypocalcemia, hypo- and hypernatremia) can occur at any age, as can infections (e.g., meningitis, encephalitis).

Pseudoseizures (psychogenic, nonepileptic) are sudden changes in behavior or mentation not associated with any physiologic cause or abnormal paroxysmal discharge of electrical activity from the brain. They are often the cause in so-called intractable seizures. Effective treatment remains elusive. A favorable outcome may be associated with an independent lifestyle, the absence of coexisting epilepsy, and a formal psychologic approach to therapy.

- 70%-90% of epileptic patients have their first seizure before age 20.

- The cause and type of epilepsy are related to age at onset.
- Head trauma is the cause of focal seizures in young adults.
- Brain tumors and vascular disease are major causes of seizure in older persons.
- Seizures occur with withdrawal from alcohol, barbiturates, and benzodiazepines.
- Seizures occur during acute use of cocaine (young adults).
- Pseudoseizures are often the basis for so-called intractable seizures.

Status Epilepticus

This is a medical emergency and a life-threatening condition. The seizure is prolonged, lasting >15-30 minutes, or there are repetitive seizures, without recovery in between. Follow the ABCs of cardiopulmonary resuscitation or trauma: airway, breathing, circulation. Draw a blood sample for glucose, electrolytes, BUN, etc. Give 50 mL of 50% dextrose with 100 mg thiamine intravenously. Slow intravenous administration of diazepam or lorazepam can be initiated. (Midazolam can also be useful, and it can be effective given intramuscularly.) You can begin with a loading dose of phenytoin or phenobarbital. If starting with benzodiazepine, then you have to go to a long-acting anticonvulsant, e.g., phenytoin or phenobarbital. Give them intravenously: phenytoin, 18-20 mg/kg (50 mg/minute), phenobarbital, 10-20 mg/kg (100 mg/minute). Consider general anesthesia or barbiturate coma if these fail.

The most common causes of status epilepticus include withdrawal of anticonvulsant agent, alcohol and "recreational" drug toxicity, and CNS infection.

Medications for status epilepticus are outlined in Table 17-8.

- Status epilepticus is life-threatening and a medical emergency.
- The seizure lasts >15-30 minutes or there are repetitive seizures without recovery.
- Give 50 mL of 50% dextrose with 100 mg thiamine intravenously.
- Slow intravenous administration of diazepam or lorazepam.
- You can begin with a loading dose of phenytoin or phenobarbital.

Anticonvulsant Therapy

Monotherapy is the treatment of choice, increasing the dose of the drug as high as necessary and as much as can be tolerated. The coadministration of antiepileptic drugs has *not* been proved to have more antiseizure efficacy than one drug without concurrently increasing toxicity. For a large population, one drug may be shown more efficacious and less toxic, but for a given patient an alternate drug may be more effective or have fewer side effects. With enzyme-inducing antiepileptic drugs (e.g., carbamazepine, phenobarbital, phenytoin, primidone), oral contraceptives may be less effective in preventing pregnancy. Valproate does not cause enzyme

Table 17-8.--Medications for Status Epilepticus

Name	Common dose (route of administration)	Effectiveness	Advantages	Disadvantages
Benzodiazepines				
Diazepam (Valium)	5-20 mg (iv)	5-15 minutes	Rapid acting	Short effective half-life
Lorazepam (Ativan)	2-8 mg (iv)	2-8 hours	Rapid acting; Longer duration of action than diazepam	May depress CNS function for hours
Midazolam (Versed)	1-10 mg (iv, im)	Minutes	Rapid acting; May be given im	Short effective half-life; Not FDA-approved for status epilepticus
Phenytoin (Dilantin)	500-1,000 mg (18 mg/kg) (iv)	24 hours	No CNS or respiratory depression	May be ineffective in status from nonidiopathic causes; Hypotension and arrhythmias at high infusion rates; Takes 20-40 min to administer
Barbiturates				
Phenobarbital (Luminal)	500-1,000 mg (iv, im)	48-120 hours	Long-lasting	Long-lasting depression of CNS function
Thiopental (Pentothal)	250-500 mg (iv)	Minutes		Short effective half-life; Respiratory depression; Respiratory arrest; Hypotension; Myocardial depression
Pentobarbital (Nembutal)	250-500 mg (iv)	Minutes		

CNS, central nervous system; im, intramuscularly; iv, intravenously.

From Slovis CM: ED management of unstable patients with status epilepticus. Updates Neurology 1991; pp 23-30. By permission of America Health Consultants.

induction and may be optimal for women using oral contraceptives.

There are special issues when dealing with epilepsy in pregnancy. Seizure control is best done with monotherapy, using the lowest possible dose of anticonvulsant and monitoring levels. There is a risk of fetal hemorrhage if the mother is taking phenytoin, phenobarbital, or carbamazepine. This risk can be minimized by the administration of vitamin K to the mother prior to delivery and to the fetus at delivery. Phenytoin, carbamazepine, primidone, and phenobarbital can all cause teratogenic abnormalities. In general, multiple drugs at high doses are associated with greater frequency of anomalies. Valproate (and probably carbamazepine) can cause failure of midline structures to close (neural tube defects). Folic acid should also be given to the mother prenatally to prevent neural tube defects.

Anticonvulsants are outlined in Table 17-9.

- The treatment of choice is monotherapy.
- Enzyme-inducing drugs may render oral contraceptives ineffective.
- Valproate may be best for women taking oral contraceptives.
- Phenytoin, carbamazepine, primidone, and phenobarbital can cause developmental abnormalities.
- Valproate may cause neural tube defects.

New Anticonvulsant Drugs

1. Felbamate. Felbamate is thought to increase seizure threshold, to prevent seizure spread, and to be useful in refractory partial seizures (with or without secondary generalization). It interacts with all other anticonvulsants and has the unusual side effects of anorexia and insomnia. However, recently, the incidence of aplastic anemia associated with its use has been higher than expected. The FDA has recommended that the use of felbamate be suspended unless, in the physician's judgment, an abrupt withdrawal would pose a more serious risk to the patient. Patients should be informed that the pharmaceutical company warns against its use except in patients whose epilepsy is so severe that the risk of aplastic anemia is acceptable in light of the benefits conferred with its use.

2. Gabapentin. The mechanism of its action is unknown. Gabapentin is effective against partial and secondary generalized tonic-clonic seizures. It is not protein-bound, has no metabolites in humans, is excreted unchanged in the urine, and does not interact with other medications. Its most troubling side effect is drowsiness. Gabapentin is available for clinical use.

3. Lamotrigine and vigabatrin. Lamotrigine decreases the release of excitatory amino acids and is effective in decreasing the frequency of partial and generalized tonic-clonic seizures. Vigabatrin is an irreversible inhibitor of GABA transaminase that results in increased GABA levels in the brain. It is effective against partial and generalized seizures.

If an epileptic patient under treatment has breakthrough seizures, consider the following: 1) compliance; 2) excessive use of alcohol and other "recreational drugs"; 3) psychologic and physiologic stress (lack of sleep, anxiety, etc.); 4) combination of 1) - 3); 5) systemic disease of any type, organ failure of any type, or systemic infection; 6) new cause of seizures (neoplasm); 7) newly prescribed medication, including other anticonvulsants (polypharmacy) and over-the-counter drugs; 8) toxic levels of anticonvulsants (with definite clinical toxicity); 9) pseudoseizures; 10) progressive CNS lesion not identified previously with neuroimaging or lumbar puncture; 11) no cause found--at this point, you must readjust anticonvulsants or replace one with another.

Surgery for Epilepsy

With improved technology, the site of seizure origin is identified more accurately, and surgical advances have made operative management safer. Of the 150,000 patients in whom epilepsy develops each year, 10%-20% have "medically intractable epilepsy." Brain surgery is an alternative therapy if antiepileptic drugs fail. However, before seizures are deemed intractable, ascertain that the correct drugs have been used in the correct amounts. Anterior temporal lobe operations and other cortical resections involve removal of the epileptic region and are performed for complex partial seizures. Corpus callosotomy (severing connections between right and left sides of the brain) is used for some types of generalized epilepsy.

- If antiepileptic drugs fail, brain surgery is an alternative treatment.
- Anterior temporal lobe operations and other cortical resections remove the epileptic region.
- Resection operations are for complex partial seizures.
- Corpus callosotomy severs the connections between the left and right sides of the brain and is used for generalized epilepsy.

HEADACHE

Cluster Headache

Cluster headache, unlike migraine, predominantly affects men. Onset usually is in the late 20s but may occur at any age. The main feature of cluster headache is its periodicity. On average, the cluster period lasts 2-3 months and typically occurs every 1-2 years. Attacks occur at a frequency of 1-3 times daily and tend to be nocturnal in more than 50% of patients. The average period of remission is about 2 years. Cluster is not associated with an aura. The pain reaches a peak in about 10-15 minutes and lasts 45-60 minutes. It is excruciating, penetrating,

Table 17-9.--Anticonvulsant Medications

Drug	Indication	Maintenance dose (range of dose), mg/kg daily	Half-life, hr	Therapeutic serum levels (range of levels), µg/mL	Minimum no. daily doses
Phenytoin	GTC, P	3-5 (4-8)	18-24	10-20	1
Phenobarbital	GTC, P	2-3 (2-5)	48-120	15-45 (10-40)	1
Primidone	GTC, P	10-25 (5-20)	6-12	5-12 (5-15)	3
Carbamazepine	GTC, P	10-20 (5-25)	12-18	4-8 (4-12)	2
Valproic acid	GTC, A, M	20-60 (10-60)	6-18	40-100 (40-100)	3
Ethosuximide	A	20-35	24-36	40-100	2
Clonazepam	A, M	0.05-0.2	20-40	20-80 (mg/mL)	2

A, absence; GTC, generalized tonic-clonic; M, myoclonic; P, simple or complex partial.

usually nonthrobbing, and maximal behind the eye and in the region of the supraorbital nerve and temples. Attacks of pain are typically unilateral. The autonomic features are both sympathetic paresis and parasympathetic overreaction. They may include 1) ipsilateral lacrimation, injection of the conjunctiva, and nasal stuffiness or rhinorrhea, 2) ptosis and miosis (ptosis may become permanent), periorbital swelling, and bradycardia. The scalp, face, and carotid artery may be tender.

- Cluster headache affects men.
- Onset is in the late 20s.
- Periodicity is the main feature.
- The cluster period lasts 2-3 months.
- Average remission is 2 years.
- Cluster is not associated with an aura.
- Pain peaks in 10-15 minutes and lasts 45-60 minutes.
- Pain is typically unilateral, excruciating, penetrating, non-throbbing, and maximal behind the eye.
- In >50% of patients, the pain is nocturnal.
- Autonomic features are present.
- Tenderness of the scalp, face, and carotid artery.

Abortive Therapy

Abortive therapy includes 1) oxygen inhalation, 5-8 L/min for 10 minutes; 2) ergotamine, especially inhalation or suppositories; 3) dihydroergotamine (DHE); 4) sumatriptan, a 5-HT$_1$ agonist; 5) corticosteroids (e.g., 8 mg dexamethasone); 6) local anesthesia (intranasal 4% lidocaine); and 7) capsaicin in the ipsilateral nostril. Surgical intervention may be indicated under certain circumstances for *chronic* cluster headache but never for episodic headache. Modified trigeminal cisternal injection of glycerol may be effectve in the treatment of chronic cluster headache.

Prophylactic Treatment

Prophylactic treatment is the mainstay of cluster headache treatment. Calcium channel blockers (verapamil) are widely used. The usual dose of lithium is 600-900 mg in divided doses. Its effectiveness is known within 1 week. Methysergide (Sansert) is most effective in the early course of the disease and least effective in later years. Ergotamine at bedtime is particularly beneficial for nocturnal attacks. Corticosteroids are helpful for short-term use, especially in patients resistant to the above drugs or to a combination of the above. The usual dose is 40 mg prednisone tapered over 3 weeks. The most effective treatment for *chronic* cluster headache is the combination of verapamil and lithium. Valproate may also be useful.

- Prophylactic treatment is the mainstay of treatment.
- Calcium channel blockers are widely used.
- Methysergide is effective early in the disease.

- Ergotamine is effective for nocturnal attacks.
- Corticosteroids are helpful short-term.
- The combination of verapamil and lithium is best for chronic cluster headache.

Migraine and Tension Headache

Psychologic and physical therapy and pharmacotherapy are components of a systemic approach to treating headache. Abortive headache medications may range from simple analgesics to anxiolytics, nonsteroidal anti-inflammatory drugs, ergots, and steroids to major tranquilizers and narcotics. Sumatriptan is an effective abortive agent for migraine headache as well as for cluster headache, but it has been associated with chest pain and possible coronary artery vasoconstriction. Prophylactic medication should not be used when the attacks occur no more than 2-3 times per month unless they are incapacitating, associated with focal neurologic signs, or of prolonged duration. When prophylactic medication is indicated, the following should be observed:

1. Begin with a low dose and increase it slowly.
2. Perform an adequate trial of medication (1-2 months).
3. Be sure that the patient is not taking drugs that might interact with the headache agent (vasodilator, estrogens, oral contraceptives).
4. Determine that the female patient is not pregnant and that she is using effective contraception.
5. Attempt to taper and discontinue prophylactic medication after the headaches are well-controlled.
6. Avoid polypharmacy.
7. Establish a strong doctor-patient relationship; emphasize that management of headache is often a team effort, with the patient playing an equal role.
8. The best medication is *no* medication.

Drugs used for prophylaxis include antiserotoninergic agents, β-blockers, calcium channel blockers, and antiprostaglandins. The antiserotoninergic agents are methysergide (Sansert), cyproheptadine (Periactin), and amitriptyline (Elavil). The most widely used β-blocker is propranolol (Inderal); others are atenolol, metoprolol, and timolol. The most useful calcium channel blocker is verapamil. Naproxen (Naprosyn and Anaprox) is the most useful antiprostaglandin medication.

Nonsteroidal anti-inflammatory drugs produce analgesia through alternate pathways that do not appear to induce dependence. They may be useful in 1) migraine, both for acute attacks and prophylaxis; 2) menstrual migraine (especially naproxen); 3) benign exertional migraine and sex-induced headache (especially indomethacin [Indocin]); 4) cluster variants (chronic paroxysmal hemicrania, episodic paroxysmal hemicrania, and hemicrania continua); 5) idiopathic stabbing headache, jabs and jolts, needle-in-the-eye, and ice-pick headaches (indomethacin is often useful); 6) muscle contraction headaches; 7) mixed headaches; and 8) ergotamine-induced headache.

- Begin with a low dose.
- Give an adequate trial, 1-2 months.
- Avoid polypharmacy.
- The best medication is no medication.
- Use nonsteroidal anti-inflammatory drugs for acute attacks and prophylaxis.

Transformation/Withdrawal Syndrome

Chronic daily headache (intractable headache) may occur de novo, probably as a form of tension headache or, more important, it may be part of an evolution from periodic migraine and/or tension headache. Chronic daily headache is often accompanied by sleep disturbances, depression, anxiety, and overuse of analgesics; 90% of the patients with this disorder have a family history of headache. Episodic migraine and other episodic benign headaches can evolve into a daily refractory intense headache. This syndrome is usually due to the overuse (>2 days/week) of ergotamine tartrate, analgesics, especially analgesics combined with barbiturates, and narcotics, and perhaps even benzodiazepines. Discontinuation of the use of these medications is necessary to control the headache. Two points have to be stressed: 1) the overuse of these medications causes daily headache, and 2) the daily use of these medications prevents other useful medications from working effectively.

The treatment of daily refractory headaches usually requires hospitalization and withdrawal of the overused medication, with repetitive intravenous administration of dihydroergotamine, intramuscular sumatriptan.

Nonsteroidal anti-inflammatory drugs, β-blocker drugs, calcium channel blocker drugs, and tricyclic antidepressants do *not* cause transformation/withdrawal syndrome. Also, non-headache patients who take large amounts of analgesics for other conditions, e.g., arthritis, do *not* develop analgesic/rebound headache. Simple withdrawal from analgesics produces significant improvement in patients with chronic daily headache. A nonprescription medication can be withdrawn abruptly. However, prescription medications (ergotamine tartrate, narcotics, barbiturates) have to be withdrawn gradually. When narcotics or compounds containing codeine and ergotamine tartrate are withdrawn, clonidine may be helpful in repressing withdrawal symptoms. Some think even simple analgesics (aspirin, acetaminophen [Tylenol]) used >2 days/week can cause daily headache syndrome.

- Associated with daily headache are sleep disturbances, depression, anxiety, and analgesic overuse.
- 90% of patients with chronic headache have a family history of headache.
- Migraine and other headaches can become a refractory intense headache.
- Overuse of medications causes daily headache and prevents the effective action of other drugs.

- Hospitalization and withdrawal of overused drugs are usually required.
- Nonsteroidal anti-inflammatory drugs, β-blockers, calcium channel blockers, and tricyclic antidepressants do *not* cause transformation/withdrawal syndrome.
- Significant improvement occurs with withdrawal of analgesics.

VERTIGO AND DIZZINESS

Accurate visual, vestibular, proprioceptive, tactile, and auditory perceptions are necessary for normal spatial orientation. These inputs are integrated in the brain stem and cerebral hemispheres. The outputs are the motor systems, extrapyramidal system, and cerebellar system. The impairment of any of these functions or of their input, integration, or output causes a complaint of "dizziness" (a sensation of altered orientation or space). Dizziness, vertigo, and disequilibrium are common complaints. The results of diagnostic tests are often normal. Diagnosis depends mainly on the medical history, with physical examination findings in some cases. Vestibular tests rarely provide an exact diagnosis. The types of dizziness are listed in Table 17-10.

Vertigo

Vertigo is an illusion of movement, usually that of rotation, and the feeling of vertical or horizontal rotation of either the person or the environment. Most patients report this as "spinning" or "rotational" feelings. Others mainly experience a sensation of staggering. In contrast to vertigo, disequilibrium is a feeling of unsteadiness or insecurity about the environment, without a rotatory sensation. Vertigo occurs when there is imbalance, especially acute, between the left and right vestibular systems. The sudden unilateral loss of vestibular function is dramatic; the patient complains of severe vertigo and nausea and vomiting and is pale and diaphoretic. With acute vertigo, the patient also has problems with equilibrium and vision, often described as "blurred vision," or diplopia. Autonomic symptoms are common--sweating, pallor, nausea, vomiting--and can cause vasovagal syncope.

Fluctuating hearing loss and tinnitus are characteristic of Meniere's syndrome. Abrupt complete unilateral deafness and vertigo occur with viral involvement of the labyrinth and/or CN VIII and with vascular occlusion of the inner ear. Patients who slowly lose vestibular function bilaterally, as with ototoxic drugs, often do not complain of vertigo but have oscillopsia with head movements and instability with walking. Even with unilateral vestibular loss, if it is slow (acoustic neuroma), patients usually do not complain of vertigo; they typically present with unilateral hearing loss and tinnitus. Vertigo invariably occurs in episodes. Common vestibular disorders with a genetic predisposition include migraine, Meniere's syndrome, otosclerosis, neurofibromatosis, and spinocerebellar degeneration.

Table 17-10.--Types of Dizziness

Vertigo
    Peripheral
    Central
Presyncopal light-headedness
    Orthostatic hypotension
    Vasovagal attacks
    Impaired cardiac output
    Hyperventilation
Psychophysiologic dizziness
    Acute anxiety
    Agoraphobia (fear and avoidance of being in public
      places)
    Chronic anxiety
Disequilibrium
    Lesions of basal ganglia, frontal lobes, and white matter
    Hydrocephalus
    Cerebellar dysfunction
Ocular dizziness
    High magnification and lens implant
    Imbalance in extraocular muscles
    Oscillopsia
Multisensory dizziness
Physiologic dizziness
    Motion sickness
    Space sickness
    Height vertigo

Benign positional vertigo is the single most common cause of vertigo. No cause is found in about half of the patients. For the other half, the most common causes are post-traumatic and postviral neurolabyrinthitis. Brief episodes of vertigo usually last <30 seconds with positional change, e.g., turning over in bed, getting in or out of bed, bending over and straightening up, and extending the neck to look up.

Typically, bouts of benign positional vertigo are intermixed with variable periods of remission. Periods of vertigo rarely last >1 minute, although after a flurry of episodes, patients may complain of more prolonged nonspecific dizziness lasting hours to days (light-headedness, swimming sensation associated with nausea). Management includes reassurance, positional exercises (vestibular exercises), and the canalith repositioning maneuver. Drugs are not very useful, but meclizine and phenergan may help with the nausea and nonspecific dizziness. Rarely, surgical treatment (section of the ampullary nerve) may be undertaken in intractable cases.

Vertigo of CNS origin is caused by acute cerebellar lesions (hemorrhages or infarcts) or acute brain stem lesions (especially, lateral medullary [Wallenberg's] syndrome). Basilar-vertebral artery disease is also a cause, but vertigo by itself is never a TIA. Other symptoms are necessary to make the diag-nosis of basilar-vertebral insufficiency--dysarthria, dysphagia, diplopia, facial numbness, crossed syndromes, hemiparesis or alternating hemiparesis, ataxia, visual field defects, etc.

Presyncopal Light-Headedness

This is best described as the "sensation of impending faint." It results from pancerebral ischemia. Presyncopal light-headedness is not a symptom of focal occlusive cerebrovascular disease, but it may indicate orthostatic hypotension, usually due to decreased blood volume, chronic use of hypotensive drugs, or autonomic dysfunction. Symptoms of vasovagal attacks are induced when such emotions as fear and anxiety activate medullary vasodepressor centers. Vasodepressor episodes can also be precipitated by acute visceral pain or sudden severe attacks of vertigo. Impaired cardiac output causes presyncopal light-headedness, as does hyperventilation. Chronic anxiety with associated hyperventilation is the common cause of persistent presyncopal light-headedness in young patients. In most subjects, only a moderate increase in respiratory rate can decrease the $PaCO_2$ level to ≤25 mm Hg in a few minutes.

Five types of syncopal attacks especially common in the elderly are:
1. Orthostatic--multiple causes.
2. Autonomic dysfunction due to peripheral (postganglionic) or central (preganglionic) involvement.
3. Reflex--such as carotid sinus syncope or cough or micturition syncope.
4. Vasovagal syncope--occurs less frequently in the elderly than in the young; however, the prognosis is worse in the elderly, with about 16% of them having major morbidity and mortality in the following 6 months compared with <1% of patients <30 years; common precipitating events in the elderly include emotional stress, prolonged bed rest, prolonged standing, and painful stimuli.
5. Cardiac syncope.

- Presyncopal light-headedness is the sensation of impending faint.
- It is not a common symptom of occlusive cerebrovascular disease.
- Vasovagal attacks occur less frequently in the elderly.
- In the young, a common cause of persistent presyncopal light-headedness is chronic anxiety with hyperventilation.
- The prognosis of vagovagal syncope is worse for the elderly; 16% have major morbidity/mortality within 6 months.
- In the elderly, vagovagal syncope is precipitated by emotional stress, bed rest, prolonged standing, and pain.

Psychophysiologic Dizziness

Patients usually describe this as "floating," "swimming," or "giddiness." They also may report a feeling of imbalance, a rocking or falling sensation, or a spinning inside the head. The symptoms are not associated with an illusion of movement or movement of the environment or with nystagmus. Commonly associated symptoms include tension headache, heart palpitations, gastric distress, urinary frequency, backache, and generalized feeling of weakness and fatigue. Psychophysiologic dizziness can also be associated with panic attacks.

Disequilibrium

Patients who slowly lose vestibular function on one side, as with an acoustic neuroma, usually do not have vertigo but often describe a vague feeling of imbalance and unsteadiness on their feet. Disequilibrium may be a presenting symptom of lesions involving motor centers of the basal ganglia and frontal lobe, e.g., Parkinson's disease, hydrocephalus, and multiple lacunar infarction syndrome. The broad-based ataxic gait of cerebellar disorders is readily distinguished from milder gait disorders seen with vestibular or sensory loss or with senile gait.

- Disequilibrium may be a presenting symptom of basal ganglia or frontal lobe lesions.

Multisensory Dizziness

This is commonly seen in the elderly and especially in patients with such systemic disorders as diabetes. A typical combination includes such things as mild peripheral neuropathy causing diminished touch and proprioceptive input, decreased visual acuity, impaired hearing, and decreased baroreceptor function. In such patients, an added vestibular impairment, as from an ototoxic drug, can be devastating.

The resulting sensation of dizziness is usually present only when the patient walks or moves and not present when the patient is supine or seated. There is a feeling of insecurity of gait and motion. The patient is usually helped by walking close to a wall, using a cane, or by holding on to another person. Drugs should *not* be used for this disorder. Instead, the use of a cane or walker is important to improve support and increase somatosensory signals.

- Multisensory dizziness is common in elderly diabetics.
- Added vestibular impairment can be devastating.
- Do not use drugs for this disorder.

NEOPLASTIC DISEASE

The most common neurologic symptoms in patients with systemic cancer are back pain, altered mental status, and headache. However, the most common neurologic complication of systemic cancer is metastatic disease, of which cerebral metastasis is the most common. In patients with back pain, epidural metastasis and direct vertebral metastasis are common, but in about 15%-20% of patients, no malignant cause is found. Nonstructural causes are the most common reasons

for headache. Some identified causes include fever, side effects of therapy, postlumbar puncture headache, metastasis (cerebral, leptomeningeal, base of skull), and intracranial hemorrhage (thrombocytopenia, hemorrhage due to intracranial metastasis). The most common cause of altered mental status is a metabolic encephalopathy, which is also the most common nonmetastatic manifestation of systemic cancer. Less common causes include intracranial metastatic disease (parenchymal and meningeal), intracranial hemorrhage, primary dementia, cerebral infarction, psychiatric disorder, known primary brain tumor, bacterial meningitis, and transient global amnesia.

Cancers that commonly cause neurologic problems are those of the lung and breast, leukemia, lymphoma, and colorectal cancer. Breast, lung, and prostate cancer are commonly associated with bony metastasis and epidural metastasis. The most common brain metastasis is from the lung. Meningeal metastases are common in lung and breast cancers, melanoma, leukemia, and lymphoma. Colorectal cancer causes local pelvic metastasis and is the most frequent cause of tumor plexopathy. Head and neck cancer are the most frequent cause of metastasis to the base of the skull. Proportionally, melanoma causes the most nervous system involvement. Gastrointestinal tract tumors (stomach, esophagus, pancreas) have the least number of neurologic complications.

Many neurologic problems in patients with cancer can be diagnosed on the basis of the medical history and findings on neurologic examination and require knowledge of both nonmetastatic- and noncancer-related neurologic illness. In general, neurologic complications of systemic cancer can be divided into the following categories:

1. Metastatic--parenchymal, leptomeningeal, epidural, subdural, brachial and lumbosacral plexuses, and nerve infiltration. This is *common.*
2. Infectious--unusual CNS infections because of immunosuppression.
3. Complications of systemic metastases--hepatic encephalopathy.
4. Vascular complications--cerebral infarction from hypercoagulable states, nonbacterial thrombotic endocarditis, radiation damage to carotid arteries, etc.; cerebral hemorrhage from such entities as thrombocytopenia and hemorrhagic metastases.
5. Systemic encephalopathies--usually from multiple causes, hypercalcemia, syndrome of inappropriate secretion of antidiuretic hormone, medications, systemic infections, etc.
6. Complications of treatment--radiation, chemotherapy, surgery: radiation necrosis of the brain, radiation myelopathy, radiation plexopathy, fibrosis of the carotid arteries, neuropathies, encephalopathies, cerebellar ataxia.
7. Nonmetastatic "remote" effect--syndromes have been described from the cerebral cortex through the central and peripheral neuraxes to muscle; they are rare.

8. Miscellaneous--various systemic and neurologic illnesses having nothing to do with the cancer.

- Cerebral metastasis is the most common neurologic complication of systemic cancer.
- Metabolic encephalopathy is the most common non-metastatic manifestation of cancer.
- The most common symptom is headache.
- Cancers commonly causing neurologic problems are lung, breast, and colorectal cancers, leukemia, and lymphoma.
- The most common brain metastasis is from lung and breast cancers, melanoma, leukemia, and lymphoma.
- The most frequent cause of tumor plexopathy is colorectal cancer.
- Proportionally, melanoma causes the most nervous system involvement.
- Common metastatic sites are parenchyma of cerebrum and cerebellum, leptomeninges, epidural and subdural spaces, brachial and lumbosacral plexuses, and nerve.
- Syndromes of nonmetastatic remote effects are rare.

Radiosurgery (gamma-knife and the LINAC-based systems) has been used to treat vascular malformations, acoustic neuromas, pituitary adenomas, and meningeal and (recently) metastatic tumors.

Primary CNS lymphoma is becoming common in both AIDS and immune competent patients. Median survival has been increased with combination therapy of radiation and chemotherapy, including hydroxyurea, procarbazine, CCNU, vincristine, cytosine arabinoside, and intrathecal methotrexate.

ABNORMAL ANTIBODIES

1. Anti-islet cell antibodies. They are found in high titer in stiff persons syndrome (anti-GAD antibodies).
2. Anti-calcium channel antibodies. They are positive in 80% of patients with Lambert-Eaton myasthenic syndrome who have primary lung cancer (small cell, squamous cell, adenocarcinoma) and in 36% who are *without* evidence of cancer. They are usually negative in patients with Lambert-Eaton myasthenic syndrome who have cancer other than lung cancer.
3. Purkinje cell antibodies (sometimes called "anti-Yo" antibodies). They are found in women with paraneoplastic cerebellar degeneration and are associated with ovarian, fallopian tube, endometrial, surface papillary and breast carcinoma, and occasionally with lymphoma. They are not found in men with paraneoplastic cerebellar degeneration or in women with gynecologic cancer without a neurologic syndrome. If these antibodies are positive in a woman who is without clinically known or laboratory proven cancer, exploratory laparotomy is probably warranted.
4. Antineuronal nuclear antibodies (ANNA). Type I ("anti-

Hu") is a marker of various neurologic disorders occurring with small cell lung cancer, including sensory and autonomic neuropathies, mixed sensory-motor neuropathies, limbic encephalopathy, cerebellar degeneration, myelopathy, radiculopathy, and motor neuropathy. Type II ("anti-Ri") is seen with a spectrum of neurologic disorders associated with breast cancer, including cerebellar ataxia, myelopathy, opsoclonus, and other brain stem disorders.
5. Acetylcholine receptor antibodies. They are rare in conditions other than myasthenia gravis (they do not occur in patients with congenital myasthenia gravis and in only about 15% of those with purely ocular myasthenia gravis). They sometimes are found in patients with amyotrophic lateral sclerosis (ALS), Lambert-Eaton myasthenic syndrome, and pernicious anemia. Striational antibodies are highly associated with thymoma and sometimes occur in Lambert-Eaton myasthenic syndrome or small cell lung carcinomas. They can occur in D-penicillamine recipients, bone marrow allografts, and autoimmune liver disorders.

- If Purkinje cell antibodies are positive in a woman who is without clinically known or laboratory proven cancer, exploratory laparotomy is probably warranted.
- Acetylcholine receptor antibodies are highly associated with thymoma.

MOVEMENT DISORDERS

Tremor

Tremor is an oscillatory rhythmical disorder. A simple classification of tremor movement disorder is as follows:
1. Rest tremor
2. Postural tremor
3. Kinetic tremor

A rest tremor is noted with the arms lying in the patient's lap while sitting or with the arms at the patient's side while walking. Rest tremor is seen in Parkinson's disease. Postural tremor is noted mainly with the arms outstretched, although there is often a kinetic component as well. Postural tremor is seen in physiologic tremor, but it is also noted pathologically in essential tremor. Kinetic tremor is seen mainly in action, as in finger-to-nose testing. This type of tremor is seen in cerebellar disease and in diseases of the cerebellar connections in the brain stem.

Essential Tremor

Essential tremor is the most common movement disorder. It is often misdiagnosed and inappropriately treated. It is a monosymptomatic condition that is manifested as rhythmic oscillations of various body parts. Middle-aged and older persons are most commonly affected, and there is often a genetic component. The hands are most affected, with the tremor present in postural position and often having a kinetic component. The head and voice are often affected. Head tremor can be either horizontal (no-no) or vertical (yes-yes). It almost never occurs in Parkinson's disease, but parkinsonian patients may have tremor of the mouth, lips, tongue, and jaw. The legs and trunk (orthostatic tremor) are affected less frequently in essential tremor.

Essential tremor is a slowly progressive condition with unknown pathophysiology. It may be due to a "central pacemaker" located in the cerebellum, motor nuclei of the thalamus, or the inferior olivary nucleus.

The agent most effective in decreasing essential tremor is alcohol. Alcoholic drinks substantially reduce the tremor for 45-60 minutes. The rate of alcoholism in patients with essential tremor is no different from that in the general population. Propranolol (80-320 mg daily) and other β-blockers and primidone (25-250 mg at bedtime) are effective. Other drugs that have been used are the benzodiazepines, especially clonazepam and lorazepam; methazolamide has also been effective in some patients, especially in head tremor. Botulinum toxin has been used recently. Stereotaxic thalamotomy can be effective in patients with severe functional disability who are unresponsive to drug therapy; surgery is probably underused.

- Movement disorders mostly in middle-aged and older people.
- Often genetic component.
- Hands are affected most.
- Head tremor almost never seen in Parkinson's disease.

Parkinson's Disease

Long-term high-dose levodopa monotherapy leads to dyskinesias and motor fluctuations. Fluctuations can be eliminated by continuous intravenous and intestinal infusions of levodopa. Other treatment strategies include using a low dose of levodopa (600 to 1,000 mg) and adding a dopamine agonist drug as well as selegiline hydrochloride and using continuous-release levodopa (Sinemet CR). When given to a patient with newly diagnosed Parkinson's disease, selegiline may delay the initiation of levodopa therapy as well as give mild symptomatic relief. Unpredictable off periods may also be helped with the use of a protein redistribution diet. Monotherapy with dopamine agonists (bromocriptine and pergolide) does not cause the motor side effects associated with levodopa, but the long-term use of a dopamine agonist is limited by its declining efficacy. There is also a tendency for these drugs to cause hallucinations, postural hypotension, and edema; bromocriptine has been associated with pulmonary and retroperitoneal fibrosis. Clozapine might be helpful in eliminating nocturnal akathesia and drug-induced psychosis.

Fetal dopamine cells transplanted into the caudate or putamen may be helpful, but this is still an experimental therapy. Stereotactic thalamotomy has been revised and can be helpful for tremor and drug-induced dyskinesia. Pallidotomy has

also been revived and may be useful for rigidity and bradykinesia. Recently, thalamic stimulation has been reported to eliminate all the symptoms of Parkinson's disease.

BOTULINUM TOXIN THERAPY

Botulinum toxin is effective therapy for cervical dystonia, blepharospasm, hemifacial spasm, spasmodic dysphonia, jaw-closing oromandibular dystonia, and limb dystonia, including occupational dystonias.

NEUROLOGY OF SEPSIS

The nervous system is commonly affected in sepsis syndrome. The neurologic conditions seen are septic encephalopathy, critical-illness polyneuropathy, septic myopathy, cachexia, and panfascicular muscle necrosis. Neurologic complications also occur in an ICU for critical medical illness. These complications include metabolic encephalopathy, seizures, hypoxic-ischemic encephalopathy, and stroke.

Septic Encephalopathy

Septic encephalopathy is brain dysfunction in association with systemic infection *without* overt infection of the brain or meninges. Early encephalopathy often begins before failure of other organs and is not secondary to single or multiple organ failure. Endotoxin does not cross the blood-brain barrier and so probably does not directly affect adult brains. Cytokines, important components of sepsis syndrome, may contribute to encephalopathy. Gegenhalten or paratonic rigidity occurs in >50% of patients and tremor, asterixis, and multifocal myoclonus occur in about 25%. Seizures and focal neurologic signs are rare.

EEG is a sensitive indicator of encephalopathy. The mildest abnormality is diffuse excessive theta low-voltage activity - (4-7 Hz). The next level of severity is intermittent rhythmic delta activity (<4 Hz). Worsening leads to delta activity becoming arrhythmic and continuous. Typical triphasic waves occur in severe cases.

Adult respiratory distress syndrome is common in severe but not mild encephalopathic cases.

- Brain dysfunction is associated with systemic infection.
- Encephalopathy precedes failure of other organs.
- Cytokines are an important part of sepsis syndrome.
- More than 50% of patients have paratonic rigidity.
- 25% of patients have tremor, asterixis, and multifocal myoclonus.
- EEG is a sensitive indicator of encephalopathy.

Critical Illness Polyneuropathy

This occurs in 70% of the patients with sepsis and multiple organ failure. There is often unexplained difficulty in weaning from mechanical ventilation. Nerve biopsy shows primary axonal degeneration of motor and sensory fibers without inflammation. Recovery from polyneuropathy is satisfactory if the patient survives sepsis and multiple organ failure.

● Nerve biopsy shows primary axonal degeneration of motor and sensory fibers without inflammation.
● Satisfactory recovery from polyneuropathy.

DEGENERATIVE DISEASE OF THE SPINE

Cervical Spondylosis

MRI combined with plain radiographs is the preferred approach for screening patients with cervical spondylosis. Surgical results for relief of the symptoms of cervical radiculopathy are better when the cause is a soft disk herniation than when spondylitic radiculopathy and myelopathy are present. In fact, surgical treatment of cervical radiculopathy due to the herniation of a soft disk is so successful that most patients and doctors prefer surgical therapy to prolonged conservative treatment. However, surgical treatment for cervical spondylitic myelopathy is much less successful, with fewer than two-thirds of patients having improvement. Cervical spondylitic myelopathy is a condition in which the spinal cord is damaged either directly by traumatic compression or indirectly by arterial deprivation or venous stasis as a consequence of proliferative bony changes in the cervical spine.

Lumbar Spine Disease

Bulging disks after the age of 30 should be considered normal and are unlikely to cause nerve root compression. Bulging disks appear round and symmetrical as opposed to herniated disks, which appear angular and asymmetrical and extend outside the disk space. The criteria for surgical treatment of lumbar disk herniations include the following: 1) presence of disk herniation on anatomical imaging, 2) dermatome-specific reflex, sensory, or motor deficits; and 3) failure of 6-8 weeks of conservative treatment.

The lateral recess syndrome (facet syndrome) is characterized by the following: 1) it produces radicular pain; 2) it is usually caused by an osteophyte on the superior articular facet; 3) the symptoms are unilateral or bilateral pain or paresthesias in the distribution of L-5 or S-1; 4) the pain is brought on by standing and walking and is relieved by sitting; and 5) the results on the straight leg raising test are usually negative.

Lumbar stenosis is characterized by the following: 1) most patients are >50 years; 2) neurogenic intermittent claudication (pseudoclaudication); 3) the symptoms are usually bilateral but can be asymmetrical or unilateral; 4) the pain usually has a dull, aching quality; 5) the whole lower extremity is generally involved; 6) the pain is provoked while walking or standing;

7) the patient is relieved by sitting or leaning forward; and 8) there is often a feeling of deadness in the legs. Decompressive operations for lumbar stenosis can be performed with low morbidity despite the advanced age of most patients. A very high initial success rate can be expected, although about 25% of patients become symptomatic in a 5-year follow-up period. On reoperation, three-fourths of the patients ultimately have a successful outcome; failures result from progression of stenosis at levels not previously decompressed or restenosis at levels previously operated on.

Musculoskeletal low back pain is best treated with a formal program of physical therapy and exercise, weight reduction, and education on postural principles.

NEUROMUSCULAR DISORDERS

A mutation in the oxygen radical detoxifying enzyme, superoxide dismutase (SOD), can cause a familial form of amyotrophic lateral sclerosis (ALS). However, no drug has been found to be effective in altering the progressive course of this disease. Recently, some beneficial effect has been noted with riluzole, especially in patients with bulbar onset of the disease. However, treating ALS with immunosuppression such as irradiation, corticosteroids, cyclophosphamide, or intravenous immunoglobulin (IVIG) is at best futile and at worst, costly harmful. However, treatment for multifocal motor neuropathy with cyclophosphamide or perhaps IVIG can be effective. This is a syndrome of purely lower motor neuron disease. It is often distal and asymmetrical, accompanied by motor conduction block on EMG, and is associated with high titers of serum antibodies to GM_1 gangliosides. However, antibody determinations are costly and have no therapeutic implication. Therefore, patients with purely lower motor neuron disease accompanied by the presence of conduction block on EMG should receive treatment with cyclophosphamide or IVIG.

Treatment strategies for myasthenia gravis include anticholinesterase, corticosteroids, azathioprine, cyclosporine, cyclophosphamide, plasma exchange, thymectomy, and IVIG. Older patients particularly derive the most benefit from azathioprine.

Prednisone, azathioprine, and methotrexate are the standard treatments for polymyositis, dermatomyositis, and inclusion-body myositis, although the latter rarely responds to treatment. Inclusion-body myositis is seen mainly in men >60 years, with symmetrical weakness of proximal and distal muscles. At times, there is asymmetric weakness, and at other times, there is a greater predominance of distal muscle involvement. Inclusion-body myositis is not associated with collagen vascular disease or neoplasms, and the creatine kinase level may be normal or slightly increased.

Plasma exchange is the treatment preferred for acute inflammatory demyelinating polyradiculopathy (Guillain-Barré syndrome), although IVIG may become the preferred treatment. In sharp contrast to AIDP, the case for steroids in CIDP is strong; plasma exchange is also effective, and corticosteroids alone or in combination with plasma exchange remain the treatment of choice. IVIG might be beneficial to some patients.

More than 60% of neuropathies associated with monoclonal gammopathy of undetermined significance (MGUS) are idiopathic, but some are associated with multiple myeloma, amyloidosis, lymphoma, and leukemia. The patients are usually >50 years and present early with symmetrical sensory radiculoneuropathy. Later, a motor polyradiculoneuropathy develops, involving mostly the legs. CSF protein is usually increased; IgM is more common than IgG or IgA. Plasma exchange can be effective therapy in patients with IgG or IgA neuropathy. They have a better response than those with IgM neuropathy. Other immunosuppressive therapy may also be effective, and even tamoxifen has reportedly been successful.

DEMYELINATING DISEASES
Idiopathic inflammatory demyelinating diseases of the CNS are as follows:
1. Multiple sclerosis
2. Isolated demyelinating syndromes--optic neuritis and transverse myelitis
3. Fulminant demyelinating diseases--acute disseminated encephalomyelitis and Marburg's variant of multiple sclerosis
4. Demyelinating syndromes with restricted distribution--Devic's syndrome (neuromyelitis optica) and Balo's concentric sclerosis (tumor-like cerebral presentation)
5. Primary progressive demyelinating diseases--chronic progressive myelopathy and progressive cerebellar syndrome
6. Asymptomatic demyelinating diseases (revealed by MRI or autopsy)

Predictors associated with a more favorable long-term course of multiple sclerosis include age <40 years at onset, female sex, optic neuritis or isolated sensory symptoms as the first clinical manifestation, and relatively infrequent attacks. Prognostic factors associated with a poor outcome include age >40 years at onset, male sex, cerebellar or pyramidal tract findings at initial presentation, relatively frequent attacks in the first 2 years, incomplete remissions, and a chronically progressive course. However, no single clinical variable is sufficient to predict the course or outcome of this disease. Acute transverse myelopathy is rarely the first sign of multiple sclerosis. Acute transverse myelopathy is usually a monophasic disorder. Abnormal MRI findings at the time of presentation of a clinically isolated syndrome suggestive of multiple sclerosis (isolated involvement of the optic nerve, brain stem, or spinal cord) is a strong predictor of the eventual clinical diagnosis of multiple sclerosis in the next 5 years. β-Interferon therapy decreases the relapse rate and intensity of relapses in patients with relapsing type of multiple sclerosis who are ambulatory.

However, the overall disability is probably not affected.

A study on steroid therapy for optic neuritis found that oral prednisone therapy was *ineffective*. The recommendation was for either a 3-day course of a high dose of intravenous methylprednisolone followed by an 11-day course of oral prednisone taper or no treatment at all.

ISCHEMIC CEREBROVASCULAR DISEASE

Pathophysiologic Mechanisms
Pathophysiologic mechanisms of ischemic cerebrovascular disease include artery-to-artery emboli (e.g., extracranial carotid bifurcation to a branch of the middle cerebral artery), cardiac embolic stroke, and lacunar infarction (small vessel disease). Other causes are hematologic disorders and states of altered coagulability (polycythemia, sickle cell anemia, thrombocytosis, severe leukocytosis, abnormalities of the cellular constituents of blood such as serologic factors like homocystinuria, deficiencies of antithrombin III, protein C, protein S, anticardiolipin antibodies, lupus anticoagulant, and mucin produced by adenocarcinomas which can cause a hypercoagulable state). Still other causes are nonarteriosclerotic vasculopathies (fibromuscular hyperplasia, granulomatous angiitis, congophilic angiopathy, systemic lupus erythematosus, etc.), dissection of the carotid or vertebral arteries, hemodynamic crisis with impairment of distal flow, mechanical compression of arteries, steal syndromes, and AIDS. "Recreational drugs" are a major risk factor for stroke in young adults.

- Pathophysiologic mechanisms of ischemic cardiovascular disease include cardiac embolic stroke, hematologic disorders, vasculopathies, and AIDS.
- In young adults, "recreational drugs" are a major risk factor for stroke.

Risk Factors
Risk factors are similar to those predisposing to coronary artery disease: hypertension, male sex, advanced age, cigarette smoking, diabetes mellitus, hypercholesterolemia, and oral contraceptives. Emboli from intracardiac mural thrombi are also an important cause of TIA and cerebral infarct. Major cardiac risk factors include left-sided chamber enlargement or aneurysm, congestive heart failure, atrial fibrillation, transmural myocardial infarction, mitral valve disease, septic emboli, paradoxical emboli, and atrial myxoma.

Hypertension is the most powerful modifiable risk factor for stroke, but other modifiable risk factors include cigarette smoking, alcohol consumption, physical activity, and cholesterol level. Although mild-to-moderate alcohol consumption appears to have a protective effect for ischemic stroke, heavy alcohol consumption increases the risk of all types of stroke, particularly intracerebral and subarachnoid hemorrhage.

TIAs

TIAs place patients at high risk for subsequent cerebral infarctions; estimates are from 4%-10% within 1 year to 33% within the patient's lifetime. Most TIAs are fleeting, usually lasting <10-15 minutes; 88% resolve within 1 hour. Infarcts, hemorrhages, and mass lesions can present like TIAs.

Amaurosis fugax is temporary, partial, or complete monocular blindness and is a classic symptom of a carotid artery TIA. It can be mimicked by glaucoma, vitreous hemorrhage, retinal detachment, papilledema, migrainous aura, temporal arteritis, and even ectopic floaters.

The long-term prognosis for patients with TIA generally follows the rules of 3s: 1/3 go on to have cerebral infarctions, 1/3 have at least one more TIA, 1/3 have no further TIAs.

- With TIAs, high risk for subsequent cerebral infarction.
- 1/3 will have cerebral infarction, 1/3 will have one more TIA, 1/3 will have no more TIAs.
- Most TIAs last <10-15 minutes.
- Infarcts, hemorrhages, and mass lesions can present like TIA.
- Amaurosis fugax is a classic symptom of a carotid artery TIA.

Carotid Endarterectomy

Carotid endarterectomy significantly lowers the risk of stroke and death in *symptomatic* patients who have 70%-99% carotid artery stenosis on angiography. For symptomatic patients with a 30%-69% stenosis, the value of carotid endarterectomy is uncertain but is being studied. Medical treatment alone is better than carotid endarterectomy in patients with 0%-29% carotid artery stenosis. Symptoms must be those of a carotid territory TIA or minor stroke and must be of recent onset (<4 months). The operation should be performed by surgeons with low rates of perioperative morbidity and mortality, and patients should be good surgical risks.

A report of a recent study (Asymptomatic Carotid Atherosclerosis Study [ACAS]) stated that patients with asymptomatic carotid stenosis ≥60% profit from carotid endarterectomy in terms of future risk for any stroke or death. All patients received proper medical treatment and aspirin. However, no stratification by degree of stenosis was provided. Important is the fact that surgeons and hospitals were particularly chosen for having past perioperative complication rates in asymptomatic patients of <3%. However, most conservative neurologists advise caution in accepting the premise that patients with asymptomatic carotid stenosis of <79% will benefit from surgical endarterectomy.

Antiplatelet Agents

Aspirin and ticlopidine are both effective in the secondary prevention of stroke. The optimum dose of aspirin is still uncertain, with ranges recommended from 30 to 1,300 mg/day. The dose of ticlopidine is 250 mg bid. Ticlopidine has been associated with neutropenia; thus the complete blood cell count must be monitored every 2 weeks for the first 3 months of treatment. It has been suggested that a subgroup of patients may profit from ticlopidine, including women, patients who have had vertebral-basilar artery symptoms, patients with cerebral ischemic symptoms while taking aspirin or receiving anticoagulation therapy, and patients with diffuse atherosclerotic disease rather than high-grade carotid artery stenosis.

Stroke Risks With Nonvalvular Atrial Fibrillation

Atrial fibrillation is associated with up to 24% of ischemic strokes and 50% of embolic strokes. The stroke rate for the entire cohort of patients with chronic atrial fibrillation is generally about 5% per year. However, patients <60 years with "lone atrial fibrillation" have a lower risk of stroke than other patients with atrial fibrillation. Stroke risk factors with atrial fibrillation include a history of hypertension, recent congestive heart failure, previous thromboembolism including TIAs, left ventricular dysfunction identified on two-dimensional echocardiograms, and the size of the left atrium identified on M-mode echocardiograms. Patients with atrial fibrillation who have one or more risk factors should receive anticoagulation therapy (low intensity anticoagulation is recommended) and those at low risk should receive aspirin.

In patients receiving anticoagulant therapy, the dominant risk factor for intracranial hemorrhage is the prothrombin time ratio (PTR). Age is another risk factor for subdural hemorrhage. A PTR of 1.3 to 1.5 (INR, 2.0-3.0) is probably an adequate level of anticoagulation for all indications except for preventing embolization from mechanical heart valves; the current recommendation is for a PTR of 1.5 to 2.0 (INR, 2.5-3.5). In general, the lowest effective intensity of anticoagulation should be used.

- Atrial fibrillation is associated with 24% of ischemic strokes and 50% of embolic strokes.
- Stroke rate is about 5% per year.
- Patients with "lone atrial fibrillation" have a lower risk of stroke.

HEMORRHAGIC CEREBROVASCULAR DISEASE

Intracranial Hemorrhage

Hypertension commonly affects deep penetrating cerebral vessels, especially ones supplying the basal ganglia, cerebral white matter, thalamus, pons, and cerebellum. Common old *misconcepts* of intracerebral hemorrhage are 1) onset is generally sudden and catastrophic, 2) hypertension is invariably severe, 3) headache is always present, 4) reduced consciousness or frank coma is usually present, 5) CSF is always bloody, and 6) prognosis is poor and mortality is high. None of these may be present, and the prognosis depends on the size and location of the hemorrhage.

- Prognosis depends on the size and site of the hemorrhage.

Surgical evacuation of intracerebral hematomas may be necessary in patients with signs of increased intracranial pressure or in those whose condition is worsening.

Cerebellar Hemorrhage

It is important to recognize this because drainage may be lifesaving. The important clinical findings are vomiting and inability to walk. Long tract signs are usually *not* present. Patients may have ipsilateral gaze palsy, ipsilateral CN VI palsy, or ipsilateral nuclear type CN VII palsy and may or may not have headache, vertigo, and lethargy. Cerebellar hemorrhage may cause obstructive hydrocephalus.

- Vomiting and inability to walk are important findings in cerebellar hemorrhage.
- Long tract signs not present.
- Cerebellar hemorrhage may cause obstructive hydrocephalus.

Subarachnoid Hemorrhage

Subarachnoid hemorrhage accounts for about 10% of strokes, including about half of those in patients <45 years, with peak age range between 35 and 65. In up to 50% of cases, an alert patient with an aneurysm may have a small sentinel bleed with a warning headache, or aneurysmal expansion may cause focal neurologic signs or symptoms, e.g., an incomplete CN III palsy. The prognosis is directly related to the state of consciousness at the time of intervention. The headache is characteristically sudden in onset and, although 1/3 occur during exertion, 1/3 also occur during rest, and 1/3 during sleep. The peak incidence of vasospasm associated with subarachnoid hemorrhage occurs between days 4 and 12 after the initial hemorrhage. Other complications include hemorrhagic infiltration into the brain, ventricles, and even subdural space, which requires evacuation; hyponatremia associated with diabetes insipidus or syndrome of inappropriate secretion of antidiuretic hormone; and communicating hydrocephalus.

In addition to the initial hemorrhage, vasospasm and rehemorrhaging are the leading causes of morbidity and mortality in patients who have subarachnoid hemorrhage.

The outpouring of catecholamines may cause myocardial damage with accompanying ECG abnormalities, pulmonary edema, and arrhythmias. Arrhythmias can be both supraventricular and ventricular and are most likely during the initial hours or days after moderate-to-severe subarachnoid hemorrhage.

- About 10% of strokes are subarachnoid hemorrhage.
- In 50% of cases, an alert patient with an aneurysm may have a small sentinel bleed.
- Prognosis is related directly to the state of consciousness at the time of intervention.
- Characteristically, headache has a sudden onset.

Hemorrhagic cerebrovascular disease is outlined in Table 17-11.

LYME DISEASE--MULTISYSTEM DISORDER

Stage I Lyme disease begins with the bite of an infected tick. Any body area may be bitten, but the thigh, groin, and axilla are common sites. Patients often cannot recall the tick bite.

Table 17-11.--Hemorrhagic Cerebrovascular Disease

Hemorrhage into parenchyma
 Hypertensive intracerebral
 Due to trauma--primarily frontal and temporal
 Hemorrhagic infarction
 Secondary to brain tumors (primary and secondary neoplasms)
 Secondary to inflammatory diseases of vasculature
 Related to disorders of blood-forming organs (blood dyscrasia, especially leukemia and thrombocytopenic purpura)
 Related to anticoagulant therapy
 Secondary to increased intracranial pressure (brain stem) (Duret hemorrhages)
 Secondary to aneurysms and congenital anomalies of blood vessels
 Early-life carotid artery occlusion
 Postsurgical
 Fat embolism (petechial)
 Hemorrhagic encephalitis (petechial)
 Undetermined cause (normal blood pressure, no other recognizable disorder)
 Amyloid angiopathy

Hemorrhage into arachnoid (subarachnoid hemorrhage)
 Trauma
 Due to aneurysm
  Saccular ("berry," "congenital")
  Fusiform (arteriosclerotic)--rarely causes hemorrhage
  Mycotic
 Due to vascular malformation
 Many of same causes as for parenchyma above

Subdural and epidural hemorrhage (hematoma)
 Mainly traumatic
 Many of same causes as for parenchyma above

Hemorrhage into pituitary (pituitary apoplexy)

Stage II disease begins weeks to months after the initial infection and is characterized by neurologic, cardiac, and ophthalmic involvement. About 15% of the patients in the U.S.A. have neurologic involvement, usually meningoencephalitis, cranial neuritis, or radiculoneuropathy. Cranial neuropathies are common, most frequently CN VII (bilaterally in 1/3 of patients). Thus, bilateral CN VII palsies in a patient from an endemic area are almost diagnostic of Lyme disease. Peripheral nervous system involvement can include the spinal roots, plexuses, and peripheral nerves.

Stage III disease marks the chronic phase and begins months to years after the initial infection. This stage is heralded by arthritic and neurologic symptoms. Any CNS symptom is possible, and there may be psychiatric symptoms and cognitive impairment. Severe fatigue is a particularly prominent feature. Rarely, a multiple sclerosis-like demyelinating illness featuring gait disturbance, urinary bladder dysfunction, spastic paraparesis, and dysarthria may develop. These symptoms may undergo exacerbations and remissions; MRI and CT reveal multifocal white matter lesions.

- Lyme disease is a multisystem disorder.
- Patients often do not recall the tick bite.
- In the U.S.A., 15% of patients have neurologic involvement.
- Cranial neuropathies, especially CN VII, are common.
- Bilateral CN VII palsies in an endemic area are diagnostic of Lyme disease.
- In stage III disease, severe fatigue is prominent.

The longer the duration of symptoms before diagnosis and effective antibiotic treatment, the greater the risk that serious symptoms will outlast the period of acute infection. Laboratory diagnosis can be difficult; ELISA can be undependable both in identifying new cases and in distinguishing acute from remote healed infection. Asymptomatic tick bites carry a less than 1% chance of Lyme infection, and treating such for Lyme disease is not cost-effective. However, typical erythema migrans accompanying either a tick bite or other typical symptoms is sufficiently diagnostic to warrant treatment following exposure in an endemic area even without abnormal serologic findings.

NEUROLOGIC COMPLICATIONS OF AIDS

The nervous system is affected clinically in up to 40% of HIV patients, and pathologic changes in the nervous system are found at autopsy in up to 90%. Neurologic features may be the presenting manifestation of the illness in 5%-10% of the patients. HIV infection is associated with various central and peripheral nervous system disorders, and multiple levels of the nervous system can be affected simultaneously. Therapy is available for many of these syndromes. HIV dementia is treated with a high dose of zidovudine (AZT). Cytomegalo-

virus encephalitis is treated with ganciclovir. A syndrome of lumbosacral polyradiculomyelopathy presenting as or manifested by progressive lumbosacral radicular symptoms (with weakness, areflexia, and sensory loss in the legs) is often due to cytomegalovirus and, thus, treated with ganciclovir. Cryptococcal meningitis is treated with amphotericin B (also flucytosine or fluconazole). CNS lymphoma in AIDS patients is treated the same as CNS lymphoma in immunocompetent patients, i.e., with radiotherapy and chemotherapy. The acute inflammatory demyelinating polyradiculoneuropathy responds well to plasma exchange or prednisone. Zidovudine-induced myopathy responds to dose reduction or withdrawal of the medication. Polymyositis is treated the same as it is in other patients, i.e., with steroid therapy.

The major HIV-related neurologic conditions are the following: 1) HIV dementia, 2) toxoplasma encephalitis, 3) CNS lymphoma, 4) progressive multifocal leukoencephalopathy, 5) cytomegalovirus encephalitis, 6) cryptococcal meningitis, 7) neurosyphilis, 8) vacuolar myelopathy, 9) distal symmetrical polyneuropathy, 10) inflammatory demyelinating polyradiculoneuropathy, 11) mononeuropathy multiplex, 12) progressive polyradiculopathy, and 13) myopathy. Toxoplasma encephalitis remains a common opportunistic infection in AIDS patients. Treatment for this infection is either pyrimethamine plus sulfadiazine or pyrimethamine plus clindamycin. However, CNS lymphoma and toxoplasma encephalitis can be difficult to differentiate because they are similar both in their clinical manifestations and CT and MRI characteristics. Therefore, patients with AIDS who present with a contrast-enhancing CNS mass lesion are treated empirically for toxoplasma encephalitis and patients undergo follow-up CT or MRI scans to see if the lesion decreases in size. Patients whose lesions do not respond to medical treatment are subjected to stereotactic biopsy to exclude other causes, including lymphoma.

Patients with AIDS dementia complex have an increased concentration of CSF β_2-microglobulin. Thus, CSF β_2-microglobulin may be a valuable marker of the severity of AIDS dementia and response to treatment. Treatment with zidovudine significantly decreases the concentration of β_2-microglobulin.

NEUROLOGIC COMPLICATIONS OF ORGAN TRANSPLANTATION

Because almost all organ transplant recipients require some degree of chronic, life-long immunosuppressive therapy, the major neurologic complications of organ transplantation are due to immunosuppression. These include direct neurotoxic side effects of immunosuppressive drugs, infections, and the development of de novo malignancies. Direct neurologic side effects:
1. Cyclosporine. Tremor is the most common side effect of cyclosporine, which also may produce various motor

syndromes such as hemiparesis, paraparesis, and quadriparesis. Cyclosporine may also produce encephalopathy and, less commonly, neuralgia and neuropathy; it is epileptogenic.

2. Corticosteroids. The side effects of corticosteroids include myopathy, steroid psychosis, withdrawal (myalgias, arthralgias, headache, lethary, nausea), and spinal cord or cauda equina compression due to epidural lipomatosis.

3. Azathioprine. It has no direct neurotoxic side effects.

CNS Infection

Infection of the CNS is relatively frequent and life-threatening. The three organisms that cause more than 80% of CNS infections are *Listeria monocytogenes*, *Cryptococcus neoformans*, and *Aspergillus fumigatus*. The greatest risk factor for CNS infection is the magnitude and duration of immunosuppression. Severe and advanced CNS infections may present with little or no clinical evidence of infection. The period of infection risk is mainly from 1-6 months after transplantation. Specific infections include: 1) acute meningitis, most often due to *Listeria*; 2) subacute or chronic meningitis, generally due to *Cryptococcus*; 3) slowly progressive dementia, frequently due to progressive multifocal leukoencephalopathy; and 4) focal brain disease due to infection usually caused by *Aspergillus*, *Toxoplasma*, *Listeria*, or *Nocardia*.

CNS Involvement by de Novo Lymphoproliferative Diseases

There is an increase in non-Hodgkin's lymphoma, especially primary CNS lymphomas. These lymphomas may be linked to infection with Epstein-Barr virus.

Other Neurologic Complications

Other complications affecting the nervous system can be classified as follows:

1. Complications arising from the underlying diseases
2. Problems resulting from the transplant procedure
3. Side effects of immunosuppression
4. Post-transplantation disorder peculiar to the specific type of transplant

The complications include compressive neuropathies, plexopathies, and radiculopathies; encephalopathy (especially with renal, liver, and heart transplants), cerebral infarctions (with bone marrow and heart transplants), and chronic graft versus host disease (especially with bone marrow transplant) involves the peripheral nervous system (but not the CNS), e.g., polymyositis, myasthenia gravis, and peripheral neuropathy including CIDP. A complication associated with liver transplantation is central pontine myelinolysis, which is manifested as altered mental status or coma, pseudobulbar palsy, and quadriplegia.

QUESTIONS

Multiple Choice (choose the one best answer)

1. Which of the following is not seen in normal healthy elderly persons?
   a. Atrophy of the small muscles of the hand
   b. Decreased ankle reflexes
   c. Decreased vibratory sensation in the legs
   d. Paratonic rigidity of the legs
   e. Decreased visual pursuit movements

2. The most common cause of hydrocephalus ex vacuo is:
   a. Alzheimer's disease
   b. Decrease in absorption of cerebrospinal fluid (CSF)
   c. Increased production of CSF
   d. Obstruction of the outflow of the fourth ventricle
   e. Physiologic cortical atrophy (aging)

3. A cerebellar syndrome manifested as a broad-based unsteady gait with heel-to-shin ataxia and relative sparing of the arms, speech, and ocular motility is most likely:
   a. A heredofamilial ataxia
   b. Sporadic parenchymatous cerebellar degeneration
   c. Alcoholic cerebellar degeneration
   d. Paraneoplastic cerebellar degeneration
   e. Toxic cerebellar dysfunction

4. All the following are characteristic of Lambert-Eaton myasthenic syndrome except:
   a. Proximal leg weakness
   b. Severe ptosis
   c. Decreased muscle stretch reflexes
   d. Mouth dryness
   e. Orthostatic hypotension

5. Lumbar puncture is contraindicated in all the following except:
   a. Idiopathic intracranial hypertension
   b. Cerebral abscess
   c. Arnold-Chiari malformation
   d. Large intracerebral hemorrhage
   e. Large ischemic cerebral infarct

6. Acute spinning vertigo accompanied by blurriness of vision, unsteady gait, nausea, and vomiting and followed by syncope is most likely due to:
   a. Acute cerebellar hemorrhage
   b. Transient ischemic attack (TIA) in the vertebrobasilar system
   c. Acoustic neuroma
   d. Acute peripheral vestibulopathy
   e. Vestibular toxin

7. All the following neurologic diseases may present and progress asymmetrically except:
   a. Parkinson's disease
   b. Motor neuron disease (amyotrophic lateral sclerosis)
   c. Subacute combined degeneration of the spinal cord
   d. Cortical-basal ganglionic degeneration
   e. Multiple sclerosis

True/False (indicate whether each answer is true or false)
8. Mononeuropathy multiplex may be seen in:
   a. Compressive neuropathy
   b. Diabetes mellitus
   c. Sarcoidosis
   d. Vasculitis

   e. Connective tissue disease
   f. Tumor infiltration

9. Regarding the neurologic complications of AIDS, the following statements are true or false:
   a. Pathologic changes in the nervous system are found at autopsy in up to 90% of cases
   b. Acute inflammatory demyelinating polyneuropathy should not be treated with plasma exchange
   c. Inflammatory myopathy should not be treated with steroids
   d. Patients presenting with contrast-enhancing CNS mass lesions should first receive treatment with pyrimethamine plus sulfadiazine
   e. The dementia complex can be treated with zidovudine
   f. A conus medullaris-cauda equina syndrome is often due to cytomegalovirus infection

10. Regarding seizure disorder, the following statements are true or false:
   a. Complex partial seizures may originate outside the temporal lobe
   b. Most adults with generalized tonic-clonic seizures begin with partial seizures
   c. Mesial temporal sclerosis is the most common pathologic condition found in temporal lobe epilepsy
   d. Addition of a second antiepileptic drug improves seizure control 25% but increases drug toxicity 40%
   e. Females with epilepsy without medication have an increased risk of fetal malformations
   f. Alcohol has an antiepileptic effect

ANSWERS

1. Answer d.

Many signs seen in the neurologic examination of normal, healthy elderly persons are not considered pathologic. These include atrophy of the small muscles of the hands, decreased ankle reflexes, decreased vibratory sensation in the legs, decreased visual pursuit movements, impairment of upward gaze, difficulty with tandem gait, difficulty balancing on one leg, and

difficulty with rapid alternating movements. There is also a decrease in the acuity of the special sensations of vision, hearing, smell, and taste. One may even elicit unusual reflexes that are often called "release signs," including snouting, palmomental, rooting, and sucking reflexes. Although elderly persons develop rigidity in the axial and appendicular muscles, including cogwheel rigidity, paratonic rigidity (gegenhalten) is a pathologic sign in an awake elderly person. Paratonia can occur in the neck and limbs in the elderly in a stuporous state of any cause.

2. Answer e.

Normal elderly persons have cerebral cortical and cerebellar atrophy with compensatory ventriculomegaly. This is a communicating hydrocephalus, but it is due simply to loss of tissue. The same pattern occurs in Alzheimer's disease, but aging is more common than Alzheimer's disease. Decreased absorption of CSF also causes a communicating hydrocephalus that can be symptomatic and lead to the triad of cognitive dysfunction, gait disorder, and urinary bladder dysfunction ("normal pressure hydrocephalus"). Increased production of CSF also leads to a communicating hydrocephalus, but it is a rare phenomenon (if it occurs at all). Obstructive hydrocephalus in any location of the ventricular system is usually due to a mass lesion.

3. Answer c.

This type of cerebellar dysfunction is called the "anterior superior vermal syndrome" or "restrictive form of cerebellar degeneration"; it is pathognomonic of alcoholic cerebellar degeneration. Although the other forms of cerebellar degeneration can begin like this, they usually progress to a more diffuse cerebellar syndrome. Toxic cerebellar dysfunction is also a diffuse syndrome, and the heredofamilial ataxias usually have other signs indicating involvement of brain stem, spinal cord, or peripheral nerve.

4. Answer b.

The Lambert-Eaton myasthenic syndrome is often associated with a small cell cancer of the lung and is manifested by proximal leg weakness and autonomic dysfunction. The muscle stretch reflexes are usually decreased or absent, but they can be elicited sometimes after exercise. As opposed to myasthenia gravis, the Lambert-Eaton myasthenic syndrome usually spares the muscles supplied by the cranial nerves. Thus, ptosis, dysarthria, and diplopia, which are more characteristics of myasthenia gravis, are rarely seen in the myasthenic syndrome.

5. Answer a.

Lumbar puncture is contraindicated with any type of mass lesion, with or without papilledema. In general, it is contraindicated in cases of increased intracranial pressure, except for idiopathic intracranial hypertension (pseudotumor cerebri). In this case, it is not only safe to perform lumbar puncture, but the lumbar puncture is diagnostic as well. When a mass lesion is present, a herniation syndrome can occur after lumbar puncture and little information is gained by analysis of the CSF.

6. Answer d.

Acute peripheral vestibulopathy is manifested as spinning vertigo accompanied by unsteady gait, blurriness of vision, and nausea and vomiting. Often, patients with this syndrome have vasovagal syncope in reaction to the vertigo. The hallmarks of acoustic neuroma are unilateral tinnitus and hearing loss, with a vague sense of unsteadiness or dizziness. A vestibular toxin does not cause vertigo but causes unsteadiness and oscillopsia. An acute cerebellar hemorrhage can lead to vertigo, unsteadiness, and nausea and vomiting, and it can progress to stupor and coma but not syncope. It is much less common than acute peripheral vestibulopathy. A diagnosis of TIA in the vertebrobasilar system requires signs of dysfunction in the cerebellum, brain stem, and occipital lobe, with or without vertigo and the accompanying signs of vertigo. The accompanying signs of spinning vertigo include unsteady gait, blurriness of vision (or sometimes double vision), and nausea and vomiting.

7. Answer c.

Diseases that are usually symmetrical in the nervous system include heredofamilial diseases, toxic and nutritional diseases, myopathies, and peripheral neuropathies including AIDP and CIDP. However, many other diseases of the nervous system may present and progress asymmetrically, including Parkinson's disease, amyotrophic lateral sclerosis, multiple sclerosis, and the unusual entity of cortical-basal ganglionic degeneration, the hallmark of which is asymmetry.

8. a, true; b, true; c, true; d, true; e, true; f, true.

Mononeuropathy multiplex (asymmetrical involvement of several nerves) suggests certain causes, including trauma, compression, diabetes, vasculitis (with or without connective tissue disease), leprosy, Lyme disease, sarcoidosis, tumor infiltration, and hereditary liability to pressure palsies.

9. a, true; b, false; c, false; d, true; e, true; f, true.

Involvement of the peripheral and central nervous systems is common in HIV patients and occurs clinically in about 40% of them, but pathologic changes can be seen in the nervous system at autopsy in up to 90% of cases. Conditions such as acute inflammatory demyelinating polyneuropathy (AIDP) and inflammatory myopathy (polymyositis) should be treated the same in AIDS patients as in immunocompetent patients. Contrast-enhancing CNS mass lesions in AIDS patients should first be treated as toxoplasma encephalitis, and if there is no response, a biopsy should be performed to look for other lesions such as lymphoma. The dementia complex can respond, at least initially, to zidovudine. A syndrome of lumbosacral polyradiculomyelopathy (conus medullaris-cauda equina syndrome) is often due to cytomegalovirus and, thus, treated with ganciclovir.

10. a, true; b, true; c, true; d, false; e, true; f, true.

Although most complex partial seizure disorders originate in the temporal lobes, they may originate in extratemporal locations; thus, the old term "temporal lobe epilepsy" has been changed to "complex partial seizures." The cause of seizures in most adults is usually a focal lesion; therefore, the seizures begin focally or partially, but they may spread throughout both cerebral hemispheres, causing secondary generalized tonic-clonic seizures. Mesial temporal sclerosis, which can be identified on MRI, is the most common pathologic condition that causes temporal lobe seizures. Although the addition of a second antiepileptic drug may improve seizure control by a small amount (perhaps 10%), toxicity increases greatly by about 90%. Whereas antiepileptic drugs can cause fetal malformations, females with epilepsy, even without treatment, have an increased risk of having a fetal malformation. Alcohol has an antiepileptic effect, and in nonalcoholic patients with epilepsy, mild drinking (1-2 drinks per day) probably does not affect seizure control. However, in epileptics who drink heavily, withdrawal from alcohol can precipitate seizures and status epilepticus.

CHAPTER 18

ONCOLOGY

Lynn C. Hartmann, M.D.

BREAST CANCER

Magnitude of the Problem

Breast cancer is the most common life-threatening malignancy in North American women (it represents one-third of all serious cancers). It will develop in approximately one in nine American women who achieve a normal life expectancy. In the United States, 180,000 new cases are diagnosed annually. The incidence is increasing, but this is a complex issue. Much of the increase is due to earlier detection. Breast cancer is the second most common cause of death due to cancer in American women (lung cancer is the most common). There are 45,000 deaths due to breast cancer in this country annually.

- Breast cancer will develop in one in nine American women.
- Incidence is increasing (largely due to screening).
- It is the second most common cause of death from cancer in American women.

Risk Factors

The risk factors for breast cancer are outlined in Table 18–1. Of note, the American Cancer Society estimates that 75% of

cases of breast cancer occur in women with no known high-risk factors.

Screening

Controlled trials performed during the past 30 years have shown that screening for breast cancer can reduce mortality from this disease. Both mammography and physical examination of the breasts by skilled examiners have been shown to contribute to this decrease in mortality (note that breast self-examination has not been appropriately evaluated in a screening study). The Health Insurance Plan (HIP) study of greater New York was the first randomized controlled trial to evaluate screening for any type of cancer.

- Screening for breast cancer can reduce mortality.
- Mammography and physical examination of breasts contribute to decreased mortality.

In 1964, 64,000 women aged 40-64 years were enrolled in the HIP study. Screening with annual mammography and clinical breast examination over 4 consecutive years was offered to 32,000 women. The randomization group included 32,000

Table 18-1.--Risk Factors for Breast Cancer

High risk: relative risk >4.0	Moderate risk: relative risk 2-4	Low risk: relative risk 1-2
Older age	Any first-degree relative with breast cancer	Menarche before age 12 years
Personal history of breast cancer		Menopause after age 55 years
Family history of premenopausal bilateral breast cancer or familial cancer syndrome	Personal history of ovarian or endometrial cancer	White race
		Moderate alcohol intake
Breast biopsy showing proliferative disease with atypia	Age at first full-term pregnancy >30 years	Long-duration (≥15 years) estrogen replacement therapy
	Nulliparous	
	Obesity in postmenopausal women	
	Upper socioeconomic class	

women (controls) who received their usual medical care. At 18 years from study entry, there were 22% fewer deaths from breast cancer in the screened group than the control group. One-third of the breast cancers detected in the screened group were found by mammography alone. Most of the benefit was derived from the physical examination, but mammography was in its infancy at that time. The reduction in mortality was noted in all age groups.

Clinical examination of the breast (i.e., by physician or nurse practitioner) and mammography are the basic screening methods; both are necessary to achieve maximal detection rates.

There is general consensus that women ≥50 years old should be screened with annual clinical examination and mammography. However, the timing for initiation of screening is controversial. Specifically, there is disagreement regarding the value of screening women aged 40-50 years. Certainly, in women deemed at high risk for breast cancer (for example, on the basis of family history), screening measures should be instituted at an appropriately earlier age, generally taken as 5 years before the earliest diagnosis of breast cancer in the family.

- Clinical examination of breast and mammography are basic detection methods.
- Women ≥50 years old need annual examination and mammography.
- There is disagreement about screening women 40-50 years old.

Currently, mammography is regarded as the most important screening test. However, about 10% of breast cancers detectable on physical examination are missed by mammography. Thus, biopsy of a suspicious palpable lump should be done despite a negative mammogram.

- Mammography is most important screening test.
- 10% of breast cancers found on physical examination are missed by mammography.
- Need biopsy for suspicious palpable lump, even if mammogram negative.

Pathology

Breast cancers are classified as ductal or lobular, corresponding to the ducts and lobules of the normal breast (Fig. 18-1). Infiltrating ductal carcinoma is the most common histologic type (70% of breast cancers). Lobular disease is more frequently multifocal and bilateral. Carcinoma in situ (CIS) refers to disease confined within the lumen of the ducts. It may be called ductal CIS (DCIS) or intraductal carcinoma. This is noninvasive disease (i.e., the basement membrane is preserved); that is, there has been no invasion of malignant cells into the stroma of the breast. Thus, there has been no access to the vasculature and no potential for spread of

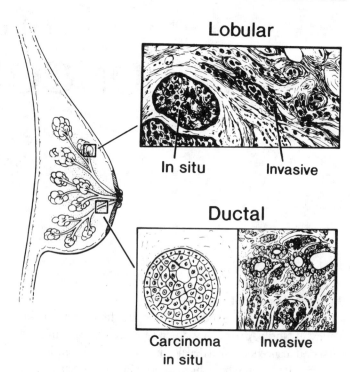

Fig. 18-1. Breast carcinomas: ductal vs. lobular, in situ vs. invasive.

disease. Thus, DCIS of the breast is treated with local measures only.

- Infiltrating ductal carcinoma is the most common histologic type.
- Lobular disease is more frequently multifocal and bilateral.
- Ductal carcinoma in situ is noninvasive disease (basement membrane preserved) and needs local therapy only.

Staging

The staging system of the American Joint Committee on Cancer is shown in Table 18-2.

Initial staging studies include 1) history and physical examination, 2) complete blood cell count, 3) chemistry panel, 4) chest radiography, 5) bilateral mammography, 6) bone scanning (stages II-IV), and 7) other imaging studies as clinically indicated.

Natural History and Prognostic Factors

Nodal Status

The number of involved axillary nodes remains the single best predictor of outcome (Fig. 18-2).

Tumor Size

After nodal status, tumor size is generally the most important prognostic factor (Table 18-3).

Table 18-2.--Staging of Breast Cancer

Primary tumor (T)

TIS   Carcinoma in situ

T1 $T = \leq 2$ cm

T2 $T = 2.1\text{-}5$ cm

T3 $T = >5$ cm

T4   T of any size with direct extension to chest wall or skin

Regional nodes (N)

N0   No involved nodes

N1   Movable ipsilateral axillary nodes

N2   Matted or fixed nodes

Distant metastasis (M)

M0   None detected

M1   Distant metastasis present (includes ipsilateral supraclavicular nodes)

Stage grouping

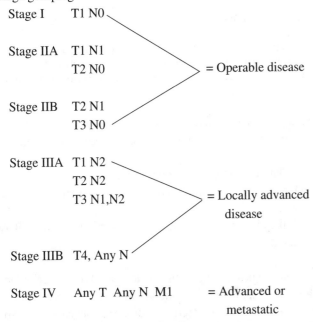

Stage I	T1 N0	
Stage IIA	T1 N1	= Operable disease
	T2 N0	
Stage IIB	T2 N1	
	T3 N0	
Stage IIIA	T1 N2	
	T2 N2	= Locally advanced disease
	T3 N1,N2	
Stage IIIB	T4, Any N	
Stage IV	Any T Any N M1	= Advanced or metastatic

Data from American Joint Committee on Cancer: Breast. *In* Manual for Staging of Cancer. Fourth edition. Edited by OH Beahrs, DE Henson, RVP Hutter, BJ Kennedy. Philadelphia, JB Lippincott Company, 1992, pp 149-154.

Hormone Receptor Status

In general, patients with estrogen-receptor-positive tumors have a better prognosis. However, the difference in recurrence rates at 5 years is only 8%-10%.

Grade

Most breast cancers are high-grade. Patients with low-grade tumors have fewer recurrences and longer survival.

- Number of involved axillary nodes is best predictor of outcome.
- After nodal status, tumor size is most important prognostic factor.
- Patients with receptor-positive tumors have better prognosis.
- Patients with low-grade tumors have better prognosis.

Treatment

Primary or Local-Regional Therapy

Primary therapy is that treatment applied to the involved breast after biopsy confirmation of breast carcinoma. The approach has changed significantly during the past 15 years. Radical surgical procedures have been replaced by lesser surgical procedures that can conserve the breast. This latter approach is combined with breast irradiation.

- Radical surgical procedures have been replaced with lesser operations.

Breast Conservation Versus Mastectomy

Several randomized controlled clinical trials have compared breast conservation (lumpectomy + axillary dissection + radiation) with mastectomy for the treatment of invasive breast cancer. All of these trials have demonstrated the therapeutic equivalence of these two options. The National Cancer Institute conducted a Consensus Conference on Early-Stage Breast Cancer in June 1990. The conclusion was that "Breast conservation treatment is an appropriate method of primary therapy for the majority of women with stage I and II breast cancer and is preferable because it provides survival rates equivalent to those of total mastectomy and axillary dissection while preserving the breast."

- Numerous trials have demonstrated therapeutic equivalence of breast conservation and mastectomy.
- Breast conservation is suitable primary therapy for most women with stage I or II breast cancer and is preferable.

Breast conservation is therapeutically equivalent to mastectomy for the primary therapy of breast cancer because the disease-free survival and overall survival rates with these two treatments have been shown to be identical. They are equivalent because the ultimate outcome of patients with breast cancer does not depend on the disease in the breast; rather, outcome depends on the presence of distant microscopic metastatic disease, which will eventually develop into clinically significant recurrent disease and death. Primary therapy does not affect distant disease.

- Distant microscopic metastatic disease determines outcome in patients with breast cancer and is not affected by the choice of primary therapy.

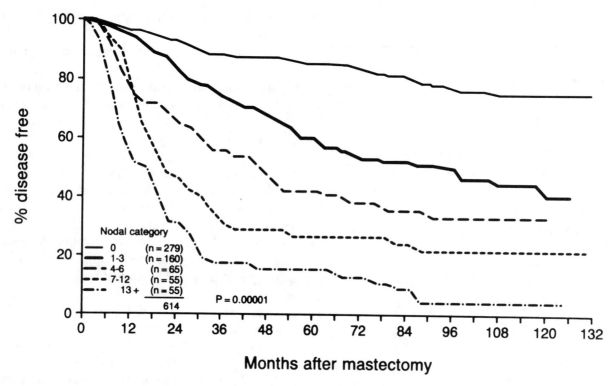

Fig. 18-2. Relation of disease-free survival to numbers of nodal metastases in more than 600 women with breast cancer treated with radical mastectomy alone in the early 1970s. (From Fisher ER, Sass R, Fisher B, and Collaborating NSABP Investigators: Pathologic findings from the National Surgical Adjuvant Project for Breast Cancers [protocol no. 4]. X. Discriminants for tenth year treatment failure. Cancer 53:712-723, 1984. By permission of American Cancer Society.)

Table 18-3.--Long-Term Results* in Patients With Node-Negative Breast Cancer Treated Surgically

Tumor size, cm	No. of patients	% free of recurrence	% dead of disease
<1	171	88	10
1.1-2.0	303	74	24
2.1-3.0	188	72	24
3.1-5.0	105	61	36

*Median duration of follow-up was 18 years.
Data from Rosen PP, Groshen S, Kinne DW: Survival and prognostic factors in node-negative breast cancer: results of long-term follow-up studies. Monogr Natl Cancer Inst 11:159-162, 1992.

Recommendations for Lumpectomy and Radiation Therapy

It is appropriate to excise the primary lesion with a normal tissue margin of approximately 1 cm. When margins are grossly involved with tumor, further resection, to achieve negative margins, is indicated. An axillary dissection is needed for all patients, whether lumpectomy or mastectomy is done. This procedure provides vital prognostic information. Megavoltage radiation therapy to the whole breast to a dose of 4,500-5,000 cGy should be used. (Lumpectomy alone, without radiation therapy, leads to a high rate of recurrences in the breast, on the order of 40%.)

Axillary irradiation after an axillary dissection is not routinely indicated and, in fact, can result in unacceptable lymphedema.

- Axillary dissection is needed for all patients.
- Megavoltage radiation therapy to whole breast should be used.
- Axillary irradiation after axillary dissection is not routinely indicated.

There are no data suggesting an increased risk of secondary malignancies, including contralateral breast cancer, resulting from breast irradiation. Certain women are not candidates for breast conservation. These include 1) women with multicentric breast malignancies, including those with more than one mass, or diffuse microcalcifications on mammography; and 2) women in whom an unacceptable cosmetic result is predicted. This includes those whose tumors are large relative to breast size and those with certain collagen vascular diseases, in whom excessive fibrosis can result after breast irradiation. Breast reconstruction is an option for interested women who have a mastectomy.

- Certain women are not candidates for breast conservation: 1) those with multicentric breast malignancies or diffuse microcalcifications on mammography or 2) those with predictable unacceptable cosmetic result.
- Breast reconstruction is option after mastectomy.

Systemic Therapy

This consists of either hormonal therapy or combination chemotherapy. It may be administered in the adjuvant setting (see this page) or for advanced disease (see page 626).

Hormonal Agents

Tamoxifen is the most widely used hormonal agent in the treatment of patients with breast cancer. Tamoxifen is a non-steroidal compound with both anti-estrogen and estrogen-like (agonist) activity. Its beneficial effects include 1) its recognized antitumor effects on breast cancer cells, 2) a decrease in new, contralateral breast cancers in women taking adjuvant tamoxifen, 3) a favorable effect on bone density (estrogen-like effect), and 4) a favorable effect on lipid profiles (estrogen-like effect). Its side effects include hot flashes, vaginal dryness, nausea, thromboembolic events (1%-2% of patients), irregular menses in premenopausal women, and an increase in the incidence of endometrial cancer (due to the estrogen-like effect on endometrial tissue).

- Tamoxifen has both anti-estrogen and estrogen-like (agonist) activity.
- Beneficial effects of tamoxifen: 1) decrease in new, contralateral breast cancer in women taking adjuvant tamoxifen; 2) favorable effect on bone density.
- Side effects of tamoxifen: 1) hot flashes, vaginal dryness, nausea, thromboembolic events; 2) increase in endometrial cancer.

Megestrol acetate is a progestational agent. Its side effects include appetite stimulation, weight gain, and fluid retention. *Fluoxymesterone* is an androgen. Side effects are those of virilization with hirsutism, male pattern baldness, deepening of the voice, and clitoromegaly. *Aminoglutethimide* suppresses adrenal steroid synthesis. Thus, addisonian symptoms are usually prevented by also giving glucocorticoid replacement. Side effects, besides adrenal insufficiency, include nausea and anorexia.

Chemotherapy

Active drugs include doxorubicin (Adriamycin, A), cyclophosphamide (C), methotrexate (M), 5-fluorouracil (F), vincristine/vinblastine, mitomycin-C, VP-16, cisplatin, and paclitaxel. Among the most commonly used combinations are CMF, CAF, and AC. Side effects of chemotherapy include reversible lowering of the blood cell counts and reversible hair loss. Severe gastrointestinal side effects are unusual. After 20 years of follow-up, no increase in second malignancies has been noted in patients who have received adjuvant chemotherapy for breast cancer.

Adjuvant Therapy

Adjuvant therapy is that administered in addition to primary localized treatment. It usually refers to systemic therapy.

In patients with *positive nodes*, the following recommendations were put forward by a 1985 National Institutes of Health Consensus Conference on Adjuvant Chemotherapy and Endocrine Therapy for Breast Cancer. Premenopausal patients with positive nodes receive chemotherapy regardless of their estrogen-receptor status (Table 18-4).

- Node-positive premenopausal patients receive chemotherapy regardless of their estrogen-receptor status.

In patients with *negative nodes*, recommendations for adjuvant therapy are less defined. Most of these women are cured with local-regional therapy alone. Nevertheless, recurrent disease develops in 25%-30% of these patients, and thus adjuvant trials have been conducted in this population to attempt to reduce disease recurrences. Several randomized trials comparing adjuvant treatment with no adjuvant treatment have been performed in node-negative breast cancer, and in general the risk of recurrence has been reduced by one-third in the treated patients. Thus, current practice has evolved to treat more and more patients who have node-negative disease. In patients with tumors ≤1 cm in diameter, however, the recurrence rate is so low that adjuvant therapy is generally not recommended.

- Most patients with node-negative breast cancer are cured with local-regional therapy alone.
- Recurrent disease develops in 25%-30% of such patients.
- Risk of recurrence in patients with node-negative disease is reduced by a third with adjuvant treatment.
- Adjuvant therapy not recommended in patients with node-negative disease whose tumors are ≤1 cm in diameter.

Table 18-5 lists general guidelines for adjuvant therapy in patients with negative nodes. These are based on clinical trials that have shown improvement in disease-free survival in treated patients compared with controls; overall survival differences, however, have not been shown with the use of adjuvant treatment in all of these subgroups.

Table 18-4.--Adjuvant Therapy: Node-Positive Breast Cancer

| | Estrogen-receptor status | |
	Positive	Negative
Premenopausal	Chemo	Chemo
Postmenopausal	Tamoxifen	Consider chemo

Chemo, combination chemotherapy.

Table 18-5.--Adjuvant Therapy: Node-Negative Breast Cancer[*]

Tumor size	Management	
≤1 cm	Observe	
>1 cm		
	Estrogen-receptor status	
	Positive	Negative
Premenopausal	Chemotherapy (occasionally tamoxifen)	Chemotherapy
Postmenopausal	Tamoxifen	Consider chemotherapy

[*]Most oncologists treat node-negative tumors ≥2 cm in size; treatment is individualized for tumors of 1-2 cm in size.

In no subset of patients, either node-positive or node-negative, is combined chemotherapy and endocrine therapy routinely recommended. This issue is being actively studied in several settings.

Therapy for Advanced Disease

We currently lack curative therapy for recurrent breast cancer. The median duration of survival in patients with recurrence is approximately 2.5 years from the time of diagnosis of recurrent disease; there is tremendous variability with this disease, however. Survival is longer with bone or soft tissue recurrence than with visceral recurrence. Hormone therapy is generally the initial systemic treatment for patients with estrogen-receptor-positive advanced disease; tamoxifen is usually the first choice, and other approaches include oophorectomy (premenopausal women), megestrol acetate, fluoxymesterone, and aminoglutethimide. Chemotherapy is used in estrogen-receptor-negative disease, rapidly progressive or life-threatening situations, or hormonally refractory disease. Radiation therapy is used for symptomatic localized disease.

- Survival with recurrent breast cancer is about 2.5 years from diagnosis of recurrence.
- Tamoxifen is usually first choice of therapy for estrogen-receptor-positive advanced disease.
- Radiation is used for symptomatic localized disease.

LUNG CANCER

Magnitude of the Problem

Approximately 170,000 new cases of lung cancer are diagnosed in the United States annually, resulting in 150,000 deaths. Thus, only approximately 10% of patients diagnosed with lung cancer survive their disease. Lung cancer is the leading cause of cancer mortality in American men and women.

Risk Factors

About 95% of lung cancers in men and about 80% of lung cancers in women result from cigarette smoking. Men who smoke 1-2 packs per day have up to a 25-fold increase in lung cancer compared with those who have never smoked. The risk of lung cancer in an ex-smoker declines with time. Passive smoking may be associated with an increased risk of lung cancer. Certain occupations (smelter workers, iron workers), chemicals (arsenic, methyl ethyl ether), and exposure to radioactive agents (radon, uranium) have been associated with increased risks for development of lung cancer. Diets high in fruit (possibly due to high β-carotene levels) may offer some protection.

- 95% of lung cancers in men and 80% in women result from cigarette smoking.
- Men who smoke 1-2 packs a day have 25-fold increase in lung cancer compared with those who never smoked.
- Passive smoking may be associated with increased risk of lung cancer.

Screening

The only readily available tools for early detection are chest radiography and sputum cytology. Data from the Mayo Lung Project concluded that "results do not justify recommending large-scale radiologic or cytologic screening for early lung cancer at this time" (Cancer 67:1155-1164, 1991). Prospective population-based studies have shown no improvement in survival by screening with chest radiography or sputum cytology. Contrary positions hold that yearly chest radiography in smokers >50 years old increases the detection rate of stage I disease and improves 5-year survival rate compared with the rates in the general population (Semin Oncol 18:87-98, 1991).

- Only readily available tools for early detection of lung cancer are chest radiography and sputum cytology.
- In prospective population-based studies, survival not improved with screening.
- In smokers >50 years old, yearly chest radiography increases detection of stage I disease.

Histologic Types and Characteristics

Adenocarcinoma typically has a peripheral location. It represents the most frequent histologic subtype found in nonsmokers. Squamous cell cancers are found centrally. They are associated with hypercalcemia (via paraneoplastic parathyroid-hormone-like peptide). They may cavitate. Small-cell carcinomas also occur centrally. They are characterized by prominent adenopathy; the primary tumor may be small. Syndrome of inappropriate antidiuretic hormone secretion and various neurologic abnormalities can occur as associated paraneoplastic syndromes with small-cell carcinomas. Large cell carcinomas may be found peripherally. They are large lesions that may also cavitate.

Staging

The "classic *Tumor-Node-Metastasis*" system is simplified in Table 18-6.

Natural History

The natural history of lung cancer, by stage, is shown in Figure 18-3.

Treatment

Non-Small-Cell Lung Cancer

The treatment of choice is surgical. Resection is safe, presuming reasonably normal cardiac, pulmonary, and other major organ function. Preoperative irradiation has shown no survival benefit in two large prospective trials, although the percentage of patients who had resection was increased. Postoperative radiation therapy has not improved survival over operation alone in any prospective trial. It definitely has no role in node-negative disease. In a prospective trial of patients with node-positive disease who had resection of squamous cell cancers, postoperative irradiation did not improve survival, even though it did significantly decrease the local recurrence rate. Postoperative adjuvant chemotherapy has not consistently improved survival in prospective trials. For nonresectable, localized, non-small-cell lung cancer, the treatment of choice is combined radiation and chemotherapy.

- For early-stage non-small-cell lung cancer, treatment of choice is surgical.
- Preoperative irradiation has shown no survival benefit.
- Postoperative irradiation has not improved survival.
- Postoperative adjuvant chemotherapy has not consistently improved survival.

Table 18-6.--Staging of Lung Cancer

Stage I	Node negative
Stage II	Hilar nodes positive
Stage III	Mediastinal or supraclavicular nodes positive or tumor extends directly into chest wall or mediastinal structures
Stage IV	Distant disease

Simplified staging system for small-cell lung cancer

Limited	Stages I-III (one hemithorax) or disease can be encompassed within one radiation port
Extensive	Metastases

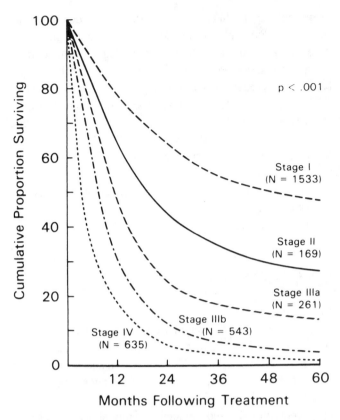

Fig. 18-3. Survival curves for patients with lung cancer by stage. (From Mountain CF: A new international staging system for lung cancer. Chest 89:225S-233S, 1986. By permission of American College of Chest Physicians.)

Small-Cell Lung Cancer

Treatment of limited-stage small-cell lung cancer consists of both chemotherapy and chest irradiation. Operation has not been shown to improve survival. For patients who have a complete response to chemotherapy and chest radiation therapy, prophylactic cranial irradiation is sometimes used to decrease the frequency of failure in the central nervous system. However, even though prophylactic cranial irradiation decreases the rate of relapse in the brain, it does not affect survival. It is associated with the risk of a delayed leukoencephalopathy, but this risk can be reduced by the administration of radiation in small-dose fractions without concomitant chemotherapy. For limited-stage small-cell disease, the median duration of survival is approximately 18 months; 30%-40% of patients survive 2 years, and 10%-20% survive 5 years.

- For small-cell lung cancer, treatment of limited-stage disease is both chemotherapy and chest irradiation.
- Prophylactic cranial irradiation decreases the risk of relapse in the brain but does not affect overall survival.
- Median survival is 18 months.

Treatment of extensive stage (stage IV) small-cell lung cancer is with chemotherapy. Combination chemotherapy is favored over single-agent therapy. Active drugs include etoposide, cisplatin, cyclophosphamide, doxorubicin, and vincristine. High-dose chemotherapy with or without autologous bone marrow transplantation or marrow colony-stimulating factors has not yet been proved superior, on a consistent basis, to standard chemotherapy. The median duration of survival is approximately 9 months; about 10% of patients survive 2 years, and ≤1% survive 5 years.

- For extensive stage small-cell lung cancer, treatment is chemotherapy.
- High-dose chemotherapy has not yet been proved superior to standard chemotherapy.
- Median survival is 9 months.

COLORECTAL CANCER

Background

Colorectal cancer is diagnosed in approximately 150,000 Americans each year and causes 60,000 deaths. Colorectal cancer is most common in North America and Europe. It is associated with high-fat, low-fiber diets. Population screening with fecal occult blood testing remains problematic. Although one recent study showed a reduction in mortality from colorectal cancer with fecal occult blood screening (N Engl J Med 328:1365-1371, 1993), it should be noted that any participants who had positive results went on to have colonoscopy. Another recent study showed that fecal occult blood tests failed to detect 70% of colorectal cancers and 80% of large (≥2 cm) polyps (JAMA 269:1262-1267, 1993). For high-risk patients, such as those with a family history of colorectal cancer or a prior colorectal cancer, structural studies of the entire large bowel, such as colonoscopy or proctoscopy plus barium enema, should be performed at appropriate intervals (e.g., every 1-3 years).

- Colorectal cancer associated with high-fat, low-fiber diets.
- For colorectal cancer, fecal occult blood testing was shown to decrease mortality in one study.
- For high-risk patients, entire large bowel should be studied at appropriate intervals.

Risk Factors

High-risk groups include persons with 1) familial polyposis syndromes (familial adenomatous polyposis--gene recently identified on chromosome 5--and Gardner's syndrome--gut polyps plus desmoid tumors, lipomas, sebaceous cysts, and other abnormalities); 2) familial cancer syndromes without polyps (hereditary nonpolyposis coli or Lynch syndromes, which are marked by colon cancer with or without endometrial, breast, and other cancers); and 3) inflammatory bowel disease.

- High-risk factors are familial polyposis syndromes, including Gardner's syndrome (gut polyps, desmoid tumors, lipo-

mas, sebaceous cysts, other abnormalities); select familial cancer syndromes; and inflammatory bowel disease.

Treatment

Surgery

Surgical resection is the preferred method of curative treatment for carcinomas of the colon or rectum. The probability of cure is highly related to stage of disease (Table 18-7), which is determined by the depth of penetration through the bowel wall and the involvement of regional nodes (Table 18-8). Cancers of the rectum tend to have a worse prognosis than cancers of the colon, stage for stage.

- Preferred treatment for colorectal cancer is surgical resection.
- Cure rate is related to stage of disease.
- Cancer of rectum has worse prognosis than cancer of colon.

Adjuvant Therapy

For *rectal cancer*, adjuvant pelvic irradiation and 5-fluorouracil are recommended for deeply invasive or node-positive lesions. For *colon cancer*, adjuvant 5-fluorouracil and levamisole are recommended for node-positive disease. Levamisole is an antihelminthic drug that has immunomodulatory activity, and it may also potentiate the cytotoxicity of 5-fluorouracil.

- For rectal cancer, adjuvant therapy includes pelvic irradiation and 5-fluorouracil.
- For colon cancer, adjuvant therapy includes 5-fluorouracil and levamisole.

Table 18-7.--Survival Rates in Colorectal Cancer, by Stage

5-year survival (surgery only), %	AJCC stage	Dukes stage
90	I	A
60-80	II	B
30-60	III	C

AJCC, American Joint Committee on Cancer.

Table 18-8.--Staging of Colorectal Cancer, by Depth of Penetration

Depth of penetration	Node	Modified Dukes stage
Mucosa	Negative	A
Into or through bowel wall	Negative	B
	Positive	C

Metastatic Disease

Select patients with minimal advanced or stage IV colorectal cancer may be candidates for an attempt at curative resection of their metastatic disease. Of carefully selected patients with limited metastatic disease to the liver or occasionally the lung, 25% will survive beyond 5 years without further evidence of disease recurrence.

The vast majority of patients with advanced or metastatic colorectal cancer are incurable with present techniques but are candidates for palliative chemotherapy. The use of leucovorin, a modulator of 5-fluorouracil, along with 5-fluorouracil is a standard approach. This yields tumor response rates ranging from 30%-40% and a 4- to 5-month longer median survival than in patients who receive 5-fluorouracil alone. The median survival is 6 months for patients treated with 5-fluorouracil alone and 10-12 months for those treated with 5-fluorouracil and leucovorin. Patients with indolent metastatic colon cancer who are asymptomatic may be observed without treatment, occasionally for prolonged periods.

- Select patients with limited disease may be candidates for curative resection.
- For patients with colorectal cancer who have metastatic disease, the vast majority are incurable.
- 5-Fluorouracil plus leucovorin is standard therapy.

Carcinoembryonic Antigen (CEA)

Proponents of CEA monitoring after operation for colorectal cancer argue that early recurrences, curable surgically, can be detected. However, CEA monitoring lacks sensitivity and specificity. It is estimated that cancer cures attributable to CEA monitoring occur in less than 1% of patients monitored (JAMA 270:943-947, 1993).

PROSTATE CANCER

Background

There are 240,000 new cases of prostate cancer annually in the United States. It is the most common cancer in men in the United States and is the second leading cause of death from cancer in men in the United States (40,000 deaths annually). The American Cancer Society recommends a digital rectal examination in men aged 40 years or older and determination of the prostate-specific antigen (PSA) value in men 50 years or older. Use of the PSA value for prostate cancer screening is a controversial issue and has not been shown to reduce mortality.

- Prostate cancer is most common cancer in men in the United States (240,000 cases annually).
- Prostate cancer is second leading cause of death from cancer in men in the United States (40,000 deaths annually).

Prognostic factors include stage of disease and grade of malignancy. The Gleason scoring system is used for grading: grading ranges from 1 (better differentiated, better prognosis) to 5 (less differentiated, worse prognosis). More than one pattern of differentiation may be present in a surgical specimen. The pathologist grades the two predominant ones individually and adds them to yield a final Gleason grade (e.g., $3 + 5 = 8$). Gleason grades 2-6 are associated with a better prognosis.

- Prognostic factors for prostate cancer are stage and grade.
- Gleason grades 2-6 have better prognosis.

Management

Management of Specific Stages

Table 18-9 simplifies the staging of prostate cancer. In general, patients with stage A1 disease are observed without treatment. Controversies surround the treatment of all other stages of this disease. For organ-confined prostate cancer (stages A2 [T1B], T1C, B [T2]), both radiation therapy and radical prostatectomy are equally viable options. Recently, some investigators have proposed observation alone and treatment with hormonal agents at the time of progression because the rate of death from prostate cancer is low for early-stage disease. A large trial is currently under way in the United States to test the value of operation compared with observation for organ-confined prostate cancer. For stage C (T3) disease (locally advanced), x-ray therapy is usually used. Some centers use androgen deprivation, and other centers use an aggressive surgical approach.

For stage D1 disease (positive pelvic nodes), the management is controversial. Divergent approaches include androgen deprivation alone, x-ray therapy with or without androgen

Table 18-9.--Staging of Prostate Cancer

Stage	Criteria
A1 (T1A)	Incidental focus of tumor in ≤ 5% of specimen
A2 (T1B)	Incidental tumor in more than 5% of tissue
T1C	Tumor identified by needle biopsy (performed because of increased PSA value)
B1 (T2A)	Involvement of half or less of one lobe
B2 (T2B)	Involvement of more than half of lobe but not both lobes
B3 (T2C)	Involvement of both lobes
C (T3)	Extracapsular local disease
D1	Pelvic nodal involvement
D2	Distant disease

deprivation, close observation with androgen deprivation at progression, or prostatectomy with androgen deprivation.

For advanced (D2) disease, bone is the most frequent site of metastatic disease. Hormonal therapy, although it is very effective and produces a response in most patients, is noncurative. The average duration of response to initial hormonal maneuver is 18 months. The average duration of survival is 2-3 years. Once the disease progresses after the initial hormonal maneuver, it is typically very refractory to secondary treatment attempts (e.g., hormonal or chemotherapy).

- Bone is the most frequent site of metastatic disease from prostate.
- Hormonal therapy is effective and produces a response, but it is noncurative.
- Average duration of survival with advanced prostatic cancer is 2-3 years.

Prostatectomy

This is reserved for patients with localized disease. The 15-year disease-specific survival rate after prostatectomy is 85%-90% for stage A2 or B disease. Impotence occurs in most patients, especially older individuals. Urinary incontinence is rare (<2% of patients).

- Prostatectomy used for localized disease.
- 15-year survival rate is 85%-90% for stage A2 or B disease.

Radiation Therapy

External beam radiotherapy is considered the equivalent of prostatectomy. It is preferred for stage C disease at most centers. Impotence can occur, but less often than with prostatectomy. A concern related to radiotherapy is that repeat biopsies after treatment have shown apparently viable tumor in >35% of patients. The clinical importance of this residual tumor is unclear, but there may be a correlation with the subsequent appearance of distant metastasis, especially with a persistent, palpable abnormality in the gland.

- External beam radiotherapy is considered the equivalent of prostatectomy at most centers.
- Impotence is less frequent with radiotherapy than prostatectomy.

Androgen Deprivation

The two sources of androgens in men are the testes (testosterone, 95%) and adrenal glands (5%). Androgen deprivation can be accomplished surgically with orchiectomy or medically. Potential agents include luteinizing hormone-releasing hormone (LHRH) agonists such as leuprolide, buserelin, and goserelin. They decrease androgen levels through continuous binding of the LHRH receptor and subsequent decrease of LH and thus testosterone. They are administered as a monthly injection of a depot preparation. LHRH agonists, on initial binding of the LHRH receptor, transiently stimulate LH release and thus cause an initial increase in the testosterone level. This explains the transient flare of prostate cancer that can occur in men with advanced disease when therapy with an LHRH agonist is first started. This possibility must be considered in patients with impending spinal cord compression or urinary obstruction.

- Androgen deprivation is accomplished with orchiectomy or medically.
- Luteinizing hormone-releasing hormone agonists depress androgen levels.
- These agonists initially stimulate a transient release of luteinizing hormone and testosterone.

Antiandrogens compete with androgens at the receptor level. Examples include cyproterone and flutamide. To effect total androgen blockade, an antiandrogen is added to therapy in patients who have had orchiectomy or who are receiving an LHRH agonist (these block testicular testosterone production but do not block adrenal androgen production). A prospective U.S. study combining an LHRH analog with flutamide versus placebo suggested an advantage for the addition of flutamide. However, other studies of total blockade have failed to show an advantage. Studies comparing orchiectomy alone with orchiectomy plus flutamide are under way in the United States. One advantage of flutamide is that it blocks the "flare" induced by LHRH agonists.

- Some physicians believe flutamide should be used in combination with orchiectomy or LHRH agonist.
- Flutamide blocks "flare" induced by LHRH agonists.

Prostate-Specific Antigen (PSA)

PSA is produced by normal and neoplastic prostatic ductal epithelium. Its concentration is proportional to the total prostatic mass. The inability to differentiate benign prostatic hyperplasia from carcinoma on the basis of the PSA level renders it inadequate as the sole screening method for prostate cancer. PSA is useful for monitoring response to therapy in cases of known prostate cancer, particularly after radical prostatectomy, when PSA should be undetectable.

- Concentration of PSA is proportional to total prostatic mass.
- The PSA test is inadequate as sole screening test for prostate cancer.
- PSA is useful for monitoring response to therapy.

OVARIAN CANCER

This disease is diagnosed annually in 20,000 American women. It is the leading cause of death due to gynecologic cancer. There are no early warning signs; most patients present with vague gastrointestinal complaints such as bloating. Most patients (75%) present with advanced disease (i.e., stages III and IV, disease spread beyond the pelvis). The term "ovarian cancer" encompasses tumors derived from the ovarian surface epithelium, not germ cell tumors.

Staging

Stage I is confined to the ovary, stage II is confined to the pelvis, stage III includes spread to the upper abdomen, and stage IV includes spread to distant sites.

- Ovarian cancer is leading cause of death due to gynecologic cancer.
- There are no early warning signs.
- Most patients (75%) present with advanced disease.

Screening

The tools evaluated thus far, namely, pelvic ultrasonography and determination of serum cancer antigen CA-125 are inadequate for screening the general female population. Screening for this disease is difficult for several reasons. The incidence of ovarian cancer is relatively low, and there are no recognized pre-invasive lesions. Moreover, pelvic ultrasonography and CA-125 lack sufficient sensitivity and specificity. However, it seems reasonable to apply these techniques on a periodic basis to women at particularly high risk of ovarian cancer, for example, those with a significant family history of the disease (two or more affected relatives). The cause of epithelial ovarian cancer is unknown. A small subset of patients (<5%) has an inherited predisposition to this disease. Generally, this occurs in families with both breast and ovarian cancer.

- Population screening for ovarian cancer is not recommended.
- Pelvic ultrasonography and CA-125 lack sufficient sensitivity and specificity.
- A small subset of patients (<5%) has an inherited predisposition to ovarian cancer and should be screened.

Treatment

The initial management of patients with epithelial ovarian cancer includes a thorough surgical staging and debulking procedure. Outcome in this disease depends on the amount of tumor tissue removed at initial operation. Subsequently, patients are treated with at least six cycles of platinum- and paclitaxel-based chemotherapy. Generally, paclitaxel and cisplatin are the favored approaches. The tumor antigen, CA-125, is expressed by approximately 85% of epithelial ovarian tumors and released into the circulation. The highest serum levels of CA-125 are found in patients with ovarian cancer, but the serum CA-125 level may also be increased in other malignancies, as well as in pregnancy, endometriosis, and menstruation. CA-125 is clearly of value for monitoring the course of ovarian cancer.

- Management of ovarian cancer includes thorough surgical staging and debulking followed by chemotherapy.
- Outcome depends on the amount of tumor tissue removed at initial operation.
- CA-125 is expressed by about 85% of epithelial ovarian tumors.
- CA-125 level may also be increased in other malignancies and in pregnancy, endometriosis, and menstruation.
- CA-125 is useful for monitoring course of disease.

TESTICULAR CANCER

Background

This cancer is diagnosed in 6,000 to 7,000 men annually. It is the most common carcinoma in males aged 15 to 35 years. It is highly curable, even when metastatic. At high risk are males with cryptorchid testes (40-fold relative risk) or Klinefelter's syndrome (also increased risk of breast cancer). Two broad categories are seminomas (40%) and nonseminomas. Types of nonseminomas include embryonal carcinoma, mature and immature teratoma, choriocarcinoma, yolk sac, and endodermal sinus tumors. There is often an admixture of several cell types within nonseminomas. Any nonseminomatous component plus seminoma is treated as a nonseminoma.

- Testicular cancer is the most common carcinoma in males 15-35 years old.
- Testicular cancer is highly curable, even when metastatic.
- High-risk factors: cryptorchid testes, Klinefelter's syndrome.
- Two categories: seminomas (40%) and nonseminomas.

Evaluation includes determination of β-human chorionic gonadotropin (hCG) and α-fetoprotein values and computed tomography of the abdomen (retroperitoneal nodes) and chest (mediastinal nodes or pulmonary nodules).

Staging

Stage I disease is confined to the testis, stage II includes infradiaphragmatic nodal metastases, stage III includes supradiaphragmatic nodal metastases, and stage IV includes extranodal metastases. About 85% of nonseminomas have elevated β-hCG or α-fetoprotein value. Approximately 10% of seminomas have increased β-hCG level. α-Fetoprotein value is never increased in pure seminoma; if it is increased, the tumor is nonseminoma and should be treated as such.

- 85% of nonseminomas have elevated β-hCG or α-fetoprotein value.
- 10% of seminomas have increased β-hCG.
- α-Fetoprotein value is never increased in pure seminoma.

Management

Radical (inguinal) orchiectomy is the definitive procedure for both pathologic diagnosis and local control. Scrotal orchiectomy or biopsy is associated with a high incidence of local recurrence or spread to inguinal nodes. After orchiectomy, the management depends on cell type (Table 18-10). Seminomas are radiosensitive. For stage I and nonbulky stage II seminoma, infradiaphragmatic lymphatic irradiation is used. The 5-year disease-free survival rate is >95%. For bulky stage II disease and stages III and IV, platinum-based chemotherapy is used. Approximately 85% of patients are cured. For stage I nonseminoma, close follow-up is often used rather than immediate retroperitoneal node dissection (a controversial issue). For stages II through IV, platinum-based chemotherapy is given. Cure rates are >95% for minimal metastatic disease, 90% for moderate bulk disease, and about 50% for bulky disease (multiple pulmonary metastases, bulky abdominal masses, liver, bone, or central nervous system metastases).

- Radical orchiectomy is the definitive initial procedure for testicular cancer.
- Early-stage seminoma is treated with x-ray therapy.
- Stage I nonseminoma may require no treatment after orchiectomy.
- Platinum-based chemotherapy is used for all other patients and results in high cure rates.

Extragonadal Germ Cell Tumor

This is uncommon. Patients present with elevated hCG or α-fetoprotein values with midline mass lesions (retroperitoneum, mediastinum, or pineal gland). No gonadal primary tumor is identifiable on examination or ultrasonography. Cisplatin-based chemotherapy is frequently curative.

MELANOMA

Background

Malignant melanoma is increasing at a rapid rate. If current trends continue, by the year 2000 approximately 1% of Americans will have a malignant melanoma. Fortunately, the 5-year survival rate has doubled from approximately 40% in the 1940s to approximately 80% now, a change attributed to earlier detection. This disease is far more common in populations living at high altitudes and those living close to the equator. Its incidence is higher in fair-skinned persons and certain families (dysplastic nevus syndrome).

- Incidence of malignant melanoma is increasing rapidly.
- 5-year survival rate has doubled as a result of earlier detection.
- Disease is related to sunlight exposure.

Diagnosis ("ABCD") and Prognosis

Keys to the diagnosis include the following:

A: Asymmetry, especially a changing lesion
B: Borders are irregular
C: Color is variable, especially with blues, blacks, and tans dispersed throughout the lesion
D: Diameter ≥6 mm

Excisional biopsy is recommended. The thickness (i.e., depth of penetration of the tumor from the epidermis into the dermis/subcutis) of a malignant melanoma is the best independent predictor of survival (Table 18-11).

Management

Surgical excision remains the principal treatment for primary malignant melanoma. The preferred approach is wide local excision to achieve a 1- to 3-cm margin. In the absence of palpable adenopathy, a lymph node dissection is not routinely performed. However, with palpable nodes, a node dissection is standard practice. Metastatic melanoma is incurable with current approaches.

PARANEOPLASTIC SYNDROMES

General

These syndromes are defined as the effects of a cancer occurring at a distance from the tumor; they are called "remote effects." They do not indicate metastatic disease. The syndromes and associated tumor types are listed in Table 18-12.

Table 18-10.--Management of Testicular Cancer

Stage	Treatment, by cell type	
	Seminona	Nonseminoma
I	XRT	? Observe
II	XRT	Chemo
III	Chemo	Chemo
IV	Chemo	Chemo

Chemo, chemotherapy; XRT, x-ray therapy.

Table 18-11.--Ten-Year Survival in Melanoma, by Depth of Tumor

Depth, mm	% alive
<0.85	96
0.85-1.69	87
1.7-3.6	66.5
>3.6	46

Data from Friedman RJ, Rigel DS, Silverman MK, Kopf AW, Vossaert KA: Malignant melanoma in the 1990s: the continued importance of early detection and the role of physician examination and self-examination of the skin. CA Cancer J Clin 41:201-226, July/Aug 1991.

Carcinoid Syndrome

This is caused by peptide mediators secreted by carcinoid tumors of the small intestine which have metastasized extensively to the liver. It is less frequent with primary carcinoids arising from other sites such as lung, thymus, or ovary. The most common symptoms are episodic flushing and diarrhea; bronchospasm may occur. Flushing and diarrhea may occur spontaneously or be precipitated by emotional factors or ingestion of food or alcohol. Carcinoid heart disease (right-sided valvular disease) is a potential late complication.

Lambert-Eaton Syndrome

This consists of muscle weakness (proximal) and gait disturbance. Strength is increased with exercise. It is associated with small-cell lung cancer.

Dermatomyositis

The female:male ratio is 2:1. Findings include muscle weakness (proximal), inflammatory myopathy, and increased creatine kinase values. Skin changes are variable and include heliotrope rash, periorbital edema, and Gottron's papules. Underlying malignancy (lung, breast, gastrointestinal) is common in patients >50 years old.

CHEMOTHERAPY

Basic Concepts

Currently, approximately 40 cytotoxic agents are available for use in North America. Taken generally, chemotherapeutic agents impair the process of cell division. Their selectivity for tumor cells is based primarily on a higher replicative rate in neoplastic cells. This selectivity for rapidly dividing cells explains the typical patterns of toxicity that occur with chemotherapy (i.e., bone marrow, gastrointestinal mucosa, and hair follicles). The general classes and mechanisms of chemotherapeutics are shown in Figure 18-4.

Table 18-12.--Classification of Paraneoplastic Syndromes

Syndrome	Mediator	Tumor type
Endocrine		
Cushing's syndrome[*]	ACTH	Small-cell lung cancer
SIADH[*]	ADH	Lung, especially small cell
Hypercalcemia[*]	PTH-like peptide	Lung, especially squamous; breast; myeloma
Carcinoid syndrome	? serotonin ? substance P	Gut neuroendocrine tumors
Hypoglycemia	Insulin Insulin-like growth factors	Gut neuroendocrine tumors; other
Neuromuscular		
Cerebellar degeneration	Anti-Purkinje cell antibodies	Lung, especially small cell; ovarian; breast
Dementia	?	Lung
Peripheral neuropathy[*]	Autoantibodies	Lung, gastrointestinal, breast
Lambert-Eaton	Antibodies to cholinergic receptor	Small-cell lung cancer
Dermatomyositis	?	Lung, breast
Skin		
Dermatomyositis	?	Lung, breast
Acanthosis nigricans	? TGF-α	Intra-abdominal cancer, usually gastric
Hematologic		
Venous thrombosis[*]	Activators of clotting cascade and platelets	Various adenocarcinomas, especially pancreatic and gastric
Nonbacterial thrombotic endocarditis	Activators of clotting cascade and platelets	Various adenocarcinomas, especially pancreatic and gastric

[*]Most common types.

ACTH, adrenocorticotropic hormone; ADH, antidiuretic hormone; PTH, parathyroid hormone; SIADH, syndrome of inappropriate secretion of antidiuretic hormone; TGF-α, transforming growth factor-α.

CHEMOTHERAPY

Fig. 18-4. General classes of chemotherapeutic agents.

Applications

The settings in which chemotherapy is used are 1) advanced disease, 2) as adjuvant therapy after definitive local treatment, and 3) as primary or "neo-adjuvant" therapy. The last application refers to situations in which patients present with a locally advanced malignancy and initial tumor reduction is needed before a primary treatment (i.e., surgery or radiation) can be applied.

Solid Tumors Sensitive to Chemotherapy

Germ cell tumors of the testis and ovary, choriocarcinomas, breast cancer, ovarian cancer, and small-cell lung cancer are in this category. In recent years, combination chemotherapy regimens have also produced impressive tumor reductions in transitional cell carcinomas of the bladder, head and neck cancer, and cervical cancer.

Why Chemotherapy Fails to Cure Most Advanced Solid Tumors

The reasons for failure are 1) tumor cell heterogeneity, including populations of cells resistant to cytotoxic agents; 2) large numbers of noncycling or resting cells; and 3) pharmacologic sanctuaries--blood-tissue barriers and blood supply-tumor barriers.

Side Effects

The most common side effects of various chemotherapeutic agents are outlined in Table 18-13.

Mechanisms of Tumor Cell Drug Resistance

The mechanisms include decreased drug uptake, increased drug efflux, decreased drug activation, increased drug inactivation, and increased production of a target enzyme.

Tumor cells may be resistant to a specific drug or they can have broad cross-resistance to structurally dissimilar drugs. This latter phenomenon is referred to as "multidrug resistance." This seems to be mediated by a large plasma membrane glycoprotein, termed the "p-glycoprotein," that functions as an energy-dependent drug-efflux pump.

● Tumor cells may be resistant to structurally dissimilar chemotherapy drugs ("multidrug resistance").

Colony-Stimulating Factors

In recent years, bone marrow colony-stimulating factors have been isolated and are now available for clinical use. These naturally occurring glycoproteins stimulate the proliferation, differentiation, and function of specific cells in the bone marrow. They may act at the level of the earliest stem cell or at

Table 18-13.--Side Effects of Chemotherapy

Class or agent	Side effects	
	Acute	Chronic
Alkylating agents	Nausea, vomiting Marrow: cytopenias	Marrow: secondary leukemias Pulmonary Gonads: decreased fertility, premature menopause

Cisplatin	Nausea, vomiting
	Renal: $\downarrow$ GFR; tubular damage
	  leads to electrolyte losses,
	  especially cations
	Peripheral neuropathy
	Tinnitus, hearing loss
		Renal: $\downarrow$ GFR; tubular damage and
		  electrolyte losses, especially cations
		
		Peripheral neuropathy
		Tinnitus, hearing loss

Doxorubicin	Nausea, vomiting
	Marrow
	Cardiac
	  Pump or conduction
	Stomatitis
		Cardiac
		  Congestive heart failure
		  Cumulative, dose-dependent, occurs in
		    1%-10% of patients receiving 550 mg/m^2

Bleomycin	Pulmonary Skin (hyperpigmentation) Fever	Pulmonary (may be aggravated by high F_{IO_2}, as in perioperative period)
Antimetabolites	Mucositis/diarrhea Marrow	
Microtubule inhibitors Vincristine	Neuropathy	Neuropathy
Taxol	Cardiac: conduction	

F_{IO_2}, fraction of inspired oxygen; GFR, glomerular filtration rate.

later mature functional cells. They differ in their specificity.

Granulocyte colony-stimulating factor (G-CSF), for example, acts fairly specifically to stimulate the production of mature neutrophils; granulocyte-macrophage CSF (GM-CSF) acts more generally, stimulating several cell lineages, including monocytes, eosinophils, and neutrophils. Both G-CSF and GM-CSF have been used to stimulate the marrow to recover after chemotherapy-induced myelosuppression. As a general rule, CSFs do not affect the depth of the leukocyte nadir but shorten the duration of neutropenia. Unfortunately, no currently available CSF reliably protects against thrombocytopenia.

ONCOLOGIC COMPLICATIONS AND EMERGENCIES

Hypercalcemia

The most common underlying causes are malignancies and primary hyperparathyroidism. Patients with primary hyperparathyroidism have elevated serum parathyroid hormone (PTH) values, but PTH is suppressed in cancer-associated hypercalcemia. Cancer-related hypercalcemia is often mediated by

a PTH-related protein secreted by the tumor. This PTH-related protein can be detected with current assays. Tumors can also cause hypercalcemia by secreting other bone-resorbing substances or by enhancing conversion of 25-hydroxyvitamin D to 1,25-dihydroxyvitamin D. Another mechanism is due to the local effects of osteolytic bone metastases.

Effects on bone and kidney contribute to hypercalcemia. Accelerated bone resorption is due to activation of osteoclasts by various mediators, primarily the PTH-like peptide. The same factors that induce osteoclast-mediated bone resorption also stimulate renal tubular reabsorption of calcium. The hypercalcemic state interferes with renal resorption of sodium and water, leading to polyuria and eventual depletion of extracellular fluid volume. This reduces the glomerular filtration rate, further increasing the serum calcium level. Immobilization tips the balance toward bone resorption, worsening the hypercalcemia.

- PTH is suppressed in cancer-associated hypercalcemia.
- This disease is often mediated by PTH-related protein secreted by a tumor.
- Bone and kidney pathophysiology lead to elevated calcium level.

Symptoms of hypercalcemia include gastrointestinal (anorexia, nausea, vomiting, constipation), renal (polyuria, polydipsia, dehydration), central nervous system (cognitive difficulties, apathy, somnolence, or even coma), and cardiovascular (hypertension, shortened QT, enhanced sensitivity to digitalis).

Cancers associated with hypercalcemia include lung (squamous cell), renal, myeloma, lymphoma, breast, and head and neck. Patients with breast cancer and those with myeloma are more likely to have bony involvement with their disease.

For treatment of hypercalcemia, the magnitude of the hypercalcemia and the degree of symptoms are key considerations. Generally, patients with a serum calcium value >14 mg/dL should be hospitalized for immediate treatment. The serum calcium value should be adjusted if the serum albumin value is abnormal. The conversion formula is 0.8 mg/dL of serum total calcium for every 1 g of serum albumin more or less than 4 g/dL. If the serum albumin value is elevated (as with dehydration), the total calcium value should be adjusted downward; if the serum albumin value is reduced (as in chronic illness), the total calcium value should be adjusted upward.

For hydration, intravenously administered normal saline (200-400 mL/hr) is initially given. Loop diuretics are used *after* volume expansion. Furosemide facilitates urinary excretion of calcium by inhibiting calcium resorption in the thick ascending loop of Henle. A loop diuretic will help correct for volume overload once the patient has been rehydrated. Specific agents are listed below:

1. Bisphosphonates (pamidronate or etidronate) are given intravenously (gastrointestinal absorption is poor). They bind to hydroxyapatite and inhibit osteoclasts.
2. Gallium nitrate (200 mg/m^2 per day) is given as continuous intravenous infusion for 5 days (unless normocalcemia is achieved earlier). It is a highly effective inhibitor of bone resorption.
3. Mithramycin (25 µg/kg) is given intravenously over 4 hours; this treatment can be repeated if necessary. Maximal hypocalcemic effect is reached at 48-72 hours. It is associated with hepatic and renal side effects.
4. Glucocorticoids have an antitumor effect on neoplastic lymphoid tissue.
5. Calcitonin is given subcutaneously or intramuscularly. It has a rapid onset of action; thus, it is useful in immediate life-threatening situations. It is a relatively weak agent with short-lived effect. Allergic reactions to salmon calcitonin are unusual, but an initial skin test with 1 unit is recommended before a full dose is given.

- Volume expansion must precede administration of furosemide.
- Furosemide inhibits calcium resorption in thick ascending loop of Henle.

- Bisphosphonates bind to hydroxyapatite and inhibit osteoclasts.
- Mithramycin has hepatic and renal side effects.
- Calcitonin is a relatively weak agent with rapid, short-lived effect.

Tumor Lysis Syndrome

This syndrome occurs as a result of the overwhelming release of tumor cell contents into the bloodstream such that concentrations of certain substances become life-threatening. It most commonly occurs in cancers with large tumor burdens and high proliferation rates which are exquisitely sensitive to chemotherapy. Examples include high-grade lymphomas, leukemia, and, much less commonly, solid tumors. The syndrome is characterized by increased uric acid, which leads to renal complications; acidosis; increased potassium, which can cause lethal cardiac arrhythmias; increased phosphate, which leads to acute renal failure; and decreased calcium, which causes muscle cramps, cardiac arrhythmias, and tetany. The syndrome can be prevented with adequate hydration, alkalinization, and administration of allopurinol before chemotherapy.

- Tumor lysis syndrome is a result of overwhelming release of tumor cell contents into bloodstream.
- It is most common in cancers with large tumor burdens and high proliferation rates exquisitely sensitive to chemotherapy.
- It is characterized by increased uric acid, increased potassium, increased phosphate, acidosis, and decreased calcium.

Febrile Neutropenia

This is defined as temperature ≥38.5°C on one occasion or three episodes ≥38.0°C plus an absolute neutrophil count ≤500 x 10^9/L (or leukocyte count ≤1,000 x 10^9/L). Management involves immediate hospitalization and institution of parenteral, broad-spectrum antibiotics. Patients usually have no infection documented, but appropriate cultures should be rapidly obtained before antibiotics are given. Use of colony-stimulating factors at the time of documentation of febrile neutropenia is not routine.

Spinal Cord Compression

Acute cord compression is a neurologic emergency. It results most commonly from epidural compression by metastatic tumor (lung, breast, prostate, myeloma, kidney). Occasionally, compression can occur from neighboring nodal involvement and tumor infiltration through intervertebral foramina (lymphoma). The locations are cervical in 10% of cases, thoracic in 70%, and lumbar in 20%. Multiple noncontiguous levels are involved in 10%-40%.

More than 90% of patients present with pain. Cervical pain may radiate down the arm. Thoracic pain radiates around the rib cage or abdominal wall; it may be described as a compressing band bilaterally around the chest or abdomen. Lumbar pain may radiate into the groin or down the leg. Pain may be aggravated by coughing, sneezing, or straight-leg raising. Focal neurologic signs depend on the level affected. Paresthesias (tingling, numbness), weakness, and altered reflexes also can be present (Table 18-14). Tenderness over the spine may help localize the level. Autonomic changes of urinary or fecal retention or incontinence may be present.

Imaging studies include bone scanning or plain radiography, which reveal vertebral metastases in approximately 85% of patients with epidural compression. Myelography or magnetic resonance imaging of the entire spine is generally recommended.

Treatment usually includes an initial bolus of 10-100 mg of dexamethasone intravenously, depending on the severity of block. Thereafter, dexamethasone is given (4 mg four times a day), although some physicians favor higher doses for a few days followed by a rapid taper. Radiation therapy is applied to the involved area(s). Operation is used in select circumstances: if no previous diagnosis of malignancy, spine instability, prior radiation to cord tolerance, and progressive neurologic decline despite radiation.

Outcome depends on the patient's neurologic function at presentation (Table 18-15).

PALLIATIVE CARE

Background

More than 70% of patients with cancer have significant pain during the course of their disease. Evaluation should include 1) a history regarding onset, quality, severity, and location of pain; exacerbating and relieving factors; associated symptoms; and 2) physical examination, which should include a complete neurologic examination. Diagnostic studies are determined by the results of the history and physical examination.

Treatment

Three-Tiered Approach

Step 1: For mild pain, administer acetaminophen or a nonsteroidal anti-inflammatory drug around-the-clock.

Step 2: When step 1 fails to provide adequate analgesia, or for moderate pain, add codeine or oxycodone.

Step 3: For severe pain or inadequate pain relief with steps 1 and 2, agents include morphine, hydromorphone, levorphanol, methadone, and fentanyl (Table 18-16).

General Principles

Choose the appropriate drug and route. Generally, the oral route is preferred. Orally administered immediate-release morphine is the usual first-line drug selected for severe pain from cancer. Begin with a low dose. Titrate the dose until analgesia is achieved or side effects occur. There is no "standard dose"; therapy must be individualized. Use around-the-clock dosing with "rescue" doses available to the patient for breakthrough pain. The fentanyl patch (a transdermal formulation) delivers drug continuously over 72 hours. It is especially useful for patients with poor tolerance of orally administered opioids or those unable to take medications orally. Adverse effects of opioids include sedation, nausea, constipation, respiratory depression, and myoclonus. No narcotic is more or less likely to result in a particular side effect profile. However, one narcotic may produce an adverse effect in a patient whereas another will not. Thus, sequential trials of different opioids may be needed to determine the one best suited for a patient.

Table 18-14.--Reflexes and Their Corresponding Roots and Muscles

Reflex	Root(s)	Muscle
Biceps	C5-6	Biceps
Triceps	C7-8	Triceps
Knee jerk	L2-4	Quadriceps
Ankle jerk	S1	Gastrocnemius

Table 18-15.--Outcome of Patients With Spinal Cord Compression, by Neurologic Status

Status at presentation	% ambulatory after radiation
Ambulatory	>80
Paraparetic	<50
Paraplegic	<10

Table 18-16.--Doses of Narcotics That Provide Equal Analgesia

Drug	Doses of equal analgesia	Half-life, hr	Peak effect, hr	Duration of effect, hr
Morphine	10 mg i.m./i.v.	2-4	0.5-1	4-6
	20-60 mg p.o.*	2-4	2	4-6
Slow-release morphine	20-60 mg p.o.*	3-4	4-6	8-12
Hydromorphone	1.5 mg i.m	2-3	0.5-1	4-6
	7.5 mg p.o.	2-3	1-2	4-6
Levorphanol	2.0 mg i.m.	12-16	0.5-1	4-6
	4.0 mg p.o.	12-16	1	4-6
Methadone	10 mg i.m.	15-150+	0.5-1.5	4-6
	20 mg p.o.	15-150+	0.5-1.5	4-6
Codeine	130 mg i.m.	2-4	1	4-6
	200 mg p.o.	2-4	1-2	4-6
Oxycodone	30 mg p.o.	2-3	1	3-6
Meperidine	75 mg i.m.	3-4	0.5-1	3-5
	300 mg p.o.	3-4	1-2	4-6
Fentanyl	0.1 mg i.v.	3-4	0.25	0.5-2
	Transdermal patch	See text	See text	72

*Relative potency of intramuscular:oral morphine changes from 1:6 to 1:2-3 with chronic dosing.
i.m., intramuscular; i.v., intravenous; p.o., oral dose.
Modified from Foley KM: The treatment of cancer pain. N Engl J Med 313:84-95, 1985. By permission of the journal.

QUESTIONS

Multiple Choice (choose the one best answer)

1. The number one cause of cancer deaths in American women is:
   a. Ovarian cancer
   b. Breast cancer
   c. Lung cancer
   d. Acute leukemia
   e. Colon cancer

2. Which of the following is the best predictor of outcome in patients with breast cancer?
   a. Age
   b. Tumor size
   c. Estrogen-receptor status
   d. Lymph node status
   e. Cathepsin-D expression

3. Which of the following is not an expected effect of tamoxifen use?

a. Hot flashes
b. Endometrial cancer
c. Stabilization of bone density
d. Thromboembolic events
e. Increase in serum cholesterol

4. A 38-year-old woman finds a lump in her right breast. A biopsy reveals infiltrating lobular carcinoma. Axillary node dissection reveals tumor in 1 of 19 nodes. The estrogen receptor is positive at 60 fmol/mg and the progesterone receptor is positive at 72 fmol/mg. The patient prefers a mastectomy; she is still menstruating regularly. The most appropriate course of action is:
   a. Six cycles of adjuvant cyclophosphamide, Adriamycin (doxorubicin), and 5-fluorouracil (CAF)
   b. Tamoxifen for 5 years
   c. Postoperative irradiation to the ipsilateral chest wall and nodal areas and tamoxifen for 5 years
   d. Oophorectomy
   e. Close follow-up every 3 months for 3 years and every 6 months for 2 additional years

5. Which of the following tumor markers is specific for ovarian cancer?
   a. CA-19-9
   b. CA-125
   c. OVCA-1
   d. BRCA-1
   e. CEA
   f. None of the above

6. A 68-year-old man had a radical prostatectomy for organ-confined prostate cancer in 1990. A routine chest radiograph reveals a 1.5-cm nodule of the right upper lobe. A computed tomography scan of the chest showed no other nodules, and fine-needle aspiration revealed adenocarcinoma. The next best step in management is:
   a. Orchiectomy
   b. Radiotherapy to the right upper lobe and mediastinum
   c. Thoracotomy
   d. Video thoracoscopy
   e. Doxorubicin-based chemotherapy

7. Which of the following is not characteristic of malignant carcinoid tumors?
   a. Diarrhea
   b. Bronchospasm
   c. Facial telangiectasia
   d. Right-sided heart failure

e. Rheumatoid arthritis

True/False (indicate whether each answer is true or false)
8. Which of the following statements regarding lung cancer are true?
   a. Malignant hypercalcemia is most commonly associated with small-cell carcinoma
   b. The relative risk for lung cancer in a smoker compared with a nonsmoker is 2.5
   c. The cell type most commonly associated with paraneoplastic syndromes is small-cell carcinoma
   d. Prophylactic cranial irradiation usually follows resection for stage I non-small-cell lung cancer
   e. Lung cancer is the second most common cause of cancer deaths in American men
   f. Screening strategies for lung cancer have not been shown to reduce mortality from this disease

9. A 42-year-old man presented with new dyspnea on exertion and was anemic (hemoglobin, 9 g/dL). Further evaluation revealed an abnormality in the transverse colon. On laparotomy, this was colonic adenocarcinoma with extension through the bowel wall and involvement of two neighboring nodes. Which of the following statements are true?
   a. Postoperative radiation and 5-fluorouracil are a standard adjuvant approach
   b. Persons with Gardner's syndrome are at high risk for this disease
   c. Persons with irritable bowel syndrome are at high risk for this disease
   d. Persons with Barrett's esophagus should be screened for colonic abnormalities
   e. If annual fecal occult blood testing in this patient is negative, no other follow-up studies are needed
   f. Multiple pulmonary nodules appearing 1 year later are unlikely to represent metastasis

10. Which of the following statements are true concerning testicular carcinoma?
    a. Males with fragile X syndrome are at high risk for this disease
    b. α-Fetoprotein value is increased only in patients with nonseminomatous germ cell tumors
    c. Nonseminomas are radiosensitive
    d. Most patients with nonseminomatous germ cell tumors have elevated values of tumor markers
    e. Ten percent of seminomas have an increased β-hCG value
    f. Bone is the most common site of metastasis from testicular carcinoma

ANSWERS

1. Answer c.

Lung cancer is the most common cause of cancer deaths in American women and men.

2. Answer d.

Numerous studies have shown, and continue to show, that nodal status remains the best prognostic factor in patients with breast cancer.

3. Answer e.

Tamoxifen is a mixed agonist or antagonist, depending on the tissue under consideration. Its estrogen-antagonist effects cause the hot flashes that are common with this agent. Its estrogen-like effects cause endometrial hyperplasia and an increased incidence of endometrial cancer, maintenance of bone density, and a slight risk of thromboembolic events (1% to 2% of patients). In general, serum cholesterol is decreased in women receiving tamoxifen.

4. Answer a.

Premenopausal patients with node-positive breast cancer receive adjuvant chemotherapy, regardless of their estrogen-receptor status. Irradiation after mastectomy is not routinely performed.

5. Answer f.

Even though CA-125 is expressed by approximately 85% of ovarian cancers, it is not specific for this malignancy; it can be increased in the setting of other cancers and certain benign conditions.

6. Answer c.

This finding could represent a new primary tumor, given the setting described, and should be resected by thoracotomy.

7. Answer e.

Rheumatoid arthritis does not occur in association with carcinomoid tumors..

8. a, false; b, false; c, true; d, false; e, false; f, true.

Small-cell carcinoma of the lung is the cell type most commonly associated with paraneoplastic syndromes, except for malignant hypercalcemia, which is associated with squamous cell carcinoma and production of the parathyroid hormone-related peptide. The relative risk for lung cancer in a smoker is 25. Prophylactic cranial irradiation is considered only for persons with limited-stage small-cell carcinoma who have a complete response to chemotherapy and thoracic irradiation. Lung cancer is the most common cause of cancer deaths in American men and women. Unfortunately, screening strategies for this disease have not shown a reduction in mortality.

9. a, false; b, true; c, false; d, false; e, false; f, false.

Most consider standard adjuvant therapy for node-positive colon cancer to be 5-fluorouracil and levamisole. 5-Fluorouracil and radiation are used after rectal cancer.

10. a, false; b, true; c, false; d, true; e, true; f, false.

Risk factors for testis cancer include cryptorchid testes and Klinefelter's syndrome. α-Fetoprotein is never expressed by seminomas. Seminomas, not nonseminomas, are radiosensitive. Testis cancer most frequently spreads to lymph nodes.

CHAPTER 19

PREVENTIVE MEDICINE

Philip T. Hagen, M.D.

DEFINITIONS

Preventive medicine is the practice of medicine that detects and alters or ameliorates 1) host susceptibility in a premorbid state (e.g., immunization), 2) risk factors for disease in a pre-disease state (e.g., increased cholesterol level), and 3) disease in the presymptomatic state (e.g., in situ cervical cancer). Not all disease is preventable because 1) not all risk factors (or all individuals at risk) are known, 2) the cost of screening everyone is not feasible, 3) barriers to medical access exist, 4) interval disease occurs, 5) characteristics of the target disease vary, 6) screening tests are imperfect, and 7) treatments are imperfect.

Primary prevention is the prevention of disease occurrence (e.g., immunization to prevent infection and blood pressure control to prevent stroke). *Secondary prevention* is the detection and amelioration of disease in a presymptomatic or pre-clinical stage (e.g., mammography detects small foci of cancer and Pap smear detects in situ cancer). *Tertiary prevention* is the prevention of future negative health effects of existing clinical disease (e.g., use of aspirin and β-blockers after myocardial infarction to prevent recurrence).

Efficacy is the potential or maximal benefit derived from applying a test or procedure under ideal circumstances (e.g., research studies with compliant patients, with ideal testing conditions, techniques, etc.). *Effectiveness* is the actual benefit that is derived from a test or procedure that is applied under usual--less than ideal--circumstances. Randomized trials in which results are analyzed by the "intention to treat" principle, i.e., all members of a group are included in the analysis whether they complied or not, give a measure of effectiveness in a population. *Cost-effectiveness* is the unit of cost incurred to achieve a given level of effectiveness. It is often expressed as the dollars spent per year of life saved. Often, the most cost-effective method of testing is not the most effective. For example, performing Pap smears every 5 or 10 years is more cost-effective, but performing them every year is more effective.

- Cost-effectiveness: cost incurred to achieve a given level of effectiveness.
- The most cost-effective test may not be the most effective test or treatment.

Years of potential life lost is one measure of the relative impact of a disease on society. This term usually refers to the years lost due to death from a disease before age 65 (or sometimes 70). For example, colon cancer kills approximately 57,000 men and women annually and breast cancer kills approximately 46,000 women. However, on average, breast cancer kills at a younger age and so has nearly 3x as many "years of potential life lost."

- Years of potential life lost: the years lost due to death from a disease before age 65 (or sometimes 70).

Incidence (rate) refers to the number of new events (deaths, diagnoses) that occur in a population in a given time (e.g., 140 cancer deaths per 100,000 people in the U.S. annually). *Prevalence* refers to the number of cases of a condition existing at a point in time in a population (e.g., currently, 1,200,000 people in the U.S. are infected with the HIV virus).

PRINCIPLES OF SCREENING FOR DISEASE

The term *mass screening* is generally applied to the relatively indiscriminate testing of a population with the intent to improve the aggregate health of the population but not necessarily of every person in the population. An example is blood pressure or cholesterol testing in a public setting such as a shopping mall.

- Mass screening: indiscriminate testing of a population to improve the aggregate health of the population.

Case finding is the technical term often used for screening conducted in the office setting. The intent is to detect asymptomatic disease and to improve the health of the person. In testing asymptomatic persons, it is important to bear in mind the dictum of "first do no harm."

- Case finding: screening conducted in the office setting to detect asymptomatic disease and to improve the health of a person.

Desirable Screening Characteristics

1. Disease characteristics: the diseases screened should be common, cause significant morbidity and mortality, have a long preclinical phase (which is curable/modifiable), have an effective treatment that is available to those screened, and have an acceptable treatment (i.e., one that is not excessively painful or disfiguring).
2. Test characteristics: the tests should be inexpensive, safe, acceptable, easy to administer, technically easy to perform, highly sensitive, and have a complementary, highly specific confirmatory test.
3. Host characteristics: the person be at risk, have access to testing, be likely to comply with follow-up testing, and have adequate overall life expectancy/functional life expectancy.

Burden of U.S. Disease

Diseases that cause the most morbidity and mortality in the U.S. may or may not be amenable to screening or case finding. Heart disease and cancer are clearly the leading causes of death in the U.S. (Tables 19-1 and 19-2). The most recent year for which actual statistics exist is 1991.

Cancer Screening

Lung Cancer

Lung cancer is a highly lethal/virulent form of cancer (it kills most of the people it afflicts) and is the leading cause of cancer death for men and women. Burden of disease (1995 estimates from the American Cancer Society): 169,900 new cases and 157,400 deaths. Peak incidence is 470/100,000 in 75-year-old men and 155/100,000 in 70-year-old women. Risk factors include 1) smoking--10x increased risk over nonsmoker and 2.5x increase over population average incidence rates; 2) age--70 years old, 10x greater risk than for 40 years old; 3) sex--male-to-female ratio is 3:1 and is primarily related to duration and intensity of smoking; 4) industrial, occupational, environmental exposure--asbestos, hydrocarbons, uranium, and radon. Tests include chest radiography and sputum cytology. Screening probably is not effective. Although the Mayo Clinic Lung Project detected more cancers, mortality was not altered in approximately 12 years of follow-up study. This may have been because of "overdiagnosis" of clinically irrelevant lesions or lead-time bias. Annual chest radiography (or sputum cytology) solely to look for treatable stage lung cancer should not be performed. Smoking is the leading preventable cause of cancer in the U.S. (and a leading cause of heart disease and stroke).

- Lung cancer: the leading cause of cancer death for men and women.
- Risk factors for lung cancer: smoking, age, sex (3:1 male-to-female ratio), and environmental exposure.
- Annual chest radiography (or sputum cytology) solely to look for treatable stage lung cancer should not be performed.
- Smoking is the leading preventable cause of cancer in the U.S.
- Physician advice to quit smoking and referral to smoke cessation counseling are probably the most cost-effective preventive measures available.

Breast Cancer

Breast cancer is the second leading cause of cancer death for women. The lifetime risk is estimated at 1 in 8 women. Burden of disease (1995 estimates from the American Cancer Society): 183,400 new cases and 46,240 deaths. Thus, breast cancer is

Table 19-1.--Mortality for Leading Causes of Death in the U.S., 1991

	No. of deaths	Death rate per 100,000 population[*]	% of total deaths
Heart diseases	720,862	219.8	33.2
Cancer	514,657	173.4	23.7
Cerebrovascular diseases	143,481	42.0	6.6
Chronic obstructive lung diseases	90,650	28.6	4.2
Accidents	89,347	32.1	4.1

[*]Age-adjusted to the 1970 U.S. standard population.
From Wingo PA, Tong T, Bolden S: Cancer statistics, 1995. CA Cancer J Clin 45:8-30, Jan/Feb, 1995. By permission of American Cancer Society.

Table 19-2.--Cancer Mortality for Women and Men, 1991 (U.S. Vital Statistics)

Age, yr					
35-54		55-74		≥75	
Women					
Breast	9,188	Lung	30,154	Lung	16,400
Lung	5,372	Breast	19,900	Colon and rectum	15,727
Colon and rectum	1,999	Colon and rectum	11,117	Breast	13,834
Uterus	1,978	Ovary	6,720	Pancreas	6,637
Ovary	1,779	Pancreas	5,669	Ovary	4,601
Men					
Lung	8,741	Lung	55,890	Lung	26,896
Colon and rectum	2,393	Colon and rectum	13,888	Prostate	20,909
Non-Hodgkin's lymphoma	1,726	Prostate	12,306	Colon and rectum	11,686
Brain and CNS	1,577	Pancreas	6,730	Pancreas	4,229
Pancreas	1,298	Esophagus	4,600	Bladder	3,698

From Wingo PA, Tong T, Bolden S: Cancer statistics, 1995. CA Cancer J Clin 45:8-30, Jan/Feb, 1995. By permission of American Cancer Society.

moderately lethal/virulent (it kills many but not most of the people it afflicts). The risk factors include 1) age--the risk increases throughout life, and the risk for an 80-year-old woman is 12x that for a 30-year-old woman; 2) family history--one first-degree relative with breast cancer, 2x-4x risk and two first-degree relatives, 3x-8x risk (if no first-degree relatives, slightly reduced risk); 3) socioeconomic status--high, increases risk 2x-4x; 4) nulliparity or age at first full-term pregnancy--if >30 years old, risk is increased 2x-4x; 5) history of benign proliferative disease--dysplastic mammographic parenchymal patterns, history of breast cancer, and high-dose radiation all increase risk approximately 2x. Risk factor analysis can define a subgroup that concentrates 85% of breast cancer in 40% of women, a relative risk of approximately 2x for the high-risk group and 0.25x for the low-risk group.

- Breast cancer: the second leading cause of cancer death for women.
- Lifetime risk: 1 in 8 women.
- One first-degree relative with breast cancer, 2x-4x risk; two first-degree relatives, 3x-8x risk.

Screening procedures include:
1. Breast self-examination: recommended to the patient, but it is not of demonstrated effectiveness.
2. Clinical breast examination: has a sensitivity of about 50%-70% and a specificity >90% and costs about $25.
3. Screen film mammography: has a sensitivity of 80%-95% for women ≥50 years old and 60%-80% for women <50 years. Specificity is 95%-99%. Positive predictive values (PPV) are about 5%-10%, with 20%-

50% of biopsies revealing cancer, depending on age (higher percentages in older women). The cost is about $100.
4. Randomized control trials worldwide have examined the effectiveness of mammography. They showed an approximate 30% decrease in mortality, but only two trials showed statistical significance. Data are conflicting or inconclusive in women younger than 50 or older than 70 years.

- Breast physical examination has a sensitivity of 50%-70% and a specificity of >90%.
- Mammography has a sensitivity of 80%-95% and a specificity of 95%-99%.
- Studies are inconclusive about the benefit of mammography for women younger than 50 or older than 70 years.

Screening risks--Radiation is estimated to produce 60 additional breast cancers in 1,000,000 women screened compared with the 93,000 cases expected to be detected. The Breast Cancer Detection and Demonstration Project showed that 2% of women were referred for surgical evaluation/aspiration, and of the 50- to 65-year-old women referred for biopsy, half were found to have cancer. About 3% of women 40-49 years old were referred for biopsy, with a smaller percentage yielding cancer.

- Radiation: 60 additional breast cancers in 1,000,000 women screened.
- Approximately 2% of screened women 50-65 years old will have biopsy and 3% of women 40-49 years old.

Cost-effectiveness: if 25% of women 40-75 years old in the U.S. were screened annually, 11,000,000/year would be screened at a cost of $1.3 billion annually for physical examination and mammography. The cost of screening and the work-up would be 100x as expensive as the costs saved by reduced treatment. Cost per year of life saved ranges from about $9,000 to $12,000, with the lower costs in the 50-year-old group and higher costs in the older age group.

- Cost of screening and work-up would be 100x as expensive as the costs saved by reduced treatment.
- Cost per year of life saved is $9,000-$12,000.

Recommendations:
1. General agreement--clinical breast examination yearly after age 40, clinical breast examination and mammography yearly for women 50-65 years old. Otherwise, recommendations vary.
2. American Cancer Society and several other groups--Clinical breast examination yearly for women ≥40 years old and mammography every 1-2 years. For women ≥50 years old, annual clinical breast examination and mammography.
3. United States Preventive Services Task Force (USPSTF)--Annual clinical breast examination for women 40-49 years old and annual clinical breast examination and mammography every 1-2 years for women ≥50 years old. Screening may begin sooner for women at high risk.
4. American College of Physicians and American Academy of Family Practice--Annual clinical breast examination for women ≥40 years old and annual mammography for women ≥50 years old (sooner if at high risk).

Colon and Rectal Cancer

Colon cancer is the second leading cause of cancer death in the U.S. Burden of disease (1995 estimates from the American Cancer Society): 138,200 new cases of colorectal cancer and 55,300 deaths due to colorectal cancer. The lifetime risk of developing colon cancer is approximately 6%. Less than 2% of colon cancers occur in people <40 years old and 90% occur in those >50 years old. The risk of developing colon cancer is approximately 2.5x greater than the risk of dying of it (which reflects potential survivability of colon cancer and the age of the population involved, i.e., there are competing causes of mortality). Colon cancer is now the second cancer for which randomized controlled trial evidence has demonstrated decreased mortality due to screening.

- Colon cancer is the second leading cause of cancer death.
- Lifetime risk is 6%.
- 90% of colon cancers are in people older than 50 years.

Natural history: cancers may develop de novo in the colon, but most of them probably develop from adenomatous polyps. The risk of a polyp becoming malignant appears to be related to time and size. Clinically significant polyps are those larger than 7 mm. The average time from formation to malignant transformation for a polyp is 7-10 years. Ten-year survival for Dukes' A or B cancer is 74%, 36% for Dukes' C, and 5% for Dukes' D.

- The risk of a polyp becoming malignant appears to be related to time and size.
- Clinically significant polyps: ones larger than 7 mm.
- The time from polyp formation to malignant transformation is 7-10 years.

The risk factors include 1) age--risk doubles every 7 years over age 50; 2) sex--risk for males is slightly greater than for females; 3) family history--if a first-degree relative has disease, the risk increases 2x-3x; 4) previous adenomatous polyps increase risk 2x-3x; 5) history of endometrial, ovarian, or breast cancer increases risk 2x; 6) familial polyposis, Gardner's syndrome--approximately 100% risk by age 40; 7) ulcerative colitis--approximately 50% risk with a 30-year history of disease; and 8) cancer family syndrome (adenocarcinoma at various locations at an early age in multiple sibs)--approximately a 50% risk.

- Risk for colon/rectal cancer doubles every 7 years over age 50.
- If first-degree relative has colon/rectal cancer, risk increases 2x-3x.
- Previous adenomatous polyps, risk increases 2x-3x.
- History of endometrial, ovarian, or breast cancer, risk increases 2x.
- Familial polyposis (Gardner's syndrome), risk is nearly 100% by age 40.
- Ulcerative colitis, about a 50% risk with a 30-year history of disease.

Tests: 1) fecal occult blood testing is 20%-30% sensitive and does not detect polyps well; 2) proctoscopy is more than 90% sensitive for the bowel visualized and could detect about 30% of cancers; 3) flexible sigmoidoscopy is also more than 90% sensitive for the bowel visualized and could detect about 60% of cancers; 4) barium enema and colonoscopy usually visualize the entire colon and are 85%-95% sensitive.

- Fecal occult blood testing is 20%-30% sensitive.
- Proctoscopy and flexible sigmoidoscopy are more than 90% sensitive for the area of the colon visualized.
- Barium enema and colonoscopy visualize the entire colon and are 85%-95% sensitive.

Recommendations--Randomized control trial data that are available show about a 30% decrease in mortality with annual fecal occult blood testing. Yet, there is little consensus about whether to screen and how to screen for colorectal cancer. Mathematical modeling suggests that annual screening with barium enema or colonoscopy might reduce mortality by 85%, but the cost would be prohibitive. The American Cancer Society recommends digital rectal examination (for prostate examination) yearly for men >40 years old and yearly for women (as part of pelvic examination) >40. Fecal occult blood testing--yearly over age 50, and sigmoidoscopy every 3-5 years over age 50. Before the recent study supporting annual fecal occult blood testing, the USPSTF concluded that the evidence was insufficient and so made no recommendation for average risk population. It recommended against colonoscopy except for a family history of two or more first-degree relatives or existence of high-risk conditions. Updated recommendations are under review. The American College of Physicians recommends fecal occult blood testing annually over age 50 and over age 40 for those at high risk. Sigmoidoscopy--every 3-5 years over age 50 or substitution of barium enema every 5 years for sigmoidoscopy. The College recommends against colonoscopy except for persons with high-risk conditions or a family history of colon cancer in a first-degree relative. The recommendation for these people is colonoscopy over age 40 every 3-5 years (air-contrast barium enema is an acceptable alternative).

- Fecal occult blood screening annually decreases mortality by 30%.
- Annual screening with barium enema or colonoscopy might reduce mortality by 85%, but the cost would be prohibitive.

Prostate Cancer

For the purposes of screening, prostate cancer is a troublesome disease, primarily because of the great difference between the "burden" of prevalent disease and the "burden" of clinical disease. The 1995 estimates from the American Cancer Society are 244,000 new cases of prostate cancer and 40,400 deaths due to it. Pathologic studies show that a small focus of prostate cancer can be found in 30%-40% of 60-year-old men. Yet in only 8%-9% of the men will prostate cancer be diagnosed, with many cases diagnosed incidentally at transurethral resection of the prostate. Currently, 80% of diagnoses are made in men older than 65 years. Relatively few men with prostate cancer die of the disease, only 2%-3% of U.S. men.

- 8%-9% of U.S. males in their lifetime will have the diagnosis of prostate cancer.
- 2%-3% of U.S. males die of prostate cancer.
- 80% of the diagnoses are made in men older than 65 years.

Natural history--Prostate cancer is a hormonally induced cancer that is generally slow growing. In most host males, it does not alter the life span or lifestyle. Growth of a tiny nidus of cancerous cells into a clinically important cancer takes 10-15 years. In elderly hosts, this process is usually halted by intervening causes of mortality. Aggressiveness and morbidity are related to size, grade, and ploidy. TA1 NxMO: Usually follow age-based mortality curve, normal survival. Mortality due to prostatic cancer is <5%. TA2 NxMO: near normal 10-year survival. TB2 or 3 NxMO: 5-year survival is about 50%.

- Prostate cancer is a hormonally induced cancer.
- It does not alter the life span or lifestyle of most host males.
- Growth into a clinically important cancer takes 10-15 years.

The risk factors include: 1) age--the risk increases exponentially after age 50; 2) race--in the U.S. blacks have 2x the risk of whites, and whites have 2x the risk of Asians; 3) family history--a first-degree relative increases the risk 3x, a brother with cancer before age 63 increases the risk 4x, and a sister with breast cancer increases the risk 2x.

- For prostate cancer in the U.S., blacks have twice the risk of whites, who have twice the risk of Asians.

Tests: 1) digital rectal examination has a PPV of 6.5%; 2) transrectal ultrasonography has a PPV of about 20% (values vary depending on population and prior screening); and 3) prostate-specific antigen (PSA) has a PPV of about 25% (values vary depending on population and prior screening). Note: because there is much undetected disease, PPV values do not have the usual meaning.

Recommendations: no good data are available from randomized controlled trials on the impact of early detection and treatment on survival. There is little agreement on recommendations for screening. Aggressive screening for prostate cancer will uncover many new cases (causing a surge in incidence) and result in many additional treatments. However, because of the natural history of the disease, screening may have minimal effect in decreasing mortality, the desired benefit. The American Cancer Society recommends digital rectal examination yearly for men >40 years old and this examination plus PSA for men ≥50 years and for men ≥40 years old at high risk. The American College of Physicians and USPSTF make no recommendations.

- There is little agreement on recommendations for screening for prostate cancer.

Several authorities have recommended *against* any form of screening--rectal examination, ultrasonography, or PSA--primarily because of concern that the impact on survival will be minimal and that the costs in detection and follow-up treatment and in deaths due to treatment (perioperative deaths) will be significant. The risk that the harm outweighs the good from detection of early stage disease exists. Screening, if performed, should be done in men likely to have a 10-year survival (the average life expectancy for a 50-year-old man is about 25 years and >10 years for a 70-year-old man).

Cervical Cancer

The 1995 estimates from the American Cancer Society are for 15,800 new cases of cervical cancer and 4,800 deaths. Cervical cancer has a bimodal risk curve divided between in situ carcinoma and invasive carcinoma. This cancer has a long preclinical phase, and progression from dysplasia to invasive cancer may take 10 to 15 years or more. A strong association exists between human papillomavirus (types 16, 18, and others) and cervical cancer. Cervical cancer may largely be a sexually transmitted disease.

- Cervical cancer: bimodal risk curve divided between in situ carcinoma and invasive carcinoma.
- It has a long preclinical phase.
- Cervical cancer is strongly associated with human papillomavirus.

The risk factors include: 1) age--the risk of invasive carcinoma increases throughout life; 2) sexual activity--early age at onset; 3) multiple sexual partners; 4) a history of sexually transmitted disease; and 5) smoking.

- Cervical cancer risk factors: early age at onset of sexual activity, multiple sexual partners, a history of sexually transmitted disease, and smoking.

Test: Pap smear has a sensitivity of 55%-80% and a specificity of 90%-99%. Experienced cytologists and pathologists and clinician sampling technique are important to test effectiveness.

- Pap smear has a 55%-80% sensitivity and a 90%-99% specificity.

Screening effectiveness--No randomized controlled trial of screening has been conducted in a general population. However, a significant body of evidence from case control studies and observational studies suggests effectiveness. Estimated overall effect of Pap smear: every 10 years, 64% reduction in invasive cancer; every 5 years, 84% reduction; every 3 years, 91% reduction; every 2 years, 92.5% reduction; and every year 93.5% reduction.

Recommendations--The general agreement is to recommend screening at the onset of sexual activity and every 1-3

years thereafter, depending on risk. The American Cancer Society recommends screening every 1-3 years for women >18 years, depending on risk factors. The American College of Physicians recommends screening every 3 years for women between 20 and 65 years old and every 2 years if they are at increased risk; for women >65 years, every 3 years if not screened within 10 years before current examination. USP-STF recommends screening every 1-3 years for women 18-65, depending on risk factors, and every 1-3 years if >65 years and if no regular screening was performed in the 10 years previously.

- General recommendation: screen at the onset of sexual activity and every 1-3 years thereafter, depending on risk.

Ovarian Cancer

Ovarian cancer is the fourth leading cause of cancer death in women. Burden of disease (1995 estimates from the American Cancer Society): 26,600 new cases of ovarian cancer and 14,500 deaths. Ovarian cancer is the leading cause of gynecologic cancer death. Age-adjusted death rates have been increasing slowly in the last 25 years.

- Ovarian cancer is the fourth leading cause of cancer death in women.
- Age-adjusted death rates have been increasing slowly.

Risk factors: 1) Lower risk--history of at least one term pregnancy has a relative risk of 0.64. The use of oral contraceptives for <1 year has the relative risk of 0.97; if used >3 years, the relative risk is 0.40. Estimated 12% decrease in risk per year of use of oral contraceptive pill up to 7 years. 2) Higher risk--family history as a risk is not well quantified, but it is an important factor if a first-degree relative has disease (only 1%-5% of ovarian cancers are familial). High fat diet, long duration of ovulatory years (i.e., late menopause), and coffee intake are possible risk factors.

- 12% decrease in risk per year with use of oral contraceptive pill up to 7 years.
- 1%-5% of ovarian cancers are familial.

Screening tests: 1) bimanual examination is insensitive; 2) ultrasonography, transvaginal or transabdominal, is more sensitive than bimanual examination but has a poor PPV; 3) CA 125 (blood test) is more sensitive than bimanual examination but also has a poor PPV. Ultrasonography or CA 125 has a significant false-positive rate. No study has been done on the impact of screening on mortality. It is estimated that 10-60 abdominal operations would have to be performed for every one cancer detected, at a cost of more than $13 billion annually to screen the 43 million woman >45 years old. An adequate study of efficacy, even with a highly sensitive and specific test, would require tens of thousands of participants.

- For ovarian cancer, bimanual examination is insensitive.
- Ultrasonography and CA 125 both are more sensitive than bimanual examination but both have a poor PPV.
- For every one ovarian cancer detected, 10-60 abdominal operations would have to be performed.

Recommendations: no randomized controlled trial screening data exist to guide recommendations. The American Cancer Society recommends bimanual palpation every 1-3 years for women age 20-40 and every year for women >40. USPSTF recommends against screening for ovarian cancer.

Tuberculosis Prevention

Burden of disease: the worldwide prevalence of tuberculosis (TB) infection (past or active) is greater than 1 billion cases, with an annual incidence rate of about 8 million. Approximately 3,000,000 people worldwide die annually of TB. The U.S. incidence is approximately 25,000 cases per year, with a mortality of 2,000 cases. The incidence decreased from 1953 to 1985, but since then TB has made a resurgence, probably because of immigration from endemic areas, HIV infection, and increased use of immunosuppressive drugs.

- TB: the U.S. incidence is approximately 25,000 cases and 2,000 deaths annually.

Natural history: infection occurs through inhalation of *Mycobacterium tuberculosis*-bearing droplets. After being infected, healthy persons are usually asymptomatic. However, it is believed that the tubercle bacillus remains viable in granulomata for many years. The risk of reactivation after asymptomatic infection (PPD conversion) is 2%/year for the first 2-3 years. A second reactivation peak occurs in the elderly with debility and disease.

- The tubercle bacillus remains viable in granulomata for many years.
- The risk of reactivation (after PPD conversion) is 2%/year for first 2-3 years after infection.
- A second reactivation peak occurs in the elderly with debility and disease.

Risk factors include: 1) foreign-born, with recent immigration; 2) institutionalization, e.g., in nursing home, 5x-30x increased risk; 3) prisoners (10x increased risk); and 4) HIV/AIDS infection. If a person is HIV-positive and has a positive PPD, the 2-year risk is 15%. If TB occurs in a young person, check his or her HIV status.

- If a person is HIV-positive and has a positive PPD, the 2-year risk is 15%.
- If TB occurs in a young person, check his or her HIV status.

Test: the PPD (Mantoux) skin test--5-tuberculin units intradermal skin test. Measure the area of induration (not erythema) at 48-72 hours. In low-risk persons, consider the reaction positive if it is >15 mm (10 mm if the person is in a high-risk group). If there has been recent contact with an infected person, 5 mm is considered positive. HIV-infected persons may be anergic and 5 mm should be considered positive. Elderly persons may be relatively anergic but can be boosted by repeating the test. Previous BCG vaccine will produce skin reactivity, but induration >15 mm should be treated as a positive reaction in an adult vaccinated as a child. Recent MMR vaccination (6 weeks) may diminish skin reactivity, and testing should be avoided during this interval. Chest radiography and sputum are not useful screening tests for conversion but may detect active disease in high-risk persons.

- Chest radiography and sputum are not useful screening tests for TB.

Preventive measures: 1) Primary prevention is with BCG vaccine, an attenuated species of *Mycobacterium bovus*. It may be as much as 80% effective when used properly. It is indicated in high-risk areas because it is inexpensive, requires a single shot, and has a low risk (only 100 fatalities in 2 billion administrations). BCG vaccine is not indicated in low-prevalence areas because it confuses interpretation of PPD response. Another primary preventive measure is environmental controls, especially in a health-care environment, with respiratory isolation, high-efficiency filter masks, and special venting of rooms/wards with TB cases.

- BCG vaccine is 80% effective when used properly.
- Its use is not indicated in low-prevalence areas.

2) Secondary prevention is with isoniazid (INH) treatment. Its use is indicated for recent converters (<2 years), contacts of infected persons with >5 mm PPD, history of TB with inadequate treatment, positive skin tests with abnormal but stable chest radiographic findings, and positive PPD (of any duration) if <35 years old. The dosage is 5-10 mg/kg daily, up to a maximum of 300 mg daily (the usual adult dose) in a single oral dose. Treatment should continue for 6-12 months (the longer the treatment, the greater the efficacy). Primary side effects are liver toxicity and peripheral neuropathy. Peak toxicity is in persons >50 years (2%-3%). Side-effect monitoring is generally through symptoms only, except in older persons (because of higher risk for toxicity) in whom serum levels of

AST or ALT (liver function testing) should be determined every 6 weeks.

- Isoniazid: 5-10 mg/kg daily up to maximum of 300 mg daily.
- Treatment should continue for 6-12 months.
- Peak toxicity is in persons older than 50 years (2%-3%).

IMMUNIZATIONS

One of the greatest successes of modern medicine for preventing disease and for extending life has been immunization. Adults have continuing immunization needs throughout life. Physicians who administer vaccines are required by law to keep permanent vaccine records (National Childhood Vaccine Act of 1986) and to report adverse events through the vaccine adverse event reporting system (VAERS). Service in the military may be considered verification of vaccination to measles, rubella, tetanus, diphtheria, and polio. Providers are now required to give patients "vaccine information pamphlets" before vaccination as a mechanism for informed consent.

Immunity may be of two types. Passive immunity--preformed antibodies are provided in large quantities to prevent or to diminish the impact of infection or associated toxins (e.g., tetanus immunoglobulin [TIG] and hepatitis B immunoglobulin [HBIG]). Passive immunity lasts for up to 3 months. Active immunity--an antigen is presented to the host immune system that in turn develops antibodies (e.g., hepatitis or tetanus) or specific immune cells (e.g., BCG). Active immunity generally lasts from years to a lifetime. Active immunity may be induced by live virus vaccines (e.g., measles), killed virus vaccines (e.g., influenza), or refined antigen vaccines (e.g., pneumococcal).

Live virus vaccines are important primarily for *who should not receive them*. In general, pregnant women, people with immune-deficiency diseases, leukemia, lymphoma, generalized malignancy, or those who are immune-suppressed because of therapy with corticosteroids, alkylating drugs, antimetabolites, or radiation should *not* be given live virus vaccines. HIV-infected persons who are immune-competent and leukemia patients who have been in remission for ≥3 months after chemotherapy generally may be vaccinated with live virus vaccines. Live virus vaccines include measles, mumps, rubella, smallpox, varicella zoster, yellow fever, and polio. Inactivated virus vaccines include enhanced inactivated polio (eIPV), hepatitis B, influenza, and rabies. Inactivated bacterial vaccines include cholera, hemophilus influenza B, meningococcal, plague, and pneumococcal.

Recently, a childhood immunization schedule has been developed and endorsed by several groups (Table 19-3). Of note is the addition of hepatitis B as a routine vaccine.

Specific Vaccines/Chemo-Prevention

Diphtheria

Diphtheria is a rare disease primarily because of vaccination. However, up to 40% of adults lack protective antibody levels. Recommendation: vaccination in combination with tetanus toxoid (see tetanus), as Td.

Tetanus

Approximately 50 cases of tetanus are reported each year; most are in adults who are either unvaccinated or inadequately vaccinated. Vaccination is nearly 100% effective. Recommendations: primary series, a three-dose series, should be completed before adulthood, usually in early childhood. Primary series consists of Td (DTP in childhood [Table 19-3]) followed in 4 weeks or more by Td followed in 6-12 months or more by another Td. The last childhood dose is usually a booster at age 15. For adults who have had a primary series, vaccinate every 10 years (e.g., mid-decade is easy to remember; if last childhood dose at 15, vaccinate at ages 25, 35, 45, etc.). Clean, minor wounds received in the 10-year interval require no further vaccination. However, for a contaminated wound, the patient should get a booster if it has been more than 5 years since the last booster. If immune status is unknown or lacking (specifically, no primary series) both toxoid and TIG should be given (250 units i.m.). Td is the preferred toxoid in an emergency setting as well as for routine vaccination. Td and TIG when given in the emergency setting should be given in separate syringes at separate locations, but they may be given at the same time.

- Tetanus vaccination: the primary series is a three-dose series.
- Adults who have had a primary series should receive a booster every 10 years.
- For a contaminated wound, the patient should get a booster if it has been more than 5 years since the last booster.

Side effects: Td may be given in pregnancy, although it is desirable to wait until the second trimester. Maternal antibodies are passed to the infant transplacentally and confer passive immunity for a few months after birth.

- Maternal antibodies are passed to the infant transplacentally.

A history of neurologic reaction, urticaria, anaphylaxis, or other severe hypersensitivity reaction is a contraindication to the readministration of toxoids. Skin testing may be performed if necessary. In the emergency setting, if other than a clean minor wound is sustained, TIG may be used when T or Td is contraindicated. Arthus-type hypersensitivity, a severe local

Table 19-3.--Recommended Childhood Immunization Schedule*—U.S., January 1995

Vaccine	Birth	2 Months	4 Months	6 Months	12 Months†	15 Months	18 Months	4-6 Years	11-12 Years	14-16 Years
Hepatitis B‡	HB-1	HB-2		HB-3						
Diphtheria, Tetanus, Pertussis§		DTP	DTP	DTP	DTP or DTaP at ≥ 15 months			DTP or DTaP	Td	
H. influenzae type b//		Hib	Hib	Hib	Hib					
Poliovirus		OPV	OPV	OPV				OPV		
Measles, Mumps, Rubella¶					MMR			MMR or MMR		

*Recommended vaccines are listed under the routinely recommended ages. Shaded bars indicate range of acceptable ages for vaccination.

†Vaccines recommended in the second year of life (i.e., 12-15 months of age) may be given at either one or two visits.

‡Infants born to hepatitis B surface antigen (HBsAg)-negative mothers should receive the second dose of hepatitis B vaccine between 1 and 4 months of age, provided at least 1 month has elapsed since receipt of the first dose. The third dose is recommended between 6 and 18 months of age. Infants born to HBsAg-positive mothers should receive immunoprophylaxis for hepatitis B with 0.5 mL Hepatitis B Immune Globulin (HBIG) within 12 hours of birth, and 0.5 mL of either Merck Sharpe & Dohme (West Point, Pennsylvania) vaccine (Recombivax HB) or of SmithKline Beecham (Philadelphia) vaccine (Engerix-B) at a separate site. In these infants, the second dose of vaccine is recommended at 1 month of age and the third dose at 6 months of age. All pregnant women should be screened for HBsAg during an early prenatal visit.

§The fourth dose of diphtheria and tetanus toxoids and pertussis vaccine (DTP) may be administered as early as 12 months of age, provided at least 6 months have elapsed since the third dose of DTP. Combined DTP-Hib products may be used when these two vaccines are administered simultaneously. Diphtheria and tetanus toxoids and acellular pertussis vaccine (DTaP) is licensed for use for the fourth and/or fifth dose of DTP in children aged ≥15 months and may be preferred for these doses in children in this age group.

//Three H. influenzae type b conjugate vaccines are available for use in infants: 1) oligosaccharide conjugate Hib vaccine (HbOC) (HibTITER, manufactured by Praxis Biologics, Inc. [West Henrietta, New York], and distributed by Lederle-Praxis Biologicals [Wayne, New Jersey]); 2) polyribosylribitol phosphate-tetanus toxoid conjugate (PRP-T) (ActHIB, manufactured by Pasteur Mérieux Sérums & Vaccins, S.A. [Lyon, France], and distributed by Connaught Laboratories, Inc. [Swiftwater, Pennsylvania], and OmniHIB, manufactured by Pasteur Mérieux Sérums & Vaccins, S.A., and distributed by SmithKline Beecham); and 3) Haemophilus b conjugate vaccine (Meningococcal Protein Conjugate) (PRP-OMP) (PedvaxHIB, manufactured by Merck Sharpe & Dohme). Children who have received PRP-OMP at 2 and 4 months of age do not require a dose at 6 months of age. After the primary infant Hib conjugate vaccine series is completed, any licensed Hib conjugate vaccine may be used as a booster dose at age 12-15 months.

¶The second dose of measles-mumps-rubella vaccine should be administered either at 4-6 years of age or at 11-12 years of age.

From Advisory Committee on Immunization Practices, American Academy of Pediatrics, and American Academy of Family Physicians: Recommended childhood immunization schedule—United States, January 1995. MMWR 43:959-960, 1995.

reaction occurring 2-8 hours after injection and often with fever and malaise, may occur in persons who have received multiple boosters. These people have very high levels of antitoxin and do not need boosters, even in the emergency room setting, more frequently than every 10 years.

Measles

Vaccination has reduced the number of cases of measles from 500,000 yearly (with 500 deaths) to 3,600 cases yearly in the mid-1980s. A disease resurgence has occurred, and in 1990, there were 27,000 cases. The risk of encephalitis with measles infection in an adult is approximately 1 in 1,000. Infection in pregnancy may induce abortion, premature labor, and low birth weight. Malformation does not appear to be as much of a problem as with rubella.

- A resurgence in measles has occurred.

- The risk of encephalitis with measles infection in an adult is approximately 1 in 1,000.

Target: Adults born after 1956 who have no medical contraindication and who have no dated documentation of at least one dose of live measles vaccination on or after their first birthday, physician-documented disease, or documented immune titers should receive vaccination. Persons with expected exposure to measles should consider revaccination or titer measurement because 10% of persons born before 1957 are not immune. Persons at risk include travelers to endemic areas, those in school settings, and health care workers. They should have documented two doses of measles vaccine on or after their first birthday. MMR is the preferred vaccine. If they have never been vaccinated, they should receive two doses given at least 1 month apart.

Exposure precautions: If the person exposed is unvaccinated, vaccinate within 72 hours if possible and give immunoglobulin if the person is not a vaccine candidate (0.5 mL/kg i.m., up to 15 mL). Health care workers should remain away from work for days 5-21 after exposure if they are not immune.

Side effects: 1) fever, temperature >103°F usually occurs on day 5-12 in 5%-15% of those vaccinated; 2) rash occurs in 5%; 3) encephalitis is rare, if it occurs at all; 4) a local reaction occurs especially in those having received killed vaccine. No apparent increase in side effects occurs with a second vaccination. Contraindications are immunoglobulin or blood products given within the previous 3 months, pregnancy, egg or neomycin allergy, and others as noted above for live virus vaccines.

Mumps

A highly effective vaccination program has reduced the number of cases of mumps from approximately 200,000 yearly to 3,000-5,000 yearly. Side effects of rash, pruritus, and purpura are uncommon, and central nervous system problems and parotitis are rare. There is no increased risk with revaccination. The contraindications are the same as for measles.

Rubella

Infection with rubella in the first trimester results in congenital rubella syndrome in up to 80% of infected fetuses. The goal of vaccination is to prevent the occurrence of this disease. Vaccination is highly effective, and there is no evidence of transmission of vaccine virus to close household contacts. The target population includes all women of childbearing age, all health care workers, and travelers to endemic areas. The side effects include: arthralgias in 25% and transient arthritis in 10%, usually 1-3 weeks postvaccination. Vaccination rarely causes chronic joint problems, certainly much less frequently than natural infection. Contraindications are immunoglobulin given within the previous 3 months (but not blood products, e.g., $Rh_0(D)$ immune globulin [RhoGAM]), pregnant women or women likely to become pregnant within 3 months (although there are no documented cases of congenital rubella syndrome in vaccinated pregnant women), and allergy to neomycin but not to egg (as prepared in a diploid cell culture).

Influenza

Since 1957, 19 influenza epidemics, with more than 10,000 excess deaths each, have occurred, and 80%-90% of the deaths occurred in persons ≥65 years old. Peak incidences occur in mid to late winter (i.e., after December). Influenza A is classified by two surface antigens: hemagglutinin (subtypes H1, H2, H3) and neuraminidase (subtypes N1, N2). Because of differing subtypes and antigenic drift, infection or vaccination more than 1 year previously may not give protection the following year. Influenza B is antigenically more stable but

still has moderate drift. Control is with vaccination (both influenza A and B) and/or chemoprophylaxis (for influenza A only).

The vaccine is an inactivated (killed) virus vaccine (virus grown in egg culture). Each year it contains three viruses, two A-type viruses and one B-type virus. Vaccines may contain whole virus, subvarion, or purified surface antigen. Subvarion and purified antigen are used in children to decrease febrile reaction. All forms may be used in adults. Ideally, vaccination should be given in October and November.

The side effects include 1) local soreness (occurs in <1/3); 2) fever, malaise, myalgia (occurs 6-12 hours postvaccination and may last 1-2 days); and 3) anaphylactic reaction (probably due to egg protein). The target population includes 1) persons ≥65 years old who reside in a nursing home or chronic care facility; 2) persons with chronic pulmonary or cardiovascular disease, including asthma, chronic metabolic diseases such as diabetes mellitus, renal dysfunction, immunosuppression; and 3) health care workers. Consideration may be given to persons in vital roles, institutional settings, or who travel to the southern hemisphere between April and September. Contraindications are 1) first trimester of pregnancy, except for those at high risk because of underlying disease, and 2) egg allergy.

Chemoprophylaxis against type A influenza is currently available in two forms, amantadine hydrochloride and rimantadine hydrochloride. These drugs interfere with the replication cycle of influenza A. In healthy populations, they are 70%-90% effective if given daily throughout the epidemic. For treatment of disease, they decrease fever and other symptoms if given within 48 hours of disease onset. These agents are used to control influenza outbreaks, usually in institutions, and are given to all unvaccinated workers and residents. They may be given regardless of vaccine status to individuals at high risk. Workers should continue taking the medication until 2 weeks after vaccination or indefinitely during the period of risk if the vaccine is contraindicated. The dosage in healthy adults is 200 mg daily.

- Amantadine and rimantadine are used for influenza A only.
- They are 70%-90% effective.
- They are used to control influenza outbreaks, usually in institutions, and are given to all unvaccinated workers and residents.

The side effects are usually minor, occurring in 5%-10% of vaccinees, and may abate with continued use. Rimantadine has less frequent central nervous system side effects than amantadine. Central nervous system side effects are nervousness, anxiety, insomnia, and decreased concentration, and those of the gastrointestinal system include anorexia and nausea. Serious side effects are seizure and confusion, usually seen in the elderly or in those with renal or hepatic disease. In these groups, the dose should be decreased in accordance with the recommendations made in the package inserts.

Hepatitis B

The lifetime risk of acquiring hepatitis B is 5% for the general population; 300,000 cases occur annually in the U.S., resulting in 10,000 hospitalizations and 250 deaths. Of the patients affected, 90% are ≥20 years old; 5%-10% become carriers, and one-quarter of these have chronic active hepatitis. Annually, 4,000 persons die of hepatitis B virus-related cirrhosis and 800 die of hepatitis B virus-related liver cancer.

- The lifetime risk of acquiring hepatitis B is 5% for the general population.
- 5%-10% become carriers.
- Annually, 4,000 persons die of hepatitis B virus-related cirrhosis and 800 die of hepatitis B virus-related liver cancer.

The current vaccine is yeast recombinant, developed from the insertion of a plasmid into *Sacchromyces cerevisiae*, which produces the copies of the surface antigen. Human-purified vaccine is no longer made. The target population includes 1) adults at increased risk, i.e., homosexual males, i.v. drug users, heterosexual persons with multiple sexual partners, and those with a history of other sexually transmitted diseases; 2) household and sexual contacts of hepatitis B virus carriers; 3) workers in health-related and public safety occupations involving exposure to blood or body fluids; 4) hemodialysis patients; 5) recipients of concentrates of clotting factors VIII and IX; 6) morticians and their assistants; and 7) travelers who will be living for extended periods in high-prevalence areas or who are likely to have sexual contacts or contact with blood in the endemic areas (especially in eastern Asia and sub-Sahara Africa).

Vaccination--Normally, vaccination consists of three doses at 0, 1 month, and 6 months. An alternative dosing schedule to induce immunity more rapidly, e.g., after exposure, involves 4 doses, the first three given 1 month apart and a fourth dose at 12 months. Postexposure prophylaxis consists of HBIG given in a single dose of 0.06 mL/kg or 5 mL for adults. It should be administered along with the vaccine in separate syringes at separate sites, but they may be administered at the same time. Current evidence suggests that for most vaccinees the vaccination has a duration of ≥7 years. Currently, revaccination is not routinely recommended. For persons who receive the vaccine in the buttock or whose management depends on knowledge of immune status (e.g., surgeons or venipuncturists), periodic serologic testing may be valuable. Those with titers <10 mIU should be revaccinated. Revaccination with a single dose is usually effective.

- Currently, revaccination for hepatitis B is not routinely recommended.

The most common side effect of hepatitis B vaccination is localized soreness. Guillain-Barré syndrome (0.5 per 100,000) was associated with human-derived hepatitis B vaccines. Comparable information is not available for the recombinant vaccination. Vaccination in pregnancy is considered advisable for women who are at risk for hepatitis B infection. The risk of hepatitis B virus infection in pregnancy far outweighs the risk of vaccine-associated problems.

- Guillain-Barré syndrome (0.5 per 100,000) was associated with human-derived hepatitis B vaccines.

Pneumococcal vaccine--Two-thirds of persons with serious pneumococcal disease have been hospitalized in the previous 5 years (a missed opportunity to vaccinate). The risk of bacteremia for persons ≥65 years old is 50 per 100,000. The current vaccine is a purified capsular material of 23 different serotypes of streptococcus pneumonia. In most healthy adults, titers persist for ≥5 years. Persons who have received a 14-valent vaccine need not be routinely revaccinated. However, persons at highest risk for pneumococcal infections, such as asplenic patients, should be revaccinated with the 23-valent vaccine if it has been >6 years since the previous dose. Patients with nephrotic syndrome and renal failure and transplant patients should be revaccinated every 3-5 years because of waning immunity.

The target population is persons ≥65 years old, adults with chronic disease states such as cardiovascular or pulmonary disease, or persons at higher risk for pneumococcal infection, e.g., because of alcoholism or cerebrospinal fluid leak. The target population also includes immunocompromised persons (such as those who are asplenic) and patients with Hodgkin's disease, lymphoma, multiple myeloma, chronic renal failure, nephrotic syndrome, HIV infection, or organ transplant. The side effects are erythema and localized pain, which occur in about 50% of all vaccinees. Other side effects such as fever, myalgia, and severe local reactions occur in <1%. Five per 1,000,000 of those vaccinated develop anaphylaxis. Revaccination within approximately 1 year is associated with increased local reaction.

- The target population is persons ≥65 years old or adults with chronic disease.

Smallpox (vaccinia)--In May 1980, WHO declared the world free of smallpox. Vaccination is no longer indicated except for persons working directly with the orthopoxviruses.

- Smallpox vaccination is no longer indicated except for persons working directly with the orthopoxviruses.

Polio--Polio is a low-risk disease in the U.S. There are OPV (live virus) and eIPV (killed virus) vaccinations. A primary series with either one has >95% effectiveness. Polio vaccination is not recommended for persons >18 years old unless they plan to travel to an endemic area and have no history of a previous primary series. For these persons, use eIPV because of the slightly lower risk of paralysis. The primary series consists of eIPV followed in 4-8 weeks by eIPV, followed in 6-12 months by eIPV. If it is <4 weeks before travel, give a single dose of either OPV or eIPV. If the primary series is incomplete, complete it despite the interval since the previous dose. If the person previously received IPV, give one dose of OPV or eIPV. For OPV, the risk of paralysis is approximately 1 in 1,000,000 after the first dose, and for susceptible household contacts, it is approximately 1 in 2,000,000.

● Polio vaccination is not recommended for persons >18 years old unless they plan to travel to an endemic area.

Rabies--Preexposure prophylaxis is recommended for animal handlers, lab workers, persons traveling to endemic areas for >1 month, or those with vocations/avocations with exposure to skunks, raccoons, and bats as well as other animals. The reservoir of infection includes carniverous animals, particularly skunks, raccoons, foxes, and bats in the U.S. Except for woodchucks, rodents are rarely infected.

QUESTIONS

Multiple Choice (choose the one best answer)
1. Tertiary prevention refers to detection and elimination or amelioration of:
   a. Recurrent disease, such as tamoxifen treatment after breast cancer
   b. Disease in a presymptomatic (preclinical) stage
   c. Risk factors before they have led to a disease state
   d. Need for immunization updates
   e. Asymptomatic, previously undetected cancer, such as malignant colon polyp

2. Desirable features of a screening test include which of the following?
   a. It is highly specific, and a highly sensitive follow-up test is available
   b. It requires a high level of expertise to be performed correctly
   c. It is a blood test
   d. It causes significant morbidity, but is highly specific
   e. It is highly sensitive even if some specificity is sacrificed

3. Randomized, controlled trial evidence of reduced mortality now supports which one of the following?
   a. Lung cancer screening (sputum cytology)
   b. Prostate cancer screening (prostate-specific antigen)
   c. Colon cancer screening (occult blood)
   d. Pelvic examinations every 3 years
   e. Ovarian cancer screening (CA 125)

4. In regard to breast cancer screening, which statement is false?
   a. There is general agreement that mammography and a clinical breast examination are appropriate between the ages of 40 and 65
   b. Randomized, controlled trial evidence suggests that mammography will decrease mortality by about 30%
   c. Having two first-degree relatives with breast cancer increases one's risk 3 to 8 times
   d. Screen film mammography has a positive predictive value of <20%
   e. Broad use of mammography will likely induce a small and insignificant number of cancers

5. In the U.S., heart disease is the leading cause of death, but it is on the decline. Cancer is the second leading cause of death, in part because people are living longer. The third leading cause of death is:
   a. Cerebrovascular disease
   b. Accidents
   c. Chronic obstructive lung disease
   d. Homicide
   e. Cirrhosis

6. All are true of purified protein derivative (PPD) skin testing except:
   a. In persons at low risk, a positive skin test is 15 mm of induration
   b. 10 mm of induration or 15 mm of erythema is considered positive
   c. 5 mm is considered positive in HIV-infected persons
   d. Relative anergy may occur with age, but may be overcome by the booster effect of repeat testing
   e. Reactivity can be affected by recent MMR vaccination

7. Ovarian cancer is the fourth leading cause of cancer death in women. Evidence supports a decreased risk of cancer in women:
   a. Who smoke
   b. Who avoid pregnancy
   c. Who have early onset of menses and late onset of menopause
   d. Who work with analine dyes
   e. Who use oral contraceptive pills for more than 1 year

True/False (indicate whether each answer is true or false)

8. Smoking is a risk factor for:
   a. Lung cancer
   b. Breast cancer
   c. Colon cancer
   d. Cervical cancer
   e. Prostate cancer
   f. Ovarian cancer

9. With regard to the prevention of influenza:
   a. The vaccine includes antigens for both influenza A and B
   b. Most health care workers should be vaccinated
   c. Amantadine and, recently, rimantadine are available as chemoprophylactic agents for influenza B
   d. Influenza vaccine is an inactivated (killed) virus vaccine
   e. For eligible people, vaccination should be administered in August and September
   f. Because vaccination is not 100% effective, amantadine and rimantadine may be given to high-risk persons without regard to their vaccine status

10. A pregnant (first-trimester) operating room nurse was stuck 3 days ago with a suture needle from a patient who is a hepatitis B carrier. On review of her immunization status, you discover she has had no shots since her school days 20 years ago. On testing, she is immune to rubella but not measles or mumps. She is not immune to hepatitis B either. Appropriate measures are the following:
    a. Tetanus booster shot
    b. Hepatitis B immune globulin (HBIG)
    c. Hepatitis B vaccine
    d. Measles vaccine
    e. Measles, mumps, rubella (MMR) vaccine
    f. Refer her to an obstetrician

ANSWERS

1. Answer a.

Primary prevention is done *before* the existence of disease, secondary prevention is done *after* disease occurs but before it is symptomatic, and tertiary prevention is done after the diagnosis *and* initial treatment of clinical disease. Thus, answer a is correct because it refers to the prevention of recurrent disease; answers b and e refer to secondary prevention, and answers c and d refer to primary prevention.

2. Answer e.

Ideally, a screening test is inexpensive, easy to perform correctly, and highly sensitive, i.e., it detects most cases of disease. Often, it is the case that maximizing sensitivity decreases specificity by labeling people without disease as having positive test results. For example, lowering the threshold of what a positive prostate-specific antigen blood test is from 4.0 to 3.0 will net more cancer cases, but it also will label as "positive" more men who do not have cancer. Thus, a highly specific follow-up test is ideal.

3. Answer c.

Only breast cancer and colon cancer screening have been shown to decrease mortality in large randomized, controlled trials. Lung cancer screening has not proved to be effective. Prostate and ovarian cancer are currently being evaluated, but results will not be available for several years. Pelvic examination is an accepted screening practice, but it has not been evaluated by controlled trial for effectiveness.

4. Answer a.

There is general agreement that mammography should be performed between the ages of 50 and 65 because several randomized, controlled trials have shown it to be effective in decreasing mortality by about 30%. The use of mammography in the 40s remains controversial, although clinical breast examination is more generally accepted. Because the incidence of breast cancer in asymptomatic women is relatively low, even a fairly sensitive screening test like mammography has a low positive predictive value. Because mammography uses x-ray radiation and broad-based routine screening will expose a large number of women to this radiation, it will likely induce a few breast cancers. However, relative to the number of cancers detected and lives saved, this is a truly insignificant number.

5. Answer a.

Cerebrovascular disease, primarily stroke, is a distant third to cancer and heart disease. Preventable risk factors for stroke include smoking and hypertension. In some age groups, for example, young adults (both men and women), accidents and homicide are leading causes of death.

6. Answer b.

PPD skin testing is used in the United States as a screening measure for exposure to *Mycobacterium tuberculosis* infection. Standard testing includes intradermal injection of 5 transdermal units and assessment of the reaction at 48-72 hours. Only the size of the induration is considered in assessing the reaction, thus answer b is incorrect. In a low-risk population, 15 mm of induration is now considered positive (the previous cutoff of 10 mm was complicated by cross-reacting mycobacterial species). In a high-risk population (recently exposed to tuberculosis or infected with human immunodeficiency virus), 5 mm of induration is considered a positive reaction. Recent (6 weeks) administration of the MMR vaccine may suppress a PPD reaction.

7. Answer e.

Screening the general population for ovarian cancer with the currently available tests is not feasible and might result in many women without cancer undergoing an exploratory operation. Women at high risk--those with a first-degree relative (mother or sister) who has disease--may be candidates for screening. Things that interrupt or decrease the number of ovulation cycles a woman goes through seem to reduce the risk of ovarian cancer. These include pregnancies, late onset of menses, and early onset of menopause. The most con-

vincing "negative" risk factor is the use of oral contraceptive pills for more than a year. For each year of oral contraceptive use, the risk of ovarian cancer decreases by about 12% for up to 7 years. Smoking does not appear to be a risk factor for ovarian cancer. Exposure to analine dyes is a risk factor for bladder cancer but not for ovarian cancer.

8. a, true; b, false; c, false; d, true; e, true; f, false.

Many diseases are associated with smoking in a causal way. However, several common cancers do not appear to be. Lung cancer clearly is related to smoking. Cervical cancer appears to be, and a history of smoking approximately doubles the risk. Breast, colon, prostate, and ovarian cancer do not appear to be related to smoking.

9. a, true; b, true; c, false; d, true; e, false; f, true.

An effective vaccine for both influenza A and B exists. It contains inactivated (killed) virus, whole or subviron particles, for two type A and for one type B viruses. Candidates for vaccination include the elderly, institutionalized persons, chronically ill persons, and (in recent years) health care workers. The vaccine usually becomes available in October and should be administered in October and November. Chemoprophylaxis includes drugs that interfere with the viral replication cycle of the influenza A virus. In an epidemic or outbreak situation, either of these drugs may be administered to high-risk persons whether or not they have been vaccinated.

10. a, false; b, true; c, true; d, false; e, false; f, false.

Answer a (tetanus booster) is false because of her first-trimester status. She does need a booster, however, and should get it after the baby is born; answers d and e are false because they are live virus vaccines and generally contraindicated in pregnancy; answer f is false because she needs rapid assessment and treatment. Certainly the physician following the pregnancy should be told of the treatment; answers b and c are true because she is at high risk for hepatitis B, a significant threat to her pregnancy. As a health care worker, she should have received her hepatitis immunization. However, because she has not, she should receive both immune globulin to counter the immediate threat of infection and the vaccination to provide casting immunity. They should be given in separate syringes at separate sites.

CHAPTER 20

PSYCHIATRY

Deborah C. Newman, M.D.

Many psychiatric symptoms are as nonspecific as fever. Some signify problems of severe magnitude, whereas others are much less significant. Generally, the symptoms can be and should be investigated further before simply recommending symptomatic relief. The current paradigm of psychiatric assessment is the biopsychosocial model in which the biologic, psychologic, and social factors contributing to the patient's clinical presentation are evaluated.

Psychiatric disorders are divided into major diagnostic groups. A simplified way to conceptualize these groups is to look at the major symptomatic features of the patient's presentation: 1) mood--depression or mania; 2) anxiety--situational stress, panic disorder, generalized anxiety, others; 3) thought--psychotic process, acute (drug-induced, metabolic/toxic) versus chronic (schizophrenic process).

Any of the above diagnostic groups can be altered by alcohol or substance abuse/dependence, delirium, or dementia. The common psychiatric disorders seen by general physicians in outpatient settings are anxiety disorders, mood disorders, substance abuse, psychophysiologic disorders, and adjustment disorders. In the general hospital setting, the common psychiatric groups are mood disorders, adjustment disorders, substance abuse, delirium, and dementia. (The term "organic mental disorders" has been removed from the latest edition of *The Diagnostic and Statistical Manual* [DSM IV] *of the American Psychiatric Association 1994* and replaced by a category called "delirium, dementia, amnestic and other cognitive disorders.") The descriptions of the psychiatric disorders in this syllabus are based on the criteria described in DSM IV.

- Common psychiatric disorders seen by general physicians in an outpatient setting: anxiety disorders, mood disorders, substance abuse, psychophysiologic disorders, and adjustment disorders.
- Common psychiatric groups in a general hospital setting: mood disorders, adjustment disorders, substance abuse, delirium, and dementia.

MOOD DISORDERS

The prevalence of mood disorders in the general population of the U.S. is estimated at 5%-8%; however, in the general medical setting, the rate may be as high as 5%-15%.

Although the essential feature of mood disorders is a disturbance of mood, it is accompanied by related cognitive, psychomotor, vegetative (sleep, appetite, etc.), and interpersonal difficulties. Fluctuations in mood are a normal occurrence. It is only when the frequency and/or intensity of these changes is extreme and accompanied by the other features described that a formal mood disorder is diagnosed. The five major groups of mood disorders cover the range from mild to severe depression to the opposite extreme of mania. Three groups relate to depression: adjustment disorder with depressed mood, dysthymia, and major depression. Two groups relate to problems with mood fluctuations between various degrees of depression and mania: cyclothymia and bipolar disorder. Each of these five major groups has several subgroups. Another important group includes mood disorders due to a general medical condition and mood disorders that are substance-induced. The clinical presentation may be similar to that of a depressive or manic episode, but the cause may be related more specifically to a general medical condition or a particular substance(s) that can then be listed. The clinical phenomenology is similar to that of a manic or depressive episode.

- Mood disorders: the essential feature is disturbance of mood.
- They are accompanied by related cognitive, psychomotor, vegetative, and interpersonal difficulties.
- Mood disorders may also be related to a general medical condition or be substance-induced.

Adjustment Disorder With Depressed Mood

Adjustment disorder with depressed mood is a reaction that develops in response to an identifiable psychosocial stressor(s), e.g., divorce, job loss, or family or marital problems. It can occur any time in anyone if the psychosocial stressors are severe. The severity of the adjustment disorder (degree of impairment) does not always parallel the intensity of the precipitating event. The critical factor appears to be the relevance of the event or stressor to the individual and his or her ability to cope with the stress. In general, these reactions are relatively transient. Although they generally can be managed by an empathic primary care physician, the development of extreme withdrawal, suicidal ideation, or failure to improve as the circumstances improve may prompt psychiatric referral. Treatment includes supportive psychotherapy, psychosocial interventions, and, sometimes, use of antidepressant agents.

Dysthymia

Dysthymia is a form of chronic depression that may have either an early or late onset, as defined by onset before or after, respectively, age 21. It can be disabling for the person because the depressed mood is present most of the time during at least a 2-year period. Many of the patients have some associated vegetative signs such as disturbance of sleep and appetite, but they also often feel inadequate, have low self-esteem, and struggle with interpersonal relationships. If onset is in late adolescence, the dysthymia may become intertwined with the person's personality, behavior, and general attitude toward life. Treatment is usually a combination of psychotherapy (insight-oriented, cognitive, or interpersonal), behavioral therapy, and pharmacotherapy. Psychopharmacotherapy may be particularly useful in patients with a family history of mood disorders or in those who have the early onset form of dysthymia. In patients with dysthymia, major depressive episodes may develop. Also, some are prone to turn to alcohol or other substance abuse to "treat" their dysphoria.

- Dysthymia: a form of chronic depression.
- Depressed mood is present most of the time during at least a 2-year period.
- Treatment is usually a combination of psychotherapy and pharmacotherapy.
- Major depressive episodes may develop in patients with dysthymia.

Major Depression

Major depression is a serious psychiatric disorder that is set apart from adjustment disorder and dysthymia by the severity of the mood and cognitive disturbances and the presence of significant somatic symptoms. The primary symptoms of major depression include: depressed mood, diminished interest or pleasure in all or almost all activities, significant weight loss or weight gain (>5% of body weight in a month), decrease or increase in appetite, insomnia or hypersomnia, psychomotor agitation or retardation, fatigue or loss of energy, feelings of worthlessness or of excessive or inappropriate guilt, diminished ability to concentrate, recurrent thoughts of death or suicidal ideation, or a suicide attempt. If delusions or hallucinations are also present, then it would be classified as "major depression with psychotic features." Another severe form of major depression is the melancholic type. In addition to the symptoms listed above, this form is characterized by the lack of reactivity to pleasurable stimuli (does not feel better even temporarily if involved in what is usually a pleasurable activity), diurnal mood variation (depression regularly worse in the morning), and early morning awakening (at least 2 hours before usual time of awakening).

- Major depression: symptoms are depressed mood, diminished interest or pleasure in all or almost all activities, and significant weight loss or weight gain.
- Melancholic type: characterized by lack of reactivity to pleasurable stimuli, diurnal mood variation, early morning awakening.

Every year about 10 million Americans have a depressive episode but about only 20% usually seek treatment. Of those who seek treatment from a physician, as many as one-third are not diagnosed or are sometimes misdiagnosed because they often present with somatic complaints. As our population ages and more elderly patients seek medical care, diagnosing and treating their mood disorders are becoming more complicated because these patients often have overlapping medical and neurologic problems. Sometimes they present with the combination of a dementing process and depression, which if treated can help manage some of the other problems. The prevalence of depression in women is twice as high as in men. The peak age of onset of depression in women is 33-45 years and in men, >55 years.

- Of persons seeking treatment for major depression, as many as one-third are not diagnosed or are misdiagnosed.
- In elderly patients, diagnosing and treating mood disorders are becoming more complicated.
- Prevalence of depression in women is twice as high as in men.

Seasonal Affective Disorder

Seasonal affective disorder is a form of depression usually characterized by the onset of depression in the fall or winter. It occurs twice as commonly in women as in men and is associated with psychomotor retardation, hypersomnia, overeating (carbohydrate craving), and weight gain. To make the diagnosis, this has to be a recurrent pattern for 2-3 consecutive years. Treatment has relied primarily on phototherapy, using a full-spectrum light source of 2,500 lux for 2 hours/day at a distance of 30 inches from the eyes or 10,000 lux sources, which can be used for 30 minutes/day. Newer sources of lights are being investigated, as are more specific details about the cause of this disorder. It appears that the antidepressant agents that selectively block serotonin reuptake may also be helpful in treating this disorder.

- Seasonal affective disorder: onset of depression in the fall and winter.
- It is twice as common in women as in men.
- It is associated with psychomotor retardation, hypersomnia, and overeating.
- Treatment: primarily phototherapy.

Depressions are heterogeneous in their clinical presentation and so probably do not have a single etiologic agent. It appears that depression is more related to alterations of several neurotransmitter systems and neuropeptides, effects on presynaptic and postsynaptic receptors, neurohormonal alterations, and, in general, an alteration in the overall balance of these systems that are so interdependent on one another.

Treatment of Depression

There are four major groups of treatment modalities for depression: psychotherapy, pharmacotherapy, electroconvulsive therapy, and circadian rhythm manipulation such as sleep deprivation or phototherapy. Generally, they are used in some combination.

Psychotherapy: There are multiple forms of psychotherapy, many of which can be used in the treatment of depression. However, the two forms that have been used extensively for treating depression are cognitive therapy and interpersonal therapy. Cognitive therapy strives to help patients have a better integration of cognition (thoughts), emotion, and behavior. This therapy is based on the premise that our thoughts have a profound impact on our emotions, which have an impact on our behavior. If we can learn more adaptive ways of thinking, it may improve our general outlook and ultimately our behavior, with an increase in a sense of worth and improved self-esteem. Interpersonal therapy focuses on current interpersonal functioning. It is based on the concept that depression is associated with impaired social relationships that either precipitate or perpetuate the disorder.

- Cognitive therapy: to help patients have a better integration of cognition (thoughts), emotion, and behavior.
- Interpersonal therapy: focuses on current interpersonal functioning.

Pharmacotherapy: The selection of medication is based on the side-effect profile of the medication and the clinical profile of the patient. Dose--Start slowly and titrate to a therapeutic dose based on clinical judgment and blood levels (when available). Duration of treatment--Usually a minimum of 6 months, counting from the time the patient attained significant improvement. Often, patients may benefit from extended use of antidepressant agents, especially if they have had multiple episodes of depression. Antidepressant agents generally should be tapered rather than abruptly stopped when their use is discontinued. If the response to the first antidepressant agent is minimal or none, consider the addition of lithium carbonate or synthetic thyroid (T_3 or T_4), change to a different class of drug, or use electroconvulsive therapy, which is still probably the most consistently effective treatment for severe depression.

Cyclothymia

Cyclothymia can be thought of as a less severe form of bipolar disorder. By definition, it is a chronic disorder that usually appears in the late teens or early twenties and involves multiple hypomanic and depressive episodes that are not severe enough to meet criteria for mania or depression and do not generally cause significant impairment of occupational or social functioning. About 20% of patients with cyclothymia have a family history of bipolar disorder. About half of the patients report improvement while taking lithium.

- Cyclothymia: a less severe form of bipolar disorder.
- It is a chronic disorder that usually appears in the late teens to early twenties.
- It generally does not cause significant impairment of occupational or social functioning.

Mania and Bipolar Disorder

The essential features of a manic episode are the presence of an abnormally euphoric, expansive, or irritable mood associated with some of the following: inflated self-esteem or grandiosity, decreased need for sleep, pressured speech, flight of ideas, distractibility, increase in goal-directed activity or psychomotor agitation, and excessive involvement in pleasurable activities that have a high potential for painful consequences (e.g., unrestrained buying sprees, sexual indiscretions, or inappropriate financial investments). To make the diagnosis of a bipolar disorder, the patient must have had episodes of both depression and mania.

- Mania: essential feature is an abnormally euphoric, expansive, or irritable mood.
- The prevalence of bipolar disorder is estimated to be about 1%.
- Bipolar disorder seems to occur at about the same frequency in women and men.
- The usual age at onset is from the teens to age 30.
- Patients generally have a family history of bipolar or other mood disorder.

Treatment is aimed at mood stabilization and improved social and occupational functioning. The primary pharmacologic treatment is lithium carbonate (see below). Other agents that are helpful include carbamazepine and valproic acid. Lithium may take up to 5-10 days to be effective. During this waiting period, the judicious use of antipsychotic agents or clonazepam is helpful in controlling the acute symptoms.

- Treatment of mania and bipolar disorder: aimed at mood stabilization and improved social and occupational functioning.
- Primary pharmacologic treatment: lithium carbonate.

Mood Disorders Due to a General Medical Condition

The essential feature of mood disorders due to a general medical condition is a disturbance of mood that is attributable to the physiologic effects of a specific medical condition. The clinical presentation may resemble that of a major depressive or manic episode, but the full criteria for one of these episodes need not be met. Medical conditions that may cause mood symptoms include endocrinopathies (Cushing's syndrome, Addison's disease, hyper- and hypothyroidism, and hyper- and hypoparathyroidism), certain malignancies (occult cancers, lymphomas, pancreatic carcinoma, gliomas), neurologic conditions (Parkinson's disease, Huntington's disease), autoimmune conditions (systemic lupus erythematosus), and infections (hepatitis, encephalitis, mononucleosis, HIV).

- Mood disorders due to a general medical condition: essential feature is a disturbance of mood attributable to the physiologic effects of a specific medical condition.
- Many medical conditions can induce mood changes.

Substance-Induced Mood Disorders

The essential feature of a substance-induced mood disorder is a disturbance of mood that is judged to be due to the direct physiologic effects of a substance. Many substances can induce mood changes, including medications, toxin exposure, or substances of abuse. The mood symptoms may occur during the use of or exposure to the substance or during withdrawal from the substance. Medications that have been implicated in inducing mood disturbances include steroids, reserpine, methyldopa, propranolol, carbonic anhydrase inhibitors, stimulants, sedative-hypnotics, benzodiazepines, and narcotics and the chronic use or abuse of alcohol or hallucinogens.

- Substance-induced mood disorders: essential feature is a disturbance of mood due to the physiologic effects of a substance.
- Many medications and drugs of abuse may induce mood changes.

PSYCHOTIC DISORDERS

"Psychosis" is a generic term used to describe behavior marked by a break from reality. Psychotic symptoms can occur in various medical, neurologic, and psychiatric disorders. Many psychotic reactions seen in medical settings are associated with the use of recreational or prescription drugs (Table 20-1). Some of these drug-induced psychotic reactions are nearly indistinguishable from schizophrenia (e.g., amphetamine and phen-cyclidine [PCP] psychoses). Other reactions may manifest as more nonspecific psychotic syndromes. Many brain regions may be involved with the production of psychotic symptoms, but abnormalities in the frontal, temporal, and limbic regions are more likely than others to produce psychotic features.

- Psychosis: a generic term describing behavior marked by a break from reality.
- Many psychotic reactions may be associated with use of recreational or prescription drugs.
- Some drug-induced psychotic reactions are nearly indistinguishable from schizophrenia.

There are disorders throughout the lifespan that may be associated with schizophrenia-like psychoses. These include genetic abnormalities, intrauterine events, neonatal brain injury, childhood neurologic insults, adolescent neuroendocrine changes, adult neurologic disorders, medical and metabolic diseases (e.g., infections, inflammatory disorders, endocrinopathies, nutritional deficiencies, uremia, hepatic encephalopathy), drug abuse, and psychologic stressors.

Schizophrenia in particular may also have a multifactorial cause. Current diagnostic criteria are divided into inclusion and exclusion criteria. Inclusion criteria include 1) presence of delusions and hallucinations; 2) marked decrement in functional level in areas such as work, school, social relations, and self-care; and 3) continuous signs of the disturbance for at least 6 months. Exclusion criteria include 1) absence of a consistent mood disorder component and 2) lack of evidence of an organic factor that produces the symptoms.

- Schizophrenia may have a multifactorial cause.

The five subtypes of schizophrenia are catatonic, disorganized, paranoid, undifferentiated, and residual.

Table 20-1.--Classes of Drugs That Can Produce Psychotic Symptoms

Stimulants
Hallucinogens
Phencyclidine (PCP)
Catecholaminergic drugs
Anticholinergic drugs
Central nervous system depressants
Glucocorticoids
Heavy metals (lead, mercury, manganese, arsenic, thallium)
Others (digitalis, disulfiram, cimetidine, bromide)

ANXIETY DISORDERS

This group of disorders includes some of the ones seen most frequently in the outpatient setting. Anxiety symptoms may be misinterpreted as those of medical illness because many of the symptoms overlap, e.g., tachycardia, diaphoresis, tremor, shortness of breath, nausea, abdominal pain, and chest pain. Autonomic arousal and anxious agitation in a medically ill patient can also be quickly attributed to stress or anxiety when it may represent pulmonary embolus or cardiac arrhythmia. Common sources of anxiety in the medical setting relate to fears of death, abandonment, loss of function, loss of a body part, pain, dependency, and loss of control. When to treat or to seek psychiatric consultation depends on the assessment of the degree of anxiety--is it at a level "expected" under the circumstances or is it unrealistic.

- Anxiety symptoms may be misinterpreted as those of medical illness.
- Common sources of anxiety in the medical setting relate to fears of death, abandonment, loss of function, loss of a body part, etc.

Adjustment Disorder With Anxious Mood

Adjustment disorder with anxious mood is a maladaptive reaction to an identifiable environmental or psychosocial stress, accompanied primarily by symptoms of anxiety that interfere with the patient's usual functioning. Treatment may include supportive counseling and help with identifying the stressor. However, in some cases the anxiety may be so severe as to require short-term use of anxiolytic agents. However, they should be used with caution to avoid problems of long-term use and possible dependence.

- Adjustment disorder with anxious mood: a maladaptive reaction to an identifiable environmental or psychosocial stress accompanied by symptoms of stress.
- It may require short-term use of anxiolytic agents.

Panic Disorder With or Without Agoraphobia

Panic disorder is recurrent, discrete episodes of extreme anxiety accompanied by various somatic symptoms such as dyspnea, unsteady feelings, palpitations, paresthesias, hyperventilation, trembling, diaphoresis, chest pain or discomfort, or abdominal distress. Agoraphobia refers to extreme fear of being in places or situations from which escape may be difficult (or embarrassing). This may lead to avoidance of such situations as driving, travel in general, being in a crowded place, and many other situations, ultimately causing severe limitations in daily functioning for the person. Panic disorder is more common in women than in men; the usual age at onset is from the late teens to the early thirties. A history of childhood separation anxiety is reported in 20%-50% of patients. The incidence is higher in first- and second-degree relatives. Most patients (78%) describe their first panic attack as spontaneous. They generally go to an emergency room after the first attack, believing they are having a heart attack or some severe medical problem.

- Panic disorder: recurrent, discrete episodes of extreme anxiety accompanied by various somatic symptoms.
- Agoraphobia: extreme fear of being in places or situations from which escape may be difficult.
- Agoraphobia is more common in women than in men.
- Patients generally go to an emergency room after their first panic attack, believing they are having a heart attack or some severe medical problem.

Some medical diagnostic groups to consider are 1) endocrine disturbances: hyperthyroidism, pheochromocytoma, and hypoglycemia; 2) gastrointestinal disturbances: colitis and irritable bowel syndrome; 3) cardiopulmonary disturbances: pulmonary embolism, exacerbation of chronic obstructive pulmonary disease, and acute allergic reactions; and 4) neurologic conditions: those associated with paresthesias, faintness, or dizziness.

Patients with panic attacks may also be prone to major episodes of depression. Alcohol use may temporarily reduce some of the distress of the panic attack and the interim anticipatory anxiety but may soon yield to rebound symptoms and potentially lead to alcohol overuse. Benzodiazepines may similarly be abused.

- Patients with panic attacks may be prone to episodes of major depression.
- Alcohol: may reduce distress of panic attacks but symptoms may rebound, potentially leading to alcohol abuse.
- Benzodiazepines may similarly be abused.

Post-Traumatic Stress Disorder

Post-traumatic stress disorder can be a brief reaction that soon follows an extremely traumatic, overwhelming, or catastrophic experience or it may be a chronic condition that produces severe disability. The syndrome is characterized by intrusive memories, flashbacks, nightmares, avoidance of reminders of the event, and often a restricted range of affect. It may occur in children. There is increased comorbidity with substance abuse, depression, and other anxiety disorders. Patients may be more prone to impulsivity, including suicide. As for other anxiety disorders, treatment is usually a combination of behavioral, psychotherapeutic, and, if necessary, pharmacologic interventions.

- Post-traumatic stress disorder: may be a brief reaction or a chronic condition that produces severe disability.
- Patients may be prone to impulsivity, including suicide.

Generalized Anxiety Disorder

Generalized anxiety disorder is characterized by chronic excessive anxiety and apprehension about life circumstances accompanied by somatic symptoms of anxiety, such as trembling, restlessness, autonomic hyperactivity, and hypervigilance. Treatment is usually a mixture of behavioral, progressive muscle relaxation, psychotherapeutic, and adjunctive psychopharmacologic modalities.

Obsessive-Compulsive Disorder

Obsessive-compulsive disorder is characterized by recurrent obsessions or compulsions that are severe enough to disrupt daily life. The obsessions are distressing thoughts, ideas, or impulses experienced as unwanted. Compulsions are repetitive, intentional behaviors usually performed in response to an obsession. The obsessions cause marked anxiety or distress, and the compulsions serve to neutralize the anxiety. Prevalence rates are about 2%-3% and occur about equally in men and women. The onset of this disorder is usually in adolescence or early adulthood. Obsessive traits are often present before onset of the disorder. The predominant neurobiologic theory for the cause of obsessive-compulsive disorder involves dysfunction of brain serotonin systems. Pharmacologic treatment of this disorder uses antidepressants that are more selective for effects on the serotonin transmission system. These include clomipramine, selective serotonin reuptake inhibitors (fluvoxamine, fluoxetine, and sertraline), monoamine oxidase inhibitors (especially for patients who may also have panic attacks), and occasionally lithium augmentation of any of the preceding agents. In very severe, debilitating cases for which other treatments have failed, psychosurgery such as cingulotomy, stereotactic limbic leukotomy, or anterior capsulotomy may be of some benefit. The effectiveness of these procedures is thought to be related to disruption of the efferent pathways from the frontal cortex to the basal ganglia. Behavioral therapies and some forms of psychotherapy can also be helpful adjunctive therapies. As with the treatment of many psychiatric disorders, it is a combination of treatments that is most often used. With obsessive-compulsive disorder, the pharmacologic treatments are generally not as effective as with major depressive episodes. Also, higher doses of the antidepressants may be needed for longer trial periods to see effectiveness in reducing symptoms of the obsessive-compulsive disorder.

- Obsessive-compulsive disorder is characterized by recurrent obsessions (distressing thoughts) and compulsions (repetitive behaviors) that are recognized as unreasonable but irresistible.
- Treatment consists primarily of antidepressants (with serotonergic activity) and behavioral therapy.

SOMATOFORM DISORDERS, FACTITIOUS DISORDERS, AND MALINGERING

Each of these disorders represents illness behaviors but differ with regard to whether the symptoms and motivations for their persistence are conscious or unconscious.

Somatoform Disorders

These include somatization disorder, conversion disorder, hypochondriasis, somatoform pain disorder (chronic pain syndromes), and body dysmorphic disorder.

Somatization Disorder

Somatization disorder is a polysymptomatic disorder that begins in early life and is characterized by recurrent multiple somatic complaints and an overwhelmingly positive review of symptoms. It mostly affects women. This disorder is often best managed with collaborative work with an empathic primary care physician and mental health professional. Regularly scheduled appointments with the primary care physician seem to lessen "doctor shopping" and frequent emergency room visits.

- Somatization disorder: begins in early life; characterized by recurrent multiple somatic complaints.
- It mostly affects women.
- "Doctor shopping" and frequent emergency room visits.

Conversion Disorder

Conversion disorder is a loss or alteration of physical functioning suggestive of a medical/neurologic disorder, but it cannot be explained on the basis of known physiologic mechanisms. The person is not conscious of intentionally producing the symptom. The disorder is not limited to pain or sexual dysfunction. It most often is seen in the outpatient setting. Patients frequently respond to any of several therapeutic modalities that suggest hope of a cure. If it becomes more of a chronic conversion disorder, it carries a poorer prognosis and is difficult to treat. Treatment focuses on management of the symptom rather than cure, much as in somatization or somatoform pain disorders.

- Conversion disorder: loss or alteration of physical functioning.
- It cannot be explained by known physiologic mechanisms.
- It is usually seen in the outpatient setting.
- Treatment focuses on management of the symptoms.

Somatoform Pain Disorder

Somatoform pain disorder (chronic pain syndromes) may occur at any age but most often starts in the 30s or 40s. It is diagnosed twice as often in women as in men and is characterized by preoccupation with pain for at least 6 months. No organic lesion is found to account for the pain, or if there is a related organic lesion, the complaint of pain or resulting interference with usual life activities is in excess of what would be expected from the physical findings. Treatment is usually multidisciplinary and focused on helping the patient manage or live with the pain rather than continuing with the expectation of "cure." Avoidance of long-term dependence on addictive substances is a general goal.

- Somatoform pain disorder: chronic pain syndromes that occur at any age but usually start in the 30s or 40s.
- It is diagnosed twice as often in women as in men.
- It is characterized by preoccupation with pain for at least 6 months.
- Treatment: usually multidisciplinary.

Hypochondriasis

Hypochondriasis is an intense preoccupation with the fear of having or the belief that one has a serious disease despite the lack of physical evidence to support the concern. It tends to be a chronic problem for the patient.

Factitious Disorders

Factitious disorders are characterized by the voluntary production of signs or symptoms of disease. The diagnosis of these disorders requires that the physician be highly suspicious. The most extreme form of the disorder is Munchausen syndrome, which is characterized by the triad of simulating disease, pathologic lying, and wandering. These cases have frequently involved men of lower socioeconomic class who have had a lifelong pattern of poor social adjustment. However, the common form generally occurs among "socially conforming young women of a higher socioeconomic class who are intelligent, educated, and frequently employed in a medically related field." The possibility of a coexisting medical disorder or intercurrent illness needs to be appreciated in the diagnostic and therapeutic management of these difficult cases. Factitious disorders are often found in patients with a history of childhood emotional traumas. These patients through their illness may be seeking to compensate for childhood traumas and secondarily to escape from and make up for stressful life situations.

- Factitious disorders: voluntary production of signs or symptoms of disease in order to assume the sick role.
- Munchausen syndrome: most extreme form of factitious disorder; characteristic triad of simulating disease, pathologic lying, wandering.
- Common form: occurs among socially conforming young women of a higher socioeconomic class.
- Factitious disorders: often in patients with a history of childhood emotional traumas.

Malingering

The essential feature of malingering is the intentional production of false or exaggerated physical or psychologic symptoms. It is motivated by external incentives such as avoiding military service or work, obtaining financial compensation or drugs, evading criminal prosecution, or securing better living conditions. Malingering should be suspected in cases in which 1) a medicolegal context overshadows the clinical presentation, 2) a marked discrepancy exists between the person's claimed stress or disability and the objective findings, 3) there is lack of cooperation during the diagnostic evaluation and in compliance with prescribed treatments, and 4) there is presence of an antisocial personality disorder. The person who is malingering is much less likely to present his or her symptoms in the context of emotional conflict, and the presenting symptoms are less likely to be symbolically related to an underlying emotional conflict.

- Malingering: intentional production of false or exaggerated physical or psychologic symptoms.
- It is motivated by external incentives.

DELIRIUM AND DEMENTIA

The primary distinguishing feature between dementia and delirium is the retention and stability of alertness in dementia.

Delirium

Delirium is characterized by a fluctuating course of an altered state of awareness and consciousness. Although the onset usually is abrupt, it may occasionally be insidious. It may be accompanied by hallucinations (tactile, auditory, visual, or olfactory), illusions (misperceptions of sensory stimuli), delusions, emotional lability, paranoia, alterations in the sleep-wake cycle, and psychomotor slowing or hyperactivity. Delirium is usually reversible with correction of the underlying cause. It often is related to an external toxic agent, medication side effect, metabolic abnormalities, central nervous system abnormality, or withdrawal of a medication or drug. Delirium is relatively common in medical/surgical inpatients older than 65 years (range, 10%-30%). The diagnosis is primarily made by clinical assessment and changes in the patient's mental status examination. High-risk groups include 1) elderly patients with medical illnesses (especially congestive heart failure, urinary tract infections, hyperkalemia, hyponatremia, malnutrition, dehydration, strokes); 2) postcardiotomy patients; 3) patients with brain damage; 4) patients in drug withdrawal; 5) burn patients; and 6) patients with AIDS.

- Delirium: fluctuating course of an altered state of awareness and consciousness.

- It is usually reversible with correction of the underlying cause.
- It is often related to: external toxic agent, medication side effect, metabolic abnormalities, central nervous system abnormality, or withdrawal of a medication or drug.
- Delirium is relatively common in medical/surgical patients older than 65 years.

The commonest cause of delirium in the elderly probably is intoxication with psychotropic drugs, especially drugs with sedative and anticholinergic side effects. Treatment initially can be separated by whether the cause is known. If it is, treating the underlying cause is most beneficial. If the cause is unknown and the patient's behavior interferes with his or her safety and medical care, several categories of intervention can be considered. Management aspects include 1) medical: monitor vital signs, electrolytes, fluid balance, etc.; 2) pharmacologic: neuroleptic agents in parenteral form are helpful, such as haloperidol given intravenously; 3) environmental supports: to help with orientation, use calendars, clock, windows (family and others with orientation information are also helpful); 4) psychosocial supports: family or other care providers can be helpful.

- Commonest cause of delirium in the elderly: intoxication with psychotropic drugs.

Dementia

Dementia is a syndrome of acquired persistent impairment of mental function involving at least three of the following five domains: memory, language, visuospatial skills, personality or mood, and cognition (including abstraction, judgment, calculations, and executive function). Some of the more common types of dementia are the following:
1. Cortical dementia--The common form is Alzheimer's disease; other types include Pick's disease and Creutzfeldt-Jakob disease. The overall prevalence is estimated at 2%-10% of the population over 65 and 15%-20% of those older than 85.
2. Subcortical dementia--Patients with this type of dementia often have an associated gait disturbance. The common type is multi-infarct dementia; other forms include normal-pressure hydrocephalus, Huntington's disease, and Parkinson's disease.
3. HIV-related dementia.
4. Dementias associated with multiple sclerosis, amyotrophic lateral sclerosis, vitamin B_{12} deficiency, hypothyroidism, and Wilson's disease.

- Cortical dementia: the common form is Alzheimer's type.
- Subcortical dementia: the common type is multi-infarct dementia.

Dementia is distinguished from delirium by intact arousal, more preserved attention, and persistence of the cognitive changes. Some forms may be reversible, as in dementia related to hypothyroidism, and some may be "treatable" without reversing the intellectual deficits, e.g., preventing further ischemic injury in patients with vascular dementia. The dementia may be a chronic progressive form in which treatment is generally related to improved control of the behavioral disturbances.

PSYCHOLOGIC ASPECTS OF AIDS

From the early to the terminal phases of AIDS and its sequelae, many psychiatric symptoms and complications are possible. The organic mental disorders associated with this process can be primary (directly induced by HIV infection), secondary (related to the effects of the HIV infection leading to immunodeficiency and opportunistic infections or tumors systemically or within the central nervous system), or iatrogenic (resulting from the treatment of HIV or its sequelae). The delirium of AIDS often has a multifactorial cause, similar to delirium in general, i.e., electrolyte imbalance, encephalopathy from intracranial or systemic infections, hypoxemia, or medication side effects. HIV itself causes encephalopathy. The dementia of AIDS can result from the chronic sequelae of most of the causes of delirium. However, direct cerebral infection with HIV probably causes much of the dementia. Other psychiatric symptoms are more nonspecific, such as anger, depression, mania, psychosis, and the general problems of dealing with a terminal illness. Also, all of these might be complicated by undiagnosed and, thus, untreated alcohol or drug dependence, especially in the early phases of the disease.

- AIDS: many possible psychiatric symptoms and complications.
- Organic mental disorders can be primary (due to HIV infection), secondary (due to immunodeficiency and opportunistic infections), or iatrogenic.
- Delirium in AIDS is multifactorial.
- Dementia in AIDS: can result from chronic sequelae of most of the causes of delirium.

THE SUICIDAL PATIENT

Suicide is not an uncommon consequence of mental illness. It occurs in all psychiatric diagnostic categories. Emergency medicine physicians are often the first to deal with patients who have either completed suicide, attempted suicide, or have suicidal ideation. The recognition of risk factors for suicide and the acute medical management of the patient are important. Although the person who overdoses with a benzodiazepine may be more serious about the intent, the person who overdoses on aspirin may be at more risk for serious medical complications.

- Suicide: occurs in all psychiatric diagnostic categories.
- Recognition of the risk factors for suicide is important.

Recognition of a suicidal gesture is important in evaluating a patient in an emergency room. Although drug overdoses are the commonest form, alcohol intoxication, single vehicle accidents, and falls from heights at times merit further investigation. Many suicidal patients saw a physician the week before the attempt. Some of the risk factors to be aware of include: older divorced or widowed men, Caucasians, unemployment, poor physical health, past suicide attempts, family history of suicide (especially if parent), psychosis, alcoholism or drug abuse, chronic painful disease, sudden life changes, living alone, and anniversary of significant loss. Almost without exception, patients who come to an emergency room with intense suicidal ideation or gestures should not be sent home alone.

- In evaluating patients in an emergency room, recognition of a suicidal gesture is important.
- Many suicidal patients saw a physician the week before the attempt.
- Patients who come to an emergency room with intense suicidal ideation or gestures should not be sent home alone.

EATING DISORDERS

The two common eating disorders are anorexia nervosa and bulimia. Both are more prevalent in women than in men. The onset is usually in the teenage or young adult years but can start prepubertally or after age 40. These disorders are now found across all income, racial, and ethnic groups. Both disorders have a primary symptom of preoccupation with weight and a desire to be thinner. The disorders are not mutually exclusive, and about 50% of patients with anorexia nervosa also have bulimia. Many patients with bulimia previously had at least a subclinical case of anorexia nervosa.

- The two common eating disorders: anorexia nervosa and bulimia.
- They are more prevalent in women than in men.
- Primary symptom: preoccupation with weight and a desire to be thinner.

Anorexia Nervosa

To meet the diagnostic criteria of anorexia nervosa, weight loss must be 15% below that expected for age and height. However, weight loss of 30%-40% below normal is not uncommon and leads to medical complications of starvation, such as depletion of fat, muscle wasting (including cardiac muscle in severe cases), bradycardia and other arrhythmias, ventricular tachycardia and sudden death, constipation, abdominal pain, leukopenia, hypercortisolemia, osteoporosis, and, in extreme cases, development of lanugo, and metabolic alterations to conserve energy (thyroid--low levels of T_3, cold intolerance, and difficulty maintaining core body temperature; reproductive--marked decrease or cessation of LH and FSH secretion and secondary amenorrhea).

Bulimia

The patients always feel as though their eating is out of control; many patients may have a concurrent depressive or anxiety disorder. Physical complications of the binge-purge cycle may include fluid and electrolyte abnormalities, hypochloremic-hypokalemic alkalosis, esophageal and gastric irritation and bleeding, large bowel abnormalities due to laxative abuse, marked erosion of dental enamel with associated decay, parotid and salivary gland hypertrophy, and hyperamylasemia (25%-40% more than normal). If bulimia is untreated, it often becomes chronic. Some patients have a gradual spontaneous remission of some symptoms.

- Patients with bulimia may have a concurrent depressive or anxiety disorder.
- The binge-purge cycle causes physical complications.

ALCOHOLISM AND SUBSTANCE ABUSE DISORDERS

Alcoholism and substance abuse disorders are a major concern in all age groups and across all ethnic, socioeconomic, and racial groups. Despite national and international efforts to curb the problem and to make treatment more readily available, many people go undiagnosed and fewer than 10% of addicted people are involved in some form of treatment, either self-help groups or with professional supervision. The lifetime incidence of alcohol and drug abuse approaches 20% of the population. These disorders have devastating effects on families and significant others and contribute to other social problems such as motor vehicle accidents and fatalities, domestic violence, suicide, and increasing health care costs. Untreated alcoholics have been estimated to generate twice the general health care costs of nonalcoholics. Patients with addictive disorders are a heterogeneous group. They may present in many different ways. What may be most critical is improvement in the diagnostic skill in recognizing addictive disorders. The current definition of alcoholism approved by the National Council on Alcoholism and Drug Dependence may also be applicable to other drugs of abuse: alcoholism is a primary, chronic disease with genetic, psychosocial, and environmental factors influencing its development and manifestations.

The disease is often progressive and fatal. It is characterized by continuous or periodic impaired control over drinking, preoccupation with the drug alcohol, use despite adverse consequences, and distortions in thinking, most notably denial.

- Fewer than 10% of addicted people are involved in some form of treatment.
- Lifetime incidence of alcohol and drug abuse approaches 20% of the population.
- Untreated alcoholics generate twice the general health care costs of nonalcoholics.
- Patients with addictive disorders are a heterogeneous group.

The adverse consequences of alcoholism and substance abuse disorders cross over into several domains:
1. Physical health--Alcohol withdrawal syndromes, liver disease, gastritis, anemia, and neurologic disorders.
2. Psychologic functioning--Impairment in cognition and changes in mood and behavior.
3. Interpersonal functioning--Marital problems and child abuse and impaired social relationships.
4. Occupational functioning--Scholastic or job problems.
5. Legal, financial, and spiritual problems.

The substance abuse disorders are divided into ten major groups: alcohol; amphetamine; cannabis; cocaine; hallucinogens; inhalants; nicotine; opioids; phencyclidine; and benzodiazepines, sedative hypnotics, and anxiolytics. Some things are specific to each of these groups, but what may be surprising is that they probably have more similarities than differences when it comes to diagnosing a problem of abuse and/or dependence. In Table 20-2, these drugs are grouped according to their perceived effects. The descriptive titles of the groups give an idea of the physiologic and psychologic activity of the drug when taken. If one thinks of the converse of these states, the withdrawal states can be partly determined. As an example, if in the group of "downers," heart rate, blood pressure, and general autonomic functions slow down when they are used, the opposite reaction would be expected with withdrawal from the substance. Another significant point is that within the group of "downers" there is considerable potential for crossover addictions.

Table 20-2.--Drugs Grouped According to Their Perceived Effects

Uppers	Downers	"All arounders"
Cocaine	Alcohol	Cannabis
Amphetamine	Opioids	Hallucinogens
Caffeine	Benzodiazepines	Inhalants
Nicotine	Sedative-hypnotics	Phencyclidine
	Barbiturates	

- Within the group of "downers," there is considerable potential for crossover addictions.

Alcoholism

Alcoholism is defined above. Medical data from physical examination and laboratory tests can be helpful. However, most of the pertinent findings are not apparent until after several years (often up to 5 years) of alcohol use and so are more reflective of middle-to-late stages of the disease. Two of the earlier detectable signs are increases of serum γ-glutamyltransferase and increased mean corpuscular volume. In both men and women, the combination of increased γ-glutamyltransferase levels and mean corpuscular volume can identify up to 90% of alcoholics. Other abnormal laboratory findings include increased levels of alkaline phosphatase, bilirubin, uric acid, and triglycerides. However, because of the number of false-negative results, it is not practical to rely on laboratory data alone for the diagnosis of alcoholism. Alcohol withdrawal can range from mild to quite severe, with the occurrence of withdrawal seizures and/or delirium tremens. The medical complications of alcoholism can affect nearly every organ system, but the central nervous system, liver, gastrointestinal tract, pancreas, and cardiovascular system are particularly sensitive to the effects of alcohol.

- Increased γ-glutamyltransferase levels and mean corpuscular volume can identify up to 90% of alcoholics.
- It is not practical to rely on laboratory data alone to make the diagnosis of alcoholism.
- Medical complications of alcoholism can affect nearly every organ system.

Benzodiazepines, Sedative-Hypnotics, and Anxiolytics

In contrast to many of the other groups, benzodiazepines, sedative-hypnotics, and anxiolytics are widely used in many areas of medicine, so that the addictions that are often seen are iatrogenic. However, five characteristics may help distinguish medical use from nonmedical use: 1) Intent--What is the purpose of the use? 2) Effect--What is the effect on the user's life? 3) Control--Is the use controlled by the user only or does a physician share in the control? 4) Legality--Is the use of the drug legal or illegal? Medical drug use is legal. 5) Pattern--In what settings is the drug used?

These same characteristics can also be used to distinguish medical from nonmedical use of opioids. Withdrawal from use of benzodiazepines and barbiturates, in particular, can be serious because of the increased risk of withdrawal seizures.

- Withdrawal of use of benzodiazepines and barbiturates, in particular, can be serious because of the increased risk of withdrawal seizures.

PSYCHOPHARMACOLOGY

The use of a pharmacologic treatment for a psychiatric disorder or the use of psychoactive medications in other disorders is a decision that generally is made after considering multiple factors in the case. Medication alone is rarely the sole treatment for a psychiatric disorder but rather a component of a broader treatment plan. Because psychoactive medications are used in various circumstances for many different indications, the major groups of these medications--antidepressants, antipsychotics, antimanic agents, anxiolytics, and sedative drugs--are discussed below in general terms rather than for treatment of specific disorders. The choice of a medication generally is based on its side-effect profile and the clinical profile of the patient. There are many effective drugs in each of the major groups, but they differ in terms of pharmacokinetics, side effects, and available routes of administration.

- Medication alone is rarely the sole treatment for a psychiatric disorder.
- The choice of a medication generally is based on its side-effect profile and the clinical profile of the patient.

Antipsychotic Agents

The several classes of antipsychotic agents can be categorized by chemical structure: phenothiazines (including their derivatives and peperidines and piperazines), thioxanthenes, butyrophenones, dibenzoxazepine, indole derivatives, pimozide, and dibenzodiazepine (Clozaril). The choice of medication is based on the patient's clinical situation, side-effect profile of the chosen agent, history of previous response, and issues related to compliance. The prevailing theory about the mechanism of action of these agents is that they cause blockade of dopamine postsynaptic receptors. This relates to both the antipsychotic activity and other side effects, depending on which dopamine pathways in the brain are affected and which of the several types of dopamine receptor is preferentially affected. If the nigrostriatal dopaminergic system (involved with motor activity) is affected, extrapyramidal symptoms may result. Blockade of the dopamine pathways in the pituitary and hypothalamus causes increased prolactin release and changes in appetite and temperature regulation. The effects of these drugs on the limbic system, midbrain tegmentum, septal nuclei, and mesocortical dopaminergic projections are thought to be responsible for their antipsychotic action.

- The theory about the mechanism of action of antipsychotic agents is that they cause blockade of dopamine postsynaptic receptors.
- The antipsychotic effects of these agents are due to their action on the limbic system, midbrain tegmentum, septal nuclei, and mesocortical dopaminergic projections.

Side Effects: Extrapyramidal Reactions

Acute dystonic reactions occur within hours or days after initiating treatment with antipsychotic drugs. These reactions are characterized by uncontrollable tightening of the face and neck muscles with spasms. The effect on the eyes may cause an oculogyric crisis, and the effect on the laryngeal muscles may cause respiratory or ventilatory difficulties. Treatment is usually with intravenous or intramuscular administration of an anticholinergic agent, followed by the use of an oral anticholinergic agent for a few days (antipsychotic agents have long half-lives).

- Acute dystonic reactions: occur within hours or days after initiating treatment with antipsychotic drugs.
- Reactions: uncontrollable tightening of the face and neck muscles with spasms.
- Treatment: intravenous or intramuscular administration of an anticholinergic agent.

1. Parkinsonian syndrome has a more gradual onset and can be treated with oral anticholinergic agents and/or decreased doses of the antipsychotic agent.
2. Akathisia is an unpleasant feeling of restlessness and the inability to sit still. It often occurs within days of initiating therapy with antipsychotic agents. Akathisia is sometimes mistaken for exacerbation of the psychosis. Treatment, if possible, is to decrease the dose of the antipsychotic agent or to try using a β-adrenergic blocking agent such as propranolol, if not contraindicated.
3. Akinesia is characterized by diminished spontaneity, few gestures, and apathy. It may be mistaken for a depressive reaction. This condition usually can be treated with an anticholinergic agent.

- Akathisia: unpleasant feeling of restlessness and the inability to sit still.

Tardive dyskinesia consists of involuntary movements of the face, trunk, or extremities. The most consistent risk factor for its development is older age. Prevention is the most important aspect of management, because no reliable treatment is available. It is best if treatment with the antipsychotic agent can be discontinued, although there may be a temporary increase in the symptoms of tardive dyskinesia.

- Tardive dyskinesia: involuntary movements of the face, trunk, or extremities.
- Prevention: the most important aspect of management.

Neuroleptic malignant syndrome is a potentially life-threatening disorder that may occur after the use of any antipsychotic agent, although it is generally more common with the high-potency antipsychotics. Its clinical presentation is characterized by severe rigidity, fever, leukocytosis, tachycardia, tachypnea, diaphoresis, blood pressure fluctuations, and marked increase in CPK levels due to muscle breakdown. Treatment consists of discontinuing the use of the antipsychotic agent and providing life-support measures (ventilation, cooling, etc.). Pharmacologic interventions may include the use of dantrolene sodium, which is a direct-acting muscle relaxant, and/or bromocriptine, which is a centrally acting dopamine agonist. Often, one of the most effective treatments is electroconvulsive therapy.

- Neuroleptic malignant syndrome: potentially life-threatening.
- It may occur after the use of any antipsychotic agent.
- Characteristics: severe rigidity, fever, leukocytosis, tachycardia, tachypnea, diaphoresis, blood pressure fluctuations, marked increase in CPK levels (muscle breakdown).

Other, non-extrapyramidal side effects of antipsychotic agents are listed in Table 20-3.

Newer Antipsychotics

Two relatively new antipsychotics now available are clozapine and risperidone. They are significantly different from their predecessors in terms of potential mechanisms of action and their side-effect profiles. Both of these agents are less likely to cause bothersome extrapyramidal side effects, and their potential for causing tardive dyskinesia may be less. The evidence for the latter will take time to establish because the onset of the symptoms is delayed and the drugs have not been widely used long enough to determine the risk of tardive dyskinesia. Neuroleptic malignant syndrome has been reported to occur with both of these agents. Clozapine has a 1%-2% risk of producing agranulocytosis, which is reversible if use of the medication is withdrawn. Because of this serious potential side effect, there is a specific requirement for performing regular blood cell counts (weekly in the first 6-18 months and then possibly less often). Risperidone seems to be well tolerated in terms of producing minimal extrapyramidal side effects at therapeutic doses. No other serious side effects have been reported to occur frequently, but the drug has not been in use long enough for us to be aware of the degree of drug interactions with other prescribed medications. Clozapine and risperidone are also significantly more expensive than their predecessors.

Antianxiety Medications

These drugs are used most appropriately to treat time-limited anxiety or insomnia related to an identifiable stress or change in sleep cycle. If used long term (>2-3 months), benzodiazepines and related substances should be tapered rather than be discontinued abruptly to avoid any of the three "discontinuation syndromes."

Table 20-3.--Side Effects of Antipsychotic Agents Aside From Extrapyramidal Effects

Anticholinergic
Orthostatic hypotension--related to α-adrenergic receptor blockade
Hyperprolactinemia--gynecomastia possible in men and women, galactorrhea (rare), amenorrhea, weight gain, breast tenderness, decreased libido
Sexual dysfunction
Dermatologic--pigmentary changes in the skin and photosensitivity
Decreased seizure threshold--caused by most antipsychotic agents

1. Relapse--Return of the original anxiety symptoms, often after weeks to months.
2. Rebound--Intensification of the original symptoms; it usually lasts several days and appears within hours to days after abrupt cessation of drug use.
3. Withdrawal--May be mild to severe and includes autonomic and central nervous system symptoms that are different from the original presenting symptoms of the disorder.

Benzodiazepines are well-absorbed orally but have unpredictable availability with intramuscular use, except for lorazepam. There is great variability among the benzodiazepines in terms of their pharmacokinetics. Many of these drugs have metabolites with very long half-lives. Therefore, much smaller doses need to be used in the elderly, in patients with brain damage, and in children--all these patient groups are prone to the paradoxical reactions (anxiety, irritability, aggression, agitation, insomnia), especially patients with known brain damage.

- Benzodiazepines: great variability in terms of their pharmacokinetics.

Buspirone is a non-benzodiazepine anxiolytic drug whose mechanism of action is not known. However, the drug has effects on many neurotransmitter systems, especially the serotonergic and dopaminergic systems. Cross-tolerance does not exist between the benzodiazepines and buspirone. It generally takes 2-3 weeks for the drug to become effective.

- Buspirone: a non-benzodiazepine anxiolytic drug.
- It takes 2-3 weeks for the drug to become effective.

Antidepressant Agents

More than 20 antidepressant agents are available in the U.S. to treat depression, and there are at least two other drugs that are antidepressants but are approved for use in this country primarily for the treatment of obsessive-compulsive disorder (clomipramine and fluvoxamine). The first-generation antidepressant agents included the tricyclics and monoamine oxidase inhibitors. The newer generation antidepressant agents are not easily grouped by their chemical structure or function but rather are a diverse group of compounds. Currently, the most widely used of this group of agents are the selective serotonin reuptake inhibitors.

Although the early generation antidepressant agents were effective in treating depression, they were associated with significant side effects, which limited their use in certain groups of patients, especially those with other medical problems. In particular, tricyclics are associated with orthostatic hypotension, anticholinergic side effects, and cardiac conduction defects. Monoamaine oxidase inhibitors are effective antidepressants but require special dietary restrictions and special attention to interactions with other medications. Because the newer generation antidepressants have fewer potential side effects and drug interactions, they are prescribed more widely, but they are not effective for everyone.

1. Tricyclics--Tertiary amines, including imipramine, amitriptyline, doxepin, and trimipramine, and secondary amines, including desipramine, nortriptyline, and protriptyline.
2. Monoamine oxidase inhibitors--Phenelzine, isocarboxazid, tranylcypromine, and pargyline.
3. Newer generation antidepressants--Maprotiline, amoxapine, trazodone, bupropion, fluoxetine, sertraline, paroxetine, fluvoxamine, venlafaxine, and nefazadone.

The mechanism of action is their effect on the catecholaminergic and serotonergic systems of the central nervous system. The various cyclic antidepressant agents block the reuptake of norepinephrine and/or serotonin, increasing the amount of these neurotransmitters at the synapse. Monoamine oxidase inhibitors block the catabolism of several biogenic amines (norepinephrine, serotonin, tyramine, phenylephrine, and dopamine), thereby increasing the amount of these neurotransmitters available for synaptic release.

- Antidepressant agents affect the catecholaminergic and serotonergic systems of the central nervous system.
- Monoamine oxidase inhibitors block the catabolism of several biogenic amines.

Antidepressant agents are primarily approved for use in the treatment of depression. However, they are useful in several other disorders, including panic disorder, obsessive-compulsive disorder, enuresis, chronic pain, migraine headache, bulimia, and attention-deficit disorder. Because they are so widely used, familiarity with the basics of their use, side effects, and drug interactions may be helpful. The choice of which antidepressant agent to use is often based on the side-effect profile

of the drug and the clinical presentation of the patient. The side effects of the major groups of antidepressant agents are listed in Table 20-4.

A complete trial of antidepressant medication consists of 6 weeks of therapeutic doses before considering refractoriness. If some improvement has occurred with the initial trial but the condition is not yet back to baseline, it may be worthwhile to try augmenting therapy with lithium carbonate before changing the medication to another class of antidepressant. Another alternative is a trial of thyroid hormone (T3) supplementation before switching use of antidepressant medications. After clinical improvement is noted, the medication may need to be maintained for an extended period of time.

- A complete trial of antidepressant medication: 6 weeks of therapeutic doses.
- Augmenting therapy with lithium carbonate may be worthwhile before changing the medication to another class of antidepressant.

Monoamine Oxidase Inhibitors

Most clinical concerns about the use of monoamine oxidase inhibitors relate to reactions from the ingestion of tyramine, which is not metabolized because of the inhibition of intestinal monoamine oxidase. Tyramine may act as a false transmitter and displace norepinephrine from synaptic vesicles. Patients should be instructed in a tyramine-restricted diet, especially to avoid aged cheeses, smoked meats, pickled herring, beer and red wine (generally all alcohol should be restricted), yeast extracts, fava beans, and overripe bananas and avocadoes. Certain general anesthetics and drugs with

Table 20-4.--Side Effects of the Major Groups of Antidepressant Agents

Orthostatic hypotension--The cardiovascular side effect that most commonly results in serious morbidity, especially in the elderly
Anticholinergic effects--Dry mouth, blurred vision, urinary retention, etc.; beware of these side effects in patients with prostatic hypertrophy and narrow-angle glaucoma. Drugs with more anticholinergic side effects also seem to be the more sedating, e.g., tertiary amine tricyclics
Cardiac conduction effects--Most of the tricyclics prolong PR and QRS intervals. Therefore, these drugs need to be used with caution in patients with preexisting heart block, such as second-degree heart block or markedly prolonged QRS and QT intervals. The tricyclics are potent antiarrhythmic agents because of their quinidine-like effect. Newer generation antidepressants have far fewer cardiac interactions.
Sedating types--Tertiary amine tricyclics and trazadone
Potentially more stimulating types--Secondary amine tricyclics, bupropion, fluoxetine, sertraline, and paroxetine

sympathomimetic activity should be avoided; especially beware of over-the-counter cough and cold preparations, decongestants, and appetite suppressants. Meperidine (Demerol) is absolutely contraindicated because of its potentially lethal interaction with monoamine oxidase inhibitors.

- Clinical concerns about monoamine oxidase inhibitors: reactions due to ingestion of tyramine, which is not metabolized.
- Tyramine: a false neurotransmitter that displaces norepinephrine from synaptic vesicles.
- Meperidine (Demerol): absolutely contraindicated because of its potentially lethal interaction with monoamine oxidase inhibitors.

Treatment of hypertensive reactions relies on administering drugs with α-adrenergic blocking properties, such as intravenous administration of phentolamine. This should be done in an emergency room. Patients may take nifedipine (10 mg sublingually) before reaching an emergency room if they have moderate-to-severe occipital headache while taking a monoamine oxidase inhibitor.

ANTIMANIC DRUGS

Lithium carbonate is the drug of choice for treating bipolar disorders. It can also be effective in patients with recurrent unipolar depressions and as an adjunct for maintenance of remission of depression after electroconvulsive therapy. Acute manic symptoms usually respond to treatment with lithium within 7-10 days. While waiting for this effect, the adjunctive use of antipsychotic agents may be helpful. Lithium is well absorbed from the gastrointestinal tract, with peak levels in 1-2 hours. Its half-life is about 24 hours. Levels are generally checked 10-12 hours after the last dose. Relatively common side effects include fine hand tremor, diarrhea, polyuria, polydipsia, thirst, and nausea, which is often improved by taking the medication on a full stomach. Lithium is contraindicated in the first trimester of pregnancy, because of its potential for causing defects in the developing cardiac system. Renal effects generally can be reversed with discontinuation of treatment with lithium. The most noticeable renal effect is the vasopressin-resistant effect leading to impaired concentrating ability and nephrogenic diabetes insipidus with polyuria and polydipsia. Most patients who take lithium develop some polyuria but not all develop more severe manifestations of nephrogenic diabetes insipidus. Renal function should be followed in all patients receiving maintenance lithium therapy. However, whether lithium has significant nephrotoxic effects is a matter of controversy. A hematologic side effect is a benign leukocytosis. Hypothyroidism may occur in as many as 20% of patients taking lithium, because of the direct inhibitory effects on thyroid hormone

production or increased antithyroid antibodies.

- Lithium carbonate: drug of choice for treating bipolar disorders.
- Common side effects: hand tremor, diarrhea, polyuria, polydipsia, thirst, and nausea.
- Renal effects generally can be reversed with discontinuation of treatment with lithium.
- Most noticeable renal effect: impaired concentrating ability.
- Hypothyroidism occurs in as many as 20% of patients receiving lithium.

Because the range between the therapeutic and toxic levels of lithium in the plasma is narrow, patients and physicians should be familiar with conditions that may increase or decrease lithium levels and with the signs and symptoms of lithium toxicity so it can be recognized and treated promptly (Tables 20-5 and 20-6).

Other Antimanic Agents

The anticonvulsants carbamazepine and valproic acid are effective in the treatment of acute manic episodes and for prophylactic maintenance therapy of bipolar disorders. The mechanism of action for their mood-stabilizing effects is not clear. Carbamazepine has a chemical structure similar to that of the tricyclic antidepressants and has a quinidine-like effect. The side effect of most concern with valproic acid is hepatotoxicity, which has occurred mostly in children receiving treatment with multiple anticonvulsants. Other antimanic agents being investigated include verapamil, a calcium channel blocker, and clonazepam, the benzodiazepine anticonvulsant.

- The anticonvulsants carbamazepine and valproic acid are effective for the treatment of acute mania and maintenance treatment of bipolar disorders.

ELECTROCONVULSIVE THERAPY

Electroconvulsive therapy is the most effective treatment for severely depressed patients, especially those with psychotic features. It is also helpful in treating catatonia and mania and may be used in children and adults. Also, electroconvulsive therapy can be administered to pregnant women. It may be effective in patients with overlapping depression and Parkinson's disease and/or dementia. Electroconvulsive therapy is administered with the patient under barbiturate anesthesia, with succinylcholine or a similar muscle relaxant to minimize peripheral manifestations of the seizure. An anticholinergic agent such as atropine is generally given to decrease secretions and to prevent bradycardia caused by central stimulation of the vagus nerve. A usual course of treatment is 6-12 sessions given over a 2-4-week period. Therapy is often initiated with

Table 20-5.--Conditions That Increase or Decrease Lithium Levels in the Plasma

Increase levels	Decrease levels
Dehydration	Increased caffeine consumption
Overheating and increased perspiration with exercise and/or hot weather	Theophylline
Nonsteroidal anti-inflammatory drugs	
Thiazide diuretics	
Angiotensin-converting enzyme inhibitors	
Certain antibiotics--tetracycline, spectinomycin, and metronidazole	

Table 20-6.--Signs and Symptoms of Lithium Toxicity

Mild-to-moderate toxicity (plasma levels, 1.5-2.0 mEq/L)	Moderate-to-severe toxicity (plasma levels, 2.0-2.5 mEq/L)	Severe toxicity (plasma levels, >2.5 mEq/L)
Vomiting	Persistent nausea and vomiting	Generalized seizures
Abdominal pain	Anorexia	Oliguria and renal failure
Dry mouth	Blurred vision	Death
Ataxia	Muscle fasciculations	
Slurred speech	Hyperactive deep tendon reflexes	
Nystagmus	Delirium	
Muscle weakness	Convulsions	
	Electroencephalographic changes	
	Stupor and coma	
	Circulatory system failure	
	Lowered blood pressure	
	Cardiac arrhythmias	
	Conduction abnormalities	

Modified from Silver JM, Hales RE, Yudofsky SC: Biological therapies for mental disorders. *In* Clinical Psychiatry for Medical Students. Edited by A Stoudemire. Philadelphia, JB Lippincott Company, 1990, pp 459-496. By permission of publisher.

unilateral, nondominant electrode placement to minimize memory loss. If satisfactory results cannot be obtained with this method, bilateral electrode placement is used.

- Electroconvulsive therapy: most effective treatment for severely depressed patients, especially those with psychotic features.
- It is also helpful in treating catatonia and mania.
- It can be given to pregnant women.
- It may be helpful in cases of overlapping depression and Parkinson's disease and/or dementia.

Mechanism of action--Electroconvulsive therapy induces changes in several transmitter-receptor systems, particularly acetylcholine, norepinephrine, dopamine, and serotonin. It downregulates β-adrenergic receptors and may decrease calcium levels in the cerebrospinal fluid. It may also affect neuropeptides and electrical conduction systems (similar to those studied by cardiac electrophysiologists).

- Electroconvulsive therapy induces changes in acetylcholine, norepinephrine, dopamine, and serotonin transmitter-receptor systems.
- It downregulates β-adrenergic receptors.
- It may decrease calcium levels in the cerebrospinal fluid.

No longer are there any absolute contraindications to electroconvulsive therapy, although there are several relative contraindications. Previously, the only absolute contraindication was the presence of an intracranial space-occupying lesion and increased intracranial pressure. Serious complications or mortality is generally reported as less than 1 per 10,000, which makes this therapy one of the safest interventions that uses general anesthesia. Morbidity and mortality usually are due to cardiovascular complications, such as arrhythmia, myocardial infarction, or hypotension. The major risks are those associated with the brief general anesthesia. Medical evaluations performed before giving the therapy should pay particular attention to

cardiovascular function, pulmonary function (because positive pressure respiration is used during anesthesia), electrolyte balance, and the patient's previous experiences with anesthesia.

- Electroconvulsive therapy: no longer any absolute contraindications.
- There are several relative contraindications.
- Morbidity and mortality are usually due to cardiovascular complications.

QUESTIONS

Multiple Choice (choose the one best answer)
1. You are asked to see a 75-year-old widowed woman who lives alone to evaluate changes in her usual personality and decline of her personal hygiene. She has no known previous psychiatric history and the relative accompanying her to the appointment brings "a bag of pills" she found in the patient's kitchen cupboard. Differential diagnoses may include all the following except:
   a. A developing dementia
   b. Schizophrenia
   c. Medication-induced reaction
   d. Increased alcohol use
   e. A depressive disorder

2. You are asked to come to the Emergency Room to evaluate a 34-year-old married mother of a 2-month-old infant. The mother presents with palpitations, tachycardia, diaphoresis, tremulousness, sensation of shortness of breath, anterior chest discomfort, lightheadedness, and intense fear. Differential diagnoses may include all of the following except:
   a. Hyperthyroidism
   b. Panic attack
   c. Cardiac arrhythmia
   d. Post-partum psychosis
   e. Increased use of caffeine

3. Major depression may be manifested by all the following except:
   a. Decreased appetite with associated weight loss
   b. Decreased need for sleep
   c. Early morning awakening
   d. Loss of interest in usually pleasurable activities
   e. Sense of hopelessness

4. A nurse in the Intensive Care Unit calls to let you know that your 63-year-old male patient who 2 days earlier had cardiac valve replacement is more agitated, seems to be having visual hallucinations, is more disoriented than yesterday, is tremulous, and is beginning to be verbally abusive to the nursing staff. He has no known past psychiatric treatment. Differential diagnoses may include all the following except:
   a. "Intensive care unit syndrome"
   b. Onset of possible delirium tremens
   c. Schizophrenia
   d. Delirium of uncertain cause
   e. Reaction to analgesic agents

5. When diagnosing alcohol dependence, the least reliable part of the history is usually:
   a. Descriptions of family members being upset by the drinking
   b. Previous driving violations for driving while intoxicated

c. The reported quantity and frequency of drinking

d. Increased gamma-glutamyltransferase and serum glutamic-oxaloacetic transaminase levels

e. Previous attempts to cut down

6. Medical complications associated with eating disorders may include all the following except:
   a. Reduced thyroid metabolism
   b. Cold intolerance
   c. Loss of cardiac muscle
   d. Increased chance of multiple birth pregnancies
   e. Salivary gland enlargement

7. Antidepressants are sometimes used for the treatment of all the following except:
   a. Panic disorder
   b. Obsessive-compulsive disorder
   c. Fibromyalgia
   d. Munchausen syndrome
   e. Bipolar disorder

True/False (indicate whether each answer is true or false)

8. Neuroleptic malignant syndrome is:
   a. Potentially life threatening
   b. Reported to be a potential problem after the use of any antipsychotic agent
   c. Characterized by hallucinations, rambling incoherent speech, and disorientation
   d. Characterized by severe rigidity, fever, leukocytosis, tachycardia, and marked increase in CPK levels

e. Often effectively treated with life-support measures and electroconvulsive therapy

9. A 54-year-old man with chronic obstructive pulmonary disease, hypertension, and bipolar disorder develops an exacerbation of his chronic obstructive pulmonary disease. His current medications include: theophylline, two inhalers (Atrovent and albuterol), lithium carbonate, and Dyazide. His physician recommends adding a short course of corticosteroids (prednisone) to his program. These medications and dietary recommendations will have the following effects on his lithium level.
   a. Theophylline will decrease the lithium level
   b. Inhalers will increase the lithium level
   c. Prednisone will not affect the lithium level
   d. Thiazide diuretics will increase the lithium level
   e. Low sodium diet will increase the lithium level

10. With regard to antidepressant agents:
    a. Serotonin selective reuptake inhibitors are most likely to cause orthostatic hypotension
    b. Tricyclic antidepressant overdoses are potentially lethal because of the cardiac arrhythmias they induce
    c. They are used to treat various psychiatric disorders in addition to depression
    d. A therapeutic trial of an antidepressant is considered 1 to 2 weeks
    e. Older patients may safely be given the same doses as younger patients

ANSWERS

1. Answer b.
The onset of schizophrenia usually occurs in the 2nd to 4th decades of life.

2. Answer d.
Although this is still within the postpartum period, there is not mention of psychotic symptoms. Panic attacks have symptoms that may also be produced by various medical disorders. (DSM IV technically identifies the postpartum period as 4 weeks.)

3. Answer b.
Although patients may have insomnia when depressed, they generally need their usual or increased amount of sleep. Decreased need for sleep is described by patients in a manic phase.

4. Answer c.
There is acute onset of the symptoms described in a person in his 60s, which would be an unusual time for the onset of schizophrenia. However, delirium is often associated with psychotic symptoms.

5. Answer c.

The report of the amount of alcohol used and the frequency of drinking is the most variable and least reliable part of the history, especially the history obtained from the patient.

6. Answer d.

Patients with eating disorder often develop problems with the reproductive system, but in women, the problem is related more to amenorrhea than to pregnancy.

7. Answer d.

Antidepressants are used to treat a wide variety of disorders, but Munchausen syndrome is a factitious disorder not treated with medication.

8. a, true; b, true; c, false; d, true; e, true.

Hallucinations, rambling incoherent speech, and disorientation are not hallmark features of neuroleptic malignant syndrome.

9. a, true; b, false; c, true; d, true; e, true.

Theophylline increases renal clearance, which will decrease the lithium level. The inhalers and prednisone will not specifically affect the lithium level; however, corticosteroids may induce further mood disturbance. Thiazide diuretics increase the lithium level, as does a diet too low in sodium. Because the latter two are frequently used treatments of hypertension, this should be kept in mind when a person is taking lithium and requries treatment for hypertension.

10. a, false; b, true; c, true; d, false; e, false.

Selective serotonin reuptake inhibitors are the *least* likely to cause orthostatic hypotension. Antidepressants are used to treat a wide variety of disorders and are often prescribed for patients of nearly all ages. As with other medications, children, adolescents, and elderly patients require appropriate dose adjustments. A duration of 4 to 6 weeks of therapeutic levels of an antidepressant is a more appropriate trial because it usually takes 2 to 4 weeks just to see the *initial* effects of an antidepressant.

CHAPTER 21

PULMONARY DISEASES

Udaya B. S. Prakash, M.D.

SYMPTOMS AND SIGNS

Cough

Cough can be voluntary or reflex. The afferent arm of the reflex consists of the sensory branches of the trigeminal, glossopharyngeal, superior laryngeal, and vagus nerves. The efferent limb includes the recurrent laryngeal and spinal nerves. Lesions in the following organs can cause cough: nose, ears, pharynx, larynx, bronchi, lungs, pleura, and abdominal viscera. Types of cough include brassy (tracheal involvement), barking (epiglottitis), wheezy (asthma), nocturnal (reflux), and positional (abscess or tumors).

- Lesion (inflammatory, mechanical, chemical, or thermal) in any part of the afferent limb of the reflex can cause cough.
- Cough can be the presenting or only manifestation of asthma.
- Positional cough occurs with lung abscess, obstructing lesions (tumors), and nocturnal reflux.

Chronic cough is defined as cough lasting ≥3 weeks without an obvious cause. Evaluation should include ear-nose-throat examination, esophagography and/or acid reflux test, pH monitoring, and methacholine inhalation challenge to exclude asthma. Nonpulmonary diseases (temporal arteritis, rheumatoid bronchiolitis, Sjögren's syndrome, and reflux esophagitis) may present with cough. Bronchoscopy in the absence of chest roentgenographic (CXR) abnormalities carries a low (4%) diagnostic yield. In nearly 6% of patients taking angiotensin converting enzyme (ACE) inhibitors, cough develops as a complication. Cross-reactivity is present among different ACE inhibitors.

- The most common causes of chronic cough: postnasal drip, asthma, reflux, and postinfectious.
- Complications of cough: cough syncope, rib fractures, and pneumothorax.

- Cough syncope: hard cough produces increased intrathoracic pressure, which causes a decrease in cardiac output and cerebral perfusion.
- Bronchoscopy has a low diagnostic yield if CXR findings are normal.
- Nonpulmonary diseases can present with cough.
- ACE inhibitors can cause cough.

Sputum

Purulent sputum occurs in bronchiectasis and lung abscess. Frothy pink sputum is seen in pulmonary edema. Expectoration of bronchial casts, mucous plugs, or thin strings occurs in asthma, bronchopulmonary aspergillosis, and mucoid impaction syndrome, and expectoration of stone (lithoptysis) occurs in broncholithiasis. Bronchorrhea (expectoration of thin serous fluid >100 mL/day) is seen in 20% of patients with diffuse alveolar cell carcinoma. Expectoration of worms is found in parasitic infections (*Ascaris*).

- Bronchorrhea occurs in diffuse alveolar cell carcinoma.
- Histoplasmosis is the most common cause of broncholithiasis.
- Sputum microscopy for eosinophils, Charcot-Leyden crystals, and Curschmann's spirals in asthmatics.

Hemoptysis

Hemoptysis is the expectoration of blood or blood-streaked sputum. Bleeding from bronchial circulation is seen in chronic bronchitis, bronchiectasis, malignancies, broncholithiasis, and foreign bodies. Bleeding from pulmonary arterial circulation is seen in pulmonary arteriovenous malformations, fungus ball, tumors, vasculitis, pulmonary hypertension, and lung abscess. Bleeding from a pulmonary alveolocapillary location occurs in mitral stenosis, left ventricular failure, pulmonary infarction, vasculitis, Goodpasture's syndrome, and idiopathic pulmonary hemosiderosis. A fistula between airways and

673

blood vessels (tracheoinnominate) can cause massive hemoptysis. Massive hemoptysis is $\geq$200 mL/24 hours, but the underlying lung dysfunction determines outcome.

- Hemoptysis must be differentiated from pseudohemoptysis (expectoration of blood previously aspirated into airways or lungs from the gastrointestinal tract, nose, or supraglottic areas).
- History, examination, and CXR are important in the diagnosis.
- The most common cause of streaky hemoptysis is chronic bronchitis or postinfectious.
- Almost all patients with hemoptysis should undergo bronchoscopy.
- Cause of death in massive hemoptysis is asphyxiation, not exsanguination.

Dyspnea

Dyspnea is the symptom (or awareness) of breathlessness. The causes include disorders of the pulmonary, cardiac, skeletal (kyphoscoliosis, etc.), endocrine, metabolic, neurologic, and hematologic systems. Other causes are physiologic dyspnea of pregnancy, drugs, psychogenic, deconditioning, and obesity. Severity is assessed clinically by grading: grade 0, no dyspnea except with strenuous exercise; grade 1, slight dyspnea on hurrying on a level surface or walking up a hill; grade 2, dyspnea while walking on a level surface and being unable to keep up with peers and having to stop to catch a breath; grade 3, dyspnea on walking 100 yards or after a few minutes and the need to stop for breath; grade 4, dyspnea on dressing or undressing or minimal exertion; and grade 5, dyspnea at rest.

- Every major organ system is a potential source for the cause of dyspnea.
- Cardiopulmonary diseases are the most common causes.
- Initial clinical grading of dyspnea is helpful in planning further tests.

In most cases, dyspnea is the result of the increased work of breathing. Other mechanisms include abnormal activation of respiratory centers, voluntary hyperventilation, and Cheyne-Stokes breathing. Clinical history, physical examination, CXR, and cardiopulmonary physiologic testing are important. Orthopnea: dyspnea in the supine posture (associated with congestive heart failure, bilateral diaphragmatic paralysis, severe chronic obstructive disease [COPD], asthma, sleep apnea, and severe reflux). Paroxysmal nocturnal dyspnea: nocturnal episodes of dyspnea resulting in frequent waking up (associated with left ventricular failure and asthma).

- Tachypnea >20 breaths/minute and bradypnea <10 breaths/minute.

- Trepopnea: dyspnea in the left or right lateral decubitus position (associated with heart disease, tumors of mainstem bronchi, unilateral pleural effusion, and post-pneumonectomy).
- Platypnea: dyspnea in the upright posture (due to increased right-to-left shunt in lung bases; seen in liver disease, severe lung fibrosis, and after pneumonectomy).
- Orthodeoxia: oxygen desaturation in the upright position (seen with platypnea).

Chest Pain

Pulmonary causes of chest pain are often difficult to distinguish from cardiac and other causes. Tightness of the chest and dyspnea are also described as chest pain by patients. Pleuritic pain is encountered in pleuritis, pleuropericarditis, pericarditis, pneumothorax, pleural effusion, mediastinitis, pulmonary embolism/infarction, esophageal diseases, aortic dissection, and chest wall trauma. Subdiaphragmatic diseases that produce chest pain include pancreatitis, cholecystitis, and colonic distension.

Cyanosis

Cyanosis is the bluish discoloration of the skin and mucous membranes that occurs when the capillary content of reduced hemoglobin is >5 g/dL. Clinically, it may be difficult to detect. Cyanosis may occur when arterial hemoglobin is unsaturated or when tissue extraction is high. Causes of central cyanosis: severe hypoxia (PaO_2 is usually <55 mm Hg), anatomical shunts, mild hypoxia with polycythemia, shock, abnormal hemoglobin, methemoglobinemia, and sulfhemoglobinemia. Anemia, even when severe, does not cause cyanosis unless reduced hemoglobin is >5 g/dL. Peripheral cyanosis results from decreased peripheral perfusion with increased O_2 extraction.

- Cyanosis occurs when reduced hemoglobin is >5 g/dL.
- It is important to distinguish central from peripheral cyanosis.
- Cherry-red flush (not cyanosis) is caused by carboxyhemoglobinemia.
- Polycythemia vera causes "red cyanosis."
- Argyria (from silver nitrate) and hemochromatosis may cause "pseudocyanosis."

Clubbing

Clubbing is the bulbous enlargement of the distal segment of a digit (fingers or toes) caused by increased soft tissue mass. Mechanisms include neurogenic, humoral/ hormonal, hereditary, and idiopathic. A vagally mediated mechanism is perhaps the most common mechanism. It can be the presenting manifestation of lung cancer, mesothelioma, and infective endocarditis. Causes of CLUBBING include C (cyanotic heart diseases), **L** (lung cancer, lung abscess, or lung fibrosis), **U** (ulcerative colitis), **B** (bronchiectasis), **B** (benign mesothelioma), **I** (infective endocarditis, idiopathic or inherited), **N** (neurogenic tumors), and **G** (gastrointestinal diseases, e.g., cirrhosis and regional enteritis).

- Clubbing may precede the onset of lung cancer.
- Common causes of clubbing include pulmonary fibrosis, congenital heart disease with right-to-left shunt, cystic fibrosis, and idopathic.
- Differential diagnosis includes items in the mnemonic CLUBBING and hypertrophic pulmonary osteoarthropathy.

Hypertrophic Pulmonary Osteoarthropathy

Hypertrophic pulmonary osteoarthropathy consists of clubbing, painful periosteal hypertrophy of long bones, and symmetrical arthralgias of large joints (usually the knees, elbows, and wrists). Other manifestations include gynecomastia, fever, and an increased erythrocyte sedimentation rate (ESR). Mechanisms of hypertrophic pulmonary osteoarthropathy include neurogenic (vagal afferents), hormonal, and idiopathic. The most common cause is bronchogenic carcinoma, usually adenocarcinoma or large cell carcinoma. Roentgenographs of long bones reveal thickness and raised periosteum. Bone scans show increased uptake of radionuclide by the affected periosteum. If resection of the tumor does not relieve the hypertrophic pulmonary osteoarthropathy, ipsilateral vagotomy is performed.

- Hypertrophic pulmonary osteoarthropathy: adenocarcinoma and large cell carcinoma of the lung are the common causes.
- Radionuclide bone scans show characteristic changes.
- Perform ipsilateral vagotomy if resection of the primary tumor does not resolve the condition.

Horner's Syndrome

Horner's syndrome encompasses ipsilateral miosis, anhidrosis, and ptosis on the side of the lesion. It is seen as a complication of superior sulcus tumor (Pancoast's tumor) of the lung and is most frequently caused by squamous cell carcinoma.

- Horner's syndrome: ipsilateral miosis, anhidrosis, and ptosis.
- It is a complication of superior sulcus tumor (Pancoast's tumor).

Superior Vena Cava Syndrome

Superior vena cava syndrome is caused by obstruction of blood flow through the superior vena cava. Common causes include lung cancer (particularly small cell cancer), Hodgkin's lymphoma, and other tumors. Mediastinal fibrosis, radiation fibrosis, and large tumors in the upper anterior mediastinum are other causes. Facial edema, fullness of the head, and prominent venous channels over the chest are often noted.

Other Signs and Symptoms

Conjunctival suffusion is seen in severe hypercarbia, superior vena cava syndrome, and conjunctival sarcoidosis. Asterixis is seen in severe acute or subacute hypercarbia. Telangiectasia of the skin and mucous membranes occurs in patients with pulmonary arteriovenous malformation. Skin lesions of various types can be seen in patients with pulmonary involvement by eosinophilic granuloma (histiocytosis X), tuberous sclerosis, sarcoidosis, or lung cancer.

HISTORY AND EXAMINATION

An approach to history taking and physical examination in patients with pulmonary disease is outlined in Table 21-1.

Percussion and auscultation findings associated with various pulmonary conditions are listed in Table 21-2.

DIAGNOSTIC TESTS

Roentgenology

CXR, plain tomography, computed tomography (CT), magnetic resonance imaging (MRI), bronchography, pulmonary angiography, and bronchial angiography are among the tests used in the diagnosis of chest diseases.

Plain Chest Roentgenography

Every internist should become familiar with interpreting the common abnormalities depicted by the plain CXR. Even if the CXR is obtained for "routine" purposes, it is better to view the films so as to develop the routine habit of reading the CXR. Although many of the "roentgenologic" diagnoses such as pneumothorax, pleural effusion, and lung nodule can be established by the CXR, it is essential to correlate the clinical and other laboratory data with CXR findings.

It is important to compare the most recent film with the previous films. This is of great significance in assessing the seriousness of any "newly" identified abnormality. It is also important to assure that the present and earlier sets of films belong to the same patient who is being evaluated. It is unlikely that a normal CXR will be shown in the American Board of Internal Medicine examination. Subtle abnormalities, if shown, will be easy to identify, if the candidate knows how to detect an abnormality. A lateral CXR is of great help in identifying retrocardiac and retrodiaphragmatic abnormalities.

- Develop the habit of reading CXRs.

Table 21-1.--History and Physical Examination in Patients With Pulmonary Disease

History
  Smoking
  Occupational exposure
  Exposure to infected persons or animals
  Hobbies and pets
  Family history of diseases of lung and other organs
  Past malignancy
  Systemic (nonpulmonary) diseases
  Immune status (suppressed, receiving chemotherapy, etc.)
  History of trauma
  Previous chest radiography
Examination
  Inspection
    Respiratory rate
    Respiratory rhythm (apneustic, Biot's, Cheyne-Stokes, Kussmaul's, parkinsonian)
    Accessory muscles of respiration in action (FEV_1 <30%)
    Postural dyspnea (orthopnea, platypnea, trepopnea)
    Intercostal retraction
    Paradoxical motions of abdomen/diaphragm
    Cough (type, sputum, blood)
    Wheeze (audible with or without stethoscope)
    Pursed lip breathing/glottic wheeze (patients with chronic obstructive pulmonary disease)
    Cyanosis
    Conjunctival suffusion (CO_2 retention)
    Clubbing
    Thoracic cage (anteroposterior diameter, kyphoscoliosis, pectus, etc.)
    Trachea, deviation
    Superior vena cava syndrome
    Asterixis, central nervous system status
    Cardiac impulse, jugular venous pressure, pedal edema (signs of cor pulmonale)
  Palpation
    Clubbing
    Tibial tenderness (hypertrophic pulmonary osteoarthropathy)
    Motion of thoracic cage (hand or tape measure)
    Chest wall tenderness (costochondritis, rib fracture, pulmonary embolism)
    Tracheal deviation, tenderness
    Tactile (vocal) fremitus
    Subcutaneous emphysema
    Succussion splash (effusion, air-fluid level in thorax)
  Percussion
    Thoracic cage (dullness, resonance)
    Diaphragmatic motion (normal, 5-7 cm)
    Upper abdomen (liver)
  Auscultation
    Tracheal auscultation
    Normal breath sounds
    Bronchial breath sounds
    Expiratory slowing (time it in seconds)
    Crackles
    Wheezes
    Pleural rub
    Mediastinal noises (mediastinal crunch)
    Heart sounds
    Miscellaneous (muscle tremor, etc.; see section on Other Signs and Symptoms)

- Obtain earlier CXRs for comparison.
- The lateral CXR is important for visualizing retrocardiac and retrodiaphragmatic abnormalities.

The identification of normal roentgenologic anatomy is necessary to be able to identify abnormal findings (Fig. 21-1). In interpreting any CXR, a routine step-by-step method should be developed so that subtle abnormalities are not missed. The CXR should be "eye-balled" as a single unit, without focusing on any one area or abnormality. This is to assure that the technique of CXR is adequate and the patient identification markers as well as orientation of the CXR (identification of left and right sides) are proper. Next, the extrapulmonary structures should be viewed. For instance, detection of the destructive arthritis of a shoulder joint seen on the CXR may be the result of rheumatoid arthritis and may prompt the CXR reader to look for pulmonary manifestations of this disease. An absent breast shadow on the CXR, particularly in a female patient, should remind the CXR reader to look for signs of pulmonary metastases. The visualization of a tracheostomy stoma and/or cannula on the CXR may indicate the possibility of previous laryngeal cancer and, thus, provide a hint to the attendant pulmonary complications such as aspiration, metastases, and secondary infection from *Pseudomonas aeruginosa*. Infradiaphragmatic abnormalities such as calcifications in the spleen, displacement of gastric bubble and the colon, and signs of upper abdominal surgery (metal sutures, feeding tubes, etc.) may be involved in the etiology of a pleuropulmonary process.

- Look at the entire CXR as a single picture at first (do not focus on localized abnormalities).
- Look for absent breast shadow, infradiaphragmatic abnormalities, and extrapulmonary skeletal abnormalities.

Table 21-2.--Percussion and Auscultation Findings

	Chest expansion	Fremitus	Resonance	Breath sounds	Egophony	Bronchophony
Pleural effusion	Decreased	Reduced	Reduced	Decreased	Absent>>present	Absent>>present
Consolidation	Decreased	Increased	Reduced	Bronchial	Present	Present
Atelectasis	Decreased	Reduced	Reduced	Decreased	Absent>present	Absent>present
Pneumothorax	Variable	Reduced	Increased	Decreased	Absent	Absent

Note: Trachea is shifted ipsilaterally in atelectasis and contralaterally in effusion. Whispered pectoriloquy is present in consolidation.

The skeletal thorax should be viewed to exclude rib fracture, osteolytic and other lesions of the ribs, rib notching, missing ribs, and vertebral abnormalities. Changes from a previous thoracic surgical procedure such as coronary artery bypass grafting, thoracotomy, lung resection, or esophageal surgery may provide clues to the pulmonary disease. Next, the intrathoracic but extrapulmonary structures such as the mediastinum (great vessels, esophagus, heart, lymph nodes, and thymus) should be assessed. The superior mediastinum should be viewed to see whether the thyroid gland extends into the thoracic cage. A calcified mass in the region of the thyroid almost always indicates a goiter. The esophagus can produce significant abnormalities in the CXR. A large esophagus, as in achalasia, may mimic a mass or a large hiatal hernia with an air-

fluid level may mimic a lung abscess. The aortopulmonary window (a notch below the aortic knob on the left just above the pulmonary artery), if obliterated, may indicate tumor or lymphadenopathy. Right paratracheal and paramediastinal lymphadenopathy can be subtle. Hilar regions are difficult to interpret. Lymphadenopathy, vascular prominence, and tumor may make the hila appear larger. The retrocardiac region may show hiatal hernia with an air-fluid level; this may be helpful in the diagnosis of reflux or aspiration. A lateral CXR is important in assessing the retrocardiac and retrodiaphragmatic regions.

- Look for rib lesions: osteolytic, expansile, notching, or absence of a rib.

Fig. 21-1. Normal CXR. *A*, Posteroanterior and *B*, lateral.

- Note changes from previous surgical procedures.
- Assess mediastinal structures: esophagus, thyroid, thymus, and the great vessels.

The pleural regions should be examined for pleural effusion, pleural thickening (particularly in the apices), blunting of costophrenic angles, pleural-based lesions such as pleural plaques or masses, and pneumothorax. A tiny pneumothorax, especially in the apical regions, is easy to miss. A lateral decubitus film may be necessary to confirm the presence of free fluid in the pleural space. Air bronchogram depicting the major airways should be viewed to identify large tumors, deviation of airways, and signs of compression or stenosis, and the relationship of the major airways to the esophagus. Finally, the lung parenchyma should be evaluated. Nearly 15% of the pulmonary parenchyma is located behind the heart and diaphragm; a lateral CXR will help in this situation. It is important *not* to overinterpret increased interstitial lung markings. Oligemia of lung fields is difficult to assess because the clarity of the film depends on the duration of the exposure of the film. Generally, bronchovascular markings should be visible throughout the lung parenchyma. Complete absence of any markings within the lung parenchyma should suggest bulla or an air-containing cyst. Apical areas should be evaluated carefully for the presence of pleural thickening, pneumothorax, small nodules, and subtle infiltrates. If the apices cannot be visualized properly with a standard CXR, a lordotic view should be obtained.

- Look for a small pneumothorax, nodules, and large airway lesions.
- Examine the apices for thickening, pneumothorax, nodules, and subtle infiltrates.
- Examine the lung parenchyma behind the heart and diaphragm.

Some of the common CXR abnormalities are depicted in the following pages (Fig. 21-2–21-23).

Tomography

Plain tomography is useful in evaluating solitary lung nodule. Calcification, location of the lesion, margins of the nodule, cavitation, and presence of adjacent nodules (satellite lesions) can be discerned with tomography (Fig. 21-24–21-29). Even though plain tomography is less expensive than CT, the latter has greatly replaced plain tomography in the assessment of solitary lung nodule.

Fluoroscopy

Fluoroscopy is useful in localizing lesions during biopsy and aspiration procedures. It is also valuable in assessing diaphragmatic motion and in diagnosing diaphragmatic paralysis by the sniff test. Paradoxic motion of the diaphragm suggests diaphragmatic paralysis.

Fig. 21-2. Collapsed left upper lobe. *A*, PA CXR and *B*, lateral CXR. The ground glass haze over left hemithorax is typical of partially collapsed left upper lobe. In a little over one-half of patients with collapsed lobes, there is evidence of loss of volume. In this situation, left hemidiaphragm is elevated, mediastinum is shifted to left, and left hilus is pulled cranially. Also, left mainstem bronchus deviates cranially. The calcification in left hilar mass represents unrelated old granulomatous infection. In *B*, the density from left hilus down toward anterior portion of chest represents the partially collapsed left upper lobe. The radiolucency substernally is right lung.

Fig. 21-3. Collapsed left lower lobe. *A*, PA CXR and *B*, lateral CXR. This is example of no evidence of loss of volume despite almost complete collapse of a large lobe. Note that rib detail and lung markings cannot be seen behind the heart due to the collapsed left lower lobe, with the border paralleling left border of heart. Lateral CXR shows wedge-shaped density of collapsed left lower lobe, but in a moderate number of cases the only evidence may be seemingly increased density over the vertebrae without wedge-shaped infiltrate being so obvious.

Fig. 21-4. Collapsed left lower lobe. *A*, PA CXR and *B*, lateral CXR. Nodule in left mid-lung field plus collapsed left lower lobe, as can be seen with a density behind the heart. This entity represents two separate primary lung cancers, viz., synchronous bronchogenic carcinomas. Do not stop with the first evident abnormality, such as nodule in mid-lung field, without carefully looking at all other areas. *B* demonstrates finding of increased density over lower thoracic vertebrae without any obvious wedge-shaped infiltrate, as in Figure 21-3. Over anterior portion of hemidiaphragm, the small wedge-shaped infiltrate is not fluid in left major fissure, because left major fissure is pulled away posteriorly. Instead, it is an incidental normal variant of fat pushed up into right major fissure.

Fig. 21-5. Collapsed right upper lobe. *A*, PA CXR and *B*, lateral CXR. *A*, This is classic "reversed S" of mass in right hilus with partial collapse of right upper lobe. Loss of volume is evident with the elevation of the right hemidiaphragm. In *B*, the partially collapsed right upper lobe can be faintly seen in the upper anterior portion of hemithorax (*arrow*).

Fig. 21-6. Collapsed right lower lobe. *A*, PA CXR and *B*, lateral CXR. *A*, This 75-year-old smoker had hemoptysis for 1½ years; his CXR had been read as "normal" on several occasions. Note linear density (*arrows*) projecting downward and laterally along right border of heart. It projects below diaphragm and is not a normal line. Also, right hilus is not evident; it has been pulled centrally and downward because of carcinoma obstructing bronchus of right lower lobe. Note very slight shift in mediastinum to the right, indicative of some loss of volume. In spite of significant collapse of right lower lobe, only subtle increased density over lower thoracic vertebrae represents this collapse.

Fig. 21-7. *A,* "Elevated right hemidiaphragm" that is really infrapulmonic effusion, as seen on decubitus film. *B,* For reasons unknown, a meniscus is not formed in some people with infrapulmonic pleural effusion. Thus, any seemingly elevated hemidiaphragm should be examined with suspicion that it could be an infrapulmonic effusion. Decubitus CXR or ultrasonography would disclose the free fluid.

Fig. 21-8. *A,* Normal, pre-pulmonary embolism on PA CXR; *B,* pulmonary embolism. CXR is read as normal in 20%-30% of patients with angiographically proved pulmonary embolism. In comparison with *A, B* shows subtle elevation of right hemidiaphragm. In *A,* right and left hemidiaphragms are equal. Elevated hemidiaphragm is the most common finding with acute pulmonary embolism in some series. Also, note plumpness of right pulmonary artery, prominent pulmonary outflow tract on left (*arrow*), and subtle change in cardiac diameter. This 28-year-old man was in shock at the time of CXR from massive pulmonary emboli as result of major soft tissue trauma produced by a motorcycle accident 7 days earlier.

Fig. 21-9. Abnormal CXR, *A*, in 68-year-old asymptomatic man. *Small arrows* outline areas of pleural calcification, particularly on right hemidiaphragm. This is tip-off to prior asbestos exposure. The process in left mid-lung was worrisome (*large arrow*), perhaps indicating a new process such as bronchogenic carcinoma in this smoker. However, CT, *B*, disclosed rounded atelectasis (*small arrow*). The comma extending from this mass is characteristic of rounded atelectasis, which is result of subacute-to-chronic pleural effusion resolving and trapping some lung as it heals. Also note pleural calcification in *B* (*large arrow*).

Fig. 21-10. Panlobular emphysema at the bases consistent with diagnosis of α$_1$-antitrypsin-deficiency emphysema. Emphysema should not be read into CXR, because all it usually represents is hyperinflation that can occur with severe asthma as well. However, in this setting there are markedly diminished interstitial markings at the bases, with radiolucency. Also, there is increased blood flow to the upper lobes because that is where most of the viable lung tissue is. Note flattening of hemidiaphragms from hyperinflation. In early stages, this is a treatable disease.

Fig. 21-11. Left pleural effusion, with loss of volume toward instead of away from effusion. This implies loss of volume on the left side for unexplained reasons, because there was no previous injury or surgical procedure in left hemithorax. The cause of left pleural effusion is collapsed left lower lobe from bronchogenic carcinoma (effusion was exudate with negative findings on cytology). Lateral CXR did not help show collapsed left lower lobe. Radiodensity over right hemithorax is shrapnel.

Fig. 21-12. *A*, *B*, and *C*, PA CXR. *A* and *B*, Coarctation with tortuous aorta, mimicking mediastinal mass. This occurs in about 1/3 of patients with coarctation. *C*, Coarctation without mediastinal abnormality. Most important is the rib notching that is very evident on the inferior borders of only a few of the ribs (*arrows* in *B* and *C*).

Fig. 21-13. Advanced cystic fibrosis, showing hyperinflation with low-lying hemidiaphragms, bronchiectasis (*small arrows* on parallel lines), and microabscesses (*large arrows*) representing small areas of pneumonitis distal to mucous plug that has been coughed out. For reasons unknown, cystic fibrosis almost always begins in upper lobes.

Fig. 21-14. Miliary tuberculosis. CXR shows miliary pattern of relatively discrete micronodules, with little interstitial (linear or reticular) markings. Disseminated fungal disease has similar appearance, as does bronchioalveolar cell carcinoma; however, these patients do not usually have the systemic manifestations of miliary tuberculosis. Other, less common differential diagnoses include lymphoma, lymphocytic interstitial pneumonitis, and pulmonary edema. *Pneumocystis carinii* pneumonia usually has more interstitial reaction.

Fig. 21-15. Histiocytosis X, or eosinophilic granuloma, shows extensive change but predominantly in upper two-thirds of lung fields. Eventually 25% of these patients have pneumothorax, as seen on this CXR. The honeycombing, also described as microcysts, is characteristic of advanced histiocytosis X.

Fig. 21-16. Sarcoidosis in 35-year-old patient. This CXR shows the predominant upper 2/3 parenchymal pattern seen in many patients with stage II or III sarcoidosis. The pattern can be interstitial, alveolar (which this one predominantly is), or a combination. There probably is some residual adenopathy in hila and right paratracheal area.

Fig. 21-17. *A*, CXR of 30-year-old woman with stage I pulmonary sarcoidosis with subtle bilateral hilar and mediastinal adenopathy, particularly right paratracheal and left infra-aortic adenopathy. *B*, CXR 1 year later, after spontaneous regression of sarcoidosis.

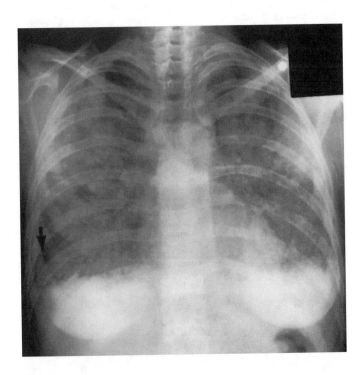

Fig. 21-18. Lymphangitic carcinoma in 27-year-old woman with 6-week history of progressive dyspnea and weight loss. Because of her young age, neoplasm was not considered. Yet, features present on this CXR should have suggested it, viz., bilateral pleural effusions, Kerley's B lines as evident in right base (*arrow*), and mediastinal and hilar lymphadenopathy in addition to diffuse parenchymal infiltrate.

Fig. 21-19. *A* and *B*, Two examples of Kerley's B lines that can be helpful in interpreting CXRs. *A*, Kerley's B lines in a 75-year-old man with colon cancer. *B*, Kerley's B lines are from metastatic adenocarcinoma of the colon and were tip-off that parenchymal process in this patient was due to metastatic carcinoma and not to primary pulmonary process such as pulmonary fibrosis, which was the working diagnosis.

Fig. 21-20. CXR of 55-year-old woman who had had right mastectomy for breast carcinoma now shows subtle but definite right paratracheal (*arrow*) and right hilar adenopathy from metastatic carcinoma of breast.

Fig. 21-21. Nodule in left mid-lung field is technically not "solitary pulmonary nodule" because of another abnormality in thorax that might be related to it, viz., left infra-aortic adenopathy. The differential would be bronchogenic carcinoma with hilar nodal metastasis or, as in this case, acute primary pulmonary histoplasmosis. Had this patient been in an area with coccidioidomycosis, that would also be in differential diagnosis.

Fig. 21-22. Pancoast tumor. Subtle asymmetry at apex of the right lung was more obvious 3 1/2 years later, at which time the diagnosis of Pancoast lesion (primary bronchogenic carcinoma) was made. The patient was symptomatic at time of initial CXR, with symptoms attributed to cervical disk.

Fig. 21-23. The adage that "not all that wheezes is asthma" should be remembered every time you encounter an asthmatic whose condition does not seem to improve. In the case shown here, A, wheezes were predominant over the left hemithorax. A forced expiration film, B, showed air trapping in left lung. Tomography, C, confirmed a lesion in left mainstem bronchus that was a bronchial carcinoid at bronchoscopy.

Fig. 21-24. *A*, Solitary pulmonary nodule evident below right hemidiaphragm, where at least 15% of lung is obscured. *B*, Tomography shows nodule has discrete border but is noncalcified. It was not present 18 months earlier. This is an adenocarcinoma.

Fig. 21-25. *A*, Solitary infiltrate in left upper lobe with air bronchogram, as evident on tomography or CT. *B*, Air bronchogram should be considered sign of bronchioalveolar cell carcinoma or lymphoma until proved otherwise.

Fig. 21-26. Popcorn calcification of hamartoma. This can also be seen in granuloma and represents a benign process.

Fig. 21-27. *A* and *B*, Bull's-eye calcification characteristic of granuloma in solitary pulmonary nodule. They occasionally enlarge but even then almost never warrant removal.

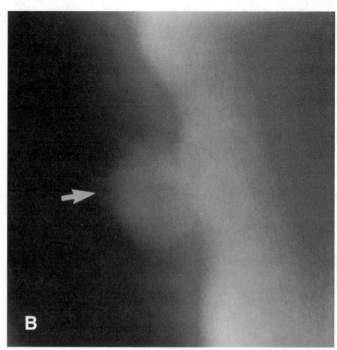

Fig. 21-28. *A* and *B*, Tomography of solitary pulmonary nodules showing satellite nodules (*arrows*). This is characteristic of granulomas.

Fig. 21-29. Tomography of solitary nodule showing spiculation, or sunburst effect, characteristic of primary bronchogenic carcinoma. Spicules represent extension of tumor into septa. CT shows similar appearance.

Computed Tomography

CT is useful in the staging of lung cancer and in assessing mediastinal and hilar lesions, diffuse lung disease, and pleural processes. It has become valuable in diagnosing diffuse lung diseases. High-resolution CT (HRCT) is capable of revealing greater details of pulmonary parenchyma. Characteristic HRCT findings are found in pulmonary eosinophilic granuloma (nodular-cystic spaces in the upper lung fields), lymphangioleiomyomatosis (well-defined cystic spaces in the upper lung zones), idiopathic pulmonary fibrosis (subpleural honeycombing), and lymphangitic pulmonary metastasis (interlobular septal enlargement and nodularity).

- Characteristic CT findings in pulmonary eosinophilic granuloma (histiocytosis X), lymphangioleiomyomatosis, idio-

pathic pulmonary fibrosis, and lymphangitic pulmonary metastasis.
- CT is helpful in the staging of lung cancer.
- CT is useful in evaluating the presence of multiple lung nodules (metastatic) and calcification in the nodule(s).
- HRCT is good for assessing pulmonary parenchyma but not the entire chest.

Conventional CT and HRCT are required for the overall assessment of the thorax. Abnormal signs that indicate diffuse lung disease include abnormal interfaces, thickened interlobular septa, nodules, and airspace opacification ("ground-glass" appearance). HRCT findings in pulmonary fibrotic diseases are >90% accurate; honeycombing is seen in 90% of patients, as compared with 30% on traditional CXR. Other diseases in which HRCT is suggestive of the underlying pulmonary process are certain cases of asbestosis, sarcoidosis, pulmonary alveolar phospholipoproteinosis, chronic eosinophilic pneumonia, and bronchiolitis obliterans.

- Clinical correlation with HRCT findings is important.
- HRCT is excellent for diagnosing bronchiectasis.

Magnetic Resonance Imaging

MRI is recommended for the initial evaluation of superior sulcus tumor (Pancoast's tumor), suspected lesions of the brachial plexus, and paraspinal masses that on CXR appear most consistent with neurogenic tumors. MRI is superior to CT in the evaluation of chest wall masses and in the search for small occult mediastinal neoplasms such as ectopic parathyroid adenomas. MRI may be useful in patients with renal failure or contrast allergy when CT is likely to require administration of a contrast agent. MRI may be superior to CT in evaluating pulmonary sequestration, arteriovenous malformation, and tumor recurrence in patients with total pneumonectomy. It is also useful in imaging the vascular structures in the thorax.

Bronchography

Bronchography is used infrequently because of the ability of HRCT in detecting bronchiectasis. Bronchography is indicated 1) if HRCT findings are doubtful in the presence of clinical features of bronchiectasis, 2) if better mapping of bronchiectatic areas is needed before lung resection for the disease, 3) in certain cases of bronchial strictures, and 4) in very young children in whom HRCT is not possible.

- HRCT has almost replaced bronchography for diagnosing bronchiectasis.

Pulmonary Angiography

The main indication for pulmonary angiography is to detect pulmonary emboli. Although the accuracy of detecting emboli in the major vessels is good, peripheral pulmonary embolism may not be seen. Anticoagulation is not a contraindication to the test. Pulmonary angiography is useful in the diagnosis of pulmonary arteriovenous fistula and malformations, and it is usually a prerequisite if embolotherapy is planned.

- Pulmonary angiography: the main indication is pulmonary thromboembolism.
- Pulmonary angiography may not detect peripheral or tiny pulmonary embolism.
- It is helpful in detecting pulmonary arteriovenous malformations and fistula.

Bronchial Angiography

Bronchial angiography is used to determine whether the bronchial arteries are causing massive pulmonary hemorrhage or massive hemoptysis. It is a prerequisite if bronchial arterial embolotherapy is planned. Complications include neurologic deficits if the spinal artery, a branch of the bronchial artery, is accidentally embolized.

- Complication of bronchial arterial embolotherapy: spinal artery embolization resulting in neurologic defects.
- Both pulmonary and bronchial angiography may be needed for some patients with massive hemoptysis.

Radionuclide Lung Scan

Ventilation-perfusion ($\dot{V}/\dot{Q}$) scan, quantitative $\dot{V}/\dot{Q}$ scan, and gallium lung scan are used in diagnosing various lung diseases.

Perfusion ($\dot{Q}$) Scan

The $\dot{Q}$ scan is commonly used in diagnosing pulmonary embolism. The likelihood of pulmonary embolism in a scan that shows "high probability" and a scan that shows "low probability" is >90% and <5%, respectively. An "intermediate probability" scan usually requires documentation of pulmonary embolism by pulmonary angiography.

Quantitative $\dot{V}/\dot{Q}$ Scan

The quantitative $\dot{V}/\dot{Q}$ scan is used to assess unilateral and regional pulmonary function by measuring $\dot{V}/\dot{Q}$ relationships. It is indicated in patients who are poor surgical candidates for lung resection because of their underlying pulmonary dysfunction. If the lung region to be resected shows minimal or no lung function by the quantitative $\dot{V}/\dot{Q}$ scan, the resection is unlikely to impair further the patient's pulmonary reserve.

Gallium Scan

Gallium (Ga 67) citrate is of minimal or no use in the diagnosis of diffuse lung diseases. The test lacks specificity and is expensive.

- Low or intermediate probability results of $\dot{V}/\dot{Q}$ scan may require further clinical evaluation and tests.
- Quantitative $\dot{V}/\dot{Q}$ scan is used to assess unilateral or regional pulmonary function; it is useful in assessing lung resectability in patients with poor lung function.
- [67]Ga scan has no clinical role in the diagnosis of diffuse lung disease.

Sputum Microscopy

Simple microscopy using a "wet" slide preparation is important in evaluating sputum eosinophilia and Charcot-Leyden crystals, particularly in asthmatics. Gram's staining of sputum should be used to evaluate bacterial infections. However, routine examination with Gram's stain is unnecessary in all patients with COPD who present with acute exacerbations. Induced sputum is helpful in identifying mycobacteria, fungi, *Pneumocystis carinii*, and malignant cells. Gastric washings are used to identify mycobacteria and fungi.

- Simple microscopy using a "wet" slide preparation is an inexpensive method to evaluate sputum eosinophilia and to identify Charcot-Leyden crystals.
- Hemosiderin-laden macrophages in sputum indicate blood ingested by alveolar macrophages.
- Smokers have a significant number of hemosiderin-laden macrophages.
- Induced sputum is excellent for identification of *Pneumocystis carinii*.

Pulmonary Function Tests

The major indication for pulmonary function tests (PFTs) is dyspnea. PFTs do not diagnose lung disease but assess the mechanical function of the respiratory system and quantitate the loss of lung function. These tests are used to separate obstructive from restrictive phenomena and to detect latent bronchospastic disease (hyperreactive airway disease) by using provocation inhalation challenge (methacholine, carbachol, or histamine). Results of previous PFTs are helpful in following the course of lung disease.

- Obstructive disease usually indicates obstruction to outflow of air from the lungs because of airway narrowing during expiration; both flow rates and volumes are affected.
- Inflow and outflow of air are limited in asthma because of bronchoconstriction throughout respiration.
- Increase in flow rates after bronchodilator therapy suggests reversible airway disease.
- Restrictive disease indicates limitation to full expansion of the lungs because of disease in the lung parenchyma, chest wall, or diaphragm. Volumes are diminished but flow rates are normal.
- A combination of obstructive and restrictive patterns is also possible (e.g., COPD with pulmonary fibrosis).

Provocation Inhalation Challenge

Provocation inhalation challenge tests are performed by inhalation challenge of methacholine, carbachol, histamine, industrial irritants suspected of causing occupational asthma, exercise, isocapneic hyperventilation, or cold air. The results define the level of nonspecific airway hyperreactivity in those suspected to have asthma. A 20% decrease in forced expiratory volume in 1 second (FEV_1) from baseline is considered a positive test. These tests are useful when the diagnosis of asthma or hyperactive airway disease is uncertain. Many normal subjects exhibit positive inhalational challenge without symptoms of asthma.

- A 20% decline in FEV_1 from baseline (before challenge) represents a positive test.

Interpretation of Pulmonary Function Tests

A step-by-step approach is helpful:

1. Evaluate volumes and flows as separate groups.
2. Total lung capacity (TLC), functional residual capacity (FRC), and residual volume (RV) indicate volumes. TLC = VC (vital capacity) + RV. Increases in TLC and RV generally suggest hyperinflation, as in COPD and bullae. If TLC and VC are decreased, consider restrictive lung disease (e.g., fibrosis) or loss of lung volume (e.g., surgery, diaphragmatic paralysis, or skeletal problems).
3. VC measured during a slow–not forced–expiration is not affected by airway collapse in COPD. Forced VC may be low with forced expiration because of airway collapse. In normal subjects, VC equals forced VC (i.e., VC = FVC).
4. FEV_1 and forced expiratory flow between 25% and 75% of VC indicate flow rates. Flow rates are characteristically diminished in COPD, but smaller decreases in flows can be seen in the presence of low lung volumes. When FEV_1 expressed as a percentage of the FVC is low, it indicates obstructive pulmonary disease.
5. Maximal voluntary ventilation (MVV) test involves rapid inspiratory and expiratory maneuvers and, thus, tests airflow through major airways and muscle strength. Patients with severe COPD may have low MVV, whereas those with restrictive lung diseases have normal MVV (because there is no obstruction to airflow). MVV also tests muscle strength. Neuromuscular diseases may lead to decreased MVV.

- Normally, MVV is decreased in obstructive disease (i.e., MVV = FEV_1 x 33).
- If MVV is low and flow rates are normal (i.e., no airway obstruction), consider weakness of the respiratory muscles, especially the diaphragm.
- MVV is also significantly decreased in major airway lesions.
- A good clinical estimate of respiratory muscle strength is obtained by measuring maximal inspiratory and expiratory pressures (Pi_{max} and Pe_{max}).
- Flow rates are normal or near normal in pure restrictive lung disease.
- Clinical features (symptoms and signs) should be correlated with the results of PFTs.

6. Diffusing capacity (DLCO) is dependent on the thickness of the alveolocapillary membrane (DM), hemoglobin level (θ), and pulmonary capillary volume (Vc). ($\frac{1}{DLCO} = \frac{1}{DM} + \frac{1}{\theta Vc}$). Diffusing capacity is low in anatomical emphysema ($\downarrow$Vc), anemia ($\downarrow\theta$), restrictive lung diseases ($\uparrow$DM), pneumonectomy ($\downarrow$Vc), pulmonary hypertension, and recurrent pulmonary emboli ($\downarrow$Vc). Diffusing capacity is increased in supine posture ($\uparrow$Vc), after exercise ($\uparrow$Vc), in polycythemia ($\uparrow\theta$), obesity ($\uparrow$Vc), left-to-right shunt ($\uparrow$Vc), and in some asthmatics. Isolated low diffusing capacity (with normal results on PFTs) is seen in pulmonary hypertension, multiple pulmonary emboli, and anemia.

- DLCO is decreased in anatomical emphysema but not in bronchitis or asthma.
- Isolated (meaning normal volumes and flows) decrease in DLCO is seen in pulmonary hypertension, multiple pulmonary emboli, and severe anemia.

Table 21-3.--Try to Interpret These Results of Pulmonary Function Tests Before Reading the Explanations*

Patient	1	2	3	4	5	6	7	8	9	10
Age (yr) and sex	73 M	43 M	53 F	43 M	50 M	20 M	58 F	40 M	28 F	44 M
Weight, kg	52	53	50	63	73	80	59	75	52	148
Tobacco	63PY	NS	NS	NS	20PY	NS	NS	NS	NS	NS
Total lung capacity, %	140	128	84	118	110	100	56	68	108	90
Vital capacity, %	52	75	86	78	82	95	62	58	106	86
Residual volume, %	160	140	90	110	112	90	65	80	98	90
FEV_1, %	35	38	82	48	80	90	85	42	112	96
FEV_1/FVC, %	40	34	80	40	60	85	88	50	85	78
FEF_{25-75}	18	14	80	35	75	88	82	24	102	88
Maximal voluntary ventilation, %	62	48	40	60	105	120	108	62	88	90
Diffusing capacity	9	10	20	28	26	32	8	8	6	40
(normal)	(22)	(28)	(20)	(28)	(27)	(34)	(26)	(28)	(32)	(28)

*Values of 80%-120% of predicted are considered normal.
FEF_{25-75}, forced expiratory flow between 25%-75% of vital capacity; FEV_1, forced expiratory volume in 1 second; FVC, forced vital capacity; NS, non-smoker; PY, pack-years of smoking.

- Decrease in hemoglobin by 1 g diminishes DLCO by 7%.
- Flow-volume curves are helpful in distinguishing between intrathoracic and extrathoracic obstructive lesions in the major airways.

Explanations of Table 21-3

Patient 1. The typical features of hyperinflation are indicated by high values for TLC and RV. VC is low because of high RV (TLC - RV=VC). Flow rates are extremely low and MVV is moderately reduced. The very low DLCO suggests parenchymal damage. Without knowing the response of spirometric variables to inhalation of bronchodilator, it is not possible to tell whether the patient has a bronchospastic component. Diagnosis: moderately severe obstructive disease with severe anatomical emphysema.

Patient 2. Young nonsmoker with features of hyperinflation (high TLC and RV). Flow rates and MVV are also severely decreased. These features suggest obstructive lung disease. The low DLCO suggests parenchymal damage (emphysema). Diagnosis: severe COPD (emphysema) caused by familial deficiency of α_1-antitrypsin.

Patient 3. Airflows and lung volumes are slightly decreased but within normal limits. Note the severely decreased MVV (this test requires rapid inspiratory and expiratory movements by the patient). In this patient, maximal inspiratory and expiratory pressures were severely decreased, suggesting muscle weakness. Diagnosis: severe thyrotoxicosis with proximal muscle weakness (thyrotoxic myopathy). This pattern of results on PFTs can be seen in neuromuscular diseases such as amyotrophic lateral sclerosis and myasthenia gravis.

Patient 4. A young nonsmoker with slightly increased but normal TLC and slightly diminished VC. Flow rates, however, are moderately decreased. This patient has mild-to-moderate obstructive phenomenon. Normal DLCO excludes anatomical emphysema or other parenchymal problems. Bronchodilator testing showed improvement in lung volumes and flow rates. Diagnosis: typical asthma.

Patient 5. A middle-aged patient and 20-pack-year smoker with mild hyperinflation (increased TLC and RV). Because these are within normal limits (80%-120% of predicted), true hyperinflation is not present. Flow rates show slight reductions, and MVV and DLCO are normal. Bronchodilator inhalation showed no improvement. Note the slightly diminished FEV_1/FVC ratio. This together with slightly diminished FEF_{25-75} suggests a mild obstructive lung disease of a nonasthmatic type. Because of normal DLCO, significant anatomical emphysema can be excluded. Diagnosis: nonasthmatic bronchitis.

Patient 6. A 20-year-old nonsmoker with normal lung volumes and flows (80%-120% of predicted normal). This patient used to be a "super athlete" and recently noted cough and chest tightness after exertion. Results from previous PFTs were unavailable. Important points from this example are: 1) in a young, otherwise healthy patient, the lung volumes and flow rates are usually "supernormal," more so in an athlete. 2) This patient may have had very high volumes and flow rates in the past, but without the results of previous PFTs, no comparison can be made (if earlier PFT results were available, the present results might represent a severe decrease in pulmonary function). 3) The medical history suggests the possibility of exercise-induced asthma, and spirometry after a treadmill exercise test showed 28% reduction in flow rates 5-10 minutes after termination of exercise. 4) Note the relatively high DLCO in this patient. Asthmatic patients, for some unknown reason (some believe as a result of increased $\dot{V}/\dot{Q}$ distribution in the lungs), show increased DLCO. Diagnosis: exercise-induced asthma.

Patient 7. A middle-aged nonsmoker with moderately severe decrease in lung volumes and normal flow rates. MVV is within normal limits, but DLCO is severely diminished. These suggest severe restrictive lung disease with significant parenchymal disease. The slightly diminished flow rates are a secondary phenomenon related to decreased lung volumes. Diagnosis: biopsy-proved idiopathic pulmonary fibrosis. Classic example of restrictive lung disease. Note that the FEV_1/FVC ratio is usually higher in true restrictive lung disease. Patients who have had lung resection also have diminished lung volumes and decreased DLCO.

Patient 8. A relatively young man with moderately decreased lung volumes. Flow rates are also diminished more than expected from the decreases in lung volumes. Reduction in the FEV_1/FVC ratio suggests the presence of obstructive lung disease. MVV is also reduced, and DLCO is severely decreased. Compared with patient 7, this patient has obstructive disease in addition to severe restrictive lung disease. Very low DLCO suggests parenchymal disease. CXR disclosed bilaterally diffuse nodular interstitial changes, especially in the upper two-thirds of the lungs. Bronchoscopic examination revealed extensive endobronchial sarcoid granulomas. Diagnosis: severe restrictive lung disease from pulmonary parenchymal sarcoidosis and obstructive airway disease secondary to endobronchial sarcoidosis.

Patient 9. A young woman with normal lung volumes and flow rates. MVV is slightly reduced but within normal limits. DLCO is very low. PaO_2 was 56 mm Hg. Diagnosis: primary pulmonary hypertension.

Patient 10. A relatively young man with normal lung volumes and flow rates. Previous PFT results were not available for comparison. DLCO is abnormally high. This patient was extremely obese, and all the abnormal results on PFTs can be explained on the basis of this. Obese patients show diminished lung volumes because of poor effort made during testing. Abnormally high DLCO is reported to be a result of increased pulmonary capillary volume. In an otherwise healthy but obese person, slightly diminished or diminished DLCO should suggest a primary pulmonary problem rather than obesity-related pulmonary dysfunction. Diagnosis: obesity-related pulmonary dysfunction.

Preoperative Evaluation of Lung Functions

Every pneumonectomy patient should be evaluated with PFTs. A patient can tolerate pneumonectomy if FEV_1 is >50% of predicted, MVV is >50% of predicted, RV/TLC is 50% of predicted, and DLCO is >50% of predicted value. If values are worse than any of the above, use split ventilatory functions and/or quantitative differential $\dot{V}/\dot{Q}$ scan. Pulmonary preparation will decrease the rate of postoperative pulmonary complications. Increased morbidity and mortality are associated with severe COPD, $PaCO_2$ >45 mm Hg (hypoxemia is not a reliable indicator), and if pulmonary artery pressure (intraoperatively) is >30 mm Hg with temporary unilateral occlusion of a pulmonary artery. Upper abdominal operations (gallbladder and abdominal aortic aneurysm repair) carry higher rates of pulmonary complications.

Exercise Test

Exercise testing can assess cardiopulmonary function. Indications for exercise testing include unexplained dyspnea or effort intolerance, ability/disability evaluation, quantitation of severity of pulmonary dysfunction, separation of cardiac from pulmonary causes of disability, evaluation of progression of a given disease process, estimation of operative risks before cardiopulmonary surgery (lung resection, heart-lung, or lung transplantation), rehabilitation, and evaluation of need for supplemental oxygen. Special equipment and expertise are required to perform an optimal exercise study.

Blood Gases and Oximetry

The interpretation of blood gas abnormalities is discussed in Chapter 5.

Bronchoscopy

Common diagnostic indications for bronchoscopy include persistent cough, hemoptysis, suspected cancer, lung nodule, atelectasis, diffuse lung disease, and lung infections. Therapeutic indications include atelectasis, retained secretions, tracheobronchial foreign bodies, airway stenosis (dilatation), and obstructing lesions (laser therapy, stent placement). Bronchoscopy is valuable in the staging of lung cancer. Complications from bronchoscopy are minimal and include bleeding from biopsy, pneumothorax (from lung biopsy), and hypoxemia. The risk of bleeding is increased in patients with renal failure, thrombocytopenia, and other bleeding diatheses.

- Bronchoscopy is safe in most patients with relatively few contraindications.
- Low diagnostic yield in pleural effusion without other CXR findings.
- Bronchoscopy is valuable in the diagnosis and staging of lung cancer.
- Bronchoscopy carries a low risk of complications.

Bronchoalveolar Lavage

Bronchoalveolar lavage (BAL) is performed by wedging a flexible bronchoscope into a segmental bronchus and instilling 100-150 mL of normal saline into the distal (abnormal) segments of the lung. The instilled saline is aspirated back via the bronchoscope and can be analyzed for cell counts, morphology, and typing. Protein and constituents can be measured in the lavage. The cells obtained represent the cell population in the alveoli. BAL effluent in normal subjects shows pulmonary alveolar macrophages ($93\% \pm 3\%$) and lymphocytes ($7\% \pm 1\%$). Other types of leukocytes are rarely found in normal nonsmokers. Because several of the diffuse lung diseases are reported to result from the inflammatory and immune cells, the presence of these cells may help in understanding the pathogenesis.

- BAL can quantify and identify cell morphology at the alveolar level.
- Normal subjects show macrophages (93%), lymphocytes (7%), and neutrophils (<1%).

An increased number of neutrophils with normal lymphocytes is reported in idiopathic pulmonary fibrosis, familial pulmonary fibrosis, and asbestosis. An increased number of lymphocytes without neutrophilia has been noted in sarcoidosis and hypersensitivity pneumonitis. Variable cell counts are seen in other diffuse lung diseases. BAL should be considered a research tool to study the pathogenesis of lung diseases. Currently, BAL has no value in the diagnosis of sarcoidosis or idiopathic pulmonary fibrosis. However, it may be helpful in diagnosing alveolar proteinosis, some infections, histiocytosis X, and lymphangitic pulmonary metastasis. The CD4/CD8 ratio is reversed in BAL obtained from patients with AIDS complicated by lymphocytic interstitial pneumonitis and in many patients with hypersensitivity pneumonitis. BAL is extremely helpful in the diagnosis of *Pneumocystis carinii*, tuberculosis, mycoses, and other infections.

- BAL has a limited role in the diagnosis of sarcoidosis and idiopathic pulmonary fibrosis.
- BAL is diagnostic of malignancy in 60% of patients with lymphangitic carcinomatosis of the lungs.
- BAL is helpful in diagnosing opportunistic lung infections.

Lung Biopsy

Lung biopsy can be performed via bronchoscopy, thoracoscopy, or thoracotomy. The indications for lung biopsy in diffuse lung disease should be based on the clinical features, treatment planned, and risks from biopsy and risk from treatment without a pathologic diagnosis. Bronchoscopic lung biopsy provides a higher diagnostic yield in sarcoidosis, histiocytosis X, eosinophilic pneumonitis, lymphangioleiomyomatosis, infections, pulmonary alveolar proteinosis, lymphangitic carcinomatosis, drug-induced lung disease, and hypersensitivity pneumonitis.

OBSTRUCTIVE LUNG DISEASES

A common pathophysiologic feature of obstructive lung diseases is the obstruction to flow of air. Under this heading are included emphysema, bronchitis, asthma, bronchiectasis, cystic fibrosis, bronchiolitis, bullous lung disease, and strictures and stenoses. The term "chronic obstructive pulmonary disease" (COPD) is used to describe the common obstructive lung diseases, i.e., emphysema, bronchitis, and asthma. Nearly 80% of patients with COPD have features of all three diseases. Nevertheless, it is important to differentiate the salient features of each disease (Table 21-4). The prevalence and mortality rates for COPD have increased during the past decade. COPD is the fifth leading cause of death in the U.S.

Etiology

Tobacco smoking is the major cause of COPD. Nearly 10% of smokers exhibit an accelerated rate of decline in FEV_1. Smokers have 10x the risk of nonsmokers of dying of chronic bronchitis and emphysema. Pipe and cigar smokers have between 1.5x and 3x the risk of nonsmokers. Smoking increases the risk of developing COPD in people with α_1-antitrypsin deficiency. Smokers have increased incidence of COPD, lung carcinoma, atherosclerosis, carcinoma of the pancreas, and skeletal chest pains. The decline in FEV_1 is proportional to the number of pack years of smoking. Other diseases associated with or aggravated by smoking: asthma; pulmonary fibrosis; carcinoma of the bladder, esophagus, larynx, and pancreas; calcification of pleural plaques in asbestosis; pulmonary alveolar phospholipoproteinosis; pulmonary eosinophilic granuloma; and alveolar hemorrhage in Goodpasture's syndrome. Passive smoking (second-hand smoke) is carcinogenic in adults. Other increased risks (particularly in children) include lower respiratory tract infections, fluid collection in the middle ear, decreased lung function, increased severity of preexistent asthma, and increased risk of developing asthma.

- Nearly 10% of smokers exhibit an accelerated rate of decline in FEV_1.
- Pulmonary eosinophilic granuloma (histiocytosis X) and pulmonary alveolar proteinosis are more common in smokers.
- Passive smoking (second-hand smoke) is carcinogenic in adults.
- Passive smoking increases the risks of lung problems, particularly in children.

Air pollution caused by oxidants, oxides of nitrogen, hydrocarbons, and sulphur dioxide has a significant role in exacerbations of COPD. Occupational exposures, heredity (α_1-antitrypsin deficiency), infections, allergy (in asthma), and other factors are also involved in the cause of COPD.

Table 21-4.--Salient Differential Features of Bronchial Asthma, Chronic Bronchitis, and Emphysema*

Differential Feature	Bronchial asthma	Chronic bronchitis	Emphysema
Onset	70% <30 yr old	≥50 yr old	≥60 yr old
Cigarette smoking	0	++++	++++
Pattern	Paroxysmal	Chronic, progressive	Chronic, progressive
Dyspnea	0 to ++++	+ to ++++	+++ to ++++
Cough	0 to +++	++ to ++++	+ to +++
Sputum	0 to ++	+++	+, ++
Atopy	50% (adult)	15%	15%
Infections	↑Symptoms	↑↑↑ Symptoms	↑Symptoms
Chest roentgenogram	Usually normal	↑ Marking	Hyperinflation
$Paco_2$	Normal or ↓ in attack	Increased	Normal or increased
Pao_2	Normal or ↓ in attack	Low	Low
DLCO	Normal	Normal or slight decrease	Decreased
FEV_1,%	↓↓ in attack or normal	↓↓	↓↓
Total lung capacity	Normal or ↑ in attack	Normal or slight ↑	↑↑↑
Residual volume	Normal or ↑ in attack	Normal or slight ↑	↑↑↑
Cor pulmonale	Rare	Common	Rare
Hematocrit	Normal	Normal or increased	Normal or increased

*↑ indicates increase; ↓, decrease; ↑↑, increased more; ↓↓, decreased more; ↑↑↑, increased greatly; ↓↓↓, decreased greatly; +, present; ++, bothersome; +++, major problem; ++++, significant problem; $Paco_2$, partial arterial carbon dioxide pressure; Pao_2, partial arterial oxygen pressure; DLCO, diffusion capacity:total lung capacity ratio; and FEV_1,%, percentage of vital capacity expired in 1 second.
From Kaliner M, Lemanske R: Rhinitis and asthma. JAMA 268:2807-2829, 1992. By permission of the American Medical Association.

Pathology

Obstruction of the airways can result from five basic mechanisms: airway collapse during expiration (COPD), bronchospasm (many causes), mucosal inflammation and edema (bronchitis, asthma, etc.), mucous gland hypertrophy (bronchitis, asthma, etc.), and extrinsic compression. The airway collapse during expiration typically occurs in emphysema, bullous lung disease, chronic bronchitis, long-standing asthma, and other obstructive lung diseases. The airway collapse occurs as a result of greatly increased intrathoracic pressure during expiration and the loss of elastic recoil of the lung (which normally prevents excessive collapse of the airways during expiration). The premature collapse of airways leads to air-trapping and hyperinflation of the lungs (barrel chest). Bronchospasm occurs as a result of increased bronchomotor tone in the smooth muscles of the bronchial tree. Bronchospasm can occur as a result of many underlying complex mechanisms mediated by the vagus nerve, extrinsic allergens, release of intrinsic chemicals, external physical and chemical injury, hypothermia of airways, and other factors. Mucous gland hypertrophy occurs in chronic bronchitis, asthma, and other airway diseases as a result of direct or indirect stimulation of mucous glands. Extrinsic compression is usually due to tumors pressing on the airways. The physiologic effect of bronchoconstriction is the narrowing of airways and resultant limitation in air flow. FEV_1 and other variables of airflow will diminish. Increased bronchomotor tone can be elicited by using provocation inhala-tion challenge tests. These tests are useful when the diagnosis of asthma or hyperactive airway disease is uncertain. Many normal subjects exhibit positive inhalational challenge without symptoms of asthma. Histologically, centrilobular emphysema is the most common type and usually starts in the upper lobes; most patients with COPD have this. The panlobular type usually starts in the lower lobes. It is seen in classic anatomical emphysema and in patients with α_1-antitrypsin deficiency.

- Causes of airway obstruction: expiratory collapse of airways, bronchospasm, mucosal inflammation, and mucous gland hypertrophy.
- Centrilobular emphysema is more common than the panlobular type.

Physiology

Decreased flow rates are characteristic of COPD. Lung compliance is increased in emphysema, and elastic recoil is decreased (the opposite occurs in restrictive lung disease). Diffusing capacity for carbon monoxide is diminished in emphysema as well as most restrictive lung diseases. Hyperexpansion is manifested by increased total lung capacity and residual volume. Retention of CO_2 (hypercarbia) is more common in bronchitic patients. Hypocarbia is more common in restrictive lung disease (due to tachypnea/hyperventilation). Hypercarbia is a poor prognostic sign in restrictive lung disease. Normal lung compliance = 0.2 L/cm H_2O.

Chronic Bronchitis

Chronic bronchitis is defined as cough with sputum for 3 months or more per year for 2 or more consecutive years. Pathologically, the Reid index (i.e., the ratio of bronchial mucous glands to bronchial wall thickness) is increased. Chronic bronchitis is a common problem. Cigarette smoking is the most common cause of chronic bronchitis. Occupational exposure and air pollution also contribute to the exacerbations. Patients exhibit productive cough, have a tendency to retain CO_2, have lower PaO_2, have a tendency toward cyanosis ("blue bloaters"), and tend to be slightly overweight. Most patients with "COPD" have a combination of chronic bronchitis and emphysema.

- Chronic bronchitics (blue bloaters) tend to retain CO_2, cough, and develop cor pulmonale sooner than emphysematous patients (pink puffers).

Emphysema

Emphysema is characterized by enlargement of the airspaces distal to the terminal bronchioles accompanied by destruction of the alveolar walls. The definition implies histologic documentation, but this is impractical in clinical practice. HRCT of the lungs is excellent for documentation of emphysema and bullous lung disease. Pure anatomical emphysema is not as common as chronic bronchitis. Emphysematous patients are thin, maintain near normal PaO_2 by increasing the work of breathing, and look adequately oxygenated. Hence, they are known as "pink puffers." A relatively common finding is severe weight loss in some patients. Carbon dioxide retention is not seen until late in the disease.

- Pink puffers have emphysema, lose weight, and do not retain CO_2 until late in the course of the disease.

Bullous Lung Disease

Small apical bullae are present in many normal persons. Bullous lung disease can be congenital or acquired. Lack of communication with bronchi may cause air-trapping. Complications include pneumothorax, COPD, infection and formation of lung abscess, bleeding into a bulla, and compression of adjacent normal lung. Surgical therapy may improve lung function by 5%-10% in 10%-15% of patients.

- Panlobular emphysema may look like a bulla.
- Bullous changes may be seen in Marfan's and Ehlers-Danlos syndromes, burnt-out sarcoidosis, and cadmium exposure.

α1-Antitrypsin Deficiency

Synthesis of α_1-antitrypsin, a secretory glycoprotein, by hepatocytes is determined by the α_1-antitrypsin gene on chromosome 14. α_1-Antitrypsin inhibits many proteolytic enzymes and, thus, protects the lungs from destructive emphysema. It is an autosomal recessive disease. Phenotypes = normals (P_IMM), heterozygote (P_IMZ), homozygote (P_IZZ), and null (P_INull). The threshold for disease is set at <11 µmol/L. Prevalence of P_IZZ in the U.S. is 1:1,670-1:3,000. From 5% to 10% of patients with P_IZZ α_1-antitrypsin deficiency escape lung disease. Smoking hastens the onset of emphysema. Signs and symptoms appear during the 3rd or 4th decade of life. α_1-Antitrypsin deficiency is associated with neonatal liver disease (hepatitis, cryptogenic cirrhosis, periportal fibrosis), respiratory distress syndrome, and in certain hemorrhagic syndromes (platelet dysfunction, disseminated intravascular coagulation, and clotting disturbances in infants). α_1-Antitrypsin derived from human plasma has been used as replacement therapy (very expensive), but data so far do not show that this prevents progression of disease.

- Smoking hastens the onset of emphysema.
- Basal emphysema on CXR, absence of perfusion to bases, absence of α_1-globulin on protein electrophoresis, patient with COPD, and family history of COPD.
- Hepatic cirrhosis develops in 1%-3% of patients.
- Young patients with clinical features of COPD: asthma, α_1-antitrypsin deficiency, cystic fibrosis, ciliary dyskinesia, and bronchiectasis due to congenital or acquired immunoglobulin deficiency or other diseases.

Asthma

Asthma or asthmatic bronchitis is an acute or chronic disease characterized by recurrent episodes of reversible bronchospasm (wheezing) leading to paroxysmal obstruction of the airways. Asthma is primarily an inflammatory disease. Therefore, inhaled corticosteroids are now considered the first line of therapy by many physicians. Controversy remains about the purported increase in mortality rate in asthmatics. Cough can be the only presenting symptom of bronchial asthma. Exercise-induced asthma is more common in younger people and presents as chest tightness or cough after termination of exercise. Many patients have normal results on PFTs during an asymptomatic period or show excellent bronchodilator response during spirometry. More detailed discussion on asthma can be found in Chapter 2.

- All that wheezes is not asthma and not all asthmatics wheeze.
- Drug-induced bronchospasm: β-blockers, prostaglandin inhibitors (acetylsalicylic acid, indomethacin), ultrasonic nebulizers, acetylcysteine, ascaris antigen, and occupational exposures.
- Provocation inhalation challenge may be needed to detect airway reactivity.

Treatment of COPD

The therapeutic approach to COPD consists of identifying the type of COPD, quantification of pulmonary dysfunction and response to bronchodilator therapy, selection of appropriate bronchodilators, anticipation and appropriate treatment of complications, and initial as well as continued education of the patient and family regarding long-term therapy. A rehabilitation program is equally important.

Bronchodilators

Bronchodilator drugs are administered to reverse the bronchoconstriction, thereby providing symptomatic relief to patients with COPD. The drugs used may be broadly classified into adrenergic agonists (sympathomimetics), β-adrenergic agonists (β_2-selective agonists), phosphodiesterase inhibitor (theophylline), anticholinergics (ipratropium, etc.), mast cell inhibitors (cromolyn sodium, etc.), antihistamines, anti-inflammatory agents (corticosteroids and methotrexate), and other agents (troleandomycin, γ-globulin, mucolytics, etc.). The usefulness (or uselessness) of these drugs is usually determined by the airway lesion responsible for airway obstruction.

Adrenergic Agonists (Sympathomimetics)

Drugs in this group include epinephrine, isoproterenol, ephedrine, and isoetharine. Epinephrine acts on both α and β receptors of effector cells. It is still used in the treatment of acute asthma. In adults, a dose of 0.1-0.3 mg (0.1-0.3 mL of a 1:1,000 dilution) is commonly used. The injection method is commonly used. A maximum of 3 doses (each 15 minutes apart) is recommended. Isoproterenol (Isuprel) has a rapid onset of action (<5 minutes) and a duration of action of 2 hours. Isoetharine (Bronkosol) is administered as an aerosol (0.5 mL diluted with 2.5 mL saline). Currently, ephedrine is rarely used in the treatment of asthma. Adverse reactions associated with adrenergic agonists include anxiety, headache, palpitations, cardiac arrhythmias, skin flushing, tremor, diaphoresis, and paradoxic bronchospasm. In the current practice, adrenergic agonists have been replaced by β-adrenergic (selective) agonists.

- Sympathomimetics are useful in the treatment of acute bronchospasm.

Short-Acting β-Adrenergic (β_2-Selective) Agonists

These are the most commonly used bronchodilators. Drugs in this group of bronchodilators include albuterol, terbutaline, metaproterenol, pirbuterol, and bitolterol. The basic mechanism of bronchodilatation is by stimulation of cyclic AMP production through activation of adenyl cyclase in the cell membrane. The cyclic AMP produced within the cell causes relaxation of smooth muscle by influencing several processes, including the sequestration of calcium. In most patients, single doses of these agents produce clinically significant bronchodilatation within 5 minutes, a peak effect 30-60 minutes after inhalation, and an effect lasting for 3-4 hours. Many of these agents are available in inhaled form (metered dose

inhalers) as well as tablet, powder, syrup, and injection forms. The standard dose for inhalation therapy is 2 inhalations four times daily. It is essential to tailor the dosages of these drugs on the basis of the clinical features and the potential side effects. Adverse effects are more common with oral preparations than with aerosols and include tremor, anxiety, restlessness, tachycardia, palpitations, increased blood pressure, and cardiac arrhythmias. Patients with prostatism may develop exacerbation of symptoms. Paradoxic bronchospasm may result from tachyphylaxis (a rapidly decreasing response to a drug after a few doses) or from exposure to preservatives, sulfites, emulsifying agents, and propellants. Tolerance is another phenomenon observed in patients receiving long-term bronchodilator therapy. Side effects are more likely in the elderly; in the presence of cardiovascular, hepatic, or neurologic disorders; and in those taking other medications for nonpulmonary diseases (β-blockers for cardiac disease, etc.). Normal therapeutic dosages of theophylline and β-agonists in combination are not usually associated with serious side effects.

- Stimulation of cyclic AMP.
- Standard dose: 2 inhalations *four times a day*.
- Side effects: tremor, anxiety, restlessness, tachycardia, palpitations, increased blood pressure, and cardiac arrhythmias.

Long-Acting β-Adrenergic (β_2-Selective) Agonists

The drugs in this group include salmeterol, fenoterol, and formoterol, but salmeterol is the only drug currently available in the U.S. Salmeterol is selective for β_2-adrenoreceptors compared with isoproterenol, a short-acting bronchodilator, which has approximately equal agonist activity on β_1- and β_2-adrenoreceptors. Albuterol has a β_2- to β_1-adrenoreceptor selectivity ratio of 1,400. Salmeterol is at least 50 times more selective for β_2-adrenoreceptors than albuterol. Salmeterol is highly lipophilic (albuterol is hydrophilic) and, hence, the depot effect in tissues along with high affinity and efficacy. These agents have prolonged duration of action (10-12 hours). The bronchodilating effects of salmeterol persist for at least 6 hours, whereas the effect of albuterol lasts for 1.5 hours. In addition to relaxing the bronchial smooth muscles by increasing intracellular cyclic AMP, these drugs also inhibit the release of proinflammatory and spasmogenic mediators from the cells in the lung tissue. Salmeterol has a persistent effect at inhibiting histamine release for up to 20 hours, as opposed to the short duration of action of isoproterenol, albuterol, and formoterol. Salmeterol and formoterol also inhibit the infiltration of inflammatory cells into the lung. These drugs are also effective in preventing exercise-induced asthma, methacholine-induced bronchospasm, and allergen challenge. The dosage of these agents is 2 inhalations (100 μg) twice daily. The longer duration of action may aid in the management of nocturnal asthma. The side effects are similar to those encountered with other β-adrenergic agents. However, tachyphylaxis associated with short-acting β$_2$-agonists is distinctly uncommon with long-acting β$_2$-agonists. Caution: salmeterol and other β-adrenergic bronchodilators may potentiate the actions of monoamine oxidase inhibitors and tricyclic antidepressants.

- Salmeterol is lipophilic (albuterol is hydrophilic).
- Long-acting bronchodilator (>12 hours).
- Dose: 2 inhalations (100 μg) twice daily.

Phosphodiesterase Inhibitor

Theophylline (methylxanthine) is the main drug in this group. Theorized mechanisms of action include inhibition of cyclic GMP, augmentation of adrenergic terminal output to airway smooth muscle, adenosine receptor antagonism, and stimulation of endogenous catecholamine. The result is a decrease in smooth muscle free calcium levels resulting from calcium ion entry into the cell or transfer or mobilization of calcium ions from storage in the sarcoplasmic reticulum. Recently, the role of theophylline in COPD and asthma has been questioned. Overall, its use has diminished and β-agonists are being used more often in its place. Theophylline is a good drug in combination with β$_2$-agonists in the management of moderate and severe asthma. Withdrawal of theophylline from patients with severe COPD has a deleterious effect on lung function. Theophylline increases respiratory muscle contractility in a dose-related fashion. The clearance of theophylline is shown in Table 21-5.

The recommended blood level is 10-15 μg/mL. The main side effects include tremors, aggravation of prostatism, tachycardia, and arrhythmias. Tobacco smoke decreases the efficacy (half-life) of theophylline. The loading dose of theophylline is 6 mg/kg (range, 5-7 mg); the maintenance dose

Table 21-5.--Theophylline Clearance

Increased by	Decreased by
β-Agonists	Allopurinol
Carbamazine	Antibiotics (macrolides)--
Dilantin	ciprofloxacin, norfloxacin,
Furosemide	isoniazid
Hyperthyroidism	β-Blocker--propranolol
Ketoconazole	Caffeine
Marijuana	Cirrhosis
Phenobarbital	Congestive cardiac failure
Rifampin	H$_2$ blocker--cimetidine
Tobacco smoke	Mexiletine
	Oral contraceptives
	Viral infection

is 0.5 mg/kg per hour or 1.15 g/24 hours. The normal adult dose is usually <1,000 mg/day. Longer acting preparations may be given in a single dose of 300-600 mg. The dosage should be decreased by 50% if the patient has received theophylline in the preceding 24 hours or if the patient has heart failure, severe hypoxemia, hepatic insufficiency, or seizures. Each dosage should be increased by 50-100 mg if the therapeutic effect is suboptimal and in smokers who can tolerate the increased dose. Each dose should be decreased by 50-100 mg if toxic effects develop or if progressive cardiac or liver failure develops. The maintenance dose for children can be larger because they tolerate the drugs better than adults.

- Tobacco smoking decreases the half-life of theophylline.
- The recommended blood level is 10-15 μg/mL.
- Frequent measuring of serum theophylline levels is unnecessary in clinical practice.

Anticholinergic Agents

Anticholinergic agents (ipratropium, atropine, etc.) are thought to prevent the increase in intracellular concentration of cyclic GMP caused by the muscarinic receptors in bronchial smooth muscle. These drugs inhibit vagally mediated reflexes by blocking the effects of acetylcholine. Their use is indicated in patients with chronic bronchitis and asthmatic bronchitis, but their role in the management of pure emphysema remains unclear. Ipratropium is a synthetic quaternary ammonium congener of atropine. As a single agent, ipratropium is not effective in the management of acute or chronic airway disease. However, it seems efficacious in the treatment of mild-to-moderate asthma, particularly if used with β-adrenergic agents and theophylline. The efficacy of the combination (ipratropium plus β-agonist) is equal to or greater than the efficacy of the medications administered separately. Ipratropium produces significant bronchodilatation and prevents bronchoconstriction caused by cholinergic agents such as methacholine and carbachol. However, ipratropium does not protect against bronchoconstriction produced by irritants such as tobacco smoke, citric acid, sulfur dioxide, or carbon dust. Allergen-induced bronchospasm also responds poorly to ipratropium therapy. Unlike atropine, ipratropium has no effect on mucus production, mucus transport, or ciliary activities. The usual dose is 2 inhalations four times daily. No more than 12 inhalations should be permitted in 24 hours. The duration of action is 3-5 hours. Side effects are minimal with ipratropium and include nervousness, headache, gastrointestinal upset, dry mouth, and cough. The drug may aggravate narrow-angle glaucoma, prostatic hypertrophy, and bladder neck obstruction.

- Ipratrapium inhibits vagally mediated reflexes by blocking the effects of acetylcholine.

- Minimal or no benefit in the management of pure emphysema.
- Not very effective if used alone.

Mast Cell Inhibitors

Cromolyn and nedocromil stabilize the cell membrane by coating it externally and blocking the release of IgE-mediated mast cell mediators, histamine, and other bronchoconstrictor mediators. Nedocromil is 4x-10x more potent than cromolyn. These are preventive drugs and not therapeutic agents to be used in a full-blown asthmatic episode. They are available as powdered preparations (spinhaler) or liquids for aerosolization. They are excellent drugs for exercise-induced asthma and in asthmatics with known allergens. The duration of action is 4-6 hours. There is no known interaction between these and other drugs. The dosage is 2 inhalations three to four times daily. For exercise-induced asthma, treatment is given 15-20 minutes before exercise. The side effects include irritation of the throat, hoarseness, and dryness of the mouth.

- These drugs do not directly relax (dilate) bronchial smooth muscle.
- Mast cell inhibitors should be used to prevent extrinsic asthma.
- Excellent for exercise- and allergen-induced asthma.

Corticosteroids

Corticosteroid is the most effective anti-inflammatory drug available for the treatment of asthma. Because asthma is considered an inflammatory disease, inhaled corticosteroid is considered by many to be the first-line drug in the treatment of mild asthma. β_2-Agonists are not substitutes for corticosteroids. The mechanism of action of corticosteroids (inhaled and systemic) is unclear. Corticosteroid aerosols rarely cause side effects of systemic (oral) steroid therapy. Inhaled steroids can be used in conjunction with systemic (oral) corticosteroids, especially during the weaning period of long-term or high-dose systemic (oral) corticosteroids. The most common side effect with aerosolized corticosteroids is oral candidiasis. Presently, asthmatic patients are being instructed to use up to 20 inhalations per day. The dosages of oral or injectable corticosteroids is dependent on the severity and duration of asthma. Corticosteroids have no bronchodilating effect in emphysematous patients. Bronchitics, however, may benefit from the anti-inflammatory action. Short- or long-term systemic corticosteroid therapy is an important aspect of treating moderate-to-severe asthma. However, systemic corticosteroid therapy in nonasthmatic COPD has a limited role; only about 15% of patients show improvement. Systemic corticosteroid therapy may contribute to muscle weakness in COPD. Inhaled corticosteroids include beclomethasone (Vanceril, Beclovent,

Becotide, and Becloforte), betamethasone (Bextasol), budesonide (Pulmicort), flunisolide (Aerobid and Bronalide), and triamcinolone acetonide (Azmacort).

- Corticosteroid is considered by many to be the first-line drug in the treatment of asthma.
- Oropharyngeal candidiasis is a complication of aerosolized corticosteroids.
- Systemic corticosteroid therapy is an important aspect of treating asthma.

Non-Steroidal Anti-Inflammatory ("Steroid-Sparing") Agents

Methotrexate, an antineoplastic drug, has been used as a steroid-sparing agent in patients taking high doses of systemic corticosteroids. The efficacy and safety of methotrexate remain controversial. Adjuvant therapy with methotrexate may have a steroid-sparing effect in asthma but beneficial responses are not consistent. Therefore, methotrexate should not be considered a standard antiasthma drug. Gold salts have been used as anti-inflammatory agents in asthmatic patients. The bronchodilator effect may not be apparent until a daily dose of 1,500 mg is administered for 6-12 months. Troleandomycin, a macrolide antibiotic, has shown a steroid-minimizing effect by decreasing the elimination of steroid. It works best with methylprednisolone rather than with prednisone or prednisolone. The normal dose is 250 mg four times daily. Other agents in this group include cyclosporine, hydroxychloroquine, and dapsone. High-dose immunoglobulin therapy has been tried in some refractory cases.

- Limited role for steroid-sparing agents in the management of asthma.
- Some steroid-sparing agents (methotrexate and gold) can produce lung toxicity.

Antihistamines

Asthma is provoked in many patients by the release of histamine and histamine analogues. Therefore, antihistamines have been used by some physicians to treat asthma. Newer agents such as astemizole (10 mg once daily) and terfenadine (60 mg twice daily) are effective in preventing pollen-induced asthma. H_1 antagonists produce bronchodilatation without inducing sedation. These drugs can produce prolongation of the QT_c interval on ECG. This may lead to ventricular tachycardia. This serious side effect is more likely in patients with liver or heart disease and if the patient is taking ketoconazole or macrolide antibiotics.

- Antihistamines are not standard antiasthmatic drugs.
- Astemizole: prolongation of QT_c interval on ECG.

Adjuvant Therapy

Expectorants and mucolytics (acetylcysteine, guaifenesin, iodinated glycerol, and potassium iodide) are used to treat the symptoms rather than the underlying bronchospasm. They are not standard therapy of asthma. Individualizing these agents based on clinical features is important. Antibiotic therapy is helpful in patients with symptoms suggestive of bacterial infection. Desensitization therapy in patients with proven extrinsic allergies may prevent acute asthmatic attacks on exposure to known allergens. Maintenance of good oral hydration, avoidance of tobacco smoking and other respiratory irritants, annual influenza vaccination, and prompt treatment of respiratory infections are equally important.

Oxygen

Nocturnal low-flow O_2 (<2 L/minute) therapy is recommended when PaO_2 is ≤55 mm Hg, PaO_2 is ≤59 mm Hg with polycythemia or clinical evidence of cor pulmonale, or SaO_2 is ≤88%. The lack of CO_2 retention should be ascertained before recommending oxygen. Continuous oxygen therapy is more useful than nocturnal treatment alone. Oxygen therapy is indicated for patients with persistent polycythemia, recurrent episodes of cor pulmonale, severe hypoxemia, and central nervous system symptoms induced by hypoxemia. The need for chronic or indefinite oxygen therapy should be reassessed after 3 months of treatment. For each liter of oxygen administered, the fraction of inhaled oxygen (F_IO_2) increases by 3%. Exercise therapy improves exercise tolerance and maximal oxygen uptake and may diminish desaturation, but exercise does not improve the results of PFTs.

- Oxygen therapy is recommended if PaO_2 ≤55 mm Hg and/or SaO_2 ≤88%.
- F_IO_2 increases by 3% for each liter of supplemental oxygen.
- An exercise program does not improve results of PFTs.

The practical aspects of managing COPD are outlined in Table 21-6.

Complications and Causes for Exacerbation of COPD

The complications and causes (unrelated to COPD but may adversely affect lung function) for exacerbation of COPD include viral and bacterial respiratory infections (common bacteria include *Haemophilus influenzae*, *Moraxella catarrhalis*, and *Streptococcus pneumoniae*), cor pulmonale, myocardial infarction, cardiac arrhythmias, pneumothorax, pulmonary emboli, bronchogenic carcinoma, environmental exposure, oversedation, neglect of therapy, excessive oxygen use (suppression of hypoxemic drive), and excessive use of β_2-agonist (tachyphylaxis). Nocturnal oxygen desaturation is common in blue bloaters, as are premature ventricular contractions

Table 21-6.--Practical Aspects of Managing COPD

Steps in management
　Identify the type of COPD
　Identify pathophysiology
　Assess lung dysfunction
　Eliminate causative/exacerbating factors
　Aim drug therapy at underlying pathophysiology
　Anticipate and treat complications
　Rehabilitation program
　Education of patient and family
Stepped care approach (especially in asthma)
　Mild asthma (FEV_1 >65% of predicted): inhaled steroids; β_2-agonists as needed
　Moderate asthma (FEV_1 36%-65% of predicted): inhaled steroids and theophylline; β_2-agonist as needed
　Severe asthma (FEV_1 <35% of predicted): inhaled steroids, theophylline, β_2-agonist regularly and as needed, and oral (or parenteral) steroids
Miscellaneous
　Anticipate timing of asthmatic attacks and timing of therapy
　Long-term maintenance therapy important to prevent asthmatic attacks
　Bronchodilator use in active smokers is counterproductive
　Do not change drug or drugs without good reason
　A combination of drugs is superior to a single drug in stable COPD
　Document (clinical, spirometry) need for multiple drugs
　Better to increase dose of metered-dose-inhaler steroids than β-agonist
　Avoid β-blockers and ACE-inhibitors
　Sputum culture on a routine basis is unnecessary
　Begin antimicrobials at start of respiratory infections
　Teach technique and dosing of metered-dose inhalers
　Consider pulmonary rehabilitation
　Continued education of patient

and episodic pulmonary hypertension. Decrease in SaO_2 correlates with an increase in pulmonary artery pressure. Severe weight loss, sometimes >50 kg, is noted in 30% of patients with severe COPD.

- Infections in COPD are caused by *H. influenzae*, *M. catarrhalis*, and *S. pneumoniae*.
- Nocturnal oxygen desaturation is common in blue bloaters.
- Decrease in SaO_2 correlates with increase in pulmonary artery pressure.
- Severe weight loss is seen in 30% of COPD (emphysema) patients.

Other Topics in COPD

Nicotine gum and patch help maintain nicotine blood levels while a smoker tries to cope with the psychologic and other aspects of addiction. Nearly 25% of smokers require treatment of more than 12 months to remain tobacco-free. Nicotine from gum is absorbed more slowly from the buccal mucosa and stomach than from the airways with inhaled smoke. Side effects include mucosal burning, light-headedness, nausea, stomachache, and hiccups. The patch causes a rash in a significant number of patients. Use of the nicotine patch with continued smoking aggravates cardiac problems. Pursed-lip breathing is helpful in patients with severe air-trapping. Intermittent positive pressure breathing in COPD has no advantage over metered-dose inhalers or compressed nebulizer therapy. Furthermore, it is more expensive than a simple nebulizer or compressed nebulizer. Intermittent positive pressure breathing may be helpful in selected situations such as postoperative atelectasis, cystic fibrosis, and bronchiectasis. Lung volume reduction surgery (lung shaving procedure) is being tested as a treatment for patients with severe emphysema. Surgical resection of 20%-30% of peripheral lung parenchyma in emphysematous patients appears to improve pulmonary functions during short-term follow-up. The benefit is thought to be the result of regaining normal or near-normal mechanical function (of thoracic cage) that was compromised by the severe hyperinflation of the lungs. Currently, this therapy should be considered experimental.

- Nicotine gum and patch are important aspects of a tobacco cessation program.
- Simultaneous use of cigarette and nicotine products aggravates cardiac problems.
- Lung volume reduction surgery is experimental.

Cystic Fibrosis

Cystic fibrosis is the most common lethal autosomal recessive disease among whites in the U.S. The locus of the responsible gene is on the long arm of chromosome 7. Cystic fibrosis develops in 1 in 2,000-3,500 live births among whites; about 1 in 20 (2%-5%) whites is a heterozygous carrier. There is no sex predominance. Occurrence in blacks is 1 in 17,000 and 1 in 90,000 in Asians. Both parents of a child with cystic fibrosis must be heterozygotes; siblings of such a child have a 50%-65% chance of being heterozygotes. The pathogenesis of cystic fibrosis is unknown, although all exocrine glands seem affected. The diagnosis is made in 80% of patients before the age of 10 years; in 10%, the diagnosis is not made until adolescent years. Obstruction of exocrine glands, with the exception of sweat glands, by viscous secretions causes almost all the clinical manifestations. Mucociliary clearance is normal in the patients with minimal pulmonary dysfunction and is decreased in those with obstructive phenomena. Secretion

of mucous glycoproteins is increased in cystic fibrosis and is responsible for forming viscoelastic gels.

- Cystic fibrosis: the most common lethal autosomal recessive disease among whites.
- In 10% of patients, the diagnosis is not made until adolescent years.
- Siblings of children with cystic fibrosis have a 50%-65% chance of being heterozygotes.
- All exocrine glands, except sweat glands, are affected.

Patients with cystic fibrosis and heterozygous carriers demonstrate nonspecific airway responses similar to those in asthmatics. Patients with cystic fibrosis have an increased susceptibility to asthma and atopy, and many of them exhibit type I and type III hypersensitivity reactions to an assortment of antigens. Positive findings on serologic testing to *Aspergillus* species and *Candida albicans* occur with higher frequency in cystic fibrosis patients than in asthmatics. Allergic bronchopulmonary aspergillosis has been noted in 10% of cystic fibrosis patients.

- Patients with cystic fibrosis and carriers exhibit increased airway response.
- Patients have increased susceptibility to develop asthma and atopy.
- Allergic bronchopulmonary aspergillosis occurs in 10% of patients with cystic fibrosis.

There is no evidence for a primary defect in sodium transport. However, there is indication that epithelial cells in cystic fibrosis patients are poorly permeable to chloride ions. A discrete chloride channel has not been identified. The potential difference across a membrane is normally negative but becomes more negative (because of chloride impermeability) in cystic fibrosis. This phenomenon may indeed represent the genetic defect in cystic fibrosis.

- No evidence for a primary defect in sodium transport in cystic fibrosis.
- Epithelial cells in cystic fibrosis patients are poorly permeable to chloride ions.
- Marked increase in the electrical potential difference across the nasal and tracheobronchial epithelium in comparison with that of normal subjects and heterozygote relatives.

Quantitative pilocarpine iontophoresis is helpful in diagnosis; abnormal results on at least two tests are necessary for the diagnosis. Other conditions that are associated with high levels of sweat sodium/chloride include smoking, chronic bronchitis, malnutrition, hereditary nephrogenic diabetes insipidus, adrenal insufficiency, and ectodermal dysplasia. The concentration of sweat sodium/chloride increases with age. Heterozygotes may have normal sweat sodium/chloride values. False-negative test results are common in the edematous states. Abnormal sweat chloride: adult, >80 mEq/L; child, >60 mEq/L. It is important to recognize that normal sweat chloride values do not exclude the diagnosis of cystic fibrosis. When sweat chloride levels are normal in a patient in whom cystic fibrosis is highly suspected, alternative diagnostic tests (nasal transepithelial voltage measurements, genotyping, etc.) should be considered.

- Diagnosis in adults requires ≥3 of the following: clinical features of cystic fibrosis, positive family history, sweat chloride ≥80 mEq/L, and pancreatic insufficiency.
- Respiratory manifestations: sinusitis, nasal polyps, progressive cystic bronchiectasis, purulent sputum, atelectasis, hemoptysis, and pneumothorax.
- *Pseudomonas aeruginosa* is the dominant organism and is impossible to eradicate.
- Increased incidence of *Pseudomonas cepacia* in the respiratory secretions; presence of *P. cepacia* is associated with rapid deterioration in lung function.

Cystic fibrosis is the most common cause of COPD and pancreatic deficiency in the first three decades of life in the U.S. Males constitute 55% of the adult patients with cystic fibrosis. The diagnosis is made after the age of 15 years in 17%-25% of patients. In adults (≥17 years), COPD is the major cause of morbidity and mortality. Adults with cystic fibrosis show a higher incidence of minor hemoptysis (60% of patients), major hemoptysis (71%), pneumothorax (16%), and sinusitis and nasal polyposis (48%). Pancreatic insufficiency is present in 95% of patients, but it is seldom symptomatic. Intussusception and fecal impaction (similar to meconium ileus) are more frequent (21%) in adults than in children. Hyperinflation of lungs on CXR and lobar atelectasis are both less frequent in adults than in children. Mean age at onset of massive hemoptysis is 19 years, and median survival from the initial episode of hemoptysis is about 3.5 years. Mean age of occurrence of pneumothorax in adults is 22 years. Azoospermia is seen in 95%.

- COPD is present in 97% of adults with cystic fibrosis and is the major cause of morbidity and mortality.
- In adults with cystic fibrosis: minor hemoptysis (60%), major hemoptysis (71%), pneumothorax (16%), and sinusitis and nasal polyposis (48%).
- Pancreatic insufficiency in 95%; it is seldom symptomatic.

Treatment of cystic fibrosis includes management of obstructive lung disease, chest physiotherapy, postural drainage, immunization against influenza, hydration, and aggressive antibiot-

ic therapy. Newer antibiotics are effective against *P. aeruginosa*. Intravenous administration of antibiotics at home on a short-term basis is now an accepted treatment. Lung transplant is an option for advanced cases. Amiloride in aerosolized form blocks the reabsorption of sodium by the respiratory epithelium and, thus, is thought to improve hydration of the respiratory secretions. Sputum in patients with cystic fibrosis contains high concentrations of extracellular DNA, a viscous material released by leukocytes. Aerosolized recombinant human DNase I (dornase alfa) reduces sputum viscosity by degrading the DNA. Results of DNase I therapy have shown reduced risk of lung infections, improvement in FEV_1, and reduced antibiotic requirement. The usual dose is 2.5 mg once a day via nebulizer; patients older than 21 years may benefit from 2.5 mg twice a day. Serum antibodies to dornase alfa develop in about 2%-4% of patients, but anaphylaxis has not been noted. Side effects of dornase alfa have included voice alteration, hoarseness, rash, chest pain, pharyngitis, and conjunctivitis. Controversial issues in the therapy of cystic fibrosis include nebulized antibiotic therapy, domiciliary long-term intravenous antibiotic therapy, systemic corticosteroids, repeated sputum culture, hospitalization for acute exacerbation, and frequent bronchoscopy to clear airways.

- Nearly 50% of patients with cystic fibrosis survive to age 25.
- The overall survival rate for cystic fibrosis patients older than 17 years is closer to 50%.
- Poor prognostic factors: female sex, residence in a nonnorthern climate, pneumothorax, hemoptysis, recurrent bacterial infections, presence of *P. cepacia*, and systemic complications.

Bronchiectasis

Bronchiectasis is ectasia, or dilatation, of bronchi due to the irreversible destruction of bronchial walls. The reversible type of bronchiectasis is seen in patients with severe bronchitis, acute pneumonia, and allergic bronchopulmonary aspergillosis. Bronchiectasis most commonly occurs in lower lung fields. Mild cylindrical bronchiectasis seen in many heavy smokers with chronic bronchitis may be diffuse. Distal bronchial segments are involved in most cases of bronchiectasis. An exception to this is the proximal bronchial involvement in allergic bronchopulmonary aspergillosis. In most cases of bronchiectasis, second- to fourth-order bronchi are involved. Disease is bilateral in 30% of all bronchiectatic cases.

- Reversible bronchiectasis in allergic bronchopulmonary aspergillosis, acute pneumonia, and chronic bronchitis.
- Upper lobe involvement in cystic fibrosis, allergic bronchopulmonary aspergillosis, and chronic mycotic and mycobacterial infections.

Most cases are diagnosed on clinical grounds (chronic cough productive of purulent sputum). Some patients with "dry bronchiectasis" caused by tuberculosis do not have productive cough but episodes of significant hemoptysis may develop. Many mildly symptomatic or asymptomatic patients with atelectatic segments of the right middle lobe and lingular segments of the left upper lobe have minor degrees of bronchiectasis. CXR shows increased markings in the bases, crowding of bronchi, segmental atelectasis, honeycombing with cystic spaces measuring <2.0 cm, loss of lung volume, and air-fluid levels (if cystic bronchiectasis is present). Chest HRCT findings include signet-ring shadows (dilated bronchus with bronchial artery forming the "stone"), bronchial wall thickening, dilated bronchi extending to the periphery, bronchial obstruction due to inspissated purulent secretions, loss of volume, and air-fluid levels if cystic or saccular changes are present. Bronchography is the most accurate diagnostic test and should be considered if surgical resection is planned.

- Nonpulmonary symptoms include fetor oris, anorexia, weight loss, arthralgia, clubbing, and hypertrophic pulmonary osteoarthropathy.
- HRCT of the chest has replaced bronchography (in most cases) in the diagnosis.
- Pulmonary function tests usually show obstructive phenomena.

Causes and Associations of Bronchiectasis

Infections
Most cases of bronchiectasis in adults are related to viral (adenovirus types 7 and 21) and/or bacterial infections (measles, influenza, or pertussis) in childhood. Tuberculosis is a common cause of bronchiectasis, particularly in the upper lobes.

- "Dry bronchiectasis" with episodes of significant hemoptysis without sputum is usually due to bronchiectasis in an area of old tuberculous damage.
- Bronchiectasis may result from chronic mycoses.

Ciliary Dyskinesia (Immotile Cilia) Syndrome
Cilia occur in the following locations (clinical problems associated with ciliary dysfunction are mentioned in parentheses): nasal mucosa (nasal polyps), paranasal sinuses (chronic sinusitis), eustachian tube (inner ear infection, deafness), tracheobronchial tree (chronic bronchitis, bronchiectasis), olfactory receptor cells (reduced olfactory function), vestibular sensory nerves (unknown), fallopian tubes (infertility?), ependymal lining of the spinal cord and brain ventricles (recurrent headache and depression), corneal inner surface (corneal deformities), vas deferens (infertility?), sperm tails (immotile sperm), and visceral primordial cells (situs inversus). Many

types of ciliary abnormalities (loss of radial spokes, eccentric tubules, absent tubules, adhesion of multiple cilia, etc.) are described. Even though the term "immotile cilia" is commonly used, the cilia do move, but their motion is abnormal and dyssynchronous.

- Many ciliary abnormalities have been described.
- Ciliary dyskinesia, rather than ciliary immotility, is the major abnormality.

The immotile cilia syndrome (Kartagener's syndrome) is an autosomal recessive disorder. Loss of the dynein arm—the fundamental defect—is an inherited abnormality involving a single protein. The prevalence of the disorder is 1 in 20,000 to 40,000 persons. Nearly 50% of patients have the triad of situs inversus, sinusitis, and bronchiectasis or at least bronchitis. Loss of the dynein arm results in sinusitis and otitis (less common in adults), nasal polyposis, bronchiectasis (in 75% of adults), situs inversus, and infertility in males. Infertility is not a universal phenomenon and, in fact, women with immotile cilia syndrome are often fertile. Kartagener's syndrome accounts for 0.5% of the cases of bronchiectasis and 15% of the cases of dextrocardia.

- Ciliary dyskinesia (Kartagener's syndrome) is an autosomal recessive disorder.
- Loss of the dynein arm is the fundamental defect.
- Situs inversus, sinusitis, and bronchiectasis are seen in 50% of cases.

Deficiency of radial spokes may result in sinusitis, nasal polyposis, otitis, mastoiditis, recurrent bronchitis, and infertility in both sexes. The diagnosis depends on the clinical features and documentation of ciliary abnormalities by electron microscopic examination of nasal mucosa, bronchial mucosa, or semen. At least 20 types of axonemal defects have been described. Ciliary defects are not always inherited; acquired forms of ciliary dyskinesia are seen in smokers and patients with bronchitis, viral infections, or other pulmonary diseases.

- Ciliary defects are not always inherited.
- Acquired ciliary defects occur in smokers, in patients with bronchitis, and after viral infections.

Hypogammaglobulinemia
Congenital (or Bruton's X-linked) agammaglobulinemia predisposes to recurrent bacterial infections and bronchiectasis. Bacteria isolated in these patients include *H. influenzae*, *S. aureus*, and *S. pneumoniae*. Acquired agammaglobulinemia (common variable) may be manifested as sinopulmonary infections in the second or third decade. Selective IgA deficiency is the most common immunoglobulin deficiency; most of these

patients are asymptomatic. IgA deficiency is frequently associated with IgG subclass (IgG2 and IgG4) deficiency. Despite the inability to form antibody, most patients have a normal number of circulating B cells, which fail to dedifferentiate into plasma cells that make immunoglobulins. Unusual bacteria (*M. catarrhalis*) may be isolated from some patients.

- The overall incidence of bronchiectasis in hypo/agamma-globulinemia is about 10%.
- Selective IgA deficiency is the most common immunoglobulin deficiency; most of these patients are asymptomatic or minimally symptomatic.
- IgA deficiency is frequently associated with IgG subclass (IgG2 and IgG4) deficiency.

Right Middle Lobe Syndrome

Right middle lobe syndrome is recurrent atelectasis of the right middle lobe in the absence of endobronchial obstruction. Isolated bronchiectasis is limited to segments of the right middle lobe. Mechanisms include compression of the middle lobe bronchus by lymph nodes, acute angulation of the origin, narrow opening of the bronchus, lengthy bronchus, and lack of collateral ventilation. CXR usually points to the diagnosis, although many patients remain asymptomatic.

- CXR shows chronic atelectasis and loss of volume in the right middle lobe (look for blurring or obliteration of the right cardiac border).
- Diagnosis is frequently made on incidental CXR finding.
- Most patients are asymptomatic.

Allergic Bronchopulmonary Aspergillosis

Allergic bronchopulmonary aspergillosis is discussed in more detail below with eosinophilic pulmonary diseases. It occurs most commonly in extrinsic asthmatics. Allergic bronchopulmonary aspergillosis develops in nearly 10% of patients with cystic fibrosis. Central bronchiectasis is present in 85% of patients with this disease at the time of initial diagnosis and has been used as a diagnostic criterion of the disease. Central bronchiectasis tends to affect the upper lung regions. Even though CXR may indicate this diagnosis, HRCT of the chest is diagnostic. However, it is not indicated in all patients.

- Central bronchiectasis involving upper lung regions.
- Bronchiectasis is reversible with treatment with high doses of systemic corticosteroids.

Yellow Nail Syndrome

The yellow nail syndrome consists of the triad of yellow to yellow-green discoloration of the nails with a thickened and curved appearance in all extremities, lymphedema of the lower extremities, and lymphocyte-predominant pleural effusion.

Bronchiectasis is seen in about 20% of patients. Some of the patients have sinusitis. Lymphedema may affect the breasts. Raynaud's phenomenon is noted in some patients. The cause is unknown, but lymphangiography has revealed lymphatic hypoplasia and atresia. Patients may present with chronic and insidious edema of the extremities. Pleural effusions occur in 35%-40% of patients, and recurrent pleural effusions are noted in about one-third. Pleural effusions may appear years after the nail changes occur and tend to be bilateral and small-to-moderate in amount. Exudates and transudates both are described.

- Triad of yellow discoloration of nails, lymphedema of lower extremities, and pleural effusion.

Obstructive Azoospermia (Young's Syndrome)

Obstructive azoospermia denotes primary infertility in males who have normal spermatozoa in the epididymis but none in the ejaculate. This is different from the ciliary dysmotility syndromes and cystic fibrosis. The following pulmonary abnormalities have been noted: grossly abnormal sinus roentgenograph (59% of patients), sinusitis (56%), repeated otitis media (32%), chronic bronchitis (35%), abnormal CXR findings (53%), and bronchiectasis (29%). The reason for the relationship between obstructive azoospermia and lung disease is unknown.

- Obstructive azoospermia and bronchiectasis.
- Pulmonary and ENT symptoms in 30% of patients.

Unilateral Hyperlucent Lung Syndrome (Swyer-James or Macleod Syndrome)

Normally, the diagnosis of this syndrome is by incidental CXR. Hyperlucency and hyperinflation of the lung (usually left) are found in conjunction with a small pulmonary artery. Bronchiectasis is seen in 25% of patients but most are asymptomatic. The cause is unknown, but congenital atresia of the pulmonary artery or acquired bronchiolitis soon after birth is postulated. Panacinar emphysema is found in the affected lung.

- Unilateral hyperlucent lung syndrome: unilateral hyperlucency of the lung with small ipsilateral pulmonary artery.
- Bronchiectasis in 25%; most patients are asymptomatic.

Miscellaneous Causes and Associations

Nearly 10% of bronchiectatic patients may demonstrate an abnormal α_1-antitrypsin phenotype with serum levels <66% of normal. Other entities include rheumatoid arthritis (Felty's syndrome), toxic chemicals, recurrent aspiration, heroin, inflammatory bowel disease, foreign body, sequestrated lung, relapsing polychondritis, chronic tracheoesophageal fistula, heart-lung transplantation, chronic granulomatous disease of childhood, and postobstructive (tumors, long-standing foreign body, stenosis, etc.).

- Uncommon causes of bronchiectasis include α_1-antitrypsin deficiency, Felty's syndrome, toxic inhalation, chronic tracheobronchial stenosis.

Complications of Bronchiectasis

Complications include hemoptysis (in 50% of patients), progressive respiratory failure with hypoxemia and cor pulmonale, and secondary infections by fungi and noninfectious mycobacterioses. The presence of these organisms usually represents a saprophytic state, but active infection has to be excluded. The most commonly isolated bacterium in bronchiectasis is *P. aeruginosa*. As in cystic fibrosis, it is impossible to eradicate this bacterium. Routine culture of respiratory secretions is not warranted in all patients.

- Source of bleeding in bronchiectasis is the bronchial (systemic) circulation and, hence, can be brisk.
- Presence of mycobacteria and fungi may represent saprophytic growth.

Treatment

Treatment of bronchiectasis is aimed at controlling the symptoms and preventing complications. Predisposing conditions should be sought and treated aggressively (gamma globulin injections, removal of foreign body or tumor, control of aspiration, and treatment of infections of paranasal sinuses, gums, and teeth). Postural drainage, chest physiotherapy, humidification, bronchodilators, and cyclic antibiotic therapy are effective in many patients. Surgical treatment is reserved for patients with troublesome symptoms, localized disease, and severe hemoptysis.

Bronchiolitis Obliterans With Organizing Pneumonia

Bronchiolitis obliterans with organizing pneumonia (BOOP) is a nonspecific diagnosis. It is a pathologic diagnosis. The main abnormality is the presence of intraluminal fibrosis in the distal airways, alveolar ducts, and perialveolar spaces. This condition is seen in patients with rheumatoid arthritis, systemic lupus erythematosus, polymyositis-dermatomyositis, mixed connective tissue disease, and silo filler's lung and after exposure to noxious gases, bleomycin, amiodarone, cytomegalovirus, influenza virus, bacteria (*Legionella, Nocardia*), *Mycoplasma, Cryptococcus,* and *Pneumocystis carinii*. BOOP also occurs after heart and bone marrow transplants and in chronic eosinophilic pneumonia and is observed as a secondary phenomenon in Wegener's granulomatosis, infarcts, granulomas, and neoplasms. CXR usually shows a patchy and diffuse ground-glass infiltrate or features similar to idiopathic pulmonary fibrosis and chronic eosinophilic pneumonia (peripheral alveolar infiltrate). Diagnosis of idiopathic BOOP is one of exclusion. Treatment consists of excluding offending agents and high doses of systemic corticosteroids.

- BOOP is a nonspecific pathologic diagnosis.
- BOOP has many causes.

Sleep Apnea

Apnea is defined as cessation of all airflow at the nose and mouth for at least 10 seconds. Sleep apnea syndrome is present if at least 30 episodes of apnea occur during a 7-hour sleep. Central sleep apnea is the cessation of airflow accompanied by an absence of respiratory effort. Obstructive sleep apnea is the cessation of airflow with continued respiratory effort. Mixed apnea is the cessation of airflow that typically begins with no respiratory effort but ends with increasing respiratory effort. Although most patients referred for evaluation of sleep apnea syndrome have a predominantly obstructive pattern, the mixed type is the most common form. In obstructive sleep apnea, the upper airway obstruction occurs either at the level of the soft palate or posterior to the base of the tongue. The occlusion is exaggerated by large neck circumference, increased size of the uvula, and pharyngeal mucosal edema (from long-term snoring).

- Central sleep apnea: cessation of airflow accompanied by an absence of respiratory effort.
- Obstructive sleep apnea: cessation of airflow with continued respiratory effort.
- Mixed sleep apnea: cessation of airflow that typically begins with no respiratory effort but ends with increasing respiratory effort.

Obstructive sleep apnea is present in 1%-2% of the population. Its clinical features include: sonorous snoring, abnormal motor behavior during sleep, daytime somnolence, personality changes, intellectual deterioration, systemic hypertension, loss of libido, abnormal behavioral outbursts, morning headaches, nightmares, hypnogogic hallucinations/automatic behavior, memory deficit, depression, nocturnal enuresis, and systemic hypertension. Male sex, older age, obesity, genetic factors, COPD, and use of sedative drugs or alcohol may contribute to or exacerbate obstructive sleep apnea syndrome. It is important to obtain a sleep history from the patient's spouse or relatives. Polysomnography (Fig. 21-30) establishes the diagnosis and is necessary to detect and quantitate obstructive sleep apnea. In obstructive apnea, there is apnea, but contraction by thoracoabdominal muscles is seen. In central apnea, in addition to apnea, there is no contraction by respiratory muscles. Severe oxygen desaturation develops during sleep (clinically significant desaturation is a decrease of $\geq 4\%$ from the baseline). Sinus arrhythmia is seen in 90% of patients. Other forms of cardiac rhythm problems include second-degree block, premature ventricular contractions (threefold increase when $SaO_2 <60\%$), and ventricular tachycardia. The incidence of cerebrovascular disease/accidents is increased in chronic obstructive sleep apnea.

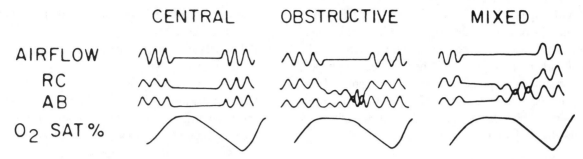

Fig. 21-30. Polysomnography in sleep apnea; airflow is absent in all forms of sleep apnea. Rib cage (RC) and abdominal (AB) movements are absent in central apnea but present in obstructive apnea. (From Strohl KP, Cherniack NS, Gothe B: Physiologic basis of therapy for sleep apnea. Am Rev Respir Dis 134:791-802, 1986. By permission of American Lung Association.)

- Clinical features: sonorous snoring, apneic episodes, and abnormal motor behavior during sleep.
- Important to obtain a sleep history from a sleep observer.
- Polysomnography is helpful in making the diagnosis and in identifying different types of sleep disorders.

Pulmonary hypertension is episodic in the early stages of significant sleep apnea but can be sustained later on. The site of airway obstruction in obstructive sleep apnea is the oropharynx; here, the tone of the genioglossus muscle and pharyngeal abductors (geniohyoid) decreases, and the resulting pharyngeal collapse produces obstruction. Before polysomnography is performed, patients should have an ENT examination, thyroid function testing, and PFTs, because similar symptoms are seen in patients with myxedema, ENT abnormalities, and COPD. Sleep apnea is also seen in "bird-like facies syndrome," cordotomy, poliomyelitis, Shy-Drager syndrome, sudden infant death syndrome, adenotonsillar hypertrophy, and severe altitude-related polycythemia. During rapid eye movement sleep in COPD, diminished tone of the intercostal muscles, decreased function reserve capacity, increased $\dot{V}/\dot{Q}$ mismatch, increased right-to-left intrapulmonary shunts, and prolonged desaturation have been demonstrated.

- Site of airway obstruction in obstructive sleep apnea is the oropharynx.
- Exclude hypothyroidism, ENT causes, narcolepsy, and severe COPD before performing polysomnography.
- COPD can produce disordered breathing, apnea, hypopnea, and periodic breathing.

Treatment of obstructive sleep apnea includes weight loss (in obese patients), nasal constant positive airway pressure, tracheostomy, and uvulopalatopharyngoplasty. The treatment of choice is nasal constant positive airway pressure. It produces a pneumatic splinting of the upper airway and increases its volume and cross-sectional area. Compliance rate with nasal constant positive airway pressure is 75%-90%. In patients with predominantly central sleep apnea, respiratory stimulants

such as medroxyprogesterone acetate have been tried. Other drugs used in both obstructive and central sleep apnea include methylphenidate (Ritalin), protriptyline, clonidine (α_2-adrenoreceptor antagonist), and fluoxetine (serotonin antagonist). In severe cases of obstructive apnea with congestive heart failure, polycythemia, bizarre behavior, and cardiac arrhythmias, treatment should include weight loss, treatment of the congestive heart failure, oxygen therapy, and consideration of tracheostomy (if nasal constant positive airway pressure is ineffective or cannot be used). The pickwickian syndrome constitutes only 5% of all sleep apnea cases. Patients are usually morbidly obese, hypersomnolent, cyanotic, plethoric, and polycythemic. In late stages, right ventricular failure is followed by left ventricular failure. Hypoxemia and hypercarbia are common. The efficiency of respiratory muscles is reduced to 60%-70% of normal.

- Nasal constant positive airway pressure is the treatment of choice for obstructive sleep apnea.
- Respiratory stimulants may relieve central sleep apnea.
- Pickwickian syndrome constitutes only 5% of all sleep apnea cases.

DIFFUSE LUNG DISEASE

Diffuse lung disease usually refers to an infiltrative process affecting most of the segments of both lungs. The term generally is not used to describe infectious or neoplastic diseases. "Diffuse lung disease" usually implies interstitial and/or alveolar filling defects. It is the result of injury to structures in the alveolar space, interstitial space, or both. The interstitial space is located between the alveolar lining cells and the capillary endothelium. The interstitium contains reticular and elastic fibers, alveolar interstitial cells (alveolar cells and histiocytes), small lymphocytes, arterioles, and a capillary network.

Pathology

Alveolar cell injury is often associated with altered permeability and resultant alveolar exudation, followed by invasion of the alveolar spaces by various cell types. This alveolitis produces an "alveolar" infiltrate on CXR. Infiltration of interstitial spaces by mononuclear cells, neutrophils, and other cells (interstitial inflammation) increases the thickness of the pulmonary interstitium. Capillary damage causes increased permeability and edema formation within interstitial spaces or alveolar spaces or both. In chronic cases, deposition of fibrous tissue in the interstitium (interstitial fibrosis) contributes to the interstitial infiltrate seen on CXR.

Physiology

Lung volumes are generally decreased in most diffuse lung diseases. TLC, VC, and RV decrease with disease progression. This is commonly referred to as a "restrictive defect." The loss of lung volumes is best correlated with interstitial fibrosis, although it can be marked in some alveolar diseases. Early in the disease, lung volumes may be normal. Airflow rates are usually normal until late in the course of the disease, when marked reduction in the volumes can be associated with mild-to-moderately reduced flow rates. The static compliance is decreased, but airway resistance is normal. The "stiff lung" increases the work of breathing, and patients typically exhibit rapid, shallow breathing to overcome this. Gas-exchange abnormality (exercise-induced hypoxemia and decreased DLCO) is the earliest change to occur in interstitial lung disease. Hypocarbia is common and caused by rapid, shallow breathing. Carbon dioxide retention is noted in late stages of the disease and is due to "respiratory exhaustion." Carbon dioxide retention is a poor prognostic sign.

● Decreased lung volumes (restrictive pattern).
● Flow rates are near normal.
● Lung compliance is decreased and elastic recoil is increased; lungs are stiff.
● DLCO is decreased early in the course.
● Exercise-induced hypoxemia.
● Hypocarbia in most patients (from hyperventilation); hypercarbia in late disease.

Roentgenology

Typical CT findings in diffuse lung diseases are described above. The main abnormalities seen on CXR can be classified into alveolar (air space) and interstitial patterns. Many diseases demonstrate both patterns. The alveolar pattern is limited to a smaller number of diseases, e.g., pulmonary edema (cardiogenic and noncardiogenic), alveolar sarcoidosis, uremic lung, intra-alveolar hemorrhage, aspiration pneumonia, pulmonary alveolar (phospholipo)proteinosis, certain bacterial pneumonias, desquamative pneumonia, certain viral and protozoal pneumonias, diffuse alveolar cell carcinoma, and diffuse pulmonary lymphoma.

● The alveolar pattern is seen in most entities that include the the word "alveolar."
● Pulmonary edema is the most common cause of alveolar pattern seen on CXR.

Because the interstitial pattern includes many diseases, it is convenient to group them into the following categories: idiopathic pulmonary fibrosis, systemic diseases (e.g., rheumatologic diseases), occupational lung diseases (including pneumoconioses and toxic exposures), drug-induced lung diseases (including radiation pneumonitis), granulomatous lung diseases (sarcoidosis, etc.), lymphangitic pulmonary metastasis, chronic mycotic and mycobacterial infections, unusual diseases (histiocytosis X, lymphangioleiomyomatosis, and tuberous sclerosis), and others (chronic bronchiectasis, cystic fibrosis, etc.).

● Grouping of interstitial pattern is helpful in considering the differential diagnosis in diffuse interstitial lung diseases.
● Lymphangitic lung metastasis is an important cause of interstitial lung disease.

The combination of alveolar-interstitial patterns and diffuse micronodular changes is also common. The anatomical distribution of the infiltrates is an important clinical consideration because certain diseases predominantly affect the upper lung zones. Other diseases may involve lower zones. These entities may produce an interstitial, alveolar, or a combination of alveolar-interstitial pattern on CXR.

● Bilateral upper lobe process: silicosis, coal workers' pneumoconiosis, sarcoidosis, mycoses, mycobacterioses, cystic fibrosis, pulmonary eosinophilic granuloma (histiocytosis X), and pulmonary lymphangioleiomyomatosis.
● Alveolar infiltrates are seen in: pulmonary edema, hematogenous metastases, acute respiratory distress syndrome, noxious gas exposure, alveolar hemorrhage syndromes, diffuse alveolar cell carcinoma, pulmonary alveolar phospholipoproteinosis, desquamative interstitial pneumonitis, early rheumatoid lung disease, amyloidosis, and alveolar microlithiasis.

Classification of Diffuse Pulmonary Diseases

Many of the diffuse pulmonary processes are classified on the basis of morphological features. Many of the diffuse pulmonary diseases have identical clinical and pathophysiologic features; yet, they are classified by different terms and abbreviations. The number of abbreviations used to describe these (see below) has resulted in significant confusion for practicing physicians; the abbreviations are listed in Table 21-7.

Table 21-7.--Abbreviations Used in the Literature to Describe Diffuse Pulmonary Diseases

BIP	Bronchiolitis-interstitial pneumonitis (a form of bronchiolitis obliterans with organizing pneumonia)
BOOP*	Bronchiolitis obliterans with organizing pneumonia
CIPF	Classic interstitial pneumonitis-fibrosis
DAD*	Diffuse alveolar damage (as in adult respiratory distress syndrome)
DIP	Desquamative interstitial pneumonitis (thought to predispose to idiopathic pulmonary fibrosis)
GIP	Giant cell interstitial pneumonitis (very rare)
HRS	Hamman-Rich syndrome
IAF	Idiopathic alveolar fibrosis (same as idiopathic pulmonary fibrosis)
IPF*	Idiopathic pulmonary fibrosis
LIP*	Lymphocytic interstitial pneumonitis (many causes)
PIP	Plasma cell interstitial pneumonitis (uncommon)
RAD	Regional alveolar damage
UIP	Usual interstitial pneumonitis (an earlier term for idiopathic pulmonary fibrosis)

*For clinical purposes (as well as for the ABIM examination), these entities are important because they constitute >90% of all of the above.

Idiopathic Pulmonary Fibrosis

Idiopathic pulmonary fibrosis is the most common cause of chronic diffuse interstitial lung disease. The diagnosis is based on clinical features, which include gradually progressive interstitial process (CXR typically shows a bibasilar interstitial process that eventually spreads upward), progressive dyspnea, clubbing (>70% of patients), Velcro crackles, positive rheumatoid factor (30%), antinuclear antibody (35%), or polyclonal gammopathy (>50%). HRCT shows subpleural honeycombing and an interstitial process in the basal areas. Pulmonary function tests show restrictive pulmonary dysfunction, low diffusing capacity, hypoxemia worsened by exercise, and hypocapnia. Other causes (see below) of an interstitial process should be excluded. Lung biopsy shows nonspecific interstitial fibrosis without granuloma formation. The response is poor to steroids (<20% of patients show measurable improvement) and immunosuppressive drugs. Hypoxemic patients benefit from supplemental oxygen. Gradual progression leads to cor pulmonale. The 5-year survival rate is <30%.

- Clubbing, Velcro crackles, and abnormal immunologic findings (rheumatoid factor, antinuclear antibody).
- Restrictive lung dysfunction.
- Hypoxemia, low diffusing capacity, and hypocapnia.
- Poor response to steroids and other agents.

Differential Diagnosis of Idiopathic Pulmonary Fibrosis

Many disease entities can produce nonspecific lung fibrosis, and at times, it is difficult to differentiate idiopathic pulmonary fibrosis from these diseases. Important ones to consider in this group are rheumatoid lung, scleroderma lung, late stages of sarcoidosis, certain drug-induced lung diseases (e.g., nitrofurantoin), radiation pneumonitis, end-stage hypersensitivity pneumonitis, certain pneumoconioses (asbestos), noxious gases, paraquat, recurrent pulmonary edema, end-stage histiocytosis X, end-stage cystic fibrosis and bronchiectasis, chronic aspiration pneumonia, and recurrent intra-alveolar hemorrhage (e.g., mitral stenosis, pulmonary hemosiderosis, and Goodpasture's syndrome).

- Rheumatoid lung and scleroderma lung can mimic idiopathic pulmonary fibrosis.
- Any end-stage diffuse lung disease can mimic idiopathic pulmonary fibrosis.

Sarcoidosis

Sarcoidosis is a multisystemic granulomatous disease of unknown cause. It affects persons in the 25-45 year age group. Sarcoidosis is characterized by widespread noncaseous epithelioid cell granulomas, depression of delayed type hypersensitivity and a decreased number of T lymphocytes, proliferation of B lymphocytes, and frequently positive Kveim skin test (rarely used).

- Sarcoidosis: multisystemic disease.
- Diminished number of T lymphocytes and increased number of B lymphocytes.
- Presence of noncaseous granuloma by itself is not diagnostic of sarcoidosis.
- Other granulomatous diseases with noncaseous granulomas: mycobacterioses (noncaseous in early stages), leprosy, mycoses, syphilis, mononucleosis, carcinoma, silicosis, hypersensitivity pneumonitis, zirconium, berylliosis, talcosis, Bakelite exposure, Crohn's ileitis, primary biliary cirrhosis, cat-scratch disease, foreign-body granulomas, hypogammaglobulinemia, and granulomatous arteritis.

Clinical Staging

Clinical staging of sarcoidosis is based on CXR findings rather than clinical severity, even though the CXR changes roughly parallel the clinical disease. Five types (formerly known as stages) of disease are seen. Type 0: normal CXR findings, with noncaseous granulomas in other sites (e.g., conjunctival, hepatic, lymphoid tissue, etc.). Type I: bilateral hilar and paratracheal lymphadenopathy (40%-50% of all patients, erythema nodosum in 3%-30%, iridocyclitis in 5%-8%). Type II: bilateral hilar and paratracheal lymphadenopathy with pulmonary parenchymal involvement (40%-50% of patients). Type III: diffuse pulmonary parenchymal disease without lymphadenopathy (14%-16% of patients). Type IV: end-stage pulmonary fibrosis with bullous changes (<5% of patients).

- Note that bilateral hilar lymphadenopathy is seen in sarcoidosis, Hodgkin's and non-Hodgkin's lymphoma, metastatic carcinoma, histoplasmosis, coccidioidomycosis, tuberculosis, berylliosis, etc.
- Most diseases that produce noncaseous granulomas also produce hilar lymphadenopathy.

Clinical Features of Sarcoidosis

Intrathoracic disease is present in 90% of patients, but almost all organs can be involved. Generalized lymphadenopathy occurs in 25% of patients, skin (lupus pernio, nodules) excluding erythema nodosum in 25%, eyes (lacrimal enlargement, corneal band opacities, iridocyclitis, glaucoma, and choroidoretinitis) in 25%, liver involvement in 25%, splenomegaly in 14%, endobronchial involvement in 11%, central nervous system involvement (paralysis of seventh cranial nerve, chronic meningitis, hypopituitarism) in 7%, bone cysts in 6%, and kidney involvement in 5%. Other manifestations include salivary gland involvement (uveoparotid fever or Heerfordt's syndrome) in 6%, nasal mucosal lesions, keloid in areas of surgical scars, diffuse arthralgias of small joints, heart (arrhythmias) in 5%, persistent violaceous skin plaques, transient vesicular eruptions on fingers, and persistent scars of old trauma on the knees. Initial complaints are lymphadenopathy (8%-70% of patients), cough (30%), dyspnea (28%), weight loss (20%-28%), fatigue (20%-27%), skin lesions (14%-25%), visual complaints (10%-21%), and fever (10%-15%). Asymptomatic disease is seen in 12%-34% of the patients.

- Almost any organ can be affected by sarcoidosis.
- Band keratopathy, lupus pernio.
- Cystic bone lesions in terminal phalanges.
- Cranial nerve VII involvement.

Laboratory Tests

Complete or partial anergy to skin tests (PPD and others) is seen in 60% of patients, positive Kveim test (not used anymore) in 95%, increased CD4/CD8 ratio, high serum level of antibodies to mycoplasma viruses (Epstein-Barr virus, rubella, parainfluenza, herpes simplex), autoantibodies to rheumatoid factor, antinuclear antibody, and T cells. Hypercalcemia results from increased sensitivity to vitamin D and increased gastrointestinal absorption of calcium (15% of patients). Other findings include hypercalciuria in 40%, increased IgG (50%), IgA (25%), IgM (12%), and alkaline phosphatase (15%). Serum levels of ACE are applicable only to adults (>20 years), because children and teenagers have high and widely variable

levels. Nearly 80% of patients with active sarcoidosis have increased serum levels of ACE, 70% with type I disease, 80% with type II, and 90% with type III. Serum levels of ACE are increased in 5% of normal subjects. Changes in levels may correspond to the activity of sarcoidosis. Some physicians use serum levels of ACE to monitor disease activity, but the clinical usefulness of this practice is limited because increased levels occur in many granulomatous diseases, including primary biliary cirrhosis, Gaucher's disease, leprosy, atypical mycobacteriosis, miliary tuberculosis, acute histoplasmosis, silicosis, and histiocytic lymphoma.

- Negative PPD in 60% of patients (because of suppressed T lymphocytes).
- Increased antibodies to viruses and hyperglobulinemia (because of increased B lymphocytes).
- Serum levels of ACE are increased in 70%-80% of patients with sarcoidosis.
- Increased ACE levels do not establish the diagnosis of sarcoidosis.
- ACE serum levels are also increased in mycobacterioses, mycoses, and Gaucher's disease.

Biopsy

Noncaseous granulomas can be identified in nearly 100% of biopsy specimens from mediastinal nodes, lung, nasal mucosal lesions, and subcutaneous nodules. Diagnostic rates of 80%-90% can be obtained from biopsy specimens of skin lesions, palpable scalene nodes, bronchial lesions, conjunctival lesions, and liver. Diagnostic accuracy decreases to <65% with biopsy specimens from bone marrow, scalene fat pad, and normal-appearing bronchial mucosa.

- Biopsy of involved organs provides a high diagnostic rate.
- Common areas for biopsy: mediastinal nodes, lung, and tracheobronchial mucosa.
- Noncaseous granuloma is not diagnostic of sarcoidosis.
- It is important to obtain cultures of biopsy specimens to exclude infectious causes of noncaseous granuloma.

Treatment

Systemic corticosteroids are indicated in progressive or symptomatic type II and type III disease, ocular sarcoidosis, persistent hypercalcemia or calciuria, progressive or disfiguring skin lesions, neurosarcoidosis, myocardial sarcoidosis, and progressive systemic disease. Phenylbutazone and antimalarial drugs have been tried in sarcoidosis refractory to treatment with steroids. Patients with sarcoidosis are sensitive to vitamin D (increased absorption of calcium from the small intestine).

- Systemic corticosteroids for progressive or symptomatic type II and type III disease.

● Avoid vitamin D and calcium supplements.

Lymphocytic Interstitial Pneumonitis

The diagnosis of lymphocytic interstitial pneumonitis is based on lung biopsy demonstration of diffuse interstitial infiltration by lymphocytes. Lymphocytic interstitial pneumonitis may result from Hodgkin's lymphoma, non-Hodgkin's lymphoma, early lymphomatoid granulomatosis, chronic lymphocytic leukemia, Waldenström's macroglobulinemia, angioimmunoblastic lymphadenopathy, Sézary syndrome, pseudolymphoma, acquired immune deficiency syndrome (AIDS), graft-versus-host disease, and congenital agammaglobulinemia. Idiopathic lymphocytic interstitial pneumonitis is a diagnosis of exclusion, although current understanding is that almost all cases of the disease represent low-grade B-cell lymphoma.

● Most lymphoproliferative diseases can produce lymphocytic interstitial pneumonitis.
● Lymphocytic interstitial pneumonitis is a pulmonary complication in AIDS and graft-versus-host disease.
● Most cases of lymphocytic interstitial pneumonitis represent low-grade B-cell lymphoma.

Eosinophilic Pulmonary Diseases

Eosinophilic pulmonary diseases, also known as pulmonary infiltrates with eosinophilia (PIE syndromes), are a heterogeneous group of disorders, except for the presence of CXR abnormality and blood eosinophilia. The presence of eosinophils in the peripheral blood may provide a clue to the diagnosis if clinical circumstances are suggestive of a PIE syndrome. Lung biopsy or bronchoalveolar lavage may be needed in some patients to document the diagnosis. Almost all entities under the classification of PIE syndrome require systemic corticosteroid therapy for prolonged periods. The following is a classification of PIE syndrome.

Asthma

Asthma is the most common cause of PIE syndrome. Eosinophilic bronchitis is characteristic of typical asthmatic episodes. The pulmonary infiltrate is usually caused by lung infection, and the eosinophilia results from exacerbation of asthma. The eosinophil count is usually 15%-20%. Peripheral blood and bronchoalveolar lavage eosinophil counts correlate with the degree of airflow obstruction. Appropriate therapy of infection and asthma produces full resolution. However, systemic corticosteroid therapy is indicated in many patients.

Simple Pulmonary Eosinophilia

Simple pulmonary eosinophilia, also known as Löffler's syndrome, is characterized by migratory peripheral (subpleural) pulmonary infiltrates (alveolar or interstitial or combined), peripheral eosinophilia, and minimal or no respiratory symptoms. In the original series, most patients had parasitic infections. Diagnosis of Löffler's syndrome requires exclusion of parasitic infection and drug reaction. The prognosis is excellent.

● One-third of patients have no cause.
● Should exclude parasitic infection or drug reaction.

Allergic Bronchopulmonary Aspergillosis

Allergic bronchopulmonary aspergillosis is often difficult to distinguish from the above, but the eosinophilia is more severe (30%) and longer lasting. The overall prevalence is 6%. More than 95% of patients with this disease have extrinsic asthma, and the disease develops in 10% of patients with extrinsic asthma. Allergic bronchopulmonary aspergillosis also occurs in about 10% of patients with cystic fibrosis. The disease is caused by both IgG- and IgE-mediated immune responses directed at *Aspergillus* species growing in the airways. Type I (bronchospasm), type III (pulmonary destructive changes), and type IV (parenchymal granuloma and mononuclear cell infiltrates) reactions are involved. Asthma previously under control that becomes refractory to treatment with nonsteroidal bronchodilators, expectoration of brownish mucus plugs, segmental atelectasis, and increasing eosinophilia and serum IgE are indicators of allergic bronchopulmonary aspergillosis. Major criteria: asthma, blood esosinophilia >1,000/mm^3, immediate skin reactivity (type I reaction—IgE dependent) to *Aspergillus* antigen, IgG antibodies (type III reaction) to *Aspergillus* antigens, high IgE (>1,000 ng/mL), transient or fixed pulmonary infiltrates, and central bronchiectasis (seen in 85% of patients). A normal IgE level in a symptomatic patient virtually excludes allergic bronchopulmonary aspergillosis. Minor criteria: presence of *Aspergillus* in sputum, expectoration of brownish mucus plugs, and late-phase (Arthus) skin test reactivity to *Aspergillus* antigen. CXR: fleeting infiltrates ("gloved finger" sign, "tramtrack line" lesions, and "toothpaste shadows") in 85% of patients, mucoid impaction in 15%-40%, atelectasis, and central bronchiectasis. Although generally associated with *Aspergillus fumigatus*, allergic bronchopulmonary mycosis can be caused by *Candida albicans*, *Aspergillus terreus*, *Curvularia lunata*, *Helminthosporium* species, and *Stemphyllium lanuginosum*.

● Allergic bronchopulmonary aspergillosis is seen almost always in patients with refractory extrinsic asthma.
● Allergic bronchopulmonary aspergillosis may develop in patients with cystic fibrosis.
● Types I, III, and IV immune reactions may be involved.
● Increased IgE level is the most useful laboratory test.
● Presence of *A. fumigatus* is only a minor criterion for the diagnosis.

- Systemic steroid therapy for >6 months is required in most patients. Therapy consists of long-term systemic corticosteroids.

Acute Eosinophilic Pneumonia

Acute eosinophilic pneumonia is relatively uncommon and is characterized by acute febrile illness of <5 days' duration; hypoxemic respiratory failure; diffuse alveolar or mixed alveolar-interstitial infiltrates; bronchoalveolar lavage eosinophilia (>25%); absence of parasitic, fungal, or other infection; and prompt and complete response to corticosteroids. Many patients require mechanical ventilatory support. Bilateral pleural effusions are common. The cause is unknown. Treatment consists of systemic corticosteroids.

- Adult respiratory distress syndrome, with fever, diffuse infiltrates, and eosinophilia.
- No recurrence after corticosteroid therapy.

Chronic Eosinophilic Pneumonia

Chronic eosinophilic pneumonia is a serious illness that requires long-term corticosteroid therapy. The female-to-male ratio is 2:1, and the median age is 50 years. The onset is insidious, and the duration of symptoms before the diagnosis is made is 7 months. More than 50% of patients have asthma of <5 years' duration. Symptoms include cough (90% of patients), fever (85%), dyspnea (60%), wheezing (35%), and weight loss (56%). Patients may present with severe respiratory distress, fever, and very high peripheral (>40%) and tissue eosinophilia. IgE levels are increased in 65% of patients. The ESR is high in most patients. CXR usually shows peripheral alveolar infiltrates ("negative image of pulmonary edema"). CT scan of the lungs shows ground-glass type of peripheral infiltrates. The pathologic features include tissue eosinophilia and bronchiolitis obliterans with organizing pneumonia. Biopsy is not required in most patients. Therapy consists of high doses of systemic corticosteroids for months to years. Recurrences are common if corticosteroid therapy is <6 months.

- Chronic illness of middle-aged patients (female:male = 2:1).
- May present as ARDS, with fever and high ESR.
- CXR: "negative" image of pulmonary edema.
- Recurs if corticosteroid therapy is <6 months.

Churg-Strauss Syndrome

Churg-Strauss syndrome is an uncommon vasculitis that is also known as "allergic angiitis-granulomatosis." Most patients have significant asthma. The eosinophil count is high (>50%). Diffuse feathery-type infiltrates are described on CXR. The prognosis is poor in those who respond poorly to high doses of systemic corticosteroids. This entity is discussed below with respiratory vasculitides.

Parasitic Infections

Almost all parasitic infections encountered in the tropics are known to cause eosinophilic lung disease. In the U.S., the most commonly encountered parasites are: *Strongyloides stercoralis*, *Ascaris* species, and *Toxocara canis*. In strongyloidosis, the clinical features include peripheral blood eosinophilia, skin rash, and transient lung infiltrates. Pulmonary infiltrates occur before ova can be detected in the stool. Chronic, recurrent strongyloidosis can last for several years. Ascariasis produces skin rash, nonproductive cough, chest pain, and, occasionally, hemoptysis. CXR: bilateral discrete densities several centimeters large in perihilar regions. Respiratory symptoms resolve over 8-10 days. *Toxocara* causes visceral larva migrans.

- In the U.S.: strongyloidosis, ascariasis, and *Toxocara* infection are common causes of PIE syndrome.
- Skin rash, eosinophilia, and patchy lung infiltrates.

Drug Reactions

Many drugs can induce pulmonary infiltrate with eosinophilia. The important ones include sulfasalazine, nitrofurantoin, aspirin, ampicillin, cromolyn, ibuprofen, iodinated contrast dye, methotrexate, minocycline, naproxen, para-aminosalicylic acid, penicillin, inhaled pentamidine, phenytoin, sulindac, tamoxifen, tetracycline, desipramine, clofibrate, chlorpromazine, bleomycin, and interleukin-2. Many other drugs have been reported to cause PIE syndrome.

- Drug-induced pulmonary infiltrate with eosinophilia is important to remember.

Neoplasms

Pulmonary neoplasms (adenocarcinoma, lymphoma, and other tumors) are associated with peripheral eosinophilia. The mechanism is unknown, although an eosinophilic chemotactic factor secreted by the tumors is thought to be responsible.

- Pulmonary neoplasms may be associated with peripheral eosinophilia.

Tropical Eosinophilia

The cause of tropical eosinophilia is unclear, although parasitic infestation from *Wuchereria bancrofti* and *Brugia malayi* most likely are responsible. Repeated laboratory examinations may be required to rule out parasitic infection as the cause of PIE syndrome. Symptoms include nocturnal cough, dyspnea, wheezing, fever, weight loss, and malaise. An asthmalike illness develops in many patients. Eosinophil count ranges from 20% to 50%. CXR may be normal or show diffuse reticulonodular infiltrates. Diethylcarbamazine citrate (Hetrazan) is the drug of choice.

- Very high eosinophilia.
- Diethylcarbamazine citrate is the drug of choice.

Hypereosinophilic Syndrome

Idiopathic hypereosinophilic syndrome (sometimes called "eosinophilic leukemia") is a rare and often fatal disease of unknown cause manifested by peripheral eosinophilia >1,500/μL for >6 months, absence of obvious reasons for eosinophilia, and signs of end-organ damage directly related to the eosinophilia. Most patients are in their third or fourth decade, and the male-to-female ratio is 7:1. Symptoms include cough, fever, weight loss, night sweats, anorexia, and pruritus. The leukocyte count is usually >10,000/μL, with eosinophil counts of 30% to 70%. The lung is involved in 40% of patients, and CXR shows interstitial nodular infiltrates, with 50% of patients demonstrating pleural effusions. Bronchoalveolar lavage may reveal >70% eosinophils. Pulmonary fibrosis may develop in chronic cases. Other serious complications include endocardial fibrosis, restrictive cardiomyopathy, mural thrombus formation, arterial thromboembolic disease, deep venous thrombosis, cerebrovascular lesions, and peripheral neuropathy.

- Very high eosinophilia in men in their third or fourth decade.
- Lung involvement in 40% of patients.
- Cardiac involvement is the most serious complication.

Bronchocentric Granulomatosis

Bronchocentric granulomatosis is not a well-defined syndrome. Surgical biopsy is required for diagnosis. Histologically, there is granulomatous and necrotizing replacement of the bronchial epithelium. It is a diagnosis of exclusion because similar pathologic features can be encountered in Wegener's granulomatosis, fungal and mycobacterial infections, aspiration, and rheumatoid lung disease. One-third of patients have tissue eosinophilia and tend to have asthma, peripheral eosinophilia, and positive sputum cultures for *Aspergillus* species. CXR may show nodular masses (60%) or pneumonic infiltrates (20%). Upper lobe and unilateral involvement is more common. Corticosteroids and cyclophosphamide have been tried.

- An ill-defined clinical entity; a diagnosis of exclusion.
- One-third of patients have asthma and eosinophilia.

Pulmonary Eosinophilic Granuloma (Histiocytosis X)

Pulmonary eosinophilic granuloma (also known as Langerhans cell granulomatosis) belongs to the reticuloendothelioses, a group of diseases of unknown cause in which an abnormal proliferation of histiocytes occurs. Histologic features consist of proliferation of histiocytes in sheet-like masses with numerous eosinophils interspersed. Pulmonary eosinophilic granuloma is uncommon and only about 1,500 cases have been reported. Most of the patients are smokers. It is more frequent in Caucasians and rare in blacks. Nearly 30% of the patients have nonspecific symptoms: fatigue, fever, and weight loss. Dyspnea is observed in 40% of patients and may result from a spontaneous pneumothorax or an osteolytic rib lesion. Physical findings are unhelpful in diagnosis. PFTs show a restrictive type of defect, with decreased lung volumes, normal flow rates, and decreased diffusing capacity. It is usual to see good pulmonary function even when CXR reveals extensive abnormalities. HRCT of chest shows characteristic cystic, nodular changes. As the disease progresses, fibrosis replaces the granulomatous process, with formation of characteristic honeycomb cysts. Typically, the involvement is diffuse, bilateral, and most pronounced in the upper two-thirds of the lung fields. Spontaneous resolution is seen in a significant number of patients. In progressive disease, corticosteroids and *Vinca* alkaloid derivatives have been used.

- More than 95% of the patients are smokers.
- It commonly is limited to the lungs or bones or both.
- Spontaneous pneumothorax is common (25%) and may be the presenting symptom.
- Young patient with spontaneous pneumothorax and honeycomb changes on CXR.
- Clinical course is usually benign, despite the persistence of severe abnormalities on CXR.

Pulmonary Alveolar Phospholipoproteinosis

Pulmonary alveolar phospholipoproteinosis, a rare disease of unknown cause, affects mostly young adults. The alveoli contain a granular eosinophilic material that is strongly PAS-positive. The alveolar material contains large amounts of dipalmytoil lecithin (surfactant). Similar pathologic features are found in patients with silica exposure, mycobacterial infections, fungal infections, leukemia, and pneumocystis infection. The pathogenesis is likely related to excessive production of surfactant and/or diminished clearance of surfactant by alveolar macrophages. It is more common in smokers. The male-to-female ratio is 3:1. An initial febrile episode is followed (after an interval of weeks to months) by progressive dyspnea with productive cough, low-grade fever, chest pain, and weight loss. CXR shows alveolar filling defect in the lower two-thirds of the lung field. Infections by *Nocardia* occur with a higher frequency. Restrictive pattern seen on PFTs in combination with decreased diffusing capacity is typical. Lung biopsy may be needed to make the diagnosis. CXR features resemble those of pulmonary edema, but the costophrenic angles are spared. Spontaneous resolution occurs in one-third of patients. Treatment of symptomatic patients consists of alveolar lavage to remove the intraalveolar material.

- Most patients are smokers.
- Alveolar infiltrates in the lower two-thirds of the lung fields.
- PAS-positive intra-alveolar material in biopsy specimens.
- Treatment: therapeutic alveolar lavage.

Pulmonary Alveolar Microlithiasis

Pulmonary alveolar microlithiasis is a rare, often familial (autosomal recessive) disorder of unknown cause. CXR is characterized by fine, sand-like mottling distributed uniformly through both lungs and extensive intra-alveolar deposition of calcium bodies. This disease is relatively asymptomatic, but cor pulmonale may be seen in some patients. Most patients are between 30 and 50 years old, with an equal male-to-female ratio. Siblings are commonly affected in familial cases. The lungs are solid and sink in water, and "onion-skin" bodies in the alveoli and fibrosis are seen on sectioning. Dyspnea is a major complaint in advanced cases, but most patients are asymptomatic. There is no known therapy.

- Fine, well-defined, sand-like infiltrates (due to calcispherites) on CXR.
- No known cause or treatment.

Lymphangiomyomatosis

Lymphangiomyomatosis is an uncommon progressive disorder of women of childbearing age. It is characterized by nodular and diffuse interstitial proliferation of the smooth muscle in the lungs, lymph nodes, and thoracic duct. Dyspnea, hemoptysis, and spontaneous pneumothorax are common. Two-thirds of the patients have chylous pleural effusion and chylous ascites may develop in many of them because of obstruction of the thoracic duct. CXR may show diffuse nodular-interstitial infiltrates with multiple small cystic areas. HRCT of chest is characteristic (cystic spaces). PFTs show obstructive features and decreased diffusing capacity. Rapidly progressive airway disease occurs in a significant number of patients. This condition is thought to be a forme fruste of tuberous sclerosis (see below). Treatment includes hormonal therapy, oophorectomy, and lung transplantation.

- Lymphangiomyomatosis: women of childbearing age with recurrent pneumothorax, chylous effusion, doughy abdomen, and hemoptysis.
- Obstructive pattern on PFTs, with low diffusing capacity, hypoxemia.
- Hyperinflated lungs with reticulonodular/nodular infiltrates.

Tuberous Sclerosis

Tuberous sclerosis, an inherited disease of mesodermal development, is characterized by epilepsy, mental retardation, congenital tumors, and malformations of the brain, skin, and viscera. Pulmonary involvement occurs in a small number

(≤8%) of patients, most of whom are women. Onset of the respiratory symptoms is between the ages of 18 and 34 years. Pulmonary pathologic features, CXR findings, and pulmonary function abnormalities are similar to those in lymphangioleiomyomatosis. Spontaneous pneumothorax is common. Pulmonary tuberous sclerosis is usually accompanied by involvement of other organs.

- Tuberous sclerosis is identical to lymphangioleiomyomatosis with regard to CXR, pulmonary dysfunction, and lung histology.
- Several diseases reveal diffuse interstitial/alveolar/nodular changes on CXR, but PFTs show an obstructive instead of a restrictive pattern. Examples: pulmonary lymphangioleiomyomatosis, histiocytosis X, tuberous sclerosis, cystic fibrosis, bronchiectasis, sarcoidosis with endobronchial involvement, and rheumatoid lung.

Neurofibromatosis of von Recklinghausen

Neurofibromatosis is a relatively common disease of dominant inheritance. It is manifested clinically by café-au-lait spots, freckling, and neurofibromas of the skin and internal organs. Pulmonary fibrosis is seen in ≤10% of the patients. The interstitial fibrosis is usually seen in the basal areas of the lungs, whereas the bullous lesions occur in the apical areas. Clinical manifestations are mild, usually consisting of only exertional dyspnea, but a restrictive pattern on PFTs and decreased diffusing capacity may be observed. Intrathoracic neurofibromas and meningoceles may occur. Pulmonary manifestations become evident in adulthood.

- Neurofibromatosis of von Recklinghausen: common disease of dominant inheritance.
- Pulmonary fibrosis, bullous lung disease, and intrathoracic meningiomas.

Hereditary Hemorrhagic Telangiectasia (Osler-Weber-Rendu Disease)

Hereditary hemorrhagic telangiectasia is an inherited disorder characterized by telangiectasia of the skin and mucous membranes and intermittent bleeding from vascular abnormalities. About 20% of the patients have pulmonary arteriovenous malformations/fistulas, which are located in the lower lobes and are multiple in one-third of the patients. On CXR, the arteriovenous malformations appear as oval or round homogeneous nodular lesions, from a few millimeters to several centimeters in diameter. Tomograms of the lesion usually disclose an artery entering the fistula and a vein leaving it. Pulmonary angiography confirms the diagnosis in virtually all patients. Symptoms depend on the degree of shunting. Paradoxical embolism is a potential complication. Central nervous system symptoms related to paradoxical embolic phenomenon are present in 30%

of patients. Most arteriovenous malformations are diagnosed in the third and fourth decades of life; the male-to-female ratio is 1:2. Dyspnea is present in nearly 60% of patients, but hemoptysis is the most common presenting symptom. Physical examination reveals cyanosis, clubbing of the nails, and a bruit or a continuous murmur over the site of the arteriovenous malformation. Catheterization studies: decreased PaO_2 and SaO_2 but normal pulmonary artery pressure. In almost all cases, therapeutic embolization or surgical resection of the malformation is recommended.

- Hereditary hemorrhagic telangiectasia: pulmonary arteriovenous malformation is seen in 20% of patients and is multiple in 35%.
- Symptoms depend on the degree of right-to-left shunt.
- Central nervous system complications due to paradoxical embolism occur in 30% of patients.
- Embolotherapy or surgical resection is indicated in most cases.

Marfan Syndrome

Marfan syndrome is a heritable, generalized disorder of connective tissue. Pulmonary abnormalities are seen in about 10% of the patients in the form of emphysema, bullous disease, generalized honeycombing, spontaneous pneumothorax (most common, seen in 5% of patients), and bronchiectasis. Spontaneous pneumothorax and bullae are causally related to Marfan syndrome. Upper lobe fibrosis is also described in this syndrome.

- Marfan syndrome: bullous lung disease.
- Spontaneous pneumothorax in 5% of patients.

OCCUPATIONAL LUNG DISEASES

Among the occupational lung diseases, the following are important: asbestos-induced lung diseases, silicosis, coal workers' pneumoconiosis, hypersensitivity pneumonitis, and gaseous inhalational diseases due to toluene diisocyanate and oxides of nitrogen.

Asbestos

Prolonged exposure to asbestos fibers may cause parietal pleural plaques, pleural thickening, pleural effusions, pulmonary fibrosis (asbestosis), malignant mesothelioma (both pleural and peritoneal), gastrointestinal cancer, and laryngeal carcinoma. The interval between exposure and increase in the number of deaths is 15-35 years for bronchogenic carcinoma, and 30-40 years for malignant mesothelioma. The annual death rate from malignant mesothelioma is 1,200 (smoking has no effect on death rate in this group) and 100 deaths from asbestosis (smokers have a 3x higher death rate).

- The majority of asbestos-related deaths are due to bronchogenic carcinoma.
- Prolonged exposure is necessary to develop asbestos-induced malignant mesothelioma.

Pleural Plaque (Hyalinosis Simplex)

The most common asbestos-related disorder is pleural plaque. It usually represents exposure that occurred more than 20 years earlier. It is neither harmful nor precancerous, but it tends to progress and to calcify over a long period (with 20-30 years' exposure, 10% of patients have calcification and with >40 years, 60% have calcification). The disease is bilateral and symmetrical, and in one-third of patients, it is associated with asbestosis (see below).

- Pleural plaque is the most common asbestos-related disorder.
- It is not precancerous.
- Calcified diaphragmatic pleura on CXR is almost always diagnostic of asbestos (other causes include ankylosing spondylitis and old tuberculous pleurisy).

Thickened Pleura (Hyalinosis Complicata)

Thickened pleura is an uncommon complication. Progressive calcification involves both visceral and parietal pleurae, lung apices, and pericardium. A recurrent acute inflammatory phase is associated with fever and exudative pleural effusion. Restrictive disease can lead to cor pulmonale.

Pleural Effusion

Pleural effusion is seen in association with asbestosis, hyalinosis complicata, and malignant mesothelioma. It is always an exudate, unilateral or bilateral, or recurrent, and in 70% of patients, it is bloody, with red blood cells exceeding 100,000/dL. Malignant mesothelioma has to be excluded.

- Bloody effusion; recurrent, unilateral or bilateral.
- It is difficult to differentiate from malignant mesothelioma.

Asbestosis

Asbestosis represents pulmonary fibrosis as well as fibrosis of visceral pleura; progressive fibrosis and honeycombing can lead to cor pulmonale. Progressive massive fibrosis is a complication. The pathogenesis is unknown, but many patients exhibit rheumatoid factor and antinuclear antibody in their sera. This is presumed to represent immune mechanisms. Early massive exposure produces severe disease. Asbestosis is clinically similar to idiopathic pulmonary fibrosis. Asbestosis affects the lower lung zones.

- Asbestosis: similar to idiopathic pulmonary fibrosis.
- Presence of antinuclear antibody and rheumatoid factor in the serum.

Bronchogenic Carcinoma

Nearly 2.5% of all lung carcinomas may be asbestos related. Carcinogenicity from asbestos exposure is not well understood, but tobacco smoking greatly compounds the risk. The lower lobes-to-upper lobes ratio is 2:1. Tumors are peripheral and frequently involve the pleura. Adenocarcinoma is more common than squamous cell carcinoma.

- Tobacco smoking + asbestos exposure = synergistic effect on carcinogenicity.
- Peripheral adenocarcinoma in the lower lobes.

Malignant Mesothelioma

Malignant mesothelioma is not always related to asbestos. All types of asbestos fibers have been implicated in the cause. There is no correlation with smoking. Initial exposure: more than 40 years before the tumor is diagnosed; incidence: 60 cases/million persons per year. It is more common in older patients. Insulation workers are at greatest risk. Common symptoms are chest pain and dyspnea. It presents as a painful exudative pleural effusion, followed by pleural nodules or masses.

- Malignant mesothelioma is not always related to asbestos exposure.
- It is not related to smoking.
- It is detected many years (>40 years) after exposure to asbestos.

Silicosis

Silicon dioxide exposure occurs in mines, quarries, sandblasting areas, road building, stone finishing, foundry, ceramics, etc. There is no increase in the risk of malignancy after silica exposure. Four clinical problems can be seen.

1. Acute silicosis is rare and has progressively fatal course (months to years). Ceramic workers, silica fluoro/soap workers, and tunneling operators are at risk. CXR shows ground glass or alveolar (upper lung fields) or fibrotic-appearing infiltrates. The pathologic features are sometimes akin to those of pulmonary proteinosis (silicoproteinosis).

2. Chronic simple silicosis: silicotic nodules of varying sizes (from millimeters to <1.5 cm) occur predominantly in the upper lung zones. The nodules may enlarge, coalesce, and produce mass-like changes (progressive massive fibrosis). The number and size of nodules increase with increased exposure. Eggshell calcification of hilar nodes is common. Findings on PFTs are normal or minimally abnormal.

3. Complicated silicosis, or progressive massive fibrosis: progressive massive fibrosis, less common than in coal workers' pneumoconiosis, is disabling and life-threat-

ening. It starts as simple silicosis and gradually produces bilateral symmetrical pulmonary masses (>1 cm) in the upper lung fields. Compensatory emphysema with both obstructive and restrictive lung functions produces hypoxemia, which in turn causes cor pulmonale. An autoimmune mechanism is postulated because of the high prevalence of abnormal immunologic laboratory data (antinuclear antibody, rheumatoid factor, etc.). Caplan's syndrome (rheumatoid lung nodules with silicosis) may be a more benign form of progressive massive fibrosis.

4. Silicotuberculosis: silica is toxic to pulmonary alveolar macrophages, which, therefore, are unable to ingest and kill mycobacteria. The risk of tuberculosis is 4x-6x higher in those with silicosis. CXR abnormalities are such that it is difficult to differentiate tuberculosis from silicosis-induced changes. The relapse rate of tuberculosis is high, and longer-than-usual antituberculous therapy may be needed. Mycobacteria involved include *M. tuberculosis*, *M. kansasii*, and *M. avium* complex. Patients with silicosis should be tested (PPD) annually. Patients with silicosis or an old fibrotic lesion on CXR who have a positive PPD should receive 4-month therapy with isoniazid and rifampin, although 12 months of isoniazid alone is an acceptable alternative.

- Silicosis does not increase the risk of developing lung cancer.
- Eggshell calcification of hilar lymph nodes is seen in silicosis and sarcoidosis.
- High prevalence of positive rheumatoid factor and antinuclear antibody in progressive massive fibrosis.
- In a patient with silicosis and fever with or without weight loss, consider silicotuberculosis.

Coal Workers' Pneumoconiosis

Because of the increased mechanization of coal extraction, coal workers' pneumoconiosis is becoming less common. A coal macule is usually <4 mm in size and consists of macrophages, fibroblasts, and reticulin and collagen fibers. Collections of these macules around small airways cause bronchiolar dilatation and focal spongy emphysema. CXR shows tiny nodular infiltrates in the upper lung zones; these may become profuse and lead to progressive massive fibrosis. Roentgenologically, nodules are classified into micronodules (<7 mm diameter) and macronodules (>7 mm diameter). Unless the patient smokes, the PFTs are normal. Nonspecific bronchitis may occur on inhalation of large amounts of coal dust. Melanoptysis, expectoration of black sputum, is sometimes seen in coal workers' pneumoconiosis. Slight decrease in FEV_1 may be related to centrilobular emphysema, but significant pulmonary dysfunction is uncommon in the absence of smoking.

- PFT abnormalities are usually caused by smoking.
- Coal workers' pneumoconiosis does not increase the risk of malignancy or tuberculosis.

Byssinosis

Byssinosis is an occupational lung disease caused by the inhalation of cotton, flax, or hemp dust. In cotton mills, cardboard rooms provide the greatest exposure. The mechanism of the lung injury is unknown; IgE is not involved. Affected persons complain of cough, paroxysmal wheezing, dyspnea, and chest tightness on the first day of work, with gradual resolution of symptoms as the work-week progresses. Decline in FEV$_1$ occurs on the first day, and lung functions improve during the week. Persistent exposure results in clinical disease indistinguishable from COPD. Treatment includes prevention of exposure and cessation of smoking.

- The mechanism of the lung injury is unknown; IgE is not involved.
- Symptoms are worse on the first day of exposure.

Berylliosis

Acute beryllium exposure (ceramic workers, beryllium processors, and certain aerospace workers) by inhalation may cause tracheobronchitis and chemical pneumonitis. Chronic berylliosis is the result of delayed-type hypersensitivity reaction that results in the formation of sarcoid-like granulomatous disease. Clinically, physiologically, and roentgenologically, chronic berylliosis resembles sarcoidosis. In suspected cases, the diagnosis can be established by performing beryllium lymphocyte transformation test. Symptomatic patients should receive treatment with corticosteroids.

- Clinically, chronic berylliosis resembles sarcoidosis.

Hypersensitivity Pneumonitis

Hypersensitivity pneumonitis, also known as extrinsic allergic alveolitis, is an immune-mediated lung disease. Many fungal precipitins and several avian proteins (pigeon-breeder's lung), animal proteins, chemicals (isocyanates), and metals (trimellitic anhydride and phthalic anhydride) are known to cause this condition. Acute (classic) and chronic forms of hypersensitivity pneumonitis are well described. Acute farmer's lung is the prototype of the acute form. Mycopolyspora faeni and *Thermoactinomyces vulgaris* are usually responsible. Symptoms appear 4-6 hours after exposure and include fever, chills, sweats, dry cough, and dyspnea. On examination, tachypnea and basal crackles without wheezing are the findings. Leukocytosis, hyperglobulinemia, and precipitating antibody can be demonstrated. Symptoms resolve rapidly (within 18-24 hours) and recur on reexposure. CXR may show increased bronchovascular markings and fine reticular and nodular defects. Biopsy (rarely indicated) may show bronchiolitis obliterans with organizing pneumonia.

- Symptoms in classic farmer's lung start 6-8 hours after exposure to causative precipitin; some patients show biphasic (immediate and late) reaction.
- Respiratory distress of varying intensity; wheezing is not a feature.
- Symptoms resolve within 18-24 hours and recur on reexposure.

Chronic farmer's lung results from repeated exposure to precipitins. Symptoms are insidious in onset, eventually resulting in progressive fibrosis. A decrease in lung volumes, compliance, and diffusing capacity and exercise-induced hypoxemia are typical in late stages. Clinically, this disease is identical to idiopathic pulmonary fibrosis. Lung biopsy usually reveals granulomatous reaction with round cell infiltrates, epithelioid cells, and septal swelling with lymphocytes and plasma cells. In pigeon-breeder's lung disease, the histologic features consist of foamy macrophages along with interstitial granulomas. Positive serologic findings are not diagnostic because 20% of asymptomatic farmers and 40% of asymptomatic pigeon breeders have positive precipitins, and 10% of symptomatic farmers have negative precipitins. The treatment for symptomatic patients is to avoid exposure to causative precipitins and use of corticosteroids.

- Obtaining a good history is important in establishing the diagnosis of chronic hypersensitivity pneumonitis.
- Most cases of hypersensitivity pneumonitis are due to fungal precipitins.
- Pigeon-breeder's lung disease is due to avian proteins.
- Typically restrictive lung dysfunction.

The points to remember about occupational lung diseases are summarized in Table 21-8.

DRUG-INDUCED LUNG DISEASE

Mechanisms of drug-induced lung disease include hypersensitivity, direct damage from toxic metabolites and oxygen radicals, alkylation of pulmonary tissue macromolecules, antigen-antibody reaction (type III), and type-I immune reactions. Table 21-9 lists different types of pulmonary problems caused by various drugs.

Drug-Induced Systemic Lupus Erythematosus

Older Caucasians are more prone to drug-induced systemic lupus erythematosus. Clinical features include arthralgias and arthritis (90% of patients) and fever and malaise (40%). Abnormal test results for antinuclear antibody (100% of

Table 21-8.--Pulmonary Diseases: Causes and Associations

Pulmonary disease	Causes and associations
Progressive massive fibrosis	Silicosis, coal, hematite, kaolin, graphite, asbestosis
Autoimmune mechanism	Silicosis, asbestosis, berylliosis
Monday morning sickness	Byssinosis, bagassosis, metal fume fever
Metals and fumes producing asthma	Bakers' asthma, meat wrappers' asthma, printers' asthma, nickel, platinum, toluene diisocyanate, cigarette cutters' asthma
Increased incidence of tuberculosis	Silicosis, hematite lung
Increased incidence of carcinoma	Asbestos, hematite, arsenic, nickel, uranium, chromate
Welder's lung	Siderosis, pulmonary edema, bronchitis, emphysema
Centrilobar emphysema	Coal, hematite
Generalized emphysema	Cadmium
Silo filler's lung	Nitrogen dioxide
Farmer's lung	*Thermoactinomyces, Micropolyspora*
Asbestos exposure	Mesothelioma, bronchogenic cancer, gastrointestinal tract cancer
Eggshell calcification	Silicosis, sarcoid
Sarcoid-like disease	Berylliosis
Diaphragmatic calcification	Asbestosis (also ankylosing spondylitis)
Nonfibrogenic pneumoconioses	Tin, emery, antimony, titanium, barium
Minimal abnormality in lungs	Siderosis, baritosis, stannosis
Bullous emphysema	Bauxite lung
Occupational asthma	Toluene diisocyanate, laboratory animals, grain dust, biologic enzymes, gum acacia, tragacanth, silkworm, anhydrides, wood dust, platinum, nickel, formaldehyde, Freon, drugs

patients), lupus erythematosus cell clot (75%), rheumatoid factor (33%), and low complement level (70%). It is caused by cardiac drugs (procainamide, quinidine, and practolol), antibiotics (nitrofurantoin, penicillin, griseofulvin, sulpha, and tetracycline), anticonvulsant agents (phenytoin, mephenytoin, and carbamazepine), antihypertensive drugs (hydralazine, methyldopa, and L-dopa), antituberculous drugs (isoniazid, streptomycin, and para-aminosalicylic acid), phenothiazines (chlorpromazine and promethazine), and miscellaneous agents (D-penicillamine, methysergide, oral contraceptives, phenylbutazone, propylthiouracil, tolazamide, etc.).

- More common in older Caucasians.
- Drug-induced systemic lupus erythematosus: pleural effusion in 50% of patients and pulmonary infiltrates in 30%.
- Procainamide, nitrofurantoin, phenytoin, hydralazine, isoniazid.

Narcotic Abuse

Heroin, morphine, methadone, and propoxyphene cause pulmonary edema, adult respiratory distress syndrome, pneumonia (in 30% of heroin addicts), bronchiectasis, and talc granulomas. Pulmonary edema is the most common complication of heroin and morphine overdose; it is usually seen within hours and resolves within 24-48 hours. Capillary endothelial damage is the most likely cause of narcotic-associated pulmonary edema. Pneumonia may be secondary to aspiration of gastric contents and septic emboli from endocarditis. Methadone produces similar pulmonary problems. Talc granuloma is the result of intravenous use of crushed analgesic tablets, talc contamination, and cotton fibers used as filters. Cornstarch (used as an adulterant) also causes granulomas.

- Noncardiogenic pulmonary edema is due to capillary damage.
- Narcotic abuse: adult respiratory distress syndrome, pneumonia, endocarditis, and talc granulomas.

Nitrofurantoin

Nitrofurantoin is the drug most commonly reported to produce pulmonary abnormalities. The acute reaction (from 3 hours to 3 months) includes dyspnea (90% of patients), cough (66%), fever (70%), crackles (65%), wheezes (40%), eosinophilia (30%), patchy process (30%), and effusions (10%-20%). Chronic cases (6 months to 7 years) are uncommon but show similar features, although a diffuse process is more common. Average dose, 150 mg/day. Pulmonary functions in acute reactions may reveal obstructive phenomena, whereas

Table 21-9.--Drug-Induced Pulmonary Diseases

Interstitial pneumonitis/fibrosis
    Chemotherapeutic agents
    Nitrofurantoin (chronic)
    Drug-induced systemic lupus erythematosus
    Gold
    Talc (intravenous use)
    Aspirated oil
    D-Penicillamine
    Pituitary snuff
    Radiation
    Oxygen
    Sulfasalazine (Azulfidine)
    Cromolyn sodium
    Methysergide
    Hexamethonium, pentolinium, mecamylamine

Noncardiac pulmonary edema
    Heroin, methadone, morphine
    Acetylsalicylic acid
    Nitrofurantoin (acute)
    Chlordiazepoxide (Librium)
    Ethchlorvynol (Placidyl)

Pleural effusion
    Nitrofurantoin (acute)
    Methysergide (chronic)
    Drug-induced systemic lupus erythematosus
    Chemotherapeutic drugs
    Radiation
    Dantrolene

Drug-induced pulmonary infiltrate with eosinophilia
    Sulfonamides
    Sulfasalazine (Azulfidine)
    Penicillin
    Isoniazid
    Aminosalicylate

    Nitrofurantoin (acute)
    Leukoagglutinin
    Methotrexate
    Procarbazine
    Carbamazepine (Tegretol)
    Imipramine (Tofranil)
    Salicylates
    Cromolyn sodium
    Methylphenidate (Ritalin)
    Dantrolene

Drug-induced hilar and mediastinal widening
    Corticosteroids
    Methotrexate
    Phenytoin (Dilantin)

Bronchospasm
    Propranolol, other β-blockers
    Acetylsalicylic acid
    Indomethacin
    Fenoprofen
    Mefenamate
    Isuprel
    Drugs that produce pulmonary infiltrate with eosinophilia
    Nebulized medications

Pulmonary hypertension
    Oral contraceptives
    Aminorex
    15-Methyl-prostaglandin-F_2

Pulmonary granulomas
    Talc
    Mineral oil
    Methotrexate
    Cromolyn sodium
    Cotton fibers (intravenous drug use)

chronic cases usually show a restrictive type of pulmonary dysfunction. Most patients recover after the drug is withdrawn.

- Acute reaction within 3 hours to 3 months; average dose 150 mg/day.
- Cough, wheeze, pleural effusion, and eosinophilia.

Chemotherapeutic Agents

    The mechanism of pulmonary reaction to chemotherapeutic agents is not clear. Many chemotherapeutic drugs produce cytotoxic changes characterized by "bizarre-appearing" type II pneumocytes. Nonspecific changes are common. Symptoms include cough, dyspnea, and fever. Fever is present in most patients and may precede the onset of dyspnea or CXR abnormalities. PFTs reveal a restrictive pattern. Arterial oxygen desaturation is common. Busulfan (Myleran) causes "busulfan lung" in about 8% of patients. Findings on PFTs may be abnormal without clinical or CXR evidence of disease.

Pulmonary reaction is usually seen after 6 months of therapy. CXR shows diffuse interstitial and alveolar infiltrates. Death may occur despite stopping the use of the drug and using steroids. Cyclophosphamide (Cytoxan) produces (but less commonly) similar reactions. However, changes are seen earlier than with busulfan. Bleomycin has a 10% incidence of pulmonary toxicity, which increases with increasing age (>70 years) and increasing dosage (>450 units). Simultaneous use of a high concentration of the inhaled oxygen increases the risk of pulmonary toxicity. Acute hypersensitivity reaction with eosinophilia has been reported in some patients. Chlorambucil (uncommonly) produces complications similar to those caused by busulfan, cyclophosphamide, and bleomycin. Carmustine produces pulmonary reactions in 1% of patients within 8 months, similar to those seen with other chemotherapeutic agents. A higher incidence of pneumothorax has been noted. Methotrexate is the only antimetabolite known to produce pulmonary disease that is self-limiting and is frequently associated with peripheral eosinophilia. Most pulmonary reactions reported have been in children treated for acute lymphatic leukemia; symptoms begin within a few days to several weeks after the initiation of therapy. CXR shows diffuse fine interstitial infiltrates, hilar adenopathy, or pleural effusion in 10% of patients.

- Cough, dyspnea, fever, and patchy lung infiltrates.
- Bizarre type II pneumocytes in most cases except in those treated with methotrexate.
- "Busulfan lung" occurs in 8%-10% of patients, usually after 6 months of therapy.
- Bleomycin lung toxicity occurs in 10% of patients; dose- (>450 units), age- (>70 yr) related, and if high FIO_2 is used.
- Methotrexate produces eosinophilia, hilar adenopathy, and pleural effusion.

Radiation

Type II pneumocytes and pulmonary capillary endothelial cells are initially affected by radiation. Radiation effects may be cumulative; the rate at which it is given is most important. A second or third course of radiation to the lung is more likely to result in a pneumonitis that can occur earlier and be devastating. During the acute phase, type II pneumocyte changes and an inflammatory process can be seen. In the chronic stage, nonspecific fibrosis is common. Symptoms of radiation pneumonitis begin insidiously 1-3 months after completion of radiation. Cough, fever, and dyspnea may precede the onset of CXR changes. The late phase begins after 6 months of radiation therapy. Dyspnea is usually out of proportion to the CXR changes. Steroid therapy has produced varying responses.

- Capillary endothelial damage has a major role in radiation-induced lung disease.
- Radiation pneumonitis is not dependent on the dose, rate,

or the volume of lung radiated.

- The concomitant use of bleomycin and cyclophosphamide and the withdrawal of steroid therapy increase the risk of radiation pneumonitis.
- The acute phase occurs about 1-3 months after radiation, and the chronic phase is seen after 6 months.
- The earlier the onset, the worse the prognosis.

Corticosteroids

Patients receiving high doses (>1 mg/kg per day) of corticosteroids are more likely to have opportunistic infections from *Nocardia asteroides*, cytomegalovirus, *Mycobacterium tuberculosis, Aspergillus fumigatus, Candida albicans*, and *Cryptococcus neoformans*. Mediastinal lipomatosis in the mid and anterior mediastinum results from excessive deposition of fat in these areas. CT of the mediastinum is diagnostic. Rapid withdrawal of steroid therapy may enhance the onset of radiation pneumonitis.

- Mediastinal lipomatosis is diagnosed with CT.

Analgesic Agents

Salicylates produce bronchospasm in aspirin-sensitive patients, pulmonary infiltrates with eosinophilia, and noncardiogenic and pulmonary edema (when blood level is >50 mg/dL). Pulmonary edema occurs within 1-2 hours after ingestion; CXR changes may persist for a week or longer. Gold sodium thiomalate and aurothioglucose produce pulmonary toxicity in 3%-5% of patients. CXR shows a diffuse interstitial process. Symptoms include cough, fever, and dyspnea. The histologic features are lymphocytic and plasma cell infiltrates. Pulmonary reactions to the use of other analgesics include bronchospasm (naproxen, indomethacin, ibuprofen, and mefenamate) and pulmonary edema (phenylbutazone and oxyphenbutazone).

- Bronchospasm occurs with acetylsalicylic acid but not with all salicylates.
- Respiratory alkalosis is followed by metabolic acidosis in salicylate overdose.
- With gold therapy, the lung reaction can be acute or insidious and is usually dose-related, with most patients having received >300 mg.

Oxygen

Oxygen toxicity can be avoided if the FIO_2 is kept below 0.5. If the duration of FIO_2 of 1.0 exceeds 24 hours or if FIO_2 of 0.6 exceeds 72 hours, the risk of pulmonary damage increases. Oxygen-induced adult respiratory distress syndrome is not amenable to any treatment, and the patients usually succumb to lung failure. Histologic features include an early exudative phase followed by an irreversible proliferative and fibrotic phase.

Oil Aspiration

With the aspiration of oil, abnormalities range from solitary nodules to various types of infiltrates, especially in the dependent lower lung fields. Mineral oil for softening stools, oily nose drops, ophthalmic drops, and other oily preparations are used frequently. Bronchographic medium has the potential to induce bronchospasm and transient changes in pulmonary functions.

● Aspiration of oil: a common but frequently overlooked cause of pulmonary infiltrates.
● It is important to obtain the history of the use of these agents.

Inhaled Medications

Inhaled medications cause bronchospasm, irritation of the upper airways, and cough in some patients. Cromolyn sodium, used in asthmatics, can produce bronchospasm, pulmonary infiltrates with eosinophilia, and nonspecific upper airway irritation.

● Cromolyn can produce bronchospasm, eosinophilia, and lung infiltrates.
● Ultrafine nebulized aerosols can cause cough and bronchospasm.

Blood Products

Leukoagglutinins in the blood may produce acute pulmonary edema. The exact mechanism is unknown, but a hypersensitivity reaction has been postulated. There is acute onset of fever, chills, cough, and dyspnea. Pulmonary infiltrates may persist for several days. Eosinophilia is seen in some patients. CXR shows a varying picture of pulmonary edema. HIV transmission from transfusion of blood or blood products.

● Blood products: pulmonary edema, eosinophilia, lung infiltrates, and HIV transmission.

Miscellaneous

β-Blockers (propranolol, metoprolol, nadolol, and timolol) may aggravate asthma; amiodarone causes interstitial pneumonitis in 1%-4% of patients. The lung pathologic reaction is dose-related and is seen usually with a dose >400 mg/day. Dyspnea and cough are noted 2-3 months after starting therapy with the drug. ACE inhibitors cause cough in 6%. D-Penicillamine provokes four types of pulmonary reaction: bronchiolitis obliterans, a Goodpasture's syndrome-like illness, diffuse alveolitis, and drug-induced systemic lupus erythematosus. Paraquat is a potent weed killer, and most cases of illness induced by it are due to accidental ingestion. Bronchiolitis, adult respiratory distress syndrome, and severe pulmonary fibrosis are common. Lung changes can be acute.

L-Tryptophan-induced eosinophilia-myalgia syndrome is related to a contaminant in the manufacturing process. The result is myalgia, eosinophilia, pulmonary infiltrates, pleural effusion, and pulmonary hypertension. Iodized contrast media produce pulmonary infiltrates, restrictive dysfunction, and low diffusing capacity. A "stippling" type of CXR changes is seen with lymphangiographic examinations. Methysergide (Sansert) may cause insidious onset of pleuropulmonary fibrosis; pleural effusion is seen in nearly 50% of patients with pleuropulmonary fibrosis.

● β-Blockers aggravate asthma and COPD.
● Amiodarone causes diffuse lung infiltrates; dose usually >400 mg/day.
● ACE inhibitors cause cough in 4%-6% of patients.
● Penicillamine can cause bronchiolitis and drug-induced systemic lupus erythematosus.

EFFECTS OF ALTITUDE, DIVING, AND DROWNING

Effects of High Altitude

Acute Mountain Sickness

Physiologic changes at high altitude are the result of reduced barometric pressure. PIO_2 decreases by 4-5 mm Hg for each 1,000 feet in elevation. The ventilatory response varies with time. Acute high altitude-induced hypoxia increases minute ventilation and reduces $PaCO_2$. This reaction is mediated by peripheral chemoreceptors. It can be reversed rapidly by oxygen inhalation. After 5-10 days, there is a further increase in ventilation and a greater decrease in $PaCO_2$, which an ambient PO_2 fails to correct. Acute ascent to high altitude increases hemoglobin concentration due to diuresis; a transient increase in the serum level of erythropoietin occurs. Acute mountain sickness affects 25%-50% of lowlanders 6-90 hours after ascent to >7,000 ft, producing lethargy, insomnia, headache, nausea, vomiting, and dyspnea. It is exacerbated by alcohol, sedatives, or overexertion soon after ascent. Cyanosis and signs of cerebral edema can occur. Prophylactic diuretic (acetazolamide is the drug of choice) therapy (before ascent) prevents acute mountain sickness. Dexamethasone is recommended by some physicians.

● Acute mountain sickness affects lowlanders 6-90 hours after ascent.
● Lethargy, insomnia, headache, nausea, vomiting, and dyspnea.
● Preventive diuretic therapy before ascent is recommended.
● Cerebral edema occurs in severe form of acute mountain sickness.

High-Altitude Pulmonary Edema

High-altitude pulmonary edema is noncardiogenic in origin and occurs after rapid ascent to >14,000 ft. It is thought to be the result of hypoxic pulmonary vasoconstriction. The incidence among mountaineers is 0.5%-10%, but susceptible individuals have a 60% incidence on reexposure to high altitude. Cold weather and exertion contribute to this condition. A time lag from 24 to 36 hours is common. Typically, symptoms appear after 36 hours and consist of dyspnea, cough, fatigue, altered mental status, and somnolence. Clinically, high-altitude pulmonary edema is similar to acute pulmonary edema from other causes, but left ventricular failure is not a feature. CXR shows patchy infiltrates. These disappear 6-48 hours after return to sea level or after therapy with high doses of oxygen.

- High-altitude pulmonary edema is a type of noncardiogenic pulmonary edema.
- Individual susceptibility increases the risk of the condition on reexposure to high altitude.

Chronic Mountain Sickness

Highlanders adapt to physiologic changes and ventilate less than acclimatized lowlanders and maintain a higher $Paco_2$ and a lower Pao_2. The respiratory drive is lost and primary alveolar hypoventilation develops. Chronic mountain sickness (Monge's disease) is the result of progressive loss of acclimatization to high altitude. Susceptible highlanders develop chronic malaise, headache, dizziness, easy fatigability, paresthesias, somnolence, and diminished mental activity. Marked cyanosis, clubbing of the fingers, polycythemia, oxygen desaturation, and cardiac enlargement occur, but the lung fields appear normal on CXR. Pulmonary arterial pressure is twice as high as that of a healthy dweller at altitude.

- Chronic mountain sickness is the result of progressive loss of acclimatization to high altitude.
- The most serious complication of chronic mountain sickness is the irreversible pulmonary hypertension.

Air Travel

Because most commercial aircraft (pressurized) cruise at high altitudes (10,000-55,000 ft), the reduced Fio_2 within the aircraft is similar to that at an altitude of 6,000 ft to 8,500 ft. As a result, patients with underlying hypoxemic pulmonary diseases may have exacerbation of their symptoms. Long flights, reduced humidity, undue exertion on board, and smoking (by other passengers) in the cabin add to the problems. If Pao_2 is <50 mm Hg (Sao_2 <85%) at rest, supplemental oxygen should be prescribed.

- Supplemental O_2 is recommended if Pao_2 is <50 mm Hg (Sao_2 <85%) at rest.

Drowning and Barotrauma

Drowning

Drowning is the fourth leading cause of accidental deaths in the U.S. Most drowning accidents occur in children (<5 years), young adults (15-29 years old), males, blacks, and in southern states. Two-thirds of drownings occur in fresh water. The greatest risk factor for drowning in adults and teenagers is alcohol consumption (in 45% of adult victims). Although hypothermia by itself is rarely the actual cause of death, it can have a significant effect on the prognosis of near-drowning victims. Aspiration occurs in about 85% of drowning or near-drowning victims; the other 15% have laryngospasm and, thus, do not have signs of aspiration. The duration of hypoxemia caused by drowning is more important in predicting mortality rather than fresh water versus salt water drowning or the electrolyte imbalance. Pulmonary complications such as adult respiratory distress syndrome and aspiration pneumonia are more common in those who aspirate. Other physiologic abnormalities include metabolic and respiratory acidosis, secondary arrhythmias, cerebral edema, shock-induced acute tubular necrosis, and hypothermia.

- Alcohol consumption is a major risk factor for drowning in adults.
- Pulmonary complications are more common in those who aspirate.

Barotrauma

Barotrauma is more common in divers and is caused by the contraction or expansion of gas that occurs because of changes in barometric pressure after a descent or ascent. Barotrauma sustained during ascent can be life-threatening. Arterial gas embolism is an important cause of death among scuba divers. Within minutes after surfacing, an afflicted diver will have neurologic symptoms ranging from focal motor, sensory, or visual deficits to unconsciousness and death. Characteristic marbling over the upper torso and focal pallor of the tongue may be seen. Pulmonary complications that result from overdistention include pneumothorax (in 10% of barotrauma victims), pneumomediastinum, mild hemoptysis, chest pain, and interstitial emphysema.

- Arterial gas embolism is an important cause of death among scuba divers.
- Interstitial emphysema is more common than pneumothorax in deep sea divers.

PULMONARY NEOPLASMS

Solitary Pulmonary Nodule

A solitary pulmonary nodule is defined as a solitary lesion seen on plain CXR. It is <4 cm and is round, ovoid, or slightly lobulated. The lesion is located in lung parenchyma, is at least moderately circumscribed, and uncalcified on plain CXR. It is not associated with satellite lesions or other abnormalities on plain CXR. Common causes include carcinoma of the lung (15%-50% of patients), mycoses (5%-50%), tuberculosis, unidentified granulomas, resolving pneumonia, hamartoma, and metastatic lesions. Uncommon causes include carcinoid, bronchogenic cyst, resolving infarction, rheumatoid and vasculitic nodules, and arteriovenous malformation.

- Solitary pulmonary nodule: pleural, skin, and other extrapulmonary lesions should be excluded.
- Granulomas and hamartomas make up 40%-60% of all solitary pulmonary nodules and 90% of nonmalignant solitary pulmonary nodules.
- Hamartomas alone comprise <10% of nonmalignant nodules.

History

The following aspects are important in the evaluation of solitary pulmonary nodules: age of patient, availability of previous CXR, smoking history, previous malignancy, exposure to tuberculous patients, travel to areas endemic for mycoses, recent respiratory infection, recent pulmonary infarction, recent trauma to chest, asthma, mucoid impaction, systemic diseases (congestive heart failure, rheumatoid arthritis, etc.), ENT symptoms (Wegener's vasculitis), mineral oil, oily nose drops, immune defense mechanisms, and family history (arteriovenous malformation).

- History: old CXR, age, smoking history, previous malignancy, and exposure history are important.

Diagnosis

Physical examination, routine complete blood cell count, chemistry group, and the exclusion of obvious causes (congestive heart failure, vasculitis, rheumatoid arthritis, etc.) are important for making the diagnosis. Obtain earlier CXR for comparison. Generally, sputum cytology, skin tests, serologic studies, and cultures on a routine basis are unrewarding in asymptomatic patients. Localized tomograms identify the location of a solitary pulmonary nodule, calcification, cavitation, satellite lesions, and margins. Chest CT is helpful in assessing calcification, density, multiple nodules (particularly in evaluating metastatic malignancy), and staging of lung cancer.

- In asymptomatic patients with a single pulmonary nodule, extensive studies (gastrointestinal tract series, intravenous pyelography, scans of bone, brain, liver, bone marrow, etc.) are not indicated because of the low diagnostic yield (<3%).
- CT detects 30% more nodules than CXR, but the role of CT in differentiating benign from malignant lesions is not established.
- Bronchoscopic brush and biopsy has about a 60% diagnostic yield in cancer.
- Transthoracic needle aspiration (CT- or fluoroscopy-guided) has an 85% diagnostic yield in cancer and a 20% risk of pneumothorax.

Decision Making

General guidelines for decision making are given in Table 21-10. If a benign cause cannot be firmly established after complete clinical, imaging, culture, and biopsy evaluations, the following two decisions advocate surgical resection: 1) the solitary pulmonary nodule is probably malignant, because little or no other clinical information is available to indicate a benign diagnosis or 2) the nodule may be benign but must be resected now because the benign nature cannot be established. If the clinical information firmly indicates a benign cause, follow-up CXR is recommended.

- If there is no change in the size or shape of the solitary pulmonary nodule for over 2 years, repeat CXR every 6-12 months.

Table 21-10.--Likelihood of Benign or Malignant Single Pulmonary Nodule According to Clinical and Radiographic Variables

Clinical factor, radiographic result	More likely benign	More likely malignant
Age	<35 yr	>35 yr
Sex	Female	Male
Smoking	No	Yes
Symptoms	No	Yes
Exposure to tuberculosis, cocci, etc.	Yes	No
Previous malignancy	No	Yes
Nodule size	<2.0 cm	>2.0 cm
Nodule age	>2 yr	<2 yr
Doubling time	<30 days	>30 days
Nodule margins	Smooth	Irregular
Calcification	Yes	No
Satellite lesions	Yes	No

- If the patient is a poor surgical risk or if surgeon or patient refuses the operation, repeat CXR every 3 months (enlargement of lesion may convince patient/surgeon to consider resection).

Primary Lung Cancer

Lung cancer is the most common malignant disease and the most common cause of cancer death in the U.S. The 1995 estimated incidence of new lung cancer cases is 14% (of all cancers) for men (prostate, 36%; colon and rectum, 10%; and urinary tract, 8%) and 13% for women (breast, 32%; colon and rectum, 12%; and uterus, 8%). The 1995 estimated rate of cancer deaths from lung cancer in the U.S. is 33% for men (prostate, 14% and colon and rectum, 9%) and 24% for women (breast, 18% and colon and rectum, 11%). The male-to-female ratio is 2:1. More than 150,000 new cases of cancer and >110,000 lung cancer deaths per year are predicted for the next several years. The risk factors include cigarette smoking (25% of cancers may result from passive smoking), other carcinogens, cocarcinogens, radon daughters (uranium mining), arsenic (glass workers, smelters, and pesticides), asbestos (insulation, textile, and asbestos mining), coal dust (coke oven, road work, and roofer), chromium (leather, ceramic, and metal), vinyl chloride (plastic), chloromethyl methyl ether (chemical), and chronic lung injury (idiopathic pulmonary fibrosis and COPD).

The WHO classification of pathologic types of pulmonary neoplasms is given in Table 21-11 and the TNM classification for staging of non-small-cell lung cancer, in Table 21-12.

Table 21-11.--WHO Classification of Pulmonary Neoplasms

Type	Histologic type
I	Squamous cell carcinoma
II	Small cell carcinoma
	Oat cell carcinoma
	Intermediate cell carcinoma
	Combined oat cell carcinoma
III	Adenocarcinoma
	Acinar adenocarcinoma
	Papillary adenocarcinoma
	Bronchoalveolar carcinoma
	Solid carcinoma with mucus formation
IV	Large cell carcinoma
	Giant cell carcinoma
	Clear cell carcinoma
V	Combined cell types
VI	Carcinoid tumors
VII	Bronchial gland tumors
	Cylindroma
	Mucoepidermoid
VIII	Papillary tumors

Small cell cancer is staged as follows:
1. Limited: single hemithorax, mediastinum, ipsilateral supraclavicular nodes.
2. Extensive: anything beyond limited stage.

Overall Survival

Overall survival rate for patients with occult and in situ cancers is >70%. Overall survival for other stages is as follows: stage I, 50%; stage II, <20%; and stage III, <10%. One-year survival for stage I cancer is >80%. In small cell cancer, the median survival is <12 months; 5-year survival for limited stage cancer is 15%-20% and for extensive disease, 1%-5%.

Cell Types and Clinical Features

Most patients are >50 years old. Only 5% of lung cancer patients are asymptomatic. The presentation is highly variable and depends on cell type, location, rate of growth, paraneoplastic syndromes, systemic symptoms, and other factors. Cough is the most frequent symptom and is more likely in squamous cell carcinoma and small cell cancer. Hemoptysis occurs in 35%-50% of patients and is more common with squamous cell, small cell, carcinoid, and endobronchial metastases. Wheezing is due to intraluminal tumor or extrinsic compression. Dyspnea depends on the extensiveness of the tumor, COPD, degree of bronchial obstruction, etc. Persistent chest pain may suggest rib metastasis, local extension, or pleural involvement. Superior vena cava syndrome may suggest small cell carcinoma, lymphoma, squamous cell carcinoma, or Pancoast's tumor. Horner's syndrome is indicative of Pancoast's tumor. Fever, postobstructive pneumonitis, nonthoracic skeletal pains, central nervous system symptoms, and abdominal pain/discomfort and hepatomegaly are indicative of possible distant metastases. Central nervous system metastasis is found in 15% of patients with squamous cell carcinoma, in 25% with adenocarcinoma, in 28% with large cell carcinoma, and in 30% with small cell carcinoma.

- Cough and hemoptysis are more common in squamous cell carcinoma and carcinoid.
- Chest pain may indicate pleural effusion, pleural metastasis, or rib lesion.
- Nonpulmonary symptoms may indicate distant metastases.
- Paraneoplastic syndromes are more common in patients with lung cancers.
- Central nervous system metastasis is more common with small cell carcinoma.

Squamous Cell Carcinoma

More than 65% of squamous cell carcinomas arise in the proximal tracheobronchial tree (first four subdivisions). They

Table 21-12.--Staging of Lung Cancer: TNM Classification

T, primary tumor

T0	No evidence of primary tumor
TX	Cancer cells in respiratory secretions; no tumor on chest radiographs or at bronchoscopy
Tis	Carcinoma in situ
T1	Tumor ≤3 cm in greatest dimension, surrounded by lung tissue; no bronchoscopic evidence of tumor proximal to lobar bronchus
T2	Tumor >3 cm in diameter, or tumor of any size that involves visceral pleura, or associated with atelectasis extending to hilum (but not involving entire lung); must be ≥2 cm from main carina
T3	Tumor involves chest wall, diaphragm, mediastinal pleura, or pericardium, or is <2 cm from main carina (but does not involve it)
T4	Tumor involves main carina or trachea, or invades mediastinum, heart, great vessels, esophagus, or vertebra, or malignant pleural effusion

N, nodal involvement

N0	No demonstrable lymph node involvement
N1	Ipsilateral peribronchial or hilar lymph nodes involved
N2	Metastasis to ipsilateral mediastinal lymph nodes, or to subcarinal lymph nodes
N3	Metastasis to contralateral mediastinal and/or hilar lymph nodes, or to scalene and/or supraclavicular lymph nodes

M, metastasis

M0	No known distant metastasis
M1	Distant metastasis present (specify site or sites)

TNM subsets for staging lung cancer

Stage 0	Tis
Stage I	T1 N0 M0
	T2 N0 M0
Stage II	T1 N1 M0
	T2 N1 M0
Stage IIIa	T3 N0 M0
	T3 N1 M0
	T1-3 N2 M0
Stage IIIb	Any T N3 M0
	T4 Any N M0
Stage IV	Any T Any N M1

also may arise in the upper airway and esophagus. Symptoms appear early in the course of the disease because of proximal bronchial involvement and consist of cough, hemoptysis, and lobar/segmental collapse with postobstructive pneumonia. CXR: atelectasis (23% of patients), obstructive pneumonitis (13%), hilar adenopathy (38%), and cavitation (5%). One-third of cases present as peripheral masses. Sputum cytology and bronchoscopy are indicated in almost all patients. One-third of squamous cell carcinomas have thick-walled irregular cavities. Treatment is with resection, radiation, and chemotherapy. Laser bronchoscopy and endobronchial brachytherapy are palliative measures.

- Squamous cell carcinoma: proximal airway disease in 66%; peripheral mass in 33%.
- Sputum cytology and bronchoscopy are important tests.
- One-third of the masses show cavitation.

Adenocarcinoma

Most adenocarcinomas arise in the periphery and, thus, remain undetected until they have spread locally or distally. Adenocarcinoma is the most common type of peripheral primary lung cancer. It may not produce pulmonary symptoms early in the course of the disease because of peripheral location. This means the chance of dissemination to extrapulmonary sites is higher for these tumors. Sputum cytology has a low yield in those without pulmonary symptoms. Advanced stages are more common in symptomatic patients; however, incidentally detected peripheral carcinomas tend to be in an early stage. The most common presentation is as a solitary peripheral nodule. A small number cavitate. Clubbing and hypertrophic pulmonary osteoarthropathy are more common than in other kinds of primary lung cancer. The response to radiation and chemotherapy is generally poor.

- Adenocarcinoma: most arise as a solitary pulmonary nodule in the periphery and, hence, are usually asymptomatic.
- Symptomatic stage usually denotes advanced disease.
- Sputum cytology has a low diagnostic yield in the absence of cough and hemoptysis.
- Clubbing and hypertrophic pulmonary osteoarthropathy are more common than in squamous cell carcinoma.

Bronchoalveolar Cell Carcinoma

Bronchoalveolar carcinoma is thought to arise from alveolar type 2 pneumocytes and/or Clara cells. The tumor presents in two forms: as a localized solitary nodular lesion and as a diffuse alveolar process. The solitary form has the best prognosis of all types of lung cancer, with a 1-year survival rate of >80%. The diffuse variety has a mean survival rate of <6 months. Bronchorrhea (>100 mL of thin serous mucus secretion/24 hours) is seen in 20% of patients. CXR shows a solitary nodule, localized infiltrate with vacuoles on tomography, and pneumonic lesions. Both forms of bronchoalveolar cell carcinoma can mimic ordinary pneumonia. Because of slow growth, the chronic course of the disease may suggest a benign process; thus, close surveillance is imperative. Treatment for a solitary lesion is resection. The response to radiation and chemotherapy is poor, although bronchorrhea seems to respond to radiation in some patients.

- Bronchoalveolar cell carcinoma: unrelated to tobacco smoking.
- The solitary form has a slow growth; it may mimic a benign pulmonary nodule.
- The solitary (localized) form has >80% 1-year survival rate after resection.
- The diffuse form has a mean survival rate of <6 months.
- Bronchorrhea occurs in 20% of patients (usually diffuse form).

Large Cell Carcinoma

In large cell carcinoma, large cells are seen on histologic examination, and CXR shows large masses. Large cell carcinoma grows more rapidly than adenocarcinoma. Cavitation is seen in 20%-25% of patients. Clubbing and hypertrophic pulmonary osteoarthropathy are more common than in other

tumors except for adenocarcinoma. Treatment is surgical. The response to radiation and chemotherapy is poor.

- Large cell carcinoma: large, rapidly growing lung mass; cavitation in 25% of patients.
- Clubbing and hypertrophic pulmonary osteoarthropathy are common.

Small Cell Carcinoma

Small cell carcinoma, which accounts for 25% of all bronchogenic carcinomas, is also called "oat cell (ovoid cells) carcinoma." The tumor originates from neuroendocrine cells (Kulchitsky cells). The tumor invades the tracheobronchial tree and spreads submucosally. Later, it breaks through the mucosa and produces changes similar to those seen in squamous cell carcinoma. CXR shows a unilateral, rapidly enlarging hilar or perihilar mass or widening of the hila/mediastinum. Less than 20% of these tumors are peripheral. Bronchoscopy may show heaped-up or thickened mucosa. This tumor responds better to radiation and chemotherapy than do other lung tumors. Prophylactic brain radiation is standard at many medical centers; this decreases the frequency of brain metastasis but does not prolong survival. Peripheral nodules that are found to be small cell carcinoma after resection should be treated as any small cell carcinoma.

- Small cell carcinoma: smokers and uranium miners are more prone.
- Positive antineuronal antibody in blood.
- Small cell carcinoma may be associated with many paraneoplastic syndromes: syndrome of inappropriate antidiuretic hormone, ACTH production, and myasthenic syndrome.
- Surgical treatment is not a standard therapeutic option; radiation and chemotherapy are.

Carcinoid

Carcinoid arises from the same cells as small cell carcinoma, but its clinical behavior is different. Typically, carcinoid presents with cough, with or without hemoptysis, in young adults. CXR may show a solitary nodule or segmental atelectasis. Paraneoplastic syndromes develop from hormonal secretion (ACTH and PTH). Treatment is surgical resection of the tumor without lung resection. The diagnosis of malignant carcinoid is based on the extent of spread noted at resection or clinical behavior.

- Carcinoid: young adult with cough and hemoptysis.
- Symptoms may be related to production of ACTH (Cushing's syndrome, hypertension) and PTH (hypercalcemia).
- Carcinoid "syndrome" is rare, occurring in <1% of patients with bronchial carcinoid.

Bronchial Gland Tumors

Cylindroma and mucoepidermoid tumors usually are located centrally and cause cough, hemoptysis, and obstructive pneumonia. Distant metastasis is unusual. Surgical treatment is used for major airway obstructive lesions. The response to radiation and chemotherapy is poor.

- Cylindroma arising in salivary glands can metastasize to the lungs after many years.

Mesenchymal Tumors

This group of tumors includes lymphoma, lymphosarcoma, carcinosarcoma, fibrosarcoma, mesothelioma (discussed above), and soft tissue sarcomas. Many of these present as large peripheral masses, homogeneous densities, and cavitated lesions.

Lymphoma

Pulmonary involvement occurs in 65% and 45% of patients with Hodgkin's and non-Hodgkin's lymphoma, respectively. CXR findings include bilateral hilar adenopathy, chylous pleural effusion, segmental atelectasis from endobronchial lesions, diffuse nodular process, fluffy infiltrates, and diffuse interstitial/alveolar infiltrates. Pseudolymphoma is a collection of abnormal lymphocytes and presents as a slow-growing lung mass; currently, it is considered a low-grade malignancy. Similarly, many of the patients thought to have lymphocytic interstitial pneumonitis currently are considered to have low-grade lymphomas that have a good response to chemotherapy. These tumors originate from the mucosa-associated lymphoid tissue.

- Intrathoracic involvement is common in Hodgkin's lymphoma.
- Bilateral hilar lymphadenopathy and chylous pleural effusion occur in young adults.
- Hodgkin's lymphoma can produce any type of CXR abnormality.

Diagnostic Tests

The results of sputum cytology are positive in 60% of patients with squamous cell carcinoma, in 21% with small cell carcinoma, in 16% with adenocarcinoma, and in 13% with large cell carcinoma. CXR is used to diagnose more tumors than sputum cytology but is not recommended as a surveillance tool for all patients. Bronchoscopy is helpful in diagnosing the cell type, in assessing staging and resectability, in using laser treatment for large airway tumors, and in brachytherapy. Transthoracic needle aspiration has an 85%-90% yield, but the incidence of pneumothorax is 25%, with most patients requiring chest tube drainage. CT scan is helpful in assessing the number of nodules in patients with pulmonary metastasis and in examination of the hila and mediastinum. Positive results on pleural fluid cytology establish stage III disease. Mediastinoscopy and mediastinotomy (Chamberlain procedure) are staging procedures that are often used before thoracotomy is performed.

- CXR helps diagnose more lung tumors than sputum cytology.
- Sputum cytology findings are positive in 60% of patients with squamous cell cancer.
- Routine surveillance of all susceptible persons (heavy smokers) with CXR and sputum cytology is not recommended.

Paraneoplastic Syndromes

As a group, primary lung tumors are the most common cause of paraneoplastic syndromes. The presence of a paraneoplastic syndrome does not indicate metastatic spread of lung cancer. The mechanism for the production of these syndromes varies. In clinical practice, it is more helpful to consider paraneoplastic manifestations based on each organ system, as described below.

- Primary lung tumors cause most of the paraneoplastic manifestations.
- Paraneoplastic syndrome does not indicate metastatic spread of lung cancer.

Endocrine

Small cell carcinoma is associated with syndrome of inappropriate antidiuretic hormone and adrenocorticotropic hormone (ACTH) production. Hypokalemia, muscle weakness, and CXR abnormality should suggest ACTH production. Note that these patients do not live long enough for typical Cushing's syndrome to develop. The ACTH levels are high and are not suppressed by dexamethasone. The overall frequency of hypercalcemia is 13%, with squamous cell cancer causing it in 25% of patients, large cell carcinoma in 13%, and adenocarcinoma in 3%. Hypercalcemia is not associated with small cell carcinoma. Bony metastasis can also cause hypercalcemia. Hyperpigmentation from melanocyte-stimulating hormone (MSH) occurs in small cell carcinoma. Calcitonin is secreted in 70% of patients with small cell carcinoma and in adenocarcinoma. Syndrome of inappropriate antidiuretic hormone is also seen in some patients with alveolar cell carcinoma and adenocarcinoma. Hypoglycemia with insulin-like polypeptide is found in patients with squamous cell carcinoma and mesothelioma. The human chorionic gonadotropin (hCG), luteinizing hormone (LH), and follicle-stimulating hormone (FSH) secreted by adenocarcinoma and large cell carcinoma may be responsible for gynecomastia.

- Abnormal CXR findings in hyponatremia: small cell carcinoma (syndrome of inappropriate antidiuretic hormone).
- Abnormal CXR findings, hypokalemia, and muscle weakness: small cell carcinoma (ACTH).

- ACTH is also produced by bronchial carcinoid.
- Hypercalcemia: squamous cell carcinoma and carcinoid.
- Calcitonin: small cell carcinoma and adenocarcinoma.
- Gynecomastia: adenocarcinoma or large cell carcinoma (FSH).

Central Nervous System

The mechanism for encephalopathy, myelopathy, sensory-motor neuropathies, and polymyositis is unknown but may include toxic, nutritional, autoimmune, and infectious causes. Cerebellar ataxia is similar to alcohol-induced ataxia and is more common with squamous cell carcinoma. Myasthenic syndrome (Lambert-Eaton syndrome) is closely associated with small cell carcinoma; there is initial weakness in the proximal muscles, but strength returns to normal with repeated stimulation. Focal neurologic signs should suggest central nervous system metastasis. Acute and rapidly progressive lower extremity signs should indicate spinal cord compression by tumor.

- Myasthenic syndrome may precede clinical detection of small cell carcinoma.
- Cerebellar ataxia (similar to alcohol-induced ataxia) is more common in squamous cell carcinoma.
- Focal neurologic signs should indicate central nervous system metastasis.

Skeletal

Hypertrophic pulmonary osteoarthropathy indicates periosteal bone formation and is associated with clubbing and symmetrical arthralgias. Other features include fever, gynecomastia, and increased ESR. Proposed mechanisms: neural (vagal afferents), hormonal, and others. Hypertrophic pulmonary osteoarthropathy is more common in adenocarcinoma and large cell carcinoma and may precede detection of the tumor by months. Clubbing alone can be the only feature. Removal of the tumor relieves the hypertrophic pulmonary osteoarthropathy.

- Hypertrophic pulmonary osteoarthropathy is more common in adenocarcinoma and large cell carcinoma.
- Ipsilateral vagotomy is indicated if the hypertrophic pulmonary osteoarthropathy persists after resection of tumor.

Others

Other paraneoplastic manifestations include: malignant cachexia, marantic endocarditis, increased incidence of thrombophlebitis, fever, erythrocytosis, leukocytosis, lymphocytopenia, eosinophilia, thrombocytosis, leukemoid reaction, disseminated intravascular coagulation, dysproteinemia, fever, acanthosis nigricans (adenocarcinoma), epidermolysis bullosa (squamous cell carcinoma), and nephrotic syndrome.

Pulmonary Metastases

Nearly 30% of all cases of malignant disease from extrapulmonary sites metastasize to the lung. More than 75% present with multiple lesions and the rest may present as a solitary pulmonary nodule, diffuse process, lymphangitic spread (breast, stomach, thyroid, pancreas, and the lung itself), and endobronchial metastases (kidney, colon, Hodgkin's lymphoma, and breast). Solitary metastases are more common with carcinoma of the colon, sarcoma, kidneys, testis, breast, and melanoma. The estimated occurrence of pulmonary metastasis by primary tumor is as follows: choriocarcinoma, 80%; osteosarcoma, 75%; kidney, 70%; thyroid, 65%; melanoma, 60%; breast, 55%; prostate, 45%; nasopharyngeal, 20%; gastrointestinal malignancies, 20%; and gynecologic malignancies, 20%.

PLEURA

Pleural Effusion

The normal volume of pleural fluid is 0.1 to 0.2 mL/kg of body weight. Excess pleural fluid collects in the pleural space when fluid collection exceeds removal by normal mechanisms. Hydrostatic, oncotic, and intrapleural pressures regulate fluid movement in the pleural space. Any of the following mechanisms can produce pleural effusion: changes in capillary permeability (inflammation), increased hydrostatic pressure, decreased plasma oncotic pressure, impaired lymphatic drainage, increased negative intrapleural pressure, and movement of fluid (through diaphragmatic pores and lymphatic vessels) from the peritoneum. The principal causes of pleural effusion are listed in Table 21-13.

Transudate Versus Exudate

The effusion is a transudate if the protein content is <3 g, specific gravity is <1.016, fluid lactic dehydrogenase is <60% of serum (fluid/serum <0.6), and serum-effusion albumin gradient (serum minus effusion albumin) is >1.2 g/dL. It is an exudate if the protein content is >3 g, fluid/serum protein is >0.5, specific gravity is >1.016, and fluid lactic dehydrogenase is >60% of serum lactic dehydrogenase or fluid lactic dehydrogenase is >200 units. Increased lactic dehydrogenase in fluid is nonspecific, but it is increased in pulmonary embolism, rheumatoid effusion, and most exudative effusions.

- It is not necessary to perform all the above tests to differentiate a transudate from an exudate.
- Clinically, it is more useful to classify cause by considering the source (organ system) of the fluid (see Table 21-13).
- Classification of pleural fluid into transudates and exudates does not permit consideration of all causes.
- The most common cause of transudate is congestive heart failure (pulmonary artery wedge pressure >25 mm Hg).

Table 21-13.--Principal Causes of Pleural Effusion

Osmotic-hydraulic*
    Congestive cardiac failure
    Superior vena caval obstruction
    Constrictive pericarditis
    Cirrhosis with ascites
    Hypoalbuminemia
    Salt-retaining syndromes
    Peritoneal dialysis
    Hydronephrosis
    Nephrotic syndrome
Infections[†]
    Parapneumonic (bacterial) effusions
    Bacterial empyema
    Tuberculosis
    Fungi
    Parasites
    Viruses and mycoplasma
Neoplasms[†]
    Primary and metastatic lung tumors
    Lymphoma and leukemia
    Benign and malignant tumors of pleura
    Intra-abdominal tumors with ascites
Vascular disease[†]
    Pulmonary embolism
    Wegener's granulomatosis
Intra-abdominal diseases[†]
    Pancreatitis and pancreatic pseudocyst
    Subdiaphragmatic abscess
    Malignancy with ascites
    Meigs' syndrome*
    Hepatic cirrhosis with ascites*
Trauma[†]
    Hemothorax
    Chylothorax
    Esophageal rupture
    Intra-abdominal surgery
Miscellaneous
    Drug-induced effusions[†]
    Uremic pleuritis[†]
    Myxedema*
    Yellow nail syndrome[†]
    Dressler's syndrome[†]
    Familial Mediterranean fever[†]

*Usually a transudate.

[†]Usually an exudate.

- The most common cause of exudate is pneumonia (parapneumonic effusion).

Glucose and pH

Pleural fluid hypoglycemia (<60 mg/dL or fluid/plasma glucose <0.6) is seen in rheumatoid effusion, malignant mesothelioma, empyema, systemic lupus erythematosus, esophageal rupture, and yellow nail syndrome. The pH of pleural fluid is <7.20 in empyema, esophageal rupture, rheumatoid effusion, tuberculosis, carcinoma, and trauma. If the pH is low (<7.20) and clinical suspicion is high for infection, drainage with a chest tube should be considered.

- Pleural fluid glucose concentration and pH usually go together (i.e., if glucose is low, so is pH).
- Low glucose levels in rheumatoid effusion, malignant mesothelioma, and empyema.
- Empyema caused by *Proteus* species produces pH >7.8 (because of ammonia production).

Amylase

Pleural fluid amylase concentration increases in pancreatitis, pseudocyst of pancreas, rupture of abdominal viscera, and esophageal rupture. The amylase level in the fluid remains higher for longer periods than that in the serum.

- Increased concentration of pleural fluid amylase in esophageal rupture is due to leakage of salivary amylase.
- In any unexplained left-sided effusion, consider pancreatitis and measure the amylase level in the pleural fluid.

Chylous Effusion

Chylous effusion cannot be diagnosed on the basis of the color or appearance of the fluid. More than 90% of true chylous effusions contain triglyceride levels >100 mg/dL, and a triglyceride level <50 mg/dL is less likely to be chylous. Make sure that the serum level of triglyceride is normal. Chylous effusion can occur in conditions listed below as well as in Kaposi's sarcoma with mediastinal adenopathy, after Valsalva maneuver during childbirth, esophagectomy, esophageal sclerotherapy, and thrombosis of the superior vena cava, innominate, or subclavian veins. Cholesterol effusions (fluid cholesterol >250 mg/dL) are not true chylous effusions. They are seen in old tuberculous effusions and rheumatoid effusions and in some cases of nephrotic syndrome.

- Chylous effusion seen in the "5 Ts," i.e., **T**horacic duct **T**rauma, **T**umor (lymphoma), **T**uberculosis, **T**uberous sclerosis (lymphangiomyomatosis).
- True chylous effusion contains chylomicrons.
- Cholesterol effusions are not true chylous effusions.

Complement

Total, C3, and C4 components in the pleural fluid are decreased in systemic lupus erythematosus (80% of patients), rheumatoid arthritis (40%-60% of patients), carcinoma, pneumonia, and tuberculosis. Increased pleural fluid ANA (>1:160) is strongly suggestive of lupus erythematosus. Rheumatoid factor is >1:320 in rheumatoid pleural effusion.

- Low complement level in pleural fluid in systemic lupus erythematosus (including in drug-induced form).
- Presence of lupus erythematosus cells in pleural fluid is diagnostic of systemic lupus erythematosus.

Blood Cell Counts

An erythrocyte count >100,000/dL in the pleural fluid produces a "bloody effusion." This is seen in trauma, tumor, asbestos effusion, pancreatitis (60%), pulmonary embolism with infarctions, etc. A leukocyte count >20,000/dL is seen in parapneumonic effusions, empyema, and leukemic effusions (rare). Pleural fluid eosinophilia is nonspecific and occurs in trauma, pulmonary infarction, psittacosis, drug-induced effusion, pulmonary infiltrate with eosinophilia-associated effusions, and pneumothorax. Pleural fluid lymphocytosis occurs in tuberculosis, chronic effusions, lymphoma, and some collagenoses.

- Bloody effusion, even if cytologic results are negative, in the presence of lung tumor usually denotes pleural metastasis.
- Eosinophilia in pleural fluid is nonspecific.
- Differential leukocyte count in pleural fluid is generally unhelpful.

Cytology

Cytologic examination should be conducted on most effusions in adults if the clinical features do not suggest an obvious benign cause. Cytologic findings are positive in 60% of all malignant effusions. Pleural biopsy results are positive in <50% of all malignant effusions. Cytologic examination and biopsy give a slightly higher yield than either one does alone. Cytologic examination is less helpful in malignant mesothelioma, and an open biopsy is often necessary. Positive fluid cytologic findings in primary lung carcinoma mean unresectability (stage III).

- Cytologic examination is an important test in most adults with an "unknown" effusion.
- Overall yield from cytologic examination is 60%; less in cases of mesothelioma and lymphoma.

Cultures

Tuberculous effusions (fluid alone) yield positive cultures in <15% of cases. Pleural biopsy (histology and culture) has a higher (>75%) diagnostic yield. Culture is of value in effusions due to actinomycosis and *Nocardia* infection, but it is less helpful in other mycoses. However, if fungal infection of the pleural space is suspected, cultures should be obtained. Cultures for viruses (influenza A, ornithosis, coxsackievirus B, and mycoplasma) are often negative. Paragonimiasis causes pleural effusion.

- In tuberculosis, it is important to culture pleural biopsy specimens.
- Poor yield in viral infections.

Pleural Biopsy

Pleural biopsy is indicated if tuberculous involvement of the pleural space is suspected. The diagnostic rate from pleural biopsy in tuberculosis is >75%, whereas pleural fluid alone has a much lower yield (<15%). The overall diagnostic yield in malignant pleural effusions is about 50%. Diagnostic rates are low (<30%) in malignant pleural mesothelioma.

- Pleural biopsy is indicated if tuberculous pleural disease is suspected.

Miscellaneous

At least 350-400 mL of fluid has to be present to be seen on CXR. Look for subpulmonic effusions, for elevated hemidiaphragms, and blunting of the costophrenic angle. When in doubt, obtain a lateral decubitus CXR. Ultrasonography is helpful in tapping small amounts of fluid and loculated fluid collections. Look for signs of trauma (rib fracture), abdominal surgery, acute abdomen, pancreatitis, cirrhosis, etc. Asbestos-induced effusions are notorious and frequently mimic malignant pleural mesothelioma, with pain, bloody fluid, and recurrence. Mesothelioma should be excluded by repeated thoracentesis, pleural biopsy, or thoracotomy.

- Small effusions are common after abdominal operations and normal labor of pregnancy; almost all resolve spontaneously.
- Drug-induced pleural effusion: nitrofurantoin, methysergide, drug-induced systemic lupus erythematosus, and busulfan.
- Nearly 20% of all effusions are undiagnosed despite extensive studies, including open pleural biopsy.

Complications

Complications of thoracentesis include pneumothorax (in 3%-20% of patients), hemothorax, pulmonary edema, intrapulmonary hemorrhage, hemoptysis, vagal inhibition, air embolism, subcutaneous emphysema, bronchopleural fistula, empyema, and puncture of liver or spleen.

Pneumothorax

Spontaneous pneumothorax occurs more commonly in young, previously healthy adults. The incidence of primary spontaneous pneumothorax is 9 cases/100,000 persons per year, with a male-to-female ratio of 6:1. Many are caused by the rupture of apical bullae. Smoking increases the risk of spontaneous pneumothorax. Secondary spontaneous pneumothorax occurs most frequently in COPD, with an annual incidence of 4 cases/100,000 patients and a male-to-female ratio of 3:1. Other causes of spontaneous secondary pneumothorax include histiocytosis X, asthma, emphysema, bullous lung disease, cystic fibrosis, lung tumors, end-stage fibrosis and honeycombing of the lungs, Marfan's disease, and during the menses in young females (catamenial pneumothorax). Iatrogenic pneumothorax may be seen after thoracentesis, trauma, esophageal rupture, tracheal fracture, subclavian needle sticks, high positive end-expiratory pressure, transtracheal aspiration, severe Valsalva maneuver, and secondary to pneumoperitoneum. Treatment of spontaneous pneumothorax includes chest tube drainage, chemical pleurodesis (tetracycline or other chemicals), talc pleurodesis, and, occasionally, surgical decortication.

- Spontaneous pneumothorax occurs in histiocytosis X, peripheral lung tumors, lymphangioleiomyomatosis, bullous lung disease, and COPD.
- In younger females with pleuritic chest pain during menses, consider catamenial pneumothorax.
- CXR obtained after full expiration is better for identifying a small pneumothorax.

Pleurodesis

Pleurodesis is indicated in the treatment of recurrent pneumothorax or pleural effusion. If repeated therapeutic thoracentesis fails to relieve symptoms, then chemical pleurodesis with tetracycline (15 mg/kg in 30 mL saline), doxycycline (10 mg/kg), minocycline (5 mg/kg), or talc (2.5-10 g) is instilled into the pleural space through a chest tube. Talc pleurodesis is > 90% effective, whereas other chemicals are 65% effective. Surgical pleurodesis may be indicated if these agents do not accomplish closure of the pleural space.

- Antibiotic pleurodesis is 65% effective.
- Talc pleurodesis is > 90% effective.

Empyema

Empyema is the collection of pus in the pleural space. For clinical purposes, the presence of bacteria in the pleural fluid is also considered empyema. Empyema is caused by bacterial pneumonia in >50% of patients (empyema develops in about 2% of patients with pneumonia), bacteremia in <10%, compromised host in <10%, trauma in 5%-15%, thoracic surgery in 10%-25%, and by esophageal perforation, lung abscess, and infarction. Bacteria that commonly are isolated are *S. aureus* (25%-35% of patients), anaerobes (15%-35%),

gram-negative bacilli (15%-30%), and *S. pneumoniae* and other streptococci (12%-15%). In one-third of the cases of anaerobic empyema, cultures of the fluid are positive, whereas <5% of parapneumonic effusion due to *S. pneumoniae* is positive on culture. Treatment consists of systemic antibiotics, chest tube drainage, thoracostomy, and decortication. Mortality is higher in older patients and in those with multiple bacterial isolates, gram-negative bacilli, serious illnesses, and hospital-acquired empyema.

- Chest tube is indicated if: purulent effusion, positive Gram stain, pH <7.00, or glucose <40 mg and LDH >1,000 U/L.

MEDIASTINUM

Mediastinal Lesions

Clinically, it is useful to divide mediastinal lesions into their location, namely, anterior, middle, and posterior mediastinum. The anterior compartment contains the thymus, ascending aorta, innominate artery and vein, superior vena cava, fat, and lymph nodes. More than 50% of mediastinal tumors are located in this compartment, and 60% of them are thymic tumors, lymphomas, and germ cell tumors. The middle mediastinum contains the cardiac chambers, pericardium, aortic arch and its branches, trachea and bronchi, esophagus, and mediastinal nodes. Most of the tumors in this compartment are cystic and 25% are metastatic malignancies. The posterior compartment contains the lower esophagus, descending aorta, sympathetic chain, and intercostal nerves. Nearly 25% of all mediastinal tumors are in the posterior compartment, and 70% of them are neurogenic tumors.

- Nearly 30% of mediastinal masses are malignant.
- Anterior mediastinum: the "6 Ts"—**T**hymoma, **T**eratoma, **T**umor (lymphoma and carcinomas), **T**horacic aortic aneurysm, **T**rauma (hematoma or aneurysm), and **T**hyroid.
- Posterior mediastinum: neurogenic tumors make up 70% of the tumors.
- Middle mediastinum: one-fourth are metastatic tumors.

Thymoma is the most common tumor in the anterior mediastinum and is associated with myasthenia gravis, red cell aplasia, and collagenoses. Neurilemoma and neurofibroma are the most common tumors in the posterior mediastinum. In adults, <4% of these tumors are malignant. Up to 40% of patients with neurofibromas have von Recklinghausen's disease. MRI may be required to exclude intraspinal extension of a mediastinal neurogenic tumor.

- Thymoma: 15%-45% of them are associated with myasthenia gravis.

- 10%-15% of patients with myasthenia gravis have thymoma.
- Thymoma is also associated with red cell aplasia, hypogammaglobulinemia, and Cushing's syndrome (ACTH from thymic carcinoid).
- Malignant changes are uncommon in posterior mediastinal tumors in adults.

Mediastinitis

Usually, an acute infection of the mediastinal space produces mediastinitis. Acute mediastinitis is an acute medical/surgical emergency. One of the most common causes is esophageal rupture caused by iatrogenic trauma (instrumentation) or tumor necrosis in the mediastinum. Fever, dyspnea, neck and thoracic paraspinal pain, dysphagia, and odynophagia are frequent. CXR almost always reveals pleural effusion and may show air in the neck or mediastinum (pneumomediastinum). Contrast imaging of the esophagus may be necessary to document the process. Immediate surgical drainage and intensive antibiotic therapy are required in all patients. Mortality is high (>50%) if diagnosis is delayed by >24 hours.

- Acute mediastinitis is caused most commonly by esophageal perforation.
- It has a high mortality rate if not diagnosed and treated within 24 hours.

Mediastinal Fibrosis/Granuloma

Mediastinal fibrosis, also known as fibrosing mediastinitis, represents an exuberant fibrotic reaction in the mediastinum. In the U.S. it is caused most commonly by histoplasmosis. Other causes include tuberculosis, autoimmune process, drugs (methysergide), and idiopathic. It represents an unusual reaction to the fungal infection. Most patients with mediastinal fibrosis do not have active histoplasmosis at the time of their diagnosis. Special stains of fibrotic tissue may show nonviable histoplasma organisms. Granuloma formation may also be seen. Extensive calcification of hilar and mediastinal lymph nodes may be seen in some patients. Calcified tissue may erode into the bronchial lumen, causing broncholithiasis. The excessive fibrotic process may encircle the airways, esophagus, major veins, and arteries in the hilar region and cause compression and sometimes occlusion of these structures. The clinical features depend on the extent of involvement of intrathoracic organs.

- Mediastinal fibrosis/granuloma is caused most often by histoplasmosis.
- Active infection is not present in patients with mediastinal fibrosis.
- The fibrotic process encircles mediastinal organs and causes symptoms.

VASCULAR DISEASES

Pulmonary Embolism

Pulmonary embolism is the major cause of death in 15% of patients dying in general hospitals and is detected in 25%-30% of routine autopsies. Nearly 200,000 deaths/year are said to result from pulmonary embolism. Antemortem diagnosis is made in <30%. In about 90% of patients who die of pulmonary embolism, death occurs within 1-2 hours. Pulmonary embolism and deep vein thrombosis frequently occur together.

Etiology

Although most (>95%) of pulmonary embolisms arise from the thrombi of the lower extremities, deep vein thrombosis is detected in only 40% of all cases of pulmonary embolism. About 60% of patients with pulmonary embolism have lower extremity deep vein thrombosis that is asymptomatic, and approximately 45% of femoral and iliac deep vein thromboses embolize. Other sources of emboli include upper extremity thrombi, right ventricular thrombi, and indwelling catheters. Larger veins (usually popliteal veins or above the level of popliteal veins) are the source of larger emboli. From 5%-15% of deep vein thromboses from the calves propagate to the thigh and iliac veins, and 5%-15% of superficial thrombophlebitis is associated with deep vein thrombosis. Factors predisposing to deep vein thrombosis include congestive heart failure, shock, estrogens, dysproteinemias, neoplasms, surgical procedures, prolonged immobilization, obesity, trauma, varicose veins, previous deep vein thrombosis, pregnancy, deficiencies of antithrombin III, proteins S and C, and the presence of lupus anticoagulant (antiphospholipid antibodies). The incidence of deep vein thrombosis in various clinical circumstances is as follows: major abdominal surgery, 14%-33%; thoracic surgery, 25%-60%; gynecologic surgery, <3% (patients <40 years old), 10%-40% (patients >40 years old), and 40%-70% (patients >40 years old with other added risks); urologic surgery, 10%-40%; hip surgery, 50%-75%; post-myocardial infarction, 20%-40%; congestive heart failure, 70%; stroke with paralysis, 50%-70%; postpartum, 3%; and trauma, 20%-40%. Idiopathic deep vein thrombosis, particularly when recurrent, may indicate the presence of neoplasm in 10%-20% of patients.

- Deep vein thrombosis is detected in only 40% of cases of pulmonary embolism.
- 20%-40% increased risk of deep vein thrombosis in patients with history of previous deep vein thrombosis.
- Among predisposing factors for deep vein thrombosis and pulmonary embolism, consider deficiencies of antithrombin III, proteins S and C, and the presence of lupus anticoagulant.
- Idiopathic, recurrent deep vein thrombosis: look for an occult neoplasm.

Deep vein thrombosis is diagnosed in only 50% of clinical cases. A diagnosis based on physical examination findings is unreliable. Homans' sign (pain and tenderness on dorsiflexion of the ankle) is elicited in <40% of cases of deep vein thrombosis, and false-positive Homans' sign occurs in 30% of high-risk patients. Impedance plethysmography and duplex ultrasonography together are the most commonly used tests and have a diagnostic accuracy of 90%-95% in detecting iliac and femoral deep vein thromboses. They are noninvasive methods and can be performed at the bedside. Serial impedance plethysmography studies are useful in detecting extension of calf vein thrombi because up to 15% of proximal deep vein thromboses are detected after the initial negative study. Both impedance plethysmography and compression ultrasonography are inaccurate for the detection of calf vein thrombosis. Many medical centers now use Doppler ultrasonography as the procedure of choice. Serial (daily) impedance plethysmography studies or duplex ultrasonography (or both) is performed in high-risk patients. Venography remains the best diagnostic test for deep vein thrombosis. In patients in whom recurrent deep vein thrombosis is questioned, venography may help differentiate a new thrombosis from an old one.

- Homans' sign is unreliable in the diagnosis of deep vein thrombosis.
- Impedance plethysmography and duplex ultrasonographic examinations have a diagnostic accuracy of >90%.
- Venography is the best test for diagnosing deep vein thrombosis.

Clinical Features

Pulmonary embolism has no typical clinical symptom and sign. Tachypnea and tachycardia are observed in nearly all patients. Other symptoms include dyspnea (80% of patients), pleuritic pain (up to 75%), hemoptysis (<25%), pleural friction rub (20%), and wheezing (15%). The differential diagnosis of pulmonary embolism includes myocardial infarction, pneumonia, congestive heart failure, pericarditis, esophageal spasm, asthma, exacerbation of COPD, intrathoracic malignancy, rib fracture, pneumothorax, pleurisy from any cause, pleurodynia, and nonspecific skeletal pains. Acute cor pulmonale occurs if >60%-75% of the pulmonary circulation is obstructed by emboli.

- No typical symptoms and signs for diagnosing pulmonary embolism.
- Dyspnea, tachypnea, and pleuritic pain are common.

Diagnostic Tests

ECG changes (nonspecific) are noted in 80% of patients, ST and T changes in 65%, T inversion in 40%, S_1Q_3 pattern in 15%, right bundle branch block in 12%, and left axis deviation in 12%. CXR may show diaphragmatic elevation in 60% of patients, infiltrates in 30%, focal oligemia in 10%-50%, pleural effusion in 20%, enlarged pulmonary artery in 20%, and no abnormalities in 30%. Lactic dehydrogenase levels are increased in 12% of patients. PaO_2 may be normal but $(A-a)O_2$ gradient will be widened. Normal $(A-a)O_2$ does not exclude pulmonary embolism. It should be emphasized that clinical examination, CXR, blood gas abnormalities, and ECG changes are not reliable in the diagnosis of pulmonary embolism. Clinical suspicion, however, is important in steering the clinician toward appropriate tests to diagnose the condition.

- CXR is normal in 30% of patients; ECG shows S_1Q_3 pattern in 15%.
- PaO_2 may be normal, but $(A-a)O_2$ gradient is usually widened.

The plasma level of D-dimer, a specific fibrin degradation product, is increased in patients with deep vein thrombosis and pulmonary embolism. However, high levels by themselves do not establish the diagnosis. Levels <300 µg/L (by ELISA) or <500 µg/L (by latex agglutination) are considered to reliably exclude pulmonary embolism in patients with an abnormal but not high-probability perfusion $(\dot{Q})$ lung scan. Normal levels of D-dimer do not exclude either deep venous thrombosis or pulmonary embolism. Increased levels of D-dimer have no positive predictive value for pulmonary embolism and should be followed with ultrasonography and/or pulmonary angiography, depending on the clinical situation. The combination of D-dimer measurement and ultrasonography may reduce the requirement for pulmonary angiography in 30% of patients with inconclusive $\dot{Q}$ scans and intermediate clinical probability of pulmonary embolism.

- High D-dimer levels by themselves do not diagnose pulmonary embolism.
- Normal or low D-dimer levels do not exclude deep vein thrombosis or pulmonary embolism.
- Increased D-dimer levels have no positive predictive value for pulmonary embolism.

Perfusion $(\dot{Q})$ scan is commonly used in the diagnosis of pulmonary embolism. In patients with proven deep vein thrombosis, this scan is recommended to exclude asymptomatic pulmonary embolism. A high probability lung scan has a sensitivity of 41% and a specificity of 97%. The likelihood of pulmonary embolism in a scan that shows "high probability" (≥2 large segmental mismatches, ≥2 large segmental matches > ventilation defect, 1 large and ≥2 moderate mismatches, or ≥4 moderate mismatches) is 90%. A "low probability" lung scan excludes the diagnosis of pulmonary embolism in >85% of patients. A normal lung scan excludes pulmonary embolism in 100%, whereas "near normal" scan excludes it in >95% of patients. An "intermediate or indeterminate probability" scan is associated with pulmonary embolism in 21%-30% of patients. Therefore, patients with an "intermediate probability" lung scan usually require pulmonary angiography to document pulmonary embolism. However, clinical suspicion is very important in deciding whether to proceed with pulmonary angiography, anticoagulation, or observation. "Intermediate" scans are encountered in 60% of patients with COPD and in 43% of patients with any previous cardiac or pulmonary disease. Pulmonary angiography is the best diagnostic test; ideally, it should be performed within 24-48 hours after onset of symptoms. False-negative results are observed in 1%-2% of pulmonary angiograms in patients with pulmonary embolism. In a patient in whom the suspicion is high for pulmonary embolism, heparin treatment should be started before starting diagnostic tests.

- Normal results on a perfusion scan exclude pulmonary embolism in >95% of patients.
- Intermediate probability scan requires pulmonary angiography in most patients.
- Patients in whom pulmonary embolism is strongly suspected should be given heparin before other diagnostic tests are performed.
- A "low probability" lung scan excludes pulmonary embolism in >85% of patients.
- Pulmonary angiography is the best diagnostic test.

Treatment

In acute deep vein thrombosis and/or pulmonary embolism, heparin therapy and warfarin therapy can be initiated simultaneously unless there is a contraindication to the use of warfarin. For patients with acute deep vein thrombosis, heparin therapy is initiated with an intravenous bolus of 5,000-10,000 U. For pulmonary embolism, a dose of 15,000 to 20,000 U is recommended (bolus dose 80 U/kg). Immediately after this, sustained therapy is begun with heparin, 1,200 U/hour by continuous intravenous infusion (maintenance dose 18 U/kg per hour) or subcutaneously, 15,000 to 20,000 U twice daily, to maintain an activated partial thromboplastin time >1.5 times control. For maintenance therapy, heparin, 5,000 U subcutaneously twice daily, or warfarin, at a dosage to achieve a prothrombin time of 1.3 to 1.5 times control or an INR ratio of 2 to 3 is begun. Heparin blocks fibrin formation promptly and broadly. In uncomplicated and nonrecurrent deep vein thrombosis and pulmonary embolism, anticoagulant therapy with warfarin for 3 to 6 months should suffice. Patients with recurrent and complicated cases (coagulopathies, etc.) may require life-long anticoagulation and other measures such as plication of the inferior vena cava (see below).

- Heparin and warfarin can be initiated simultaneously unless

there is a contraindication to the use of warfarin.
- In uncomplicated pulmonary embolism, the activated partial thromboplastin time and prothrombin time should be maintained at >1.5 times control and at an INR ratio of 2 to 3, respectively.

Thrombolytic agents (streptokinase, urokinase, and tissue plasminogen activator [tPA]) are used in massive pulmonary embolism and massive iliofemoral thrombosis. The indications are controversial, although they are generally indicated in patients with massive deep vein thrombosis and/or pulmonary embolism. These agents should be given within 24 hours of pulmonary embolism, and following the loading dose, maintenance therapy is given for 6 hours. Dosages for streptokinase: the loading dose of 250,000 IU is infused over 30 minutes, followed by a maintenance dose of 100,000 U/hour for up to 24 hours. For urokinase: the loading dose is 4,400 IU/kg infused over 10 minutes, followed by continuous infusion of 4,400 IU/kg per hour, for 12-24 hours. For tPA: a total dose of 100 mg (a bolus of 15 mg given intravenously) over a 2-hour period. Adequacy of thrombolytic therapy is monitored with thrombin time. Contraindications to the use of thrombolytic agents include a recent (within 10 days) surgical procedure, intra-arterial procedures, renal or liver biopsies within the preceding 14 days, ulcer disease, recent cerebrovascular accident, hemorrhagic diathesis, and pregnancy.

- Definite indications for thrombolytic agents are controversial.
- Pulmonary angiography is recommended before using thrombolytic agents.

The incidence of bleeding complications due to heparin is 3%-8% and to warfarin, 4%. The cumulative incidence of fatal bleeding is 1% at 1 year and 2% at 3 years among those receiving chronic warfarin therapy. Age, reason for anticoagulation, use of interfering drugs, and hypertension are not associated with bleeding in patients receiving chronic warfarin therapy. Hemorrhagic risk does not appear to be related to heparin dosage or activated partial thromboplastin time. Drugs that prolong the effect of warfarin include salicylate, heparin, estrogen, antibiotics, clofibrate, quinidine, and cimetidine. Drugs that decrease the effect of warfarin include glutethimide, rifampin, barbiturates, and ethchlorvynol. Inferior vena caval plication or umbrella insertion is indicated in recurrent deep vein thrombosis in a patient who recently had a massive pulmonary embolism, presence of a bleeding disorder, or contraindication to anticoagulant therapy or failure of anticoagulant therapy. Inferior vena caval plication does not replace anticoagulant therapy; many patients require both. Recurrence of pulmonary embolism after inferior vena caval interruption is noted in 5% of patients. Vena caval occlusion occurs in 3%-5% of patients.

- Bleeding complications due to heparin are 3%-8% and to warfarin, 4%.
- Inferior vena caval plication does not replace anticoagulation therapy; many patients require both.

Prophylaxis

Prophylaxis against deep vein thrombosis and/or pulmonary embolism includes early ambulation postoperatively or after immobilization, intermittent pneumatic compression of the lower extremities, active and passive leg exercises, and a low dose (10,000-15,000 U/day) of heparin given subcutaneously. The use of low-molecular-weight heparin (LMWH) has been approved in the U.S. for prophylaxis against deep vein thrombosis and pulmonary embolism after total hip arthroplasty. LMWH has a rapid onset of action and may supersede standard heparin in the future. LMWH is safe and about 50% more effective than standard heparin. Because of a more predictable dose response to LMWH, the need to monitor the dose and activated partial thromboplastin time is not as important. A once daily dose may lead to outpatient treatment without laboratory monitoring. The risk of heparin-induced thrombocytopenia is decreased significantly with LMWH.

Complications

Pulmonary infarction is a complication of pulmonary embolism, but this problem does not develop in every patient with pulmonary embolism. The exact incidence is unknown. Complications of pulmonary infarction include secondary infection, cavitation, pneumothorax, and hemothorax. Recurrent pulmonary embolism is a common cause of secondary pulmonary hypertension. Mechanical obstruction of one-half to two-thirds of the pulmonary vascular bed by emboli is necessary for this complication to develop (see below).

Pulmonary Hypertension

Pulmonary hypertension exists when pulmonary artery pressure at rest is >30/10, with a mean of ≥20 mm Hg. It can be classified broadly into primary and secondary forms.

Primary

Primary pulmonary hypertension is a rare disease of unknown cause manifested by various degrees of precapillary pulmonary hypertension. By definition, identifiable causes of pulmonary hypertension have to be ruled out before primary pulmonary hypertension can be diagnosed. Usually, it is a disease of young females (female-to-male ratio is from 10:1 to 2:1); nearly 10% of patients with primary pulmonary hypertension are >60 years old. Familial association is fairly common. Dyspnea, fatigue, and frequent syncope are common symptoms. Angina-like pain may be present, and Raynaud's phenomenon is frequent. Loud pulmonic second sound, right-sided third heart sound, and tricuspid regurgitation may be present. Exercise-induced hypoxemia and

decreased diffusing capacity are important findings. CXR may show prominent central pulmonary arteries and decreased peripheral pulmonary vasculature. Pulmonary artery pressure measurement is most helpful in making the diagnosis. Most patients die within 5-6 years after diagnosis (5- and 10-year mortality rates of 63% and 85%, respectively); the mortality rate during pregnancy may be as high as 50%. Right ventricular failure is the primary determinant of prognosis. Vasodilators (calcium channel blockers) and long-term anticoagulation prolong life. High-dose calcium-channel blockers, continuous intravenous prostacycline, and inhaled nitric oxide are the newer treatments under investigation. Oxygen therapy is necessary to relieve hypoxemia. Lung transplantation is a therapeutic option.

- Primary pulmonary hypertension: young women with normal findings on PFTs and low diffusing capacity.
- Exertional dyspnea, fatigue, and syncopal episodes.
- Nearly 10% of patients are >60 years old.

Secondary

Causes of secondary pulmonary hypertension include recurrent pulmonary embolism, COPD (cor pulmonale), scleroderma, chronic mitral stenosis, chronic mountain sickness, sleep apnea, drug-induced (aminorex, L-tryptophan, and tainted rapeseed oil), pulmonary veno-occlusive disease, and others. Recurrent pulmonary embolism is a relatively common cause of secondary pulmonary hypertension. Mechanical obstruction of one-half to two-thirds of the pulmonary vascular bed by emboli is necessary for pulmonary hypertension to develop. It is often difficult to distinguish pulmonary hypertension caused by recurrent pulmonary emboli from primary pulmonary hypertension. A significant number (10%) of patients have underlying coagulopathies (deficiencies of antithrombin III, proteins S and C, and presence of lupus anticoagulant). The gradual onset of dyspnea and signs of pulmonary hypertension and right ventricular strain are the presenting symptoms. Exercise-induced hypoxemia is common. Perfusion scans may not be entirely reliable if emboli are small and peripheral. Even pulmonary angiography may not provide definite clues. Clinical suspicion, hemodynamic measurements, $\dot{V}/\dot{Q}$ scan, pulmonary angiography, pulmonary angioscopy, and lung biopsy may be needed in some cases for the documentation. In progressive disease, surgical therapy (pulmonary thromboendarterectomy) may be indicated. Palliative therapy includes life-long anticoagulant therapy, calcium channel blockers, and supplemental oxygen.

- Difficult to distinguish pulmonary hypertension caused by pulmonary emboli from primary pulmonary hypertension.
- High incidence (10%) of underlying coagulopathies.
- Surgical thromboendarterectomy is indicated in selected patients.

- Life-long anticoagulation after inferior vena caval interruption is required for many patients.

Pulmonary Veno-Occlusive Disease

Pulmonary veno-occlusive disease is a disease of young men. It is uncommon and has no known cause, although mycoplasma infection, chemotherapy, and toxins may be responsible. Common findings are the gradual onset of exertional dyspnea associated with diffuse mottling and Kerley's B lines on CXR, hypoxemia, and low diffusing capacity. Without lung biopsy, the diagnosis cannot be firmly established. This is a rapidly fatal condition, with death within 2 years after diagnosis. Treatment is symptomatic.

- Pulmonary veno-occlusive disease: young males with rapidly progressive pulmonary hypertension.
- Kerley's B lines and diffuse mottling on CXR.

Other Causes of Pulmonary Hypertension

Mitral stenosis, left atrial myxoma, obstruction to left ventricular outflow, pulmonary arterial tumor emboli, schistosomiasis, severe chronic hypoxemia (COPD, sleep apnea, etc.), mixed connective tissue disease, scleroderma, systemic lupus erythematosus, eosinophilia-myalgia syndrome, chronic liver disease, sickle cell disease, and Raynaud's phenomenon are associated with pulmonary hypertension. Diagnosis of these entities is based on clinical suspicion, and treatment is aimed at the underlying causes.

Pulmonary Vasculitides

The vasculitides are a heterogeneous group of disorders of unknown cause characterized by varying degrees of inflammation and necrosis of the arteries and, sometimes, veins. Immunologic factors, absence or deficiency of certain chemical mediators in the body, and infectious processes caused by mycoses, particularly *Aspergillus* and *Mucor*, are associated with vasculitis. The common vasculitides and their incidence in North America are as follows: giant cell (temporal) arteritis, 26.5%; polyarteritis nodosa, 14.6%; Wegener's granulomatosis, 10.5%; Schönlein-Henoch purpura, 10.5%; Takayasu's arteritis, 7.8%; and Churg-Strauss syndrome, 2.5%. The rest of the vasculitides are due to collagen diseases and nonspecific causes.

Giant Cell (Temporal) Arteritis

Giant cell arteritis is a vasculitis of unknown cause, but it has been described in association with polymyalgia rheumatica. It usually affects persons of middle age and older. The clinical illness appears gradually, with nonspecific constitutional symptoms (low-grade fever, malaise, and weight loss) followed by specific symptoms such as claudication of the jaw and sudden loss of vision. Headache is the most common symptom. Pulmonary involvement in giant cell arteritis may present with cough, sore throat, and hoarseness. Nearly 10% of patients with giant cell arteritis have prominent respiratory symptoms, and the respiratory symptoms are the initial manifestation in 4%. Giant cell arteritis should be considered in older patients with a new cough or throat pain without obvious cause. Pulmonary nodules, interstitial infiltrations, pulmonary artery occlusion, and aneurysms have been described.

- Giant cell arteritis: elderly persons with cough, low-grade fever, malaise, weight loss, headache, and polymyalgia.
- Nearly 10% of patients have prominent respiratory symptoms.
- Cough, sore throat, and hoarseness may be the presenting features of giant cell arteritis.

Wegener's Granulomatosis

Wegener's granulomatosis is a distinct type of systemic vasculitis characterized by necrotizing granulomatous vasculitis of the upper and lower respiratory tract, glomerulonephritis, and variable degrees of small vessel vasculitis. The term "limited Wegener's granulomatosis" is used to describe the disease involving the lungs only, but patients with this "limited" form show kidney involvement if renal biopsy specimens are obtained. Histologic features include discrete or confluent granulomatosis, necrotizing granuloma in combination with vasculitis, fibrinoid necrosis, microabscesses, focal vasculitis, thrombosis, and fibrous obliteration of the vascular lumen. Eosinophilic infiltrates are seen in tissue samples, but peripheral blood eosinophilia is not a feature of Wegener's granulomatosis.

- Wegener's granulomatosis is a systemic disease with major respiratory manifestations.
- Renal involvement with focal segmental glomerulonephritis is characteristic.

The mean age at onset of symptoms is 45.2 years (the male-to-female ratio is 2:1); 91% of the patients are Caucasian. Initial symptoms are nonspecific: fever, malaise, weight loss, arthralgias, and myalgias. The organs affected are the skin (40%-50% of patients), eyes (43%), and central nervous system (25%). Arthralgias occur in 58% of patients and frank arthritis in 28%. ENT symptoms are the initial complaints in 90% of patients (rhinorrhea, purulent or bloody nasal discharge, sinus pain, nasal mucosal drying and crust formation, epistaxis, and otitis media).

- Major organs affected: "ELKS," i.e., **E**NT, **L**ungs, **K**idney, and **S**kin.
- ENT symptoms are the initial complaints in 90% of patients.
- Nasal septal perforation and ulceration of the vomer bone

are two important signs.
- Differential diagnosis of "saddle-nose" deformity: Wegener's granulomatosis, relapsing polychondritis, and leprosy.

Ulcerated lesions of the larynx and trachea occur in 30% of untreated patients and subglottic stenosis in 8%-18% of treated patients. The pulmonary parenchyma is affected in more than 60% of patients. Symptoms include cough, hemoptysis, and dyspnea. The clinical manifestations can range from subacute to rapidly progressive respiratory failure. Most patients with pulmonary symptoms have associated nodular infiltrates on CXR. Hemoptysis is seen in 98% of patients and CXR abnormalities in 65%, including unilateral (55% of patients), bilateral (45%), infiltrates (63%), nodules (31%), infiltrates with cavitation (8%), and nodules with cavitation (10%). CXR shows rounded opacities (from a few millimeters to several centimeters large). The nodules are usually bilateral and one-third cavitate. Solitary nodules occur in 30%-40% of patients. Pneumonic infiltrates, lobar consolidation, and pleural effusions are also seen. Typical interstitial infiltrates are uncommon. Massive pulmonary alveolar hemorrhage is occasionally a life-threatening emergency. Benign stenoses of the tracheobronchial tree are more likely in chronic cases and in patients whose disease is stable. Because opportunistic infection by *Pneumocystis carinii* is common in patients receiving corticosteroid therapy for Wegener's granulomatosis, chemoprophylaxis against this organism is recommended for these patients.

- Hemoptysis in almost all patients.
- CXR: multiple nodules or masses with cavitation in 35% of patients.
- Diffuse alveolar infiltrates indicate alveolar hemorrhage; diffuse alveolar hemorrhage found in 5%-45% of biopsy/autopsy-documented cases.
- Tracheobronchial stenosis occurs in 15%.

Laboratory Findings

Laboratory findings in Wegener's granulomatosis include an increased ESR, normochromic normocytic anemia, thrombocytosis, positive rheumatoid factor, and increase in immunoglobulin and circulating immune complexes. The identification of antineutrophil cytoplasmic antibodies in most of the patients with Wegener's granulomatosis has helped to establish the diagnosis in atypical or unusual cases of systemic vasculitis. Two main patterns of cytoplasmic fluorescence are recognized: granular with central-accentuated cytoplasmic (c-ANCA) and perinuclear (p-ANCA). The c-ANCA pattern is highly specific for Wegener's granulomatosis. When a restrictive definition of Wegener's granulomatosis is used (i.e., one that requires documented granulomatous inflammation of the lungs), c-ANCA is present in >90% of patients with untreated active disease. Its sensitivity is only about 65% pos-

itive in patients with granulomatous disease limited to the upper or lower respiratory tract or to both areas. In patients who are in remission, the sensitivity is about 30%.

- Wegener's granulomatosis: routine laboratory findings are nonspecific.
- c-ANCA is generally considered specific for Wegener's granulomatosis
- Titers of c-ANCA correlate with activity of the disease.

p-ANCA is positive in various diseases, including inflammatory bowel disease, autoimmune liver disease, rheumatoid arthritis, and many other vasculitides. p-ANCA with specificity against myeloperoxidase has been reported to be closely associated with microscopic polyangiitis, mononeuritis multiplex, leukocytoclastic vasculitis of the skin, pauci-immune necrotizing-crescentic glomerulonephritis, and other vasculitides affecting small vessels. Some cases of Churg-Strauss syndrome reportedly demonstrate p-ANCA with specificity for myeloperoxidase.

- p-ANCA has been noted in other vasculitides and collagen diseases.
- p-ANCA with specificity for myeloperoxidase should suggest small vessel vasculitis (microscopic polyangiitis).

Treatment

Corticosteroids with cyclophosphamide therapy are highly effective in Wegener's granulomatosis. A complete response is seen in >90% of patients. In milder cases, corticosteroid therapy alone may suffice. Many patients require prolonged treatment with smaller doses of corticosteroid and/or cyclophosphamide. Some physicians have observed resolution of Wegener's granulomatosis after treatment with an antimicrobial agent, trimethoprim-sulfamethoxazole. Subglottic stenosis may require surgical therapy.

- Cyclophosphamide and corticosteroids are effective.

Churg-Strauss Syndrome

Churg-Strauss syndrome, also known as "allergic granulomatosis and angiitis," is among the least common vasculitides. It is characterized by pulmonary and systemic vasculitis, extravascular granulomas, and eosinophilia, which occur exclusively in patients with asthma or a history of allergy. Allergic rhinitis, nasal polyps, nasal mucosal crusting, and septal perforation occur in >70% of the patients. Nasal polyposis is a major clinical finding. The chief pulmonary manifestation is asthma, which is noted in almost all patients. CXR abnormalities are noted in >60% of patients: patchy and occasionally diffuse alveolar-interstitial infiltrates in the perihilar area, with a predilection for the upper two-thirds of the lung fields.

A dramatic response can be expected with high doses of systemic corticosteroids.

- Refractory asthma and progressive respiratory distress should suggest Churg-Strauss syndrome.
- Allergic rhinitis, nasal polyps, nasal mucosal crusting, and septal perforation occur in >70% of patients.
- Tissue and blood hypereosinophilia and elevation of IgE are common.

Behçet's Disease

Behçet's disease is a chronic relapsing multisystemic inflammatory disorder characterized by aphthous stomatitis along with two or more of the following: aphthous genital ulcerations, uveitis, cutaneous nodules or pustules, synovitis, and meningoencephalitis. Occlusion of major vessels and aneurysms have been observed in 10%-37% of patients. Superficial and deep vein thromboses of the upper and lower extremities and thrombosis of the inferior and superior venae cavae occur in 7%-37% of patients. Pulmonary vascular involvement produces major hemoptysis. Serious hemoptysis, initially responsive to therapy with corticosteroids, tends to recur; death is due to hemoptysis in 39% of patients. CXR may show lung infiltrates, pleural effusions, prominent pulmonary arteries, and pulmonary artery aneurysms.

- Behçet's disease: major hemoptysis is the cause of death in 39% of patients.
- Fistula between the airway and vascular structures is common.
- High incidence of deep vein thrombosis and pulmonary thromboembolism.

Takayasu's Arteritis

Takayasu's arteritis, or "pulseless disease," is a chronic inflammatory disease of unknown cause that primarily affects the aorta and its major branches, including the proximal coronary arteries and renal arteries and the elastic pulmonary arteries. Pulmonary artery involvement is seen in >50% of patients, with lesions in the medium- and large-sized arteries. Early abnormalities occur in the upper lobes, whereas the middle and lower lobes are involved in later stages of the disease. Perfusion lung scans have shown abnormalities in >75% of patients.

- Takayasu's arteritis: pulmonary artery involvement in >50% of patients.

Urticarial Vasculitis

Urticarial vasculitis is manifested by urticarial lesions, pruritus, and arthralgias in 60% of the patients, arthritis in 28%, abdominal pain in 25%, and glomerulonephritis in 15%. Many of the pulmonary complications described have been in patients with the hypocomplementemic variety of the disease. Pulmonary vasculitis has not been demonstrated in patients with urticarial vasculitis. However, many of these patients have COPD, and up to 62% of patients with hypocomplementemic urticarial vasculitis acquire COPD. Many of these patients have been smokers.

- Higher incidence of COPD in patients with hypocomplementemic urticarial vasculitis.

Eosinophilia-Myalgia Syndrome

Dietary ingestion of L-tryptophan tablets was linked to an epidemic of eosinophilia-myalgia syndrome in 1989. Clinical manifestations of this syndrome included myalgias, fatigue, muscle weakness, arthralgias, edema of the extremities, skin rash, oral and vaginal ulcers, scleroderma-like changes, ascending neuropathy, and peripheral blood eosinophilia. About 60% of the patients had pulmonary complications: pulmonary infiltrates associated with severe pulmonary distress and progressive hypoxemia, pleural effusion, diffuse bilateral reticulonodular infiltrates, and pulmonary hypertension.

- Eosinophilia-myalgia syndrome is caused by a contaminant in L-tryptophan preparations.
- Features: pulmonary hypertension, interstitial granulomas, and respiratory distress.
- Identical etiopathologic mechanisms in eosinophilia-myalgia syndrome and Spanish toxic oil syndrome.

Essential Mixed Cryoglobulinemia

Essential mixed cryoglobulinemia is characterized by recurrent episodes of purpura, arthralgias, weakness, and multiorgan involvement. Histologic features are comparable to those of leukocytoclastic vasculitis. Increases in rheumatoid factor and cryoglobulin are frequent findings. Pulmonary insufficiency, Sjögren's syndrome-like illness with lung involvement, fibrosing alveolitis, and bronchiectasis have been described in isolated cases.

Polyarteritis Nodosa

Polyarteritis nodosa is characterized by a necrotizing arteritis of small- and medium-sized muscular arteries that involves multiple organ systems. It is important to recognize that this disease rarely affects the lungs. Although the earlier literature described vasculitis in the bronchial and pulmonary vasculature, many of the patients had granulomatous lesions with eosinophilic infiltrates. In retrospect, it appears that most of the patients with the diagnosis of pulmonary polyarteritis nodosa indeed had Churg-Strauss syndrome.

Secondary Vasculitis

Many of the rheumatologic diseases (e.g., systemic lupus erythematosus, rheumatoid arthritis, and scleroderma) demonstrate secondary vasculitic processes in the tissues involved. Certain infectious processes, particularly mycoses, may cause secondary vasculitis. When confronted with vasculitic lesions, the well-known etiologic agents such as drugs and chemicals should be considered.

Alveolar Hemorrhage Syndromes

Diffuse hemorrhage into the alveolar spaces is called "alveolar hemorrhage syndrome." Disruption of the pulmonary capillary lining may result from damage caused by different immunologic mechanisms (e.g., Goodpasture's syndrome, renal-pulmonary syndromes, glomerulonephritis, and systemic lupus erythematosus), direct chemical/toxic injury (toxic or chemical inhalation, trimellitic anhydride), physical trauma (pulmonary contusion), and increased vascular pressure within the capillaries (mitral stenosis, severe left ventricular failure). The severity of hemoptysis, anemia, and respiratory distress depends on the extent and rapidity with which bleeding occurs in the alveoli.

- Alveolar hemorrhage syndrome is caused by different mechanisms.
- Hemoptysis is not always present in alveolar hemorrhage syndrome.
- CXR may show a diffuse alveolar process, but this is not typical.
- Serial measurement of diffusing capacity is not a reliable test for continued intra-alveolar bleeding.
- The presence of hemosiderin-laden macrophages in bronchoalveolar lavage or sputum is not a dependable test for diagnosing alveolar hemorrhage syndrome.

Goodpasture's Syndrome

Goodpasture's syndrome is a classic example of cytotoxic (type II) disease. The Goodpasture antigen (located in type IV collagen) is the primary target for the autoantibodies of patients with Goodpasture's syndrome or anti-glomerular basement membrane disease. The highest concentration of Goodpasture antigen is in the glomerular basement membrane. The alveolar basement membrane is affected by cross-reactivity with the glomerular basement membrane. Lung biopsy reveals diffuse alveolar hemorrhage and intra-alveolar hemosiderin-laden macrophages. Immunofluorescent microscopy shows linear deposition of IgG and complement (in contrast to the "lumpy-bumpy" deposition seen in systemic lupus erythematosus) along basement membranes. Anti-glomerular basement membrane (GBM) antibody is positive in >90% of patients with Goodpasture's syndrome, but it is also present in persons exposed to influenza virus, hydrocarbons, and peni-cillamine and in some patients with systemic lupus erythematosus, polyarteritis nodosa, and Schönlein-Henoch purpura. Some patients are reported to exhibit p-ANCA with and without anti-GBM antibody. The male-to-female ratio is 7:1, with an average age of 27 years at the time of diagnosis. Recurrent hemoptysis from intra-alveolar hemorrhage, pulmonary insufficiency, renal involvement, and anemia are the main features. CXR shows a diffuse alveolar filling process. Treatment consists of high doses of corticosteroids and plasmapheresis.

- Goodpasture's syndrome: example of a type II (cytotoxic) immune reaction.
- Anti-GBM antibody is present in >90% of patients with Goodpasture's syndrome.
- Anti-GBM antibody is not specific for Goodpasture's syndrome.
- Smoking increases the risk of bleeding.

Glomerulonephritis

Nearly 50% of the patients with alveolar hemorrhage syndromes caused by a renal mechanism do not have anti-GBM antibody. The mechanism of alveolar hemorrhage in these patients is mediated by immune-complex disease. Several vasculitic syndromes belong to this group. The alveolar hemorrhage syndrome in systemic lupus erythematosus and other vasculitides is discussed elsewhere.

Vasculitides

Diffuse alveolar hemorrhage is sometimes seen in patients with vasculitides. Alveolar hemorrhage is rare as an initial symptom of Wegener's granulomatosis and is more common in Churg-Strauss syndrome and Schönlein-Henoch purpura. Alveolar hemorrhage is much more common in Behçet's disease than in other vasculitides. Pulmonary capillaritis is a distinct histologic lesion, characterized by extensive neutrophilic infiltration of the alveolar interstitium. Subclinical alveolar hemorrhage may occur in patients with this disease. This pathologic lesion can be seen in various vasculitides such as Wegener's granulomatosis, microscopic polyarteritis, systemic lupus erythematosus, and other collagen diseases. p-ANCA with specificity to myeloperoxidase may be positive in patients with pulmonary capillaritis.

Mitral Valve Disease

Diffuse alveolar hemorrhage is a well-known feature of mitral stenosis, even though the possibility is rarely considered in clinical practice. Severe mitral insufficiency can also produce alveolar hemorrhage. In surgically untreated patients, recurrent episodes of alveolar hemorrhage may lead to chronic hemosiderosis of the lungs, fibrosis, and punctate calcification/ossification of the lung parenchyma.

- Mitral stenosis is an important cause of alveolar hemorrhage syndrome.

Idiopathic Pulmonary Hemosiderosis

Idiopathic pulmonary hemosiderosis is a rare disorder of unknown cause. It is manifested as recurrent intra-alveolar hemorrhage, hemoptysis, and secondary iron deficiency anemia. Most cases begin in childhood. Although this disease is often fatal, a prolonged course is common. In childhood, the male-to-female ratio is 1:1; in adults, it is 3:1. Pathologic features include hemosiderin-laden macrophages. No autoimmune phenomena are noted. Some patients have cold agglutinins. The iron content in the lung depends on the duration of the disease. Clinical features are chronic cough with intermittent hemoptysis, iron deficiency anemia, fever, and weight loss. CXR shows transient, blotchy, perihilar alveolar infiltrates in the mid and lower lung fields. Small nodules, fibrosis, and cor pulmonale may also be found. Treatment is repeated blood transfusions, iron therapy, corticosteroids, and, possibly, cytotoxic agents. A 30% mortality rate within 5 years after disease onset has been reported. Idiopathic pulmonary hemosiderosis is a diagnosis of exclusion.

- Idiopathic pulmonary hemosiderosis: chronic cough with intermittent hemoptysis and iron deficiency anemia.
- Generalized lymphadenopathy in 25% of patients, hepatosplenomegaly in 20%, and clubbing in 15%.
- The kidneys are not involved.
- Eosinophilia occurs in 10% of patients.

Toxic Alveolar Hemorrhage

Fumes or dust of trimellitic anhydride (a component of certain plastics, paints, and epoxy resins) act as a hapten to cause acute rhinitis and asthmatic symptoms if exposure is minor. With greater exposure, alveolar hemorrhage probably occurs by a different immunologic mechanism. The trimellitic anhydride-hemoptysis anemia syndrome occurs after "high-dose exposure" to fumes. Antibodies to trimellitic anhydride, human proteins, and erythrocytes have been found in these patients. Other toxins known to cause alveolar hemorrhage syndromes are penicillamine and mitomycin C.

LUNGS IN NONPULMONARY DISEASES

Rheumatoid Arthritis

"Rheumatoid lung" indicates diffuse interstitial pneumonitis and fibrosis associated with rheumatoid arthritis. It is the most serious pleuropulmonary complication of the disease. CXR shows this process in 1.6%-4.5% of patients, whereas the results of PFTs suggest a restrictive lung process in more than 30%. Clinical, physiologic, and histologic features mimic those of idiopathic pulmonary fibrosis. CXR reveals a bibasilar interstitial process, micronodules, or (in late stages of the disease) honeycombing.

Rheumatoid (necrobiotic) nodules occur in the lung parenchyma. These are more common in men and in those with seropositive rheumatoid arthritis. The nodules may precede the arthritic symptoms. Rheumatoid nodules produce minimal symptoms. They are from a few millimeters to several centimeters in size, are usually bilateral, and occur near pleuropulmonary surfaces. Two-thirds of them cavitate. Rheumatoid pneumoconiosis (Caplan's syndrome) is pneumoconiosis associated with rheumatoid nodules. It is found in persons with silicosis, asbestosis, aluminosis, and other conditions. This syndrome is characterized by pulmonary nodules (1-5 cm in diameter) that evolve rapidly and may undergo cavitation.

Rheumatoid pleurisy is the most common thoracic manifestation of rheumatoid arthritis. In clinical practice, its incidence is 8% in males and 1.6% in females with rheumatoid arthritis. One-third of the patients with rheumatoid pleurisy remain asymptomatic. Pleural effusion may precede the onset of arthritic symptoms by months. Pleural fluid analysis shows that the effusion is typically an exudate, usually yellow and rarely bloody. Chronic effusions appear opalescent green because of a high cholesterol content ("pseudochylothorax"). The glucose level is very low (<30 mg/dL) in >80% of patients.

Obstructive airway disease is seen in one-third of patients with rheumatoid arthritis. Histologic findings include follicular bronchiolitis and bronchitis. The combination of rheumatoid arthritis and smoking is associated with a much higher prevalence of obstructive lung disease than is either of these conditions alone. A genetic predisposition to obstructive lung disease may be a contributing factor.

- Pulmonary manifestations are more common in males with rheumatoid arthritis.
- Pleural involvement occurs in up to 10% of patients; fluid has low glucose levels and high cholesterol levels.
- Rheumatoid lung mimics idiopathic pulmonary fibrosis.
- Obstructive airway disease is seen in 34% of patients with rheumatoid arthritis.

Systemic Lupus Erythematosus

Pleural involvement is the most common and, often, the presenting feature of systemic lupus erythematosus in 50%-83% of patients. Painful pleurisy is observed in 50% of patients. Pleural effusions are small to moderate and bilateral in 50% of patients. The fluid is almost always an exudate, and the glucose level is normal or high. Levels of C50 as well as of C3 and C4 are decreased in 80% of patients. Lupus erythematosus cells have been found in 0 to >85% of effusions. The presence of these cells is specific for lupus pleuritis. Diffuse interstitial pneumonitis is distinctly uncommon in systemic lupus erythematosus. Patchy and irregular areas of interstitial pneumonitis and fibrosis develop in 15%-45% of patients with systemic lupus erythematosus. Plate-like or discoid atelectasis is more common and occurs in the lower two-thirds of the lung fields. Infectious processes, particularly in patients receiving immunosuppressive therapy for systemic lupus erythematosus, are the most common cause of pulmonary parenchymal infiltrates. PFTs usually reveal a restrictive dysfunction.

Pulmonary hemorrhage is an important complication that is noted in up to 10% of patients. Renal disease from systemic lupus erythematosus enhances the risk of alveolar hemorrhage. Pulmonary hemorrhage may range from subclinical to massive. Significant hemoptysis is observed in 8%-15% of patients. CXR reveals bibasal, patchy, alveolar infiltrates. The mortality from systemic lupus erythematosus-induced alveolar hemorrhage is >50%, with patients dying within several days after the onset of hemoptysis.

Pulmonary embolism is more common than in other collagenoses in systemic lupus erythematosus because of the lupus anticoagulant syndrome (manifested by a prolonged activated partial thromboplastin time, normal clotting and platelet counts, presence of anticardiolipin antibody, and false-positive results on the VDRL test). Long-term anticoagulation therapy is required to prevent venous thromboembolic phenomena. Pulmonary hypertension is rare in systemic lupus erythematosus. Lupus pneumonitis, a rare feature of systemic lupus erythematosus, is characterized by acute dyspnea, high fever, and cough with occasional hemoptysis. Diaphragmatic dysfunction has been described in some patients, but the clinical significance of this finding is unclear, even though it may account for the "unexplained dyspnea." Drug-induced systemic lupus erythematosus is described above.

- Pleural involvement is common in systemic lupus erythematosus; low complement level in pleural fluid.
- Diffuse pulmonary infiltrates and fibrosis are very uncommon.
- Alveolar hemorrhage is seen in 10% of patients; significant hemoptysis in 10%.
- Pulmonary embolism is relatively common (due to lupus anticoagulant).
- Lupus pneumonitis is rare.
- Pleural effusion is more common with procainamide- and hydralazine-induced systemic lupus erythematosus than with other drug-induced forms of the disease.

Scleroderma (Progressive Systemic Sclerosis)

Diffuse pulmonary fibrosis is seen in up to 80% of patients at post mortem, even though many patients are minimally symptomatic during life. Chronic progressive pulmonary fibrosis is seen in two-thirds of patients and is the most common respiratory complication. The pathologic features are identical to those of idiopathic pulmonary fibrosis. One-third of patients have abnormal CXR, but >50% complain of exertional dyspnea and exhibit low diffusing capacity. Pulmonary involvement is more severe in the CREST (Calcinosis, Raynaud's phenomenon, Esophageal involvement, Sclerodactyly, and Telangiectasia) variant of scleroderma. The most common abnormality on PFTs is the slow but progressive restrictive dysfunction with low diffusing capacity. The earliest abnormality is the decreased diffusing capacity; deterioration in PFT results is an important predictor of mortality. Aspiration pneumonia results from the esophageal dysfunction and reflux that are extremely common in scleroderma. Pulmonary hypertension is common in scleroderma, especially in the CREST variant, and is a major cause of mortality and morbidity. The pathogenic mechanisms include chronic hypoxemia due to pulmonary fibrosis and/or medial hypertrophy of the pulmonary arteries. The latter mechanism, which is independent of the arterial changes caused by hypoxia, is responsible for pulmonary hypertension in 35%-60% of patients.

- Diffuse lung fibrosis (similar to that of idiopathic pulmonary fibrosis) is seen in most patients.
- Aspiration pneumonia: due to esophageal dysfunction and reflux.
- Pulmonary hypertension: major cause of morbidity and mortality.
- All pulmonary complications are more severe in CREST syndrome.
- Pleural disease, pleural effusion, obstructive disease, and hemoptysis are uncommon in scleroderma.

Polymyositis-Dermatomyositis

Interstitial pneumonitis and fibrosis, occurring in the basal areas of the lungs, are the most common pulmonary abnormalities and are seen in 5%-10% of patients. Pulmonary disease caused by polymyositis may present as acute pneumonitis with alveolar or mixed alveolar-interstitial infiltrates. There is no relationship between the severity and progression of the myositis and the severity of respiratory disease. More than 50% of patients with anti-Jo1 antibody exhibit interstitial pulmonary disease. Not all patients demonstrate this antibody in their serum. In 35% of patients, pulmonary disease precedes the skin and/or myopathic features by 1-24 months. Pulmonary disease presents as dyspnea, cough, and hypoxemia; symptoms related to gastroesophageal reflux may be the initial manifestation in some patients. Aspiration pneumonitis is a common feature because of esophageal involvement. A restrictive type of lung dysfunction is present in nearly 50% of patients. Poor cough strength due to weakness of respiratory muscles augments the progression of aspiration pneumonia, which is the cause of death in 10% of patients. Hypoventilation results from proximal myopathy. Progressive hypoventilation and respiratory failure manifested by increasing hypercarbia are poor prognostic signs. Paraneoplastic variant of polymyositis-dermatomyositis (see Lung Cancer) should be differentiated from the idiopathic or autoimmune types of the disease discussed here. When elderly patients present with polymyositis-dermatomyositis, an underlying malignancy must be excluded before considering the diagnosis of autoimmune polymyositis-dermatomyositis.

● Polymyositis-dermatomyositis: interstitial pneumonitis and fibrosis in up to 10% of patients.
● >50% of patients with anti-Jo1 antibody in their serum have interstitial pulmonary disease.
● Aspiration pneumonia due to esophageal dysfunction causes death in 10% of patients.
● Hypoventilation due to proximal myopathy is the leading cause of death.
● Weakness of proximal muscles and a characteristic skin rash (heliotrope hue).

Mixed Connective Tissue Disease

Patients with mixed connective tissue disease have the clinical features of systemic lupus erythematosus, scleroderma, and polymyositis-dermatomyositis and high titers of a specific circulating antibody to an extractable nuclear ribonucleoprotein antigen. Most of the patients are women, and the average age at time of diagnosis is 37 years. Renal disease occurs in 10%-20% of patients, and pulmonary involvement is observed in 20%-80%. Many of the clinical and pathophysiologic pleuropulmonary manifestations are similar to those observed in systemic lupus erythematosus, scleroderma, and polymyositis-dermatomyositis. Abnormal findings on PFTs and CXR have been observed in 69% of asymptomatic patients, impaired diffusing capacity in 67%, and restrictive lung volumes in 50%. Pleurisy is one of the common manifestations of the disease, with an incidence of 6%-40%. Pleural fluid shows the same characteristics as that in systemic lupus erythematosus. The effusions are usually small and resolve spontaneously. Pulmonary hypertension is the most serious complication of mixed connective tissue disease and is noted in up to 67% of patients.

● Mixed connective tissue disease: clinical features of systemic lupus erythematosus, scleroderma, and polymyositis-dermatomyositis.
● Features: pulmonary fibrosis, pleural effusion, aspiration pneumonia, and pulmonary hypertension.

Ankylosing Spondylitis

Ankylosing spondylitis is a chronic disorder of unknown cause characterized by progressive inflammatory disease involving the axial spine and adjacent soft tissues. The sacroiliac, hip, and shoulder joints are commonly affected. It is distinctly a disease of males. Pulmonary involvement is reported in 2%-70% of the patients. Pulmonary problems include chest wall restriction due to ankylosis of the costovertebral joints, fibrosis of the lung apices, and, rarely, apical cavitations. The most common abnormality is the fibrobullous apical lesion, which is noted in 14%-30% of cases. Bullous changes, mycetomas, parenchymal fibrosis, and bronchiectasis are other complications. The cavitated lesions may occasionally become infected by *Aspergillus, M. avium* complex, or *M. kansasii.* Pleural effusion is rare. Fixation of the cricoarytenoid with respiratory distress, calcification and ossification of cartilaginous structures in the upper airways, ankylosing hyperostosis of cervical spines, and bilateral vocal cord paralysis with airway obstruction have been described. Costovertebral ankylosis seldom produces pulmonary symptoms even though PFTs show diminished total lung capacity, vital capacity, and diffusing capacity. Increased residual volume and functional residual capacity are common findings.

● In clinical practice, <5% of patients with ankylosing spondylitis have pulmonary problems.
● Fibrobullous lesions in the lung apices; they may become infected secondarily.
● Diaphragmatic calcification develops in a small number of patients.

Sjögren's Syndrome

Pulmonary complications are seen in both the primary and secondary forms of Sjögren's syndrome and occur in 1.5%-75% of patients. These complications include desiccation of the upper respiratory tract (xerotrachea), obstructive process involving both large and small airways, localized infiltrates, bronchiectasis, pleurisy, and pleural effusion. The diffuse interstitial process in Sjögren's syndrome (seen in 1% of patients) usually represents lymphocytic interstitial pneumonitis. Both primary and secondary forms of Sjögren's syndrome are associated with lymphoproliferative diseases in the respiratory system. Pulmonary involvement by lymphoma is associated with the syndrome in 15%-20% of patients. Hilar lymphadenopathy or masses should also suggest the likelihood of lymphoma. Most of these lymphomas are of B-cell origin and respond favorably to therapy.

● Sjögren's syndrome: diffuse lung infiltrate usually represents lymphocytic interstitial pneumonitis.
● The most serious complication is lymphoma.
● Cough is common, due to xerotrachea.

Lymphomatoid Granulomatosis

Lymphomatoid granulomatosis is a lymphoproliferative disease and not a vasculitis, even though it is characterized by prominent vascular infiltrates and necrosis along with granulomatosis. In the same patient, the histologic features form a spectrum from benign-appearing lymphocytic interstitial pneumonitis to frank lymphoma. Lymphoma develops in more than 50% of patients. Multisystem involvement is common. CXR findings are similar to those in Wegener's granulomatosis, with patchy ill-defined infiltrates and multiple nodules. Nearly one-third of the nodules cavitate. The presence of hilar lymphadenopathy suggests lymphomatous changes. Mean age at diagnosis for males is 48 years; the male-to-female ratio is 1.7:1. Cough, dyspnea, hemoptysis, fever, weight loss, malaise, central nervous system symptoms, and peripheral neuropathy are common. Dermal lesions occur in 30% of patients. The prognosis is poor.

- Lymphomatoid granulomatosis is a lymphoproliferative disease.
- The clinical features may resemble those of Wegener's granulomatosis.

Relapsing Polychondritis

Relapsing polychondritis, a rare disease of unknown cause, affects cartilage throughout the body. It is an autoimmune disease and has been described in association with Wegener's granulomatosis, systemic lupus erythematosus, cryptogenic cirrhosis, and hydralazine therapy. Even though the involvement of the tracheobronchial cartilage is a late phenomenon, >50% of deaths are due to respiratory involvement. Diagnosis is made by noting inflammation of two or more cartilaginous sites. Other manifestations are iritis, episcleritis, hearing deficit, cataracts, aortic valvular insufficiency, anemia, increased ESR, and liver dysfunction. Treatment with high doses of corticosteroids is reportedly beneficial.

- Relapsing polychondritis: expiratory collapse of the major airways.
- Features: recurrent lung infections and respiratory distress.

Leukemia

The lungs are commonly involved in late leukemia. Infection is the most common cause of death. Mediastinal and hilar adenopathy are seen in 25% of patients (especially in chronic lymphocytic leukemia), parenchymal involvement in 25% (especially in acute monomyelocytic leukemia and chronic lymphocytic leukemia), pleural effusion in 20%, and pulmonary hemorrhage in 6%.

- Leukemic lung infiltrates are uncommon.
- The most common cause of infiltrates is infection.

- Patients who are receiving chemotherapy and develop prolonged (>3 weeks) granulocytopenia are most likely to have disseminated aspergillosis.

Plasma Cell Dyscrasia

Amyloidosis involving the lungs is common in the primary form of amyloidosis. The diffuse type has a poor prognosis. Tracheobronchial amyloidosis produces diffuse submucosal infiltration and hemoptysis. Solitary amyloidoma presents as a lung mass. Myeloma is seen as a direct extension of a rib lesion, plasmacytoma, parenchymal infiltrates (rare), or as a pleural effusion (rare). Waldenström's macroglobulinemia produces effusion in 50% of patients and may also produce parenchymal infiltrates.

- Amyloidosis is also associated with sleep apnea (macroglossia).
- Secondary amyloidosis associated with chronic bronchiectasis and other chronic lung diseases is a pathologic finding with minimal clinical problems.

Transfusion Reactions

Transfusion-related acute lung injury is a form of noncardiogenic pulmonary edema. It is caused by the passive transfer of granulocyte or lymphocyte antibodies in the donor serum. HLA-specific antibodies are identified in the donor sera of 65% of patients who have this reaction. Acute respiratory distress occurring within 4 hours (after 2 hours in most) after transfusion is typical. Clinical manifestations include chills, fever, tachycardia, dry cough, and blood eosinophilia. CXR shows perihilar patchy opacities. Recovery is rapid and complete in almost all patients.

- Consider transfusion-related reaction if CXR findings suggest pulmonary edema.

Hemoglobinopathies

Sickle cell anemia is the most important entity. Pulmonary infections are seen in >50% of patients; *S. pneumoniae* is frequently implicated. Acute chest syndrome is a life-threatening complication of sickle cell anemia characterized by chest pain, fever, prostration, and CXR abnormalities. Pulmonary infarctions are common in adults. Lung functions in chronic cases show a restrictive pattern. Recurrent pulmonary embolism and infarction may produce pulmonary hypertension. Pneumovax is indicated for all patients with sickle cell disease. Hydroxyurea significantly decreases the frequency of acute chest syndrome and other complications.

- Recurrent lung infections (*S. pneumoniae*).
- Pneumovax is important (asplenia or hyposplenia).
- Acute chest syndrome: chest pain, fever, prostration, and

CXR abnormalities.

- Recurrent pulmonary embolism and secondary pulmonary hypertension.

Methemoglobinemia

Methemoglobinemia occurs when >1% of blood hemoglobin is oxidized to the ferric form. Physicians should check for asymptomatic cyanosis, normal Pa_{O_2}, low Sa_{O_2}, and a history of drug ingestion.

- Methemoglobinemia: normal Pa_{O_2}, low Sa_{O_2}.

Renal Diseases

Many pulmonary complications are seen in renal diseases. "Uremic lung" is a form of noncardiogenic pulmonary edema that occurs in acute and chronic renal failure. "Butterfly" shadows (alveolar infiltrates limited to the inner two-thirds of both lungs, with sparing of peripheral areas) seen on CXR should suggest this diagnosis. The CXR changes are proportional to the degree of azotemia and acidosis in acute renal failure. Pleural effusion is common in acute and chronic renal failure, uremia, and nephrotic syndrome and in patients receiving peritoneal and hemodialysis. In most cases, the fluid is a transudate. Pulmonary calcification occurs in chronic renal failure, especially in patients receiving chronic maintenance hemodialysis, and in secondary hyperparathyroidism. It is due to "metastatic calcification" of the lungs. CXR shows soft infiltrates that resemble pulmonary edema. The diagnosis is made by demonstrating pulmonary uptake of [99]technetium diphosphonate in radionuclide scans. Hypoxemia during dialysis is the result of hypoventilation to compensate for the loss of CO_2 through the dialysis membrane. Pulmonary-renal syndromes, sometimes called "lung purpura," consist of those entities in which the lungs and kidneys are affected by the same pathologic process. Examples include Goodpasture's syndrome, Wegener's granulomatosis, Schönlein-Henoch purpura, Churg-Strauss syndrome, systemic lupus erythematosus, scleroderma, and drug-induced vasculitis.

- Uremic lung (pulmonary edema) is proportional to degree of azotemia; it produces a "butterfly" alveolar pattern on CXR.
- Subdiaphragmatic pleural effusions (small transudates) are common in renal diseases.
- Pulmonary calcification occurs with chronic hemodialysis.
- Hypoventilation (thus, low Pa_{O_2}) during hemodialysis is due to the loss of CO_2 through the dialysis membrane.

Gastrointestinal Diseases

It is important to look for hiatal hernia and air-fluid level behind the heart on CXR. Check for a history of aspiration. Aspiration pneumonia should be considered in any patient with esophageal problems or symptoms. Peptic ulcer disease and COPD frequently exist together, perhaps because gastric hypersecretion is stimulated by increased arterial P_{CO_2} and decreased P_{O_2}. Gastrectomy patients have an increased incidence of pulmonary tuberculosis. Celiac sprue is reported in association with pulmonary hemosiderosis and fibrosis. Chronic ulcerative colitis and Crohn's ileitis are associated with an increased incidence of asthma, obstructive airway disease, bronchiectasis, and upper airway involvement. Whipple's disease is associated with cough (50% of patients), hilar adenopathy, and pleuropericardial effusions.

- Hiatal hernia and other esophageal problems should be considered in determining the cause of aspiration pneumonia and other lung problems.
- Tuberculosis occurs in postgastrectomy patients.

Hepatic Diseases

Pleural effusion is found in 6% of patients with hepatic cirrhosis; it is usually right-sided and almost always associated with ascites. The fluid is identical in character to ascitic fluid. Uninfected fluid is usually a transudate. A large amount of peritoneal fluid may push both hemidiaphragms superiorly, causing respiratory distress. Unless ascites is treated adequately, pleural fluid continues to accumulate despite repeated thoracentesis. Arterial hypoxemia is common in hepatic cirrhosis and is the result of venoarterial shunting in the basal regions of the lungs. Orthodeoxia (desaturation in the upright posture) and platypnea (dyspnea in the upright posture) are due to increased right-to-left shunting from gravitational forces. α_1-Antitrypsin deficiency may be associated with cirrhosis of the liver, especially in children.

- Ascites: right-sided pleural effusion; usually a transudate.
- Pleural fluid persists unless ascites is treated adequately.
- Dyspnea (platypnea) and hypoxemia (orthodeoxia) are made worse by standing.
- α_1-Antitrypsin deficiency is associated with cirrhosis.

Pancreatic Diseases

Acute pancreatitis can produce adult respiratory distress syndrome, pulmonary edema, left-sided pleural effusion, elevation of hemidiaphragm, and basal atelectasis. The incidence of pleural effusion is 3%-15%; effusion is left-sided in 95% of patients. The pleural fluid exhibits increased amylase and exudative levels of proteins. Pulmonary edema (adult respiratory distress syndrome) is seen in 20%-50% of patients with acute pancreatitis. It is related to the diminished production of lecithin, the main constituent of the surfactant dipalmitoyl lecithin. Massive effusions and pleurocutaneous fistulae are seen in chronic pancreatitis.

- Adult respiratory distress syndrome is the most serious pulmonary complication of pancreatitis.
- Pleural effusion (exudate) is left-sided in 95% of patients; bloody in 30%.

Endocrine Diseases

Acromegaly is associated with sleep apnea. Thyroid goiter causes tracheal deviation and cough; stridor and superior vena cava syndrome are rare. Of intrathoracic goiters, 85% are anterior to the trachea and present as anterior mediastinal masses. The other 15% arise from the posterior aspect. Thyrotoxicosis is seen in some patients. Intrathoracic extension of goiter does not predispose to malignant changes. Calcification within the mass is common. Thyrotoxicosis commonly produces exertional dyspnea; this is related to myopathy, increased work of breathing, and increased oxygen uptake. Asthma is difficult to manage in thyrotoxicosis because of more sensitive bronchomotor tone and rapid metabolism of bronchodilators. Myxedema may be associated with pleural effusions that are small and transudates. Both central and obstructive sleep apnea occur in myxedema, and both resolve with treatment of myxedema. Diabetes mellitus is associated with an increased incidence of bronchitis, tuberculosis, and mucormycosis. Cushing's syndrome and excessive steroid therapy may produce mediastinal lipomatosis and widening (chest CT is diagnostic). Electrolyte imbalances can affect respiratory function. Severe hypophosphatemia can cause respiratory muscle weakness and respiratory failure. Hypokalemia and hypomagnesemia can also cause respiratory weakness.

- No increased risk of malignant transformation with intrathoracic goiters.
- Thyrotoxic dyspnea is common and is related to myopathy and increased work of breathing.
- Obstructive and central sleep apnea are seen in myxedema; both resolve with treatment of myxedema.
- Severe metabolic alkalosis can present as hypercarbic respiratory acidosis (due to compensatory hypoventilation).

Pregnancy

Dyspnea occurs during the second (in 50% of pregnant women) and third (in 75%) trimesters. Increased resting ventilation is common. Hiatal hernia (moderately symptomatic) occurs in 60% of pregnant women. Pulmonary edema occurs in eclampsia, toxemia, and amniotic fluid embolism and with the use of tocolytics (β_2-agonists). Amniotic fluid embolism accounts for 8% of maternal deaths. Varicella pneumonia and coccidioidomycosis carry higher morbidity and mortality in pregnant women. Sarcoidosis resolves during pregnancy (perhaps because of estrogens) but recurs post partum. Molar pregnancy is associated with trophoblastic embolization into the lungs in 10% of women undergoing evacuation of hydatidi-

form mole. Choriocarcinoma metastasizes to the lung in 65% of cases.

Gynecology

Catamenial (associated with menses) pneumothorax is responsible for 5% of the cases of spontaneous pneumothorax in women ≤50 years. The cause is unclear, although diaphragmatic defects and endometriosis have been proposed. Almost all cases of pneumothorax are right-sided. Thoracic endometriosis may cause hemoptysis, atelectasis, and catamenial pneumothorax. In Meig-Salmon syndrome, ascites and pleural effusion occur in association with ovarian fibroma and other benign tumors. The effusions are frequently right-sided transudates. The effusion resolves with resection of the ovarian tumor.

Neurologic Diseases

Central (neurogenic) hypoventilation is usually from acquired causes such as narcotic overdosage, cerebral edema, central nervous system infections, myxedema, syringomyelia, and, in some cases, Parkinson's disease. Central hyperventilation is a regular, rapid breathing that keeps the rate of respiration in the range of 3-6 times normal for hours or days. Although the arterial oxygen level of these patients is normal, they are reported to have a high mortality rate. Neurogenic pulmonary edema is a complication of catastrophic cerebrovascular accidents, trauma to the head, epileptic seizures, and acute trauma to the spinal cord. This form of noncardiogenic pulmonary edema is thought to occur when increased intracranial pressure stimulates hypothalamic centers that release an excessive α-adrenergic discharge. This reaction produces increased systemic and pulmonary vascular resistance, severe hemodynamic alterations, and pulmonary edema. CXR shows asymmetrical, hazy, diffuse changes that persist even after pulmonary hemodynamics return to normal. Coma and loss of consciousness result in loss of airway protection, which in turn may lead to aspiration pneumonia. In chronic cases, recurrent pulmonary infections and pulmonary thromboembolism are serious threats to life.

Spinal cord disorders cause several lung problems. In patients with quadriplegia, lung volumes (total lung capacity and vital capacity) may be diminished by 33%-55% of predicted normal values. Most deaths associated with quadriplegia are due to pulmonary complications, such as hypoventilation, aspiration, ineffective cough, recurrent infections, and pulmonary emboli. Neuromyopathies that affect the respiratory system include myasthenia gravis, myasthenic syndrome, amyotrophic lateral sclerosis, polymyositis, periodic paralysis, acid maltase deficiency, hypokalemia, and hypophosphatemia. In myasthenia gravis, the risk of respiratory failure is increased by surgical procedures, infections, corticosteroid therapy, and the use of aminoglycosides. In addition to decreased static lung volumes, patients with neuromyopathies may have decreased inspiratory and expiratory forces. Testing of maximal inspiratory and expiratory pressures is a sensitive way to assess respiratory muscle weakness. Anterior horn cell disorders such as acute febrile polyneuritis (Guillain-Barré syndrome) and acute poliomyelitis produce hypoventilatory respiratory failure. Patients with myotonic dystrophy or progressive muscular dystrophy may have insidious chronic respiratory failure. Autonomic nervous system disorders such as familial dysautonomia can diminish the response to hypoxia and hypercapnia. Autonomic dysfunction due to diabetes mellitus, amyloidosis, and syringomyelia may progress to respiratory failure. Obstructive sleep apnea and central sleep apnea have been reported in autonomic disturbances.

- Neurogenic pulmonary edema is a form of noncardiogenic pulmonary edema caused by increased intracranial pressure.
- Aspiration pneumonia, recurrent pulmonary infections, and pulmonary thromboembolism occur in comatose and unconscious patients.
- In myasthenia gravis, the risk of respiratory failure is increased by surgical procedures, infections, corticosteroid therapy, and the use of aminoglycosides.
- Measurement of maximal inspiratory and expiratory pressures is a sensitive way to assess respiratory muscle weakness.
- Obstructive sleep apnea and central sleep apnea occur in diseases of the autonomic nervous system.
- In middle-aged or elderly persons with progressive respiratory deterioration, hypercapnia, and aspiration (with or without fasciculations), look for amyotrophic lateral sclerosis.

Diaphragmatic Paralysis

Unilateral diaphragmatic paralysis decreases total lung capacity by 35% and vital capacity and maximal voluntary ventilation by 20%. Bilateral diaphragmatic paralysis diminishes vital capacity by 50% in the upright position and perhaps by 60%-75% in the supine position. In patients with bilateral diaphragmatic paralysis, orthopnea is a major problem. Ipsilateral diaphragmatic dysfunction is frequently associated with hemiplegia. A sniff test (to demonstrate paradoxical motion) or diaphragmatic electromyography may be necessary to document diaphragmatic paralysis.

- Acute dyspnea in the supine posture should suggest the possibility of bilateral diaphragmatic paralysis.
- Diaphragmatic fluoroscopy (sniff test) is useful, but 6% of normal subjects have positive findings on this test.
- Chronic diaphragmatic paralysis (>6 months) usually is idiopathic in origin.
- Acute unilateral diaphragmatic paralysis should be evaluated; hilar mass should be excluded.

Skeletal Diseases

Kyphoscoliosis is the most common spinal deformity associated with pulmonary complications. The causes of scoliosis include congenital, neuropathic (poliomyelitis, cerebral palsy, and syringomyelia), myopathic (muscular dystrophy, amyotonia, and Friedreich's ataxia), and traumatic causes. It also occurs in mesenchymal disorders and in association with neurofibromatosis. Idiopathic scoliosis is the most common variety seen in clinical practice. A familial type is also reported. The curvature or angulation of a scoliotic spine is best measured by Cobb's scoliotic angle. Pulmonary symptoms are noted when the angle is >70 degrees. Angulation increases during younger life, and pulmonary symptoms appear during the fourth and fifth decades. The most common pulmonary abnormality is a decrease in static lung volumes: total lung capacity and vital capacity. There is an inverse correlation between the angle and vital capacity, total lung capacity, functional residual capacity, residual volume, and compliance. Although arterial hypoxemia is often present in symptomatic patients, $Paco_2$ is normal in most cases. Hypoventilation and $\dot{V}/\dot{Q}$ mismatch are mainly responsible for hypoxia. Pulmonary hypertension and cor pulmonale are serious complications. Pectus excavatum ("funnel chest"—caving in of the sternum and the anterior ends of the cartilages and ribs) is associated with pulmonary sequestration, Marfan syndrome, and *M. avium* complex infection. Pectus carinatum ("pigeon breast"—bulging or protrusion of the sternum and anterior cartilages and ribs) is associated with congenital heart disease.

- Pulmonary symptoms begin when the scoliotic angle is >70 degrees.
- Respiratory symptoms appear during the fourth and fifth decades.
- Although arterial hypoxemia is often present in symptomatic patients, $Paco_2$ is normal in most patients.
- Static lung volumes are diminished; an inverse relationship between scoliotic angle and lung volumes.
- Pectus deformities may be associated with congenital cardiac disorders.

PULMONARY INFECTIONS

Viral Infections

One-third of upper respiratory tract infections are caused by the rhinovirus group. The common cold is caused by rhinovirus, parainfluenza virus, adenovirus, respiratory syncytial virus, and coxsackievirus A21. Coxsackieviruses are a more frequent cause of viral respiratory tract infections in the summer and autumn. The virus cannot be isolated in 40% of respiratory tract infections presumed to be caused by a virus. Ciliary abnormalities with microtubular alterations (dysmorphic cilia) is a common acquired (transient) problem during acute viral illness. Therefore, temporary interference with mucociliary clearance may increase the risk of other infections. Viral respiratory tract infections constitute 83% of all acute infectious problems, and these infections are highly contagious. They have a seasonal variation: 50% of people have a viral respiratory tract infection during December-February and only 20% in June-August.

- Coxsackieviral infections are more frequent in the summer and autumn.
- Ciliary abnormalities are common (acquired and transient) during acute viral illness.

Viral Pneumonia

Viral pneumonia is caused by respiratory syncytial virus; parainfluenza virus types 1, 2, 3; adenovirus types 1, 2, 3, 5, 7; and influenza virus A and B. In adults, it is caused by influenza virus and adenovirus. Respiratory syncytial virus is the common cause of respiratory problems in children, and parainfluenza virus types 1 and 3 cause bronchiolitis. In adults, varicella pneumonia is a severe illness. Resolution of the disease may be followed by nodular pulmonary calcification. Herpesvirus may cause pneumonia in an immunocompromised host or in patients with extensive burns. Cytomegalovirus, a member of the herpesvirus group, is found in almost all body secretions of infected patients. This virus is seen more commonly in immunocompromised and transplant patients and in cases of lymphoreticular malignancy, cardiopulmonary bypass, and multiple blood transfusions and in association with *Pneumocystis carinii* infection (AIDS). Cytomegalovirus is the second most common infection in patients with AIDS. Diffuse, small nodular, or hazy infiltrates are seen on CXR in 15% of patients with pneumonia caused by cytomegalovirus, but interstitial pneumonia due to cytomegalovirus is seen in 50% of bone marrow graft recipients. Findings of inclusion bodies and high titers of cytomegalovirus may help in making the diagnosis.

- Viral pneumonia in nonimmunocompromised adults is caused by influenza virus and adenovirus.
- Varicella (chickenpox) pneumonia is more common in adults than in children and results in diffuse pulmonary calcification.
- Cytomegalovirus infection is more common in immunocompromised patients and in patients with AIDS.
- Isolation of cytomegalovirus from respiratory tract secretions does not always establish infection.

Influenza

Influenza is responsible for >50% of diagnosed viral pneumonias in adults. Influenza A pneumonia is a major cause of morbidity and mortality during the winter months in the U.S. Influenza B is more endemic than influenza A and is responsible for 20%-30% of influenza infections. Parainfluenza viruses are responsible for 15% of all viral pneumonias. Nearly all patients with influenza A pneumonia have underlying heart disease, usually rheumatic valvular disease. Clinical features are high fever, dyspnea, cyanosis, fluffy or nodular infiltrates in the mid lung fields, and respiratory failure. Annual (in the autumn) influenza vaccination is recommended for high-risk individuals (COPD, heart disease, diabetes mellitus, kidney disease, debilitated condition, >60 years old, and immunocompromised patients). Overall protection rates are 70%.

- Patients at risk for influenza infection: heart disease, COPD, kidney disease, diabetes mellitus, chronic anemia, and immunosuppressed.
- Secondary bacterial pneumonia is common.
- Coxsackievirus B causes pleurodynia (Bornholm disease or "devil's grip"): fever, headache, malaise, and severe pleuritic pain lasting from several days to weeks.

Hantavirus Pulmonary Syndrome

Hantavirus pulmonary syndrome, first recognized in the southwestern U.S. in May 1993, is caused by an RNA virus (family, Bunyaviridae; genus, *Hantavirus*). The rodent reservoir for this virus is the deer mouse (*Peromyscus maniculatus*). Through October 1993, 42 cases (from 12 states, all west of the Mississippi River) of this syndrome had been reported to the Centers for Disease Control. Subsequently, the disease has been diagnosed in nearly half the states and as far east as New York. The overall mortality rate has been 62%. Clinical features: median age of patients, 32 years (range, 12-69 years), males (52%), and Native Americans (55%). The illness is characterized by a prodrome of fever, myalgia, headache, abdominal pain, nausea or vomiting (or both), and cough, followed by the abrupt onset of respiratory distress. Bilateral pulmonary infiltrates that occur within 48 hours of onset of illness have been reported in all patients. Hemoconcentration in 71% and thrombocytopenia in 71%. Fever, hypoxia, and hypotension occur after hospitalization. For those in shock and who have lactic acidosis, the prognosis is poor. No sequelae have been reported in survivors. Autopsy has routinely revealed serous pleural effusions and heavy edematous lungs, with interstitial mononuclear cells in the alveolar septa, alveolar edema, focal hyaline membranes, and occasional alveolar hemorrhage. *Hantavirus* antigens are detected with immunohistochemistry. Serologic (*Hantavirus*-specific immunoglobulin M or increasing titers of IgG), polymerase chain reaction, and other studies are available through the Centers for Disease Control. Ribavirin trials are being conducted.

- The reservoir for *Hantavirus* is the deer mouse.
- The syndrome is more common in southwestern U.S.
- Features: febrile illness, unexplained respiratory distress, bilateral pulmonary infiltrates, and pleural effusion.
- Hemoconcentration, thrombocytopenia, shock, and hypoxemia.

Mycoplasma

Because humans are the only reservoir for *Mycoplasma*, spread is from person to person. Thus, infections occur in epidemic and endemic form and outbreaks occur in closed populations (e.g., military camps and colleges). Epidemics are more common in the summer and autumn. Illness is more common in school-aged children and young adults. The incubation period is 2-3 weeks. The predilection is for the respiratory tract. Clinical features include fever (85% of patients), coryza, pharyngitis (50%), bullous myringitis (20%), tracheobronchitis, cough (>95%), pleural effusion, hemolytic anemia, erythema multiforme, hepatitis, thrombocytopenia, and Guillain-Barré syndrome. Nearly 20% of all community-acquired pneumonias and 50% of all pneumonias in healthy young adults in close living quarters (e.g., military recruits and dormitory students) may be caused by *M. pneumoniae*. Pneumonia occurs in only 3%-10% of infected persons and is more likely in younger adults (military recruits or summer camps); it causes interstitial pneumonia and acute bronchiolitis. CXR shows unilateral bronchopneumonia, lower lobe involvement (65% of patients), and pleural effusion (5%). Cold agglutinins (>1:64 in 50% of patients) appear during the 2nd-3rd week after the onset of symptoms and the titer decreases to insignificant levels by 4-6 weeks. Complement fixation serology—a fourfold increase in titer noted in 50%-80% of patients. The organism can be cultured from respiratory tract secretions, the middle ear, and the cerebrospinal fluid.

- Epidemic and endemic forms in closed populations.
- Bullous myringitis, hemolytic anemia, erythema multiforme, and Guillain-Barré syndrome.
- Causes interstitial pneumonia and acute bronchiolitis.
- Cold agglutinins (>1:64 in 50% of patients) appear during 2nd-3rd week.

Bacterial Infections

Sinusitis

Most bacterial infections of sinuses occur after an acute viral infection of the nasal mucosa. Bacteria in acute (A) and chronic (C) sinusitis are: pneumococci (A, 20%-35% of patients; C, 5%-15%), *H. influenzae* (A, 15%-30%; C, 3%-10%), *Streptococcus,* anaerobes and aerobes (A, 5%-35%; C, 10%-25%), *S. aureus* (A, 3%-6%; C, 5%-15%), and no growth (A, 2%-25%; C, 25%-60%). *M. catarrhalis* is also frequently involved. The maxillary sinus is commonly involved, and nearly 10% of the cases of maxillary sinusitis are related to odontogenic infections. CT scans of the sinuses are better than traditional roentgenographs for detecting sinusitis.

- Sinus involvement is also seen in asthma, chronic bronchitis, bronchiectasis, cystic fibrosis, Kartagener's syndrome, and Wegener's granulomatosis.
- Fungal sinusitis is more common in granulocytopenic patients.

Otitis Media

The relationship between otitis media and common viral infections is strong, especially in children. Nearly 10% of children with measles have otitis media. Bacteria are isolated in 70%-80% of patients with otitis media and include pneumococci (25%-75% of patients), *H. influenzae* (15%-30%), anaerobes (peptococci and propionibacteria) (20%-30%), group A streptococci (2%-10%), and *S. aureus* (1%-5%). Ampicillin-resistant *H. influenzae* is found in 15%-40% of patients.

- Otitis media in adults occurs in severe diabetes mellitus and cystic fibrosis.

Pharyngitis

Pharyngitis is caused by group A *S. pyogenes* (>30% of patients), *N. gonorrhoeae, C. diphtheriae,* and *M. pneumoniae* (5%). Sore throat is also caused by adenovirus, Epstein-Barr virus, and other viruses.

Pneumonia

Streptococcal Pneumonia

Streptococcus pneumoniae is responsible for 90% of the cases of pneumonia in adults. It is most common in infants and the elderly. The incidence peaks in the winter and spring, when carrier rates in the general population may be as high as 70%. People at high risk include those with cardiopulmonary disease (especially pulmonary edema), viral respiratory infections, hemoglobinopathy, and hyposplenism and immune-suppressed patients. Many patients are elderly, alcoholic, or immunocompromised. The incidence of bacteremic pneumonia in hospitalized patients is 25% and carries a mortality rate of 20%. Bacteremic pneumonia in the elderly is not associated with fever in 30% but is associated with minimal respiratory symptoms in 50%, altered mental state in 50%, and volume depletion in 50%. Leukocytosis of 10,000-30,000/mm^3 is common. Sputum may be blood streaked or rusty. Early in the disease, CXR findings may be normal, but later, they may show classic lobar pneumonia. Pleurisy/effusion is common and cavitation is rare. About 20% of pneumococci are resistant to tetracycline and trimethoprim-sulfamethoxazole.

- A mortality rate of about 30% in bacteremic patients >50 years old.
- Mortality is associated with pneumococcal meningitis in 20%.

The pneumococcal vaccine consists of a mixture of highly purified capsular polysaccharide from the 23 most prevalent or invasive pneumococcal types accounting for at least 90% of pneumococcal pneumonias. It offers as much protection against drug-resistant as drug-sensitive pneumococci. The vaccination decreases serious complications of pneumococcal infection by about one-half and reduces the carrier state among the general population. Pneumococcal vaccination is recommended for elderly persons (>65 years) and for patients with diabetes mellitus, significant heart and lung diseases, renal insufficiency, hepatic insufficiency, sickle cell anemia, asplenia or hyposplenia, hematologic and other malignancies, chemotherapy, alcoholism, cerebrospinal fluid leakage, immune deficiency states, organ transplants, or AIDS. Some physicians recommend pneumococcal vaccination in all adults, especially in health care workers. Those who received the 13-valent vaccine should be revaccinated with the 23-valent vaccine. Even though the efficacy does not decline with increasing interval after vaccination in younger immunocompetent subjects, the pneumococcal antibody levels appear to wane with time. Primary vaccination and revaccination 6 or more years after a first dose of pneumococcal vaccine stimulate comparable mean antibody levels. Some institutions (American College of Physicians) recommend repeat vaccination every 10 years. Patients with nephrotic syndrome and other protein-losing nephropathies rapidly lose pneumococcal antibody and, thus, should receive pneumovax every 5-6 years. Pneumococcal vaccination should be given to pregnant women only if clearly needed.

- Overall efficacy of pneumococcal vaccine is 60%.
- Efficacy rates for certain diseases vary (diabetes mellitus, 84%; coronary artery disease, 73%; congestive heart failure, 69%; COPD, 65%; and anatomic asplenia, 77%).
- Pneumovax decreases the incidence of pneumonia by 79%-92%.

Staphylococcus Pneumonia

S. aureus occurs in the nasal passages of 20%-40% of normal adults, but pneumonia is uncommon. *S. aureus* pneumonia is more likely to occur in patients with severe diabetes mellitus, immunocompromised status, dialysis, drug abusers, and those with influenza or measles. In drug addicts, it may begin as septic emboli with right-sided endocarditis. It is one of the nosocomial types of pneumonia. Consolidation, bronchopneumonia, abscess with air-fluid level, pneumatocele, empyema, and a high mortality rate characterize staphylococcal pneumonia.

- Present in nasal passages of normal subjects.
- Immunocompromised, diabetics, and drug abusers.
- Lung abscess and pneumatoceles are more common.

Pseudomonas aeruginosa

P. aeruginosa is a ubiquitous organism commonly isolated from patients with cystic fibrosis and bronchiectasis. Pneumonia may occur in patients with COPD, congestive heart failure, diabetes mellitus, kidney disease, alcoholism, tracheostomy, prolonged ventilation, postoperative status, and compromised hosts. *Pseudomonas* pneumonia results in microabscess, alveolar hemorrhage, and necrotic areas. CXR may show bilateral, patchy infiltrates.

- *P. aeruginosa*: difficult to distinguish colonization from true infection.
- Important organism in cystic fibrosis, bronchiectasis, malignant otitis media, and ventilator patients.

Klebsiella pneumoniae

Pneumonia due to *K. pneumoniae* is more likely in alcoholics, diabetics, and hospitalized patients. Also, it is more common in males. Dependent lobes are affected more frequently. In lobar pneumonia caused by *K. pneumoniae*, CXR may show a "bulging fissure." Complications include abscess and empyema.

- *K. pneumoniae*: more likely to cause pneumonia in alcoholics, diabetics, and hospitalized patients.
- Bulging fissure sign.

Haemophilus influenzae

Unencapsulated strains of *H. influenzae* are present in the sputum of 30%-60% of normal adults and in 58%-80% of patients with COPD. In contrast, bacteremia is almost always associated with encapsulated strains. Both strains cause pulmonary infections and otitis, sinusitis, epiglottitis, and pneumonia. Most patients with pneumonia have underlying COPD or alcoholism, even though *H. influenzae* pneumonia develops in healthy military recruits. The amount of sputum production is significant. Pneumonia is seen in the lower lobes more often than in the upper lobes. CXR findings are typical for bronchopneumonia or lobar pneumonia. Pleural effusions occur in 30% of patients, and cavitation is rare.

- *H. influenzae*: both unencapsulated and encapsulated strains cause lung infections.
- Pleural effusion in 30% of patients with pneumonia; cavitation is rare.
- More common in those with COPD and alcoholism and in military recruits.

Moraxella (Branhamella) catarrhalis

M. catarrhalis is a gram-negative diplococcus that is part of the normal flora. Colonization is more common in the winter. It causes sinusitis, otitis, and pneumonia. The latter is more likely in patients with COPD, alcoholism, diabetes mellitus, and immunocompromised status. Bacteremia is rare. Infection produces segmental patchy bronchopneumonia in the lower lobes. Cavitation and pleural effusion are rare. These bacteria produce β-lactamase, and most are resistant to penicillin and ampicillin.

- *M. catarrhalis*: formerly known as *Branhamella*.
- COPD, immunocompromised status, and alcoholics.
- Most strains produce β-lactamase.

Legionella pneumophila

More than 20 species of *Legionella*, a gram-negative bacillus, have been identified. Water is its natural habitat. Disease results from inhalation of aerosolized organisms. Epidemics have occurred because of contaminated air-conditioning cooling towers, construction or excavation in contaminated soil, and contaminated hospital showers. Risk factors include COPD, smoking, cancer, diabetes mellitus, immunosuppression, and chronic heart and kidney diseases. Almost all cases of pneumonia are caused by *L. pneumophila* (85% of patients) and *L. micdadei* (10%). Bacteria can be demonstrated in tissue with Dieterle's stain and fluorescent antibody staining. Most cases occur in the summer and early autumn. Men older than 50 years are more likely to be infected than younger people. The incubation period is 2-10 days. Symptoms, in decreasing order of frequency, are: abrupt onset of cough (hemoptysis in 30% of patients), chills, dyspnea, headache, myalgia, arthralgia, and diarrhea. Common signs include fever, relative bradycardia, and change in mental status. The diagnosis is established by fluorescent antibody stain (FA stain), which is positive in the sputum in 20% of serologically positive patients. Bacteria can be cultured from tissue or other samples. Serology takes from 1 to 3 weeks before a titer of 1:64 is seen; peak titer is reached in 5-6 weeks. A titer of 1:128 is suspicious and a fourfold increase in titer is diagnostic.

- Risk factors: COPD, smoking, cancer, diabetes mellitus, immunosuppression, chronic heart and kidney diseases.
- Features: hyponatremia and hypophosphatemia in 50% of patients, lobar consolidations in 50%, leukocytosis (>10,000) in 60%, proteinuria in 20%, and increased SGOT in 60%.
- False-positive titer can be seen in plague, tularemia, leptospirosis, and adenovirus infections.
- *Legionella* serology titer of 1:128 is suspicious and a fourfold increase in titer is diagnostic.

Anaerobic Bacteria

Bacteroides melaninogenicus, Fusobacterium nucleatum, anaerobic cocci, and anaerobic streptococci are responsible for most cases of anaerobic pneumonia. *Bacteroides fragilis* is recovered from 15%-20% of patients with anaerobic pneumonia. Most of these anaerobes reside in the oropharynx as saprophytes. Common factors responsible for aspiration of anaerobes include altered consciousness, tooth extraction, poor dental hygiene, oropharyngeal infections, and drug overdose. Anaerobic bacterial infections may complicate underlying pulmonary problems (cancer, bronchiectasis, foreign body, etc.). Foul-smelling sputum is found in >50% of patients. Patchy pneumonitis in dependent segments may progress to lung abscess and empyema.

- Aspiration of anaerobes is associated with: altered consciousness, tooth extraction, poor dental hygiene, oropharyngeal infections, and drug overdose.
- Cavitated lung abscess in dependent lobes and empyema.

Community-Acquired "Atypical" Pneumonia

Organisms causing "atypical" community-acquired pneumonia include *Mycoplasma pneumoniae, Chlamydia psittaci, Chlamydia pneumoniae, Coxiella burnetii*, tularemia, and *Legionella* species. Mycoplasma pneumonia and legionellosis are discussed above. Community-acquired "typical" pneumonias are caused by *Streptococcus pneumoniae* (45% of patients), gram-negative bacilli (15%), and *Haemophilus influenzae* (15%).

- Community-acquired "atypical" pneumonia caused by *M. pneumoniae, C. psittaci, C. pneumoniae, C. burnetii*, and *Legionella* species.

Chlamydia pneumoniae (TWAR strain)

Chlamydia pneumoniae is confined to the human respiratory tract; no reservoirs are known. Person-to-person spread occurs among schoolchildren, family members, and military recruits. The incubation period is 10-65 days (mean, 31 days). Reinfection may be common, with cycles of disease every few years. About 15% are symptomatic and their clinical features include pharyngitis (90% of the patients), pneumonia (10%), bronchitis (5%), and sinusitis (5%). Pharyngeal erythema and wheezing are common. Among older adults, 40% of community-acquired cases of pneumonia are due to *C. psittaci*. CXR shows unilateral segmental patchy opacity. Complement fixation test is not sensitive and nonspecific.

- *C. pneumoniae*: person-to-person spread among schoolchildren, family members, and military recruits.
- Causes pneumonia in 10% of patients and bronchitis in 5% of symptomatic patients.
- Pneumonia caused by *C. pneumoniae* is separate from psittacosis (see below).

Chlamydia psittaci

C. psittaci causes psittacosis (ornithosis) in humans. The organism is found in psittacine birds (parrots and lories), turkeys, pigeons, and other birds. Infected birds have anorexia, weight loss, diarrhea, ruffled feathers, inability to fly, conjunctivitis, and rhinitis. In humans, the incubation period is 1-6 weeks. Clinical features include myalgias, fever, headache, pharyngitis, lethargy, confusion, delirium, neutropenia (in 25% of patients), and splenomegaly (in 1%-10%). Pulmonary symptoms are late and mild. CXR shows patchy unilateral or bilateral lower lobe pneumonia and an occasional small pleural effusion. Laboratory findings include normal leukocyte count, increased CPK level, and a fourfold increase in complement fixation test over >2 weeks.

- Psittacosis: caused by exposure to sick birds that harbor *C. psittaci*.
- Clinical features: myalgias, fever, headache, lethargy, confusion, delirium, and splenomegaly (1%-10% of patients).
- Note the differences: chlamydia pneumonia (human-to-human transmission of virus), psittacosis (birds-to-human transmission of virus), and pigeon-breeder's or bird fancier's lung (hypersensitivity pneumonitis caused by immune reaction to avian proteins).

Coxiella burnetii

C. burnetii is a rickettsia shed in the urine, feces, milk, and birth products of sheep, cattle, goats, and cats. It causes Q fever. Humans are infected by inhalation of dried aerosolized material. The incubation period is 10-30 days. Clinical features: fever, myalgias, chills, nausea, vomiting, chest pain, and cough (late). CXR findings may be normal or show unilateral bronchopneumonia and small pleural effusions. Lobar consolidation is seen in 25% of patients. Hepatitis and endocarditis can occur. The leukocyte count is normal, but liver enzyme levels may increase; complement fixation serology is positive.

- *C. burnetii*: rickettsial illness (Q fever).
- Inhalation of dried inoculum from urine, feces, milk, and birth products of sheep, cattle, goats, and cats.
- Bronchopneumonia and pleural effusion.
- Endocarditis is a late complication.

Francisella tularensis

F. tularensis is a gram-negative bacillus transmitted to man from wild rabbits, squirrels, and other wild animals and by bites of ticks or deer flies. The incubation period is 2-5 days. Cutaneous ulcer and lymphadenopathy are common features. Cough, fever, and chest pain are frequent, but many patients are asymptomatic. CXR shows unilateral lower lobe patchy infiltrates (bilateral in 30% of patients) and pleural effusion in 30% of patients. The leukocyte count is normal; the organism is

not seen with Gram staining of the sputum. Serology (agglutinins): fourfold change (titer >1:160).

- *F. tularensis*: a gram-negative bacteria; causes tularemia.
- Transmitted from wild rabbits, squirrels, and other wild animals.
- Bronchopneumonia and pleural effusion.

Yersinia pestis

Y. pestis is a gram-negative bacillus that causes plague. It is more prevalent in New Mexico, Arizona, Colorado, and California than in other states. It is spread from wild rodents (occasionally, cats), either directly or by fleas, usually in May-September. The incubation period is 2-7 days. Clinical features are fever, headache, bubo (groin or axilla), cough, and tachypnea. Pneumonia occurs in 10%-20% of the patients. Bilateral lower lobe alveolar infiltrates are found on CXR. Pleural effusion is common and nodules and cavities can occur. Leukocyte count is 15,000-20,000/mL; the organism is seen with Giemsa staining and in cultures or direct fluorescent antibody from blood, lymph node, sputum. Serology is positive.

- *Y. pestis*: more prevalent in southwestern U.S.
- It is spread from wild rodents (occasionally, cats), either directly or by fleas.
- Pneumonia in 10%-20% of patients; pleural effusions are common.

Hospital-Acquired (Nosocomial) Pneumonia

Almost 60% of the cases are caused by gram-negative bacilli, 10% by *S. aureus*, 10% by *S. pneumoniae*, and the rest by anaerobes, *Legionella* species, etc. Risk factors include coma, hypotension, shock, acidosis, azotemia, prolonged treatment with antibiotics, major surgical operations, lengthy procedures, mechanical ventilation, and immunosuppressive therapy.

- Hospital-acquired pneumonia: nearly 60% of cases are caused by gram-negative bacilli, 10% by *S. aureus*, 10% by *S. pneumoniae*.
- In hospital outbreaks involving a single type of organism, consider contaminated respiratory equipment.

Aspiration Pneumonitis

Two separate types of aspiration pneumonitis are acute and chronic. The acute type usually results from aspiration of a volume >50 mL with a pH <2.4. It produces classic aspiration pneumonia. Predisposing factors include nasogastric tube, anesthesia, coma, seizures, central nervous system problems, diaphragmatic hernia with reflux, and tracheoesophageal fistula. Hospitalized patients in whom aspiration pneumonia develops are infected by *E. coli*, *S. aureus*, *K. pneumoniae*, and *P. aeruginosa*. Community-acquired cases of aspiration pneumonia are caused by infections due to anaerobes (*B. melaninogenicus*, *F. nucleatum*, and gram-positive cocci).

Multiple antibiotics may be needed. Preventive measures are important. Chronic aspiration pneumonia results from recurrent aspiration of small volumes. Examples of this type include patients with diaphragmatic hernia and reflux and mineral oil granuloma. Unexplained chronic cough, patchy lung infiltrates, and nocturnal wheeze and cough are the symptoms.

- Acute aspiration pneumonia usually results from the aspiration of a volume >50 mL with a pH of <2.4; it may cause adult respiratory distress syndrome.
- Chronic aspiration pneumonia results from the aspiration of small volumes on a chronic recurrent basis, as in diaphragmatic hernia with reflux and mineral oil granuloma.

Lung Abscess

A parenchymal suppurative process is usually caused by bacteria. CXR shows a cavitary lesion, often with an air-fluid level. The three clinical groups of lung abscesses are primary, opportunistic, and hematogenous. Primary lung abscesses are associated with oral sepsis; aspiration accounts for up to 90% of all abscesses. Common causes include alcohol, drugs, anesthesia, seizures, stroke, coma, esophageal disorders, endobronchial obstruction (cancer, foreign body), and postpneumonic necrosis. Lung abscesses caused by opportunistic infections are seen in newborn infants with prematurity or congenital cardiopulmonary disorders, in elderly patients with blood dyscrasia, and in cancer of the lung or oropharynx. The infections may be nosocomial and occur with steroid therapy and postoperatively. Hematogenous lung abscesses occur with septicemia, septic embolism, and sterile infarcts (3% of patients). A history of any of these conditions in association with fever, cough with purulent or blood sputum, weight loss, and leukocytosis suggests the diagnosis. CXR is helpful in making the diagnosis. The abscess may rupture into the pleural space and cause empyema or flood other areas of the lung, causing adult respiratory distress syndrome. Bronchoscopy should be performed in selected patients to obtain cultures, to drain the abscess, and to exclude obstructing lesions. Treatment includes drainage (physiotherapy, postural, and bronchoscopic), antibiotics for 4-6 weeks, and surgical treatment if medical therapy fails.

- Primary lung abscess: associated with oral sepsis; aspiration accounts for up to 90% of all abscesses.
- Opportunistic lung abscesses are more common in elderly patients with blood dyscrasia and in association with cancer of the lung or oropharynx, steroid therapy, postoperative status, and nosocomial pneumonia.
- Hematogenous lung abscess is seen in septicemia, septic embolism, and sterile infarcts (3%).
- Bacteria responsible include anaerobic cocci (30%-40% of patients), anaerobic bacilli (30%-50%), aerobic gram-pos-

itive cocci (25%), and aerobic gram-negative bacilli (5%-12%).

Mycobacterioses

Mycobacterium tuberculosis

M. tuberculosis causes the most common type of human-to-human chronic infection by mycobacteria worldwide. The most common mode of transmission of infection is by inhalation of droplet nuclei from expectorated respiratory secretions. Diagnosis of active infection is by demonstrating the organism in respiratory secretions or other body fluids or tissues. The diagnostic yield from sputum is 25%-30%; induced sputum, 28%-55%; laryngeal swab, 25%; and gastric washings, 10%-34%. Bronchoscopically obtained specimens have a 30% greater yield, as compared with induced sputum and gastric washings. Culture of pleural fluid only has a low yield (<20%), but culture of pleural biopsy specimens has a >70% diagnostic yield.

- Positive tuberculin skin test, using purified protein derivative (PPD), indicates exposure to mycobacteria and not active infection.
- Diagnosis of active infection is by demonstration of the organism in respiratory secretions or other body fluids or tissues.
- Bronchoscopically obtained specimens have a 30% greater yield, as compared with induced sputum and gastric washings.

The tuberculin skin test (PPD) is an example of delayed (T-cell-mediated) hypersensitivity reaction. About 25% of patients with active tuberculosis are PPD negative. False-negative PPD is also seen in infections with viruses, bacteria (typhoid, brucella, and leprosy), live virus vaccinations, chronic renal failure, nutritional deficiency, diseases of lymphoid organs (Hodgkin's disease, sarcoidosis, and chronic lymphocytic leukemia), drugs (steroids and immunosuppressive agents), extremes of age (newborn or old), recent or overwhelming infection with mycobacteria, and acute stress. PPD skin testing should use a 5-TU (intermediate strength) preparation; the widest induration is read at 48 and 72 hours.

- PPD reaction represents a delayed type of hypersensitivity reaction.
- PPD becomes positive within 4 weeks after exposure to tubercle bacilli.
- PPD is negative in 25% of patients with active tuberculosis.

Indications for PPD include persons with signs and symptoms suggestive of current tuberculous infection, recent contacts with known or suspected cases of tuberculosis, abnormal CXR findings compatible with past tuberculosis, patients with diseases that increase the risk of tuberculosis (silicosis, gastrectomy, diabetes mellitus, immune suppression, and HIV infection), and groups at high risk of recent infection with *M. tuberculosis* (immigrants, long-time residents and workers in hospitals, nursing homes, prisons, and inner city or skid-row populations). The following criteria are used (based on skin reaction to PPD and clinical information) to determine a "positive" PPD skin test.

- ≥5 mm: adults and children with HIV infection, close contact with infectious cases, and those with fibrotic lesions on CXR.
- ≥10 mm: other at-risk adults and children, including infants and children <4 years of age.
- ≥15 mm: any person without a defined risk factor for tuberculosis.
- Recent PPD skin test converters: ≥10 mm increase within a 2-year period for those <35 years old, ≥15 mm increase for those ≥35 years old, and infants and children <4 years old with ≥10 mm skin reaction.

Tuberculosis of the pleura is common and is usually encountered in younger (<40 years) patients. In the U.S., 4% of all tuberculous patients have pleural involvement, and pleural tuberculosis constitutes 23% of cases with extrapulmonary tuberculosis. Effusions usually occur 3-6 months after primary infection. Acute presentation (cough, fever, and pleuritic chest pain) is more common in younger patients. Bilateral effusions (almost always exudates) occur in 5%-8% of patients, and the PPD is positive in >66%. Low pleural fluid glucose (<50 mg/dL) and low pH occur in 20% of patients. Pleural biopsy is positive for caseous granulomas in 50%-80% of patients and cultures in >75%. Pleural fluid culture is positive in only 15% of patients and sputum is positive in 40%. Bronchopleural fistula is a complication.

- Tuberculous pleuritis seen in younger (<40 years old) patients.
- Effusion occurs 3-6 months after primary infection.

Definitive therapy is indicated for all patients with culture-positive tuberculosis. Usually, treatment should include multiple drug (>2 drugs) therapy in all patients with active tuberculosis (Tables 21-14 and 21-15).

Extrapulmonary tuberculosis can be treated effectively with either a 6- or 9-month regimen. However, miliary tuberculosis, bone/joint tuberculosis, and tuberculous meningitis in infants and children should be treated for 12 months. Systemic corticosteroid therapy may be useful in prevention of pericardial constriction, neurologic complication from tuberculous meningitis, tuberculous bronchial stenosis, and adrenal insuf-

ficiency caused by tuberculosis. In pregnant women with tuberculosis, streptomycin should be avoided.

- Miliary, skeletal, and meningeal tuberculosis may require 12 months of therapy.
- Systemic corticosteroids are helpful in extrapulmonary tuberculosis.
- Tuberculosis is not an indication for therapeutic abortion.
- Avoid streptomycin in pregnancy.

Prophylactic therapy (standard prophylaxis consists of isoniazid, 300 mg orally once a day for 12 months) should be considered for the following persons (regardless of age) with a positive PPD: persons with HIV infection, persons at risk for HIV infection with unknown HIV status, close contacts of sputum-positive persons with newly diagnosed infectious tuberculosis, newly infected persons (recent PPD converters), and persons with increased risk of developing tuberculosis (diabetes mellitus, corticosteroid therapy, immunosuppressive therapy, intravenous drug use, hematologic and reticuloendothelial malignancies, end-stage renal disease, and clinical conditions associated with rapid weight loss or chronic undernutrition, silicosis, and postgastrectomy status). Preventive therapy is indicated for the following persons with a negative PPD: children who have close contacts with infectious persons and anergic HIV-infected adults at increased risk of tuberculosis. Preventive therapy is also suggested for persons <35 years old without the above risk factors but who belong to the following groups: foreign-born persons from high-prevalence countries, medically underserved low-income persons from high-prevalence populations (blacks, Hispanics, and Native Americans), and residents of long-term care facilities (correctional institutions, nursing homes, and mental institutions). The recommended duration of prophylactic therapy (usually isoniazid, 300 mg/day) for PPD-positive persons is outlined below (from Am J Respir Crit Care Med 149:1359-1374, 1994):

- Adults without HIV infection: at least 6 months.
- Adults and children with HIV infection: 12 months of prophylaxis.
- Children without HIV infection: 9 months.
- Silicosis or old fibrotic lesion on CXR without active tuberculosis: 4-month therapy with isoniazid and rifampin, although 12 months of isoniazid alone is an acceptable alternative.
- Persons suspected to be infected with isoniazid-resistant organisms should receive treatment with rifampin rather than isoniazid.
- *Bacille Calmette-Guérin* (BCG) vaccine is recommended (in the U.S.) for PPD-negative infants and children: 1) who are at high risk of intimate and prolonged exposure to per-

Table 21-14.--Regimen Options for Initial Treatment of Tuberculosis Among Children and Adults

TB without HIV infection			TB with HIV infection
Option 1	Option 2	Option 3	
Administer daily INH, RIF, and PZA for 8 weeks followed by 16 weeks of INH and RIF daily or 2-3 times/week* in areas where the INH resistance rate is not documented to be <4%. EMB or SM should be added to the initial regimen until susceptibility to INH and RIF is demonstrated. Continue treatment for at least 6 months and 3 months beyond culture conversion. Consult a TB medical expert if the patient is symptomatic or smear or culture positive after 3 months.	Administer daily INH, RIF, PZA, and SM or EMB for 2 weeks followed by 2 times/week* administration of the same drugs for 6 weeks (by DOT), and subsequently, with 2 times/week administration of INH and RIF for 16 weeks (by DOT). Consult a TB medical expert if the patient is symptomatic or smear or culture positive after 3 months.	Treat by DOT, 3 times/week* with INH, RIF, PZA, and EMB or SM for 6 months.[†] Consult a TB medical expert if the patient is symptomatic or smear or culture positive after 3 months.	Option 1, 2, or 3 can be used, but treatment regimens should continue for a total of 9 months and at least 6 months beyond culture conversion.

DOT, directly observed therapy; EMB, ethambutol; INH, isoniazid; PZA, pyrazinamide; RIF, rifampin; SM, streptomycin; TB, tuberculosis.

*All regimens administered 2 times/week or 3 times/week should be monitored by DOT for the duration of therapy.

[†]The strongest evidence from clinical trials is the effectiveness of all four drugs administered for the full 6 months. There is weaker evidence that SM can be discontinued after 4 months if the isolate is susceptible to all drugs. The evidence for stopping PZA before the end of 6 months is equivocal for the 3 times/week regimen, and there is no evidence of the effectiveness of this regimen with EMB for less than the full 6 months.

From Centers for Disease Control and Prevention: Initial therapy for tuberculosis in the era of multidrug resistance. Recommendations of the Advisory Council for the Elimination of Tuberculosis. MMWR 42(No. RR-7):1-8, 1993.

sistently untreated or ineffectively treated patients with infectious pulmonary tuberculosis, cannot be removed from the source of exposure, and cannot be placed on long-term prophylactic therapy, or 2) who are exposed continuously to persons with tuberculosis who have bacilli resistant to both isoniazid and rifampin. BCG vaccination is also recommended for PPD-negative infants and children in groups in which the rate of new infections is >1% per year and for whom the usual surveillance and treatment programs have been attempted but are not operationally feasible.

Mycobacterium avium Complex

M. avium complex, a noncontagious mycobacterium, is distributed widely in the environment. It may exist as a saprophyte in the lungs of persons living in rural areas and in patients with underlying COPD, bronchiectasis, prior tuberculosis, reflux esophagitis, or silicosis. M. avium complex may assume a pathogenic role in patients with AIDS and hairy cell leukemia and in other immunocompromised states. It is a relatively common cause of noncontagious tuberculosis involving the lymph nodes and bone. Nearly 30% of patients with M. avium

complex isolates have active disease. A clinically significant infection from atypical mycobacteria is diagnosed if the same organism is isolated repeatedly from the same source, if clinical features suggest active infection, and if tissue samples show active granuloma formation and organisms. In patients with AIDS, M. avium complex has been isolated from bone marrow, sputum/pulmonary tissue, blood, lymph node, gastrointestinal tract, and liver. A marked granulomatous response usually is not seen because of a severe decrease in the number of T lymphocytes. Patients with AIDS suspected to have infection with M. avium complex should have their blood, bone marrow, lymph nodes, stool, and small bowel biopsy and bronchoscopic specimens cultured. Lung infection caused by M. avium complex may produce patchy nodules or infiltrates; the latter more closely resembles M. tuberculosis on CXR. Repeated sputum cultures and tissue sampling may be necessary to make the diagnosis of active infection.

● M. avium complex exists as a saprophyte in persons with COPD, bronchiectasis, prior tuberculosis, reflux esophagitis, or silicosis.

Table 21-15.--Antituberculosis Drugs, Dosages, and Major Toxicities

Drug	Adult dosage (daily)	Pediatric dosage (daily)	Main adverse effects
Isoniazid (INH)*[†]	300 mg PO, IM	10-20 mg/kg (max. 300 mg)	Hepatic toxicity, peripheral neuropathy
Rifampin *[‡] (Rifadin, Rimactane)	600 mg PO, IV	10-20 mg/kg (max. 600 mg)	Hepatic toxicity, flu-like syndrome
Pyrazinamide[§]	1.5 to 2.5 g PO	15-30 mg/kg (max. 2 g)	Arthralgias, hepatic toxicity, hyperuricemia
Ethambutol[//](Myambutol)	15-25 mg/kg PO	15-25 mg/kg PO	Optic neuritis
Streptomycin[¶]	15 mg/kg IM	20-30 mg/kg	Vestibular toxicity, renal damage
Combinations			
Rifamate (isoniazid 150 mg, rifampin 300 mg)	2 tablets	Not recommended	
Rifater (isoniazid 50 mg, rifampin 120 mg, pyrazinamide 300 mg)	≤44 kg: 4 tablets 45-54 kg: 5 tablets ≥55 kg: 6 tablets	Not recommended	
Second-line drugs			
Capreomycin (Capastat)	15 mg/kg IM	15-30 mg/kg	Auditory and vestibular toxicity, renal damage
Kanamycin (Kantrex, and others)	15 mg/kg IM, IV	15-30 mg/kg	Auditory toxicity, renal damage
Amikacin (Amikin)	15 mg/kg IM, IV	15-30 mg/kg	Auditory toxicity, renal damage
Cycloserine[#] (Seromycin, and others)	250-500 mg bid PO	10-20 mg/kg	Psychiatric symptoms, seizures
Ethionamide (Trecator-SC)	250-500 mg bid PO	15-20 mg/kg	Gastrointestinal and hepatic toxicity, hypothyroidism
Ciprofloxacin (Cipro)	500-750 mg bid PO	Not recommended	Nausea, abdominal pain, restlessness, confusion
Ofloxacin (Floxin)	300-400 mg bid or 600-800 mg/day PO	Not recommended	Nausea, abdominal pain, restlessness, confusion
Aminosalicylic acid (PAS; Teebacin)	4-6 g bid PO	75 mg/kg bid	Gastrointestinal disturbance

*Intravenous preparations of isoniazid and rifampin are available.

[†]For intermittent use after a few weeks to months of daily therapy, dosage is 15 mg/kg (max. 900 mg) twice/week for adults. Pyridoxine 10 to 25 mg should be given to prevent neuropathy in malnourished or pregnant patients and in those with HIV infection, alcoholism, or diabetes mellitus.

[‡]For intermittent use after a few weeks to months of daily therapy, dosage is 600 mg twice/week.

[§]For intermittent use after a few weeks to months of daily therapy, dosage is 2.5 to 3.5 g twice/week.

[//]Usually not recommended for children less than 6 years old because visual acuity cannot be monitored. Some clinicians use 25 mg/kg per day during first 1-2 months or longer if organism is isoniazid-resistant. Decrease dosage if renal function diminished. For intermittent use after a few weeks to months of daily therapy, dosage is 50 mg/kg twice/week.

[¶]Available from Pfizer (800-254-4445) free of charge to physicians, clinics, or hospitals. When oral drugs are given daily, streptomycin is generally given 5 times per week (15 mg/kg, or a maximum of 1 g per dose) for an initial 2 to 12 week period, and then (if needed) 2 to 3 times per week (20 to 30 mg/kg, or a maximum of 1.5 g per dose). For patients > 40 years old, dosage is reduced to 500 to 750 mg 5 times per week and 20 mg/kg when given twice per week. Some clinicians change to lower dosage at 60 rather than 40 years old. Dosage should be decreased if renal function is diminished.

From Drugs for tuberculosis. The Medical Letter. 37:67-70, Aug 4, 1995. By permission of The Medical Letter.

- It can become a pathogen in patients with AIDS, hairy cell leukemia, silicosis, immunosuppression, or prosthetic devices and in the post-transplantation state.
- *M. avium* complex major cause of mortality and morbidity in patients with AIDS.

M. avium complex is highly resistant to medical treatment. For the usual "moderately severe" case of pulmonary disease, initial therapy should consist of isoniazid, rifampin, and ethambutol for 18-24 months, with streptomycin during the initial 2-3 months. For patients (immunologically intact) with a solitary pulmonary nodule, chemotherapy need not be given after resection. For patients with rapidly progressive (particularly AIDS) and highly symptomatic pulmonary disease, a more aggressive initial therapy is indicated—one using regimens of 5-6 drugs, including ethionamide, cycloserine, and kanamycin as well as the agents listed in Table 21-15 and below. Currently, it is generally agreed that every regimen to treat *M. avium* complex should contain either azithromycin or clarithromycin. Initial chemotherapy with 5-6 drugs is also indicated for patients with life-threatening disseminated disease. For patients with localized pulmonary disease and adequate cardiorespiratory reserve, resection in combination with chemotherapy may offer a better outcome than chemotherapy alone.

- *M. avium* complex is usually resistant to antituberculous therapy.
- For the usual case, initial therapy should consist of isoniazid, rifampin, and ethambutol for 18-24 months, with streptomycin during the initial 2-3 months.
- For more serious infections, 5-6 drugs for a prolonged time (>18 months) may be required.
- The addition of azithromycin or clarithromycin is recommended.

Patients with HIV infection and <100 CD4+ T lymphocytes/mL should be administered prophylaxis (rifabutin, 300 mg/day orally) against *M. avium* complex. Prophylaxis should be continued for the patient's lifetime. Disseminated infection should be treated with at least two agents, and every regimen should contain either azithromycin or clarithromycin. Therapy should be continued for the patient's lifetime.

Other Mycobacteria

M. kansasii is also likely to infect previously damaged lungs. Clinically, it can resemble *M. tuberculosis* infection. The response to 3-drug therapy is good, with cure rates >85%. *M. kansasii* (as well as *M. avium* complex and *M. scrofulaceum*) is involved most commonly in cervical lymphadenopathy. Excision of the nodes is sufficient therapy in most cases. Mycobacteria that are easy to treat include *M. haemophilum, M.*

kansasii, M. marianum, M. szulgai, M. ulcerans, and *M. xenopi*.

- Mycobacteria that are difficult to treat: *M. avium* complex, *M. chelonei, M. fortuitum, M. scrofulaceum*, and *M. simiae*.
- Rarely pathogenic mycobacteria: *M. asiaticum* and *M. malmoense*.
- Nonpathogenic species: *M. flavescens, M. gordonae, M. nonchromogenicum, M. parafortuitum, M. phlei, M. smegmatis, M. terrae* complex, *M. triviale*, and *M. vaccae*.

Toxicity From Antituberculous Drugs

When streptomycin is not included in treatment regimens lasting 6-9 months, the incidence of adverse reactions is about 3%. The addition of streptomycin increases the frequency of side effects to 8%. Patient compliance improves and the risk of monotherapy (emergence of resistant organisms) diminishes when fixed-dose drug combinations are used. In adults, it is important to perform a baseline assessment of liver function creatinine, complete blood cell count, platelet count, uric acid (if pyrazinamide is used), and ophthalmic examination (if ethambutol is used) before antituberculous therapy is begun. All patients should be monitored periodically for adverse reactions to the drugs.

Isoniazid

Isoniazid, the most commonly used antituberculous drug, can cause hepatitis. The incidence of hepatitis is age-dependent: rare in patients <20 years old, 0.3% between 20 and 34 years, 1.2% between 35 and 49 years, and 2.3% for those older than 50. The overall incidence is <1%. Hepatic dysfunction develops in 46% of patients within the first 2 months, in 36% during the 2nd month, and in 54% after the 3rd month. Middle-aged and black females are at higher risk. Hepatitis is more likely in patients who are rapid acetylators, and neuritis is more likely in patients who are slow acetylators. The rate of acetylation is determined genetically. Phenytoin toxicity is higher in slow acetylators. Isoniazid also causes skin rash, purpura, drug-induced systemic lupus erythematosus, and arthritis. The addition of pyridoxine is recommended for those with neuropathy (diabetes mellitus, uremia, alcoholism, and malnutrition), pregnancy, and seizure disorder. Patients older than 35 years who are receiving preventive therapy with isoniazid should have their liver function monitored, with levels of transaminase being measured at 1, 3, 6, and 9 months; however, tests of liver function should not replace careful clinical assessment.

- The incidence of isoniazid-induced hepatitis is age-dependent; it is more likely in older persons.
- It may cause peripheral neuropathy by interfering with the metabolism of pyridoxine.
- The interaction of isoniazid and phenytoin increases the serum concentration of both drugs.

Rifampin

Rifampin has an overall incidence of serious side effects of 1%. The most common reaction to rifampin is gastrointestinal upset. A transient increase in SGOT is common. Hepatitis is worse with isoniazid therapy. Therapy with intermittent, larger doses (>10 mg/kg) of rifampin is associated with thrombocytopenia, flu-like syndrome, hemolytic anemia, and cholestatic jaundice. Rifampin causes a harmless orange discoloration of body secretions. It also increases the metabolism of contraceptive pills, corticosteroids, warfarin, oral hypoglycemic agents, theophylline, anticonvulsants, ketoconazole, cyclosporine, methadone, and antiarrhythmic drugs (digitalis, quinidine, verapamil, and mexiletine); therefore, dosages of these drugs may have to be increased.

- The most common side effect of rifampin: gastrointestinal upset.
- Hepatitis is worse with isoniazid therapy.
- Rifampin induces hepatic microsomal enzymes; this may accelerate the clearance of drugs metabolized by the liver.

Ethambutol

Ethambutol is a bacteriostatic drug. In doses >25 mg/kg, it causes retrobulbar neuritis in <1% of patients; symptoms usually are observed 2 months after therapy is begun. Because ophthalmoscopic findings are normal in these patients, symptoms are important (blurred vision, central scotoma, and red-green color blindness). These symptoms precede changes in visual acuity.

- Retrobulbar neuritis (dose-related) is the most frequent and serious side effect.
- Renal failure prolongs the half-life of the drug and increases the frequency of ocular toxicity.

Pyrazinamide

Pyrazinamide is bactericidal for *M. tuberculosis* in an acid environment. It is active against mycobacteria in macrophages and penetrates well into tissues, including the cerebrospinal fluid. The most serious adverse reaction is hepatic damage. Hyperuricemia is common but gout is not, although arthralgias are reported occasionally. Skin rash and gastrointestinal upset are sometimes encountered.

- Pyrazinamide is effective in an acid environment (macrophages and nodules).
- Its most serious adverse reaction is hepatic damage.

Streptomycin

Streptomycin is bactericidal in an alkaline environment. It must be administered parenterally. It is excreted by the kidneys. The dosage should be decreased in those with renal insufficiency. The most common adverse side effect is vestibular toxicity, which causes vertigo. Hearing loss may also occur. These side effects are more likely in the elderly. Ototoxicity and nephrotoxicity are related to both the cumulative dose and the peak serum concentration.

- Streptomycin is bactericidal in an alkaline environment (cavities).
- It produces vestibular toxicity.
- Nephrotoxicity and vestibular toxicity are more common in persons >60 years.

Other Drugs

Other drugs used in the treatment of tuberculosis include para-aminosalicylic acid, ethionamide, cycloserine, capreomycin, kanamycin, thiacetazone, amikacin, and quinolones (ofloxacin and ciprofloxacin), rifabutin, clofazimine, β-lactamase antibiotics (amoxicillin) and β-lactamase inhibitors (clavulanic acid), and new macrolides (azithromycin and clarithromycin). These drugs are not first-line agents in the treatment of infection caused by *M. tuberculosis*. Rifabutin (rifamycin spiropiperidyl derivative) shows activity against certain rifampin-resistant strains of *M. tuberculosis*. The side effects are similar to those of rifampin. The role of macrolides in the treatment of *M. avium* complex is discussed above.

Pulmonary Mycoses

Serious fungal infections are found at autopsy in 2% of patients overall, in 5%-10% of those with solid tumors, and in 20%-40% of those dying of leukemia. Renal transplantation patients (15%) have a fungal infection at some time in their post-transplantation course. Almost all mycoses produce granulomas. The saprophytic state of fungi is a common problem, particularly with aspergillus species.

Histoplasmosis

Histoplasma capsulatum causes histoplasmosis. This infection is more common in the Mississippi, Ohio, and St. Lawrence River valleys than in other areas. Infection is by inhalation of fungal spores. A large number of infectious spores are present in chicken coops, dusty areas, starling roosts, bat-infested caves, and decayed wood. Clinical forms include asymptomatic infection, symptomatic infection (similar to viral upper respiratory tract infection), disseminated (immunocompromised host), chronic cavitary (structural defects), mediastinal granuloma, mediastinal fibrosis, pulmonary nodules, and calcified lesions on CXR. Disseminated disease may occur in patients with AIDS. Hilar adenopathy may be seen. Skin testing is not useful in clinical practice. More than 80% of the population in endemic areas have positive findings on skin test. Skin test may produce positive serologic findings. Complement fixation titer >1:32 is not diagnostic but strongly supportive of active disease and may help as a prognostic indicator. Immunodiffusion shows that the H-band is the last to come and the first to go and the M-band is the first to come and the last to go. Recovery of the organism from body fluids, bone marrow, or tissue is diagnostic. The serum level of ACE may be increased in histoplasmosis. There is no need to treat acute disease (self-limiting). Progressive or disseminated disease requires therapy with antifungal agents. Erythema nodosum and pericarditis may occur.

- Histoplasmosis: exposure to chicken coops, dusty areas, starling roosts, bat-infested caves, and decayed wood.
- Histoplasmin skin test should not be used to diagnose infection.
- The chronic cavitary form clinically mimics chronic tuberculosis.
- Mediastinal fibrosis, pulmonary calcification, broncholithiasis, and superior vena cava syndrome.
- Histoplasmosis is the most common cause of mediastinal granuloma.

Coccidioidomycosis

Coccidioides immitis causes coccidioidomycosis. The endemic zone extends from northern California to Argentina. Infections are more common when dry windy conditions exist, with epidemics occurring in the dry hot months after the rainy season, often after the soil is disturbed. Clinical forms include mildly symptomatic pulmonary infection (flu-like illness in 40% of patients), asymptomatic nodules or thin-walled cavities, coccidioidal pneumonia, chronic cavitary form, disseminated, and "valley fever" (erythema nodosum, erythema multiforme, arthralgia, arthritis, and eosinophilia). CXR may show lobar infiltrates (70% of patients), scattered patchy areas, atelectasis, hilar adenopathy (25%), pleural effusion (3%), cavities (8%), nodules (5%), and normal findings (3%). Filipinos, African-Americans, and Mexicans are at greater risk for dissemination and death. Infection acquired late during pregnancy is associated with higher maternal and fetal mortality. The coccidioidin (mycelial phase) skin test (used previously) does not affect coccidioidomycosis serology but may produce serologic findings positive for histoplasmosis. Thirty percent more cases are diagnosed with spherulin (parasitic phase) skin testing (currently used) than with coccidioidin. The incidence of positive skin reaction in disseminated cases is higher (>60%). A violent reaction occurs if given to patients with erythema nodosum. Latex particle agglutination (IgM) serologic testing is positive in 71% of patients within 2 weeks and in 90% within 4 weeks. The false-positive rate is 6%-10%; it has no value in detecting antibody in the cerebrospinal fluid. Titer is not helpful in follow-up evaluation. Complement fixation (IgG) serologic results become positive later than the results of the latex test; <10% are positive within the first 10 days, and 80% become positive in 4-6 weeks. Titer is very helpful in diagnosis and prognosis: a rapidly increasing titer is associat-

ed with a poor prognosis; a titer >1:16 is significant, and a titer <1:8 may persist for years. Positive cerebrospinal fluid titer confirms infection in the central nervous system.

- Coccidioidomycosis: southwestern U.S.; epidemics occur in the dry hot months after the rainy season.
- Clinical forms: asymptomatic nodules, thin-walled cavities, coccidioidal pneumonia, chronic cavitary form, and disseminated.
- Spherulin (parasitic phase) skin test (currently used) diagnoses 30% more cases than coccidioidin.
- Complement fixation serologic findings are helpful in diagnosis and prognosis.

Blastomycosis

Blastomyces dermatitidis causes blastomycosis. Miniepidemics have occurred in North Carolina, Minnesota, and Illinois. One miniepidemic involved campers in Wisconsin, "Namekagon fever." Most cases occur in the southern, south-central, and Great Lakes states. Persons in contact with soil are more likely to be infected. The male-to-female ratio is 10:1. Pulmonary forms are acute pneumonic form (resolution or progressive pulmonary involvement), asymptomatic, and insidious pulmonary or extrapulmonary dissemination. The most characteristic CXR finding is a perihilar mass that mimics carcinoma. Pleural effusion is seen in <3% of patients with the pneumonic form. The skeletal system (vertebral bodies, ribs, skull, and long bones) is the second most common site of dissemination, and the male genitourinary tract (excluding the kidneys) is the third most frequent site. The mucosa, central nervous system, adrenals, and other organs are not commonly involved. No skin test is available. Serology is unavailable.

- Blastomycosis is more pyogenic than histoplasmosis.
- Blastomycosis: contact with soil, manual laborers, and Great Lakes states.
- Most characteristic CXR finding: a perihilar mass mimicking carcinoma.
- Extrapulmonary dissemination is seen in 65% of patients; the skin is the most frequent site of dissemination.
- Serologic test is unreliable.

Cryptococcosis

Cryptococcus neoformans, the only fungus that is not dimorphic (no mycelia), causes cryptococcosis. The organism is widely distributed in the soil, foods, and excreta of pigeons and other animals. In humans, it may exist as a saprophyte in preexisting lung disease, but one-third to one-half of patients with cryptococcosis are immunosuppressed. The lung is the portal of entry, but the most common clinical presentation is subacute or chronic meningitis (the common cause of death). Diseases with which it is commonly associated are Hodgkin's and non-Hodgkin's disease, leukemia, sarcoidosis, and diabetes mellitus. The onset of central nervous system symptoms, fever, nausea, and anorexia is insidious. Pulmonary features include cough with scant sputum (15% of patients), chest pain (45%), dyspnea (25%), hemoptysis (7%), and night sweats (25%). Nodular infiltrates with cavitation, especially in the lower lobes, occasional hilar adenopathy, and a solitary mass may be found. Diagnosis can be established with positive sputum cultures (35% of patients), bronchoscopic specimens (35%), and open lung biopsy (100%). India ink preparation of the cerebrospinal fluid is positive in 30%-60% of patients. Direct testing for cryptococcal antigen in the cerebrospinal fluid is more sensitive than direct staining. In HIV-infected patients, serum cryptococcal antigen testing is highly sensitive. Serologic testing (detects polysaccharide antigen) of the cerebrospinal fluid is positive in 90% of central nervous system infections and in 30% of non-central nervous system infections. Serologic testing should be performed on blood, cerebrospinal fluid, and urine.

- *C. neoformans*: saprophytic or pathogenic state.
- Infection is more common in immunocompromised patients.
- Nodular, cavitary, and patchy infiltrates.
- The cerebrospinal fluid should be examined in almost all patients with organisms in respiratory secretions.

Aspergillosis

Aspergillus fumigatus, A. flavus, and *A. niger* are responsible for several pulmonary manifestations. The clinical forms include 1) allergic bronchopulmonary aspergillosis (discussed above), 2) hypersensitivity pneumonitis in red cedar wood workers, 3) mycetoma or fungus ball in preexisting lung disease, 4) locally invasive (chronic necrotizing) aspergillosis, 5) disseminated, 6) bronchocentric granulomatosis, and 7) saprophytic. The organism is ubiquitous and frequently colonizes the respiratory tract in patients with lung disease. Invasive aspergillosis in immunosuppressed hosts is the most serious form of infection and occurs mainly in granulocytopenic patients with hematologic malignancies. *Aspergillus* is isolated at autopsy in 10% of patients with acute leukemia. Of all patients with invasive aspergillosis (diagnosed pre or post mortem), 40% have acute lymphocytic leukemia, 20% have acute myelomonocytic leukemia, 10% have chronic myelogenous leukemia, 5% have Hodgkin's disease, and 10% have other hematologic malignancies. The presence of the organism in respiratory secretions is not diagnostic; tissue invasion should be documented. Aspergilloma is a mass of fungal hyphae in preexisting lung cavities. The major symptoms include hemoptysis, cough, low-grade fever, and weight loss. Fungus ball can be caused by *Candida, Coccidioides, Nocardia,* and *Sporotrichum*. CXR and tomograms show a meniscus of air around the fungus ball (Monod's sign), almost always in the upper lobes. Skin testing gives positive results in 20% of

patients, and serologic findings are positive in >90%. Because surgical therapy of aspergilloma carries a high morbidity and mortality, another therapeutic option is to use intracavitary instillation of amphotericin. Allergic bronchopulmonary aspergillosis shows positive skin test findings in 100% of patients and positive serology findings in >75%.

- Granulocytopenia and lung infiltrates in hematologic malignancies almost always mean disseminated aspergillosis.
- Aspergillosis is frequently accompanied by *Pseudomonas* or *Candida*.
- Aspergilloma (fungus ball) occurs in previously damaged lung; hemoptysis is a serious complication.

Zygomycosis (Mucormycosis)

Zygomycetes includes the order Mucorales (phycomycetes) and causes zygomycosis. The organisms have a worldwide distribution. Serious infections of the lungs, central nervous system, and skin are seen in patients with diabetes mellitus, hematologic malignancies, skin or mucosal injuries, and those receiving cytotoxic drugs. The organism invades blood vessels (as does *Aspergillus*) and may cause significant hemoptysis. CXR may show patchy infiltrates, consolidation, cavitation, and effusions. Bronchial stenosis is a peculiar complication of zygomycosis. The diagnosis must be established by biopsy, although sputum culture may suggest it. No serologic test is available. Zygomycosis is a nonseptate fungus.

- Zygomycosis: immunocompromised and diabetic patients.
- Propensity to invade blood vessels; hemoptysis is common.
- In a poorly controlled diabetic patient with swelling of the eyelids and a black discharge from the nose, consider zygomycosis.

Candidiasis

Candida albicans causes candidiasis and is responsible for about 75% of serious infections. This is a ubiquitous organism that is present in the oropharynx of 30% of normal persons, in the gastrointestinal tract in 65% of normal persons, and in the vagina of 30%-70% of women. Systemic candidiasis is found at autopsy in as many as 25% of patients with leukemia. Other risk factors are diabetes mellitus, cancer, cirrhosis, renal failure, blood dyscrasia, cytotoxic therapy, intravenous or urinary catheters, antibiotics given intravenously, prostheses, cachexia, burns, and HIV infection. Disseminated infection is uncommon in patients with AIDS. Lung involvement is relatively rare, and CXR shows patchy or diffuse infiltrates. *Candida* bronchitis, an occupational disease of tea tasters, is manifested by low-grade fever, cough, and patchy infiltrates.

- Candidiasis: more common in patients with hematologic malignancies.

- Prolonged granulocytopenia predisposes to disseminated infection (as in disseminated aspergillosis).
- Lung involvement is uncommon; patchy or diffuse lung infiltrates.

Sporotrichosis

Sporothrix schenckii causes sporotrichosis. The organism is a dimorphous fungus that exists as a saprophyte in the soil, plants, wood, straw, sphagnum moss, decaying vegetation, cats, dogs, and rodents. Sporotrichosis is an occupational hazard for farmers, florists, gardeners, horticulturists, and forestry workers. Infection is by cutaneous inoculation. Cutaneous nodules along lymphatics may appear in 75% of patients. Hematogenous dissemination to the lungs is rare, but inhalation-induced pulmonary disease mimics cavitary tuberculosis. The diagnosis is made by tissue examination. Latex agglutination with an increasing titer and a titer of >1:80 suggests active disease. Skin infection may be associated with negative serologic findings.

- Sporotrichosis: an occupational hazard of florists, horticulturists, and gardeners.
- Lymphangitis of the skin and subcutaneous nodules.
- Pulmonary infection mimics chronic tuberculosis.

Nocardiosis

Nocardia asteroides (also *N. brasiliensis* and *N. caviae*) causes nocardiosis. *N. asteroides* is a weakly acid-fast organism that is a saprophyte in the soil, dust, plants, and water. The lungs and central nervous system are the two organs commonly involved. Infection is more common in immunosuppressed patients and in patients with pulmonary alveolar proteinosis. Primary infection leads to necrotizing pneumonia with abscess formation. No inflammatory response or granuloma formation occurs. Infection may produce pleural effusion. Lymphohematogenous spread is seen in 20% of patients; nearly all of these have brain abscesses. The diagnosis is made at autopsy in 40% of cases. Isolation of the organism from respiratory secretions is not diagnostic of infection, because the saprophytic state is well recognized. No serologic test is available.

- Nocardiosis: immunocompromised patients and those with pulmonary alveolar proteinosis.
- Necrotizing pneumonia and lung abscess.
- Saprophytic state should be differentiated from pathogenic state.
- Central nervous system involvement is common in those with disseminated infection.

Actinomycosis

Actinomyces israelii or *A. bovis* causes actinomycosis. The organism is a fungus-like bacterium. *Actinomyces* is not found in the soil or vegetation but is easily isolated from scrapings around the teeth, gums, and tonsils. It is an opportunistic infection and becomes invasive with severe caries, tissue necrosis, and aspiration. In tissue, the organism grows into a "sulfur granule" caused by mycelial clumps in a matrix of $CaPO_4$. The disease is more common in rural areas, with a male-to-female ratio of 2:1. Infection is always mixed with anaerobes. Skin abscesses, ulcers, sinus tracts, and cervicofacial node involvement are found in 30%-40% of patients. Pulmonary involvement is seen in 20%, with cough, fever, pulmonary consolidation, pleurisy with effusion, and, eventually, draining sinuses. Serologic testing (agar double-dilution test) is positive in 90% of patients with disseminated disease and negative in those with localized infection.

- Actinomycosis: associated with severe dental caries, tissue necrosis, and aspiration; opportunistic infection.
- Sulfur granules from abscesses, fistulas, or wounds.
- Cough, fever, pulmonary lesions, pleural effusion, and fistula and sinus tracts.

Protozoal Infections

Included in protozoal infections are *Pneumocystis carinii*, toxoplasmosis, and amebiasis. *P. carinii* is either a protozoan or a fungus with trophozoite and cyst stages. The cyst stains best with methenamine silver nitrate. This organism is seen mainly in immunosuppressed patients and accounts for 40% of the cases of interstitial pneumonia in these patients. The frequency of infection increases in proportion to the intensity of immunosuppressive treatment. *P. carinii* infection is seen in 5% of patients receiving treatment with a single drug, in 28% of those receiving four drugs, and in 43% of those receiving polychemotherapy and irradiation. Patients with AIDS are in the high-risk group for *P. carinii* infection. Infection causes alveolar and interstitial inflammation and edema with plasma cell infiltrates. The organisms are found in alveolar macrophages. Clinical features include the abrupt onset of fever, tachypnea, hypoxia, cyanosis, respiratory distress, relatively normal findings on lung examination, and a patchy or diffuse interstitial/alveolar process. Routine laboratory data are unhelpful. The diagnosis can be made with induced sputum, bronchoalveolar lavage, or lung biopsy findings.

- *P. carinii* infection: respiratory symptoms and signs are more serious in non-AIDS patients.
- Induced sputum and bronchoalveolar lavage are excellent methods for diagnosis.
- The number of organisms in tissue preparations from non-AIDS patients is smaller.
- Upper lobe process seen on CXR in patients receiving pentamidine aerosol therapy.

Noninfectious Pulmonary Complications in AIDS

Infectious pulmonary complications are discussed in Chapter 14. Noninfectious complications include diffuse interstitial lung disease, lymphocytic interstitial pneumonitis, cystic lung disease, pneumothorax, pulmonary hypertension, Kaposi's sarcoma, and non-Hodgkin's lymphoma.

Nonspecific interstitial pneumonitis is a common occurrence in patients with chronic AIDS and represents 30%-40% of all episodes of lung infiltrates in these patients. More than 25% of patients with this problem have either concurrent Kaposi's sarcoma, previous experimental therapies, or a history of *P. carinii* pneumonia or drug abuse. The clinical features are similar to those of patients with *P. carinii* pneumonia. Histopathologic features of the lung in interstitial pneumonitis associated with AIDS may include varying degrees of edema, fibrin deposition, and interstitial inflammation with lymphocytes and plasma cells. There is no known therapy.

- More than 25% of patients with interstitial pneumonitis have either concurrent Kaposi's sarcoma, previous experimental therapies, or a history of *P. carinii* pneumonia or drug abuse.

Lymphocytic interstitial pneumonitis is caused by pulmonary infiltration with mature polyclonal B lymphocytes and plasma cells. It occurs in children of mothers in groups at high risk for AIDS, Haitians, and patients with AIDS. Systemic corticosteroid therapy may produce significant improvement. Lymphocytic interstitial pneumonitis is a nonspecific entity in adults with AIDS.

- Lymphocytic interstitial pneumonitis is diagnostic of AIDS when it occurs in a child <13 years old with serologic findings positive for HIV.
- Pulmonary lymphoid hyperplasia has been reported in 40% of children with AIDS.

Cystic lung disease is more common in patients with *P. carinii* infections and in those receiving aerosolized pentamidine therapy. Cystic lesions are more common in the upper and mid lung zones. Chest CT identifies these small- to medium-sized cystic lesions. Pneumothorax occurs with increasing frequency in patients with *P. carinii* pneumonia and in those receiving pentamidine aerosol therapy. Other causes of pneumothorax include Kaposi's sarcoma, tuberculosis, and other infections. Pneumothorax in patients with AIDS carries a poor prognosis.

- Cystic lung disease and pneumothorax are more common in those with *P. carinii* pneumonia receiving aerosolized pentamidine therapy.
- High incidence of bilateral synchronous pneumothoraces.

Pleural effusion is seen in 25% of hospitalized patients with AIDS. Nearly one-third of the pleural effusions are due to noninfectious causes. Hypoalbuminemia is the leading cause of these effusions. Other important noninfectious causes include Kaposi's sarcoma and atelectasis. Among the infectious causes, bacterial pneumonias, *P. carinii* pneumonia, and *M. tuberculosis* are important. Fungal infections can also produce pleural effusion. Large effusions are caused by tuberculosis and Kaposi's sarcoma.

- Pleural effusion is caused by infections in two-thirds of hospitalized patients with AIDS.
- Kaposi's sarcoma and tuberculosis cause large effusions.

Pulmonary hypertension has been found in patients with AIDS. The mechanism is not clear, but HIV is thought to affect the endothelium directly and to cause vascular changes. The clinical, physiologic, and pathologic features are identical to those seen in primary pulmonary hypertension.

- Pulmonary hypertension in AIDS is clinically identical to that in idiopathic pulmonary hypertension.

Kaposi's sarcoma occurs with a greater frequency in homosexuals with AIDS. The incidence of this sarcoma has gradually decreased. Previous or concurrent pulmonary opportunistic infections have been noted in >70% of patients. Pulmonary involvement from Kaposi's sarcoma occurs in 18%-35% of patients with this sarcoma. In most patients, pulmonary Kaposi's sarcoma is established only at autopsy. The diagnostic yield from bronchoscopy is 24% and from lung biopsy, 56%. Hemoptysis is an uncommon complication in Kaposi's sarcoma, although endobronchial metastasis develops in nearly 30% of patients. CXR may show the typical nodular infiltrates in a small number (<10%) of patients. The more nodular (as opposed to interstitial) pattern and the rather slow evolution of lung infiltrates due to Kaposi's sarcoma are different from the relatively rapidly evolving *P. carinii* pneumonia.

- Frequently, pulmonary Kaposi's sarcoma is preceded by cutaneous lesions.
- Pulmonary involvement due to Kaposi's sarcoma occurs in 18%-35% of patients with this sarcoma.
- At autopsy, lung involvement is found in nearly 50% of patients with Kaposi's sarcoma.
- Clinically, pulmonary Kaposi's sarcoma is indistinguishable from *P. carinii* pneumonia or opportunistic pneumonia.
- Multiple, discrete, raised, violaceous, or bright red tracheobronchial lesions can be seen on bronchoscopy.
- Endobronchial lesions are also caused by *M. avium* complex.

Non-Hodgkin's lymphoma involving the lungs is seen in

a small number (<10%) of patients with AIDS. The lymphoma in these patients is usually extranodal non-Hodgkin's B-cell lymphoma.

ACKNOWLEDGMENT

The contribution of chest roentgenographic figures and accompanying legends by Edward C. Rosenow III, M.D., is gratefully acknowledged.

QUESTIONS

Multiple Choice (choose the one best answer)

1. A 56-year-old man with stable cardiomyopathy is taking an angiotensin converting enzyme inhibitor and amiodarone for ventricular arrhythmia that is well controlled. A few days after this therapy was begun, significant cough without dyspnea or wheeze developed. Chest roentgenography shows stable cardiomegaly. Physical examination results indicate no evidence of congestive heart failure. Which of the following is the most likely cause of his new pulmonary symptom?
   a. Angiotensin converting enzyme inhibitor drug
   b. Amiodarone
   c. Occult pulmonary edema
   d. Upper respiratory tract infection
   e. New onset of asthma

2. A 43-year-old nonsmoker presents with progressive dyspnea (he has class II dyspnea by the New York Heart Association classification) and weight loss of 12 kg during the preceding 24 months. Chest roentgenography reveals significant hyperinflation. Pulmonary function tests show (% predicted) TLC, 128; VC, 75; RV, 140; FEV_1, 38; FEV_1/FVC, 34; MVV, 48; and DLCO, 36. There is no response to inhalation of bronchodilator. Which of the following is the most likely diagnosis?

   a. Chronic asthma
   b. Emphysema
   c. Chronic bronchitis
   d. Pulmonary fibrosis
   e. Diaphragmatic weakness

3. A 47-year-old man presents with dyspnea and diffuse lung infiltrates. A diagnostic bronchoalveolar lavage is planned. Which of the following diseases is most likely to be diagnosed by this procedure?
   a. Idiopathic pulmonary fibrosis
   b. Pulmonary parenchymal sarcoidosis
   c. *Pneumocystis carinii* pneumonia
   d. Chronic asbestosis
   e. Pulmonary lymphangioleiomyomatosis

4. A middle-aged male nonsmoker presents with progressive dyspnea of 7 months' duration. He has no cough or wheeze. The results of physical examination and chest roentgenography are normal. The results of complete pulmonary function tests, including body plethysmography and methacholine provocation challenge, are normal. The measured lung compliance is 200 mL/cm H_2O. Which of the following diseases is most likely to be responsible for his dyspnea?
   a. Pulmonary edema
   b. Extrinsic asthma

c. Progressive anatomic emphysema
d. Nonpulmonary disease
e. Pulmonary fibrosis

5. A 45-year-old asthmatic patient is evaluated for his chronic asthma, which has been relatively stable. However, he wants to try the new bronchodilator drug, salmeterol. Which of the following instructions should you include in the prescription for this drug?
   a. Two inhalations every 6 hours
   b. Two inhalations as needed for wheezing
   c. Two inhalations every 24 hours
   d. Two inhalations every 4 hours
   e. Two inhalations every 12 hours

6. A 24-year-old man with cystic fibrosis presents with several episodes of mild-to-moderate hemoptysis. Chest roentgenography reveals no changes in the chronic abnormalities. The hemoptysis subsides spontaneously. Which of the following statements best applies to this patient?
   a. Because hemoptysis is unusual in cystic fibrosis, another cause (cancer) should be excluded
   b. Recurrent pneumothorax is more likely now than when he was 12 years old
   c. Intussusception and fecal impaction are unlikely
   d. Pancreatic insufficiency is unlikely
   e. Atopy and bronchospastic disease are unlikely to occur

7. A 65-year-old man with a clinical diagnosis suspected of chronic idiopathic pulmonary fibrosis is referred for further evaluation of his pulmonary status. Of the following diagnostic tests at your disposal, which one is least likely to be helpful in diagnosis and treatment?
   a. Chest roentgenography
   b. Pulmonary function tests
   c. Arterial blood gas analysis
   d. High-resolution computed tomography of the chest
   e. Bronchoalveolar lavage

8. A 38-year-old man, a nonsmoker, presents with recent onset of mild exertional dyspnea. Physical examination results are normal. Chest roentgenography reveals bilateral upper lobe alveolar-interstitial infiltrates. Which of the following diagnoses is least likely in this patient?
   a. Pulmonary eosinophilic granuloma (histiocytosis X)
   b. Silicosis
   c. Histoplasmosis
   d. Occult malignancy with pulmonary metastases
   e. Sarcoidosis, stage III

9. A 30-year-old man, nonsmoker, presents with recent onset

of dry cough. Physical examination reveals raised erythematous nodules over both shins. Chest roentgenography shows bilateral hilar lymphadenopathy and bilateral upper lobe alveolar-interstitial infiltrates. Serum angiotensin converting enzyme level is high (4x normal). The serum level of calcium is increased at 12.4 mg/dL. Which of the following diagnostic and/or therapeutic maneuvers is inappropriate at this point?
   a. Pulmonary function testing
   b. Tuberculin (PPD) skin testing
   c. ^{67}Gallium citrate scan of the lungs
   d. Sputum culture for mycobacteria
   e. Bronchoscopic biopsy of bronchial mucosa and lung

10. A 34-year-old man presents with sudden onset of hemoptysis. He has been dyspneic for many years and his chest roentgenograms have shown multiple lower lobe, ill-defined nodular densities. Examination reveals cyanosis, telangiectasia over the lips and tongue, and a bruit over the lower lung fields. Which of the following is incorrect regarding this patient's condition?
   a. Neurologic complications are common
   b. Even if this patient has no symptoms, his lung lesions should be treated
   c. High-output cardiac failure is a complication
   d. Bronchoscopic biopsy of pulmonary lesions is indicated
   e. Hemoptysis is the most common presenting symptom

11. A 58-year-old man, 45-pack-year smoker, is found to have a 2-cm solitary peripheral right upper lobe lung nodule during his annual physical examination. The nodule was not present on a chest roentgenogram obtained 14 months earlier. The results of clinical examination and routine laboratory tests reveal no abnormalities. Computed tomography reveals that the nodule is solitary, uncalcified, and indeterminate. Which of the following approaches is most appropriate for this patient?
   a. Surgical resection
   b. Observation and repeat chest roentgenography in 4 months
   c. Brain and bone scans and upper and lower gastrointestinal tract series
   d. Bronchoscopy, if nondiagnostic, followed by transthoracic needle aspiration
   e. Tuberculin (PPD) skin test

12. A 68-year-old woman, a 60-pack-year smoker, presents with cough, hemoptysis, and a chest roentgenogram that reveals right upper lobe atelectasis. The serum level of calcium is increased at 13.2 mg/dL. Which of the following diagnostic tests is inappropriate in this patient?

a. Pulmonary function testing

b. A 24-hour urinary calcium measurement

c. Bronchoscopy

d. Radionuclide bone scan

e. Computed tomography of the chest and upper abdomen

13. Which of the following is not true about chylous pleural effusion?

a. The appearance of the fluid is characteristic

b. Chylomicrons are present in the fluid

c. The triglyceride level in the fluid is usually high (>110 mg/dL)

d. High cholesterol level in the fluid does not establish the diagnosis of chylous effusion

e. It may be caused by lymphangioleiomyomatosis

14. A 56-year-old woman presents with swelling of the left calf and tenderness of the left calf and thigh after a cross-country car trip. Before the trip, she had an upper respiratory tract infection, which continues to bother her (low-grade fever and cough productive of yellow sputum). Which of the following is most likely to provide the diagnosis?

a. Calf pain on dorsiflexion of the left ankle

b. Duplex ultrasonography of the left lower extremity

c. Perfusion lung scan

d. Pulmonary angiography

e. Cine-computed tomography of the lungs

15. During the initial evaluation of the 56-year-old woman mentioned above, left-sided pleuritic chest pain and dyspnea developed. A perfusion lung scan showed a low probability of pulmonary embolism. Which of the following tests is most likely to be diagnostic?

a. Chest roentgenography

b. Arterial blood gas analysis

c. Pulmonary angiography

d. Serial (daily) perfusion lung scan

e. Serial (daily) duplex ultrasonography of the lower extremity

16. A middle-aged man presents with fever, malaise, arthralgias, epistaxis, cavitated lung nodules, and ulcerated skin lesions. Urinalysis shows red blood cell casts. The erythrocyte sedimentation rate is 96 mm/hr, and the serum creatinine level is 2.2 mg/dL. Renal biopsy reveals focal segmental glomerulonephritis. Which of the following is incorrect regarding this patient's illness?

a. A complete response can be expected with corticosteroid and cyclophosphamide therapy

b. Major airway stricture and stenosis are potential complications

c. Alveolar hemorrhage may occur

d. Presence of cytoplasmic antineutrophil cytoplasmic antibody (c-ANCA) is most likely

e. Presence of perinuclear antineutrophil cytoplasmic antibody (p-ANCA) is most likely

17. A 30-year-old black man presents with chronic exertional dyspnea. The results of chest roentgenography suggest pulmonary hypertension. Hemoglobin is 8.8 g/dL, and a special blood smear demonstrates sickle shaped erythrocytes. Which of the following is incorrect regarding this patient's hematologic problem?

a. He is susceptible to recurrent chest infections

b. Pulmonary hypertension may result from recurrent pulmonary emboli

c. Pulmonary infections most commonly are caused by *Staphylococcus aureus*

d. Pneumonia vaccination is indicated

e. Pulmonary function testing is likely to show restrictive lung disease

18. A college student returns home with a week-long history of fever, sore throat, and cough. Bullous myringitis is noted on otoscopic examination. Which of the following is not a feature of this illness?

a. Outbreaks occur in closed populations

b. Erythema multiforme may be seen

c. Hemolytic anemia and thrombocytopenia may occur

d. Cavitated lung lesions are likely

e. Guillain-Barré syndrome may complicate the illness

19. A 25-year-old Native American man living in New Mexico has a prodrome of fever, myalgia, headache, abdominal pain, and nausea followed by cough and respiratory distress. Chest roentgenography shows bilateral lung infiltrates and pleural effusions. Which of the following is not a feature of this syndrome?

a. The reservoir for the infectious agent is the deer mouse

b. It almost exclusively affects Native Americans

c. Hemoconcentration is seen in most of the patients

d. Thrombocytopenia is present in >65% of patients

e. No sequelae are observed in survivors

20. Which of the following pairings ("connections") is incorrect?

a. Alveolar proteinosis and nocardiosis

b. Horticulturist and sporotrichosis

c. Exposure to wild animals and tularemia

d. Chronic bronchitis and allergic bronchopulmonary aspergillosis

e. Prolonged granulocytopenia and disseminated aspergillosis

21. Progressive dyspnea develops in a 32-year-old man with AIDS while he is receiving chronic therapy with inhaled pentamidine. Chest roentgenography reveals bilateral hilar vascular prominence. Bronchoalveolar lavage shows no evidence of infection. Which of the following is the most likely cause of the respiratory symptoms?
    a. Kaposi's sarcoma involving hilar lymph nodes
    b. Disseminated histoplasmosis
    c. Disseminated coccidioidomycosis
    d. Sarcoidosis
    e. Pulmonary hypertension

22. A 45-year-old man with stage IV sarcoidosis returns for follow-up examination. Chest roentgenography reveals a new cavitated lesion with a central mass in the right upper lobe. Which of the following is least likely in this patient?
    a. Significant hemoptysis
    b. Progressive weight loss, fever, and malaise
    c. Distant metastases
    d. Significant morbidity and mortality following surgical resection of the lung lesion
    e. Potential for cure with intracavitary instillation of an appropriate drug

23. Which of the following is incorrect about hypertrophic pulmonary osteoarthropathy?
    a. It consists of clubbing, painful periosteal hypertrophy of the long bones, and symmetrical arthralgias
    b. Gynecomastia, fever, and an increased erythrocyte sedimentation rate may be seen
    c. It most often is associated with non-small-cell carcinoma of the lung
    d. Ipsilateral (to the tumor) vagotomy is a therapeutic option
    e. Hypercalcemia is a common feature

24. A 30-year-old woman, a nonsmoker, with no history of asthma presents with exertional dyspnea and cough. Chest roentgenography reveals a diffuse bilateral interstitial/nodular process. Pulmonary function tests show moderately severe obstructive dysfunction. These features are not compatible with which of the following:
    a. Diffuse bronchiectasis
    b. Sjögren's syndrome
    c. Idiopathic pulmonary fibrosis
    d. Pulmonary lymphangioleiomyomatosis
    e. Pulmonary eosinophilic granuloma

25. Which of the following entities is not associated with smoking and/or aggravated by smoking?
    a. Pulmonary alveolar proteinosis
    b. Pulmonary eosinophilic granuloma

    c. Bronchoalveolar cell carcinoma
    d. Increased risk of alveolar hemorrhage in Goodpasture's syndrome
    e. Calcification of asbestos-induced pleural plaques

26. Which of the following is not associated with α_1-antitrypsin deficiency?
    a. Scleroderma
    b. Panacinar (panlobular) emphysema
    c. Emphysema affecting the lower lung zones
    d. Liver disease
    e. Panniculitis of the skin

27. Which of the following is not a feature of primary pulmonary hypertension?
    a. Usually a disease of young females
    b. Familial association is fairly common
    c. Raynaud's phenomenon is frequently seen
    d. Pulmonary artery capillary wedge pressure is increased
    e. Right ventricular failure is the primary determinant of prognosis

28. Which of the following is incorrect regarding pulmonary manifestations of systemic lupus erythematosus?
    a. Pleural involvement is the most common and often the presenting feature
    b. Diffuse interstitial pneumonitis is rare
    c. Alveolar hemorrhage is noted in up to 10% of patients
    d. Esophageal dysmotility contributes to pulmonary complications
    e. Pulmonary embolism is relatively common

True/false (indicate whether each answer is true or false)

29. Increasing asthmatic symptoms developed in a 34-year-old woman with chronic extrinsic asthma under control despite rigorous therapy with nonsteroidal bronchodilators. She has now noted expectoration of brownish-black sputum. Chest roentgenography reveals a soft patchy infiltrate in both upper lungs. With regard to this patient's new symptom complex:
    a. The serum level of immunoglobulin E is likely to be high
    b. High-resolution computed tomography of the lungs may show central bronchiectasis
    c. The presence of *Aspergillus fumigatus* in the sputum is diagnostic of the underlying condition
    d. Systemic corticosteroid therapy is indicated
    e. Long-acting β-agonist therapy is the treatment of choice
    f. Eosinophilia is usually absent

30. Bronchiolitis obliterans with organizing pneumonia (BOOP) may be associated with the following:

a. Polymyositis-dermatomyositis
b. Chronic eosinophilic pneumonia
c. Silo-filler's lung disease
d. Heart transplant recipients
e. Cystic fibrosis
f. Idiopathic pulmonary fibrosis

31. With regard to sleep apnea syndromes:
a. Central sleep apnea is the cessation of airflow accompanied by an absence of respiratory effort
b. Obstructive sleep apnea is the cessation of airflow with continued respiratory effort
c. Mixed sleep apnea is the cessation of airflow that typically begins with no respiratory effort but ends with increasing respiratory effort
d. Hypothyroidism can cause both obstructive and central sleep apnea
e. Tracheostomy is the treatment of choice for obstructive sleep apnea
f. Nasal constant airway positive pressure therapy is ineffective in obstructive sleep apnea

32. A 28-year-old woman presents to you for another opinion about systemic corticosteroid therapy recommended by her family physician for biopsy-proved sarcoidosis. Which of the following aspects of this patient's disease would require this therapy?
a. Asymptomatic and stable stage I disease
b. Stage I disease with endobronchial involvement manifested by cough and wheezing
c. Progressive stage III disease
d. Neurologic involvement
e. Hypercalcemia
f. Erythema nodosum

33. A 44-year-old man, nonsmoker, presents with progressive weakness and mild dyspnea. Chest roentgenography shows a well-defined anterior mediastinal mass. With regard to this patient's mediastinal lesion:
a. Thymoma is the most likely diagnosis
b. Red cell aplasia and hypogammaglobulinemia may occur
c. Most of these tumors are malignant
d. Myasthenia gravis is likely to be the cause of his weakness
e. The treatment of choice is external beam radiation
f. Barium esophagography is important to delineate the mass

34. A 68-year-old man, an 82-pack-year smoker, presents with hemoptysis. Chest roentgenography reveals mediastinal widening. The serum level of potassium is 2.8 mEq/L.

The following are more likely to occur in this patient:
a. Diminished serum level of sodium
b. Positive antineuronal antibody in the serum
c. Myasthenia gravis
d. Neurologic symptoms and signs
e. Typical Cushing's syndrome
f. Hypercalcemia

35. A 38-year-old man with chronic renal failure has been receiving chronic hemodialysis. However, he is not compliant with the dialysis schedule and medications. The following pulmonary complications are likely to occur:
a. Noncardiogenic pulmonary edema
b. Diffuse pulmonary calcification
c. Hypoxemia during hemodialysis
d. Pleural effusion
e. Recurrent alveolar hemorrhage
f. Pulmonary lymphoma

36. A 55-year-old man, a chronic alcoholic, presents with severe abdominal pain and dyspnea. Chest roentgenography reveals a moderate-sized left pleural effusion. The serum level of amylase is increased to 5x the normal value. With regard to the pleural effusion in this abdominal disease:
a. Pleural effusion is almost always left-sided
b. The pleural fluid is an exudate
c. The amylase level in the pleural fluid remains increased for a longer period than in the serum
d. Pleural fluid is almost always hemorrhagic
e. Adult respiratory distress syndrome may occur in this patient
f. The complement level is likely to increase in the fluid

37. A middle-aged man, a heavy smoker, presents with mild exertional dyspnea, worse in supine posture, since he recovered from coronary artery bypass grafting 5 weeks earlier. Hypothermic cardioplegia was used intraoperatively. Now, his left ventricular function is normal. Chest roentgenography reveals an elevated left hemidiaphragm. Fluoroscopy suggests paralysis of the left hemidiaphragm. The following recommendations are appropriate for this patient:
a. Computed tomography of the chest
b. Bronchoscopy
c. Diaphragmatic electromyography
d. Sleep in the semirecumbent or upright position
e. Continued observation
f. Intermittent positive pressure breathing (IPPB)

38. A tuberculin (PPD) reaction of ≥5 mm is considered positive in the following:
a. Those born in high prevalence (for tuberculosis) countries

b. Close contacts of patients with infectious tuberculosis
c. Persons with human immunodeficiency virus infection
d. Persons who exhibit fibrotic lesions on chest roentgenography
e. Intravenous drug users
f. All health care workers

39. Pulmonary coccidioidomycosis may be associated with or manifested by the following:
    a. Flu-like illness
    b. Erythema nodosum
    c. Thin-walled lung cavities
    d. Hilar lymphadenopathy
    e. Pleural effusion in >50% of patients

f. Fibrosing mediastinitis

40. A 30-year-old laborer presents with a 1-week history of fever (<101°F), cough, and progressive dyspnea. Raised erythematous nodules are noted along both shins. Chest roentgenography shows diffuse nodular (3 to 7 mm) infiltrates in both lungs. Medical history reveals that he was a member of a team that explored a bat-infested cave 4 weeks earlier. The following steps are appropriate in this patient:
    a. Close follow-up
    b. Histoplasma serologic testing
    c. Serologic test and skin test for blastomycosis
    d. Amphotericin given intravenously
    e. Triple antibacterial therapy
    f. Bronchoalveolar lavage and lung biopsy

ANSWERS

1. Answer a.

Cough develops in nearly 6% of patients taking angiotensin converting enzyme inhibitor drugs. Amiodarone is a well-known cause of pulmonary disease and frequently produces chest roentgenographic abnormalities. Pulmonary edema is unlikely because his cardiac status is stable. Cough without other symptoms is unlikely to be caused by an upper respiratory infection. New onset of asthma is less likely, although cough can be the presenting symptom of asthma.

2. Answer b.

All findings in this patient are typical of emphysema. An asthmatic patient responds to a bronchodilator. A chronic bronchitic's DLCO is usually normal. Lung functions in pulmonary fibrosis should show a restrictive pattern. In diaphragmatic weakness, MVV is diminished (out of proportion to FEV_1). Weight loss is seen in emphysema.

3. Answer c.

Bronchoalveolar lavage is excellent for the diagnosis of *Pneumocystis carinii*. It has little or no clinical role in the other diseases.

4. Answer d.

Normal lung compliance is 200 mL/cm H_2O. Therefore, this

patient's lungs are normal, and his dyspnea is nonpulmonary in origin.

5. Answer e.

Almost all aerosolized bronchodilators are generally used four times daily. It is important to know that the treatment regimen for longer acting salmeterol calls for a 12-hourly dosing.

6. Answer b.

All complications mentioned in this question are more common in adults with cystic fibrosis than in children.

7. Answer e.

As noted in the answer to question 3, bronchoalveolar lavage has no clinical role in the diagnosis of idiopathic pulmonary fibrosis. The other tests help to assess pulmonary dysfunction; computed tomography may establish the diagnosis if the clinical features indicate idiopathic pulmonary fibrosis.

8. Answer d.

In this young nonsmoker, a bilateral upper lobe process is most unlikely to represent metastatic cancer. Most primary lung cancers originate in the upper lobes, whereas metastatic disease is more common in the lower lung zones.

9. Answer c.

This patient has sarcoidosis. Even though earlier reports

used gallium scan in the diagnosis and follow-up of patients with sarcoidosis, it is no longer considered a helpful test.

10. Answer d.

The patient has hereditary hemorrhagic telangiectasia with pulmonary arteriovenous malformations. Neurologic complications are quite common in this condition, and almost all patients should undergo therapy to eliminate the pulmonary lesions. Bronchoscopic biopsy may lead to severe bleeding and should not be performed.

11. Answer a.

In this patient, primary lung cancer is the most likely diagnosis, and, thus, surgical resection is the best option.

12. Answer b.

This patient most likely has squamous cell carcinoma of the lung. The hypercalcemia may be related to paraneoplastic syndrome or metastatic bone disease. In either case, urinary calcium measurements will be of little help in management.

13. Answer a.

The appearance of pleural fluid can be misleading in the diagnosis of chylous effusion and empyema. Cholesterol pleural effusions are not true chylous effusions. The presence of chylomicrons is necessary to establish the diagnosis of chylous effusion.

14. Answer b.

The most likely diagnosis is deep vein thrombosis. She has no new symptoms to suggest pulmonary embolism (respiratory symptoms were present before the leg symptoms developed).

15. Answer c.

In spite of the results of the lung scan, the clinical suspicion at this point is high for pulmonary embolism. Pulmonary angiography is indicated.

16. Answer d.

This patient had all the characteristic features of Wegener's granulomatosis. c-ANCA is quite specific for this diagnosis. p-ANCA may be present in Wegener's granulomatosis, but not consistently so.

17. Answer c.

Pulmonary infections in patients with sickle cell anemia most often are caused by *Streptococcus pneumoniae*.

18. Answer d.

Mycoplasma pneumonia causes patchy pulmonary infil-

trates and small pleural effusions. Cavitated lung lesion is not a feature. Other complications mentioned represent some of the unusual manifestations of this infection.

19. Answer b.

Hantavirus pulmonary syndrome is not necessarily limited to Native Americans.

20. Answer d.

Allergic bronchopulmonary aspergillosis occurs in patients with asthma and cystic fibrosis. Other connections mentioned in the question and elsewhere in the text are important for board examinations.

21. Answer e.

The first four conditions are usually associated with pulmonary parenchymal lesions, even though stage I sarcoidosis is more likely to present with hilar adenopathy. In stage I sarcoidosis, almost all patients are asymptomatic and chronic dyspnea is unlikely. Pulmonary hypertension is now a well-known complication in patients with AIDS.

22. Answer c.

This patient has chronic sarcoidosis complicated by aspergilloma. Hemoptysis and systemic illness are among the indications for surgical resection, which carries a high rate of morbidity and mortality. Because of this, many pulmonologists use intracavitary instillation of amphotericin.

23. Answer e.

Hypercalcemia is not a feature of hypertrophic pulmonary osteoarthropathy; the latter is associated most often with either adenocarcinoma or large cell carcinoma of the lung.

24. Answer c.

Obstructive lung disease develops in all the conditions mentioned (even though chest roentgenography findings may suggest restrictive disease) except in pulmonary fibrosis in which the typical findings are those of restrictive lung disease.

25. Answer c.

All the conditions except bronchoalveolar cell carcinoma of the lung are associated with smoking. Note that those who smoke bleed more if they have Goodpasture's syndrome, but smoking does not predispose to the development of this disease.

26. Answer a.

All except scleroderma are associated with α_1-antitrypsin deficiency.

27. Answer d.

Pulmonary artery capillary wedge pressure is usually normal or slightly decreased in most forms of pulmonary hypertension. It may be increased in pulmonary hypertension caused by left-sided cardiac lesions such as mitral stenosis.

28. Answer d.

Esophageal dysmotility is not a feature of systemic lupus erythematosus. It is a common problem in scleroderma, mixed connective tissue disease, and polymyositis-dermatomyositis.

29. a, true; b, true; c, false; d, true; e, false; f, false.

The presence of *Aspergillus* species is only a minor criterion for the diagnosis of allergic bronchopulmonary aspergillosis. Eosinophilia is common. Systemic corticosteroid therapy for >6 months is indicated.

30. a, true; b, true; c, true; d, true; e, false; f, false.

BOOP is a pathologic diagnosis and has many causes. It is not a feature of cystic fibrosis and idiopathic pulmonary fibrosis.

31. a, true; b, true; c, true; d, true; e, false; f, false.

Nasal constant positive airway pressure breathing is the treatment of choice in obstructive sleep apnea. Tracheostomy is reserved for severe cases that do not respond to nasal constant positive airway pressure.

32. a, false; b, true; c, true; d, true; e, true; f, false.

Asymptomatic stage I sarcoidosis and erythema nodosum do not require corticosteroid therapy.

33. a, true; b, true; c, false; d, true; e, false; f, false.

Thymoma is the most common tumor in the anterior mediastinum. Most thymomas are benign. The treatment of choice is surgical resection.

34. a, true; b, true; c, false; d, true; e, false; f, false.

Syndrome of inappropriate ADH secretion in this patient with small cell carcinoma can cause hyponatremia. Myasthenic syndrome (not myasthenia gravis) is more likely in this patient,

as are neurologic problems. Patients with small cell carcinoma do not live long enough for typical Cushing's syndrome to develop.

35. a, true; b, true; c, true; d, true; e, false; f, false.

Among the many pulmonary complications in chronic renal failure, alveolar hemorrhage and pulmonary lymphoma are not included. Because of hemodialysis-induced hypocarbia during dialysis, patients hypoventilate and exhibit hypoxia. Pulmonary calcification is common in those receiving chronic hemodialysis.

36. a, true; b, true; c, true; d, false; e, true; f, false.

In pancreatitis, the pleural fluid is bloody in 30% of patients. Amylase level remains higher for longer periods in the pleural fluid. The complement level is not altered in pancreatitis.

37. a, false; b, false; c, false; d, true; e, true; f, false.

This patient has hypothermia-induced diaphragmatic paralysis ("frost-bitten phrenic") that developed during heart surgery. Diaphragmatic weakness usually resolves over 6-8 weeks. Observation and reassurance are necessary.

38. a, false; b, true; c, true; d, true; e, false; f, false.

Note the relatively new guidelines for interpretation of tuberculin (PPD) skin test result (page 753).

39. a, true; b, true; c, true; d, true; e, false; f, false.

Pleural effusion is noted in <10% of patients with coccidioidomycosis. Fibrosing mediastinitis most commonly is caused by histoplasmosis.

40. a, true; b, true; c, false; d, false; e, false; f, true.

Not all patients with acute histoplasmosis require antifungal therapy. In this patient, it is important to diagnose the infection before commencing any type of treatment. Note that there is no reliable skin test or serologic test for the diagnosis of blastomycosis.

NOTES

CHAPTER 22
RHEUMATOLOGY

Robert M. Valente, M.D.
William W. Ginsburg, M.D.

PART I
Robert M. Valente, M.D.

RHEUMATOID ARTHRITIS

Rheumatoid arthritis is a chronic systemic inflammatory disease characterized by joint destruction. It affects 0.03%-1.5% of the population worldwide. Its incidence peaks between ages 35 and 45; however, the age-related prevalence continues to increase even past age 65. The presentation of an unknown antigen to immunologically susceptible persons is believed to trigger rheumatoid arthritis. Several viruses have been implicated in chronic arthritis, including Epstein-Barr virus, HTLV-1 virus, rubella virus, cytomegalovirus, herpes simplex virus, parvovirus, and arbovirus. Mycobacterium, heat-shock proteins, and autoimmunity to such endogenous components as immunoglobulin, proteoglycans, and collagen are also implicated.

There is an immunogenetic predisposition to developing rheumatoid arthritis. Class II major histocompatibility complex (MHC) molecules on the surface of antigen-presenting cells are responsible for initiating cellular immune responses and for stimulating the differentiation of B lymphocytes into plasma cells that produce antibody. Most patients with rheumatoid arthritis have class II MHC type HLA-DR4 or HLA-DR1 or both. HLA-DR4 can be divided into five subtypes, two of which independently promote susceptibility to rheumatoid arthritis. Compared with controls, patients with HLA-DR2 are less likely to have rheumatoid arthritis. Rheumatoid arthritis patients with HLA-DR3 may have low-titer rheumatoid factor and increased toxicity to gold and D-penicillamine.

- Rheumatoid arthritis affects 0.03%-1.5% of the population.
- Most patients with rheumatoid arthritis have class II MHC type HLA-DR4 or HLA-DR1 or both.
- There is a 6x increase in concordance of rheumatoid factor-positive rheumatoid arthritis among dizygotic twins.

- There is a 30x increased risk of rheumatoid arthritis in a monozygotic twin when sibling has the disease.
- There is a 3x-5x increased risk of rheumatoid arthritis in white Americans with HLA-DR4.

The immune reaction begins in the synovial lining of the joint. The earliest pathologic changes in the disease are microvascular injury that leads to increased vascular permeability and the accumulation of inflammatory cells (CD4 lymphocytes, polymorphonuclear leukocytes, and plasma cells) in the perivascular space. Cytokines, lymphokines, and various anaphylatoxins and chemoattractants are released. Angiogenesis occurs in the synovial membrane. Patients have swelling, pain, and joint stiffness with the onset of vascular injury and angiogenesis. The warmth, swelling, pain, and limitation of motion worsen as the synovial membrane proliferates and the inflammatory reaction builds. Mediators of inflammation promote synovial cell proliferation, the accumulation of neutrophils in synovial fluid, and the maturation of B cells into plasma cells. Plasma cells in the joint locally synthesize rheumatoid factor and other antibodies that promote inflammation. The local immune response becomes self-perpetuating. The immune complexes activate the complement system, releasing chemotactic factors and promoting vascular permeability and opsonization. Increased phagocytosis leads to increased lysosomal enzyme release and the digestion of collagen, cartilage matrix, and elastic tissues. The release of oxygen free radicals injures cells. Damaged cell membranes release phospholipids that fuel the arachidonic acid cascade and promote the local inflammatory response. Proliferating synovium polarizes into a centripetally invasive pannus, destroying the weakened cartilage and subchondral bone. Chondrocytes, stimulated in the inflammatory milieu, release their own proteases and collagenases.

- Rheumatoid factor is an immunoglobulin (usually IgM) that binds other immunoglobulins (usually IgG) at their Fc components, forming immune complexes.
- The immune reaction begins in the synovial lining of the joint.
- Swelling, pain, and joint stiffness occur with the onset of vascular injury and angiogenesis.
- Immune complexes activate the complement system.
- The release of oxygen free radicals injures cells.

Clinical Features

The joints most commonly involved (>85% of patients) in rheumatoid arthritis are the metacarpophalangeal and proximal interphalangeal joints and the wrists (Fig. 22-1). The distribution of involvement is symmetrical; predominantly small joints are involved. Ultimately, the knees (80% of patients), ankles (80%), shoulders (60%), elbows (50%), hips (50%), acromioclavicular joints (50%), cervical spine (40%), and temporomandibular joints (30%) can be involved. The sternoclavicular joints, cricoarytenoid joints, and the ear ossicles are affected infrequently. Joints affected with rheumatoid arthritis are warm and swollen. The joint enlargement feels spongy and occurs with the thickening of the synovium. An associated joint effusion may make the joint feel fluctuant. Patients describe deep aching and soreness in the involved joints which are aggravated by use and can be present at rest. Prolonged morning joint stiffness and "gelling" or recurrence of this prolonged stiffness after resting are hallmarks of joint

inflammation. The patient may feel the stiffness throughout the body, not just in the involved peripherial joints. This global stiffness is one of the many constitutional features that complicate rheumatoid arthritis.

- The joints most commonly involved in rheumatoid arthritis are the metacarpophalangeal and proximal interphalangeal joints and the wrists (>85% of patients).
- The distribution of involvement is symmetrical.
- Hallmarks of joint inflammation: prolonged morning joint stiffness and "gelling" or recurrence of the prolonged stiffness after resting.

Constitutional Features

Fatigue initially affects up to 40% of patients. Weight loss, muscle pain, excessive sweating, or low-grade fever occurs in 20% of patients presenting with rheumatoid arthritis. Most patients with *active* arthritis have more than 1 hour of morning stiffness. The musculoskeletal complications of rheumatoid arthritis are listed in Table 22-1.

Musculoskeletal Complications

Cervical Spine

One-half of all patients with seropositive rheumatoid arthritis have involvement of the cervical spine. It is diagnosed with cervical flexion and extension radiographs that demonstrate subluxation. One-half of these patients have subluxation at

Fig. 22-1. Moderately active seropositive rheumatoid arthritis. The patient has soft tissue swelling across the entire row of metatarsophalangeal joints and proximal interphalangeal joints bilaterally and soft tissue swelling mounding up over the wrists. Note the nearly complete lack of change at the distal interphalangeal joints.

Table 22-1.--Musculoskeletal Complications of Rheumatoid Arthritis

---

Characteristic deformities include

Boutonnière deformity of the finger, with hyperextension of the distal interphalangeal joint and flexion of the proximal interphalangeal joint

Swan-neck deformity of the finger, with hyperextension at the proximal interphalangeal joint and flexion of the distal interphalangeal joint

Ulnar deviation of the metacarpophalangeal joints; it can progress to complete volar subluxation of the proximal phalanx from the metacarpophalangeal head

Compression of the carpal bones and radial deviation at the carpus

Subluxation at the wrist

Valgus of the ankle and hindfoot

Pes planus

Forefoot varus and hallux valgus

Cock-up toes from subluxation at the metatarsophalangeal joints

---

the atlantoaxial level, and the rest have subaxial subluxations, typically at two or more levels. The cervical instability is usually asymptomatic; however, patients may have pain and stiffness in the neck, occiput, shoulder, or interscapular areas. Patients may present with syncope, light-headedness, paresthesias of the face or limbs, or nystagmus. Occasionally, the first sign of cervical instability may be sudden ataxia, weakness of the limbs, or frank tetraplegia. Interference with blood flow in the vertebral arteries (vertebrobasilar insufficiency) explains some of the cranial nerve symptoms and the blackouts. New neurologic symptoms mandate urgent neurologic evaluation and consideration of surgical intervention. However, cervical subluxation does not usually progress to neurologic or vascular compromise. Indications for surgical treatment include neurologic or vascular compromise and intractable local symptoms. In active patients, prophylactic cervical spine stabilization is recommended when there is evidence of extreme (>8 mm) subluxation of C-1 over C-2. The probability of cervical involvement is predicted by the severity of peripheral arthritis.

- One-half of all patients with seropositive rheumatoid arthritis have involvement of the cervical spine.
- Patients with cervical spine involvement may present with syncope, light-headedness, paresthesias of face and limbs, nystagmus, ataxia, or acute myelopathy.
- Indications for surgical treatment: neurologic or vascular compromise and intractable local symptoms.
- The probability of cervical involvement is predicted by the severity of peripheral arthritis.

Popliteal Cyst

Flexion of the knee markedly increases the intra-articular pressure of a swollen joint. This pressure produces an outpouching of the posterior components of the joint space that is termed a "popliteal" or a "baker's" cyst. The cyst can rupture down into the calf or, rarely, superiorly into the posterior thigh. Rupture of the popliteal cyst with dissection into the calf may resemble acute thrombophlebitis and is called "pseudophlebitis." Fever, leukocytosis, and ecchymosis around the ankle (crescent sign) can occur with the rupture. Ultrasonographic examination of the popliteal space can be diagnostic. Popliteal cysts should be distinguished from a popliteal artery aneurysm, lymphadenopathy, and (more rarely) benign or malignant tumors. Treatment of an acute cyst rupture includes bed rest, elevation of the leg, ice massage, and an intra-articular injection of corticosteroid. Treatment of the popliteal cyst requires improvement in the knee arthritis.

- Popliteal cyst is also called "baker's" cyst.
- Rupture of a popliteal cyst may resemble acute thrombophlebitis ("pseudophlebitis").
- Ultrasonography can distinguish cysts from popliteal artery aneurysm, lymphadenopathy, and tumors.

Tenosynovitis

Tenosynovitis of the finger flexor and extensor tendon sheaths is common. It presents with diffuse swelling between the joints or a palpable grating within the flexor tendon sheaths in the palm with passive movement of the digit. Other tenosynovial syndromes in rheumatoid arthritis include de Quervain's and wrist tenosynovitis. Persistent inflammation can produce stenosing tenosynovitis, loss of function, and, ultimately, rupture of hand extensor tendons. Treatment of acute tenosynovitis includes immobilization, warm soaks, nonsteroidal anti-inflammatory drugs (NSAIDs), and local injections of corticosteroid in the tendon sheath.

- Tenosynovitis of the finger flexor and extensor tendon sheaths is common.
- Other tenosynovial syndromes in rheumatoid arthritis: de Quervain's and wrist tenosynovitis.

Carpal Tunnel Syndrome

Rheumatoid arthritis is the second most common cause of carpal tunnel syndrome (pregnancy is the number one cause). This syndrome is associated with paresthesias of the hand in a typical median nerve distribution. Discomfort may radiate up the forearm or into the upper arm. The symptoms worsen with prolonged flexion of the wrist and at night. Late complications include thenar muscle weakness and atrophy and permanent sensory loss. Other nerve entrapment syndromes, including tarsal tunnel syndrome, affect patients with rheumatoid arthritis. Treatment includes resting splints, control of inflammation, and local injection of glucocorticosteroids. Surgical release is recommended for persistent symptoms.

- Rheumatoid arthritis is the second most common cause of carpal tunnel syndrome.
- Carpal tunnel syndrome: paresthesias of the hand in a typical median nerve distribution.
- Other nerve entrapment syndromes, including tarsal tunnel syndrome, affect patients with rheumatoid arthritis.

Extra-Articular Complications of Rheumatoid Arthritis

Typically, extra-articular complications are seen in patients who have high titers of rheumatoid factor. In general, the number and severity of the extra-articular features vary with the duration and severity of disease.

Rheumatoid Nodules

From 20% to 35% of patients have rheumatoid nodules, which occur over extensor surfaces and at pressure points. They also occur in the lungs, heart, kidney, and dura mater. The nodules occur almost exclusively in patients with rheumatoid factor. They have characteristic histopathologic features. A central area of necrosis encircled by palisading fibroblasts is surrounded by a collagenous capsule and a perivascular collection of chronic inflammatory cells. Breakdown of the skin over rheumatoid nodules, with ulcers and infection, can be a major source of morbidity. The infection can spread to local bursae, infect bone, or spread hematogenously to joints.

- 20%-35% of patients have rheumatoid nodules.
- Rheumatoid nodules occur over extensor surfaces and at pressure points.
- Rheumatoid nodules have characteristic histopathologic features.

Rheumatoid Vasculitis

Rheumatoid vasculitis usually occurs in patients who have severe deforming arthritis and a high titer of rheumatoid factor. The vasculitis is mediated by the deposition of circulating immune complexes on the blood vessel wall, with activation of complement. At its most benign, it occurs with rheumatoid arthritis and nodules, with small infarcts over the nodules and at the cuticles. Proliferation of the vascular intima and media causes this obliterative endarteropathy, which has little associated inflammation. It is best managed by controlling the underlying arthritis. Leukocytoclastic or small vessel vasculitis produces palpable purpura or cutaneous ulceration, particularly over the malleoli of the lower extremities. This vasculitis can cause pyoderma gangrenosum or peripheral sensory neuropathy. Secondary polyarteritis, which is clinically and histopathologically identical to polyarteritis nodosa, can

result in mononeuritis multiplex. Occasionally, the vasculitis appears after the joint disease appears "burned out." Glucocorticosteroids do not promote vasculitis in cases of rheumatoid arthritis.

- Rheumatoid vasculitis usually occurs in patients who have severe deforming arthritis and a high titer of rheumatoid factor.
- Rheumatoid vasculitis is mediated by the deposition of circulating immune complexes on the blood vessel wall.
- Rheumatoid vasculitis comprises a spectrum of vascular disease, including rheumatoid nodules and obliterative endarteropathy, leukocytoclastic or small vessel vasculitis, and secondary polyarteritis (systemic necrotizing vasculitis).

Neurologic Manifestations

Neurologic manifestations of rheumatoid arthritis include mild peripheral sensory neuropathy. Sensory-motor neuropathy (mononeuropathy) suggests vasculitis or nerve entrapment (e.g., carpal tunnel syndrome). Cervical vertebral subluxation can cause myelopathy. Erosive changes may promote basilar invagination of the odontoid process of C-2 into the underside of the brain, causing spinal cord compression and death.

Pulmonary Manifestations

The most common form of lung disease in patients with rheumatoid arthritis is mild obstructive pulmonary dysfunction. The prevalence of obstructive change increases with the duration of the disease. It is associated with keratoconjunctivitis sicca. Pleural disease has been noted in 40% of autopsies of cases of rheumatoid arthritis. Clinically significant pleural disease is less frequent. Characteristically, rheumatoid pleural effusions are asymptomatic until they become large enough to interfere mechanically with respiration. The pleural fluid is an exudate. The concentration of glucose in the pleural fluid is low (10-50 mg/dL) because of impaired transport of glucose into the pleural space. The pleural effusion in rheumatoid arthritis has a mononuclear cell predominance and usually <5,000 cells/μL. Pulmonary nodules appear singly or in clusters. Single nodules have the appearance of a coin lesion. Nodules typically are pleural-based and may cavitate and create a bronchopleural fistula. Pneumoconiosis in rheumatoid arthritis, "Caplan's syndrome," is synergistic, producing a violent fibroblastic reaction and large nodules. Acute interstitial pneumonitis is a rare complication that may begin as alveolitis and progress to respiratory insufficiency and death. Interstitial fibrosis is a chronic slowly progressive process. It has physical findings of diffuse dry crackles on lung auscultation and a reticular nodular radiographic pattern affecting both lung fields, initially in the lung bases. A decrease in the diffusing capacity of the lung for carbon dioxide and a restrictive pattern on pulmonary function testing complicate symptomatic interstitial fibrosis. Interstitial changes are highly associated with smoking. Bronchiolitis obliterans with or without organizing pneumonia may occur with rheumatoid arthritis or its treatment. It produces an obstructive picture on pulmonary function testing.

- Obstructive airway disease is found in 35% of patients with rheumatoid arthritis.
- Rheumatoid pleural disease is common but symptomatic. The pleural fluid is remarkable for low levels of glucose.
- Rheumatoid lung nodules are pleural-based and can cause a bronchopleural fistula.
- Interstitial fibrosis is usually a chronic slowly progressive process.

Cardiac Complications

Pericarditis has been noted in 50% of autopsies of cases of rheumatoid arthritis. Rheumatoid nodules can occur in the pericardium. However, patients rarely present with pericardial symptoms. Effusive pericarditis uncommonly produces cardiac tamponade. Recurrent effusive pericarditis without symptoms occasionally evolves to chronic constrictive pericarditis. Untreated constrictive pericarditis has a 70% 1-year mortality. Rheumatoid arthritis carditis includes conduction abnormalities in the myocardium. Valve dysfunction and coronary vasculitis have also been described. Granulomatous inflammation can spread to involve the base of the aorta.

- Patients rarely present with pericardial symptoms despite frequent serous pericarditis.
- Untreated constrictive pericarditis has a 70% 1-year mortality.
- Granulomatous inflammation can spread to involve the base of the aorta.

Liver Abnormalities

Patients with rheumatoid arthritis can have increased levels of liver enzymes, particularly alkaline phosphatase. Increased levels of aspartate aminotransferase, γ–glutamyltransferase, and acute-phase proteins and decreased levels of albumin and prealbumin also occur in active rheumatoid arthritis. Liver biopsy shows nonspecific changes of inflammation or nodular regenerative hyperplasia, which may cause portal hypertension and hypersplenism. Many medications used to treat rheumatoid arthritis increase liver enzyme levels.

- Increased levels of liver enzymes, particularly alkaline phosphatase, may occur in rheumatoid arthritis.
- Nodular hyperplasia of the liver can complicate rheumatoid arthritis and lead to portal hypertension and hypersplenism.
- Many medications used to treat rheumatoid arthritis increase the levels of liver enzymes.

Ophthalmic Abnormalities

Keratoconjunctivitis sicca, or secondary Sjögren's syndrome, is the most common ophthalmic complication in rheumatoid arthritis. Episcleritis and scleritis also occur independent of the joint inflammation and are usually treated topically. Severe scleritis progressing to scleromalacia perforans causes blindness. Infrequent ocular complications of rheumatoid arthritis include episcleral nodules, palsy of the superior oblique muscle caused by tenosynovitis of its tendon sheath (Brown's syndrome), and uveitis. Retinopathy is an infrequent complication of antimalarial medication.

- Keratoconjunctivitis sicca, or secondary Sjögren's syndrome, is the most common ophthalmic complication in rheumatoid arthritis.
- Severe scleritis progressing to scleromalacia perforans causes blindness.

Laboratory Findings

Nonspecific alterations in many laboratory values are common in patients with rheumatoid arthritis. Normocytic anemia (hemoglobin in the 10-g/dL range), leukocytosis, thrombocytosis, hypoalbuminemia, and hypergammaglobulinemia are common. Rheumatoid factor (IgM) occurs in 90% of patients, but its presence may not be detected for months to years after the initial joint symptoms are noted. Rheumatoid factor is a marker of immune stimulation and occurs in various connective tissue diseases and infections, including subacute bacterial endocarditis and lymphoproliferative disorders. Diseases in bold type in Table 22-2 are most likely to have high titers of rheumatoid factor. Five percent of the normal population have a low titer of rheumatoid factor. Cryoglobulins and antinuclear antibodies are common. Eosinophilia occurs in up to 30% of patients with rheumatoid arthritis. It may be a marker for toxicity due to gold treatment or it may accompany rheumatoid vasculitis. C-reactive protein correlates with disease activity, but it is not more helpful than the erythrocyte sedimentation rate. Rheumatoid arthritis patients with active disease have low iron-binding capacity, low plasma levels of iron, and low erythropoietin levels, unless they are iron deficient.

- Normocytic anemia and leukocytosis are common in rheumatoid arthritis.
- Rheumatoid factor is neither specific nor sensitive for the diagnosis of rheumatoid arthritis.
- Cryoglobulins and antinuclear antibodies are common in patients with seropositive rheumatoid arthritis.
- Eosinophilia may be a marker for rheumatoid vasculitis or toxicity due to gold treatment.
- C-reactive protein correlates with disease activity, but it is not more helpful than the erythrocyte sedimentation rate.

Table 28-2.--Diseases That May Have Positive Rheumatoid Factor*

Rheumatoid arthritis
Sjögren's syndrome
Systemic lupus erythematosus
Scleroderma
Sarcoidosis
Idiopathic pulmonary fibrosis
Mixed cryoglobulinemia
Hypergammaglobulinemic purpura
Asbestosis
Malignancies
Infectious mononucleosis
Influenza
Chronic active hepatitis
Vaccinations
Tuberculosis
Syphilis
Subacute bacterial endocarditis
Brucellosis
Leprosy
Salmonellosis
Malaria
Kala-azar
Schistosomiasis
Filariasis
Trypanosomiasis

*Diseases that are printed in boldface type are the most likely to have high-titer rheumatoid factor.

Fig. 22-2. Radiographic features of long-standing rheumatoid arthritis. Periarticular osteoporosis is marked by decreased cortical margins and reduction in trabecular textures in the periarticular areas. There is symmetrical narrowing of the joint space at the proximal interphalangeal joints and second and third metacarpophalangeal joints. Marginal erosions are best seen at the thumb interphalangeal and metacarpophalangeal joints and at the second and third metacarpophalangeal joints. Additional destructive changes have nearly obliterated the usual margins of the carpal bones, making it difficult to distinguish them individually.

Synovial fluid is cloudy and light yellow, with poor viscosity, and typically contains 10,000-75,000 leukocytes/µL (60%-75% polymorphonuclear neutrophils). Synovial fluid levels of glucose are low. Microscopic crystals are absent. Ragocytes, phagocytic cells with intercellular immunoglobulin and cholesterol crystals, may be found.

Radiographic Findings

The radiographic findings in early rheumatoid arthritis are normal or show soft tissue swelling. Later, the characteristic changes of periarticular osteoporosis, symmetrical narrowing of the joint space, and marginal bony erosions become obvious. Radiographic changes at end-stage rheumatoid arthritis include subluxation and other deformities, joint destruction, fibrous ankylosis, and, rarely, bony ankylosis (Fig. 22-2).

- The characteristic radiologic changes in rheumatoid arthritis include: periarticular osteoporosis, symmetrical narrowing of the joint space, and marginal bony erosions.

Diagnosis of Rheumatoid Arthritis

To make the diagnosis of rheumatoid arthritis, symptoms must be present for more than 6 weeks in persons 16 years old or older. Four of the seven criteria of the American Rheumatism Association listed in Table 22-3 must be satisfied for the diagnosis to be made.

Natural History

More than one-half of patients with rheumatoid arthritis have insidious onset of the joint disease, occurring over weeks to months. However, in one-third of the patients, the onset is rapid, occurring in days or weeks. Early in the course of the disease, most patients have oligoarthritis. Their disease becomes polyarticular with time. From 10% to 20% of patients have progressive arthritis. The course may be slow, fluctuating, or rapid, but the end point is the same: disabling, destructive arthritis. The group that does not respond to therapy is small (<5% of all patients with seropositive rheumatoid arthritis). Patients with polycyclic disease have flares interrupted by

Table 22-3.--American Rheumatism Association Criteria for Making the Diagnosis of Rheumatoid Arthritis[*]

One or more hours of morning stiffness in and around the joints

Arthritis of three or more joint areas involved simultaneously

Arthritis of at least one area in the wrist, metacarpophalangeal, or proximal interphalangeal joints

Symmetrical arthritis involving the same joint areas on both sides of the body

Rheumatoid nodules

Serum rheumatoid factor

Radiographic changes typical of rheumatoid arthritis, including periarticular osteoporosis, joint-space narrowing, and marginal erosions.

---

[*]1987 revision

partial or complete remissions. They account for 70% of all patients with rheumatoid arthritis. Spontaneous remissions in the polycyclic or progressive group almost never occur after 2 years of disease. Patients who meet the 1987 American Rheumatism Association modified criteria for rheumatoid arthritis, including wrist and metacarpophalangeal involvement, are at higher risk for progressive rheumatoid arthritis. Most of the disability is determined in the first several years of disease. The relationship between disease duration and inability to work is nearly linear. After 15 years of rheumatoid arthritis, 15% of patients are completely disabled. The life span of men with rheumatoid arthritis is decreased by 7.5 years and 3.5 years for women, in comparison with their normal counterparts. Mortality is predicted by age, disease severity, comorbid cardiovascular disease, and functional status. Mortality is also influenced by educational level and socioeconomic factors.

- In one-third of patients, the onset of rheumatoid arthritis is rapid (days or weeks).
- 10%-20% of patients have progressive arthritis.
- The relationship between disease duration and inability to work is nearly linear.
- With rheumatoid arthritis, life span is decreased by 7.5 years for men and 3.5 years for women.

Treatment of Rheumatoid Arthritis

The management of patients with rheumatoid arthritis requires making the correct diagnosis, determining the functional status of the patient, and selecting goals of management with the patient. Goals of management include relieving inflammation and pain and maintaining function.

The principles emphasized by physical medicine include bed rest or rest periods, improving nonrestorative sleep, and joint protection (including modification of activities of daily life, range of motion exercises, orthotics, and splints, if they help

the pain). Exercise should begin with range of motion and stretching to overcome contracture. Strengthening and conditioning exercises should be prescribed carefully, depending on the activity of the patient's disease.

Initial treatment is with an NSAID given at anti-inflammatory doses. If the response is inadequate after 3-4 weeks, a trial of a second nonchemically related NSAID is used. Glucocorticoids may be necessary to preserve function. Disease-modifying agents of rheumatic disease are also known as second-line agents, slow-acting antirheumatic drugs, or remittive agents. Short-term studies with disease-modifying agents of rheumatic disease confirm improved quality of life. They are used sequentially. The classic indications for adding a disease-modifying, or second-line, agent include the correct diagnosis, failure of disease to respond to an NSAID, as a glucocorticoid-sparing agent, and when sufficient disease exists to justify the therapeutic risk. Six months of uninterrupted treatment with a disease-modifying agent is usually required to assess its efficacy. They augment the response to concomitantly used NSAIDs or corticosteroids given in low doses. Disease-modifying agents of rheumatic disease include:

- Methotrexate.
- Antimalarial drugs.
- Sulfasalazine.
- Intramuscular injections of gold.
- Azathioprine.
- Cyclophosphamide.

Patients receiving one of these disease-modifying agents will take it, on average, for 3-5 years before the lack of efficacy or toxicity forces discontinuation of its use. A second disease-modifying agent is substituted for the first one when a therapeutic or toxic roadblock is reached. Failure to respond to one of these agents does not predict a negative response or intolerance to the others. Clinical trials of combinations of disease-modifying agents have not documented a favorable benefit-to-toxicity ratio. (For information on individual drug indications and adverse effects, see the section at the end of this chapter on antirheumatic drugs.)

- Goals of management include relieving inflammation and pain and maintaining function.
- A disease-modifying agent is added when symptoms are inadequately controlled with NSAIDs, to reduce dependence on glucocorticoids, and when disease activity justifies the risk of the agent.
- Rheumatoid arthritis: initial treatment is with an NSAID given at anti-inflammatory doses.
- Glucocorticosteroids may be necessary to preserve function.
- Disease-modifying agent: 6 months of uninterrupted treatment is usually required to assess efficacy.

Surgery in the Treatment of Rheumatoid Arthritis

Orthopedic surgery for resistant rheumatoid arthritis remains the most significant therapeutic option for preserving or enhancing patient function. Synovectomy of the wrist and nearby tendon sheaths is beneficial when medication alone fails to control the synovitis. The operation preserves joint function and prevents the lysis of extensor tendons that can result in a loss of function. Synovectomy of the knee, either open or through an arthroscope, can delay the progression of rheumatoid arthritis from 6 months to 3 years. Removal of nodules and treatment for local nerve entrapment syndromes are also important surgical treatments for rheumatoid arthritis. Arthroplasty is reserved for patients in whom medical management has failed and in whom intractable pain or compromise in function developed because of a destroyed joint. Arthroplasty, arthrodesis (wrist), and synovectomy are important components of well-balanced rheumatology treatment programs. Total joint arthroplasty in rheumatoid arthritis patients has a slightly poorer long-term outcome than in patients with osteoarthritis. Nevertheless, joint replacement surgery has had a major impact on patient disability.

- Orthopedic surgery is the most significant advance in the treatment of medically resistant rheumatoid arthritis.
- To anticipate or to attempt to achieve complete symptomatic relief in every patient is an unrealistic and impossible goal.
- Total joint arthroplasty in rheumatoid arthritis patients has a slightly poorer long-term outcome than in patients with osteoarthritis.

CONDITIONS RELATED TO RHEUMATOID ARTHRITIS

Seronegative Rheumatoid Arthritis

Rheumatoid factor-negative (seronegative) rheumatoid arthritis is not associated with extra-articular manifestations. However, the arthritis usually is destructive, deforming, and indistinguishable from seropositive rheumatoid arthritis.

- Seronegative rheumatoid arthritis is not associated with extra-articular manifestations.

Seronegative Rheumatoid Arthritis of the Elderly

A subgroup of patients older than 60 with seronegative rheumatoid arthritis may have milder arthritis. This subgroup suddenly develops polyarticular inflammation that is controlled best with low doses of prednisone. Minimal destructive changes and deformity occur. An additional group of elderly seronegative arthritis patients (men in their 70s) present with acute polyarthritis and pitting edema of the hands and feet. They have a prompt and gratifying response to low doses of prednisone.

- Patients >60 years who suddenly develop rheumatoid factor-negative polyarticular arthritis are best controlled initially with low doses of prednisone.

Adult-Onset Still's Disease

Systemic **juvenile** rheumatoid arthritis is known as "Still's disease." It has quotidian (fever spike with return to normal all in one day) high-spiking fevers, arthralgia, arthritis, seronegativity (negative rheumatoid factor and antinuclear antibody), leukocytosis, macular evanescent rash, serositis, lymphadenopathy, splenomegaly, and hepatomegaly. Fever, rash, and arthritis are the classic triad of Still's disease.

- Systemic juvenile rheumatoid arthritis is called "Still's disease."
- Classic triad of Still's disease: fever, rash, and arthritis.

Adult-onset Still's disease has a slight female predominance. Its onset commonly occurs between ages 16 and 35. Temperature >39°C occurs in a quotidian or double quotidian pattern in 96% of the patients. The rash has a typical appearance: a macular salmon-colored eruption on the trunk and extremities. The transient rash is usually noticed at the time of increased temperature. Arthritis occurs in 95% of these patients, and in about one-third, the joint disease is progressive and destructive. Adult-onset Still's disease has a predilection for the wrist, shoulders, hips, and knees. Sixty percent of patients complain of sore throat, which can confuse the diagnosis with rheumatic fever. Weight loss is common. Lymphadenopathy occurs in two-thirds of the patients and hepatosplenomegaly in about one-half. Pleurisy, pneumonitis, and abdominal pain occur in less than one-third of the patients.

Treatment of adult-onset Still's disease includes high doses of aspirin or indomethacin. Corticosteroids may be needed to control the systemic symptoms. Half of the patients require gold salts, immunosuppressive agents, or D-penicillamine to control the systemic and articular features.

- Adult-onset Still's disease: a slight female predominance.
- Arthritis occurs in 95% of the patients.
- There is a predilection for the wrist, shoulders, hips, and knees.
- 60% of patients complain of sore throat.
- Rheumatoid factor and antinuclear antibodies are absent.

Felty's Syndrome

Felty's syndrome has the classic triad of rheumatoid arthritis, leukopenia, and splenomegaly. (Classic Felty's syndrome usually occurs after 12 years or more of rheumatoid arthritis.) It occurs in <1% of patients with rheumatoid arthritis. Splenomegaly either may not be clinically apparent or may be manifested only after the arthritis and leukopenia have been present for some time. Other features of Felty's syndrome are listed in Table 22-4. Patients with this syndrome frequently have bacterial infections, particularly of the skin and lungs. Infection related to the cytopenia is the major cause of mortality. High titers of rheumatoid factor are the rule, and a positive antinuclear antibody occurs in two-thirds of the patients. Hypocomplementemia often occurs with active vasculitis. Rarely, the hematologic abnormalities in Felty's syndrome remit spontaneously. Shortened erythrocyte survival related to the splenomegaly aggravates inflammatory-block anemia. In 40% of patients, thrombocytopenia is caused by splenic sequestration. The leukocyte count typically is less than 3,500/μL. An absolute neutropenia occurs with granulocyte counts between 500 and 1,000/μL. Bone marrow studies usually document myeloid hyperplasia, with an excess of immature granulocyte precursors suggesting maturation arrest. The marrow is rarely hypocellular. Patients often die of sepsis despite vigorous antibacterial treatment.

Treatment can include corticosteroids, gold, methotrexate, lithium, and splenectomy. There is considerable variability in the response to therapy. Recurrent infection, life-threatening infection, or life-threatening hemolytic anemia are indications for splenectomy. Felty's syndrome must be distinguished from a neoplastic disorder, large granular lymphocytosis, and nodular regenerative hyperplasia of the liver with portal hypertension and hypersplenism.

- Felty's syndrome occurs in <1% of patients with rheumatoid arthritis.
- Felty's syndrome has the classic triad of rheumatoid arthritis, leukopenia, and splenomegaly.
- High titers of rheumatoid factor are the rule.
- Patients with Felty's syndrome frequently die of infection.

Sjögren's Syndrome

Sjögren's syndrome has a triad of clinical features: keratoconjunctivitis sicca (with or without lacrimal gland enlargement), xerostomia (with or without salivary gland enlargement), and connective tissue disease (usually rheumatoid arthritis). Idiopathic Sjögren's syndrome is diagnosed predominantly in middle-aged women. Histologically, it is characterized by CD4 lymphocytic infiltration and destruction of lacrimal salivary glands. Clinically, it is manifested by dry eyes, dry mouth, and a waxing and waning polyarthritis. Additional features of primary Sjögren's syndrome are listed in Table 22-5. Most patients with Sjögren's syndrome have a polyclonal hypergammaglobulinemia. Autoantibodies typically are present, including rheumatoid factor, antinuclear antibodies, and antibodies to extractable nuclear antigens (SS-A and SS-B).

Patients can present with primary Sjögren's syndrome without any additional connective tissue disease. The primary syndrome typically has an episodic and nondeforming arthritis. More commonly, rheumatoid arthritis, systemic lupus erythematosus, scleroderma, polyarteritis nodosa, or polymyositis accompanies Sjögren's syndrome. There is no perfect definition for Sjögren's syndrome, and no test is completely diagnostic. Simple dry eyes of the aged must be distinguished from Sjögren's syndrome. When focal central nervous system abnormalities occur in Sjögren's syndrome, vasculitis or a demyelinating process similar to that of multiple sclerosis is suspected. Patients with Sjögren's syndrome have an increased risk of developing non-Hodgkin's lymphoma. Transient episodes of lymphocytic pneumonitis, lymphocytic pulmonary infiltrates, and episodes of pleuritic pain may be prominent features in a subset of patients. Some patients have diffuse interstitial pulmonary fibrosis.

Treatment of primary Sjögren's syndrome is mainly symptomatic. In addition to hydration, systemic therapy is indicated if there is evidence of systemic inflammation. A Sjögren-like syndrome has been described in patients with HIV infection.

Table 22-4.--Features of Felty's Syndrome

Classic triad
Nodular, erosive polyarthritis
Leukopenia
Splenomegaly
Other features
Recurrent fevers with and without infection
Weight loss
Lymphadenopathy
Skin hyperpigmentation
Lower extremity ulcers
Vasculitis
Neuropathy
Keratoconjunctivitis sicca
Xerostomia
Other cytopenias

Table 22-5.--Features of Sjögren's Syndrome

Malaise
Fatigue
Arthralgias
Myalgias
Low-grade episodic polyarthritis
Raynaud's phenomenon
Renal tubular acidosis
Cutaneous vasculitis
Central nervous system abnormalities
Peripheral neuropathy
Sensory
Autonomic

- Classic triad in Sjögren's syndrome: dry eyes, dry mouth, and a connective tissue disorder (usually rheumatoid arthritis).
- Sjögren's syndrome can exist by itself or with another formal connective tissue disease such as rheumatoid arthritis, systemic lupus erythematosus, scleroderma, or myositis.
- Treatment focuses on control of inflammation and symptoms of dryness.
- A Sjögren-like syndrome has been described in patients with HIV infection.

OSTEOARTHRITIS

Osteoarthritis is the failure of articular cartilage and subsequent degenerative changes in subchondral bone, bony joint margins, synovium, and para-articular fibrous and muscular structures. Osteoarthritis is the most common rheumatic disease; 80% of patients have some limitation of their activities, and 25% are unable to perform major activities of daily living. More than 10% of the population older than 60 have osteoarthritis. Half a million new patients annually develop symptomatic hip or knee osteoarthritis.

- Osteoarthritis is the most common rheumatic disease.
- More than 10% of the population older than 60 have osteoarthritis.

Pathogenesis of Osteoarthritis

Two principal changes associated with osteoarthritis are the progressive focal disintegration of articular cartilage and the formation of new bone in the floor of the cartilage lesion at the joint margins (osteophytes). Not all the mechanisms causing osteoarthritis have been identified. Current theories include: 1) changes in proteoglycan synthesis by chondrocytes, 2) enzymatic degradation of cartilage, 3) changes in the collagen framework of cartilage, 4) change in subchondral bone resilience, 5) crystal deposition in cartilage, and 6) abnormality of the bone and cartilage interface. It must be emphasized that osteoarthritis is not just the consequence of "wear and tear."

- Osteoarthritis: progressive focal disintegration of articular cartilage.
- Formation of bone in the floor of the cartilage lesion at the joint margins (osteophytes).

Clinical Features of Osteoarthritis

The pain of an osteoarthritic joint is usually described as a deep ache. The pain occurs with use of the joint and is relieved with rest and cessation of weight bearing. As the disease progresses, the involved joint may be symptomatic with minimal activity or even at rest. The pain originates in the structures around the disintegrating cartilage (there are no nerves in the cartilage). There may be stiffness in the joint with initial use,

but this initial stiffness is not prolonged as it is in inflammatory arthritis, such as rheumatoid arthritis. Although the symptoms are related predominately to the mechanical failure and motion limits, joint debris can promote mild inflammation, accumulation of synovial fluid, and mild hypertrophy of the synovial membrane. Acute inflammation can transiently occur at Heberden's nodes (distal interphalangeal joints with prominent osteophytes as a consequence of osteoarthritis) or at the knee with tearing of a degenerative meniscal cartilage.

- Osteoarthritic pain is usually described as a deep ache.
- The pain originates in the structures around the disintegrating cartilage.
- The stiffness with initial use of the joint is not prolonged in osteoarthritis as it is in inflammatory arthritis (rheumatoid arthritis).

Physical examination documents joint margin tenderness, fine crepitance, limits to motion, and enlargement of the joint. The enlargement is usually bony (proliferation of cartilage and bone to form osteophytes), but it can include effusions and mild synovial thickening. Deformity is a late consequence of the osteoarthritis and is associated with atrophy or derangement of the local soft tissues, ligaments, and muscles. Radiographic or physical examination evidence of osteoarthritis severity does not predict the patient's symptoms.

Clinical Subsets of Osteoarthritis

Primary Osteoarthritis

Primary osteoarthritis is cartilage failure without a known cause that would predispose to osteoarthritis. It almost never affects the shoulders, metacarpophalangeal joints, or ulnar side of the wrist. It is divided into several clinical patterns, as described below.

Generalized osteoarthritis involves the distal interphalangeal joints, proximal interphalangeal joints, first carpometacarpal joints, hips, knees, and spine (Fig. 22-3). It occurs most frequently in middle-aged postmenopausal women. Many of the patients have joint hypermobility. Mucous cysts are gelatinous cysts that form on the dorsolateral or dorsomedial aspect of the distal interphalangeal joints in osteoarthritis. Fluid aspirated from these cysts contains hyaluronic acid. A mucous cyst communicates with the distal interphalangeal joint space and can regress spontaneously or rupture. Joint sepsis can occur after cyst rupture. Surgical removal usually requires removal of the associated osteophyte; otherwise, the mucous cyst will recur.

Isolated nodal osteoarthritis is primary osteoarthritis that affects only the distal interphalangeal joints. It occurs predominantly in women and has a familial predisposition.

Fig. 22-3. Generalized osteoarthitis. Note prominent bony swelling at the proximal (Bouchard's nodes) and distal (Heberden's nodes) interphalangeal joints. The metacarpophalangeal joints are spared. Early hypertrophic changes are seen on profile at the first carpometacarpal joint, given a slight squaring of the hand deformity appreciated best on the left.

Isolated hip osteoarthritis is more common in men than in women. It has no clear association with obesity or activity.

Erosive osteoarthritis affects only the distal and proximal interphalangeal joints. Patients with erosive osteoarthritis have episodes of local inflammation. Mucous cyst formation is common. Painful flare-up of the disease recurs for years. Symptoms usually begin about the time of menopause. Bony erosions and collapse of the subchondral plate--features not usually seen in primary osteoarthritis--are markers of erosive osteoarthritis. Joint deformity can be severe. In many cases, bony ankylosis develops. Ankylosis is usually associated with relief of pain. The synovium is intensely infiltrated with mononuclear cells. This condition may be confused with rheumatoid arthritis. Up to 15% of the patients may later develop more classic features of rheumatoid arthritis.

Diffuse idiopathic skeletal hyperostosis is a variant of primary osteoarthritis. It occurs chiefly in men older than 50 years. It is also known as "Forestier disease," "ankylosing hyperostosis of the spine," "spondylitis ossificans ligamentosa," and "spondylosis hyperostotica." The diagnosis requires finding characteristic, exuberant, flowing osteophytosis that connects four or more vertebrae, with preservation of the disk space. Diffuse idiopathic skeletal hyperostosis must be distinguished from typical osteoarthritis of the spine with degenerative disk disease and from ankylosing spondylitis. Extraspinal sites of disease involvement

include calcification of the pelvic ligaments, exuberant osteophytosis at the site of peripheral osteoarthritis, well-calcified bony spurs at the calcaneus, and heterotopic bone formation after total joint arthroplasty. Patients with diffuse idiopathic skeletal hyperostosis are often obese and 60% have diabetes mellitus or glucose intolerance. Symptoms include mild back stiffness and, occasionally, back pain. Pathologically and radiologically, diffuse idiopathic skeletal hyperostosis is distinct from other forms of primary osteoarthritis.

- Primary osteoarthritis almost never affects the shoulders, metacarpophalangeal joints, or the ulnar side of the wrist.
- Generalized osteoarthritis involves the distal interphalangeal joints, proximal interphalangeal joints, first carpometacarpal joints, hips, knees, and spine.
- Isolated nodal osteoarthritis is primary osteoarthritis affecting only distal interphalangeal joints.
- Isolated hip osteoarthritis is more common in men than in women.
- Erosive osteoarthritis affects only the distal and proximal interphalangeal joints.
- Diffuse idiopathic skeletal hyperostosis is a variant of primary osteoarthritis.

Secondary Osteoarthritis

Secondary osteoarthritis is cartilage failure caused by some known disorder, trauma, or abnormality. Metabolic abnormalities, including ochronosis, hemochromatosis, Wilson's disease, and acromegaly, are complicated by secondary osteoarthritis. Paget's disease of bone, involving the femur or pelvis about the hip joint, can predispose to osteoarthritis. Secondary osteoarthritis frequently complicates the damage caused by inflammatory arthritis. Any patient with an unusual distribution of osteoarthritis or widespread chondrocalcinosis should be considered to have secondary osteoarthritis. Secondary osteoarthritis includes the clinical conditions mentioned below.

- Osteoarthritis involving the shoulder, metacarpophalangeal joints, isolated large joints, or with chondrocalcinosis should prompt physicians to look for secondary causes of osteoarthritis.
- Ochronosis, hemochromatosis, Wilson's disease, and acromegaly are complicated by secondary osteoarthritis.

Congenital malformations of joints. Congenital hip dysplasia and epiphyseal dysplasia lead to premature osteoarthritis. Other developmental abnormalities, including slipped capital femoral epiphysis and Legg-Calvé-Perthes disease (idiopathic avascular necrosis of the femoral head), may first present as premature osteoarthritis years after they occur.

Trauma. Injury to a joint or supporting periarticular tissues can predispose to osteoarthritis. Stress from repeated impact loading can weaken subchondral bone. Internal joint derangement with ligamentous laxity or meniscal damage alters the normal mechanical alignment of the joint. Post-traumatic osteoarthritis is the most common form of secondary osteoarthritis. Isolated large joint involvement is a clue to post-traumatic osteoarthritis. Chronic rotator cuff tear with subsequent loss of shoulder joint cartilage (cuff arthropathy) and knee osteoarthritis years after meniscal cartilage damage are examples of secondary osteoarthritis.

- Injury to a joint or supporting periarticular tissues can predispose to osteoarthritis.
- Post-traumatic osteoarthritis is the most common form of secondary osteoarthritis.
- Isolated large joint involvement is a clue to post-traumatic osteoarthritis.

Alkaptonuria/ochronosis. This is a rare disorder of tyrosine metabolism. Deficiency of the enzyme homogentisic acid oxidase leads to excretion of large amounts of homogentisic acid in the urine. Oxidized, polymerized homogentisic acid pigment collects in connective tissues ("ochronosis"). The diagnosis may go unrecognized until middle life. The first manifestation can be secondary osteoarthritis. The patient's urine darkens when allowed to stand or with the addition of NaOH. Ochronotic arthritis affects the large joints (e.g., the hips, knees, and shoulders). The radiographic

finding of calcified intervertebral disks at multiple levels is characteristic of ochronosis. Other manifestations include grayish brown scleral pigment and generalized darkening of the ear pinnae.

- Alkaptonuria/ochronosis is a rare disorder of tyrosine metabolism.
- Ochronosis: oxidized, polymerized homogentisic acid pigment collects in connective tissues.
- Ochronotic arthritis affects the large joints: the hips, knees, and shoulders.

Hemochromatosis. Arthropathy affects up to 50% of patients with hemochromatosis and generally resembles osteoarthritis; however, it involves joints not typically affected by generalized primary osteoarthritis. Hemochromatosis arthropathy involves the metacarpophalangeal joints and shoulders. Attacks of acute pseudogout arthritis may occur in relation to deposition of calcium pyrophosphate dihydrate crystals. Chondrocalcinosis is commonly superimposed on chronic osteoarthritic change in hemochromatosis. The pathogenesis of joint degeneration in hemochromatosis is not clear. Iron is present in very low quantities in the affected cartilage. Treatment is symptomatic; the underlying iron accumulation is also treated.

- Arthropathy affects up to 50% of patients with hemochromatosis.
- It involves the metacarpophalangeal joints and shoulders.
- The pathogenesis of joint degeneration in hemochromotosis is not clear.

Wilson's disease. Arthropathy occurs in 50% of adults with Wilson's disease. Arthropathy is unusual in children. The radiologic appearance varies somewhat from that of primary osteoarthritis. There are more subchondral cysts, sclerosis, cortical irregularities, and radiodense lesions, which occur centrally and at the joint margins. Focal areas of bone fragmentation occur, but they are not related to neuropathy. Although chondrocalcinosis occurs, calcium pyrophosphate dihydrate crystals have not been observed in the synovial fluid.

- Arthropathy occurs in 50% of adults with Wilson's disease.
- Arthropathy is unusual in children.

Apatite microcrystals. They are associated with degenerative arthritis and are found in patients with hypothyroidism, hyperparathyroidism, and acromegaly. They occur without an associated endocrinopathy. The role of microcrystalline disease and the progression of osteoarthritis are not clear, especially in the absence of acute recurrent flares of pseudogout.

Neuroarthropathy (Charcot's joint). Neuroarthropathy commonly affects patients with diabetes mellitus. Men and women are equally affected. Patients with diabetic neuroarthropathy have had diabetes an average of 16 years. Frequently, the diabetes is poorly controlled. Neuroarthropathy is a consequence of the peripheral neuropathy responsible for blunted pain perception and poor proprioception. Repeated microtrauma, overt trauma, and, occasionally, small vessel occlusive disease (diabetes) contribute to the cause. The foot is involved most commonly in diabetics. Involvement of the knee, lumbar spine, and upper extremity is uncommon. Classically, hip and spinal neuroarthropathy is caused by tertiary syphilis, and shoulder neuroarthropathy is associated with syringomyelia. Patients can present with an acute arthritic condition that includes swelling, erythema, and warmth. Callus formation occurs at the site of bony damage, and the callus subsequently blisters and ulcerates. Patients usually describe some pain and walk with an antalgic limp. Osteomyelitis frequently complicates diabetic neuroarthropathy. Infection can spread from skin ulcers to the bone. Diabetic neuroarthropathy begins with trauma-induced fragmentation of bone and cartilage. The tarsometatarsal joint is affected most often. The normal joint architecture is disorganized. Bone and cartilage fragments later coalesce to form characteristic sclerotic loose bodies. With joint destruction and disorganization, there is attempt at reconstruction with new bone formation. This periosteal new bone is inhibited by small vessel ischemic change in some diabetics. Diabetic osteopathy is a second form of neuroarthropathy. Osteopenia of para-articular areas, particularly the distal metacarpals and proximal phalanges, results in rapidly progressive osteolysis and juxta-articular cortical defects. As in classic neuroarthropathy, this can be associated with osteomyelitis.

- Neuroarthropathy (Charcot's joints) commonly affects patients with diabetes mellitus.
- Neuroarthropathy is a consequence of peripheral neuropathy.
- In diabetics, the foot is involved most commonly.
- Osteomyelitis is caused by skin ulcers extending to the bone.

Aseptic necrosis of the bone. Also known as avascular necrosis of bone, this may lead to collapse of the articular surface and subsequent osteoarthritis. It usually is seen in the hip after femoral neck fracture. Aseptic necrosis of the bone has various causes, including alcoholism, sickle cell disease, systemic lupus erythematosus, trauma, and caisson disease. Systemic corticosteroid therapy increases the risk of aseptic necrosis. Rare causes of osteonecrosis include Gaucher's syndrome, atherosclerotic vascular disease, and fat emboli. No underlying cause can be identified in 10%-25% of patients.

- Aseptic necrosis usually is seen in the hip after femoral neck fracture.
- Causes: alcoholism, sickle cell disease, systemic lupus erythematosus, trauma, and caisson disease.
- Systemic corticosteroid therapy increases the risk of aseptic necrosis.

Hemophilic arthropathy. Patients with hemophilia and recurrent hemarthroses are at risk for hemophilic arthropathy, a type of progressive degenerative arthropathy that is more destructive than primary osteoarthritis. Widening of the intercondylar notch of the knees is an early radiographic feature suggesting the diagnosis of this condition.

Radiographic Features of Osteoarthritis

The radiographic features of osteoarthritis do not always predict the amount of symptoms. Common radiographic features include: osteophyte formation, asymmetrical joint-space narrowing, subchondral bony sclerosis, subchondral cysts, and buttressing of angle joints. Later bony changes include malalignment and deformity (Fig. 22-4). In the spine, the radiographic finding called "spondylosis" includes anterolateral spinous osteophytes, degenerative disk disease with disk-space narrowing, and facet sclerosis. A defect in the bony structure of the posterior neural arch produces spondylolysis. With bilateral spondylolysis, subluxation of one vertebra on another may occur, a condition called "spondylolisthesis." The causes of spondylolisthesis include trauma, osteoarthritis, and congenital etiologies. No laboratory studies of blood are useful in the diagnosis of osteoarthritis.

- Common radiographic features include: osteophyte formation, asymmetrical joint-space narrowing, subchondral bony sclerosis, subchondral cysts, and buttressing of angle joints.
- No laboratory studies of blood are useful in the diagnosis of osteoarthritis.

Therapy for Osteoarthritis

Therapeutic goals include relieving pain, preserving joint motion and function, and preventing further injury and wear of cartilage. Weight loss (important in knee osteoarthritis), use of canes or crutches, correction of postural abnormalities, and proper shoe support are helpful measures. Isometric or isotonic range of motion exercises and muscle strengthening provide para-articular structures with extra support and help reduce symptoms. Relief of muscle spasm with local application of heat or cold to decrease pain can help.

Initial drug therapy should be analgesics, such as acetaminophen (1 g four times daily as needed). NSAIDs are beneficial for inflammatory flares of osteoarthritis and usually do not need to be taken in anti-inflammatory doses every day. Rarely, depot corticosteroids offer some temporary relief.

Fig. 22-4. Severe osteoarthritis. Hypertrophic changes, asymmetrical joint-space narrowing, and subchondral sclerosis are prominent at the interphalangeal joints and at the first carpometacarpal joint. Note that the metacarpophalangeal joints are completely spared, distinguishing this arthritis from rheumatoid arthritis. Also, there is joint-space narrowing and sclerosis at the base of the thumb at the first carpometacarpal joint and between the trapezium and the scaphoid. Osteoarthritis does not affect equally the entire wrist compartment. The involvement seen here is the most common. An additional interesting feature seen here is central erosions at the second and third proximal interphalangeal joints. This variant occasionally has been called "erosive osteoarthritis."

Joint arthroplasty may relieve pain, stabilize joints, and improve function. Total joint arthroplasty is very successful at the knee or hip. Table 22-6 describes the indications for total joint arthroplasty in patients with radiographically advanced osteoarthritis. Surgical treatment for osteoarthritis of the shoulder is usually reserved for patients with intractable pain. The functional outcome in total shoulder arthroplasty is less predictable. Tibial osteotomy redistributes knee-joint forces. Arthroscopy removes loose bodies and trims torn menisci to correct lockup or give way of the joint. Herniated disks or spinal stenosis may require decompression.

- Weight loss is important in knee osteoarthritis.
- Simple analgesics such as acetaminophen are the first choice for treating osteoarthritis.

Table 22-6.--Indications for Total Joint Arthroplasty

Radiographically advanced osteoarthritis
Night pain that cannot be modified by changing position
Lockup or give way of the weight-bearing joint associated with falls or near falls
Joint symptoms compromise activities of daily living

ARTHRITIS IN CHRONIC RENAL FAILURE

Up to 75% of patients undergoing chronic renal dialysis have musculoskeletal complaints after 4 years of dialysis. Erosive symmetrical polyarthritis occurs in patients who have received maintenance dialysis for more than 10 years. It can affect the interphalangeal joints, metacarpophalangeal joints, wrists, shoulders, and knees. Symmetrical joint-space narrowing and para-articular osteoporosis are prominent. There is no osteophytosis to confuse this condition with osteoarthritis. The synovial fluid is noninflammatory, and the synovitis on biopsy is nonspecific. Ischemic necrosis occasionally causes problems with large joints.

After 10 years of hemodialysis, 65% of patients have pathologic or radiologic evidence of amyloid deposition (renal failure amyloid arthropathy). The amyloid is composed of β_2-microglobulin, which has a high affinity for Congo red and is permanganate sensitive. It is arthrotropic. Serum concentrations of β_2-microglobulin are 60 times higher in long-term hemodialysis patients than in normal persons. Patients receiving peritoneal dialysis have a similar increase in β_2-microglobulin. Destructive arthropathy of large joints affects the hip, knee, shoulder, and wrist. Rapid progression to complete joint-space loss occurs over a 3- to 12-month period. β_2-microglobulin amyloid is found frequently in the synovium, large periarticular cysts, and joint erosions. Shoulder pain and stiffness syndrome and carpal tunnel syndrome are strongly related to amyloid deposition. Currently, treatment is aimed at relieving the symptoms.

- It can affect the interphalangeal joints, metacarpophalangeal joints, wrists, shoulders, and knees.
- Up to 75% of patients undergoing chronic renal dialysis develop musculoskeletal complaints after 4 years of dialysis.
- Shoulder pain, stiffness syndrome, and carpal tunnel syndrome are strongly related to amyloid deposition.

SEPTIC ARTHRITIS

Any new acute inflammatory arthritis should be considered septic or related to microcrystalline inflammation until proved otherwise. Several clinically distinct forms of septic arthritis are reviewed below.

Gonococcal Arthritis

Approximately 0.2% of patients with gonorrhea develop disseminated gonococcal infection. The male-to-female ratio is 3:1. Females present with acute gonococcal arthritis during pregnancy or within 1 week after onset of menses (related to the pH of the vaginal secretions). Typically, the patients are 15 to 30 years old. The two distinct forms of gonococcal arthritis are the first, or bacteremic, form (also called the "dermatitis tenosynovitis" form) and the second, or nonbacteremic, form. Patients with the first form have inflammatory tenosynovitis, dermatitis/pustules, and fever. About one-half of them present with a migratory inflammatory arthritis/arthralgia of the knee, wrist, or ankle. Synovial fluid effusions are uncommon. In the second form, fever, rash/pustules, or tendinitis are not noted. Blood cultures typically are negative. This form begins as a migratory polyarthralgia that subsequently localizes in one or more joints.

- Any new acute inflammatory monarthritis in a sexually active person should be considered related to gonococcal infection until proved otherwise.
- When gonococcal infection is suspected, it is essential that specimens from the throat, joint, anorectum, blood, and genitourinary tract be cultured.
- Patients who have recurrent disseminated gonococcal infection may have an associated terminal complement component deficiency.
- Disseminated gonococcal infection: develops in 0.2% of patients with gonorrhea.
- Two forms of gonococcal arthritis: bacteremic (dermatitis tenosynovitis) and nonbacteremic.
- Blood cultures typically are negative.

Synovial fluid cultures are positive in 30% of patients with known disseminated gonococcal infection. Culture of a skin papule/pustule is positive for gonococcus in 40%-60% of patients. The leukocyte count in joint fluid is often 5,000-10,000/µL, which is lower than in other septic arthropathies. The joint effusions of disseminated gonococcal infection more often are related to a reactive or postinfectious arthritis than to a classic septic arthritis. This hypersensitivity reaction in the joint may explain why synovial fluid leukocyte counts are typically low and cultures are frequently negative.

Most patients with disseminated gonococcal infection can be treated as outpatients. Treatment should include an antichlamydial antibiotic. Patients with disseminated gonococcal infection who are noncompliant and those with a purulent arthropathy should be hospitalized for intravenous administration of antibiotics for 24-48 hours, after which they may receive therapy as outpatients. Patients who have recurrent disseminated gonococcal infection may have an associated terminal complement component deficiency. Occasionally, antibiotic prophylaxis is required. Gonococcal arthritis due to penicillin-resistant organisms has been described.

- Disseminated gonococcal infection: 30% of patients have positive synovial fluid cultures.
- The joint effusions more often are related to reactive or postinfectious arthritis.
- Treatment should include an antichlamydial antibiotic.

Nongonococcal Bacterial Arthritis

Nongonococcal bacterial arthritis is caused by hematogenous spread of bacteria, direct inoculation, and extension of soft tissue infection or osteomyelitis into the joint space. The joints most commonly affected are the knees, hips, shoulders, ankles, wrists, elbows, fingers, and toes. Patients with cancer, diabetes mellitus, chronic renal failure, liver disease, or sickle cell anemia are predisposed to septic arthropathy. Patients with chronic inflammatory and degenerative arthritis also are at increased risk for septic arthritis. The possibility of septic arthritis should always be considered in patients with polyarthritis who have a single joint flare that is out of proportion to the rest of the joint symptoms. Patients who are taking immunosuppressive agents and intravenous drug abusers are also at increased risk for septic arthritis. In any patient with a septic joint, the possibility of infectious endocarditis, other septic joints, or disk-space infection should be considered.

- Nongonococcal bacterial arthritis: caused by hematogenous spread of bacteria, direct inoculation, and extension of soft tissue infection or osteomyelitis
- Most commonly affected joints: knees, hips, shoulders, ankles, wrists, elbows, fingers, and toes.
- Patients with chronic inflammatory and degenerative arthritis, patients taking immunosuppressive agents, and intravenous drug abusers are at increased risk for septic arthritis.

Bony destruction is not seen for 10 days to 3 weeks after the disease starts; therefore, radiographic findings may lag considerably behind clinical symptoms. Early features include osteoporosis, marginal erosions, and secondary osteomyelitis with periostitis. Nongonococcal septic arthritis is a rheumatologic medical emergency. Delay in either the diagnosis or the treatment of infection increases the risk of permanent disability and joint destruction. Cultures of the blood and other areas should be performed as clinically indicated. Synovial fluid should be harvested immediately. Gram staining of centrifuged synovial fluid should also be performed. Typically, patients with nongonococcal septic arthritis have >50,000/µL leukocytes in the synovial fluid. Synovial fluid levels of glucose and lactic acid are not helpful in making the diagnosis of infectious arthritis. Organisms involved in nongonococcal bacterial arthritis include *Staphylococcus aureus*, *Streptococcus* species, gram-negative bacilli, *Staphylococcus epidermidis*,

Streptococcus pneumoniae, and *Haemophilus influenzae*. In sickle cell anemia, *Salmonella* is the organism that usually causes septic arthritis. The portal of entry can predict the organism. Rheumatoid nodule breakdown and ulcer formation predispose the patient with rheumatoid arthritis to staphylococcal septic arthritis.

- Early features of nongonococcal septic arthritis: osteoporosis, marginal erosions, and secondary osteomyelitis with periostitis.
- Nongonococcal septic arthritis is a rheumatologic medical emergency.
- Synovial fluid levels of glucose and lactic acid are not helpful in making the diagnosis.

Broad-spectrum antibiotics should be used until culture results are available. The infected joint must be drained as completely as possible. Daily aspiration of the joint or joints may be required until clinical recovery is documented. The number of leukocytes in the synovial fluid should progressively decrease over a 5-7-day period, along with a decrease in the amount of synovial fluid formed. If this pattern is not observed at 5-7 days, orthopedic open drainage must be considered. Orthopedic drainage is usually indicated in joints such as the hip that are not readily accessible with closed needle drainage. Duration of treatment depends on the virulence of the organism. Antibiotics should be given intravenously for at least 2 weeks and until clinical recovery (synovial fluid does not reaccumulate) is obvious.

- Consider septic arthritis in a patient with rheumatoid arthritis who has single joint flare out of proportion to the rest of the joint symptoms.
- In sickle cell anemia, *Salmonella* commonly causes septic arthritis.
- In any patient with a septic joint, the possibility of infectious endocarditis, other septic joints, or disk-space infection should be considered.
- Surgical (open) drainage and debridement may be necessary if repeated closed drainage and antibiotics are not successful over the first 5-7 days of treatment.

Mycobacterial and Fungal Joint Infections

Mycobacteria and fungi are responsible for chronic bone and joint infections. Many months pass before focal areas of osteopenia or articular erosions develop. In weight-bearing joints, the joint space is preserved for some time (occasionally years) after erosive changes occur. A negative PPD rules out *Mycobacterium tuberculosis* monarticular arthropathy in well-fed, nonsuppressed patients. A synovial biopsy from a mycobacterial joint infection documents granulomas, with or without caseation. The absence of granulomas does not rule out fungal or mycobacterial infection.

- Mycobacteria and fungi are responsible for chronic bone and joint infections.
- The absence of granulomas does not rule out fungal or mycobacterial infection.

Rheumatic Fever and Poststreptococcal Reactive Arthritis

The incidence of acute rheumatic fever in the U.S. has been declining steadily, although scattered outbreaks have occurred among U.S. school children and armed forces personnel. One-third of patients with acute rheumatic fever deny any antecedent sore throat. It is important to consider rheumatic fever with any new polyarthritis. Arthritis affects two-thirds of all patients with rheumatic fever. In adults, arthritis occurs more frequently and may be the only feature of acute rheumatic fever. Although any joint may be affected, the arthritis usually involves the large joints, particularly the knees, ankles, elbows, and wrists. It is accompanied by the signs and symptoms of an acute febrile illness. Each joint remains inflamed for no more than 1 week, and the entire course of polyarthritis is usually severe for about 1 week. By the end of 4 weeks, it usually subsides. Flare-ups may occur in a small percentage of patients when treatment with salicylates or corticosteroids is withdrawn. Rheumatic fever never causes permanent joint damage. However, repeated attacks of rheumatic fever may result in a particular type of deformity called "Jaccoud's deformity," in which the metacarpophalangeal joints are no longer aligned correctly but are in ulnar deviation.

- Consider rheumatic fever with any new polyarthritis.
- Arthritis usually involves the large joints, particularly the knees, ankles, elbows, and wrists.
- Repeated attacks may result in Jaccoud's deformity.

Patients with mild arthralgias and no carditis can be treated with analgesics. A high dose of salicylates (3-6 g/day) is the mainstay of treatment. Corticosteroids are more potent than salicylates in suppressing acute inflammation and may be required for patients who do not respond to salicylates. Rebounds of rheumatic activity may appear when anti-inflammatory therapy is discontinued. Rebounds do not occur more than 6 weeks after stopping anti-inflammatory therapy.

- The mainstay of treatment is a high dose of salicylates.
- Corticosteroids may be required for patients not responding to salicylates.

Viral Arthritis

Arthritis accompanies several common viral diseases in humans. Viruses commonly associated with arthralgia or arthritis include HIV, hepatitis B, rubella, parvovirus, and, less commonly, mumps virus, adenovirus, herpesvirus, and enterovirus. Most viral-related arthritides have joint symptoms that occur quite suddenly, are of brief duration, and do not recur. In most cases, the arthritis is nondestructive and does not lead to any currently recognized form of chronic joint disease. Patients with arthritic symptoms related to hepatitis B infection develop an earlier than usual antibody response. Similar musculoskeletal involvement has not been demonstrated in patients with type A or type C hepatitis. Up to 25% of those with hepatitis B infection have a prodromal polyarthralgia/arthritis. Joint symptoms persist from several days to weeks before resolving with the onset of jaundice. Rubella-associated arthritis usually occurs in women 20-40 years old. Joint symptoms may occur as early as 6 days before or as long as 6 days after the appearance of the characteristic macular, papular rash of rubella. Symptoms usually evolve over a 2-week period. Arthralgias have been reported to be present for more than 1 year. A live virus vaccine for rubella has also been associated with transient arthralgia and arthritis.

- Viruses commonly associated with arthralgia or arthritis include HIV, hepatitis B, rubella, parvovirus, and, less commonly, mumps virus, adenovirus, herpesvirus, and enterovirus.
- 25% of those with hepatitis B infection have a prodromal polyarthralgia/arthritis.
- Viral arthritis presents quite suddenly, lasts days to weeks, and does not recur.

Acquired Immunodeficiency Syndrome

Many musculoskeletal conditions are associated with HIV infection, and several of them may be the first manifestations of progression to full-blown AIDS. HIV infection may be confused with diseases such as systemic lupus erythematosus and Sjögren's syndrome. The implications for the correct diagnosis are obvious. The morbidity associated with rheumatic syndromes in patients with HIV infection is considerable and often requires treatments and monitoring not typically required by their non-HIV infected counterparts. Epidemiologic studies have not concluded whether HIV infection predisposes to arthritis or whether other viral or immune mechanisms associated with HIV infection have a role in the pathogenesis of arthritis.

- HIV infection may be confused with systemic lupus erythematosus and Sjögren's syndrome.
- The morbidity associated with rheumatic syndromes in patients with HIV infection is considerable.

Rheumatologic Manifestations of HIV Infection

Reiter's Syndrome and Undifferentiated Spondyloarthropathy

A spectrum from classic psoriatic arthritis or Reiter's syndrome to more nonspecific enthesopathy and destructive arthritis occurs in the HIV-infected population. The prevalence of these conditions in HIV-infected patients varies from 0.5% to 10% of reported populations. Except for several cases of very mild sacroiliitis, axial involvement does not occur in HIV-associated arthritides. These HIV-associated spondyloarthropathies have a predisposition for HLA-B27 and frequently have severe enthesopathy and dactylitis. The foot and ankle are the common sites of inflammation/enthesopathy in Reiter's syndrome. Sometimes, the "AIDS foot" features are so severe as to be almost diagnostic. The arthritis of Reiter's syndrome in HIV infection can be additive and ultimately destructive and disabling; however, it more commonly is episodic and associated with remissions. Conjunctivitis in this population is unusual. Most HIV-positive patients with Reiter's syndrome have clinical features such as urethritis, keratoderma blennorrhagicum, circinate balanitis, or painless oral ulcers, thus fulfilling the diagnostic criteria for Reiter's syndrome. Genitourinary tract infection with *Ureaplasma* or *Chlamydia* is uncommon. However, in one-third of patients, the onset of HIV-associated Reiter's syndrome was linked to a documented infection with enteric organisms known to precipitate reactive arthritis.

- Prevalence varies from 0.5% to 10% of reported population.
- The signs and symptoms of Reiter's syndrome, psoriatic arthritis, or nonspecific enthesopathy and destructive arthritis occur before or simultaneously with the onset of full-blown AIDS in about two-thirds of reported cases.
- Sometimes, the "AIDS foot" features are so severe as to be almost diagnostic.
- Conjunctivitis is unusual.

Systemic Lupus Erythematosus-Like Illness in HIV Infection

Many of the features of systemic lupus erythematosus are similar to those found in HIV infections. These similarities can lead to diagnostic difficulties. HIV infection should be considered when the diagnosis of systemic lupus erythematosus is considered in men or in patients who practice high-risk behaviors for HIV. Antinuclear antibodies in titers >1:80 have not been observed in HIV infection, and antibodies to anti-double-strand DNA are absent in HIV infection. Patients with systemic lupus erythematosus and rheumatoid arthritis have had resolution of their inflammatory symptoms after HIV infection.

- HIV infection should be considered when the diagnosis of systemic lupus erythematosus is considered in men or in patients who practice high-risk behaviors for HIV.
- Antibodies to anti-double-strand DNA are absent in HIV infection.

HIV-Associated Vasculitis

Many vasculitic syndromes have been described in association with HIV infection. The common ones are primary angiitis of the central nervous system, angiocentric lymphoproliferative lesions related to lymphomatoid granulomatosis, and polyarteritis nodosa. It has to be proved whether the association of vasculitis and HIV infection is coincidental, related to comorbid factors (drugs or other infections), or represents a direct pathogenic role for HIV. All patients with primary angiitis of the central nervous system and lymphoproliferative angiocentric vasculopathies should be tested for HIV. Furthermore, any person with known HIV infection who presents with new mononeuritis should be evaluated for vasculitis.

- Consider HIV infection in all new cases of CNS vasculitis and angiocentric lymphoproliferative disease.
- Anyone with known HIV infection who has new mononeuritis should be evaluated for vasculitis.

NONARTICULAR RHEUMATISM

Fibromyalgia

Fibromyalgia is a uniform syndrome characterized by chronic diffuse musculoskeletal pain. Other names for this condition are fibrositis, tension myalgias, generalized nonarticular rheumatism, psychogenic rheumatism, and benign myalgic encephalomyelitis. For the diagnosis, the pain should be present for at least 3 months and should involve areas on both sides of the body above and below the waist and some part of the axial skeleton. A high tender point count is an additional obligatory criterion for classification of fibromyalgia. Fibromyalgia affects 2%-10% of all populations studied and 15% of all general medical patients seen by internists; 75%-95% of all the patients are women. It is unusual for the diagnosis to be made in a person younger than 12 or for a first episode to occur after age 60. Of the patients (or their parents), 60% recall childhood growing pains or leg pains. Fibromyalgia is the second most common reason (after the common cold) for lost work days.

- Fibromyalgia: chronic diffuse musculoskeletal pain.
- Other names: fibrositis, tension myalgias, generalized nonarticular rheumatism, psychogenic rheumatism, and benign myalgic encephalomyelitis.
- Fibromyalgia affects 2%-10% of all populations studied; 75%-95% of patients are women.

Symptoms

The patients typically describe pain all over the body and use qualitatively different descriptions of the pain and discomfort than used by patients with rheumatoid arthritis. Patients localize the pain poorly, referring it to muscle attachment sites or muscles. The discomfort is worse in the morning and can be associated with stiffness. Physical activity or changes in the weather typically aggravate the symptoms. Most patients describe nonrestorative, nonrestful sleep. Anxiety is common.

Active depression is not seen more commonly in these patients than in the general population. Articular symptoms can be prominent. Patient complaints include subjective joint swelling, hand and joint pain, prolonged morning stiffness, Raynaud-like vasospasm, and dry eyes. Headaches, paresthesias, numbness, and pseudosciatica-like pains are also common. About one-third of the patients have visceral symptoms, including urinary urgency, severe pelvic pain unexplainable as dysmenorrhea or endometriosis, and irritable bowel syndrome. The onset of fibromyalgia occurs after an acute illness, typically a viral syndrome, in more than half of the patients. In some patients, symptoms develop after trauma, such as injury on the job or motor vehicle accidents.

- Patients with fibromyalgia typically describe pain all over the body.
- Physical activity or weather changes typically aggravate the symptoms.
- Raynaud-like vasospasm, dry eyes, headaches, paresthesias, numbness, and pseudosciatica-like pains are common.
- The onset of fibromyalgia occurs after an acute illness, typically a viral syndrome, in more than half the patients.

Diagnosis

Fibromyalgia is a diagnosis of exclusion. Detailed physical examination will exclude most inflammatory and neurologic diseases. The finding of painful points at muscle attachment sites supports the diagnosis of fibromyalgia. Laboratory evaluation includes performing a complete blood cell count, erythrocyte sedimentation rate, and thyroid function studies and determining levels of electrolytes, creatinine, calcium, and phosphorus. In selected cases, creatine kinase values and pelvic and spine radiographic findings are helpful in excluding other diseases. No diagnostic test confirms the diagnosis of fibromyalgia. Muscle biopsies, electromyographic and sleep studies, and magnetic resonance imaging (MRI) are not necessary for the diagnosis.

- The finding of painful points at muscle attachment sites supports the diagnosis of fibromyalgia.
- No laboratory test confirms the diagnosis of fibromyalgia.

Natural History

Fibromyalgia is a chronic waxing and waning problem. Patients have periods of pain and dysfunction alternating with variable periods of feeling reasonably well. Over a period of years, a patient's symptoms and concerns can shift considerably from musculoskeletal concerns to fatigue to headaches or to irritable bowel. There is no increased disability in patients who have had fibromyalgia for longer periods of time in comparison with patients in whom the diagnosis is recent. The factors that may affect the presentation and perpetuation of fibromyalgia are listed in Table 22-7. Treatment includes reas-

Table 22-7.--Factors That May Influence the Presentation and Perpetuation of Fibromyalgia Syndrome

Neurophysiology	Personal traits	External factors
Poor spinal postures	Personality type	Lack of physical fitness
Sleep disorder	Self-esteem	Job satisfaction
Activated deep pain system	Cultural beliefs	Family dysfunction
	Coping skills	Substance abuse
	Pain language	Loss of control over life options

surance and education, ensuring an adequate night's sleep, establishing a cardiovascular fitness program, and better flexibility and posture. Nonsteroidal anti-inflammatory drugs have a slight synergistic effect with sedating medications.

- Fibromyalgia is a chronic waxing and waning musculoskeletal pain syndrome.
- There is no progressive disability.
- Most of the patients with fibromyalgia are not depressed.

Low Back Pain

One-third of all people over age 50 have acute low back pain. Chronic low back pain is the number-one compensable work-related injury. The many causes of low back pain include mechanical, neurologic, inflammatory, infectious, neoplastic, and metabolic causes and referred pain from the viscera. Only 3% of patients presenting with acute low back pain have an organic cause not apparent after the initial interview and physical examination. More than 80% find relief on their own or with the help of a medical practitioner within the first 2 weeks of symptoms.

- Only 3% of patients presenting with acute low back pain have an organic cause not apparent after the initial interview and physical examination.

Diagnosis

The most important consideration during the initial evaluation of acute low back pain is the possibility of severe spinal cord or cauda equina compromise. In the absence of evidence for acute spinal cord compromise or spinal infection or neoplastic involvement, immediate pursuit of a cause for the acute back pain is not appropriate. Objective leg weakness or bladder and bowel dysfunction are indications for more extensive physical examination, consideration of urgent lumbar myelography, and possible surgical decompression. Significant weight loss or pain that interferes with sleep suggests a neoplastic or infectious process. Pain that worsens with coughing, straining, or sneezing suggests irritation of the dura mater. Radiating pain, weakness, or numbness in an extremity implicates irritation of a spinal nerve root. Exertional calf or thigh cramping but normal peripheral pulses suggests pseudoclau-

dication or symptomatic lumbar stenosis. Pseudoclaudicant symptoms improve with leaning over a cart or with sitting (not standing still). Referred pain from an abdominal, pelvic, or hip area suggests an extra-axial cause. An insidious onset with prominent morning stiffness suggests an inflammatory axial arthropathy.

- Objective leg weakness or bladder or bowel dysfunction are indications for more extensive examination.
- Significant weight loss or pain that interferes with sleep suggests a neoplastic or infectious process.
- Exertional calf or thigh cramping but normal peripheral pulses suggests pseudoclaudication.
- An insidious onset with prominent morning stiffness suggests an inflammatory axial arthropathy.

In the absence of specific historical or physical examination findings, laboratory or plain radiograph findings would not suggest malignancy, infection, systemic illness, or neurologic compromise. The radiographic findings of spondylosis, single disk degeneration, facet osteoarthritis, transitional lumbosacral segments, Schmorl's nodes, spina bifida occulta, mild scoliosis, and increased lumbosacral angle are not relevant to a patient's complaints of acute back pain. The use of bone scans, electromyography, computed tomography (CT), or MRI is not necessary to evaluate routine acute low back pain. The indications for spinal radiography in patients with acute low back pain are listed in Table 22-8.

Table 22-8.--Indications for Spinal Radiography in Patients With Acute Low Back Pain

First episode of acute back pain is after age 50
History of back disease
History of back surgery
History of neoplasm
Acute history of direct trauma to the back
Fever
Weight loss
Severe pain unrelieved in any position
Neurologic symptoms or signs

Treatment

The treatment of acute nonspecific low back pain begins with reassuring the patient, because 80% of all patients with acute low back pain have significant improvement in 2 weeks. Of the 20% that continue to have significant symptoms, 80% will have improvement in another 2 weeks. Bed rest should be prescribed for all cases of acute nonspecific low back pain. Short-term use of narcotic analgesics can supplement the use of acetaminophen, NSAIDs, and muscle relaxants such as cyclobenzaprine. Physical therapy measures include local heat and ice massage. Pelvic traction and transcutaneous electrical nerve stimulation (TENS) add little to the management of acute nonspecific low back pain. Glucocorticosteroids injected epidurally are best suited to acute disk herniation, although their role is controversial. Injections into the facets are helpful occasionally, particularly if the patient describes a locking or catching as part of the pain syndrome.

- Pelvic traction and TENS add little to the management of acute nonspecific low back pain.
- In 90% of patients, acute low back pain (local or sciatic presentations) remits within 4-6 weeks.
- Clinical suspicion of acute spinal cord compromise, spinal infection, or neoplasm requires immediate evaluation and prompt therapy.

Bursitis

A bursa is a closed sac containing a small amount of synovial fluid and lined with a membrane similar to that surrounding a diarthrodial joint. Bursae are present in the areas where tendons and muscles move over bony prominences. Additional bursae form in response to irritative stimuli. Trauma to a bursal area may lead to an inflammatory response. Chronic overuse or irritation can aggravate bursal inflammation. Greater trochanteric bursitis is aggravated by tight ileotibial bands, hard mattresses, and a waddling gait. Systemic disorders such as rheumatoid arthritis or gout cause bursitis. Treatment of aseptic bursitis involves strict immobilization, ice compresses, NSAIDs, bursal aspiration, and corticosteroid injections. Glucocorticosteroids should not be given if there is clinical suggestion of sepsis. All bursal fluid should be cultured and evaluated for crystals. Acute trochanteric bursitis responds to reduced activity (especially walking), the use of a walking stick in the opposite hand, a foam mattress pad, and local modalities described above.

- Greater trochanteric bursitis is aggravated by tight ileotibial bands, hard mattresses, and a waddling gait.
- Glucocorticosteroids should not be given if there is clinical suggestion of sepsis.
- Acute trochanteric bursitis responds to reduced activity.

Septic bursitis may occur secondary to puncture wounds or cellulitis or after a local injection. At least half of the time, there is no portal of entry for infection in septic superficial bursitis (olecranon and prepatellar bursae). The organisms frequently responsible for infection are staphylococci (*aureus* and *epidermidis*) and streptococci. Patients with septic superficial bursitis present with localized pain and swelling. Erythema may be present, but it does not necessarily suggest infection. Warmth about the area of the superficial bursa should raise the possibility of a septic bursa. If there is doubt, the bursa should be aspirated with strict aseptic technique. The needle should be passed through uninvolved skin. When infection is suspected, patients should be treated empirically with antistaphylococcal and antistreptococcal oral antibiotics, pending the microbiologic results. Gram stains are positive in only 40%-60% of patients. The number of leukocytes in infected bursal fluid can be low compared with that in infected joint fluid. This may be due to the modest blood supply of the bursae compared with that of joints. Patients with more severe infections or with associated cellulitis frequently do not respond to outpatient management. They should be hospitalized and given antibiotics intravenously, and the affected part should be immobilized for 3-4 days. Repeated aspirations may be necessary until the fluid stops accumulating. Occasionally, incision and drainage are required, and in chronic cases refractory to antibiotics, bursectomy is indicated.

- Septic bursitis frequently occurs without evidence of a portal of entry.
- Bursal warmth is the best predictor of infection.
- Gram stains are positive in only 40%-60% of patients.
- The number of leukocytes in infected bursal fluid can be low.
- Patients with more severe infections should be hospitalized.

Polymyalgia Rheumatica

Polymyalgia rheumatica is a clinical syndrome usually characterized by the sudden onset of aching and morning stiffness in the proximal musculature. The definition includes an increased erythrocyte sedimentation rate. Results of rheumatologic studies, including rheumatoid factor, antinuclear antibody, and complement levels, are negative or normal. In 1%-3% of cases, patients can present with a normal erythrocyte sedimentation rate. The presence of other specific diseases such as rheumatoid arthritis, chronic infection, inflammatory myositis, or malignancy excludes the diagnosis of polymyalgia rheumatica. Some definitions of polymyalgia rheumatica require a rapid response to small doses of prednisone (10-15 mg daily). This condition is more common in whites and has a moderate female predominance. It almost never occurs in persons <50 years old. It is endemic in the population of people >50 years old, with as many as 50 new cases each year per 100,000 population.

- Polymyalgia rheumatica: sudden onset of aching and morning stiffness in the proximal musculature and increased erythrocyte sedimentation rate.
- Negative rheumatoid factor, antinuclear antibody, and complement levels.
- The presence of other specific diseases excludes the diagnosis of polymyalgia rheumatica.
- It almost never occurs in persons <50 years old.

Features and Differential Diagnosis

Patients with polymyalgia rheumatica complain of stiffness more than pain. This stiffness is most prominent in the mornings and after prolonged sitting. Because the patients have difficulty raising their arms over their heads when they awaken, they characteristically roll to the edge of the bed and allow their feet to drop when getting out of bed. They occasionally have mild constitutional symptoms, including sweats, fevers, anorexia, and weight loss. Prominent constitutional features should suggest associated giant cell arteritis. Oligoarticular synovitis can occur, particularly at the knees, wrists, and shoulders. Radionuclide joint scans in patients with active polymyalgia rheumatica confirm hip and shoulder synovitis. Polyarticular small joint arthritis is not a feature. Polymyalgia rheumatica patients without vasculitis may have granulomatous myocarditis and hepatitis. Muscles from these patients show normal tissue or mild type II muscle fiber atrophy. Table 22-9 summarizes the rheumatic syndromes and other diseases that occasionally present with a polymyalgia rheumatica-like syndrome. Depression must be considered in patients with atypical features. Clinical evaluation and screening laboratory tests usually distinguish polymyalgia rheumatica from these other conditions.

- Polymyalgia rheumatica: stiffness is more prolonged in the mornings and after prolonged sitting.
- Prominent constitutional features should suggest associated giant cell arteritis.
- Oligoarticular synovitis can occur.
- Polyarticular small joint arthritis is not a feature.

Pathogenesis and Relationship to Giant Cell Arteritis

The pathogenesis of polymyalgia rheumatica is unknown. Clinicians appreciate the close relationship between giant cell arteritis and polymyalgia rheumatica. Familial aggregation and increased incidence in patients of northern European background suggest a genetic predisposition. HLA-DR4 is associated with these conditions more commonly than would be expected by chance. Of patients with giant cell arteritis, 40% have symptoms of polymyalgia rheumatica during the course of their disease.

- Up to 15% of patients with polymyalgia rheumatica also have giant cell arteritis.

Table 22-9.--Systemic Illnesses Presenting With a Polymyalgia-Like Syndrome

Rheumatic syndromes	Other systemic illnesses
Systemic vasculitis	Paraneoplastic syndromes
Myositis	Systemic amyloidosis
Systemic lupus erythematosus	Infectious endocarditis
Seronegative rheumatoid arthritis	Hyperthyroidism
	Hypothyroidism
Polyarticular osteoarthritis	Hyperparathyroidism
Fibromyalgia	Osteomalacia
Remitting seronegative, symmetric synovitis and peripheral edema	Depression

- 40% of patients with active giant cell arteritis have symptoms of polymyalgia rheumatica.
- Polymyalgia rheumatica can begin before, appear simultaneously with, or develop after the symptoms of giant cell arteritis.

Treatment

All patients with polymyalgia rheumatica should respond completely after 3-5 days of treatment with prednisone, 10 to 20 mg/day. After giant cell arteritis has been excluded, most patients can be managed initially with prednisone doses of 15 mg/day or less. Follow the patients clinically, and when necessary, determine the erythrocyte sedimentation rate to confirm the clinical suspicion of a disease flare. Other acute-phase reactants are not superior to the erythrocyte sedimentation rate. Polymyalgia rheumatica is thought to be a self-limited disease. Prednisone treatment is discontinued in more than half the patients within 2 years.

- All patients should respond completely after 3-5 days of treatment with prednisone.
- Polymyalgia rheumatica is thought to be a self-limited disease.

VASCULITIC SYNDROMES

Introduction

Vasculitis, or angiitis, is an inflammatory disease of blood vessels. It often causes damage to the vessel wall and stenosis or occlusion of the vessel lumen by thrombosis and progressive intimal proliferation of the vessel. The pathologic consequences of vasculitis are related directly to the ischemic consequences of vascular occlusion. The distribution of the vascular lesions and the size of the blood vessels involved vary considerably in different vasculitic syndromes and in different patients with the same syndrome. Vasculitis can be transient, chronic, self-limited, or progressive. It can be the primary abnormality or secondary to another systemic process. Histopathologic classification does not distinguish local from systemic illness or secondary from primary insult. The key clinical features suggestive of vasculitis are listed in Table 22-10. Vasculitis "look-alikes," or simulators, are listed in Table 22-11. These diseases and conditions should be considered whenever the patient's condition suggests vasculitis. A scheme for diagnosing vasculitis is outlined in Table 22-12. The ability to recognize characteristic clinical patterns of involvement is very helpful to the diagnosis of vasculitis.

- The pathologic consequences of vasculitis are related directly to the ischemic consequences of vascular occlusion.
- Vasculitis can be transient, chronic, self-limited, or progressive.

Specific Vasculitic Syndromes

Giant Cell Arteritis

Giant cell arteritis, also known as "temporal arteritis," predominantly affects persons >50 years old. The prevalence exceeds 223 cases per 100,000 persons >50 years old. It is most common in persons of northern European ancestry.

Females outnumber males by a ratio of 3:1. Polymyalgia rheumatica symptoms may develop in 40%-50% of all patients with giant cell arteritis. Up to 15% of patients with polymyalgia rheumatica have temporal artery biopsies positive for giant cell arteritis. There is considerable morbidity with this disease; however, the rate of blindness is declining. The mortality rate for patients with giant cell arteritis is similar to that for the general population.

- Giant cell arteritis: most common in persons of northern European ancestry.
- Polymyalgia rheumatica develops in 40% of patients with giant cell arteritis.
- 15% of patients with polymyalgia rheumatica have temporal artery biopsies positive for giant cell arteritis.

Pathology--Giant cell arteritis involves the blood vessels originating from the arch of the aorta. However, any artery,

Table 22-10.--Clinical Features That Suggest Vasculitis

Constitutional features
Fatigue, fever, weight loss, and anorexia
Skin lesions
Palpable purpura, necrotic ulcers, livedo reticularis, urticaria, nodules, and digital infarcts
Arthralgia or arthritis
Myalgia or prominent fibrositis
Polymyalgia rheumatica symptoms
Claudication or phlebitis
Headache
Cerebrovascular accident
Neuropathy
Mononeuritis multiplex
Hypertension
Abnormal renal sediment
Pulmonary abnormalities
Pulmonary hemorrhage, pulmonary nodules with cavities
Abdominal pain or intestinal hemorrhage
Nonspecific indicators of inflammation
Anemia, thrombocytosis, low levels of albumin, elevated erythrocyte sedimentation rate, increased levels of liver enzymes, or eosinophilia

Table 22-11.--Syndromes That Mimic Vasculitis

Cardiac myxoma with embolization
Infective endocarditis
Thrombotic thrombocytopenic purpura
Atheroembolism: cholesterol or calcium emboli
Ergotism
Pseudoxanthoma elasticum
Ehlers-Danlos type 4
Neurovasculopathy secondary to antiphospholipid syndrome
Arterial coarctation or dysplasia
Infectious angiitis
Lyme disease
Rickettsial infection
HIV infection

Table 22-12.--The Diagnostic Approach to Vasculitis

Proper clinical suspicion for vasculitis[*]
Consider conditions that mimic vasculitis
Recognize clinical pattern of involvement
Define the extent and severity of disease
Narrow the diagnostic possibilities with laboratory tests
Select the confirmatory study
Efficient (highest yield study)
Safe as possible
Weigh urgency of diagnosis with risk of
Diagnostics
Therapeutics

[*]Table 22-10.

and occasionally veins, can be affected, but it is unusual for the intracranial arteries to be involved. Giant cell arteritis affects arteries in a segmental or patchy fashion. Histopathologically, extensive disruption of all layers of the vessel wall occurs, with intimal thickening and a prominent mononuclear and histiocytic infiltrate. Multinucleated giant cells infiltrate the vessel wall in 50% of cases. Fragmentation and disintegration of the internal elastic membrane, the other characteristic feature, is closely associated with the accumulation of giant cells.

- Giant cell arteritis affects arteries in a segmental or patchy fashion.

Clinical features--Early clinical features of giant cell arteritis include temporal headache, polymyalgia rheumatica symptoms, fatigue, and fever. The classic features of this disease are included in Table 22-13. Arteritis of the branches of the ophthalmic or posterior ciliary arteries causes ischemia of the optic nerve (ischemic optic neuritis) and blindness. Less often, retinal arterioles are occluded. After the visual deficit is established, it is usually permanent. When blindness occurs in an untreated person, it often occurs bilaterally within 1-2 weeks. Blindness occurs in <15% of untreated patients. Large peripheral artery involvement in giant cell arteritis occurs in about 10% of patients. Extremity claudication, Raynaud's phenomenon, aortic dissection, decreased pulses, and vascular bruits suggest large peripheral artery involvement. Patients with large peripheral artery involvement do not differ from those with more classic giant cell arteritis, either histologically or with regard to laboratory findings.

- Early clinical features: temporal headache, polymyalgia rheumatica symptoms, fatigue, and fever.
- Visual deficit is usually permanent.
- Blindness occurs in <15% of untreated patients.

Diagnosis--Positive temporal artery biopsy findings make

a search for occult malignancy unnecessary and document the long-term need for corticosteroid therapy. This is important when corticosteroid therapy toxicity becomes an issue, particularly in elderly patients. The temporal artery biopsy specimen should be 3-5 cm long to compensate for patchy involvement. Multiple histologic sections should be taken of the pathologic specimen. In 15% of patients, the biopsy is positive on the opposite side if that on the initial side is negative. Typical laboratory abnormalities in acute active giant cell arteritis include a markedly increased erythrocyte sedimentation rate, moderate normochromic anemia, and thrombocytosis. Mild increase in liver enzymes, most typically alkaline phosphatase, occurs in one-third of the patients. Liver biopsies performed in selected cases have documented granulomatous hepatitis. The erythrocyte sedimentation rate is rarely normal in patients with active giant cell arteritis. This occurs in <2% of all patients. The diagnostic criteria for giant cell arteritis are given in Table 22-14.

- The temporal artery biopsy specimen should be 3-5 cm long to compensate for patchy involvement.
- In 15% of patients, the biopsy is positive on the opposite side if that on the initial side is negative.
- Typical laboratory abnormalities: markedly increased erythrocyte sedimentation rate, moderate normochromic anemia, and thrombocytosis.

Treatment--Treatment is initiated with corticosteroids when the diagnosis of giant cell arteritis is considered and the biopsy is requested. A temporal artery biopsy specimen remains positive for disease even after 3-4 days of corticosteroid treatment. Treatment includes prednisone, typically 40-60 mg/day in a divided dose. Corticosteroids can be given parenterally in case of visual or life-threatening symptoms. Most symptoms of giant cell arteritis begin to respond within 24 hours after initiating corticosteroid therapy. Visual changes that are present for more than a few hours are invariably irreversible. Alternate-day administration of corticosteroids does not control symptoms in at least half of the patients.

Table 22-13.--Classic Clinical Features of Giant Cell Arteritis

Fever, weight loss, fatigue
Polymyalgia rheumatica symptoms
Temporal headache
Jaw or tongue claudication
Ocular symptoms
Blindness
Diplopia
Ptosis
Scalp tenderness
Dry cough
Peripheral large vessel vasculitis (10%)

Table 22-14.--Diagnostic Criteria for Giant Cell Arteritis

Temporal artery biopsy findings positive for classic giant cell arteritis
or
Four of the five following criteria:
Tender, swollen temporal artery
Jaw claudication
Blindness
Polymyalgia rheumatica symptoms
Rapid response to corticosteroids

- Treatment is initiated with corticosteroids when the diagnosis of giant cell arteritis is considered and the biopsy is requested.
- Treatment: prednisone, typically 40-60 mg/day in a divided dose.
- Alternate day administration of corticosteroids does not control initial symptoms in at least half of the patients.

Outcome--Giant cell arteritis typically has a self-limited course over a period of 2 years. In 24 months, half the patients are able to discontinue their treatment with corticosteroids. Except for penicillamine and azathioprine, the use of steroid-sparing agents has not been studied systematically. Methotrexate may be considered in patients not responding to or intolerant of corticosteroids.

- Giant cell arteritis typically has a self-limited course over a period of about 2 years.
- Methotrexate may be considered in patients not responding to or intolerant of corticosteroids.

Takayasu's Arteritis

Takayasu's arteritis is also known as "aortic arch syndrome" or "pulseless disease." Each year, about 2.6 new cases per 1,000,000 population occur. Most patients are between the ages of 15 and 40. At least 80% of them are female. This disease is more common in the Orient, Latin America, and Eastern Europe. Microscopically, its pathologic features cannot be distinguished from those of giant cell arteritis. Takayasu's arteritis affects the aorta and its primary branches. The arterial wall is irregularly thickened, with luminal narrowing, dilatations, aneurysms, and distortions. The aortic valve and coronary ostia can be involved.

- Takayasu's arteritis: most patients are between the ages of 15 and 40.
- At least 80% of patients are female.
- The aorta and its primary branches are affected.

Clinical and laboratory features--The constitutional features of fever, weight loss, fatigue, and arthralgia can precede symptoms of ischemia to the brain or claudication of the extremities. Renovascular hypertension, pulmonary hypertension, and coronary artery insufficiency can complicate Takayasu's arteritis. Cutaneous vasculitis, erythema nodosum, and synovitis occasionally occur in cases of active Takayasu's arteritis. Compromise of the cerebral vasculature can lead to dizziness, blurry or fading vision, syncope, and, occasionally, stroke. Physical examination findings confirm vascular bruits, absence of peripheral pulses, and, occasionally, fever. When the disease is active, abnormal values of laboratory studies reveal increased erythrocyte sedimentation rate, normochromic anemia, and thrombocytosis.

- Fever, weight loss, fatigue, and arthralgia can precede symptoms of ischemia.
- Physical examination findings: bruits, absence of peripheral pulses, fever (occasionally), and increased erythrocyte sedimentation rate.

Treatment and outcome--Corticosteroid therapy alone is usually adequate for controlling the inflammation. On average, patients receive corticosteroids for about 2 years. In about half of the patients, the pulse returns. Late stenotic complications are amenable to vascular surgery and bypass grafting. Survival is >90% at 10 years. Congestive heart failure from previous coronary artery involvement and cerebral vascular accidents are major causes of mortality.

- Renovascular hypertension, pulmonary hypertension, and coronary artery insufficiency can complicate Takayasu's arteritis.
- Corticosteroid therapy alone is usually adequate.
- Survival is >90% at 10 years.

Polyarteritis

Polyarteritis is a systemic necrotizing vasculitis that occurs by itself or in association with several diseases (secondary). When it occurs as a primary vasculitis, it is called "polyarteritis nodosa." A necrotizing vasculitis that is indistinguishable from polyarteritis nodosa occurs in association with rheumatoid arthritis, systemic lupus erythematosus, other connective tissue diseases, cryoglobulinemia, hepatitis-B infection, hairy-cell leukemia, and other malignant conditions. Polyarteritis nodosa occurs in one patient per year per 100,000 population. Males outnumber females 2:1. The peak incidence occurs in ages 40 to 60, although all age groups are affected. If untreated, the systemic form of polyarteritis has <15% survival at 5 years.

- Polyarteritis: systemic necrotizing vasculitis that occurs by itself or in assocation with several diseases.
- Males outnumber females 2:1.

Pathology--Polyarteritis involves small systemic muscular arteries. Histopathologically there is a focal transmural inflammation of small muscular arteries marked by fibrinoid necrosis and a pleomorphic, neutrophil-predominant infiltration. Elastic laminae are disrupted, producing a characteristic "blow out" of the vessel wall and microaneurysms. The coexistence of normal, active, and healed areas in the same vessel is unique to polyarteritis.

- Small systemic muscular arteries are involved.
- The coexistence of normal, active, and healed areas in the same vessel is unique to polyarteritis.

Clinical features--Polyarteritis is usually a systemic illness associated with prominent constitutional features, including fever, fatigue, weight loss, and, occasionally, myalgia or arthralgia. Other common features are listed in Table 22-15. Patients can have temporal artery involvement with jaw claudication. Occasionally, polyarteritis is limited to a single organ or found incidentally associated with cancer at the time of surgery. In such cases, patients may be cured with surgical removal. Polyarteritis limited to the kidney parenchyma is called "microscopic polyarteritis nodosa" and is one cause of acute renal failure. Occasionally, patients with microscopic polyarteritis nodosa have positive antineutrophil cytoplasmic antibody (ANCA), usually with a perinuclear staining pattern (p-ANCA) or myeloperoxidase-ANCA.

- Patients with polyarteritis can have temporal artery involvement with jaw claudication.
- Polyarteritis limited to the kidney parenchyma is called

microscopic polyarteritis nodosa.

- Occasionally, p-ANCA or myeloperoxidase-ANCA is positive.

Diagnosis--Abnormal laboratory findings include normocytic anemia, increased erythrocyte sedimentation rate, and thrombocytosis. Complement consumption may be evident if immune complexes are part of the abnormality. Evidence for hepatitis B infection should be sought. Evaluation should document the extent and severity of the condition. The confirmatory test typically is angiography or biopsy of involved tissue showing vasculitis. The biopsy should be of accessible symptomatic tissue. The sensitivity of confirmatory tests in symptomatic and asymptomatic sites is listed in Table 22-16. Visceral angiography, including views of the renal and mesenteric arteries, shows saccular or fusiform aneurysm formation coupled with smooth, tapered stenosis alternating with normal or dilated blood vessel (Fig. 22-5).

Table 22-15.--Clinical Features of Polyarteritis

Common features	Uncommon features
Fever, fatigue, weight loss	Coronary arteritis
Arthralgia, arthritis	Myocardial infarction
Myalgia	Congestive heart failure
Mononeuritis multiplex	Central nervous system abnormalities
Focal necrotizing glomerular nephritis	Seizures
Abnormal renal sediment	Cerebrovascular accident
Hypertension	Lung (interstitial pneumonitis)
Skin abnormalities	Eye (retinal hemorrhage)
Palpable purpura	Testicular pain
Livedo reticularis	
Cutaneous infarctions	
Abdominal pain/ischemic bowel	
Liver enzyme abnormalities	

Table 22-16.--Sensitivity of Confirmatory Tests for Polyarteritis Nodosa

Test	Symptomatic, % positive	Asymptomatic, % positive
Nerve biopsy		20
(+/- neuropathy)	70	
Testicular biopsy		20
(+/- testicular pain)	70	
Muscle biopsy		29
(+/- myalgia and positive EMG findings)	66	
Liver biopsy		-
(abnormal findings on liver enzyme tests)	20	
Kidney biopsy		-
(+ active sediment)	20	
Visceral angiography		
(+ abdominal pain/infarction)	60	

Fig. 22-5. Visceral polyarteritis nodosa. Angiography shows the classic features of smooth tapers followed by normal or dilated vessel. Note the large saccular aneurysm in the hepatic artery. (From Audiovisual Aids Subcommittee of the Education Committee of the American College of Rheumatology: Syllabus: Revised Clinical Slide Collection on the Rheumatic Diseases and 1985, 1988, and 1989 Slide Supplements. Atlanta, Georgia, American College of Rheumatology.)

- Evidence for hepatitis B infection should be sought.
- Confirmatory test: typically, angiography or biopsy of involved tissue showing vasculitis.
- Visceral angiography shows saccular or fusiform aneurysm formation coupled with smooth, tapered stenosis.

Treatment--The cornerstone of treatment is early diagnosis and corticosteroid therapy. Cytotoxic and antimetabolite drugs such as cyclophosphamide, chlorambucil, methotrexate, and azathioprine are often used in combination with corticosteroids. These agents are added when the disease is rapidly progressive particularly if polyarteritis involves an internal organ such as the kidney, gut, or heart. They also are useful as steroid-sparing agents. When confronted with possible progression of disease in the absence of markers of systemic inflammation (increased erythrocyte sedimentation rate), consider superimposed infection and noninflammatory proliferative vasculopathy. The role of antivasospastic medication and antiplatelet agents has not been well established, but they may be helpful in the vasculopathic or healing phase of polyarteritis.

- Cytotoxic and antimetabolite drugs, such as cyclophosphamide, chlorambucil, methotrexate, and azathioprine, are often used in conjunction with corticosteroids.

Outcome--In the first year after diagnosis of polyarteritis, deaths are related to the extent of disease activity, particularly gastrointestinal tract ischemia and renal insufficiency. After 1 year, complications of treatment, including infections in the immune-compromised patient, contribute most to mortality rates. Polyarteritis survival at 5 years with treatment is between 55% and 60%. This does not seem to be influenced by the addition of cytotoxic agents to corticosteroid treatment.

- In the first year after diagnosis, deaths are related to the extent of disease activity, particularly gastrointestinal tract ischemia and renal insufficiency.
- Survival at 5 years with treatment is 55%-60%.

Churg-Strauss Vasculitis

Churg-Strauss vasculitis, or Churg-Strauss syndrome, is similar to polyarteritis and usually accounts for 6%-30% of series that combine polyarteritis and Churg-Strauss syndrome. The median age at onset is about 38 years (range, 15 to 69 years). Churg-Strauss vasculitis is defined by 1) a history of or current symptoms of asthma, 2) peripheral eosinophilia ($>1.5 \times 10^9$ eosinophils/L), and 3) systemic vasculitis of at least two extrapulmonary organs. There is a slight male predominance. The histopathologic features of the disease include eosinophilic extravascular granulomas and granulomatous or nongranulomatous small vessel necrotizing vasculitis. It typically involves the small arteries, veins, arterioles, and venules.

- Churg-Strauss vasculitis: history of or current symptoms of asthma, peripheral eosinophilia ($>1.5 \times 10^9$ eosinophils/L), and systemic vasculitis of at least two extrapulmonary organs.
- It involves the small arteries, veins, arterioles, and venules.

Clinical features--There are three clinical stages of Churg-Strauss syndrome. Patients need not progress in an orderly manner from one stage to another. Usually there is a prodrome of allergic rhinitis, nasal polyposis, or asthma. Second, peripheral blood and tissue eosinophilia develops, suggesting Löffler's syndrome. Chronic eosinophilic pneumonia and gastroenteritis may remit or recur over years. The third stage is life-threatening vasculitis. Transient, patchy pulmonary infiltrates or nodules, pleural effusions, pulmonary angiitis and cardiomegaly, eosinophilic gastroenteritis, extravascular necrotizing granulomata of the skin, mononeuritis multiplex, and polyarthritis can complicate Churg-Strauss syndrome.

- Prodrome of allergic rhinitis, nasal polyposis, or asthma.
- Peripheral blood and tissue eosinophilia develops.
- Transient, patchy pulmonary infiltrates, extravascular necrotizing granulomata of the skin, and mononeuritis multiplex.

Treatment and outcome--One-year survival with Churg-

Strauss syndrome is somewhat better than for polyarteritis and is >90%. There is more cardiac involvement but fewer renal deaths than in polyarteritis. Treatment relies on corticosteroids with or without the addition of cytotoxic agents. The eosinophilia resolves with treatment. Typically, cytotoxic agents are reserved for patients with disease not controlled by corticosteroids or for those requiring a steroid-sparing agent.

- Churg-Strauss syndrome: more cardiac involvement but fewer renal deaths than in polyarteritis.
- Eosinophilia resolves with treatment.

Buerger's Disease

Buerger's disease, or thromboangiitis obliterans, occurs almost exclusively in young adult smokers, who typically present with claudication of the instep and loss of digits from ischemic injury. They occasionally require amputation of an affected limb. Buerger's disease affects the small- and medium-sized arteries and veins of the extremities. Acute vasculitis in Buerger's disease is accompanied by characteristic intraluminal thrombus that contains microabscesses. Usually, the disease is arrested when smoking is stopped.

- Buerger's disease occurs almost exclusively in young adult smokers.
- Claudication of the instep and loss of digits from ischemic injury.
- The disease is arrested when smoking is stopped.

Primary Angiitis of the Central Nervous System

Clinical features--Primary angiitis of the central nervous system, once thought to be rare, has a chronic fluctuating and progressive course. The average age of patients presenting with this disease is 45 years. It has a slight male predominance. Forty percent of the patients present with <4 weeks of symptoms; another 40% present with symptoms that have been noted for >3 months. The most common symptom is headache (mild or severe) associated with nausea or vomiting. Nonfocal neurologic abnormalities (including confusion, dementia, drowsiness, or coma) may interrupt prolonged periods of apparent remission. Acute stroke-like focal neurologic presentations are increasingly described, particularly in young, previously healthy women. Cerebral hemorrhage occurs in <4% of patients. Focal and nonfocal neurologic abnormalities coexist in half of the patients. Systemic features--fever, weight loss, arthralgia, and myalgia--are uncommon and occur in <20% of the patients; seizures occur in about 25%.

- Primary angiitis of the central nervous system: chronic fluctuating and progressive course.
- Most common symptom is headache, with nausea or vomiting.

- Nonfocal neurologic abnormalities may interrupt prolonged periods of apparent remission.
- Acute stroke-like focal neurologic presentations in young, previously healthy women.
- Cerebral hemorrhage occurs in <4% of patients.

Diagnosis--There are no reliable noninvasive tests for making the diagnosis. The mainstays of diagnosis are cerebral angiography and biopsy of central nervous system tissues, including the leptomeninges. Nearly 40% of all patients with positive biopsy findings (pathologically documented) have normal arteriographic results. At least one in four patients with angiographically documented vasculitis has false-negative biopsy findings. The typical pathologic feature of primary angiitis of the central nervous system is a granulomatous inflammatory process centered around small veins and arterioles that is more prominent in the leptomeninges than in the underlying cortex. In 15% of patients, there is no granulomatous change. Inflammation is patchy, which may explain the biopsy sampling error. Cerebrospinal fluid examination is highly sensitive for the disease. The cerebrospinal fluid is abnormal in >90% of those patients with pathologically documented primary angiitis of the central nervous system. CT examinations of the head are not specific or sensitive for the condition. MRI examinations may be sensitive but do not distinguish this primary angiitis from other vasculopathic or demyelinating lesions of the brain. MRI is not useful in following the condition. Patients with a chronic progressive course are more likely to have the diagnosis made pathologically and have abnormal results on examination of the cerebrospinal fluid.

- Mainstays of diagnosis: cerebral angiography and biopsy of central nervous system tissues, including the leptomeninges.
- 40% of all patients with positive biopsy findings have normal arteriographic results.
- Cerebrospinal fluid is abnormal in >90% of patients.

Rheumatologic syndromes that may produce a clinical picture similar to that of primary angiitis of the central nervous system include Cogan's syndrome (nonsyphilitic keratitis and vestibular dysfunction), Behçet's syndrome (uveitis, oral and genital ulcers, meningitis, and vasculitis), systemic lupus erythematosus, and polyarteritis. Drug-induced vasculopathy (particularly cocaine), demyelinating disease, HIV infection, Lyme disease, syphilis, carcinomatous meningitis, angiocentric immunoproliferative lesions, and antiphospholipid antibody syndrome are also part of the differential diagnosis of patients presenting with a syndrome suggesting primary angiitis of the central nervous system.

Treatment--The treatment for primary angiitis of the central nervous system may be influenced by the clinical subset. Younger patients with acute disease in whom the diagnosis was made with angiography have a benign course and typically respond well to a short course of corticosteroid treatment and calcium channel blockers to prevent vasospasm. Patients with a protracted course, abnormal cerebrospinal fluid, and diagnosis made with biopsy are best treated with combination therapy, including corticosteroids and cytotoxic agents. If untreated, this clinical subset has a high mortality rate.

● Short course of corticosteroids and calcium channel blockers to prevent vasospasm.

Wegener's Granulomatosis

Clinical features--Wegener's granulomatosis is a well-recognized pathologic triad of upper and lower respiratory tract necrotizing granulomatous inflammation and focal segmental necrotizing glomerulonephritis. Wegener's granulomatosis occurs in <1 person annually per 100,000 population. Peak incidence of the disease occurs in the fourth and fifth decades of life. There is a slight male predominance. Eighty-five percent of the patients have generalized disease, including glomerulonephritis; 15% can present with local inflammation involving only the upper respiratory tract or the kidneys. The clinical features of this disease are summarized by the mnemonic ELKS: involvement of Ear/nose/ throat, Lung, Kidney, and Skin. Lung involvement most commonly includes thick-walled, centrally cavitating pulmonary nodules. Alveolitis and pulmonary hemorrhage occur in up to 20% of patients. Biopsy in the patients with renal involvement shows focal segmental necrotizing glomerulonephritis and, occasionally, granulomatous vasculitis. Skin involvement may include urticaria, petechiae, papules, vesicles, ulcers, pyoderma, and livedo reticularis. Inflammatory arthritis is uncommon. Wegener's granulomatosis arthritis can appear like rheumatoid arthritis. However, the arthritis is usually oligoarticular and transient, occurring early in the clinical presentation. Nervous system involvement includes distal sensory neuropathy, mononeuritis multiplex, and cranial nerve palsies. Conjunctivitis, uveitis, and proptosis are not unusual. Neurosensory hearing loss has been described together with serous otitis and inner ear vasculitis. Wegener's granulomatosis-associated subglottic tracheal stenosis due to chondritis should be distinguished from primary polychondritis.

● Wegener's granulomatosis: triad of upper and lower respiratory tract necrotizing granulomatous inflammation and focal segmented necrotizing glomerulonephritis.
● ELKS: involvement of Ear/nose/throat, Lung, Kidney, and Skin.
● Alveolitis and pulmonary hemorrhage occur in up to 20% of patients.
● Nervous system involvement: distal sensory neuropathy, mononeuritis multiplex, and cranial nerve palsies.

Pathologic diagnosis--The diagnosis of Wegener's granulomatosis may require finding characteristic pathologic features in biopsy specimens. Biopsy of the upper respiratory tract suggests the diagnosis in 55% of patients, but only 20% show granulomata and/or vasculitis associated with necrosis. The finding of acute and chronic inflammation and necrosis without granulomata may be adequate to make the diagnosis if the rest of the clinical picture is classic. An open lung biopsy has a higher diagnostic yield than transbronchial biopsy. Renal biopsies usually document only a focal segmental necrotizing glomerulonephritis. Infrequently, renal biopsy shows vasculitis. Relevant laboratory findings in active Wegener's granulomatosis include nonspecific increase in the erythrocyte sedimentation rate and platelet count, normocytic anemia, and low levels of albumin. Further refinement in the c-ANCA test may simplify diagnosis. Currently, the c-ANCA test alone is not adequate to make the diagnosis of Wegener's granulomatosis.

● Diagnosis: may require finding characteristic pathologic features in biopsy specimens.
● Laboratory findings: nonspecific increase in erythrocyte sedimentation rate and platelet count and normocytic anemia.

ANCA--c-ANCA is directed against proteinase 3, a serine protease from azurophilic granules. c-ANCA occurs in >90% of active cases of generalized Wegener's granulomatosis, in 75% of the cases without renal involvement, and in 10%-50% of syndromes similar to Wegener's granulomatosis. These syndromes include idiopathic crescentic glomerulonephritis (30% of cases), microscopic polyarteritis nodosa (50%), and Churg-Strauss syndrome (10%). However, in a patient with only sinusitis or a pulmonary infiltrate, a positive ANCA would have only a 5% positive predictive value for vasculitis. The antibody titer correlates loosely with disease activity, although the titers can remain increased despite clinical improvement. p-ANCA is directed against myeloperoxidase and other neutrophil cytoplasmic constituents. p-ANCA (myeloperoxidase) is found in idiopathic crescentic glomerulonephritis (70% of cases), microscopic polyarteritis nodosa (50%), Churg-Strauss syndrome (70%), Wegener's granulomatosis (20%), and systemic lupus erythematosus. p-ANCA directed against leukocyte elastase, lactoferrin, and other antigens can occur in patients with various vasculitic syndromes, primary sclerosing cholangitis, ulcerative colitis, primary biliary cirrhosis, rheumatoid arthritis, and in 5% of normal subjects.

● c-ANCA occurs in >90% of active cases, in 75% of cases without renal involvement, and in 10%-50% of syndromes similar to Wegener's granulomatosis.
● p-ANCA (myeloperoxidase) is found in idiopathic glomerulonephritis (70% of cases), microscopic polyarteritis nodosa

(50%), Churg-Strauss syndrome (70%), Wegener's granulomatosis (20%), and systemic lupus erythematosus.

Treatment and outcome--If untreated, generalized Wegener's granulomatosis has a mean survival of 5 months and 95% mortality in 1 year. More than 95% of patients eventually have clinical remission with oral cyclophosphamide treatment. Intravenously given cyclophosphamide does not maintain remission as well as the drug given orally. Corticosteroids are useful initially but can be tapered quickly after the disease is controlled. The median time to achieve remission after initiating therapy is 12 months, but 50% of the patients achieving remission have a relapse. Mortality in the first year of disease is related primarily to the inflammatory process, with pulmonary hemorrhage or renal failure. In subsequent years, drug toxicity may dominate, with opportunistic infection and increasing risk of neoplasm and hemorrhagic cystitis related to the use of cyclophosphamide.

- If untreated, generalized Wegener's granulomatosis has a mean survival of 5 months.
- Cyclophosphamide has revolutionized Wegener's granulomatous treatment and dramatically altered the natural history.
- Corticosteroids are useful initially but can be tapered quickly after the disease is controlled.

Small Vessel Vasculitis

Clinical features--Small vessel vasculitis is also known as "hypersensitivity" or "leukocytoclastic vasculitis," although these terms are not exactly interchangeable. Small vessel vasculitis occurs by itself or complicates many infectious, neoplastic, and connective tissue diseases. It occurs in the skin and may be manifested by urticaria, palpable purpura, livedo reticularis, or skin ulceration. It can be associated with peripheral neuropathy, arthralgia, or synovitis. Small vessel vasculitis affects just the skin or can be a systemic process involving internal organs and nerves. Mononeuritis multiplex, diffuse pulmonary hemorrhage, and renal vasculitis are complications of systemic small vessel vasculitis. Small vessel vasculitis occurs with many illnesses; a partial listing is given in Table 22-17.

- Small vessel vasculitis: also called hypersensitivity or leukocytoclastic vasculitis.
- It occurs by itself or complicates many infectious, neoplastic, and connective tissue diseases.
- It occurs in the skin and may be manifested by urticaria, palpable purpura, livedo reticularis, or skin ulceration.

Histopathology--A neutrophilic- or (uncommonly) lymphocytic-predominant infiltrate surrounds small arteries, veins, arterioles, or venules. Immune complexes deposit in vessel walls, along with fibrin deposition, endothelial cell swelling and necrosis, and a polymorphonuclear leukocytoclasis with scattering of nuclear fragment or nuclear dust. This histopathologic picture is called "leukocytoclastic vasculitis." It is a pathologic diagnosis and does not predict the clinical condition. Palpable purpura is the classic clinical correlate of leukocytoclastic vasculitis. However, many other cutaneous presentations of leukocytoclastic vasculitis occur.

- Histopathologic picture: leukocytoclastic vasculitis.
- Classic clinical correlate of leukocytoclastic vasculitis: palpable purpura.

Diagnosis--These various conditions are distinguished clinically and pathologically. For instance, Schönlein-Henoch vasculitis has IgA deposition in vessel walls and normal complement levels. Mixed cryoglobulinemia has circulating cryoglobulins and evidence of complement consumption. Complement levels, especially C4, may be low transiently in hypersensitivity vasculitis. Hypersensitivity vasculitis is almost always a nonsystemic small vessel vasculitis temporally related to infection, ingestion of drugs, or, less commonly, malignancy. The results of other laboratory studies are nonspecific. The leukocyte count and platelet count may be increased. Eosinophilia may be present. The erythrocyte sedimentation rate is usually increased.

- It can be associated with peripheral neuropathy, arthralgia, or synovitis.

Table 22-17.--Conditions With Small Vessel Vasculitis

Systemic small vessel vasculitis
Systemic vasculitis
Wegener's granulomatosis
Polyarteritis (primary and secondary)
Churg-Strauss vasculitis
Takayasu's arteritis
Schönlein-Henoch purpura/vasculitis
Serum sickness
Goodpasture's syndrome
Nonsystemic small vessel vasculitis
Hypocomplementemic vasculitis
Leukocytoclastic vasculitis related to:
Rheumatoid arthritis
Sjögren's syndrome
Systemic lupus erythematosus
Other connective tissue diseases
Drug-induced and postinfectious angiitis
Mixed cryoglobulinemia
Malignancy-associated vasculitis
Inflammatory bowel disease
Organ transplant-associated vasculitis

- Complement levels may be low in mixed cryoglobulinemia and hypersensitivity vasculitis.
- Schönlein-Henoch vasculitis has the clinical features of purpura, arthritis, gastrointestinal hemorrhage, and nephritis. Complement levels are always normal in Schönlein-Henoch vasculitis.

Treatment and outcome--Typically, the outcome of nonsystemic small vessel vasculitis is good. Control of the infection or discontinuation of the offending drug may be all that is required. In other cases, corticosteroids or NSAIDs are beneficial. Hypersensitivity vasculitis is usually self-limited, but it may recur with repeated exposure to the antigen or drug. Control of concomitant systemic inflammation is important. For example, better control of rheumatoid arthritis, lupus, or other connective tissue disease may be required.

- Nonsystemic small vessel vasculitis: the outcome is good.
- Hypersensitivity vasculitis may recur with repeated exposure to the antigen or drug.

Cryoglobulinemia

Cryoglobulins are immunoglobulins that reversibly precipitate at reduced temperatures. They are grouped into two major categories. *Type I cryoglobulins* are aggregates of a single monoclonal immunoglobulin and are generally associated with multiple myeloma, Waldenström's macroglobulinemia, and lymphomas. They are usually found in high concentration (1-5 g/dL). Patients with type I cryoglobulins are often asymptomatic. Symptoms of type I cryoglobulinemia are usually related to increased viscosity and include headaches, visual disturbances, nosebleeds, Raynaud's phenomenon, and ischemic ulceration from occlusion of arterioles and venules by precipitated immune complexes. Vasculitis is rare.

- Type I cryoglobulins are aggregates of a single monoclonal immunoglobulin.
- Patients with type I cryoglobulins are often asymptomatic.
- Symptoms are usually related to increased viscosity.
- Vasculitis is rare.

Type II cryoglobulins consist of more than one class of immunoglobulin. Type II cryoglobulinemia (or mixed cryoglobulinemia) can occur alone (primary) or secondary to another disease. Commonly, type II cryoglobulinemia involves an IgM molecule with anti-immunoglobulin specificity (rheumatoid factor). However, not all rheumatoid factors are cryoglobulins. Other components of the immune complexes formed include hepatitis C antigen, other infectious agents, cellular/nuclear antigens, and complement. These immune complexes precipitate slowly and are present in smaller quantities (50-500 mg/dL) than type I cryoglobulins. Cooled specimens

must be kept for up to 3 days to identify type II cryoglobulins. Type II cryoglobulins have been further divided into those complexes in which one immunoglobulin is a monoclonal protein (monoclonal-mixed cryoglobulinemia). This distinction appears to have little clinical or prognostic usefulness. Type II cryoglobulins are frequently associated with chronic infections and autoimmune disorders. The infecting agent or autoimmune antigen complexed with IgG antibody probably stimulates IgM production. When the infections resolve, the cryoglobulins disappear. The immune complexes that form precipitate on endothelial cells in peripheral blood vessels and fix complement, promoting vasculitic inflammation. The size of immune complexes, ability to fix complement, persistent IgM production, and many other factors may influence the clinical presentation of mixed cryoglobulinemia. The typical presentation is that of nonsystemic small vessel vasculitis with palpable purpura, urticaria, and cutaneous ulceration. Peripheral neuropathy, arthralgia, and arthritis are common. Less commonly, mixed cryoglobulinemia occurs with hepatosplenomegaly, pneumonitis or pulmonary hemorrhage, focal segmental necrotizing glomerulonephritis, serositis (pleurisy, pericarditis), and thyroiditis.

- Type II cryoglobulins are frequently associated with chronic infections (most often hepatitis C) and immune disorders.
- Typical presentation: nonsystemic small vessel vasculitis with palpable purpura, urticaria, and cutaneous ulceration.
- Peripheral neuropathy, arthralgia, and arthritis are common.

Laboratory studies--Nonspecific laboratory indicators of inflammation are usually found in patients with type II cryoglobulinemia and small vessel vasculitis. These studies include an increased erythrocyte sedimentation rate, increased immunoglobulin levels, positive rheumatoid factor, and low levels of complement. Evidence of chronic hepatitis infection (particularly hepatitis C) is frequently identified. For cryoglobulin testing, it is important to draw blood into a warmed syringe and to keep it warm until transferred to a cryocrit tube. Serum protein electrophoresis, immunoelectrophoresis, and quantitative immunoglobulin determinations can be helpful in some cases. Hepatitis C and other viral serologies may elucidate the nature of the disease and help in decisions about therapy (therapy is discussed above in the section on small vessel vasculitis).

- Immunoglobulin levels and the erythrocyte sedimentation rate are increased, rheumatoid factor is positive, and complement levels are low.
- Evidence of chronic hepatitis infection (particularly hepatitis C) is frequently identified.

Outcome--The clinical course of nonsystemic vasculitis is mild and prolonged. In systemic small vessel vasculitis caused by mixed cryoglobulinemia, the course and prognosis depend on the organs involved. Progressive renal disease is the most common systemic complication. Pulmonary hemorrhage is life-threatening. Some patients with mixed cryoglobulinemia eventually develop cirrhosis or a lymphoproliferative disorder.

- Progressive renal disease is the most common systemic complication.

Vasculitis Associated With Connective Tissue Diseases

Obliterative endarteropathy--Vascular involvement in rheumatoid arthritis can have various presentations. A positive rheumatoid factor is invariably present in patients with vasculitis related to rheumatoid arthritis. Digital nail fold and nodule infarcts occur in some patients with active rheumatoid arthritis. Histopathologically, this is a bland, obliterative endarteropathy with intimal proliferation. Managing the rheumatoid arthritis itself is all that is needed, because these vasculopathic changes require no other therapy. A process similar to that of obliterative endarteropathy occurs in scleroderma and systemic lupus erythematosus. A renal arcuate artery vasculopathy is responsible for scleroderma renal crisis.

- Rheumatoid factor is invariably present in patients with vasculitis related to rheumatoid arthritis.

Small and medium vessel vasculitis--Small vessel vasculitis or leukocytoclastic vasculitis with palpable purpura and systemic vasculitis (polyarteritis) can occur with severe seropositive nodular rheumatoid arthritis. A systemic necrotizing vasculitis, histopathologically indistinguishable from polyarteritis nodosa, complicates some cases of seropositive rheumatoid arthritis. Renal involvement with rheumatoid arthritis-associated polyarteritis is uncommon when compared with polyarteritis nodosa. Systemic lupus erythematosus can present with leukocytoclastic vasculitis or a polyarteritis-like picture. Sjögren's syndrome uncommonly includes small vessel vasculitis, with either a polymorphonuclear leukocyte or lymphocyte predominance. This vasculitis may cause peripheral neuropathy and some of the central nervous system features of Sjögren's syndrome. Type II cryoglobulins and vasculitis may complicate many different connective tissue diseases. Cryoglobulins should be assayed in any patient with a formal autoimmune disease who develops vasculitis.

- Small vessel vasculitis or leukocytoclastic vasculitis can occur with severe seropositive nodular rheumatoid arthritis.
- Systemic lupus erythematosus can present with leukocytoclastic vasculitis or a polyarteritis-like picture.
- Cryoglobulins should be assayed in any patient with a formal autoimmune disease who develops vasculitis.

Large vessel vasculitis--Aortitis, an inflammation of the aortic root with dilatation and aortic insufficiency, occurs in a minority of patients with HLA-B27-associated spondyloarthropathies. The patients present with aortic valve insufficiency.

Atypical Vasculitic Syndromes: Differential Diagnosis

Patients may present with the classic features of one of the vasculitic syndromes described above. When they do not, a diagnostic approach to what type of vasculitis is present may prove more difficult. Some patterns suggesting vasculitic disease and their differential diagnoses are listed in Tables 22-18 and 22-19 and Figure 22-6.

Skin Lesions Associated With Vasculitis

Palpable purpura almost always suggests leukocytoclastic vasculitis, but this pathologic diagnosis does not define the clinical syndrome. Table 22-19 outlines the differential

Table 22-18.--Acute Pulmonary-Renal Syndrome: Differential Diagnosis

Common	Uncommon
Wegener's granulomatosis	Schönlein-Henoch vasculitis
Churg-Strauss syndrome	Connective tissue diseases with associated vasculitis
Systemic lupus erythematosus	Rheumatoid arthritis
Cryoglobulinemic vasculitis	Mixed connective tissue disease
Goodpasture's syndrome	Polychondritis
Systemic small vessel vasculitis	Behçet's syndrome
	Thrombotic thrombocytopenic purpura
	Thromboembolic disease
	Infectious pneumonia
	Streptococcus
	Mycoplasma
	Legionella

Table 22-19.--Palpable Purpura: Differential Diagnosis

Polyarteritis
Churg-Strauss vasculitis
Wegener's granulomatosis
Leukocytoclastic vasculitis (classic)
Schönlein-Henoch vasculitis
Connective tissue disease-associated vasculitis
Cryoglobulinemia
Hypersensitivity to drugs, infection, and malignancy

diagnosis of palpable purpura. Nodules or papules diagnosed as necrotizing granuloma on biopsy occur in Churg-Strauss syndrome, Wegener's granulomatosis, rheumatoid arthritis, and, occasionally, systemic lupus erythematosus. Other nodules or papules without necrotizing granulomata can be the sign of angiocentric lymphoproliferative disorders or sarcoid or they may be related to inflammatory bowel disease. Urticarial or pustular lesions complicate hypocomplementemic vasculitis, inflammatory bowel arthritis syndrome, and Behçet's syndrome. Livedo reticularis, which is associated with proliferative endarteropathy, occurs in connective tissue diseases and antiphospholipid antibody syndrome and in association with cholesterol emboli and many systemic necrotizing vasculitides.

- Urticarial or pustular lesions complicate hypocomplementemic vasculitis, inflammatory bowel arthritis syndrome, and Behçet's syndrome.
- Livedo reticularis occurs in connective tissue diseases and antiphospholipid antibody syndrome.

Sinusitis and Vasculitis

Included in the differential diagnosis of sinusitis and presumed vasculitis are Wegener's granulomatosis, Churg-Strauss syndrome, relapsing polychondritis, angiocentric lymphoproliferative disorders, sarcoid, nasopharyngeal carcinoma, and, occasionally, systemic bacterial or fungal infection.

ANTIRHEUMATIC DRUG THERAPIES

Nonsteroidal Anti-Inflammatory Drugs

NSAIDs are among the most commonly prescribed medications in the world. There are no clear guidelines for selecting a particular NSAID on the basis of toxicity or efficacy. Patients vary in their responsiveness to different drugs. The variety of these drugs available permits individualization of therapy. All of them are equivalent to aspirin with regard to efficacy. They are all potent cyclooxygenase inhibitors or prodrugs of cyclooxygenase inhibitors. No clinical study has consistently found greater efficacy or tolerance for any one of these medications. NSAIDs are used to treat all types of arthritis and many types of soft tissue rheumatism.

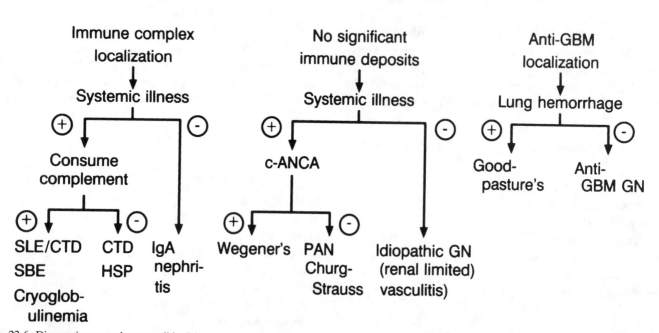

Fig. 22-6. Diagnostic approach to vasculitis. Disease pattern recognition. Focal segmental necrotizing glomerulonephritis (kidney biopsy). c-ANCA, antineutrophil cytoplasmic antibody with cytoplasmic staining; CTD, connective tissue diseases; GBM, glomerular basement membrane; GN, glomerulonephritis; HSP, Henoch-Schönlein purpura; PAN, polyarteritis nodosa; SBE, subacute bacterial endocarditis; SLE, systemic lupus erythematosus. (Modified from Rosen S, Falk RJ, Jennette JC: Polyarteritis nodosa, including microscopic form and renal vasculitis. *In* Systemic Vasculitides. Edited by A Churg, J Churg. New York, IGAKU-SHOIN Medical Publishers, 1991, pp 57-77. By permission of publisher.)

- Patients vary in their responsiveness to different drugs.
- NSAIDs are all potent cyclooxygenase inhibitors or pro-drugs of cyclooxygenase inhibitors.

Mechanisms of Action

The mechanism of the action of NSAIDs is incompletely understood. They decrease prostaglandin synthesis by inhibiting cyclooxygenase conversion of arachidonic acid to prostaglandin precursors. Prostaglandins cause vasodilatation, mediate pain, and potentiate the inflammatory effects of histamines and bradykinin. Furthermore, prostaglandins act as immunomodulators, influencing cellular and humoral immune responses. NSAIDs have potent analgesic effects that are related to their suppression of prostaglandin synthesis. Decreased levels of prostaglandin decrease the sensitivity of peripheral nerve receptors and may affect pain transmission. Acetaminophen is not a potent prostaglandin inhibitor in peripheral tissue. However, it does affect prostaglandin concentrations in neural tissue. This may explain the analgesic effect of acetaminophen. Acetaminophen, salicylates, and other NSAIDs are potent antipyretic medications.

- NSAIDs decrease prostaglandin synthesis by inhibiting cyclooxygenase conversion of arachidonic acid to prostaglandin precursors.
- Decreased levels of prostaglandin decrease the sensitivity of peripheral nerve receptors and may affect pain transmission.

Mechanisms of Toxicity of NSAIDs

Toxic reactions are primarily due to inhibition of prostaglandin production. Prostaglandins protect the gastric mucosal barrier from autodigestion. Patients with renal insufficiency or liver or cardiac disease may have prostaglandin-dependent renal blood flow. They have further decrease of renal function when NSAIDs inhibit prostaglandins. Also, NSAIDs interfere with the synthesis of thromboxane, which influences platelet aggregation and hemostasis. Blocking cyclooxygenase with NSAIDs augments conversion of arachidonic acid to leukotrienes. Leukotrienes (previously known as "slow-reacting substance of anaphylaxis") aggravate asthma, rhinitis, hives, and nasal polyps.

- Toxic reactions are due primarily to inhibition of prostaglandin production.
- NSAIDs interfere with the synthesis of thromboxane.
- Leukotrienes aggravate asthma, rhinitis, hives, and nasal polyps.

NSAIDs are bound extensively to plasma proteins. Protein binding has obvious implications for other medications that are also protein bound. Phenylbutazone and aspirin inhibit the metabolism of oral hypoglycemic agents and increase the

risk of hypoglycemia. Indomethacin, diclofenac, and piroxicam decrease lithium excretion. NSAIDs can also influence methotrexate toxicity at high doses (>50 mg/week) by interfering with the renal clearance of methotrexate.

- Phenylbutazone and aspirin inhibit the metabolism of oral hypoglycemic agents and increase the risk of hypoglycemia.
- Indomethacin, diclofenac, and piroxicam decrease lithium excretion.

Most NSAIDs attenuate the effects of antihypertensive medications. Diuretics, β-blockers, and angiotensin converting enzyme inhibitors are the drugs affected most by the influence of NSAIDs on renal prostaglandins. Aspirin irreversibly inhibits cyclooxygenase. The effect of all the other NSAIDs on cyclooxygenase is reversible. All these drugs prolong the bleeding time. The use of aspirin needs to be discontinued for up to 10 days before the bleeding time returns to normal. NSAIDs should be discontinued at least 4-drug half-lives before an invasive procedure. NSAIDs with a short half-life are best when an acute effect (e.g., treatment of acute gout) is required. The half-life is proportional to the onset of maximal clinical benefit. The common side effects of NSAIDs are listed in Table 22-20.

- Diuretics, β-blockers, and angiotensin converting enzyme inhibitors are the drugs affected most by the influence of NSAIDs on renal prostaglandins.
- Aspirin irreversibly inhibits cyclooxygenase.
- NSAIDs usually prolong the bleeding time.

Gastrointestinal Side Effects

Twenty percent of chronic users of NSAIDs have gastric ulcer noted on endoscopy, and 15%-35% report dyspepsia, but this complaint does not appear to be related to abnormal findings on endoscopy. Nausea and abdominal pain are described in up to 40% of users of nonsteroidal anti-inflammatory drugs. Stomach upset/pain forces discontinuation of these drugs in more than 10% of patients. Gastrointestinal blood loss related to these drugs is most often occult and can result in iron deficiency anemia. The true incidence of significant gastrointestinal bleeding requiring hospitalization or operation or resulting in death is unknown. However, the elderly are at greatest risk for significant gastrointestinal toxicity related to nonsteroidal anti-inflammatory drugs. Patients with significant comorbid factors--such as cardiovascular disease, previous stomach ulcer, and diabetes--and those taking corticosteroids are at higher risk. Alcohol and tobacco use also predisposes to the development of gastrointestinal toxicity.

- Of chronic users of NSAIDs, 20% have gastric ulcer and 15%-35% have dyspepsia.
- Stomach upset/pain forces discontinuation of these drugs

Table 22-20.--Common Side Effects of Nonsteroidal Anti-Inflammatory Drugs

Gastrointestinal
  Nausea
  Abdominal pain
  Constipation or diarrhea
  Occult blood loss and iron deficiency anemia
  Peptic ulcer disease
  Colitis and colonic hemorrhage
Renal
  Reduced renal blood flow
  Reduced glomerular filtration rate
  Increased creatinine clearance
  Pyuria
  Interstitial nephritis
  Papillary necrosis
  Nephrotic syndrome
  Hyperkalemia and type IV renal tubular acidosis
  Fluid retention
Hematologic
  Bone marrow suppression
    Agranulocytosis
    Aplastic anemia
  Iron deficiency anemia
  Platelet aggregating defect
Neurologic
  Delirium/confusion
  Headache
  Dizziness
  Blurred vision
  Mood swings
  Aseptic meningitis
Dermatologic
  Urticaria
  Erythema multiforme
  Exfoliative syndromes (toxic epidermal necrolysis)
  Oral ulcers
  Dermatitis
Pulmonary
  Pulmonary infiltrates
  Noncardiac pulmonary edema (aspirin toxicity)
  Anaphylaxis and bronchospasm
  Nasal polyps
Drug interactions
  Augment hemostatic defect of warfarin
  Attenuate antihypertensive effect of diuretics, β-blockers, angiotensin converting enzyme inhibitors
  Influence drug metabolism
    Methotrexate (high doses only)
    Lithium
    Oral hypoglycemic agents

in >10% of patients.
● Gastrointestinal blood loss related to these drugs is most often occult.

Other Toxic Effects of NSAIDs

Bone marrow toxicity, including agranulocytosis and aplastic anemia, can occur with all NSAIDs, most frequently with phenylbutazone. Central nervous system symptoms such as headaches, dizziness, mood alterations, blurred vision, and confusion are reported most frequently with the use of indomethacin. Ibuprofen, tolmetin, and sulindac have been associated with aseptic meningitis in patients with systemic lupus erythematosus. All the central nervous system effects resolve when the use of NSAIDs is discontinued. Rashes, urticaria, exfoliative dermatitis, erythema multiforme, and scalded skin syndrome or toxic epidermal necrolysis all occur, albeit rarely, with the use of NSAIDs. Easy bruisability is a common complaint of chronic users of these drugs. Patients may develop dependent petechiae if their platelet function is already compromised. Pulmonary infiltrates, bronchospasm, and anaphylaxis may occur with all NSAIDs, including aspirin. Although it is not IgE-mediated, anaphylaxis is seen most commonly in patients who have the classic triad of asthma, nasal polyps, and aspirin sensitivity. Combination therapy with NSAIDs should be avoided. Whereas toxicity is additive, there is no evidence that the therapeutic effect is additive.

● The elderly are especially at risk for significant gastrointestinal toxicity related to NSAIDs.
● Acetaminophen is not a potent prostaglandin inhibitor in peripheral tissue.
● Bone marrow toxicity, including agranulocytosis and aplastic anemia, can occur with NSAIDs.
● Central nervous system symptoms are reported most frequently with the use of indomethacin.

Nonacetylated Salicylates

Careful studies have not identified significant differences in efficacy of nonacetylated salicylates compared with NSAIDs. Nonacetylated salicylates minimally inhibit prostaglandin production. Although their use decreases the incidence of gastrointestinal bleeding, they do not prevent many of the gastrointestinal symptoms that influence patient compliance. Tinnitus remains a potential problem. Nonacetylated salicylates do not interfere with renal blood flow, and they do not inhibit platelet function. They usually can be prescribed for patients with aspirin allergy.

● Nonacetylated salicylates minimally inhibit prostaglandin production.
● Nonacetylated salicylates do not interfere with renal blood flow, and they do not inhibit platelet function.

Disease-Modifying Antirheumatic Drugs

Antimalarial Compounds (Hydroxychloroquine)

Open and randomized placebo-controlled studies have confirmed the benefit of hydroxychloroquine in the management of rheumatoid arthritis and systemic lupus erythematosus. The drug collects in pigmented tissues, including the pigment layer of the retina and skin. The dose typically does not exceed 4.5 mg/kg daily. Retinopathy is the major toxic effect associated with the use of hydroxychloroquine. The risk of irreversible retinopathy is small (<3%) in patients taking <4.5 mg/kg daily. The elderly may be at somewhat increased risk. Regular eye examinations can identify the premaculopathy stage of the toxic reaction, which is reversible. Permanent symptomatic retinopathy is preventable when patients have eye examinations every 6 months.

- Retinopathy is the major toxic effect associated with the use of hydroxychloroquine.
- The risk of irreversible retinopathy is small (<3%) in patients taking <4.5 mg/kg daily.

In rheumatoid arthritis and systemic lupus erythematosus, the clinical response to hydroxychloroquine does not appear before 8 weeks. Improvement may not occur until after 6 months of continuous therapy. Approximately 40%-60% of patients with rheumatoid arthritis may respond (based on established criteria for response). It is most commonly used in combination with NSAIDs or low doses of corticosteroids in patients with early or mild polyarthritis. The use of hydroxychloroquine in combination with other disease-modifying antirheumatic drugs has not been studied completely.

- The clinical response to hydroxychloroquine does not appear before 8 weeks and may not occur until after 6 months of continuous therapy.

Gold Salts

There are three preparations of gold salts: gold sodium thiomalate (Myochrysine, given intramuscularly), aurothioglucose (Solganal, given intramuscularly), and auranofin (Ridaura, given orally). Intramuscular injections of gold salts started in the first few years of disease can reduce the number of tender and swollen joints and improve grip strength. Gold treatment decreases the erythrocyte sedimentation rate and typically reduces the rheumatoid factor titer. Gold may work partly by influencing macrophage function. Adding intramuscular injections of gold to the treatment within the first 2 years of rheumatoid arthritis increases the potential for remission by approximately one-third over patients not treated with a disease-modifying antirheumatic drug. Gold given intramuscularly is also prescribed to patients with HLA-B27-associated peripheral arthritis. It has no effect on the axial (spinal)

inflammatory arthritis. Intramuscular injections of gold may cause disease flares in systemic lupus erythematosus.

- Gold treatment decreases the erythrocyte sedimentation rate and typically reduces the rheumatoid factor titer.
- No effect on axial (spinal) inflammatory arthritis.
- There is a 60% chance that patients will respond to gold given intramuscularly.

Gold therapy may be initiated if there is no history of previous gold toxicity, and the results of complete blood cell count and urinalysis are normal or stable. Gold therapy should be continued until at least 1,000 mg have been administered before a lack of response prompts discontinuation. It is important to check for any potential toxic reaction with each intramuscular injection. A complete blood cell count and urinalysis are usually performed before each injection. Patients should be questioned about any new symptoms. Adverse experiences in patients treated with injections of gold are responsible for 1-year toxicity dropout rates approaching 35%. Vasomotor responses (nitritoid reaction) occur more commonly with gold sodium thiomalate than with aurothioglucose. The nitritoid reaction occurs shortly after injection and is characterized by weakness, dizziness, nausea, vomiting, sweating, and facial flushing. Common reactions to intramuscular injections of gold include stomatitis and rashes. More than 50 types of rashes occur with gold injections. Often, the mucocutaneous reaction can be managed by changing the gold preparation or holding and later rechallenging with a lower dose. Gold therapy causes membranous glomerulonephropathy with proteinuria and nephrotic syndrome. Of the patients receiving intramuscular injections of gold, 40% have to discontinue use of the medication because of nephropathy. Hematologic disturbances occur in <2% of all patients receiving gold injections. Immunothrombocytopenia, agranulocytosis, and aplastic anemia can be life-threatening conditions.

- Gold therapy should be continued until at least 1,000 mg have been administered before a lack of response prompts discontinuation.
- One-year toxicity dropout rates approach 35%.
- Vasomotor responses occur more commonly with gold sodium thiomalate than with aurothioglucose.
- Common reactions to intramuscular injections of gold include stomatitis and rashes and less commonly, bone marrow suppression or membranous glomerulopathy.
- It is important to check for any potential toxic reaction with each intramuscular injection by questioning the patient and checking blood counts and a urinalysis.
- The nitritoid reaction occurs shortly after a gold injection and is characterized by weakness, dizziness, nausea, vomiting, sweating, and facial flushing.

Auranofin is an orally administered gold compound. About 25% of the dose is rapidly absorbed; the majority of the medication is eliminated in the feces. The medication should be continued for at least 4-6 months to assess its therapeutic potential. Meta-analysis suggests auranofin is less effective than other disease-modifying antirheumatic drugs, including gold given intramuscularly and methotrexate. The most frequent toxic effect is diarrhea.

- Auranofin is an orally administered gold compound.
- Auranofin is less effective than other disease-modifying antirheumatic drugs.
- The most frequent toxic effect is diarrhea.

D-*Penicillamine*

The mechanism of action of D-penicillamine is not completely understood. It does reduce immune complex formation. Penicillamine is a treatment for systemic sclerosis (scleroderma), rheumatoid arthritis, and, possibly, vasculitis associated with cryoglobulinemia. Penicillin allergy is not a contraindication to the use of penicillamine. The adage "go low, go slow" emphasizes dosing increments that decrease the toxic effects associated with penicillamine. It is the only rheumatologic medication that needs to be taken on an empty stomach, 1 hour before or 2 hours after meals. The medication should be tried for at least 6 months, if tolerated, to assess its potential for therapeutic benefit. Its toxicity profile is similar to that of intramuscular injections of gold, including the mucocutaneous reactions, nephropathy, and hematologic abnormalities. Several autoimmune phenomena have been described, including myasthenia gravis, polymyositis, systemic lupus erythematosus-like syndrome, and a Goodpasture-like syndrome. Penicillamine causes skin fragility and poor wound healing by inhibiting collagen synthesis.

- Penicillin allergy is not a contraindication to the use of penicillamine.
- Penicillamine needs to be taken on an empty stomach.
- Penicillamine can cause rashes, oral ulcers, nephropathy, and bone marrow suppression.
- Several autoimmune phenomena may occur secondary to treatment with D-penicillamine including myasthenia gravis, polymyositis, a lupus-like illness, and Goodpasture's syndrome.

Sulfasalazine

Enteric-coated tablets of sulfasalazine (Azulfidine-EN-tabs) have reduced some of the immediate gastrointestinal upset associated with this drug. The metabolites of sulfasalazine include 5-aminosalicylic acid and sulfapyridine. The mechanism of its action is unknown. The results of short-term randomized trials indicate significant efficacy in mild-to-moderate rheumatoid arthritis. Rheumatologists also recommend treatment with

sulfasalazine for seronegative spondyloarthropathies and psoriatic arthritis. The benefit of this drug in rheumatoid arthritis is equal to that of intramuscular injections of gold but with fewer toxic effects. Sulfasalazine treatment is usually reserved for milder cases of inflammatory polyarthritis. Although the onset of efficacy occurs as early as 8 weeks, the effect may not be documented for as many as 6 months. The toxic effects include nausea, vomiting, gastric ulcers, and, more rarely, hepatitis or cholestasis. Ten percent of patients complain of headache or sense of fatigue. Currently, this drug does not have FDA approval for management of rheumatoid arthritis.

- The mechanism of action of sulfasalazine is unknown.
- Sulfasalazine treatment: usually reserved for milder cases of inflammatory polyarthritis.
- The benefit of this drug in rheumatoid arthritis may be equal to that of intramuscular injections of gold.

Methotrexate

Methotrexate is a structural analogue of folic acid and is considered an antimetabolite rather than a cytotoxic agent. It is used extensively in rheumatoid arthritis and also has a place in the treatment of psoriatic arthritis and peripheral arthritis of seronegative spondyloarthropathies. Methotrexate may have a role in the treatment of some aspects of systemic lupus erythematosus and scleroderma. Its mechanism of action includes inhibition of folate metabolism (critical in nucleotide production), inhibition of leukotriene B4, and increasing intracellular adenosine. It has both immunomodulator and anti-inflammatory effects. Its strongest effect is on rapidly dividing cells, particularly those in the S phase of the cell cycle. Methotrexate is unique among disease-modifying antirheumatic drugs because its antirheumatic effect occurs within 4-6 weeks. Oral, subcutaneous, and intramuscular and/or intravenous routes are equally effective for low dosages.

- Methotrexate: used extensively in rheumatoid arthritis and has a place in the treatment of psoriatic arthritis, peripheral arthritis of seronegative spondyloarthropathies, and some aspects of systemic lupus erythematosus and scleroderma.
- The antirheumatic effect occurs within 4-6 weeks.

Of rheumatoid arthritis patients receiving treatment with methotrexate, 80% have a significant improvement within the first year of therapy. At 5 years, it is estimated that at least 35% of patients treated with methotrexate still take it. No other disease-modifying antirheumatic drug has this combination of efficacy and tolerability. Most patients with rheumatoid arthritis have a severe flare of their disease within 3 weeks after discontinuation of methotrexate therapy. This drug should not be used in patients with significant renal dysfunction (creatinine >2.0 mg/dL). Coadministration of trimethoprim sulfa antibiotics and methotrexate increases hematologic toxicity.

- 80% of rheumatoid arthritis patients taking methotrexate have significant improvement within the first year of treatment.
- Most rheumatoid arthritis patients have a severe flare of their disease within 3 weeks after discontinuation of methotrexate therapy.

Gastrointestinal toxic reactions are common side effects of methotrexate. Nausea and vomiting may persist for 24-48 hours after ingestion. Stomatitis and diarrhea are insurmountable problems for some patients. Methotrexate treatment should be withheld from patients with significant gastric ulceration until their ulcers have healed. Increased liver enzyme levels suggest a subclinical hepatic toxic effect due to methotrexate. Persistent increase in aspartate aminotransferase levels or decreasing albumin levels are markers for developing hepatic fibrosis and, potentially, cirrhosis. Cryptic cirrhosis may develop without liver enzyme abnormalities being detected. Stomatitis and the less common hematologic abnormalities such as leukopenia, thrombocytopenia, and pancytopenia may respond to folic acid supplementation. Pulmonary abnormalities, including chemical pneumonitis and insidious pulmonary fibrosis, may occur with methotrexate treatment. Acute pneumonitis due to methotrexate may be associated with eosinophilia. Neurologic features such as headache and seizure are uncommon. Methotrexate is teratogenic and should be withheld for 3 months before the patient attempts to conceive.

- Gastrointestinal toxic reactions are the common side effects of methotrexate.
- Methotrexate should not be used in patients with significant renal dysfunction.
- Stomatitis and diarrhea are insurmountable problems for some patients.

Azathioprine

Azathioprine and its metabolites are purine analogues. It is considered a cytotoxic agent. Azathioprine is metabolized by xanthine oxidase and thiopurine methyltransferase (TPMT). Allopurinol, an inhibitor of xanthine oxidase, delays the metabolism of azathioprine and can lead to toxic reactions if the dose of azathioprine is not decreased by 50%-66%. Thiopurine methyltransferase can be assayed; low levels of this enzyme predict the 1 in 300 patients who will develop a severe hematologic reaction to azathioprine. Controlled studies document the efficacy of azathioprine in the treatment of rheumatoid arthritis and systemic lupus erythematosus.

The most common problem with azathioprine is gastrointestinal toxic effects. An idiosyncratic, acute pancreatitis-like attack is an absolute contraindication to further treatment with this drug. Cholestatic hepatitis is rare, but if it occurs, it generally does so within the first several weeks of drug administration. If tolerated initially, hematologic toxic effects become

the most significant concern. In patients who have undergone organ transplant, azathioprine treatment increases the risk of neoplasia, particularly lymphomas, leukemias, and skin and cervical malignancies. Azathioprine does not alter fertility, but it may have some teratogenic potential. For pregnant women, azathioprine should be reserved for those with severe or life-threatening rheumatic diseases.

- Azathioprine is a cytotoxic agent.
- The most common problems with azathioprine are gastrointestinal toxic effects and cytopenias.
- Allopurinol should be avoided in patients taking azathioprine.

Cyclophosphamide

Cyclophosphamide is a potent alkylating agent. It acts on dividing and nondividing cells, interfering with cellular DNA function. It depletes T cells and B cells, causing considerable immunosuppression. Oral cyclophosphamide is well absorbed and completely metabolized within 24 hours, and most of its metabolites are excreted in the urine. Allopurinol increases the risk of leukopenia in patients taking cyclophosphamide. Short-term studies document significant efficacy of this drug in the treatment of rheumatoid arthritis at doses of 1-2 mg/kg per day. Unequivocal healing and arresting of erosive change occur. The considerable toxicity associated with chronic administration of cyclophosphamide has raised questions about whether it should be used in rheumatoid arthritis. It is the drug of choice in the treatment of generalized Wegener's granulomatosis. Intravenous administration of cyclophosphamide is efficacious in managing severe systemic lupus erythematosus, including proliferative glomerulonephritis. Short-term advantages of intravenous pulse of cyclophosphamide in patients with lupus nephritis may include fewer toxic effects on the bladder and perhaps a lower risk of infection.

- Cyclophosphamide depletes T cells and B cells, causing considerable immunosuppression.
- Allopurinol increases the risk of leukopenia in patients taking cyclophosphamide.
- Intravenous administration of cyclophosphamide is efficacious in managing severe systemic lupus erythematosus.

Dose-related bone marrow suppression is common in patients receiving cyclophosphamide and requires close laboratory monitoring. Immune suppression from treatment with cyclophosphamide increases the risk of infection. Herpes zoster infection occurs in most patients receiving the drug orally. Cyclophosphamide directly affects ovarian and testicular function. Premature ovarian failure frequently occurs in premenopausal lupus patients taking the drug. Spermatogenesis can also be affected by this drug, which causes atrophy of seminiferous tubules. Cyclophosphamide has teratogenic potential.

Alopecia, stomatitis, cardiomyopathy (with drug doses used to treat cancer), and pulmonary fibrosis may complicate cyclophosphamide therapy. The metabolites of this drug, including acrolein, accumulate in the bladder. Acrolein has direct mucosal toxic effects and causes hemorrhagic cystitis. This complication is potentially life-threatening. The chronic use of cyclophosphamide taken orally is associated with increased risk of neoplasia, including hematologic and bladder malignancies. The risk of malignancy with intravenous pulse therapy has not been established.

- Cyclophosphamide: dose-related bone marrow suppression is common.
- Cyclophosphamide directly affects ovarian and testicular function.
- The chronic use of cyclophosphamide is associated with increased risk of neoplasia.

Glucocorticosteroids

Glucocorticosteroids modify the inflammatory response dramatically. They are potent inhibitors of neutrophil function. Glucocorticosteroids suppress cellular immune activity and, to a lesser extent, inhibit the humoral response. Low doses of glucocorticosteroids (<10 mg of prednisone per day) are frequently used in the day-to-day management of the articular manifestations of rheumatoid arthritis. At least one-third of all patients with rheumatoid arthritis take glucocorticosteroids chronically. The role of glucocorticosteroids in the treatment of rheumatoid arthritis is a controversial matter. Pulse or bolus therapy cannot be recommended for the routine management of flairs of rheumatoid arthritis. High doses of glucocorticosteroids (1-2 mg of prednisone per kilogram of patient body weight) may be required for life-threatening or serious inflammatory disorders, including systemic vasculitis and complications of systemic lupus erythematosus.

- Glucocorticosteroids are potent inhibitors of neutrophil function.
- They suppress cellular immune activity and, to a lesser extent, inhibit the humoral response.
- One-third of all patients with rheumatoid arthritis take glucocorticosteroids chronically.

These drugs have many side effects, which are not idiosyncratic but actually unwanted effects of the medication. The longer patients receive them and the higher the dose that is used, determine how fast an unwanted effect appears. Many patients with rheumatoid arthritis tolerate prednisone doses in the 1-5 mg/day range for years without having serious side effects. Patient concerns about glucocorticosteroids include weight gain from increased appetite, water retention, and hirsutism. Longer-term concerns include thinning of the skin, bruising easily, progressive osteoporosis (unclear if this happens with physiologic doses of prednisone) and compression fractures, high blood pressure, glucose intolerance, cataract formation, and aggravation of glaucoma. The psychoactive potential of high doses of glucocorticosteroids is an additional factor in treating older patients. Glucocorticosteroid psychosis can complicate the diagnosis of neuropsychiatric lupus.

- Many patients with rheumatoid arthritis tolerate prednisone doses in the 1-5 mg/day range for years without having serious side effects.
- Long-term concerns: thinning of the skin, progressive osteoporosis and compression fractures, high blood pressure, glucose intolerance, cataract formation, and aggravation of glaucoma.
- Glucocorticosteroid psychosis can complicate the diagnosis of neuropsychiatric lupus.
- Glucocorticosteroids interfere with wound healing and increase risk of opportunistic infection.

PART II

William W. Ginsburg, M.D.

CRYSTALLINE ARTHROPATHIES

Gout and Hyperuricemia

Hyperuricemia has been described in 2%-18% of normal populations, but the prevalence of clinical gouty arthritis ranges from 0.1%-0.4%. There is a family history of gout in 6%-18% of patients. Genetic studies suggest a multifactorial inheritance pattern. Of patients with hyperuricemia whose uric acid level is >9 mg/dL, gout will develop in 5 years in approximately 20%.

- Hyperuricemia occurs in 2%-18% of normal populations.
- Prevalence of gouty arthritis is 0.1%-0.4%.
- 6%-18% of patients have family history of gout.
- In patients with uric acid level >9 mg/dL, gout develops in 20% in 5 years.

Hyperuricemia may result from uric acid overproduction or underexcretion, or both. Overproduction is the cause in ≤10% of patients with primary gout. Of these 10%, about 15% have one of the two X-linked inborn errors of purine metabolism: 1) hypoxanthine-guanine phosphoribosyltransferase (HGPRTase) deficiency (Lesch-Nyhan syndrome) and 2) 5-phosphoribosyl-1-pyrophosphate (PRPP) synthetase overactivity. Of the remaining 90% of patients who have overproduction, most are obese, but the cause of overproduction and the relationship between obesity and overproduction of uric acid remain unknown.

- ≤10% of patients with primary gout have overproduction of uric acid.

Underexcretion of uric acid occurs in approximately 90% of patients with gout. They have reduced filtration of uric acid, enhanced tubular reabsorption, or decreased tubular secretion.

Events leading to initial crystallization of monosodium urate in the joint after approximately 30 years of asymptomatic hyperuricemia are unknown. Trauma with disruption of microtophi in cartilage leads to release of urate crystals into synovial fluid. The urate crystals become coated with immunoglobulin and then complement. They are then phagocytosed by leukocytes with subsequent release of chemotactic protein, activation of the kallikrein system, and disruption of the leukocytes, which release lysosomal enzymes into synovial fluid.

- Events leading to initial crystallization of monosodium urate in joint after years of asymptomatic hyperuricemia are unknown.

Important Enzyme Abnormalities in Uric Acid Pathway

Lesch-Nyhan syndrome is a complete deficiency of hypoxanthine-guanine phosphoribosyltransferase. It is characterized by X-linked disorder in young boys, hyperuricemia, self-mutilation, choreoathetosis, spasticity, growth retardation, and severe gouty arthritis (Fig. 22-7).

Fig. 22-7. Purine metabolism. HGPRTase, hypoxanthine-guanine phosphoribosyltransferase; PRPP, phosphoribosylpyrophosphate; PRPP syn, phosphoribosylpyrophosphate synthetase; ⊖, feedback inhibition.

- Lesch-Nyhan syndrome characterized by X-linked disorder in young boys, self-mutilation, spasticity, severe gouty arthritis.

5-Phosphoribosyl-1-pyrophosphate (PRPP) synthetase overactivity is associated with hyperuricemia, X-linked disorder, and gouty arthritis.

Adenosine deaminase deficiency is autosomal recessive. There is a buildup of deoxyadenosine triphosphate in lymphocytes, which is toxic to immature lymphocytes. It is a combined immunodeficiency state with severe T-cell and mild B-cell dysfunction. Features of the disorder are hypouricemia, recurrent infection, chondro-osseous dysplasia, and elevated deoxyadenosine in plasma and urine. Treatment for the disorder is with irradiated frozen red blood cells or marrow transplantation.

- Adenosine deaminase deficiency is combined immunodeficiency state with severe T-cell and mild B-cell dysfunction.
- It is autosomal recessive.
- Features are hypouricemia and recurrent infection.

Xanthine oxidase deficiency is autosomal recessive. It is characterized by hypouricemia, xanthinuria with xanthine stones, and myopathy associated with deposits of xanthine and hypoxanthine.

- Xanthine oxidase deficiency is characterized by hypouricemia.
- It is autosomal recessive.

Causes of Secondary Hyperuricemia

Secondary hyperuricemia can be attributed to overproduction or underexcretion of uric acid (Table 22-21).

Causes of Hypouricemia

Increased urinary excretion of uric acid contributes to hypouricemia. It can develop in healthy persons with an isolated defect in tubular reabsorption of uric acid. It is also related to diminished reabsorption of urate, such as in Fanconi syndrome, Fanconi syndrome associated with Wilson's disease, carcinoma of the lung, acute myelogenous leukemia, light-chain disease, and use of outdated tetracycline. Malignant neoplasms, such as carcinoma, Hodgkin's disease, and sarcoma, are also associated with increased uric acid excretion. Hypervolemia caused by inappropriate secretion of antidiuretic hormone can also be a factor. Drugs involved in increased uric acid excretion are high-dose aspirin, probenecid and other uricosuric agents, and glyceryl guaiacolate. Radiographic contrast agents that can cause hypouricemia are iopanoic acid (Telopaque), iodipamide meglumine (Cholografin), and diatrizoate sodium (Hypaque). It can also occur in severe liver disease.

Table 22-21.--Causes of Secondary Hyperuricemia

Overproduction
  Myeloproliferative disorders
    Polycythemia, primary or secondary
    Myeloid metaplasia
    Chronic myelocytic leukemia
  Lymphoproliferative disorders
    Chronic lymphatic leukemia
    Multiple myeloma
  Disseminated carcinoma and sarcoma
  Sickle cell anemia, thalassemia, and other forms of chronic hemolytic anemia
  Psoriasis
  Cytotoxic drugs
  Infectious mononucleosis
  Obesity
  Increased purine ingestion
Underexcretion
  Intrinsic renal disease
    Chronic renal insufficiency of diverse cause
    Saturine gout (lead nephropathy)
  Drug-induced
    Thiazide diuretics, furosemide, ethacrynic acid, ethambutol, pyrazinamide, low-dose aspirin, cyclosporine, nicotinic acid, laxative abuse, levodopa
  Endocrine conditions
    Adrenal insufficiency, nephrogenic diabetes insipidus, hyperparathyroidism, hypoparathyroidism, pseudohypoparathyroidism, hypothyroidism
  Metabolic conditions
    Diabetic ketoacidosis, lactic acidosis, starvation, ethanolism, glycogen storage disease type I, Bartter's syndrome
  Other
    Sarcoidosis
    Down syndrome
    Beryllium disease

- Causes of increased urinary excretion of uric acid are isolated defect in tubular reabsorption of uric acid, Fanconi syndrome, carcinoma of lung, acute myelogenous leukemia, drugs (high-dose aspirin, probenecid), radiographic contrast agents, and severe liver disease.

Decreased synthesis of uric acid can also cause hypouricemia. The drug allopurinol inhibits the enzyme xanthine oxidase, causing hypouricemia. The decrease can also be caused by congenital deficiencies in enzymes involved in purine biosynthesis: 5-phosphoribosyl-1-pyrophosphate synthetase deficiency, adenosine deaminase deficiency, purine nucleoside phosphorylase deficiency, and xanthine oxidase deficiency (xanthinuria). Acquired deficiency in xanthine oxidase activity (metastatic adenocarcinoma of lung) can also cause decreased synthesis of uric acid, as can acute intermittent porphyria.

Predisposing Factors to Gout and Pseudogout

The following can predispose to an attack of gout or pseudogout: trauma, operation (3 days after), major medical illness (myocardial infarction, cerebrovascular accident, pulmonary embolus), fasting, alcohol use, and infection.

- Factors that precipitate gout and pseudogout: trauma, operation, alcohol.

Treatment of Acute Gouty Arthritis

Do not administer allopurinol or probenecid until the acute attack completely subsides. Because of severe gastrointestinal side effects, high-dose oral colchicine is rarely used for an acute attack. Intravenously administered colchicine (1-2 mg) has no gastrointestinal side effects. It has increased toxicity in patients with renal insufficiency, bone marrow depression, sepsis, and immediate prior use of oral colchicine. In patients with a history of heart failure or peptic ulcers, this is drug of choice. It can cause severe extravasation if it infiltrates into subcutaneous tissues.

- Colchicine: severe gastrointestinal side effects with oral form, no gastrointestinal side effects with intravenous administration.

Indomethacin (or other nonsteroidal anti-inflammatory drugs, NSAIDs) is one of the drugs of choice when used for 7- to 10-day course and when there is no contraindication to its use. Do not use it in patients with congestive heart failure, peptic ulcer disease, or renal insufficiency. It can have marked sodium retention properties. It should not be used in patients with nasal polyps and aspirin sensitivity because indomethacin may cause bronchospasm. Frontal headache is an uncommon side effect.

- Avoid nonsteroidal anti-inflammatory drugs in patients with congestive heart failure, peptic ulcer disease, and renal insufficiency.
- Avoid indomethacin in patients with nasal polyps and aspirin allergy.

Intra-articular or oral corticosteroids and subcutaneous ACTH are other treatments, especially in patients who have contraindications to colchicine and NSAIDs.

Treatment of Intercritical Period

Probenecid is a uricosuric. It inhibits tubular reabsorption of filtered and secreted urate, thereby increasing urinary excre-

tion of uric acid. Colchicine, 0.6 mg twice a day, is given prophylactically for 6-12 months to prevent exacerbation of acute gout. It should not be used if the patient has a history of kidney stones or if 24-hour urine uric acid value is >1,000 mg (normal, <600 mg/day). Probenecid delays renal excretion of indomethacin and thereby increases its blood level. Probenecid delays the renal excretion of acetylsalicylic acid (ASA), and ASA completely blocks the uricosuric effect of probenecid. ASA also blocks tubular secretion of urates. Do not use probenecid with methotrexate because probenecid increases methotrexate blood levels, which increase toxicity from methotrexate.

- Probenecid inhibits tubular reabsorption of filtered and secreted urate.
- Not used if patient has a history of kidney stones or if 24-hour uric acid value is >1,000 mg.
- Delays renal excretion of indomethacin.
- Delays renal excretion of ASA.
- Do not use with methotrexate.

Allopurinol is a xanthine oxidase inhibitor. It can precipitate acute gout, so colchicine, 0.6 mg twice a day, is given for 6-12 months. It is the drug of choice if the patient has a history of renal stones or renal insufficiency. If allopurinol is used, the dose of 6-mercaptopurine or azathioprine needs to be reduced by 25%. Allopurinol and probenecid are usually not used simultaneously unless the patient has extensive tophaceous gout with good renal function. Allopurinol can cause rash and a severe toxicity syndrome consisting of eosinophilia, fever, hepatitis, decreased renal function, and an erythematous desquamative rash. This usually occurs in patients with decreased renal function. Allopurinol should be given in the lowest dose possible to keep the uric acid value <6 mg/dL.

- Allopurinol is xanthine oxidase inhibitor.
- It can precipitate gout.
- It is drug of choice if patient has history of renal stones or renal insufficiency.
- Can cause severe toxicity syndrome: eosinophilia, fever, hepatitis, decreased renal function, erythematous desquamative rash.

The indications for allopurinol rather than probenecid for lowering the uric acid level are tophaceous gout, gout complicated by renal insufficiency, uric acid excretion >1,000 mg/day, history of uric acid calculi, use of cytotoxic drugs, allergy to uricosuric agents, and secondary hyperuricemia with overproduction of uric acid. Allopurinol should be used before treatment of rapidly proliferating tumors. The nucleic acid liberated with cytolysis is converted to uric acid and can cause renal failure secondary to precipitation of uric acid in collecting ducts and ureters (acute tumor lysis syndrome). Patients should also have adequate hydration and alkalinization of the urine before chemotherapy.

- Indications for allopurinol: tophaceous gout, gout complicated by renal insufficiency, history of uric acid calculi, use of cytotoxic drugs.

Renal Disease and Uric Acid

Renal function is not necessarily adversely affected by an elevated serum urate concentration. The incidence of interstitial renal disease and renal insufficiency is no greater than that in patients of comparable age with similar degrees of hypertension, arteriosclerotic heart disease, diabetes, and primary renal disease. Correction of hyperuricemia (to ≤10 mg/dL) has no apparent effect on renal function. Most rheumatologists do not treat asymptomatic hyperuricemia if the uric acid level is <10.0 mg/dL (normal, to 8.0). When hyperuricemia is associated with a urinary uric acid >1,100 mg/24 hours, which increases the risk of uric acid stones, renal function should be observed closely. Excessive exposure to lead may contribute to the renal disease found in some patients with gout.

- Renal function not adversely affected by elevated serum urate concentration.
- Correction of hyperuricemia (to ≤10 mg/dL) has no apparent effect on renal function.

Miscellaneous Points of Importance

- Positive diagnosis of a crystalline arthritis requires identification of crystal by polarization microscopy.
- Uric acid crystals are strongly negatively birefringent (needle-shaped).
- 30% of patients with chronic tophaceous gout will be positive for rheumatoid factor (usually weakly positive).
- 10% of patients with acute gout will be positive for rheumatoid factor (usually weakly positive).
- 5%-10% of patients will have simultaneous gout and pseudogout attack.
- 50% of synovial fluids aspirated from first metatarsophalangeal joints of asymptomatic patients with gout have crystals of monosodium urate.
- Up to 20% of patients with acute gout have a normal level of serum uric acid at the time of the acute attack.
- Gout in premenopausal female is very unusual.
- There have been many recent reports of superimposed gout occurring in Heberden's and Bouchard's nodes in older women taking diuretics.
- A septic joint can trigger a gout or pseudogout attack in a predisposed person. Always obtain synovial fluid analysis for crystals, Gram stain, and culture. The frequency of gout in patients who have had cardiac transplantation is high (25%). Both cyclosporine and diuretics cause hyperuricemia.

Calcium Pyrophosphate Deposition Disease

Etiologic Classification

Calcium pyrophosphate deposition disease (CPPD) is classified as idiopathic, hereditary, or associated with metabolic disease. The associated diseases include hyperparathyroidism, hemochromatosis-hemosiderosis, hypothyroidism, gout, hypomagnesemia, hypophosphatasia, Wilson's disease, and ochronosis. CPPD is also associated with amyloidosis, Bartter's syndrome, osteoarthritis, and Paget's disease.

Pseudogout

When CPPD causes an acute inflammatory arthritis, the term "pseudogout" is applied. CPPD crystals are weakly positively birefringent and are rhomboid-shaped. Pseudogout rarely involves the first metatarsophalangeal joint. It most commonly affects knees, but wrists, elbows, ankles, and intervertebral disks may be involved. It usually occurs in older individuals. Most patients with pseudogout have chondrocalcinosis on radiography. The presence of chondrocalcinosis does not necessarily mean that a patient will have pseudogout or even CPPD. Dicalcium phosphate dihydrate apatite (calcium hydroxyapatite) also can cause chondrocalcinosis to be seen on radiography, although less frequently. Persons on dialysis in whom acute arthritis or periarthritis develops frequently have calcium hydroxyapatite-induced disease. Gout, pseudogout, calcium oxalate, and infection are also possibilities in patients who undergo dialysis.

- Pseudogout is acute inflammatory arthritis caused by CPPD.
- CPPD crystals are weakly positively birefringent.
- Most commonly affects knees; wrists, elbows, ankles, and intervertebral disks can be affected.
- Chondrocalcinosis is found on radiographs in most patients with pseudogout.
- Chondrocalcinosis does not mean that patient will have pseudogout or even CPPD.

Treatment of Pseudogout

For treatment of acute attacks, NSAIDs or injection of a steroid preparation can be used. Intravenously administered colchicine is effective for acute attacks, but oral administration is not consistently effective. Prophylactic oral colchicine (0.6 mg twice to three times daily) can lead to a decrease in frequency and severity of pseudogout attacks. In patients with underlying metabolic disease, the frequency of acute attacks of pseudogout does not decrease with treatment of the underlying disease (e.g., hypothyroidism, hyperparathyroidism).

- Treatment of acute attacks of pseudogout: NSAIDs, injection of steroid preparation, or colchicine given intravenously.
- Prophylactic oral colchicine can lead to decrease in frequency and severity of attacks.

Hydroxyapatite Deposition Disease

Presentation

Clinical presentations include 1) acute inflammation (calcific tendinitis, osteoarthritis with inflammatory episodes, periarthritis/arthritis dialysis syndrome, rupture of calcinotic deposits in scleroderma) and 2) chronic inflammation (osteoarthritis and Milwaukee shoulder--glenohumeral osteoarthritis, rotator cuff tear, noninflammatory joint fluid containing hydroxyapatite).

- Hydroxyapatite deposition disease can present as acute or chronic inflammation.

Diagnosis and Treatment

Individual crystals cannot be seen on routine polarization microscopy (Table 22-22). Small, round (shiny coin) bodies 0.5 to 100 μm are seen. On electron microscopy, these represent lumps of needle-shaped crystals. Positive identification requires transmission electron microscopy or elemental analysis. Alizarin red stain showing calcium staining provides a presumptive diagnosis (if CPPD is excluded). Treatment involves NSAIDs and intra-articular steroids.

- Individual crystals not seen on polarization microscopy.
- Positive identification requires transmission electron microscopy.

Calcium Oxalate Arthropathy

This disorder occurs in patients with primary oxalosis and patients on chronic hemodialysis. It can cause acute inflammatory arthritis. Crystals are large, bipyramidal, and birefringent. Calcium oxalate can cause chondrocalcinosis or large soft tissue calcifications.

- Calcium oxalate arthropathy occurs in patients with primary oxalosis and patients on chronic hemodialysis.

Other Crystals Implicated in Joint Disease

Cholesterol crystals are a nonspecific finding and have been found in the synovial fluid of patients with various types of chronic inflammatory arthritis. Cryoglobulin crystals are found in essential cryoglobulinemia and paraproteinemia. Corticosteroid crystals are found in an arthritis flare after a corticosteroid injection, and Charcot-Leyden crystals have been found in hypereosinophilic syndromes. In patients on hemodialysis, aluminum phosphate crystals can develop.

SPONDYLOARTHROPATHIES

Conditions that form the spondyloarthropathies include ankylosing spondylitis, Reiter's syndrome, reactive arthritis, enteropathic spondylitis, and psoriatic arthritis.

Spondyloarthropathies are characterized by involvement of sacroiliac joints (uncommon in rheumatoid arthritis), peripheral arthritis (usually asymmetric oligoarticular), absence of rheumatoid factor, and an association with HLA-B27; they are enthesopathic disorders.

The human leukocyte antigen (HLA) region of the 6th chromosome contains genes of the human histocompatibility complex. Every person has two 6th chromosomes, one inherited from each parent. On each of these there is an HLA-A and HLA-B allele. Therefore, everyone has two HLA-A types and two HLA-B types. With regard to inheritance, an offspring has a 50% chance of acquiring a specific HLA-A or HLA-B antigen from a parent (Fig. 22-8). Siblings have a 25% chance of being identical for all four HLA-A and HLA-B alleles.

Frequency of HLA-B27 in control populations is as follows: whites (United States), 8%; African blacks, 0%; Asians, 1%; Haida (North American Indian), 50%.

The rheumatic diseases associated with HLA-B27 are ankylosing spondylitis (HLA-B27 in >90%), Reiter's syndrome or reactive arthritis (>80%), enteropathic spondylitis (approximately 75%), and psoriatic spondylitis (approximately 50%).

Table 22-22.--Differential Diagnosis According to Results of Synovial Fluid Analysis

Diagnosis	Leukocyte count, per mm^3	Differential	Polarization microscopy
Degenerative joint disease	<1,000	Mononuclear cells	Negative
Rheumatoid arthritis	5,000-50,000	PMNs	Negative
Gout	5,000-100,000	PMNs	Monosodium urate
Pseudogout	5,000-100,000	PMNs	CPPD
Hydroxyapatite	5,000-100,000	PMNs	Negative
Septic arthritis	≥100,000	PMNs	Negative

CPPD, calcium pyrophosphate deposition disease; PMN, polymorphonuclear leukocytes.

- Ankylosing spondylitis associated with HLA-B27 in >90% of cases.

Many theories have been proposed to explain the association between HLA-B27 and the spondyloarthropathies: B27 may act as a receptor site for an infective agent; B27 is a marker for an immune response gene that determines susceptibility to an environmental trigger; and B27 may induce tolerance to foreign antigens with which it cross-reacts.

An offspring of a person with HLA-B27 has a 50% chance of carrying the antigen. In randomly selected persons with HLA-B27, the chance of developing disease is 2%. In B27-positive relatives of B27-positive patients with ankylosing spondylitis, the risk of developing disease is 20%.

Ankylosing Spondylitis

New York Criteria of 1966

Clinical criteria include 1) limitation of motion of the lumbar spine in all three planes (anterior flexion, lateral flexion, extension), 2) history of or the presence of pain at the dorsolumbar junction or in the lumbar spine, and 3) limitation of chest expansion to 1 inch (2.5 cm) or less measured at the level of the fourth intercostal space.

Grading

Ankylosing spondylitis is graded as follows: definite ankylosing spondylitis is 1) grade 3-4, bilateral sacroiliitis with at least one clinical criterion; 2) grade 3-4 unilateral or grade 1 bilateral sacroiliitis with clinical criterion 1 (limitation of back movement in all three planes) or with both clinical criteria 2 and 3 (back pain and limitation of chest expansion). Probable ankylosing spondylitis is grade 3-4 bilateral sacroiliitis with no clinical criteria.

Features

Characteristic features of low back pain in ankylosing spondylitis are age at onset usually between 15-40 years, insidious onset, duration >3 months, morning stiffness, improvement with exercise, family history, involvement of other systems, and diffuse radiation of back pain.

- Features of low back pain in ankylosing spondylitis: age at onset between 15-40 years, insidious onset, improvement with exercise.

Findings of ankylosing spondylitis on physical examination are listed in Table 22-23.

Other physical findings in ankylosing spondylitis are listed in Table 22-24.

The radiographic findings in ankylosing spondylitis are 1) sacroiliac involvement (erosions, "pseudowidening" of joint space, sclerosis [both sides of sacroiliac joint; this finding is needed for diagnosis], fusion); and 2) spine involvement (squaring of superior and inferior margins of vertebral body, syndesmophytes, bamboo spine).

- Radiographic findings in ankylosing spondylitis: erosions, syndesmophytes, bamboo spine.

Laboratory Findings

The erythrocyte sedimentation rate may be elevated, there may be an anemia of chronic disease, rheumatoid factor is absent, and 95% of white patients are positive for HLA-B27.

Extraspinal Involvement

Enthesopathic involvement distinguishes spondyloarthropathies from rheumatoid arthritis and consists of plantar fasciitis, Achilles' tendinitis, and costochondritis. Hip and shoulder involvement are common (up to 50%), but peripheral joints can be affected, usually asymmetric involvement of the lower extremities. Some patients diagnosed with juvenile rheumatoid arthritis, especially male adolescents, really have juvenile ankylosing spondylitis in which peripheral arthri-

Fig. 22-8. Inheritance of HLA antigens.

Table 22-23.--Findings in Ankylosing Spondylitis

Characteristic	
Scoliosis	Absent
Decreased range of movement	Symmetric
Tenderness	Diffuse
Hip flexion with straight-leg raising	Normal
Pain with sciatic nerve stretch	Absent
Hip involvement	Frequently present
Neurodeficit	Absent

tis preceded the low back pain.

- Enthesopathic involvement in ankylosing spondylitis: plantar fasciitis, Achilles' tendinitis, costochondritis.
- Hip and shoulder involvement common (up to 50%).
- Some patients diagnosed with juvenile rheumatoid arthritis, especially male adolescents, have juvenile ankylosing spondylitis.

Extraskeletal Involvement

Other findings in active disease include 1) fatigue, 2) weight loss, 3) low-grade fever, and 4) iritis (25% of patients). Iritis is an important clinical clue in the diagnosis of spondyloarthropathies. It is not found in adults with rheumatoid arthritis.

- Iritis is important clue to diagnosis of spondyloarthropathies; not found in adults with rheumatoid arthritis.

Late complications can include 1) cord compression due to traumatic spinal fracture, 2) cauda equina syndrome (symptoms include neurogenic bladder, fecal incontinence, leg pain), 3) fibrotic changes in upper lung fields (cavities can develop and aspergillomas have been reported), 4) aortic insufficiency in 3%-5% of patients, 5) complete heart block, and 6) amyloidosis.

- Late complications of ankylosing spondylitis: cord compression due to traumatic spinal fractures, cauda equina syndrome, fibrotic changes in upper lung fields, aortic insufficiency.

Ankylosing Spondylitis in Men and Women

Ankylosing spondylitis has been thought to be a disease primarily of men, but it is now recognized that the incidence in women is higher than originally thought, although women have less tendency for spinal ankylosis. The ratio of men to women is approximately 3:1. Women more frequently have osteitis pubis and peripheral joint involvement.

Differential Diagnosis

The differential diagnosis includes diffuse hypertrophic skeletal hyperostosis (DISH), osteitis condensans ilii, fusion of sacroiliac joint in paraplegia, osteitis pubis, and degenerative joint disease. The clinical symptoms of DISH are "stiffness" of spine and relatively good preservation of spine motion. Patients with DISH can have dysphagia related to cervical osteophytes. It generally affects middle-aged and elderly men. Criteria for DISH are "flowing" ossification along the anterolateral aspect of at least four contiguous vertebral bodies, preservation of disk height, absence of apophyseal joint involvement, absence of sacroiliac joint involvement, and extraspinal ossifications, including ligamentous calcifications.

Osteitis condensans ilii usually affects young to middle-aged females with normal sacroiliac joints. Radiography shows sclerosis on iliac side of sacroiliac joint only. The sacroiliac joint can also be involved with 1) tuberculosis, 2) metastatic disease, 3) gout, 4) Paget's disease, or 5) infection (*Brucella, Serratia, Staphylococcus*).

Table 22-24.--Results of Testing in Ankylosing Spondylitis

Test	Method	Results
Schober	Make a mark on the spine at level of L-5 and one at 10 cm directly above with the patient standing erect. Patient then bends forward maximally and the distance between the two marks is measured	An increase of <5 cm indicates early lumbar involvement
Chest expansion	Measure maximal chest expansion at nipple line	Chest expansion of <5 cm is clue to early costovertebral involvement
Sacroiliac compression	Exert direct compression over sacroiliac joints	Tenderness or pain suggests sacroiliac involvement

- Osteitis condensans ilii usually affects young to middle-aged females; radiography shows sclerosis on iliac side of sacroiliac joint only.
- Sacroiliac joint can be involved with metastatic disease, gout, Paget's disease, infection (*Brucella, Serratia, Staphylococcus*).

Treatment

Treatment involves physical therapy (posture very important), exercise (swimming), cessation of smoking, genetic counseling, and drug therapy with NSAIDs such as indomethacin; aspirin is not effective. Sulfasalazine therapy may also provide benefit, especially in patients with peripheral joint involvement.

Reiter's Syndrome

This is a seronegative asymmetric arthropathy (predominantly affects lower extremities). One or more of the following conditions also occurs: 1) urethritis, 2) dysentery, 3) inflammatory eye disease (conjunctivitis), and 4) mucocutaneous disease (balanitis, oral ulcerations, or keratoderma). In addition, approximately 80% of patients are HLA-B27 positive. Another finding is keratoderma blennorrhagicum (characteristic skin and mucous membrane findings (skin lesions are painless). It is *indistinguishable* clinically and histologically from psoriasis. Joint predilection is for the toes and asymmetric large joints in the lower extremities. It can cause "sausage"-toe-like psoriasis. The distal interphalangeal joints in the hands can be affected also. Cardiac conduction disturbances and aortitis can develop. Sacroiliitis (sometimes unilateral) and iritis can occur. Long-term studies indicate that the disease remains episodically active in 75% of patients and that disability is a frequent outcome.

- Reiter's syndrome: seronegative asymmetric arthropathy with urethritis, dysentery, inflammatory eye disease, mucocutaneous disease.
- 80% of patients are HLA-B27 positive.
- Cardiac conduction disturbances and aortitis can develop.

Treatment is with NSAIDs (indomethacin), gold, and methotrexate. Treatment with tetracycline or erythromycin-type antibiotics may decrease the duration of illness in *Chlamydia*-triggered Reiter's syndrome.

Reactive Arthritis

This is an aseptic arthritis induced by a host response to an infectious agent rather than direct infection. HLA-B27 is associated in 80% of cases. The condition develops after infections with *Salmonella* organisms, *Shigella flexneri, Yersinia enterocolitica,* and *Campylobacter jejuni,* which cause diarrhea, and *Chlamydia* and *Ureaplasma urealyticum,* which

cause nonspecific urethritis. In addition to polyarthritis, clinical features of Reiter's syndrome, including sacroiliitis, may develop. Patients usually have self-limited disease. Joint destruction is *not* common. The condition is usually managed with NSAIDs.

- Reactive arthritis: aseptic arthritis induced by host response to infectious agent rather than direct infection.
- HLA-B27 is associated in 80% of cases.
- Develops after infections with *Salmonella, Shigella flexneri, Yersinia enterocolitica, Campylobacter jejuni, Chlamydia, Ureaplasma urealyticum.*
- Clinical features of Reiter's syndrome may develop.

Arthritis Associated With Inflammatory Bowel Disease

Two distinct types of arthritis are associated with chronic inflammatory bowel disease: 1) a nondestructive oligoarthritis of peripheral joints tending to come and go in time with the activity of the bowel disease and 2) ankylosing spondylitis (enteropathic spondylitis). The spondylitis is not a complication of the bowel disease. It is often diagnosed many years before the onset of bowel symptoms, and its subsequent progress bears little relationship to the bowel disease. Approximately 75% of patients with ankylosing spondylitis and inflammatory bowel disease are HLA-B27 positive. Patients with inflammatory bowel disease alone do not have an increased frequency of HLA-B27 and are not at increased risk for development of spondylitis.

- Patients with inflammatory bowel disease alone do not have increased frequency of HLA-B27.

Psoriatic Arthritis

Psoriatic arthritis develops in 7% of patients with psoriasis. Pitting of nails is strongly associated with joint disease. Patients with more severe skin disease are at higher risk for development of arthritis. Hyperuricemia is present in 15% of all patients with psoriasis whether or not they have arthritis. A "sausage" finger or toe is characteristic of psoriatic arthritis and is very uncommon in rheumatoid arthritis. Radiographic evidence of involvement of the distal interphalangeal joint with erosions is common in psoriasis and uncommon in rheumatoid arthritis. Psoriatic arthritis also can cause a characteristic "pencil-in-cup" deformity of the distal interphalangeal and proximal interphalangeal joints on radiography.

- Psoriatic arthritis develops in 7% of patients with psoriasis.
- Pitting of nails is strongly associated with joint disease.
- Hyperuricemia is present in 15% of all patients with psoriasis.

- "Sausage" finger or toe is characteristic.
- "Pencil-in-cup" deformity of distal and proximal interphalangeal joints is radiographic finding.

There are five clinical groups of psoriatic arthritis: 1) predominant distal interphalangeal joint involvement, 2) arthritis mutilans, 3) symmetrical polyarthritis-like rheumatoid arthritis but negative for rheumatoid factor, 4) asymmetrical oligoarthritis, and 5) psoriatic spondylitis (HLA-B27 positive in 50%-75% of cases). Treatment is with NSAIDs, gold, hydroxychloroquine, methotrexate, and azathioprine.

LYME DISEASE

Lyme disease is a tick-borne spirochetal illness with acute and chronic manifestations affecting the skin, heart, joints, and nervous system primarily. Diagnosis is important because treatment with appropriate antibiotics at an early stage of disease can prevent chronic sequelae. Even some chronic symptoms are treatable. Endemic areas in the United States include Connecticut, Delaware, Maryland, Massachusetts, New Jersey, New York, Pennsylvania, Rhode Island, Minnesota, Wisconsin, California, Nevada, Oregon, and Utah.

- Lyme disease is a tick-borne spirochetal illness.
- Acute and chronic manifestations affect skin, heart, joints, nervous system.

The Tick

Ticks that transmit Lyme disease include *Ixodes dammini* in the northeastern and midwestern United States and *Ixodes pacificus* in the western United States. *Amblyomma americanum* ("Lone Star" tick) is a possible vector in the eastern, southern, and western United States. *Ixodes scapularis* is the common deer tick. It has a wide distribution. Humans are accidental hosts.

The Spirochete

Borrelia burgdorferi was an unknown organism until isolated initially from ticks by Burgdorfer in 1983. It is similar to an organism causing relapsing fever. It apparently exists only in the digestive tract of tick vectors.

Clinical Stages of Lyme Disease

Signs and symptoms occur in stages that may overlap. Later stages may occur *without* evidence of previous disease.

Stage I

About 50% of patients experience erythema chronicum migrans. Flu-like symptoms, including fever, headache, malaise, and adenopathy, can occur. They usually occur several days to a month after the tick bite.

- In stage I, 50% of patients experience erythema chronicum migrans.

Stage II

Symptoms begin weeks to months after the initial symptoms in stage I. Disseminated infection develops and can include symptoms of the skin, musculoskeletal system, heart, and nervous system. In approximately 15% of patients, neurologic symptoms develop, including Bell's palsy, meningoencephalitis, and sensory and motor radiculoneuritis. Approximately 5% of patients have cardiac abnormalities, including heart block. About 30%-50% of patients have arthritis. This usually affects large joints, primarily the knee, and joint fluid analysis shows a leukocytosis similar to that in rheumatoid arthritis. Baker's cysts may form early and are prone to rupture in patients who have arthritis of the knees.

- In stage II, symptoms begin weeks to months after initial symptoms of stage I.
- Disseminated infection develops.
- 15% of patients have neurologic symptoms.
- 5% of patients have cardiac abnormalities.
- 30%-50% of patients have arthritis.

Stage III

This usually occurs several years after the initial onset of illness. Episodes of arthritis can develop and become chronic. Histologically, the synovium resembles that in rheumatoid arthritis, although a unique feature of Lyme arthritis is the finding of an obliterative endarteritis. Spirochetes are occasionally seen in and around the blood vessels. Patients in whom chronic joint disease develops have increased frequency of HLA-DR4, often in combination with HLA-DR2. Patients with chronic arthritis have a poor response to antibiotics.

- Stage III occurs several years after initial onset of illness.
- Episodes of arthritis can be chronic.
- Synovium resembles that in rheumatoid arthritis.
- Unique feature of Lyme arthritis is obliterative endarteritis in the synovium.
- Patients with chronic joint disease have increased frequency of HLA-DR4, often in combination with HLA-DR2.

Diagnosis

Culturing the organism is difficult and of low yield. Antibody to spirochete can be measured by several techniques. The enzyme-linked immunosorbent assay (ELISA) is most commonly performed, but this is not standardized and there is a significant frequency of false-positive and false-negative results. Patients with other autoimmune diseases can have false-positive results. Also, such results may occur in syphilis, relapsing fever, and Rocky Mountain spotted fever. Although patients with syphilis have false-positive Lyme serologic results by ELISA, patients with Lyme disease have negative results of VDRL test. Up to 25% of patients with lupus and rheumatoid arthritis have false-positive results of Lyme test by ELISA. It is important to remember that test results remain negative for up to 4 to 6 weeks after infection. Also, if patients are treated early with tetracycline or another antibiotic, the results might never be positive, although symptoms of chronic Lyme disease can result. The Western blot assay for Lyme disease is now being used as a confirmatory test if the ELISA test result is positive.

- In Lyme disease, culturing organism is difficult and of low yield.
- ELISA assay is commonly performed but is not standardized.
- Significant frequency of false-positive results with ELISA.
- False-positive results may occur in syphilis, relapsing fever, Rocky Mountain spotted fever.
- Up to 25% of patients with lupus and rheumatoid arthritis have false-positive results of Lyme test by ELISA.
- Patients treated early with tetracycline or other antibiotic may never have positive results.

Treatment

For early treatment of Lyme disease, either oral tetracycline or doxycycline, or amoxicillin in children, can prevent later complications. The optimal treatment for patients with chronic symptoms is unclear but can include the use of penicillin G, 20 million units intravenously daily for 14 days, or ceftriaxone, 2 g intravenously daily for 14 days. Patients with Lyme disease can experience worsening of symptoms analogous to the Jarisch-Herxheimer reaction and can be treated with acetaminophen.

- Early treatment of Lyme disease is either oral tetracycline or doxycycline (amoxicillin in children).

HYPERTROPHIC PULMONARY OSTEOARTHROPATHY

This syndrome is characterized by an oligoarthritis or polyarthritis that can have a presentation similar to that of rheumatoid arthritis. Patients have associated clubbing, and periosteal new bone formation at the end of long bones is noted on radiography. This finding is very unusual in rheumatoid arthritis. This syndrome is usually associated with carcinoma of the lung, but it can occur with other types of cancer. It also occurs in severe cystic fibrosis and in congenital heart disease when hypoxia is present. Other associations include bacterial endocarditis, bronchiectasis, sarcoidosis, pulmonary or intestinal tuberculosis, myxedema, amebiasis, hepatic or biliary cirrhosis, inflammatory bowel disease, subphrenic or liver abscess, and aortic aneurysm.

- Hypertrophic pulmonary osteoarthropathy has associated clubbing.
- Radiography shows periosteal new bone formation at end of long bones.
- Syndrome is usually associated with carcinoma of lung.

OSTEOID OSTEOMA

Osteoid osteoma is a benign bone tumor. It usually occurs between the ages of 5 and 30 years in males and females with equal frequency. The classic symptom is bone pain at night, which is relieved completely with aspirin or another nonsteroidal anti-inflammatory agent. Diagnosis is made by routine radiography, but often this is negative and a bone scan is needed to locate the tumor, and tomography or computed tomography can then be done for better visualization. Radiography shows a small nidus, usually less than 1 cm, varying from radiolucent to radiopaque, depending on the age of the lesion. There is usually a lucent ring around the nidus and adjacent bone sclerosis. Treatment includes excision, which is curative.

- Osteoid osteoma is a benign bone tumor.
- Bone pain at night is relieved by aspirin or other nonsteroidal anti-inflammatory agent.
- Treatment includes excision, which is curative.

NEUROPATHIC ARTHRITIS

This occurs because of loss of proprioception of affected joints. The most common cause of a neuropathic (Charcot) joint is diabetes, which characteristically affects the ankle, tarsal bones, and metatarsophalangeal joints. Tabes dorsalis affects the spine and knees, and syringomyelia characteristically affects the shoulders and elbows. Most patients experience some pain, but not as much as would be expected in a patient with degenerative arthritis without superimposed neuropathy. Radiographic changes usually show marked destruction of affected joints.

- Neuropathic arthritis occurs because of loss of proprioception of affected joints.
- Most common cause of neuropathic (Charcot) joint is diabetes.
- Diabetes characteristically affects the ankle, tarsal bones, metatarsophalangeal joints.
- Tabes dorsalis affects spine and knees.
- Syringomyelia affects shoulder and elbows.

BYPASS ARTHRITIS

This occurs in patients who have undergone intestinal bypass operations, including jejunocolic or jejunoileal. The arthritis may be acute or subacute, is usually intermittent, and can last occasionally for short periods only to recur. The most commonly affected joints include the metacarpophalangeal, proximal interphalangeal, wrists, knees, and ankles. It is commonly associated with a dermatitis, which can be pustular in nature. Circulating immune complexes composed of bacterial antigens have been found in both the circulation and the synovial fluid and are thought to be the cause of this disorder. Treatment entails NSAIDs and antibiotics such as tetracycline, but many times reanastomosis may be necessary for resolution of symptoms.

- Bypass arthritis occurs in patients who have had intestinal bypass operations.
- Most commonly affected joints: metacarpophalangeal, proximal interphalangeal, wrists, knees, ankles.
- Commonly associated with a dermatitis.

AVASCULAR NECROSIS OF BONE

Many conditions are associated with spontaneous avascular necrosis. Common associated conditions include alcoholism, steroid use, connective tissue diseases (especially lupus), and hemoglobinopathies. Other conditions include diabetes, acquired immunodeficiency syndrome (AIDS), fat embolism, gout, hyperlipidemia, immunosuppressive therapy, radiation therapy, pancreatitis, thermal injuries including burns, electrical injuries and frostbite, decompression syndrome (caisson's disease), and hematopoietic disorders including hemophilia, histiocytosis, polycythemia, and Gaucher's disease. The most commonly affected joints include the hips, shoulders, and knees.

- Conditions associated with avascular necrosis of bone: alcoholism, steroid use, connective tissue diseases (especially lupus), hemoglobinopathies.
- Most commonly affected joints: hips, shoulders, knees.

Increased interosseous pressure has been noted. Because of this, core decompression of the hip reportedly prevents further progression, but proof of this outcome has not been established. Many times, patients with avascular necrosis have bilateral disease, although they have symptoms on only one side. Early in the disease radiographs may be normal. A radiolucent crescent line can occasionally be seen; this represents a plane of cleavage or fracture. Magnetic resonance imaging is the most sensitive test to demonstrate avascular necrosis, but bone scanning can also be used. Standard treatment includes non-weight-bearing of the affected joint.

- Magnetic resonance imaging is most sensitive test for demonstrating avascular necrosis; bone scanning can also be used.

SYSTEMIC LUPUS ERYTHEMATOSUS

Systemic lupus erythematosus (SLE) is a chronic inflammatory disease of unknown cause with a wide spectrum of clinical manifestations and variable course. Antibodies that react with nuclear and cytoplasmic antigens commonly are found in patients with the disease. Genetic, hormonal, and environmental factors seem to be important in the cause. Multiple organs may be affected, and the disease course is variable and characterized by exacerbations and remissions.

- Genetic, hormonal, and environmental factors seem important in cause of SLE.
- SLE characterized by exacerbations and remissions.

Diagnosis

Four of the following findings are needed for diagnosis of SLE: malar rash; discoid lupus; photosensitivity; oral ulcers; arthritis; proteinuria (protein, >0.5 g/day) or cellular casts; seizures or psychosis; pleuritis or pericarditis; hemolytic anemia, leukopenia, lymphopenia, or thrombocytopenia; antibody to nDNA, antibody to Sm (Smith) or LE cells, or false-positive results of VDRL test; and positive results of fluorescent antinuclear antibody test.

Epidemiology

The female:male ratio is 8:1, during the reproductive years. The first symptoms usually occur between the second and fourth decades of life. The disease seems to be less severe in the elderly. In SLE with onset at an older age, the female:male ratio is equal. The frequency of SLE is increased in American blacks, Native Americans, and Asians.

- Female:male ratio in SLE is 8:1 during reproductive years.
- Increased frequency of SLE in American blacks, Native Americans, Asians.

Etiology

Type C oncornavirus is present in NZB/W mice, and both viral protein and antibody to protein are found in mouse glomeruli. Direct causal relationship has *not* been established. In human disease, viral-like particles in glomeruli of patients with SLE are also seen in other kinds of kidney damage. Attempts to isolate viruses have been unsuccessful. Patients with SLE have elevated antibody titers to a wide range of antigens without much sign of specificity for a particular viral agent.

- In SLE, elevated antibody titers to a wide range of antigens without much sign of specificity for a particular viral agent.

Genetics

Among relatives of patients with SLE, 20% have an immunologic disease. Another 25% have antinuclear antibodies, circulating immune complexes, antilymphocyte antibodies, or a false-positive result on VDRL test without clinical disease. Concordance among monozygotic twins is much greater than among dizygotic twins. Genetic and environmental factors are both important in development of SLE. Immune complex levels are much higher in persons with close contact to patient than in unexposed consanguineous relatives. The frequency of HLA-B8, HLA-DR2, and HLA-DR3 is increased.

- 20% of relatives of patients with SLE have "immunologic" disease.
- In SLE, frequency of HLA-B8, HLA-DR2, and HLA-DR3 is increased.

Immune System

There is a decrease in the cellular immune system with an absolute decrease in T-suppressor cells. There is an increase in the humoral immune system with B-cell hyperactivity resulting in polyclonal activation.

- In SLE, there is an absolute decrease in T-suppressor cells with an increase in humoral immune system with B-cell hyperactivity.

Pathogenesis

Circulating immune complexes (anti-nDNA) are responsible for glomerulonephritis and probably skin disease. Immune complexes bind complement, which initiates inflammatory process. Organ-specific autoantibodies are 1) antierythrocyte, 2) antiplatelet, 3) antileukocyte, and 4) antithyroid.

- Circulating immune complexes (anti-nDNA) are responsible for glomerulonephritis.

Late complications of SLE are related to vascular damage in relative absence of active immunologic disease. Damage to intima during active disease probably results in premature deterioration of vasculature and various thrombotic, ischemic, and hypertensive manifestations.

Clinical Manifestations

Arthritis is characteristically nondeforming and nonerosive. Avascular necrosis of bone occurs, and not only in patients taking steroids. Navicular, femoral head, and tibial plateau are most commonly affected.

Fever in SLE is usually caused by the disease, but infection *must* be ruled out. Shaking chills and leukocytosis strong-

ly suggest infection. Subacute cutaneous LE is a subset of SLE that primarily has skin involvement with psoriasiform or annular erythematous lesions. Patients may be negative for antinuclear antibodies but frequently are positive for antibodies to the extractable nuclear antigen SS-A (Ro).

- Fever in SLE is usually caused by disease, but infection must be ruled out.

Central nervous system lupus is a most variable and unpredictable phenomenon. Manifestations such as impaired organic psychiatric function, seizures, long tract signs, cranial neuropathies, and migraine-like attacks occur with little apparent relationship to each other or to other systemic manifestations. Immune complexes in the choroid plexus are *not* specific for central nervous system disease. They also occur in patients without central nervous system disease. There is no specific laboratory abnormality. Patients may have increased cerebrospinal fluid protein (IgG) and pleocytosis. C4 levels in cerebrospinal fluid are not helpful.

- Central nervous system lupus is a most variable and unpredictable phenomenon.
- Immune complexes in choroid plexus are *not* specific for central nervous system disease.

Electroencephalography can be abnormal. Brain scanning is of no help. Magnetic resonance imaging usually shows areas of increased signal in the periventricular white matter, similar to that found in multiple sclerosis. Magnetic resonance imaging findings are nonspecific and can be seen in patients who have SLE without central nervous system manifestations. Pathologic examinations of autopsy specimens usually reveal microinfarcts, nerve cell loss, vasculitis, or no detectable abnormalities. Psychosis caused by steroid therapy is probably rarer than previously thought. When in doubt about the cause of the psychosis, the steroid dose can be increased and the patient observed. Patients can have isolated central nervous system involvement and normal results of cerebrospinal fluid examination and no other organ involvement.

- Electroencephalography can be abnormal in SLE.
- Brain scanning is not helpful.
- Magnetic resonance imaging findings are nonspecific.
- Psychosis caused by steroid therapy is probably rarer than thought.

Women with SLE who become pregnant have a high prevalence of spontaneous abortion. Because abortion itself may lead to a flare of disease, therapeutic abortion ordinarily is not recommended after first trimester. Flares of disease should be treated with steroids, particularly during the postpartum period.

- High prevalence of spontaneous abortion in SLE.
- Therapeutic abortion is not recommended after first trimester.

Infants of mothers with SLE can develop thrombocytopenia and leukopenia from passive transfer of antibodies. They also can develop transient cutaneous lesions and transient complete heart block. Mothers usually have anti-SS-A (Ro), which crosses the placenta and is transiently present in the infant. Mothers usually are HLA-B8/DR3, but there is no HLA association in the child. In some affected infants, no clinical disease is present in the mother although antibodies are present.

Renal Involvement

Types of renal disease in SLE are 1) mesangial, 2) focal glomerulonephritis, 3) membranous glomerulonephritis, 4) diffuse proliferative glomerulonephritis, 5) interstitial nephritis with defects in renal tubular handling of K^+, and 6) renal vein thrombosis with nephrotic syndrome.

Treatment of renal disease depends in part on the results of renal biopsy. Patients with mesangial changes alone do not require aggressive therapy. Patients with active diffuse proliferative glomerulonephritis are treated with high-dose steroids with or without immunosuppressive agents. Immunosuppressive agents are steroid-sparing and lower the incidence of renal failure in patients with diffuse proliferative glomerulonephritis but do not improve overall survival. Appropriate treatment for focal proliferative glomerulonephritis and membranous glomerulonephritis is controversial because the prognosis is favorable. Renal biopsies can be helpful in directing therapy. Patients with high activity indices such as active inflammation, proliferation, necrosis, and crescent formation are considered for aggressive therapy. Patients with high chronicity indices such as tubular atrophy, scarring, and glomerulosclerosis are less likely to respond to aggressive therapy.

- Patients with mesangial changes alone do not require aggressive therapy.
- Active diffuse proliferative glomerulonephritis is treated with high-dose steroids with or without immunosuppressive agents.
- Renal biopsies are helpful for directing therapy.

Laboratory Findings

Anemia of chronic disease and hemolytic anemia (Coombs' positive) can occur. Leukopenia usually does not predispose to infection. Antilymphocyte antibodies cause lymphopenia in SLE. In Felty's syndrome, infection is common as a result of granulocytopenia. Idiopathic thrombocytopenic purpura with presence of platelet antibodies can be the initial manifestation of SLE. Polyclonal gammopathy secondary to hyperactivity of humoral immune system is common. The erythrocyte sedimentation rate usually correlates with disease activity.

- Hemolytic anemia (Coombs' positive) can occur in SLE.
- Idiopathic thrombocytopenic purpura can be the initial manifestation of SLE.

Hypocomplemetemia (CH_{50}, C3, C4) usually correlates with active disease. Hypocomplementemia with increased anti-nDNA antibodies usually implies renal disease (or skin disease). A total complement value too low to measure but normal C3 and C4 values suggest a hereditary complement deficiency. Familial C2 deficiency is the most common complement deficiency in SLE, but C1r, C1s, C1q, C4, C5, C7, and C8 deficiencies also have been reported.

- Hypocomplementemia usually correlates with active disease.
- Hypocomplementemia with increased anti-nDNA antibodies usually implies renal disease (or skin disease).

Patients with SLE may have false-positive results of VDRL test as a result of antibody to phospholipid, which cross-reacts with VDRL. Among patients with false-positive results on VDRL test, 80% have circulating anticoagulant. Patients with SLE also can have false-positive results of fluorescent treponemal antibody test, but this is usually of the "beaded pattern" of fluorescence. LE cells are present in approximately 70% of patients with SLE. They are caused by antibody to deoxyribonucleoprotein (DNP). Testing for this is not performed in many centers. Anti-DNP is also detected by the fluorescent antinuclear antibody test in a homogeneous pattern.

- 80% of patients with false-positive results on VDRL test have a circulating anticoagulant.
- LE cells present in about 70% of patients with SLE.

Anti-nDNA levels fluctuate with disease activity, whereas levels of other autoantibodies (i.e., ribonucleoprotein, Sm, antinuclear antibody) show no consistent relationship to levels of anti-nDNA or disease activity. Methods used to measure anti-nDNA are 1) an immunofluorescent method using *Crithidia luciliae*, an organism with a kinetoplast that contains helical native DNA free of other nuclear antigens--therefore, there is no single-stranded DNA contamination; and 2) radioimmunoassay and other techniques, which suffer from the difficulty of maintaining DNA in its native double-stranded state and so are contaminated with single-stranded DNA. All patients with lupus should have positive results of antinuclear antibody test. A positive result is by no means specific for lupus. Antinuclear antibody patterns are outlined in Table 22-25. Other autoantibodies and disease associations are outlined in Table 22-26.

Table 22-25.--Antinuclear Antibody Patterns

Fluorescent pattern	Antigen	Disease association
Rim, peripheral, shaggy	nDNA	SLE
Homogeneous	DNP	SLE, others
Speckled	ENA	MCTD, SLE, others
Nucleolar	RNA	Scleroderma

DNP, deoxyribonucleoprotein; ENA, extractable nuclear antigens; MCTD, mixed connective tissue disease; RNA, ribonucleic acid.

Table 22-26.--Autoantibodies in Rheumatic Diseases

Antibody	Disease association
Anti-ssDNA	SLE, 100%
	High frequency in other CTD; also chronic infection, CAH, interstitial lung disease
Anti-nDNA	SLE, 50%-60%
Anti-Sm (Smith)	SLE, 30%
Anti-RNP (ribonuclear protein)	MCTD, 100% high titer
	SLE, 30% titer
	Scleroderma, low frequency, low titer
Anti-SS-A	Sjögren's, 70%
	SLE, 35%
	Scleroderma + MCTD, low frequency, low titer
Anti-SS-B	Sjögren's, 60%
	SLE, 15%
Antihistone	Drug-induced SLE, 95%
	SLE, 70%
	RA, 20%
Anti-Sc1-70 (antitopoisomerase I)	Scleroderma, 25%
Anticentromere	CREST, 70%-90%
	Scleroderma, 10%-15%
Anti-PM1	PM, 50%
Anti-Jo1 (histidyl-tRNA synthetase)	PM, 30%

CAH, chronic active hepatitis; CREST, syndrome of *c*alcinosis cutis, *R*aynaud's phenomenon, *e*sophageal dysmotility, *s*clerodactyly, *t*elangiectasia; CTD, connective tissue disease; MCTD, mixed connective tissue disease; PM, polymyositis; RA, rheumatoid arthritis.

- Anti-nDNA levels fluctuate with disease activity.
- Positive result of antinuclear antibody test is by no means specific for lupus.

Treatment

Treatment should match the activity of SLE in the individual patient. Serial monitoring of organ function and appropriate immunologic evaluation (anti-nDNA, C3, erythrocyte sedimentation rate) allow rapid recognition and treatment of flares and appropriate tapering of steroid dose during periods of disease quiescence. Table 22-27 provides guidelines for treatment, and Table 22-28 outlines the complications of treatment.

Outcome

The 10-year survival rate is 90% in newly diagnosed SLE. Prognosis is worse in blacks and Hispanics than in whites. Prognosis is worse in patients with creatinine values >3.0 mg/dL. The major causes of death are 1) renal disease, 2) infection, 3) central nervous system involvement, and 4) vascular disease (e.g., myocardial infarction).

- The 10-year survival rate is 90% in newly diagnosed SLE.
- Prognosis is worse in blacks and Hispanics.

DRUG-INDUCED LUPUS

Many drugs have been implicated in drug-induced lupus. The most common drugs are listed in Table 22-29. One must differentiate between the clinical syndrome of drug-induced lupus and only a positive antinuclear antibody result without clinical symptoms. Many drugs can cause a positive antinuclear antibody result without ever causing the clinical syndrome of drug-induced lupus. Only hydralazine and procainamide have been strongly implicated in drug-induced lupus. A drug-induced lupus syndrome will develop in approximately 5% of persons taking hydralazine and in approximately 15%-25% of those who take procainamide for more than a year. Virtually all patients taking procainamide for 1 year will have a positive result of antinuclear antibody test.

- Only hydralazine and procainamide are strongly implicated in drug-induced lupus.
- Virtually all patients taking procainamide for 1 year have positive antinuclear antibody test.

Clinical Features

The clinical manifestations of drug-induced lupus are arthralgias and polyarthritis, which occur in approximately 80% of

Table 22-27.--Treatment of Manifestations of Systemic Lupus Erythematosus

Manifestation	Treatment
Arthritis, fever, mild systemic symptoms	ASA, NSAID
Photosensitivity, rash	Avoidance of sun, use of sunscreens
Rash, arthritis	Hydroxychloroquine (Plaquenil)
Significant thrombocytopenia, hemolytic anemia	Steroids
Renal disease, CNS disease, pericarditis, other significant organ involvement	Steroids
Rapidly deteriorating renal function	? Pulse therapy
CNS, renal disease	? Cytotoxic agents
Renal disease	? Plasmapheresis

ASA, acetylsalicylic acid; CNS, central nervous system; NSAID, nonsteroidal anti-inflammatory drug.

Table 22-28.--Complications of Treatment for Systemic Lupus Erythematosus

Treatment	Complication
Ibuprofen	Aseptic meningitis (headache, fever, stiff neck, CSF pleocytosis)
NSAID	Decreased renal blood flow
ASA	Salicylate hepatitis (common), benign
Cyclophosphamide	Hemorrhagic cystitis, alopecia, opportunistic lymphomas, infection, increased incidence of lymphomas (CNS)
Hydroxychloroquine (Plaquenil)	Retinal toxicity

ASA, acetylsalicylic acid; CNS, central nervous system; CSF, cerebrospinal fluid; NSAID, nonsteroidal anti-inflammatory drug.

Table 22-29.--Implicated Agents in Drug-Induced Lupus

Definite	Probable
Common	Phenytoin
Procainamide	Carbamazepine
Hydralazine	Ethosuximide
Uncommon	Propylthiouracil
Isoniazid	Penicillamine
Methyldopa	Sulfasalazine
Chlorpromazine	Lithium carbonate
Quinidine	Acebutolol
	Lovastatin

cases. Malaise is common, and fever has been reported in up to 40% of cases. Cardiopulmonary involvement is common, and approximately 30% of patients have pleural-pulmonary manifestations as their presenting symptoms. Pericarditis has been reported in approximately 20% of cases. Diffuse interstitial pneumonitis has been noted. Asymptomatic pleural effusions may be found on routine chest radiography. A few cases of pericardial tamponade have been reported. In contrast to SLE, the incidence of renal and central nervous system involvement is low in drug-induced lupus. Therefore, it is regarded as more benign than SLE. Clinical differences include a lower incidence of skin manifestations, lymphadenopathy, and myalgias in drug-induced disease.

- In drug-induced lupus, arthralgias and polyarthritis occur in about 80% of cases.
- Malaise is common; fever occurs in up to 40% of cases.
- About 30% of patients have pleural-pulmonary manifestations.
- Pericarditis reported in about 20% of cases.
- Incidence of renal and central nervous system involvement is low.

Other differences between drug-induced lupus and SLE include age and sex distribution. SLE is predominantly a disease of premenopausal females, whereas drug-induced disease has an almost equal sex distribution and occurs in an older population. This disparity in age reflects the use of hydralazine and procainamide in primarily an older population.

Laboratory Abnormalities

Virtually all patients with SLE and drug-induced lupus have antinuclear antibodies. Although patients with SLE and drug-induced lupus are serologically similar in many respects, there are notable differences. Antibodies to native DNA are found in only a small percentage of cases of drug-induced lupus but in approximately 60% of cases of SLE. Serum total hemolytic complement is usually normal in drug-induced disease, in contrast to SLE. However, antibodies such as anti-Sm, SS-B, and ribonucleoprotein are also unusual in drug-induced lupus. The frequency of antihistone antibodies in drug-induced lupus is high (>95% of cases), but these also occur in approximately 60% of cases of SLE. Other laboratory abnormalities in drug-induced lupus can include a positive LE prep, positive Coombs' test, positive rheumatoid factor, false-positive result of serologic test for syphilis, circulating anticoagulants, and cryoglobulins.

Metabolism

Drugs involved in drug-induced lupus have different chemical structures, but three of them--isoniazid, procainamide, and hydralazine--contain a primary amine or hydralazine that is acetylated by the hepatic *N*-acetyltransferase system. Persons who are taking one of these drugs and who are slow acetylators have a much higher incidence of serologic abnormalities and clinical disease than rapid acetylators. These manifestations also occur over a shorter period in slow acetylators than in rapid acetylators.

- Slow acetylators have a much higher incidence of serologic abnormalities and clinical disease.

Treatment

When possible, patients with drug-induced lupus should stop using the offending drug. Symptoms will usually subside within several weeks, although the duration for complete resolution varies depending on the drug. Serologic abnormalities can remain for years after resolution of clinical symptoms. Patients taking procainamide are most likely to have a rapid remission once use of the drug is stopped, but patients taking hydralazine might have prolonged clinical manifestations. Treatment depends on the clinical manifestations and could include aspirin or other NSAIDs or possibly prednisone if needed.

OVERLAP SYNDROMES

An overlap syndrome is a disease characterized by features of more than one connective tissue disease. Secondary Sjögren's syndrome accompanying another connective disease is not classified as an overlap syndrome.

Mixed Connective Tissue Disease

This is described as a distinct disease with variable features of SLE, polymyositis, systemic sclerosis, and rheumatoid arthritis. The incidence of renal disease is low. It is serologically characterized by a positive antinuclear antibody and by high titer of the autoantibody anti-RNP. Anti-nDNA antibodies usually are not present. Raynaud's phenomenon is common.

Undifferentiated Connective Tissue Disease

This disease does not fulfill the diagnostic criteria for definite connective tissue disease. Common symptoms include Raynaud's phenomenon, arthralgias, fatigue, and variable joint or soft tissue swelling. The antinuclear antibody may be positive, but other autoantibodies are not present. Patients need to be observed to determine whether progression to a distinct connective tissue disease occurs.

ANTIPHOSPHOLIPID SYNDROME

SLE is an autoimmune disease that is characterized by the formation of many autoantibodies. Recently, much attention has been focused on antiphospholipid antibodies, including the lupus circulating anticoagulant and various anticardiolipin antibodies that have been associated with recurrent arterial and venous thrombosis. Several studies have shown that the lupus anticoagulant is an antiphospholipid antibody of either the IgG or the IgM immunoglobulin class. The hallmark of the lupus anticoagulant is prolongation of all phospholipid-dependent coagulation tests. The anticoagulant acts at the level of the prothrombin activator complex of the clotting cascade. The complex that consists of factor V, factor Xa, calcium, and phospholipids is necessary for the conversion of prothrombin to thrombin. The lupus anticoagulant antibody is thought to interact with the phospholipid portion of the complex, interfering with the calcium-ion-dependent binding of prothrombin factor Xa to the phospholipid. The failure of normal plasma to correct the prolonged clotting time distinguishes the lupus anticoagulant from antibodies directed against specific clotting factors and from clotting factor deficiencies. In the usual coagulation screening tests, the lupus anticoagulant results in prolongation of the activated partial thromboplastin time with or without slight prolongation of the prothrombin time (Table 22-30).

- Lupus anticoagulant is antiphospholipid antibody of either IgG or IgM immunoglobulin class.
- Prolongation of all phospholipid-dependent coagulation tests is hallmark of lupus anticoagulant.
- Anticoagulant acts at level of prothrombin activator complex of clotting cascade.
- Activated partial thromboplastin time is prolonged and not corrected by adding normal plasma.

Various other tests are reported to be sensitive for detection of lupus anticoagulants, including the plasma clot time, kaolin clotting time, a platelet neutralization procedure, and modified Russell's viper venom time.

Table 22-30.--Coagulation Tests Characterizing the Lupus Anticoagulant

Screening tests
Prothrombin time (PT) normal or prolonged
Partial thromboplastin time (PTT) prolonged
Plasma clot time prolonged
Tests identifying the lupus anticoagulant
Prolonged PTT not corrected by adding normal plasma

Given 1) the long-recognized association of the lupus anticoagulant with a chronic biologic false-positive serologic test for syphilis (reagin), 2) the identification of cardiolipin (a phospholipid) as the principal antigen in the test for reagin, and 3) the demonstration of cross-reactivity of lupus anticoagulant antibodies with phospholipids, sensitive solid-phase radioimmunoassays and enzyme-linked immunosorbent assays have been developed for the detection of anticardiolipin antibodies. Anticardiolipin antibodies can be of either the IgG or the IgM immunoglobulin class. Many, but not all, patients with the lupus anticoagulant have elevated IgG or IgM anticardiolipin antibody levels. Like the lupus anticoagulant, anticardiolipin antibodies cross-react with several negatively charged phospholipids.

- Anticardiolipin antibodies can be of either the IgG or the IgM immunoglobulin class.
- Many, but not all, patients with lupus anticoagulant have elevated IgG or IgM anticardiolipin antibody levels.

The lupus anticoagulant and anticardiolipin antibodies are most commonly associated with SLE, but they have also been reported in various other autoimmune, malignant, infectious, and drug-induced diseases. Other diseases include Sjögren's syndrome, rheumatoid arthritis, idiopathic thrombocytopenic purpura, Behçet's syndrome, myasthenia gravis, and mixed connective tissue disease. The antibodies can also be found in persons who have no apparent disease but in whom recurrent thrombosis develops.

- Lupus anticoagulant and anticardiolipin antibodies have also been reported in various other autoimmune, malignant, infectious, and drug-induced diseases.

In contrast to the earliest reports of patients with lupus anticoagulants in which an association with hemorrhagic disorders has been noted, subsequent studies have shown that the risk of bleeding is rare, and when bleeding is present it is usually due to associated thrombocytopenia or prothrombin deficiency. There is a paradoxical association between the presence of the lupus anticoagulant and anticardiolipin antibodies and recurrent venous or arterial thrombosis. Thrombotic events described have included stroke, transient ischemic attacks, myocardial infarctions, brachial artery thrombosis, deep venous thrombophlebitis, retinal vein thrombosis, hepatic vein thrombosis resulting in Budd-Chiari syndrome, and pulmonary hypertension. Other manifestations include recurrent fetal loss, thrombocytopenia, positive results of Coombs' test, migraines, chorea, epilepsy, chronic leg ulcers, livedo reticularis, and progressive dementia resulting from cerebrovascular accidents. Recently, acquired valvular heart disease, especially aortic insufficiency, has been described. The mechanism or mechanisms by which antiphospholipid antibodies are associated with thromboembolic manifestations remain unclear. Blocking of the production of prostacyclin from vascular endothelial cells, inhibition of prekallikrein activity and fibrinolysis, and decreased plasminogen activator release have all been described.

- Risk of bleeding is rare; when present, it is usually due to associated thrombocytopenia or prothrombin deficiency.
- Paradoxical association between the presence of the lupus anticoagulant and anticardiolipin antibodies and recurrent venous or arterial thrombosis.
- Other manifestations: recurrent fetal loss, thrombocytopenia, positive Coombs' test, migraines, chorea, epilepsy, chronic leg ulcers, livedo reticularis, progressive dementia from cerebrovascular accidents.
- Acquired valvular heart disease, especially aortic insufficiency, has been described.

Although many patients with lupus and other diseases can have a lupus anticoagulant or anticardiolipin antibodies, of either the IgG or the IgM class, thrombosis will not necessarily develop. In general, patients with the highest levels of anticardiolipin antibodies are more prone to thrombosis than those with lower levels. Also, the IgG anticardiolipin antibody is much more strongly associated with recurrent thrombosis than is the IgM anticardiolipin antibody. If there is no history of thrombosis, most physicians are reluctant to treat the patient for a lupus anticoagulant or elevated anticardiolipin antibodies alone without clinical manifestations.

- Patients with highest levels of anticardiolipin antibodies are more prone to thrombosis.
- IgG anticardiolipin antibody is more strongly associated with recurrent thrombosis than is IgM anticardiolipin antibody.

Treatment
Treatment of patients with the lupus anticoagulant and anticardiolipin antibodies is unclear. For most patients who have recurrent thrombosis, warfarin (Coumadin) is prescribed and will need to be taken for life. Treatment with steroids decreases the lupus anticoagulant activity, but no studies suggest that they prevent recurrent thrombosis; this possibility is still undetermined.

RAYNAUD'S PHENOMENON
This is biphasic or triphasic color changes (pallor, cyanosis, erythema) accompanied by pain and numbness in hands or feet. Cold is a common precipitating agent. Associated factors are listed in Table 22-31.

- Cold is common precipitating agent for Raynaud's phenomenon.

Table 22-31.--Causes of Secondary Raynaud's Phenomenon

Chemotherapeutic agents
    Bleomycin
    Vinblastine
Toxins
    Vinyl chloride
Vibration-induced injuries
    Jackhammer use
Vascular occlusive disorders
    Thoracic outlet obstruction
    Atherosclerosis
    Vasculitis
Connective tissue diseases
    Scleroderma, 90%-100%
    Mixed connective tissue disease, 90%-100%
    Systemic lupus erythematosus, 15%
    Rheumatoid arthritis, <10%
    Polymyositis
Miscellaneous
    Cryoglobulinemia
    Cold agglutinins
    Increased blood viscosity

Raynaud's phenomenon is a possible abnormality of microvasculature with intimal fibrosis. In male patients with Raynaud's phenomenon, a rare occurrence, a connective tissue disease often develops. Although Raynaud's phenomenon is common in females, it usually is not associated with a connective tissue disease unless the patient has positive results for antinuclear antibody, which suggest that a connective tissue disease is likely to develop in the future.

Skin capillary microscopy reveals tortuous, dilated capillary loops in systemic sclerosis, mixed connective tissue disease, and polymyositis. They also may be present in patients with Raynaud's phenomenon who will go on to develop systemic sclerosis, polymyositis, or mixed connective tissue disease.

Treatment involves smoking cessation, wearing gloves, biofeedback, 2% nitrol paste, and antihypertensives (methyldopa, prazosin, dibenzyline, nifedipine). Stellate ganglion block is used if ischemia is severe. β-Adrenergic blockers increase spasm and so are not used.

To differentiate primary Raynaud's phenomenon from the secondary form (resulting from a connective tissue disease), clinical features are considered. In primary Raynaud's disease, females are usually affected, the onset is at menarche, usually all digits are involved, and attacks are very frequent. The severity of symptoms is mild to moderate, and they can be precipitated by emotional stress. Digital ulceration and finger edema are rare, as is periungual erythema. Livedo reticularis is frequent. In persons with Raynaud's phenomenon secondary to a connective tissue disease, both males and females are affected. The onset of Raynaud's phenomenon is in the mid-20s or later. It often begins in a single digit, and attacks are usually infrequent (zero to five a day). The severity is moderate to severe, and it is not precipitated by emotional stress. Digital ulceration occurs in 30%-50% of cases, and finger edema and periungual erythema are frequent. Livedo reticularis is uncommon.

SYSTEMIC SCLEROSIS (SCLERODERMA)

For diagnosis of systemic sclerosis, one major criterion or two or more minor criteria need to be present. The major criterion is symmetric induration of the skin of the fingers and skin proximal to metacarpophalangeal or metatarsophalangeal joints. The minor criteria are sclerodactyly, digital pitting scars or loss of substance from the finger pad, and bibasilar pulmonary fibrosis.

- Systemic sclerosis is characterized by symmetric induration of skin of fingers and skin proximal to metacarpophalangeal or metatarsophalangeal joints and by bibasilar pulmonary fibrosis.

Clinical Manifestations

Skin

Patients are at risk for the development of rapidly progressive acral and trunk skin thickening and early visceral abnormalities. Skin and visceral changes tend to parallel each other in severity, but not always. Some patients have rapid progression for 2-3 years and then arrestment or some improvement of the disorder.

Raynaud's Phenomenon

Raynaud's phenomenon occurs in almost all patients. It usually occurs more than 2 years before skin changes. The vasospasm in the hands can be associated with reduced perfusion to the heart, lungs, kidneys, and gastrointestinal tract. If Raynaud's phenomenon is not present, but skin findings are suggestive of scleroderma, another disease such as eosinophilic fasciitis should be considered.

Articular

Nondeforming symmetric polyarthritis similar to rheumatoid arthritis may precede cutaneous manifestations by 12 months. Patients can have both articular erosions and nonarticular bony resorptive changes of ribs, mandible, radius, ulna, and distal phalangeal tufts which are unique to systemic sclerosis. Up to 60% of patients have "leathery" crepitation of tendons of wrist.

Pulmonary

Significant decrease in CO diffusion can be present with normal chest radiograph. Diffuse interstitial fibrosis occurs in approximately 70% of patients and is most common pulmonary abnormality. Pleuritis (with effusion) is very rare. Pulmonary hypertension is more common in patients with CREST variant (see next column).

- Significant decrease in CO diffusion can be present with normal chest radiograph.
- Diffuse interstitial fibrosis occurs in about 70% of patients.
- Pleuritis very rare.

Cardiac Manifestations

Cardiac abnormalities occur in up to 70% of patients. Conduction defects and supraventricular arrhythmias are most common. Pulmonary hypertension with cor pulmonale is the most serious problem.

- Cardiac abnormalities in up to 70% of patients.
- Pulmonary hypertension with cor pulmonale is most serious problem.

Gastrointestinal

Esophageal dysfunction is the most frequent gastrointestinal abnormality. It occurs in 90% of patients and often is asymptomatic. Lower esophageal sphincter incompetence with acid reflux may produce esophageal strictures or ulcers. Antacids or cimetidine may help. Reduced esophageal motility may respond to therapy with metoclopramide, nifedipine, and methacholine alone or in combination. Small bowel hypomotility may be associated with bacterial overgrowth and malabsorption. Treatment with tetracycline may be helpful.

- Esophageal dysfunction is most frequent gastrointestinal abnormality.
- Lower esophageal sphincter incompetence with acid reflux may produce esophageal strictures or ulcers.
- Small bowel hypomotility may be associated with bacterial overgrowth.

Renal

Renal involvement frequently results in fulminant hypertension, renal failure, and death if not treated aggressively. Proteinuria, newly diagnosed *mild* hypertension, microangiopathic hemolytic anemia, vascular changes on renal biopsy, and rapid progression of skin thickening may precede overt clinical findings of renal crisis. Association of renal involvement with hyperreninemia prompted use of suppressors of renin synthesis and release (propranolol) and of angiotensin converting enzyme inhibitors. Aggressive early antihypertensive therapy can extend life expectancy.

Laboratory Findings

Antiscleroderma antibody (anti-Scl70) is found in approximately 25% of patients, and anticentromere antibody occurs in 10%-20%.

Treatment

No remissive or curative therapy is available. Retrospective studies suggest that D-penicillamine (750 mg daily) may decrease skin thickness, prevent or delay internal organ involvement, and prolong life expectancy.

- No remissive or curative therapy available.

CREST SYNDROME

This is characterized by *c*alcinosis cutis, *R*aynaud's phenomenon, *e*sophageal dysmotility, *s*clerodactyly, and *t*elangiectasias. Skin involvement progresses slowly and is limited to the extremities. Development of internal organ involvement is delayed. Lung involvement occurs in 70% of patients. Diffusing capacity is low, and pulmonary hypertension can develop. The latter is more common in CREST than in diffuse scleroderma. Onset of Raynaud's phenomenon occurs before skin changes (less than 2 years before skin changes). Anticentromere antibody is found in 70%-90% of patients and antiscleroderma-70 antibody in 10%. The incidence of primary biliary cirrhosis is increased.

- In CREST syndrome, 70% of patients have lung involvement.
- Diffusing capacity is low, and pulmonary hypertension can develop.
- Anticentromere antibody in 70%-90% of patients.
- Increased incidence of primary biliary cirrhosis.

SCLERODERMA-LIKE SYNDROMES

Disorders Associated With Occupation or Environment

This group includes polyvinyl chloride disease, organic solvents, jackhammer disease, silicosis, silicone implants (still a questionable association), toxic oil syndrome, and deteriorated urea-formaldehyde foam.

Eosinophilic Fasciitis

Clinical features of this disorder include tight bound-down skin of extremities characteristically sparing the hands and feet. Peau d'orange skin changes can develop. Onset after vigorous exercise is common. Raynaud's phenomenon does not occur, and there is no visceral involvement. Flexion contractures and carpal tunnel syndrome can develop.

- Eosinophilic fasciitis is characterized by tight bound-down skin of extremities, usually sparing hands and feet.
- No visceral involvement.

Laboratory findings are peripheral eosinophilia, increased sedimentation rate, and hypergammaglobulinemia. The diagnosis is based on the findings of inflammation and thickening of fascia on deep fascial biopsy. Treatment is with prednisone (40 mg daily). The response is usually good. Associated conditions are aplastic anemia and thrombocytopenia (both antibody-mediated) and leukemias and myeloproliferative diseases.

- Lab findings include peripheral eosinophilia.
- Treatment with prednisone provides good response.

Metabolic Causes of Scleroderma-Like Syndrome

This group includes porphyria, amyloidosis, carcinoid, and diabetes mellitus (flexion contractures of tendons in hands can develop).

Other Causes

As a manifestation of *graft-versus-host disease*, skin induration develops in up to 30% of patients who receive bone marrow transplant. *Drug-induced disorders* are caused by carbidopa, bleomycin, and bromocriptine. *Eosinophilic myalgia syndrome* is associated with ingestion of L-tryptophan. Eosinophilia, myositis, skin induration, fasciitis, and peripheral neuropathy develop. Skin changes are similar to those of eosinophilic fasciitis. A contaminant rather than L-tryptophan itself is thought to be the cause. There is a poor response to steroids. *Scleredema* frequently occurs after streptococcal upper respiratory tract infection in children. It is usually self-limiting. Swelling of the head and neck is common. In adults, diabetes mellitus is often associated. *Scleromyxedema* is associated with IgG monoclonal protein. Cocaine use and appetite suppressants also cause scleroderma-like illness.

INFLAMMATORY MYOPATHIES

Inflammatory myopathies can be classified into several categories, including polymyositis, dermatomyositis, myositis associated with malignancy, childhood-type, and overlap connective tissue disease. Polymyositis is an inflammatory myopathy characterized by proximal muscle weakness. Patients with dermatomyositis can have an associated rash that includes a heliotrope hue of the eyelids, a rash on the metacarpophalangeal and proximal interphalangeal joints (Gottron papules), and photosensitivity dermatitis of the face. Most patients have an elevated creatine kinase level, a characteristic electromyogram, and a characteristic muscle biopsy.

- Polymyositis is inflammatory myopathy characterized by proximal muscle weakness.

- Feature of dermatomyositis is rash that includes heliotrope hue of eyelids.

The electromyogram is characteristic but not diagnostic of inflammatory myopathies. It shows decreased amplitude and increased spike frequency, it is polyphasic, and conduction speed is normal. Fibrillation is not specific for inflammatory myopathies, but when present it indicates active disease. Loss of fibrillation usually means the inflammatory myopathy is under control, but if the electromyogram is still myopathic, it suggests an associated steroid myopathy caused by treatment. The muscle biopsy, which is mandatory in all patients with inflammatory myopathy, shows degeneration, necrosis, and regeneration of myofibrils and lymphocytic plus monocytic infiltrate in a perivascular or interstitial distribution.

- Electromyogram is characteristic but not diagnostic of polymyositis.

The association of polymyositis and dermatomyositis with malignancy is controversial. In patients older than 40 years, perhaps 10% of those with dermatomyositis have an associated malignancy. The antibody anti-Jo1 is associated with polymyositis and dermatomyositis in approximately 25% of cases. This antibody is associated with inflammatory arthritis, interstitial lung disease, Raynaud's phenomenon, and increased mortality primarily due to respiratory failure. The autoantibody anti-Mi-2 is associated with dermatomyositis in 2%-20% of patients.

- Perhaps 10% of patients >40 years with dermatomyositis have associated malignancy.
- Anti-Jo1 is associated with polymyositis and dermatomyositis in about 25% of cases.

Treatment of polymyositis includes prednisone (60 mg daily), usually for 1 to 2 months, until the muscle enzyme values normalize. The dosage is slowly reduced thereafter, and the clinical course and creatine kinase values are monitored. In steroid-resistant cases, either azathioprine (1-2 mg/kg per day) or methotrexate can be used.

Aspiration pneumonia can occur as a result of pharyngeal weakness. If so, a liquid diet, feeding tube, or feeding gastrostomy is needed until there is clinical improvement.

With regard to the differential diagnosis, inclusion body myositis needs to be considered. This usually occurs in the older age group. The onset of weakness is more insidious, occurring over many years. The creatine kinase value often is only minimally to several times elevated, and distal weakness and proximal weakness occur. The electromyogram, besides showing a myopathic picture, can also have an associated neuropathic picture. Diagnosis of inclusion body myositis is made from biopsy. Histopathology is indistinguishable from that of polymyositis except for the presence of eosinophilic inclusions and rimmed vacuoles with basophilic enhancement. Inclusion body myositis responds poorly to prednisone and immunosuppressive therapy, and the course is one of slow progressive weakness.

- Inclusion body myositis usually occurs in older age group.
- Diagnosis is made from biopsy.
- It responds poorly to prednisone.

QUESTIONS

Multiple Choice (choose the one best answer)
1. Inflammation in a joint is always accompanied by swelling, stiffness, and:
   a. Evidence for infection
   b. Pain on motion
   c. An elevated Westergren sedimentation rate
   d. An abnormal radiograph
   e. A positive rheumatoid factor

2. Rheumatoid factor as assayed in the clinical laboratory measures antibodies directed against:
   a. Evil humors in the joint
   b. The FC portion of IgG
   c. Sheep red blood cells
   d. Latex particles
   e. The FC portion of IgM

3. The most common cause of secondary osteoarthritis is:
   a. Obesity
   b. Osteoporosis
   c. Trauma
   d. Hemochromatosis
   e. Previous rheumatoid arthritis

4. In the acutely swollen joint, the three most important causes to consider are:
   a. Rheumatoid arthritis, osteoarthritis, gout
   b. Systemic lupus erythematosus, septic arthritis, trauma
   c. Septic arthritis, rheumatoid arthritis, trauma
   d. Trauma, microcrystalline arthritis, septic arthritis
   e. Microcrystalline arthritis, gout, pseudogout

5. Septic arthritis in young adults and teenagers is most commonly caused by:
   a. Tuberculosis
   b. *Gonococcus*
   c. *Pseudomonas*
   d. *Streptococcus*
   e. *Staphylococcus*

6. Which joints are characteristically involved in the bony hypertrophy of primary osteoarthritis and not commonly involved in the synovial inflammation of rheumatoid arthritis?
   a. Distal interphalangeal joints (DIPs)
   b. Proximal interphalangeal joints (PIPs)
   c. Metacarpophalangeal joints (MCPs)
   d. Knees
   e. Hips

7. Which of the following antirheumatic drugs should be avoided in mixed renal insufficiency (creatinine value more than 2.0 mg/dL)?
   a. Methotrexate
   b. Hydroxychloroquine
   c. Intermuscular gold
   d. Allopurinol
   e. Azathioprine

8. Which of the following genes is associated with an increased risk of progressive destructive rheumatoid arthritis?
   a. HLA-DR3
   b. HLA-DR4
   c. HLA-DR5
   d. HLA-B27
   e. HLA-A8

9. The most frequent cause of nontraumatic shoulder pain is:
   a. Thoracic outlet syndrome
   b. Osteoarthritis of the glenohumeral joint
   c. Bicipital tendinitis

d. Rotator cuff tendinitis

e. Referred pain from the neck

10. Fibromyalgia, a generalized aching condition of more than 3 months in duration, is commonly associated with:
   a. An elevated Westergren sedimentation rate
   b. Elevated creatine kinase value
   c. Positive antinuclear antibody
   d. Abnormal sleep study
   e. Multiple subspecialty evaluations with no definitive diagnosis

11. Which clinical description best characterizes Sjögren's syndrome?
   a. Neutropenia, splenomegaly, and rheumatoid arthritis
   b. Dry eyes, dry mouth, and arthritis
   c. Fever, arthritis, and rash
   d. Large granular lymphocyte proliferation
   e. Raynaud's phenomenon, sun sensitivity, and oral ulcers

12. Which of the following are useful for distinguishing giant cell arteritis from polymyalgia rheumatica?
   a. Fever, weight loss, and fatigue
   b. Chronic morning stiffness of the hip and shoulder muscle girdles
   c. Temporal headache and scalp soreness
   d. Rapid improvement with glucocorticosteroid treatment
   e. Elevated Westergren sedimentation rate

13. Classic Wegener's granulomatosis is remarkable for:
   a. Purpura, arthritis, and nephritis
   b. Sinusitis, pulmonary nodules, and nephritis
   c. Headache, jaw claudication, amaurosis fugax
   d. Purpura, mononeuritis, nephritis
   e. Iritis, oral ulcers, skin pustules

14. Cyclophosphamide and chlorambucil are two alkylating agents used to treat systemic vasculitis. They share the potential for toxic side effects, including bone marrow suppression, immunosuppression, and risk of malignancy. In what important way does the toxicity profile of cyclophosphamide differ from that of chlorambucil?
   a. Hepatitis and cirrhosis
   b. Renal failure
   c. Hemorrhagic cystitis
   d. Oral ulcers and rash
   e. Osteoporosis

15. A 45-year-old white man presents with a hot, red, swollen knee. Joint aspiration reveals monosodium urate crystals, and a diagnosis of gout is established. He considers himself otherwise in excellent health, and his past medical history has been unremarkable. Which of the following would be the most appropriate treatment for his acute gout?
   a. Oral colchicine
   b. Aspirin
   c. Probenecid
   d. Indomethacin
   e. Allopurinol

16. A 22-year-old white man presents with a 4-month history of low back pain with morning stiffness. He has a previous history of iritis. Which of the following HLA antigens might you expect to be associated with these complaints?
   a. HLA-B8
   b. HLA-DR4
   c. HLA-B27
   d. HLA-DR2
   e. HLA-B17

17. A 21-year-old college student from Connecticut has swelling of both knees. Two years previously, he had had Bell's palsy. There is no history of other joint involvement or history of a rash. The most likely diagnosis is:
   a. Rheumatoid arthritis
   b. Systemic lupus erythematosus
   c. Lyme disease
   d. Ankylosing spondylitis
   e. Reiter's syndrome

18. A 24-year-old white man presents with a 1-week history of several swollen toes. He has a past history of conjunctivitis. He also has noted some low back stiffness, most pronounced in the morning. The most likely diagnosis is:
   a. Rheumatoid arthritis
   b. Systemic lupus erythematosus
   c. Gout
   d. Lyme disease
   e. Reiter's syndrome

19. A 42-year-old woman with a 10-year history of systemic lupus erythematosus manifested by renal involvement, fever, arthritis, and pericarditis was admitted with a 2-day history of malaise, arthralgias, and fever to 38.2°C. She was receiving 10 mg of prednisone and 50 mg of cyclophosphamide. Which of the following would be least helpful in her management?
   a. Determination of sedimentation rate
   b. Urinalysis and culture
   c. Anti-nDNA and C3 testing

d. Hematology group, including differential

e. Blood cultures

20. Which of the following is the most appropriate treatment for a patient with severe Raynaud's phenomenon with digital ischemia?
    a. Plasmapheresis
    b. Metoprolol
    c. Nifedipine
    d. Gamma globulin, intravenously
    e. Biofeedback

21. Which one of the following autoantibodies is most frequently found in CREST syndrome?
    a. Rheumatoid factor
    b. Anti SS-A
    c. Anticentromere
    d. Anti SS-B
    e. Antineutrophil cytoplasmic antibodies

True/False (indicate whether each answer is true or false)

22. A family history is supportive in making the diagnosis of:
    a. Rheumatoid arthritis
    b. Systemic lupus erythematosus
    c. Ankylosing spondylitis
    d. Knee osteoarthritis
    e. Gout
    f. Wegener's granulomatosis

23. Metabolic diseases commonly associated with arthritis include:
    a. Type II diabetes mellitus
    b. Hemochromatosis
    c. Addison's disease
    d. Acromegaly
    e. Wilson's disease
    f. Ochronosis

24. Characteristic neurologic complications of rheumatoid arthritis include the following:
    a. Brachial plexopathy
    b. Cervical radiculopathy
    c. Cervical myelopathy
    d. Carpal tunnel syndrome
    e. Peripheral neuropathy and mononeuritis multiplex
    f. Seizures

25. Criteria for the diagnosis of rheumatoid arthritis include the following:
    a. Positive rheumatoid factor
    b. Joint pain for 6 or more weeks
    c. Symmetric swelling of several joints

d. Involvement of the metacarpophalangeal joints and wrist

e. Family history of rheumatoid arthritis

f. Radiographic appearance of marginal erosions

26. Adverse glucocorticosteroid effects include the following:
    a. Insomnia
    b. Osteomalacia
    c. Glucose intolerance
    d. Myopathy
    e. Cataracts
    f. Aggravation of hypertension

27. Results of the antineutrophil cytoplasmic antibody (ANCA) blood test are frequently positive in the following:
    a. Wegener's granulomatosis
    b. Mixed cryoglobulinemia
    c. Churg-Strauss syndrome
    d. Microscopic polyarteritis
    e. Schönlein-Henoch purpura
    f. Giant cell arteritis

28. The following may be associated with hypouricemia:
    a. Allopurinol therapy
    b. Low-dose aspirin
    c. Cyclosporine therapy
    d. Xanthine oxidase deficiency
    e. Adenosine deaminase deficiency
    f. Nicotinic acid therapy

29. The autoantibody anti-SSA is associated with the following conditions:
    a. Sjögren's syndrome
    b. Subacute cutaneous lupus
    c. Drug-induced lupus
    d. Congenital heart block in neonates
    e. Raynaud's phenomenon
    f. Mixed connective tissue disease

30. A 48-year-old woman with a biopsy-proven diagnosis of polymyositis has been receiving prednisone, 60 mg daily, for the past 2 months. She is still complaining of proximal muscle weakness. The following could be helpful for differentiating a steroid-induced myopathy from persistent active polymyositis at this time:
    a. Creatine phosphokinase determination
    b. Aldolase determination
    c. The finding of proximal muscle weakness on physical examination
    d. Electromyography
    e. Presence of anti-Jo1
    f. Muscle biopsy

ANSWERS

1. Answer b.

Inflammation in a joint is accompanied by pain on motion. The classic features of inflammation include swelling, redness, pain, and loss of function. Inflammation does not require the presence of infection. Many patients with inflammatory joint disease have normal sedimentation rates. Radiography of a hand with inflammatory arthritis may not show damage for many months after symptoms appear. A positive rheumatoid factor is not necessary for the diagnosis of inflammatory arthritis.

2. Answer b.

Rheumatoid factor assayed in clinical laboratories measures entemeric IgM directed against the FC portion of IgG. It is a measure of immune complexes circulating in the blood. Several chronic conditions, such as infections and malignancies, can produce immune complexes, including a positive rheumatoid factor. The rheumatoid factor therefore is not a specific marker for rheumatoid arthritis. In addition, up to 5% of the normal population will have a low-titer positive rheumatoid factor. Other rheumatoid factors exist, including IgA and IgG; however, their clinical significance is less well known, and therefore they are not clinically useful.

3. Answer c.

The most common cause of secondary osteoarthritis is trauma. Obesity is linked to osteoarthritis only at the knee in females. Osteoporosis is not a risk factor for osteoarthritis. Hemochromatosis and previous rheumatoid arthritis are conditions that predispose to osteoarthritis, but they are not nearly as common as trauma.

4. Answer d.

In the acutely swollen joint, the three most important causes to consider are trauma, microcrystalline arthritis, and septic arthritis (remember trauma, crystals, or infection).

5. Answer b.

Septic arthritis in young adults and teenagers is most commonly caused by *Neisseria gonococcus*. In fact, any new acute arthritis in sexually active teens and young adults should make the clinician think of gonococcal arthritis.

6. Answer a.

The joints characteristically involved in osteoarthritis but not rheumatoid arthritis are the distal interphalangeal joints (DIPs).

7. Answer a.

Methotrexate is the only drug in this list which should be almost always avoided in renal insufficiency when the creatinine level is 2 mg/dL or more.

8. Answer b.

HLA-DR4 defines a cell-surface heterodime responsible for presenting processed antigen to T-cell receptors. For this reason, rheumatoid arthritis is suspected to require active T-cell participation to initiate and probably propagate the inflammatory process.

9. Answer d.

The most frequent cause of nontraumatic shoulder pain is rotator cuff tendinitis. The other problems listed are also part of the differential diagnosis of shoulder pain, but 90% of all nontraumatic shoulder pain is related to rotator cuff tendinitis.

10. Answer e.

Fibromyalgia is not consistently associated with any laboratory, radiographic, or study abnormality. A strong marker for fibromyalgia in patients in tertiary care centers is the multiple subspecialty evaluation with no definitive diagnosis (other than fibromyalgia).

11. Answer b.

Sjögren's syndrome by definition involves dry eyes, dry mouth, and connective tissue disease. Neutropenia, splenomegaly, and rheumatoid arthritis are part of Felty's syndrome. Fever, arthritis, and rash should make one think of adult-onset Still's disease. Large granular lymphocyte proliferation can complicate certain subtypes of Felty's syndrome and seropositive rheumatoid arthritis. Raynaud's phenomenon, sun sensitivity, and oral ulcers should raise the possibility of systemic lupus erythematosus.

12. Answer c.

Temporal headache and scalp soreness are the only features that are unique to giant cell arteritis when compared with polymyalgia rheumatica. At least 40% of patients with giant cell arteritis have features of polymyalgia rheumatica. Conversely, 15% of patients with polymyalgia rheumatica develop features that suggest coexisting giant cell arteritis at some point during their disease.

13. Answer b.

Classic Wegener's granulomatosis is remarkable for upper and lower granulomatous respiratory tract inflammation and nephritis.

14. Answer c.

Hemorrhagic cystitis is a unique complication of cyclophosphamide treatment. This major complication predominantly occurs in patients who receive cyclophosphamide orally rather than the intravenous pulse form. It can be life-threatening.

15. Answer d.

Nonsteroidal anti-inflammatory drugs, including indomethacin, are effective in treating acute gout. High-dose oral colchicine therapy is associated with severe gastrointestinal side effects and is rarely used. Aspirin is usually not beneficial. Both allopurinol and probenecid are used to treat hyperuricemia and are given in the intercritical period. They are not helpful in the treatment of acute gout.

16. Answer c.

A history of low back pain with morning stiffness in a young person is characteristic of a spondyloarthropathy. The HLA-B27 antigen has a strong association with the spondyloarthropathies and with iritis.

17. Answer c.

Lyme disease characteristically causes an arthritis of the knees. It is also associated with Bell's palsy. The rash of erythema chronicum migrans can occur in Lyme disease but does not always occur. The arthritis usually starts several years after the tick bite. Many patients are unaware of a previous tick bite. Connecticut is an endemic state for Lyme disease. None of the other conditions listed are associated with Bell's palsy.

18. Answer e.

Reiter's syndrome characteristically occurs in young white males. Toe involvement is common. It is also associated with conjunctivitis. Nonspecific urethritis can also occur. Swollen toes are very unusual in rheumatoid arthritis, lupus, and Lyme disease. Although gout can cause swelling of toes, it is unusual in a 24-year-old man and would not be associated with conjunctivitis.

19. Answer a.

In this patient, the differential diagnosis is between an infection and active lupus. The sedimentation rate would be increased in either condition and therefore would not be helpful in management. A urinalysis and culture as well as blood cultures would be helpful to rule out infection. A hematology group study that revealed leukocytosis would also suggest infection. An elevated anti-DNA and depressed C3 level would suggest active lupus.

20. Answer c.

Nifedipine has been proved to be effective in the treatment of Raynaud's phenomenon with digital ischemia. β-Adrenergic blockers such as metoprolol can aggravate the condition. Biofeedback can be used in patients with mild Raynaud's phenomenon but would be ineffective in patients with ischemia.

21. Answer c.

Anticentromere antibodies have a strong association with CREST syndrome. They are much less frequent in patients with systemic sclerosis. Other autoantibodies can be found in patients with CREST syndrome, but these are unusual and usually in very low titer. Antineutrophil cytoplasmic antibodies are found in patients with Wegener's granulomatosis and other vasculitides.

22. a, true; b, true; c, true; d, false; e, true; f, false.

A family history is supportive of the diagnosis of rheumatoid arthritis, systemic lupus erythematosus, ankylosing spondylitis, and gout. No genetic linkage has been identified in primary knee osteoarthritis or in Wegener's granulomatosis.

23. a, false; b, true; c, false; d, true; e, true; f, true.

Hemochromatosis, acromegaly, Wilson's disease, and ochronosis are associated with secondary osteoarthritis. Type II diabetes mellitus is usually associated with soft tissue problems, including carpal tunnel syndrome, Dupuytren's contractures, and a syndrome of limited joint mobility in the hands associated with diabetic cutaneous sclerosis. Addison's disease is not commonly associated with arthritis, but on occasion it can present with symptoms that suggest fibromyalgia.

24. a, false; b, false; c, true; d, true; e, true; f, false.

Characteristic neurologic complications of rheumatoid arthritis include cervical myelopathy, carpal tunnel syndrome, and peripheral neuropathy and mononeuritis multiplex. Rheumatoid arthritis is not associated with brachial plexopathy or cervical radiculopathy. Seizures are one of the neurologic complications of systemic lupus erythematosus.

25. a, true; b, true; c, true; d, true; e, false; f, true.

Criteria for rheumatoid arthritis include positive rheumatoid factor, joint pain and swelling for more than 6 weeks, symmetric swelling of several joints, involvement of the metacarpophalangeal joints and wrist, and radiographic appearance of marginal erosions. The only criterion not mentioned is rheumatoid nodules. At least four criteria must be present for diagnosis. A family history of rheumatoid arthritis is not included in the criteria.

26. a, true; b, false; c, true; d, true; e, true; f, true.

Adverse glucocorticosteroid effects include insomnia, glucose intolerance, myopathy, cataracts, and aggravation of hypertension. The only incorrect answer is osteomalacia. Glucocorticosteroids are known to cause osteoporosis.

27. a, true; b, false; c, true; d, true; e, false; f, false.

The ANCA test is positive in many cases of Wegener's granulomatosis, Churg-Strauss syndrome, and microscopic polyarteritis. It is not positive in mixed cryoglobulinemia or Schönlein-Henoch purpura.

28. a, true; b, false; c, false; d, true; e, true; f, false.

Allopurinol is a xanthine oxidase inhibitor and is associated with hypouricemia. Low-dose aspirin is associated with hyperuricemia, whereas high-dose aspirin is associated with hypouricemia. Cyclosporine therapy also induces hyperuricemia, as does nicotinic acid. Both xanthine oxidase deficiency and adenosine deaminase deficiency are inborn errors of metabolism associated with hypouricemia.

29. a, true; b, true; c, false; d, true; e, false; f, false.

The autoantibody anti-SSA is associated with Sjögren's syndrome, subacute cutaneous lupus, and congenital heart block in neonates. Drug-induced lupus is associated with anti-histone antibody. Raynaud's phenomenon has no associated autoantibodies. Mixed connective tissue disease is associated with the autoantibody anti-RNP.

30. a, true; b, true; c, false; d, true; e, false; f, true.

An increased creatine phosphokinase or aldolase level is indicative of active muscle inflammation. Also, an electromyogram showing active fibrillation potentials would be indicative of active inflammation. A muscle biopsy, if needed, could also differentiate active polymyositis from a steroid myopathy. A steroid myopathy would show type II muscle atrophy, whereas in active polymyositis there would be an inflammatory infiltrate and muscle necrosis. The finding of proximal muscle weakness would not differentiate a steroid myopathy from active polymyositis. Also, the presence of anti-Jo1 would not differentiate active from inactive disease.

CHAPTER 23

VASCULAR DISEASES

Thom Rooke, M.D.

ANEURYSMS

Abdominal Aortic Aneurysms

Although congenital or acquired aneurysms can affect any blood vessel in the body, abdominal aortic aneurysms are the ones most commonly encountered by the general medical practitioner. In autopsy series or studies in which unselected adult patients are screened with ultrasonography, the frequency of abdominal aortic aneurysms (usually defined as a vessel diameter ≥3 cm) ranges from 1.5%-3.2%. In high-risk patients, such as those with coronary or peripheral vascular disease, the rate may be as high as 5%-10%. The growth rate of these aneurysms is typically 0.3-0.5 cm per year, and 95% are located below the origin of the renal arteries. Five percent of all aneurysms are the so-called inflammatory type. For a patient with an abdominal aortic aneurysm, the chance that a first-degree relative also has one is approximately 20%.

- Abdominal aortic aneurysms are the most common aneurysm encountered by the general practitioner.
- Frequency (vessel diameter ≥3 cm) is 1.5%-3.2%.

- In high-risk patients, frequency is as high as 5%-10%.
- Growth rate is 0.3-0.5 cm per year.
- 95% are below origin of renal arteries.
- Chance that first-degree relative has aneurysm is about 20%.

Cause

Most aneurysms are associated with atherosclerosis and hypertension, but predisposing factors such as connective tissue disease (Marfan syndrome, Ehlers-Danlos syndrome, pseudoxanthoma elasticum), infection, trauma, vasculitis, and others may also be involved.

- Most abdominal aortic aneurysms are associated with atherosclerosis and hypertension.
- Other predisposing factors: connective tissue disease (Marfan syndrome, Ehlers-Danlos syndrome), infection.

Diagnosis

Various imaging methods are used to diagnose aneurysms (Fig. 23-1).

Fig. 23-1. Aneurysms can be diagnosed and evaluated with many imaging methods. *A,* Aortogram shows multiple saccular aneurysms (*arrows*) protruding from abdominal aorta. *B,* Computed tomogram cuts through a large, inflamed abdominal aortic aneurysm (*arrow*). Eccentric layer of laminated thrombus (*arrowheads*) surrounds lumen. *C,* Ultrasound scan shows a saccular aneurysm protruding from popliteal artery (*arrow*).

Rupture

The overall mortality rate with ruptured abdominal aortic aneurysm is 80%, and 50% of patients die before they reach the hospital. Of those who survive to reach the hospital, 25% die before operation can be performed, and 40% die during or after operation. The risk of rupture is directly related to aneurysm size. For aneurysms of 5.0, 6.0, or 7.0 cm in diameter, the yearly rate of rupture is <5%, 5%-10%, and 20%, respectively.

- Overall mortality rate with ruptured abdominal aortic aneurysm is 80%.
- 50% of patients die before they reach the hospital.
- Of those who survive to reach the hospital, 25% die before operation.
- 40% of patients die during or after operation.
- Risk of rupture is related to aneurysm size.

Treatment

In the series with the best results, the surgical mortality rate for elective aneurysm resection is 3%-5%. If the operation is performed on high-risk patients, on elderly patients (>80 years), or in hospitals not specializing in vascular surgery, the mortality rate doubles to 7%-10%. A reasonable approach to management is based on the size of the aneurysm: <4.5 cm in diameter, observe; 4.5-6.0 cm, operate electively if the patient is a good surgical risk; and >6.0 cm, consider operation even if the patient is a poor surgical risk.

- Surgical mortality rate for elective resection of abdominal aortic aneurysm: 3%-5%.
- Rate in high-risk patients is 7%-10%.
- Management based on aneurysm size: <4.5 cm, observe; 4.5-6 cm, operate electively; >6.0 cm, consider operation even if patient is a poor risk.

Other Aneurysms

Other aneurysms that are occasionally encountered by the internist include popliteal aneurysms (these typically thrombose rather than rupture, and when they do so they may cause limb-threatening embolizations or acute ischemia); splenic aneurysms (these often appear in the left upper quadrant as calcified masses on radiographs of the chest or abdomen); iliac aneurysms (almost always seen in conjunction with abdominal aortic aneurysm); and thoracic aortic aneurysms (ascending or descending). Whenever an aneurysm is detected, it is essential that the clinician screen for the presence of occult aneurysms.

- Popliteal aneurysms typically thrombose rather than rupture.
- Aneurysms may cause limb-threatening embolization.
- When an aneurysm is detected, clinician must screen for occult aneurysms.

ACUTE ARTERIAL OCCLUSION

Cause

Most cases of acute arterial occlusion can be attributed to one of three causes: thrombosis, emboli, and dissection.

Thrombosis

Thrombosis in situ usually occurs at the site of an underlying vascular abnormality such as an atherosclerotic lesion (plaque rupture) or within an aneurysm. Clotting disorders are only rarely the cause of spontaneous arterial thrombosis. Both antiplatelet and anticoagulant agents may be useful in preventing arterial thrombosis.

- Thrombosis in situ that causes acute arterial occlusion occurs at the site of atherosclerotic lesion or within aneurysm.
- Antiplatelet and anticoagulant agents may prevent arterial thrombosis.

Emboli

Emboli large enough to occlude relatively large arteries usually (in >95% of cases) have a cardiac source. The most common abnormalities producing cardiac-derived emboli include ventricular mural thrombus (typically caused by an infarct or cardiomyopathy), valvular disease (native or prosthetic), and atrial disorders such as chronic or paroxysmal atrial fibrillation. Mural tumors such as atrial myxoma rarely embolize. Other unusual causes of large arterial emboli include paradoxic emboli, in which a thrombus originating in the deep venous system passes through an atrial septal defect or patent foramen ovale and enters the arterial system. Antiplatelet drugs or anticoagulants may prevent some types of emboli.

- Emboli large enough to occlude large arteries usually have a cardiac source.
- Cardiac-derived emboli result from ventricular mural thrombus, valvular disease, paroxysmal atrial fibrillation.
- An unusual cause of emboli is paradoxic emboli: thrombus passes through atrial septal defect or patent foramen ovale and enters arterial system.

Dissection

Dissections are usually associated with hypertension, atherosclerosis, aneurysms, or certain degenerative or connective tissue disorders. As invasive diagnostic and therapeutic cardiovascular interventions have become more popular, iatrogenic dissection has markedly increased in frequency. Trauma (blunt or penetrating) also accounts for a significant number of dissections.

- Dissections are usually associated with hypertension, atherosclerosis, aneurysms, or certain degenerative or connective tissue disorders.

• Iatrogenic dissection has increased in frequency.

Clinical Manifestations

Remember the six P's: 1) pulseless, 2) polar (cool), 3) pallor, 4) pain, 5) paresthesias, and 6) paralysis. It is essential to remember that when acute arterial occlusion occurs, the first abnormalities noted include pulselessness, limb coolness, and limb pallor; although these are important findings, they do not necessarily imply critical ischemia, and the limb can generally be watched as long as necessary. When pain and paresthesia occur, revascularization is necessary and should be performed at the earliest convenient opportunity. However, when motor weakness or paralysis begins to develop in a patient with acute arterial occlusion, the potential for limb loss is high, and revascularization should be performed immediately (within 2 or 3 hours if possible).

• Six P's of acute arterial occlusion: 1) pulselessness, 2) polar (cool), 3) pallor, 4) pain, 5) paresthesias, and 6) paralysis.

• When motor weakness or paralysis begins to develop, potential for limb loss is high; immediate revascularization is needed.

Treatment

Specific forms of treatment depend on the cause of the occlusion and are largely beyond the scope of this chapter. Thrombosis may be treated surgically or with lytic agents. Emboli may be treated surgically, including percutaneous removal with a Fogarty balloon catheter. Dissection typically requires operation, although in some situations a dissection may heal with conservative therapy. In most cases, anticoagulation, control of hypertension, and limb protection are indicated.

VASCULITIS (SMALL AND MEDIUM-SIZED VESSELS)

Cause

Several processes may produce vasculitis of small and medium-sized vessels; although none of these are individually common, as a group they are encountered by the internist on a regular basis. In general, immunologic or autoimmune phenomena are thought to be involved in the production of most vasculitides, although the exact mechanism(s) by which this occurs is poorly understood.

Specific Vasculitides

The most commonly encountered types of vasculitis include polyarteritis nodosa, Wegener's granulomatosis, and rheumatoid vasculitis.

Polyarteritis Nodosa

This is an acute, necrotizing vasculitis (Fig. 23-2) that affects primarily medium-sized and small arteries. It is a systemic disorder that may involve the kidneys, joints, skin, nerves, and various other tissues. The diagnosis is usually made with biopsy (the affected tissues generally show necrotizing changes and disruption of the blood vessels) or angiography (focal stenoses and microaneurysms are typical). Corticosteroids and cytotoxic agents (such as cyclophosphamide and azathioprine) are frequently effective for treatment.

• Polyarteritis nodosa: acute, necrotizing vasculitis that affects medium-sized and small arteries.

• It is a systemic disorder.

• Diagnosis is made with biopsy and angiography.

• Corticosteroids and cytotoxic agents are effective therapy.

Wegener's Granulomatosis

This granulomatous, necrotizing process can affect blood vessels in the respiratory tract and kidneys. In severe cases, surrounding structures, including the skin, may be involved.

Fig. 23-2. Necrotizing vasculitis. The constellation of findings shown here (ulcerations, livedo, petechial skin lesions) are typical of many vasculitic processes that affect small or medium-sized vessels.

The syndrome is typically fatal without treatment. The diagnosis has been aided in recent years by the ability to test for antineutrophil cytoplasmic antibodies; although they are present in many vasculitides, a typical granular pattern is seen in Wegener's granulomatosis. Treatment consists of prednisone, cyclophosphamide, and, in some cases, trimethoprim-sulfamethoxazole.

- Wegener's granulomatosis can affect blood vessels in respiratory tract and kidneys.
- Syndrome is typically fatal without treatment.
- Diagnosis is aided by testing for antineutrophil cytoplasmic antibodies.
- Treatment consists of prednisone and cyclophosphamide.

Rheumatoid Vasculitis

Blood vessels are frequently involved in rheumatoid and other collagen vascular diseases. The findings frequently resemble those of polyarteritis nodosa, although the skin is affected more often. In the United States, rheumatoid vasculitis is the third most common cause of chronic leg ulcers, after atherosclerosis and venous disorders. Prednisone is usually effective, with or without other immunosuppressive agents.

- Rheumatoid vasculitis is similar to polyarteritis nodosa, except skin is affected more often.
- It is the third most common cause of chronic leg ulcers in United States.
- Prednisone is usually effective treatment.

Other Vasculitides

A wide variety of other vasculitides may affect small and medium-sized vessels. These include allergic angiitis (Churg-Strauss syndrome), cryoglobulinemia, Schönlein-Henoch purpura, various forms of hypersensitivity vasculitis, serum sickness, and numerous nonspecific necrotizing and nonnecrotizing vasculitides. In general, most of these can be treated with corticosteroids or a steroid-sparing immunosuppressant.

BUERGER'S DISEASE

Cause

The cause of Buerger's disease (thromboangiitis obliterans) remains unknown, but its association with smoking is powerful and well known. Few, if any, cases occur in the absence of tobacco use. Pathologically, the disease resembles a vasculitis; the vessel is typically thrombosed and infiltrated with inflammatory cells. Granuloma formation and microabscesses are common.

- Cause of Buerger's disease is unknown.
- Association with smoking is powerful and well known.
- Granuloma and microabscesses are common.

Clinical Manifestations

The disease usually affects the small distal arteries first and progresses proximally if smoking is continued. Veins are also often involved; the first manifestation of Buerger's disease may be superficial phlebitis. If smoking is discontinued, the process is frequently arrested; if smoking continues, the disease almost always progresses. Interestingly, whereas other vasculitides typically demonstrate an elevated erythrocyte sedimentation rate, in Buerger's disease it is often minimally elevated or normal.

- Buerger's disease affects small distal arteries first.
- Veins are also involved.
- First manifestation may be superficial phlebitis.
- Erythrocyte sedimentation rate is minimally elevated or normal.

Diagnosis

The diagnosis is usually made on the basis of the history. The patient is typically <40 years old, has distal disease (Fig. 23-3), and has a history of cigarette use. Men were once thought to be primarily affected, but in recent years the number of women with this diagnosis has increased. Angiography shows typical findings that can aid in the diagnosis, and definitive pathologic findings can often be obtained on appropriate biopsy.

- Typical patient with Buerger's disease: <40 years old, has distal disease, has history of cigarette use.

Treatment

Cessation of smoking is an absolute necessity. Other treatments (such as pentoxifylline and sympathectomy) are of unknown benefit.

- Cessation of smoking is a necessity in Buerger's disease.

ERGOTISM

Mechanism of Action

Ergotamine and ergot derivatives are potent arterial vasoconstrictors. They are thought to produce vasoconstriction by cross-reacting with α-adrenergic (and to a lesser extent, serotonergic) receptors in the blood vessel wall. These compounds are typically given either orally or by suppository. Their major indication is for the treatment of vasomotor (migraine) headache.

Fig. 23-3. Buerger's disease. Distal portions of digits are severely ischemic. Bilateral ischemia affecting multiple digits is suggestive of Buerger's disease, thromboembolic disease, or a connective tissue disorder.

- Ergotamine and ergot derivatives are potent arterial vasoconstrictors.
- They cross-react with α-adrenergic receptors in the blood vessel wall.

Clinical Manifestations

The typical patient with ergotism is a young female with a history of headaches. The patient may complain of vasospastic phenomena such as Raynaud's disease or Prinzmetal's angina. However, the vasospasm may be so persistent and severe that it mimics or leads to arterial occlusion. Myocardial infarction, mesenteric insufficiency or infarction, limb ischemia, neurologic findings, cutaneous infarctions, and other ischemic syndromes may result from its use.

- Typical patient with ergotism: young female with history of headaches.
- Vasospastic phenomena may be present, such as Raynaud's disease or Prinzmetal's angina.

Diagnosis

The diagnosis of ergot toxicity is almost always made from the history and by exclusion. It is often difficult to elicit a history of ergot use from patients, many of whom use the compound unknowingly, fail to recognize the significance of its use, or use it in an intentionally abusive way.

- Diagnosis of ergot toxicity is almost always made from history and by exclusion.

Treatment

Discontinuing the use of ergot usually leads to relief of symptoms. Occasionally, vasodilator therapy is indicated. Sodium nitroprusside is generally effective in this regard, although calcium or α-adrenergic blockers may also be useful.

- Discontinuing use of ergot leads to relief of symptoms.
- Sodium nitroprusside is generally effective.

THORACIC OUTLET SYNDROME

Cause

Thoracic outlet syndrome occurs when the brachial plexus, subclavian artery, or subclavian vein becomes compressed in the region of the thoracic outlet (Fig. 23-4). Symptoms are thought to result from nerve compression in 90%-95% of cases; only a small number are clearly due to venous or arterial compression. Thoracic outlet syndrome is the most common cause of acute arterial occlusion in the upper extremity of adults <40 old years. Repetitive trauma to the artery can lead to intimal damage, embolization, aneurysm formation, or acute thrombosis. Thoracic outlet syndrome is also the most common

Fig. 23-4. Positional thoracic outlet obstruction is frequently due to the presence of a cervical rib (*arrow*).

cause of upper extremity acute venous occlusion in the young adult. "Stress" thrombosis, which occurs during periods of intense upper extremity activity such as lifting heavy weights, is typically the consequence of intermittent venous occlusion.

- Symptoms of thoracic outlet syndrome are thought to result from nerve compression in 90%-95% of cases.
- Thoracic outlet syndrome is most common cause of acute arterial occlusion in upper extremity of adults <40 years old.
- Thoracic outlet syndrome is the most common cause of upper extremity acute venous occlusion in young adults.

Diagnosis

When arterial compression is present, obliteration of the radial pulse is a strong indication of thoracic outlet syndrome. Nerve involvement is much more difficult to determine; electromyography and nerve conduction studies have not proved consistently useful for diagnosis. Intermittent venous compression is also difficult to document, and when it is found (on ultrasound duplex scanning or magnetic resonance imaging) its significance is uncertain. One of the most useful clinical tests is the elevated arm stress test (EAST), in which the patient raises his or her hands above the head and clenches and unclenches the fist for 1 or 2 minutes. The appearance of typical symptoms, with or without signs of vascular involvement such as delayed capillary refilling, is suggestive of the syndrome.

- Indication of thoracic outlet syndrome: obliteration of radial pulse.
- Nerve involvement is more difficult to determine.
- Useful test is elevated arm stress test.

Treatment

Conservative measures should be tried first. These include exercise, stretching activities, and avoidance of aggravating factors. When conservative measures fail and symptoms warrant, surgical resection of the first rib is curative in 80%-85% of patients. In those with significant arterial involvement (such as intimal damage or aneurysm formation), the involved section of arteries should be replaced with a graft. Patients with recent venous thrombosis can have the clot cleared preoperatively with thrombolytic therapy.

- For thoracic outlet syndrome, conservative measures should be tried first.
- Surgical resection of first rib is curative in 80%-85% of cases.

MICROEMBOLI

Cause (Fig. 23-5)

Whereas macroemboli most frequently originate in the heart, microemboli more commonly originate from the peripheral vessels, although cardiac sources can occur. The most common variety are atheroemboli, which are small thrombi or cholesterol particles given off by fragmenting atherosclerotic plaques. Malfunctioning cardiac valves (native or prosthetic), dissection flaps, intracardiac tumors, and a host of other lesions can also spawn microemboli. Plaque rupture may occur spontaneously, but it is increasingly found as a complication of invasive (catheter) procedures.

- Microemboli commonly originate from peripheral vessels.
- Most common variety are atheroemboli.
- Plaque rupture may occur spontaneously or as a complication of invasive procedure.

Clinical Manifestations

Microemboli may produce livedo, rubor, petechia, focal cutaneous necrosis, and organ ischemia or infarction. These findings depend on the distribution and extent of embolization. Diffuse microembolization from a source proximal to the renal or mesenteric vessels is a catastrophic occurrence that can lead to visceral and renal infarction and severe peripheral ischemia.

- Microemboli may produce livedo, rubor, petechia, focal cutaneous necrosis, and organ ischemia or infarction.

Treatment

The only reliable treatment of persistent microemboli is identification and removal of the embolic source. Because atherosclerosis is a diffuse process, the search for an embolic source often demonstrates widespread disease for which no

Fig. 23-5. Embolic disease. *A*, Distal infarcts and petechia. *B*, Emboli to buttocks after aortic catheterization. This patient had catheter-induced cholesterol microemboli that caused small infarctions and petechiae over back and buttocks.

simple surgical repair is readily apparent. Medical therapy, such as aspirin or anticoagulation, may help but often does not. Indeed, there is a well-recognized syndrome in which warfarin triggers or exacerbates atheroemboli. The exact mechanism of this phenomenon remains uncertain. Dipyridamole has been advocated by some, but it remains of unproven value.

● Only reliable treatment for microemboli is identification and removal of embolic source.
● There is a syndrome in which warfarin triggers or exacerbates atheroemboli.

DISSECTION

Cause

Dissection, like aneurysm formation, is a degenerative condition that can affect most large or medium-sized arteries. Dissection occurs when the intima or media separates from the remainder of the artery creating a flap that can obstruct the lumen of the vessel (Fig. 23-6). Aneurysm formation or rupture of the weakened wall may occur. Marfan syndrome, Ehlers-Danlos syndrome, cystic medial necrosis, and a host of other conditions can predispose to dissection. Hypertension is frequently present. The aorta is the artery most frequently affected by dissection. Iatrogenic dissection may occur because of invasive diagnostic or therapeutic intravascular procedures, blunt trauma, or deceleration injuries.

● Dissection is a degenerative condition affecting most large or medium-sized arteries.
● Marfan syndrome, Ehlers-Danlos syndrome, and cystic medial necrosis predispose to dissection.
● Hypertension is frequently present.
● Aorta is the artery most frequently affected by dissection.

Classification

The two most common systems for classifying aortic dissection are the Stanford and the DeBakey systems, defined as follows:

Stanford A: any dissection involving the ascending aorta regardless of the site of primary intimal tear or distal extent of propagation
Stanford B: any dissection confined entirely to the distal aorta (i.e., distal to the aortic arch)

DeBakey type 1: equivalent to Stanford A
DeBakey type 2: a dissection limited to the ascending portion of the aorta
DeBakey type 3: equivalent to Stanford B.

Fig. 23-6. Computed tomogram of abdominal aorta clearly shows a flap (*arrow*) resulting from a dissection. Dissections can also be studied with angiography or ultrasonography.

Diagnosis

The sudden onset of "tearing" chest, scapular, or abdominal pain should alert the clinician to the possibility of aortic dissection. The pain commonly migrates as the dissection extends. Evidence of arterial occlusion may be present if the dissection flap causes vascular obstruction. Care must be taken to avoid misdiagnosing dissection as myocardial infarction because the administration of thrombolytics in this setting is potentially lethal. Several tests may be used to screen for, or confirm the diagnosis of, dissection. Aortography is the historical standard, although computed tomography (conventional and ultrafast) and transesophageal echocardiography are rapidly emerging as equivalent or possibly superior technologies. Magnetic resonance imaging, digital subtraction angiography, transthoracic or abdominal duplex ultrasonography, and other similar tests are less desirable because of their limited ability to visualize the flap and their increased expense.

- Symptoms of aortic dissection: "tearing" chest, scapular, or abdominal pain.
- Pain commonly migrates as dissection extends.
- Misdiagnosis as myocardial infarction needs to be avoided.
- Aortography is the standard test.

Treatment

Dissections involving the ascending aorta (Stanford A, DeBakey type 1 or 2) should be treated with an emergency operation. The mortality rate for patients in this group who are treated medically is >90%. The perioperative mortality rate is ≤20%. When the dissection involves the aortic valve, replacement or repair of the valve is necessary. Dissections involving the descending aorta (Stanford B or DeBakey type 3) may be treated either medically or surgically. Generally, medical therapy can be attempted first (β-adrenergic blockade, reduction of blood pressure as much as tolerated), and if the pain resolves promptly the patient can be followed. Operation should be performed if pain persists or recurs, aneurysms develop or enlarge, or limb or abdominal ischemia occurs. Regardless of the treatment used, serial follow-up with computed tomography should be performed to look for enlargement or resolution of the dissection and the integrity of the graft anastomosis.

- Dissections of ascending aorta should be treated with emergency operation.
- Mortality rate with medical treatment of dissection of ascending aorta is >90%.
- Dissection of descending aorta may be treated medically or surgically.
- Operation for dissection of descending aorta is needed if pain persists or recurs, aneurysms develop, or limb or abdominal ischemia occurs.

Other Dissections

Dissections of the coronary artery can result from diagnostic catheterization or interventional therapeutic procedures such as percutaneous transluminal coronary angioplasty. Spontaneous carotid dissection can occur and is manifested by a constellation of symptoms that include unilateral headache, focal cerebral ischemic symptoms, and pulsatile tinnitus. Although there is no surgical option for this condition, spontaneous resolution is the rule. In contrast, spontaneous renal dissection is usually treated surgically. Iliofemoral dissections are usually the result of diagnostic or therapeutic catheter procedures performed through groin puncture sites.

- Carotid dissection resolves spontaneously.
- Renal dissection is usually treated surgically.

FIBROMUSCULAR DYSPLASIA

Background

Fibromuscular dysplasia (FMD) is a dysplastic disease affecting medium-sized and small arteries. Women are affected much more frequently than men. Most patients with FMD have renovascular involvement (60%-70%), and about 30% have cerebrovascular involvement. FMD can affect any layer of the arterial wall (intima, media, adventitia); the pathologic classification of this disease is usually based on the site of involvement. The most common form of FMD is medial (medial fibroplasia), which represents 70%-95% of all forms of FMD.

- FMD is a dysplastic disease of medium-sized and small arteries.
- Renovascular involvement occurs in 60%-70% of cases.
- Cerebrovascular involvement occurs in about 30% of cases.

Diagnosis

In patients with renovascular hypertension or arterial occlusive disease, an FMD-related cause can be determined by angiography. In the most common forms of dysplasia the artery has a "string-of-beads" appearance (Fig. 23-7). These beads typically represent alternating stenotic and aneurysmal regions of blood vessels. Examination of biopsy specimens, when available, can aid in the diagnosis of FMD. Pathogenically, FMD can produce stenotic lesions that may limit or occlude blood flow. It can also predispose to aneurysm formation or dissection.

- FMD is diagnosed with angiography.
- Artery has "string-of-beads" appearance.
- FMD can produce stenotic lesions or predispose to aneurysm formation or dissection.

Fig. 23-7. Fibromuscular dysplasia. This typical angiographic "string-of-beads" appearance is classic for fibromuscular dysplasia.

Treatment

FMD is best treated, when possible, by percutaneous transluminal angioplasty (PTA). Nearly two-thirds of patients with renovascular FMD will be "cured" by PTA alone. Operation should be reserved for patients in whom PTA fails, or in whom aneurysm or dissection is present. In certain patients, particularly those in whom PTA has failed and who are poor surgical risks, drug therapy alone may be adequate.

- FMD is best treated by percutaneous transluminal angioplasty.
- Almost two-thirds of patients are "cured" by angioplasty alone.
- Operation is used when angioplasty fails or when aneurysm or dissection is present.

GIANT CELL ARTERITIS

Background

Giant cell arteritis is a granulomatous vasculitic process of unknown cause. The large arteries are primarily affected. The two major syndromes of giant cell arteritis are Takayasu's arteritis and temporal arteritis.

- Giant cell arteritis is a granulomatous vasculitic process.
- Two major syndromes: Takayasu's arteritis and temporal arteritis.

Takayasu's Arteritis

Takayasu's arteritis (Fig. 23-8) affects primarily the aorta and its major branches, particularly those of the aortic arch. It is more common in females than in males. Also known as pulseless disease, it frequently leads to complete occlusion of the brachiocephalic vessels. Patients are almost always <50 years old. Affected arteries may occasionally form aneurysms. The diagnosis is usually made from the history, examination, and arteriography. Angiographic findings include tapered narrowings (such as the "string" sign) of the brachiocephalic vessels; these occasionally go on to produce occlusion. When necessary, or when tissue is available, the diagnosis can be made from biopsy. The erythrocyte sedimentation rate is almost always increased in patients with active Takayasu's arteritis, and it can serve as an index of disease activity. Other acute-phase reactants, such as C-reactive protein, are occasionally useful.

- Takayasu's arteritis is more common in females.
- Patients are almost always <50 years old.

Fig. 23-8. Angiogram of abdominal aorta in a patient with Takayasu's arteritis shows multiple areas of stenosis involving distal aorta, iliac arteries, and renal arteries. Narrowed regions represent areas of the artery which have undergone inflammation or scarring.

● Diagnosis is made from the history, examination, and arteriography.

Therapy primarily involves the use of prednisone. High-dose prednisone (50-100 mg daily in single dose or divided doses) is usually instituted for 3-6 weeks, or until the sedimentation rate has stabilized in the normal range. Slow taper (2.5-5.0 mg every 2-4 weeks) is the rule, with the taper slowing to as little as 1 mg per month once the daily dose reaches 10 mg. The rate of taper should be modified according to the sedimentation rate and the clinical picture. In some cases, low-dose prednisone may be needed for prolonged periods or even indefinitely. Occasionally, vessels that were stenotic during the active phase of the disease will "reopen" during treatment. When surgical correction is necessary, efforts should be made to hold off until the disease has been adequately treated, or preferably until it is "burned out."

● Treatment of Takayasu's arteritis is with high-dose prednisone that is slowly tapered.

Temporal Arteritis

Temporal arteritis primarily affects people >50 years old. It predominantly affects secondary or tertiary branches from the aorta. Like Takayasu's arteritis, its systemic manifestations may include fatigue, malaise, fever, and myalgias. It is pathologically indistinguishable from Takayasu's arteritis. Temporal arteritis should be suspected in any patient with systemic symptoms and pain or tenderness localized to the temporal arteries. As with Takayasu's arteritis the erythrocyte sedimentation rate is typically increased, and the degree of increase can be used to monitor the activity of the disease. Although angiography can be used to make the diagnosis, biopsy is much more commonly used because of the accessibility of the temporal artery. Biopsy should include as long a piece of the temporal artery as possible, and it may need to be performed bilaterally before the disease can be excluded.

● Temporal arteritis primarily affects people >50 years old.
● Systemic manifestations: fatigue, malaise, fever, myalgias.
● Temporal arteritis is pathologically indistinguishable from Takayasu's arteritis.
● Diagnosis should be suspected in any patient with pain or tenderness localized to the temporal arteries.

Like Takayasu's arteritis, the treatment of temporal arteritis involves the use of corticosteroids. A typical program is 50-100 mg of prednisone per day, and treatment is usually maintained for 3-6 weeks or until the erythrocyte sedimentation rate has stabilized in the normal range. The relapse rate during taper is higher than that for Takayasu's arteritis, and in some series it approaches 50%. Longer-term, higher-dose corticosteroid programs may be necessary.

If the diagnosis of temporal arteritis is being seriously considered, treatment with prednisone should begin immediately. This approach prevents the sudden, unexpected complication of blindness due to occlusion of the central retinal artery. Biopsy results remain accurate if biopsy is performed within several days after starting treatment with corticosteroids.

● For temporal arteritis, treatment with prednisone should begin immediately to prevent sudden, unexpected blindness due to occlusion of the central retinal artery.

RAYNAUD'S PHENOMENON

Background

Raynaud's phenomenon refers to any inappropriate or excessively intense episode of cutaneous, digital, or limb vasoconstriction. It most commonly affects the upper limb. Females are affected far more commonly than males. Attacks are usually triggered by exposure to the cold or by emotional stress. The disease can be divided into two categories, primary and secondary, depending on cause.

● Raynaud's phenomenon is inappropriate or excessively intense episode of cutaneous, digital, or limb vasoconstriction.

Primary Raynaud's Phenomenon

The cause of primary Raynaud's phenomenon is unknown. Episodes are usually bilateral. Digital ulcerations are rare but may occur occasionally. The symptoms are usually stable and may be related to abnormalities in adrenergic function, blood viscosity, or endothelial disorders.

● Episodes of primary Raynaud's phenomenon are usually bilateral.
● Digital ulcerations are rare.

Secondary Raynaud's Phenomenon

This refers to Raynaud's phenomenon occurring as the result of some other underlying abnormality. Predisposing factors include atherosclerosis, arteritis, cancer, collagen vascular disease, thoracic outlet syndrome, embolic occlusions, occupational disease, certain drugs (β-adrenergic blocker, nicotine, ergotamine), and various other conditions. Secondary Raynaud's phenomenon is occasionally unilateral (perhaps affecting a single digit) and may produce skin breakdown.

● Secondary Raynaud's phenomenon is the result of some other underlying abnormality.

Diagnosis

The diagnosis of Raynaud's phenomenon is made primarily on clinical grounds. Provocative testing to document and assess normal vasoconstriction is often of limited value because of the difficulty in reliably reproducing symptoms in the laboratory setting.

● Diagnosis of Raynaud's phenomenon is made on clinical grounds.

Treatment

The treatment of Raynaud's phenomenon is often difficult. In cases of secondary Raynaud's phenomenon, treatment of the underlying condition should be attempted whenever possible. Simple conservative measures such as dressing warmly, avoiding unnecessary exposure to the cold, and intermittent hand warming may improve the condition substantially. Biofeedback is effective in certain cases. Drugs with a potential for causing vasoconstriction should be avoided. Occasionally it is necessary to move to a warmer climate to achieve complete relief. Certain vasodilators, especially nifedipine, prazosin, and other calcium or α-adrenergic blockers, may help in selected cases. Interruption of the sympathetic nerves, either through ganglionic injection or surgical sympathectomy, is often useful in patients with severe symptoms.

● Simple treatment for Raynaud's phenomenon: dressing

warmly, avoiding exposure to cold, intermittent hand warming.
● Certain vasodilators may help in selected cases.

ACUTE DEEP VENOUS THROMBOSIS

Cause

The factors predisposing to deep venous thrombosis (DVT) include those of Virchow's triad: stasis, trauma, and hypercoagulability. Underlying conditions that can predispose to DVT include cancer, inflammatory bowel disease, pregnancy or estrogen use, obesity, age, surgery or trauma, congestive heart failure, previous DVT, and a host of others.

● Factors in DVT include Virchow's triad: stasis, trauma, hypercoagulability.

Clinical Manifestations

Acute DVT is notoriously difficult to diagnose on clinical grounds only. Swelling, pain, discoloration, positive Homans' sign, cord palpation, and other typical features can suggest the diagnosis but are frequently misleading. In many cases extensive DVT may be minimally symptomatic or even asymptomatic, whereas in others the proximal DVT is so massive that the leg becomes mottled, cyanotic, markedly tender, and ischemic; this condition is referred to as phlegmasia cerulea dolens.

● DVT is notoriously difficult to diagnose on clinical grounds only.

Diagnosis

Venography has long been the standard method for definitively diagnosing DVT, but duplex scanning (with or without color flow) is rapidly emerging as an equivalent method for the diagnosis of proximal DVT. Nonimaging (functional) methods such as impedance plethysmography and continuous-wave Doppler remain reliable, cost-efficient methods for detecting proximal DVT. They are unreliable for excluding below-knee thrombus. Fortunately, the embolic potential of below-knee thrombus is extremely low, and in many clinical situations it is safe to follow patients who have negative results of functional studies such as impedance plethysmography.

● Venography is standard method to diagnose DVT.
● Duplex scanning is an equivalent method for diagnosis of proximal DVT.

Treatment

Patients with acute, proximal DVT should be hospitalized and treated with intravenously administered heparin. The activated partial thromboplastin time should be kept at 2.0-2.5

times the control value throughout heparinization. In the past, warfarin was not given until 5-7 days into treatment; newer programs are now administering warfarin at the time of admission and discontinuing the use of heparin when the prothrombin time is therapeutic and stable. In any case, the patient should remain hospitalized until the prothrombin time is therapeutic (1.5-2.0 times control value, or INR of 2-3) and the patient is able to ambulate without pain. Use of warfarin should be maintained for at least 3 months. In most cases of DVT, an elastic compression stocking should be prescribed and worn during treatment with warfarin.

- Treatment for DVT: hospitalization, intravenously administered heparin.
- Patient is hospitalized until prothrombin time, while receiving warfarin, is therapeutic.
- Warfarin is used for at least 3 months.

Unprecipitated DVT

In patients with unprecipitated DVT, be sure to search for an underlying, occult disorder that may be predisposing the patient to clot formation.

- For unprecipitated DVT, search for underlying disorder.

PULMONARY EMBOLISM

Background

Pulmonary embolism is a major cause of death in the United States and may cause as many as 250,000 fatalities per year. It is estimated that up to 80% of significant pulmonary emboli escape detection and that 50% of patients suspected of having pulmonary emboli on clinical grounds actually do not. The mortality rate is between 20% and 35% for untreated pulmonary emboli, and it is 8% when the condition is properly diagnosed and treated.

- Mortality rate with untreated pulmonary emboli: 20%-35%.

Pathophysiology

The risk factors for pulmonary emboli are the same as those for deep venous thrombosis (see page 845). Emboli are most likely to originate in the large, deep veins of the lower extremity (iliofemoral system), although 10% of pulmonary emboli come from the upper extremity. Thrombi in the superficial veins or deep venous system distal to the knee do not commonly embolize.

- Emboli most likely to originate in large, deep veins of lower extremity.
- 10% of emboli come from upper extremity.

Signs and Symptoms

There is generally poor correlation among symptoms, clinical findings, and the presence or absence of pulmonary emboli. Most pulmonary emboli occur silently. When signs and symptoms occur, they are highly variable. In the Urokinase Pulmonary Embolism Trial, the most common signs and symptoms included tachypnea (respiration rate >16 per minute), 92%; dyspnea, 85%; pleuritic chest pain, 74%; apprehension, 59%; rales, 58%; and cough, 53%. Phlebitis was clinically apparent in only 32%. Other common findings included an accentuated second heart sound, tachycardia, fever, hemoptysis, diaphoresis, and syncope. Massive pulmonary embolism may cause syncope, cor pulmonale, cardiogenic shock, and cardiac arrest with electromechanical dissociation. Chronic pulmonary emboli may lead to pulmonary hypertension and the development of cor pulmonale.

- Correlation is poor among symptoms, clinical findings, and presence or absence of pulmonary emboli.
- Most pulmonary emboli occur silently.
- Chronic pulmonary emboli may lead to pulmonary hypertension.

Screening Tests

The most common electrocardiographic abnormality noted in pulmonary embolism is sinus tachycardia. Classic electrocardiographic findings such as an S_1, Q_3, T_3 pattern, right bundle branch block, right-axis deviation, and increased P wave are present in only one-fourth of patients. Chest radiography is likewise nonspecific; findings include pleural effusion in 50%, right-sided cardiomegaly, pulmonary infarction, elevation of the hemidiaphragm, and atelectasis. The arterial blood gas may show decreased Po_2 and Pco_2.

Specific Tests

Ventilation-perfusion scanning is one of the most widely used tests to screen for pulmonary embolism. It should be viewed as a useful test when the findings suggest either a high probability or normal results. Intermediate- or low-probability results should be viewed as nondiagnostic. Pulmonary angiography remains the standard diagnostic method. Computed tomography, especially ultrafast, is also a useful diagnostic tool.

- Ventilation-perfusion scanning is widely used to screen for pulmonary embolism.
- Pulmonary angiography is standard diagnostic method.

Treatment

Anticoagulation is the mainstay of treatment for acute pulmonary embolism. It should be started immediately with heparin, which is usually given for 5-10 days. The regimen is then switched to warfarin, which should be maintained for 3-6 months. In cases of massive pulmonary embolism, thrombolytic therapy should be considered. Streptokinase, urokinase, and tissue-plasminogen activator are all potentially useful agents. In patients with massive, life-threatening pulmonary embolism who have contraindications to thrombolytic therapy or who have not responded to an attempt at lysis, or in whom severe, chronic pulmonary embolism is present, surgical embolectomy can be considered. Patients who cannot tolerate anticoagulation should be considered for a caval filter to prevent recurrent, possibly lethal, pulmonary embolism.

CHRONIC DEEP VENOUS INSUFFICIENCY (POSTPHLEBITIC SYNDROME)

Background

Chronic deep venous insufficiency (DVI) is among the most common causes of leg ulcer in the United States (Fig. 23-9). The condition develops when veins become chronically obstructed, or when venous valvular incompetence develops. These recurrences are usually caused by deep venous thrombosis. Although the exact mechanism by which venous insufficiency produces chronic changes is unknown, it appears that chronically increased venous pressure is the culprit.

- DVI is one of the most common causes of leg ulcer in the United States.
- Recurrences are usually caused by deep venous thrombosis.

Clinical Manifestations

DVI may lead to limb swelling, pigmentation (from hemosiderin deposition in the perivascular tissues), induration and cellulitis, dermatitis, and ulceration. The most commonly

Fig. 23-9. Leg of a man with severe deep venous insufficiency. Persistently elevated venous pressure produces changes including swelling, inflammation, and hemosiderin deposition. The extensive region of discoloration is due to hemosiderin that has been deposited in the skin.

affected area of the leg is the medial malleolus, although any portion of the lower part of the leg may be involved.

- DVI most often affects the medial malleolus.

Diagnosis

The diagnosis is made from the clinical history, physical findings, and objective testing. Specific tests for DVI include continuous-wave Doppler (with or without duplex imaging), various types of plethysmographic studies, and descending venography.

Treatment

DVI is treated primarily with measures to control swelling. The leg should be elevated whenever possible, and long periods of standing or sitting should be avoided. Elastic compression, either in the form of stockings or wrap, is essential. The compression must be graduated and of sufficient magnitude to prevent swelling. If stockings are to be used, the swelling should be maximally reduced before fitting. Additional compression can be supplied by the use of elastic pads. Dermatitis and other forms of inflammation are often improved by the use of corticosteroid cream. Antibiotics should be reserved for situations in which infection is apparent. Anticoagulation is not necessary unless recurrent clotting has developed or is likely. Venous stripping or perforator ligation may be useful in a limited number of cases with refractory ulcers. The stripping of superficial veins should be avoided if deep venous obstruction is present, because the superficial veins may be acting as collaterals. Occasionally a chronic arteriovenous fistula may mimic DVI. This possibility should be considered when penetrating trauma, surgical procedures, or other causes of fistula are present.

- Elastic compression is essential for DVI.
- Venous stripping or perforator ligation is useful in a limited number of cases.
- Chronic arteriovenous fistula may mimic DVI.

LYMPHEDEMA

Background

Lymphedema is the result of hypoplasia, dysfunction, or obstruction of the lymphatic vessels (Fig. 23-10). As a result, lymphatic fluid accumulates in the interstitial space and the extremity becomes swollen. Pitting edema is present early in the disease, but in chronic cases the subcutaneous tissues become fibrotic and hyperplastic, producing woody nonpitting edema.

- Lymphedema results from hypoplasia, dysfunction, or obstruction of lymphatic vessels.
- Pitting edema occurs early in disease.

Cause

Lymphedema may be primary (due to a congenital abnormality or predisposition) or secondary (due to trauma, infection, cancer, and other disorders). Primary lymphedema most commonly becomes manifest at puberty (lymphedema praecox) and may be familial in about 15% of cases. Secondary lymphedema is a worldwide problem of major proportion. In tropical countries, the most common causes of lymphedema are filarial disorders, and the lymphedema produced can be severe (elephantiasis). In Western or industrialized countries, tumors (such as breast, prostate, gynecologic) and recurrent infections are the most common causes. The treatment of breast cancer commonly produces edema of the upper extremity. The likelihood and severity of lymphedema depend on the type and extent of operation and the use of adjuvant therapy such as radiation or chemotherapy.

● Primary lymphedema manifests at puberty (lymphedema praecox) and may be familial.
● In tropical countries, common causes of lymphedema are filarial disorders.
● In Western countries, tumor and recurrent infections are most common causes of lymphedema.

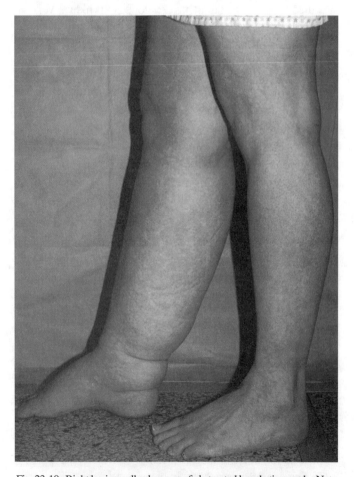

Fig. 23-10. Right leg is swollen because of obstructed lymphatic vessels. Note that the dorsum of the foot is involved in this process.

Diagnosis

The diagnosis of lymphedema can usually be made from the history and physical examination. When a confirmatory study is necessary, the best technique is lymphoscintigraphy. In this test, a small amount of radiolabeled colloid is injected in the web space between the digits, where its progress through the lymphatics is followed with nuclear scanning. The patency of lymphatics can thus be determined. Lymphangiography has been considered the standard, but it should be avoided whenever possible because of its invasive nature and tendency to cause lymphangitis, which may worsen lymphedema.

● Lymphoscintigraphy is best diagnostic technique for lymphedema.
● Lymphangiography should be avoided because of its invasive nature.

Treatment

In most cases, lymphedema is incurable but treatable. Good hygiene and protection from trauma are among the most important elements of care. The limb should be elevated as often as possible to drain the tissue and keep swelling to a minimum. Elastic compression stockings (often with pressures as high as 50 or 60 mm Hg) are the mainstay of treatment. Sequential compression pumps capable of generating pressures of 80-100 mm Hg can be used to "milk" lymphatic fluid out of the legs. Antibiotics should be used liberally to treat or provide prophylaxis against bacterial infection. In some cases, surgical techniques to reduce the size of the limb or bypass blocked lymphatics are possible.

● Elastic compression stockings are mainstay of treatment for lymphedema.

ARTERIOVENOUS MALFORMATION OR FISTULA

Background

Arteriovenous malformation or fistula (Fig. 23-11) may be acquired or congenital. Acquired cases are generally due to penetrating trauma, iatrogenic processes such as surgery or catheterization, or spontaneous degeneration of blood vessels. Congenital malformation or fistula may involve primarily arterial, venous, capillary, or lymphatic tissues; at times the lesions are mixed and involve elements of all four.

● Arteriovenous malformations may be acquired or congenital.

Consequences

Arteriovenous malformations may be of cosmetic significance only, or they can produce pain, tissue destruction, or limb hypertrophy, especially when the flow is high. In some

Fig. 23-11. Arteriovenous malformation. This extensive congenital malformation has led to venous volume and pressure overload. As a result, many of the clinical findings are similar to those of chronic venous insufficiency. If blood flow is high enough, heart failure may develop.

patients, congestive heart failure has occurred as a result of the high demand for blood flow associated with these lesions.

Treatment

The treatment of many arteriovenous malformations is difficult because the malformation may involve deep or vital structures and make resection impossible; vessels feeding or draining the lesion may be difficult to identify, reach, and ligate; the lesion has a propensity to redevelop after resection; and successful treatment may produce ischemia in regions distal to the malformation. Thus, conservative measures are frequently used. When pain, swelling, congestive heart failure, the possibility of malignancy, or other problems force a consideration of interventional therapy, surgery or embolization is

usually attempted. Catheter-directed embolization is showing increasing utility in this regard.

- Treatment of arteriovenous malformation is difficult.

ULCERS

Types

Vascular ulcers can be divided into four categories: ischemic, venous, arteriolar, and neurotrophic.

Ischemic

Ischemic ulcers (Fig. 23-12) result from arterial occlusive disease (large or small vessels) that reduces blood flow below the level necessary for maintaining skin viability. The ulcers tend to be distal (digits or foot) and may be triggered by trauma, including mild abrasion from shoes. They often become infected. Ischemic ulcers are usually painful unless associated neuropathy is present.

- Ischemic ulcers result from arterial occlusive disease.
- Ischemic ulcers tend to be distal (digits or foot).
- Ulcers are usually painful.

Venous

Venous ulcers (Fig. 23-13) were discussed on page 847. They result from skin breakdown associated with chronic venous insufficiency. Other signs or symptoms of venous stasis are usually present around the ulcer, including swelling, pigmentation, and indurated cellulitis. Trauma is often a precipitating factor. The ulcers are usually located over the medial malleolus, but they may occur on any part of the leg. They are typically painful, but not as painful as ulcers caused by ischemia.

Fig. 23-12. Ischemic ulcer located distally on foot. There was poor wound granulation, and the ulcer was very painful.

Fig. 23-13. Venous ulcer. Note location over medial malleolus and surrounding hyperpigmentation and cellulitis.

- Venous ulcers are associated with chronic venous insufficiency.
- Venous ulcers are not as painful as ischemic ulcers.

Arteriolar

Also known as "hypertensive" ulcers, arteriolar ulcers (Fig. 23-14) result from small-vessel occlusion. They tend to have punched-out or irregular (serpiginous) borders and are usually extremely painful. A wide variety of processes can lead to the small-vessel occlusion producing arteriolar ulcers; these include hypertension, vasculitis, and collagen vascular diseases.

- Arteriolar ulcers result from small-vessel occlusion.
- They have punched-out or irregular (serpiginous) borders.
- They are extremely painful.

Fig. 23-14. Arteriolar (vasculitis) ulcer. This case has a clean, punched-out appearance.

Neurotrophic

Patients with neuropathy, particularly those who are diabetic, frequently develop neurotrophic ulcers (Fig. 23-15) as a result of chronic trauma. The ulcers are painless and pale and typically have associated thick edges and callous formation. They are almost always present over pressure points or sites of repetitive trauma.

- Neurotrophic ulcers often develop in patients with neuropathy (diabetes).
- Ulcers are painless and pale and have thick edges and callous formation.

LOOK-ALIKES

Several processes can produce leg ulcers that may mimic vascular lesions. These include pyoderma gangrenosum, Kaposi's sarcoma, various infections, cutaneous tumors, lipedema (mimicking lymphedema), myxedema, trauma, and various other problems.

Fig. 23-15. Neurotrophic ulcers over pressure points on insensitive foot.

WARFARIN NECROSIS

This rare entity occurs in <1% of patients receiving the medication. It usually develops 3-6 days after initiation of therapy (more often in women) and is characterized by the sudden development of erythematous or hemorrhagic skin lesions. These eventually become gangrenous, and the overlying skin sloughs. Areas of skin with underlying fatty deposits (e.g., breasts, buttocks) are most commonly affected. The exact cause of this reaction is unknown, but a decreased level of protein C may be involved. When it occurs, the use of warfarin should be discontinued immediately.

- Warfarin necrosis occurs in <1% of patients receiving the medication.
- It develops 3-6 days after therapy.
- It is characterized by erythematous or hemorrhagic skin lesions that become gangrenous.
- Use of warfarin should be discontinued immediately.

HEPARIN-INDUCED THROMBOCYTOPENIA

The frequency of heparin-induced thrombocytopenia is probably 1% or 2%, but estimates as high as 30% have been reported. It typically begins 5-10 days after the initiation of heparin therapy. Patients with this condition are frequently asymptomatic but may develop hemorrhagic or thrombotic complications. The cause probably involves an antigen/antibody interaction, but the exact mechanism is poorly understood. Treatment consists of discontinuing use of heparin when the problem is identified.

- Heparin-induced thrombocytopenia occurs in 1% or 2% of patients receiving the medication.
- It begins 5-10 days after initiation of therapy.
- Cause involves antigen/antibody interaction.

IATROGENIC VASCULAR DISEASE AND TRAUMA

Vascular trauma is an increasingly common occurrence. Interventional procedures such as catheterization can produce occlusion, dissection, or bleeding. Other common sources of trauma include penetrating injuries, acceleration injuries, and blunt trauma.

QUESTIONS

Multiple Choice (choose the one best answer)

1. Which of the following statements about aneurysms is incorrect?
   a. Most abdominal aortic aneurysms are associated with atherosclerosis or hypertension
   b. The diameter of an abdominal aortic aneurysm usually enlarges at a rate of 1-2 cm per year or more
   c. Small aneurysms are less likely to rupture than large ones
   d. Popliteal aneurysms usually do not rupture
   e. Abdominal aortic aneurysms <4.5 cm in diameter can usually be observed

2. Choose the best answer.
   a. Arterial thrombosis is usually associated with a specific clotting disorder
   b. The most common type of embolization is a paradoxical emboli
   c. The increased use of invasive diagnostic and therapeutic cardiovascular interventions has led to a marked decrease in the frequency of iatrogenic dissections, largely because the equipment is becoming safer and the operators are more skilled
   d. The sudden loss of a pulse in a limb implies critical ischemia
   e. Acute arterial thrombosis may be treated surgically or, in some cases, with lytic therapy

3. Which of the following statements is *false*?
   a. Most vasculitides are thought to be due to immunologic or autoimmune phenomena, although in most cases the exact mechanism is poorly understood
   b. Vasculitis can be diagnosed with either biopsy or angiography
   c. Steroids are rarely used for the treatment of vasculitis, because newer immunosuppressive drugs are effective and can avoid many of the side effects associated with steroids
   d. Cryoglobulinemia can be associated with vasculitis

e. Buerger's disease may affect both the arteries and the veins

4. Which of the following statements about the thoracic outlet syndrome is *false*?
   a. Most cases are clearly due to venous or arterial compression
   b. Thoracic outlet syndrome is the most common cause of acute arterial occlusion in the upper extremities of adults <40 years old
   c. Thoracic outlet syndrome is the most common cause of upper extremity venous occlusion in the young adult
   d. Cervical ribs are frequently associated with thoracic outlet syndrome
   e. It is difficult to document nerve involvement in patients with thoracic outlet syndrome

5. Which of the following statements is *true*?
   a. The arteries most often affected by dissection are the carotid arteries
   b. Hypertension is rare in patients with dissection
   c. Stanford type B dissections may be treated either medically or surgically
   d. Stanford type A dissections should be treated only surgically when there is evidence of impending aortic rupture
   e. Carotid dissections should be treated immediately with operation

6. Which of the following statements about arteriovenous (AV) malformations or fistula is *true*?
   a. AV fistula almost always occurs on a congenital basis
   b. Congenital AV malformations can be large enough to cause heart failure, but acquired fistulae never do
   c. Congenital AV malformations are always painless
   d. Congenital AV malformations may involve arteries, veins, capillaries, or lymphatic tissues
   e. Almost all congenital AV malformations can be resected and cured surgically

7. Which of the following statements is *false*?
   a. Lymphedema usually spares the feet, but lipedema does not
   b. Skin malignancies may mimic vascular ulcers

c. Skin infections may mimic vascular ulcers
d. Traumatic skin lesions may mimic ulcers
e. Thyroid disease may mimic vascular disease

True/False (indicate whether each answer is true or false)
8. Which of the following statements are true?
   a. Women are affected by fibromuscular dysplasia more frequently than men
   b. Fibromuscular dysplasia can produce stenosis, aneurysms, or dissection
   c. Because of the potential for aneurysm formation, fibromuscular dysplasia should be treated surgically whenever possible
   d. Temporal arteritis is associated with giant cells (hence the frequent reference to giant cell arteritis), but Takayasu's arteritis is not
   e. Takayasu's arteritis may cause blindness if it is not promptly treated
   f. Takayasu's arteritis is almost exclusively a disease of males

9. Which of the following statements are true?
   a. Digital ulcerations are common in primary Raynaud's phenomenon
   b. Deep vein thrombosis is notoriously difficult to diagnose on clinical grounds alone
   c. Most pulmonary emboli occur silently
   d. Deep venous insufficiency is a common cause of leg ulceration in the United States
   e. The most common cause of lymphedema in the United States is filarial infection
   f. The most common cause of neurotrophic leg ulcers is diabetes

10. Patients with Buerger's disease (thromboangiitis obliterans) usually:
    a. Have an increased sedimentation rate
    b. Smoke
    c. Are female
    d. Have aortic involvement
    e. Have granulomas or other evidence of vasculitis in involved vessels
    f. Improve with steroids and vasodilation, even if they still smoke

ANSWERS

1. Answer b.

Most abdominal aortic aneurysms enlarge at a rate of 0.3-0.5 cm per year. A rate of 1-2 cm per year is much faster than one would normally expect. Small aneurysms (less than 4.5 cm) usually do not rupture and therefore can be observed. Popliteal aneurysms may rupture, but more commonly they thrombose or serve as a source of embolus.

2. Answer d.

Either thrombolysis (with a lytic agent such as streptokinase, urokinase, or tissue plasminogen activator) or operation may be used to treat an acutely thrombosed artery, depending on the situation. Most arterial thrombi do not occur in patients with identifiable clotting disorders, but instead they are associated with, for example, atrial fibrillation, aneurysm, or atherosclerosis. The increased use of invasive procedures contributes to an increase in iatrogenic complications. The sudden loss of a pulse does not necessarily imply critical (limb-threatening) ischemia, because collateral blood vessels may keep the pulseless limb viable.

3. Answer c.

Steroids remain the mainstay of treatment in most types of vasculitis such as temporal arteritis, polyarteritis nodosa, and Takayasu's arteritis.

4. Answer a.

Most patients with symptomatic thoracic outlet syndrome have symptoms attributable to positional nerve compression. Only a minority have definite arterial or venous involvement.

5. Answer c.

Stanford type A dissections (i.e., dissections involving the ascending thoracic aorta) should always be treated surgically. Stanford type B dissections may, in selected cases, be managed conservatively with nonsurgical methods.

6. Answer d.

Fistulae frequently occur because of trauma or operation (including renal dialysis fistulae) and therefore not all are congenital. When large, acquired AV fistulae can cause heart failure. Many AV malformations are associated with significant pain. AV malformations are frequently unsuitable for surgical resection, especially when they are large or deep.

7. Answer a.

Lymphedema generally involves the toes and feet, whereas lipedema usually spares these regions. Skin malignancies, infections, and trauma can all mimic vascular ulcers. Myxedema, due to thyroid disease, frequently resembles edema of vascular origin.

8. a, true; b, true; c, false; d, false; e, false; f, false.

Fibromuscular dysplasia affects more women than men, and it can cause arterial stenosis, aneurysms, or dissection; however, only rarely does it progress to cause significant arterial aneurysms, so treatment is generally limited to symptomatic lesions and is not performed as prophylaxis. Takayasu's disease has giant cells and a predilection for women, but it does not typically cause blindness, as does temporal arteritis.

9. a, false; b, true; c, true; d, true; e, false; f, true.

Digital ulcers are uncommon in primary Raynaud's phenomenon and usually reflect significant underlying disease processes. Deep vein thrombosis is difficult to diagnose on clinical grounds alone and must be evaluated with objective testing. Venous ulcers are the usual vascular ulcers in the United States, and neurotrophic ulcers are most commonly caused by diabetes. Filarial disease is the most common cause of lymphedema worldwide, but it is uncommon in the United States.

10. a, false; b, true; c, false; d, false; e, true; f, false.

Patients with Buerger's disease are usually men with normal erythrocyte sedimentation rates. They almost always use tobacco in some form. Aortic involvement is distinctly uncommon. The pathologic findings are typically those of vasculitis (with or without granulomas). No therapy is truly effective in these patients if they continue to use tobacco.

NOTES

INDEX

Note: Page numbers in italics refer to color plates; page numbers followed by "t" refer to tables.

in treatment of myocardial
infarction, 85
Assist-control mode (mechanical
ventilation), 135
Assistive devices for elderly, 380
Astemizole, 23
Asterixis, 675
Asthma
allergic, 9
assessment of mild, moderate,
or severe symptoms, 9
characteristics, 697
drugs provoking asthma, 13, 16
as eosinophilic lung disease, 711
histologic hallmarks, 11
intrinsic, 9
management of, 12-15
medications for, 12-13
nonallergic, 10
occupational, 16
spirometry flow-volume curve,
10
Ataxia, Friedreich, 363-364
Ataxia-telangiectasia, 156
Atheromatous disease, 9
Atherosclerosis
abdominal aortic aneurysms
associated with, 835
mechanism of, 76-77
stiff vascular tree with, 450
Atrial fibrillation
associated with ischemic and
embolic strokes, 614
diagnosis and treatment, 68-70
in Wolff-Parkinson-White
syndrome, 72
Atrial flutter, 68
Atrial septal defect
primum, 43
secundum, 42-43
sinus venosus, 43
Atrioventricular (AV) block, 65-67
Atropine
in digitalis toxicity, 123-124
poisoning signs and symptoms,
115
Autoimmune disorders
See also bullous diseases,
autoimmune
autoimmune hepatitis (AH),
314-315
familial endocrine disorders, 263
Graves' disease, 190
hemolytic anemia as, 402-403
polyglandular autoimmune
disorders, 263
Autonomy of patient, 551-552

Autosomal aneuploidy syndromes,
353
Autosomal dominant inheritance,
356-363, 366, 423
Autosomal recessive diseases,
363-367
Autosomes, 353
AVP. See arginine vasopressin
(AVP)
Axillary dissection, 624
Axillary irradiation, 624
Azathioprine, 807
Azoles
fluconazole, 526
itraconazole, 526
ketoconazole, 525
AZT. See antiretroviral therapy;
zidovudine
Aztreonam, 521

B

Bacillary angiomatosis, 470
Bacilli, gram-negative
Bordatella pertussis, 477
brucellosis, 477
Capnocytophaga, 478
Escherichia coli, 475
Haemophilus influenzae, 476-
477
Klebsiella, Enterobacter, and
Serratia infections, 475
Legionella micdadei, 478
legionnaires' disease, 477-478
Pasteurella multocida, 478
plague, 478
Proteus, Morganella, and
Providencia infections, 475
Pseudomonas infections, 476
Salmonella typhi, 476
Stenotrophomonas maltophilia,
476
tularemia, 478
Bacilli, gram-positive
anthrax, 478
cutaneous diphtheria, 479
diphtheria, 479
Erysipelothrix rhusiopathiae,
479
Listeria monocytogenes, 478
Rhodococcus equi, 479
Bacillus cereus, 293
Back pain
diagnosis and treatment,
789-790
in lumbar spine disease, 612

treatment of acute lower back
pain, 349-350
Back symptoms, nonspecific, 349
Bacteremia, catheter-related, 139
Bacteria, anaerobic
aspiration pneumonitis, 751-752
bacteroides infections, 480
Chlamydia pneumoniae
(TWAR strain), 750
Chlamydia psittaci, 751
clostridial infections, 480-481
Clostridium botulinum, 480-481
community-acquired
pneumonia, 750
Coxiella burnetii, 751
Francisella tularensis, 751
hospital-acquired (nosocomial)
pneumonia, 751
lung abscess, 752
Peptococcus, 480
tetanus, 480
Yersinia pestis, 751
Bacterial infections
See also antibacterial agents
anaerobic bacteria, 750-752
otitis media, 748
pharyngitis, 748
pneumonia, 748-750
sinusitis, 748
Bacterial overgrowth, 291-292
Barbiturates, 116
Barium radiography, 280
Barium swallow fluoroscopy,
272-275
Barotrauma, 722
Barrett's esophagus, 271-272, 275
Basement membrane disease, 576
Basophils, 10
Bayes' theorem, 79
Becker muscular dystrophy, 367-368
Behçet's disease, 738
Belladonna alkaloid, 115
Benign biliary tract strictures, 324
Benzodiazepines
See also buspirone
as antianxiety medications, 666
antidote, 119
distinguishing medical from
nonmedical use, 664
effects and treatment of
overdose, 125
Bernstein test (esophageal), 276
Berylliosis, 717
β-Adrenergic blockers
after myocardial infarction, 75
responsiveness of asthmatics,
9-10

treatment, 85-86
ventricular arrhythmias during, 75
Myocardial ischemia, perioperative monitoring, 338
Myocardial necrosis, 84-85
Myocardium, stunned, 84
Myoneural junction
  clinical syndromes of lesions of, 596-597
  disease, 598
Myopathy
  causes, 597
  classification of, 597
  defined, 597
Myositis, 612
  See also dermatomyositis; polymyositis
Myotonia, 597
Myotonic dystrophy, 360-361, 597
Myxedema crisis, 197
Myxoma, cardiac, 53

N

N-acetylcysteine, 121
Nails
  in systemic disease, 161
  yellow nail syndrome, 705
NAME syndrome, 155
Narcotics
  antidote, 119
  pulmonary disease induced by abuse, 718
Native valve infective endocarditis, 501-502
Naxalone (Narcan), 117
Necrobiosis lipoidica diabeticorum, 160, *166*
Necrobiotic xanthogranuloma, 160
Necrosis
  acute tubular, 562-565
  avascular necrosis of bone and joint infections, 819
  of the bone and joint infections, 783
  myocardial, 84-85
  papillary, 578
  warfarin, 851
Necrotizing vasculitis, 837-838
Nedocromil, 10, 12
Negative predictive value (NPV), 33-34
Neoplasms
  associated with eosinophilia, 712
  of parathyroid, 262

primary cardiac, 54
pulmonary, 723-728
Neoplastic disease
  in AIDS, 537
  neurologic symptoms in, 609-610
Nephritic syndrome, 570-571
Nephritis, interstitial
  acute, 577
  acute tubulointerstitial, 577
  analgesic chronic, 577-578
  chronic interstitial, 577-578
  electrolyte and toxin-induced, 578
  other renal diseases presenting with, 578
Nephropathy
  analgesic, 577-578
  diabetic, 214-215
  IgA, 572
  minimal change, 573
  stages of diabetic, 574
Nephrotic syndrome
  caused by focal glomerular sclerosis, 573
  caused by membranous glomerulopathy, 573-574
  caused by minimal change nephropathy, 573
  defined, 570
Nerve disease, peripheral, 598
Nerve root lesions, 595
Neuralgia
  glossopharyngeal, 593-594
  trigeminal, 593-594
Neuroarthropathy (Charcot's joint), 783
Neurofibromatosis
  clinical manifestations, 157, *165*
  I and II autosomal dominant disorder, 361-362
  of von Recklinghausen, 714
Neuroleptic malignant syndrome, 665-666
Neurologic conditions
  emergency, 636-637
  HIV-related, 616
  related to organ transplant, 616-617
Neurologic examination, 591-592
Neurologic symptoms
  of patients with cancer, 609-610
  principles for interpreting, 599-600
Neurology of sepsis, 611-612
Neuromuscular disorders, 612-613

Neuropathic arthritis, 818-819
Neuropathy
  causes, 595-596
  of diabetes mellitus, 215-216
  motor polyneuropathy, 596
  sensory polyneuropathy, 596
  venous ulcers in patients with, 850
Neutropenia
  causes and incidence, 431
  febrile, 636
Nicotinic acid, 347-348
NIDDM. *See* diabetes mellitus
Nifedipine, 217
Nitrates, 95
Nitrites, 119
Nitrofurantoin, 718-719
Nitroglycerin, 85
Nocardiosis, 486, *539*
Nocturnal myoclonus, 393
Nodal status (breast cancer), 622-623
Nonalcoholic steatohepatitis, 316
Non-Hodgkin's lymphoma
  in AIDS, 410
  classification, 412-413
  cure rates, 412-413
  treatment, 413, 415
Nonsteroidal anti-inflammatory drugs (NSAIDs)
  arthritis, septic antirheumatic drug therapy, 802-804
  association with peptic ulcer, 277
  in treatment of COPD, 700
Noonan's syndrome, 245
Normochromic-normocytic anemias, 399
Norwalk virus, 512
NPV. *See* negative predictive value (NPV)
NSAIDs. *See* nonsteroidal anti-inflammatory drugs (NSAIDs)
Nutrient absorption, 288-289
Nutrition, pre- and perioperative, 341

O

Oaths reflecting beliefs and principles, 551
Obsessive-compulsive disorder
  antidepressant agents in treatment of, 667
  described, 660
Obstructive azoospermia (Young's